IHSS	idiopathic hypertrophic subaortic stenosis	**PO**	orally, by mouth (*per os*)
I & O	intake and output	**PRN**	when required (*pro re nata*)
IM	intramuscular	**PT**	prothrombin time
IOP	intraocular pressure	**PTT**	partial thromboplastin time
IPPB	intermittent (or inspiratory) positive pressure breathing	**PVC's**	premature ventricular contractions
IV	intravenous	**q**	each, every (*quaque*)
JVP	jugular venous pressure	**qd**	every day (*quaque die*)
kg	kilogram	**qid**	four times a day (*quater in die*)
L	liter or liters	**R**	rate, usually with reference to respiratory rate
LAV	lymphadenopathy-associated virus	**RBC**	red blood cell
lbs	pounds	**RDA**	recommended daily dietary allowance
LDH	lactic dehydrogenase	**RDS**	respiratory distress syndrome
LDL	low density lipoproteins	**REM**	rapid eye movement
LE	lupus erythematosus	**RNA**	ribonucleic acid
LH	luteinizing hormone	**RSV**	respiratory syncytial virus
LH-RH	luteinizing hormone-releasing hormone	**SBE**	subacute bacterial endocarditis
LRI	lower respiratory tract infection	**SA**	sinoatrial
m	meter	**SC**	subcutaneous
MAO	monoamine oxidase	**SGOT**	serum glutamic-oxaloacetic transaminase (now often called AST)
MAOI	monoamine oxidase inhibitor	**SGPT**	serum glutamic-pyruvic transaminase (now often called ALT)
μg	microgram	**SIADH**	syndrome of inappropriate antidiuretic hormone secretion
mg	milligram		
MI	myocardial infarction	**SLE**	systemic lupus erythematosus
min	minute(s)	**SMA-12**	sequential multiple analysis-12
ml	milliliter	**SRS-A**	slow-reacting substance of anaphylaxis
ng	nanogram		
NMS	neuroleptic malignant syndrome	**T**	temperature
npo	nothing by mouth (*nihil per os*)	**T$_{1/2}$**	half-life
NSAID	nonsteroidal anti-inflammatory drug	**T$_3$**	triiodothyronine
OC	oral contraceptive	**T$_4$**	thyroxine (tetraiodothyronine)
OTC	over the counter	**TB**	tuberculosis
P	pulse	**TCA**	tricyclic antidepressant
PABA	par-aminobenzoic acid	**TCID**	tissue culture infectious doses
PAT	paroxysmal atrial tachycardia	**TIA**	transient ischemic attack
PBG	porphobilinogen	**tid**	three times a day (*ter in die*)
PBI	protein-bound iodine	**U**	units
PCWP	pulmonary capillary wedge pressure	**UPG**	uroporphyrinogen
PDA	patent ductus arteriosus	**URI**	upper respiratory (tract) infection
PE	pulmonary emboli	**UTI**	urinary tract infection
PG	prostaglandin	**VMA**	3-methoxy-4 hydroxymandelic acid
pH	hydrogen ion concentration	**VLDL**	very low density lipoproteins
PID	pelvic inflammatory disease	**WBC**	white blood cell
PMS	premenstrual syndrome	**WBCT**	whole blood clotting time

1996
Lippincott's Nursing Drug Guide

1996
Lippincott's Nursing Drug Guide

Amy M. Karch, RN, MS

Director of Applied Science/Lecturer
Nazareth College
Rochester, NY

J.B. Lippincott Company
Philadelphia

Acquiring Editor: Margaret Belcher
Coordinating Editorial Assistant: Emily Cotlier
Project Editor: Sandra Cherrey Scheinin
Design Coordinator: Melissa Olson
Interior Designer: Anne O'Donnell
Cover Designer: William T. Donnelly
Production Manager: Helen Ewan
Production Coordinator: Kathryn Rule
Compositor: Port City Press, Inc.
Printer/Binder: R. R. Donnelley & Sons Company/Crawfordsville
Cover Printer: Lehigh Press Lithographers

Copyright (©) 1996, by J. B. Lippincott Company. All rights reserved. No part of this book may be used or reproduced in any manner whatsoever without written permission except for brief quotations embodied in critical articles and reviews. Printed in the United States of America. For information write J. B. Lippincott Company, 227 East Washington Square, Philadelphia, Pennsylvania 19106.

6 5 4 3 2 1

ISSN: 1081-857X

ISBN: 0-397-55148-7

Any procedure or practice described in this book should be applied by the health-care practitioner under appropriate supervision in accordance with professional standards of care used with regard to the unique circumstances that apply in each practice situation. Care has been taken to confirm the accuracy of information presented and to describe generally accepted practices. However, the authors, editors, and publisher cannot accept any responsibility for errors or omissions or for any consequences from application of the information in this book and make no warranty express or implied, with respect to the contents of the book.

Every effort has been made to ensure drug selections and dosages are in accordance with current recommendations and practice. Because of ongoing research, changes in government regulations and the constant flow of information on drug therapy, reactions and interactions, the reader is cautioned to check the package insert for each drug for indications, dosages, warnings and precautions, particularly if the drug is new or infrequently used.

Consultants

Clinical Consultants

Marion J. Anema, RN, PhD
Professor & Dean, School of Nursing
Tennessee State University
Nashville, Tennessee

Jean Bartek, RN, PhD, CARN
Associate Professor
University of Nebraska Medical Center
Colleges of Nursing and Medicine
Omaha, Nebraska

Patricia Brown-Dominguez, RN, MSN
Assistant Professor
Houston Baptist University
College of Nursing
Houston, Texas

Sarah Connor, RNCS, BSN, MSN, EdD
Assistant to Vice President and Dean of Faculty
Armstrong State College
Savannah, Georgia

Elizabeth Fisk, RN, MS
Associate Professor
Nursing Department
Fitchburg State College
Fitchburg, Massachusetts

Sally Scavone, RN, BSN, MS
Assistant Professor
Nursing Department
Erie Community College/City Campus
Erie, New York

Theresa Schumacher, RN, BSN, MSN
Area Chairperson, Level 4
School of Nursing
Good Samaritan Hospital
Cincinnati, Ohio

Pharmacology Consultants

Jeffrey Baldwin, BS (Pharm), PharmD, RPh
Associate Professor of Pharmacy Practice and (courtesy) Pediatrics
University of Nebraska Medical Center
College of Pharmacy
Omaha, Nebraska

James Fenner, PharmD, BCPS
Clinical Coordinator, Infectious Disease
Buffalo General Hospital
Department of Pharmacy
Buffalo, New York

Barbara Kesler, RPh
Instruction Coordinator
El Paso Community College
Staff Pharmacist
Thomson General Hospital
El Paso, Texas

Robert Stanton, MBA, PharmD
Clinical Pharmacist
Cabell Huntingdon Hospital
Assistant Professor
Marshall University
Huntingdon, West Virginia

Patricia Warunek, RN, PhD
Professor, Department of Biology
Farleigh-Dickinson University
Teaneck, New Jersey

Preface

How To Use This Drug Guide

The number of clinically important drugs increases every year, as does the nurse's responsibility for drug therapy. No nurse can memorize all the drug information needed to provide safe and efficacious drug therapy. The *1996 Lippincott's Nursing Drug Guide* provides the drug information nurses need in a concise, ready-access format, and presents nursing considerations related to drug therapy in the format of the nursing process—a framework for applying basic pharmacologic information to patient care. It is intended for the nurse who is just learning how to apply pharmacologic data in the clinical situation, as well as for the busy practicing professional nurse who needs a quick, easy-to-use guide to the clinical use of drugs. This book provides broad coverage of the drugs commonly encountered by nurses and of drugs whose use commonly involves significant nursing intervention. Commonly used medical abbreviations are found throughout the book. All abbreviations are defined in the list of Commonly Used Medical Abbreviations, located on the inside front cover and facing page.

The first section of this book provides a concise review of the nursing process and its application to pharmacologic situations. A review of selected drug classifications provides a convenient, complete summary of the drug information pertinent to all drugs.

Drug information is presented in monograph form, with the monographs arranged alphabetically by generic name. If the generic name of a drug is not known, it may be found quickly by checking the comprehensive index at the back of the drug guide, using *whatever* name is known. The index provides the generic name—the key to finding the appropriate monograph—for most drug brand names, for commonly used chemical names, and for any commonly used "jargon" names (such as "IDU" for idoxuridine). In addition, the index lists drugs by clinically important classes. Chlorpromazine, for example, is indexed by its generic name, by its brand names, and by classes such as an antipsychotic drug (a therapeutic classification), a phenothiazine (a chemical classification), and a dopaminergic blocking drug (a classification by postulated mechanism of action). Each page of the book contains guide words at the top, much like a dictionary, to facilitate easy access to any drug. The right hand edge of the book contains letter guides, again to facilitate finding a drug as quickly as possible.

Each drug monograph is complete in itself—that is, it includes all of the clinically important information that a nurse needs to know to give the drug safely and effectively. Every monograph begins with the drug's generic (nonproprietary) name, an alphabetical list of the most common brand names, including common brand names found only in Canada (noted by the designation CAN), a notation indicating if the drug is available as an OTC drug, its pregnancy category classification, and its schedule (if it is a controlled substance).

Commonly accepted pronunciation (after *United States Adopted Names [USAN] and the United States Pharmacopeia [USP] Dictionary of Drug Names, 1987*) is provided to help the nurse feel more comfortable discussing the drug with other members of the health care team. The clinically important drug classes of each drug are indicated to put the drug in appropriate context. The pharmacokinetic profile of the drug is given in table form to allow easy access to such information as half-life, peak levels, distribution, and so forth. The therapeutically useful actions of the drug are described, including, where known, the mechanism(s) by which these therapeutic effects are produced; no attempt is made to list *all* of the drug's known actions here. A description of the therapeutically useful actions is followed by a list of the clinical indications for the drug, including important non-FDA approved or "unlabeled" indications, as well as orphan drug uses where appropriate. This is followed by a listing of the contraindications to drug use and cautions that should be considered.

Dosage information is listed next, including adult, pediatric, and geriatric, and dosages for different indications when these differ. Details of drug administration that must not be overlooked for the safe administration of the drug (eg, "Dilute before infusing," or "Infuse *slowly* over 30 minutes") are included in the dosage section, but other aspects of drug administration (eg, directions for reconstituting a powder for injection) are presented under "Implementation" in the next section of the monograph. If there is a treatment for the overdose of this drug, that information is indicated in a separate section. A pharmacokinetics table offers a quick reference to how the drug is handled in the body. The **IV Facts** section will give concise, important information that is needed for drugs given IV—dilution, flow rate, compatibilities—making it unnecessary to have a separate IV handbook.

This section is followed by commonly encountered adverse effects. The adverse effects are listed by body system, and the most commonly encountered adverse effects appear in italics to make it easier to assess the patient for adverse effects and to teach the patient about what to expect. Adverse effects that are potentially life-threatening are in bold for easy access. Adverse effects that have been reported, but appear less commonly or rarely, are also listed to make the drug information as complete as possible. Clinically important interactions are listed separately for easy access—drug-drug, drug-food, and drug-laboratory test interferences to consider when using the drug and any nursing action that is necessary because of this interaction.

The remainder of each monograph is concerned with nursing considerations, which are presented, as stated above, in the format of the nursing process. The steps of the nursing process are given slightly different names by different authorities; this drug guide considers: assessment (history and physical), implementation, and drug-specific teaching points for each of the drugs presented.

1. ***Assessment:*** Outlines the information that should be collected before administering the drug. This section is further divided into two subsections:
- *History:* Includes those underlying conditions that constitute contraindications/cautions for use of the drug.
- *Physical:* Provides data by organ system that should be collected before beginning drug therapy, both to allow detection of conditions that are contraindications/cautions to the use of the drug and to provide baseline data to allow detection of adverse reactions to the drug.
2. ***Implementation:*** Lists in chronologic order, those nursing activities that should be undertaken in the course of caring for a patient who is receiving the drug. This includes interventions related to drug preparation and administration, the provision of comfort and safety measures, and drug levels to monitor, as appropriate.
3. ***Drug-Specific Patient Teaching Points:*** Includes specific information that is needed for teaching the patient who is receiving this drug. This information can be transferred to the type of sample Patient Teaching Guide that is found in the appendices and used as written information cards for the patient to take home.

The appendices contain information that is useful to nursing practice but may not lend itself to the monograph format—combination drugs, biologicals, topical drugs, vitamins, laxatives, ophthalmic preparations, adjuncts to general anesthesia, peripheral vasodilators, general anesthetics, topical corticosteroids—as well as pregnancy categories, schedule of controlled substance, formulas for dosage calculations, pediatric nomograms, a list of nursing diagnoses, a guide for injections, a recommended immunization schedule, equianalgesic dosages for narcotics, common cancer chemotherapy combinations, a guide for immunizations, guides to drug compatibility and drug compatibility in syringes, and the sample patient teaching guide referred to earlier. A suggested bibliography follows the appendices.

It is hoped that the overall organization and concise, straightforward presentation of the material in this *1996 Lippincott's Nursing Drug Guide* will make it a clinically useful reference for the nurse who needs easily accessible information to facilitate drug therapy within the framework of the nursing process. It is further hoped that the thoroughness of the additional sections of the book will make it an invaluable reference that will replace the need for several additional references.

Amy M. Karch, RN, MS

Acknowledgments

I would like to thank the many people who have helped to make this book possible: My students and colleagues, past and present, who have helped me learn how to make pharmacology useable in different areas of nursing practice and who have so generously shared their experience to make this book even more clinically useful; my editor at J.B. Lippincott Company, Margaret Belcher, who believed in this project and provided encouragement and humor when it was needed most, and who mastered all of the minute details and kept things in order; Diana Intenzo, for being the constant that is so badly needed in this business; Emily Cotlier, who kept all of us on our toes; Mark Jacobson and Tim Morgan, who spent hours working to get this project computer compatible; Sandy Cherrey Scheinin for organizing and mediating all of the editing process; my husband, Dr. Fred E. Karch, who was able to share his wonderful understanding and knowledge of pharmacology, medicine, and computers, and who offered support and encouragement and tolerated the long nights and late dinners; my children Timothy, Mark, Cortney, and Kathryn for their encouragement and begrudging tolerance and smiles; and Cider who provided endless hours of company and who always answered all problems and frustrations with a happily wagging tail that kept everything in perspective.

Contents

Part I

1 **Nursing process guidelines related to drug administration** 3

2 **Pharmacologic drug classification** 7

Part II

Alphabetical listing of drugs by generic name 57

Appendix A
Drug tables 1151
 Anorexiants 1151
 General anesthetics 1152
 Local anesthetics 1158
 Commonly used biologicals 1157
 Other biologicals 1177
 Chemotherapeutic regimens 1177
 Commonly used fixed-combination drugs: Dosages 1177
 Laxatives 1202
 Peripheral vasodilators 1202
 Vitamins 1206
 Topical agents 1207
 Topical corticosteroids 1207

Appendix B
Recommended immunization schedule 1223

Appendix C
Formulae for calculating pediatric dosages 1224

Appendix D
FDA pregnancy categories 1226

Appendix E
DES schedules of controlled substances 1227

Appendix F
NANDA-approved nursing diagnoses 1228

Appendix G
Narcotic equianalgesic dosages 1231

Appendix H
Injections information 1232

Appendix I
Patient teaching guide   1237

Appendix J
Adjuncts to anesthetics   1238

Appendix K
Ophthalmic agents   1240

Appendix L
Drug compatibility guide   1244

Appendix M
Quick check: Compatibility of drugs in syringe   1246

Bibliography   1249

Index   1251

Part I

I

Nursing Process Guidelines Related to Drug Administration

The delivery of medical care today is in a constant state of change and sometimes in crisis. The population is aging, resulting in more chronic disease and more complex care issues. The population is transient, resulting in unstable support systems, fewer at-home care providers and helpers. At the same time, medicine is undergoing a technological boom (eg, CAT scans, NMRIs, experimental drugs). Patients are being discharged earlier from the acute care facility or not being admitted at all for procedures that used to treated in the hospital with follow-up support and monitoring. Patients are becoming more responsible for their own care and for following complicated medical regimens at home.

Nursing is a unique and complex science and a nurturing and caring art. In the traditional sense, nurses have always been seen as ministering and soothing the sick. In the current state of medical changes, nursing also has become more technical and scientific. Nurses have had to assume increasing responsibilities involved with not only nurturing and caring, but with assessing, diagnosing, and intervening with patients to treat, prevent, and educate to help people cope with various health states.

The nurse deals with the whole person—the physical, emotional, intellectual, and spiritual aspects—considering the ways that a person responds to treatment, disease, and the change in lifestyle that may be required by both. The nurse is the key health care provider in a position to assess the patient—physical, social, and emotional aspects—to administer therapy and medications, teach the patient how best to cope with the therapy to ensure the most effectiveness, and evaluate the effectiveness of therapy. This requires a broad base of knowledge in the basic sciences (anatomy, physiology, nutrition, chemistry, pharmacology), the social sciences (sociology, psychology) and education (learning approaches, evaluation).

Although all nursing theorists do not completely agree on the process that defines the practice of nursing, most include certain key elements in the nursing process. These elements are the basic components of the decision-making or problem-solving process: assessment (gathering of information), diagnosis (defining that information to arrive at some conclusions), intervention (eg, administration, education, comfort measures), and evaluation (determining the effects of the interventions that were performed). The use of this process each time a situation arises ensures a method of coping with the overwhelming scientific and technical information confounding the situation and the unique emotional, social, and physical aspects that each patient brings to the situation. Using the nursing process format in each instance of drug therapy will ensure that the patient receives the best, most efficient, scientifically based holistic care.

Assessment

The first step of the nursing process is the systematic, organized collection of data about the patient. Because the nurse is responsible for holistic care, these data must include information about physical, intellectual, emotional, social, and environmental factors. They will provide the nurse with information needed to plan discharge, plan educational programs, arrange for appropriate consultations, and monitor physical response to treatment or to disease. In actual clinical practice, this process never ends. The patient is not in a steady state but is dynamic, adjusting to physical, emotional, and environmental influences. Each nurse develops a unique approach to the organization of the assessment, an approach that is functional and useful in the clinical setting and that makes sense to that nurse and that clinical situation.

Drug therapy is a complex, integral, and important part of health care today, and the principles of drug therapy need to be incorporated into every patient assessment plan. The particular information that is needed and that should be assessed will vary with each drug, but the concepts involved are similar and are based on the principles of drug therapy. Two important areas that need to be assessed are history and physical assessment.

History

Past experiences and past illnesses impact the actual effect of a drug.

Chronic Conditions: These may be contraindications to the use of a drug or may require that caution be used or that drug dosage be adjusted.

Drug Use: Prescription drugs, OTC drugs, street drugs, alcohol, nicotine, and caffeine all may have an impact on the effect of a drug. Patients often neglect to mention OTC drugs, not considering them actual drugs, and should be asked specifically about OTC drug use.

Allergies: Past exposure to a drug or other allergen can predict a future reaction or note a caution for the use of a drug, food, or animal product.

Level of Education: This information will help to provide a basis for patient education programs and level of explanation.

Level of Understanding of Disease and Therapy: This information also will direct the development of educational information.

Social Supports: Patients are being discharged earlier than ever before and often need assistance at home to provide care and institute and monitor drug therapy.

Financial Supports: The financial impact of health care and the high cost of medications need to be considered when prescribing drugs and depending on the patient to follow through with drug therapy.

Pattern of Health Care: The way that a patient seeks health care will give the nurse valuable information to include in educational information. Does this patient routinely seek followup care or wait for emergency situations?

Physical Assessment

Weight: Weight is an important factor when determining if the recommended dosage of a drug is appropriate. The recommended dosage is based on the 150-lb adult male. Patients who are much lighter or much heavier will need a dosage adjustment.

Age: Patients at the extremes of the age spectrum—pediatric and geriatric—often require dosage adjustments based on the functional level of the liver and kidneys and the responsiveness of other organs.

Physical Parameters Related to the Disease State or Known Drug Effects: Assessment of these factors before beginning drug therapy will give a baseline level with which future assessments can be compared to determine the effects of drug therapy. The specific parameters that need to be assessed will depend on the disease process being treated and on the expected therapeutic and adverse effects of the drug therapy. Because the nurse has the greatest direct and continual contact with the patient, the nurse has the best opportunity to detect the minute changes that will determine the course of drug therapy and therapeutic success or discontinuation because of adverse or unacceptable responses.

The monographs in this book include the specific parameters that need to be assessed in relation to the particular drug being discussed. This assessment provides not only the baseline information needed before giving that drug, but the data needed to evaluate the effects of that drug on the patient. The information given in this area should supplement the overall nursing assessment of the patient, which will include social, intellectual, financial, environmental, and other physical data.

Nursing Diagnoses

Once data have been collected, the nurse must organize and analyze that information to arrive at a nursing diagnosis. A nursing diagnosis is simply a statement of the patient's status from a nursing perspective. This statement directs appropriate nursing interventions. A nursing diagnosis will show actual or potential alteration in patient function based on the assessment of the clinical situation. Because drug therapy is only a small part of the overall patient situation, the nursing diagnoses that are related to drug therapy must be incorporated into a total picture of the patient. In many cases the drug therapy will not present a new nursing diagnosis, but the desired effects and adverse effects related to each drug given should be considered in the nursing diagnoses for each patient. The North American Nursing Diagnosis Association (NANDA) list of accepted nursing diagnoses is included as Appendix F.

Interventions

The assessment and diagnosis of the patient's situation will direct specific nursing interventions. Three types of interventions are frequently involved in drug therapy: drug administration, provision of comfort measures, and patient/family teaching.

Drug Administration

Drug: Ensuring that the drug being administered is the correct dose of the correct drug at the correct time, and is being given to the correct patient, is standard nursing practice.

Storage: Some drugs require specific storage environments (eg, refrigeration, protection from light).

Route: Determining the best route of administration is often determined by the prescription of the drug. Nurses can often have an impact on modifying the prescribed route to determine the most efficient route and the most comfortable one for the patient based on his or her specific situation. When establishing the prescribed route, it is important to check the proper method of administering a drug by that route.

Dosage: Drug dosage may need to be calculated based on available drug form, patient body weight or surface area, or kidney function.

Preparation: Some drugs require specific preparation before administration. Oral drugs may need to be shaken, crushed; parenteral drugs may need to be reconstituted or diluted with specific solutions; topical drugs may require specific handling before administration.

Timing: Actual administration of a drug may require coordination with the administration of other drugs, foods, or physical parameters. The nurse, as the caregiver most frequently involved in administering a drug, must be aware and juggle all of these factors and educate the patient to do this on his or her own.

Recording: Once the nurse has assessed the patient, made the appropriate nursing diagnoses, and delivered the correct drug by the correct route, in the correct dose, and at the correct time, that information needs to be recorded in accordance with the local requirements for recording medication administration.

Each monograph in this book contains pertinent guidelines for storage, dosage, preparation, and administration of the drug being discussed.

Comfort Measures

Nurses are in the unique position to help the patient cope with the effects of drug therapy as they impact him or her.

Placebo Effect: The anticipation that a drug will be helpful (placebo effect) has been proved to have tremendous impact on actual success of drug therapy, so the nurse's attitude and support can be a critical part of drug therapy. A back rub, a kind word, a positive approach may be as beneficial as the drug itself.

Side Effects: These interventions can be directed at decreasing the impact of the anticipated side effects of the drug and promoting patient safety. Such interventions include environmental control (eg, temperature, lighting), safety measures (eg, avoiding driving, avoiding the sun, using side rails), physical comfort (eg, skin care, laxatives, frequent meals).

Lifestyle Adjustment: Some drug effects will require that a patient change his or her lifestyle to cope effectively. Diuretic users may have to rearrange the day to be near toilet facilities when the drug works.

MAOI users have to adjust their diet to prevent serious drug effects.

Each monograph in this book will include a list of pertinent comfort measures appropriate to that particular drug.

Education

With patients becoming more responsible for their own care, it is becoming essential that they have all of the information necessary to ensure safe and effective drug therapy at home. Many states now require that the patient be given written information. Key elements that need to be included in any drug education include the following:

1. Name, dose, and action of drug: With many people seeing more than one health care provider, this information is important for ensuring safe and effective drug therapy.
2. Timing of administration: Patients need to know specifically when to take the drug with regard to frequency, other drugs, and meals.
3. Special storage and preparation instructions: Some drugs require particular handling that the patient will need to have spelled out.
4. Specific OTC drugs to avoid: Many people do not consider OTC drugs to be actual drugs and may inadvertently take them and cause unwanted or even dangerous drug-drug interactions. Spelling out particular problems of which to be aware will help the patient avoid these situations.
5. Special comfort or safety measures that need to be considered: Alerting the patient to ways to cope with anticipated side effects will prevent a great deal of anxiety and noncompliance with drug therapy. The patient also may need to be alerted to the need to return for followup tests or evaluation.
6. Safety measures: All patients need to be alerted to keep drugs out of the reach of children. They also need to be reminded to tell any health care provider whom they see that they are taking this drug. This can prevent drug-drug interactions and misdiagnosing based on drug effects.
7. Specific points about drug toxicity: Warning signs of drug toxicity of which the patient should be aware should be listed. He or she can be advised to notify the health care provider if any of these effects occur.
8. Specific warnings about drug discontinuation: Some drugs with a small margin of safety and drugs with particular systemic effects cannot be stopped abruptly without dangerous effects. Patients taking these drugs need to be alerted to the problem and encouraged to call immediately if they cannot take their medication for any reason (eg, illness, financial).

Each drug monograph in this book lists specific teaching points that relate to that particular drug. The appendix presents a basic patient teaching guideline that can be used in conjunction with the drug-specific teaching points to provide the patient with a compact, written drug card.

Evaluation

Evaluation is part of the continual process of patient care that leads to changes in assessment, diagnosis, and intervention. The patient is continually evaluated for therapeutic response, the occurrence of drug side effects, and the occurrence of drug-drug or drug-laboratory test interaction. The efficacy of the nursing interventions and the education program must be evaluated. In some situations, the nurse will evaluate the patient simply by reapplying the beginning steps of the nursing process and analyzing for change. In some cases of drug therapy, particular therapeutic drug levels need to be evaluated as well.

Monographs in this book list specific evaluation criteria as they apply to each drug. Regular evaluation of drug effects, side effects, and so forth will not be specifically listed but can be deduced from information in the monograph regarding therapeutic effects and adverse effects.

II

Pharmacologic Drug Classification

☐ Alkylating Agents

Pregnancy Category D

Therapeutic actions
Alkylating agents are cytotoxic: they alkylate cellular DNA, interfering with the replication of susceptible cells and causing cell death. Their action is most evident in rapidly dividing cells.

Indications
- Palliative treatment of chronic lymphocytic leukemia; malignant lymphomas, including lymphosarcoma, giant follicular lymphoma; Hodgkin's disease; multiple myelomas; testicular cancers; brain tumors; pancreatic cancer; ovarian and breast cancers
- Often used as part of multiple agent regimens

Contraindications/cautions
- Alkylating agents are contraindicated in the presence of hypersensitivity to the drugs, concurrent radiation therapy, hematopoietic depression, pregnancy, lactation.

Adverse effects
- CNS: *Tremors, muscular twitching, confusion,* agitation, ataxia, flaccid paresis, hallucinations, seizures
- GI: Nausea, vomiting, anorexia, **hepatotoxicity**
- Respiratory: Bronchopulmonary dysplasia, pulmonary fibrosis
- Hematologic: *Bone marrow depression,* hyperuricemia
- GU: Sterility
- Dermatologic: Skin rash, urticaria, alopecia, keratitis
- Other: *Cancer, acute leukemia*

■ Nursing Considerations

Assessment
- *History*: Hypersensitivity to drug, radiation therapy, hematopoietic depression, pregnancy, lactation
- *Physical*: Temperature; weight; skin—color, lesions; R, adventitious sounds; liver evaluation; CBC, differential, hemoglobin, uric acid, renal and liver function tests

Implementation
- Arrange for blood tests to evaluate hematopoietic function before beginning therapy and weekly during therapy.
- Do not give full dosage within 4 wk after a full course of radiation therapy or chemotherapy because of the risk of severe bone marrow depression.
- Ensure that patient is well hydrated before treatment.
- Arrange for small, frequent meals and dietary consultation to maintain nutrition if GI upset occurs.
- Arrange for skin care as appropriate for rashes.

Drug-specific teaching points
- Know that the following side effects may occur: nausea, vomiting, loss of appetite (dividing the dose may help; small, frequent meals also may help; try to maintain your fluid intake and nutrition while on this drug; drink at least 10–12 glassses of fluid each day); infertility (from irregular menses to complete amenorrhea; men may stop producing sperm; this may be an irreversible problem; discuss your feelings with your nurse or physician);

Adverse effects in *Italics* are most common; those in **Bold** are life-threatening.

Amy M. Karch: Lippincott's Nursing Drug Guide. ©1996 J. B. Lippincott Company

this drug can cause severe birth defects; it is advisable to use birth control methods while on this drug.
- Report unusual bleeding or bruising; fever, chills, sore throat; cough, shortness of breath; yellowing of the skin or eyes; flank or stomach pain.

Representative Drugs
busulfan
carboplatin
carmustine
chlorambucil
cisplatin
cyclophosphamide
ifosfamide
lomustine
mechlorethemine
melphalan
streptozocin
thiotepa
uracil mustard

Alpha₁-Adrenergic Blockers

Pregnancy Category C

Therapeutic actions
Alpha-adrenergic blockers selectively block postsynaptic alpha₁-adrenergic receptors, decreasing sympathetic tone on the vasculature, dilating arterioles and veins, and lowering both supine and standing blood pressure; unlike conventional alpha-adrenergic blocking agents (eg, phentolamine), they do not also block alpha₂ presynaptic receptors, so they do not cause reflex tachycardia.

Indications
- Treatment of hypertension (alone or in combination with other agents)
- Treatment of BHP (terazosin)
- Unlabeled uses: management of refractory CHF and Raynaud's vasospasm, treatment of prostatic outflow obstruction

Contraindications/cautions
- Alpha-adrenergic blockers are contraindicated in the presence of hypersensitivity to any alpha₁-adrenergic blocker, lactation. They should be used with caution in the presence of CHF, renal failure, pregnancy.

Adverse effects
- CNS: *Dizziness, headache, drowsiness, lack of energy, weakness,* nervousness, vertigo, depression, paresthesia
- GI: *Nausea,* vomiting, diarrhea, constipation, abdominal discomfort or pain
- CV: *Palpitations,* sodium and water retention, increased plasma volume, edema, dyspnea, syncope, tachycardia, orthostatic hypotension
- GU: Urinary frequency, incontinence, impotence, priapism
- EENT: Blurred vision, reddened sclera, epistaxis, tinnitus, dry mouth, nasal congestion
- Dermatologic: Rash, pruritus, alopecia, lichen planus
- Other: Diaphoresis, lupus erythematosus

Clinically important drug-drug interactions
- Severity and duration of hypotension following first dose of drug may be greater in patients receiving beta-adrenergic blocking drugs (eg, propranolol), verapamil

Nursing Considerations

Assessment
- *History*: Hypersensitivity to alpha₁-adrenergic blocker, CHF, renal failure, lactation
- *Physical:* Body weight; skin—color, lesions; orientation, affect, reflexes; ophthalmologic exam; P, BP, orthostatic BP, supine BP, perfusion, edema, auscultation; R, adventitious sounds, status of nasal mucous membranes; bowel sounds, normal output; voiding pattern, normal output; kidney function tests, urinalysis

Implementation
- Arrange to administer, or have patient take, first dose just before bedtime to lessen likelihood of first dose effect (syncope), believed due to excessive postural hypotension.

Adverse effects in *Italics* are most common; those in **Bold** are life-threatening.

- Place patient in recumbent position, and treat supportively if syncope occurs; condition is self-limiting.
- Monitor patient for orthostatic hypotension, which is most marked in the morning, is accentuated by hot weather, alcohol, exercise.
- Monitor edema, body weight in patients with incipient cardiac decompensation, and arrange to add a thiazide diuretic to the drug regimen if sodium and fluid retention, signs of impending CHF occur.
- Ensure ready access to bathroom facilities if GI effects occur.
- Provide small, frequent meals, frequent mouth care if GI effects occur.
- Establish safety precautions if CNS, hypotensive changes occur (eg, side rails, accompany patient).
- Arrange for analgesic as appropriate for patients experiencing headache.
- Provide appropriate consultations to help patient to cope with sexual dysfunction and priapism.

Drug-specific teaching points

- Take this drug exactly as prescribed. Take the first dose just before bedtime. Do not drive a car or operate machinery for 4 h after the first dose.
- Avoid OTC drugs (eg, nose drops, cold remedies) while you are taking this drug; these could cause dangerous effects. If you feel that you need one of these preparations, consult your nurse or physician.
- Know that the following side effects may occur: dizziness, weakness (these are more likely to occur when you change position, in the early morning, after exercise, in hot weather, and when you have consumed alcohol; some tolerance may occur after you have taken the drug for awhile, but you should avoid driving a car or engaging in tasks that require alertness while you are experiencing these symptoms; change position slowly, and use caution in climbing stairs; lie down for a while if dizziness persists); GI upset (frequent, small meals may help); impotence (you may want to discuss this with your nurse or physician); dry mouth (sucking on sugarless lozenges, ice chips may help); stuffy nose. Most of these effects will gradually disappear with continued therapy.
- Report frequent dizziness or faintness.

Representative Drugs
doxazosin
prazosin
terazosin

☐ Aminoglycosides

Pregnancy Category C

Therapeutic actions
Aminoglycosides are antibiotics that are bactericidal. They inhibit protein synthesis in susceptible strains of gram-negative bacteria, which appear to disrupt the functional integrity of bacterial cell membrane, causing cell death. Oral aminoglycosides are very poorly absorbed and are used for the suppression of GI bacterial flora.

Indications
- Short-term treatment of serious infections caused by susceptible strains of *Pseudomonas* species, *Escherichia coli*, indole-positive *Proteus* species, *Providencia* species, *Klebsiella-Enterobacter-Serratia* species, *Acinetobacter* species
- Suspected gram-negative infections before results of susceptibility studies are known
- Initial treatment of staphylococcal infections when penicillin is contraindicated or when infection may be caused by mixed organisms
- Neonatal sepsis when other antibiotics cannot be used (often used in combination with penicillin-type drug)
- Unlabeled uses: as part of a multidrug regimen for treatment of *Mycobacterium avium* complex (a common infection in AIDS patients) and orally for the treatment of intestinal amebiasis; adjunctive treatment of hepatic coma and for suppresssion of intestinal bacteria for surgery

Contraindications/cautions

- Aminoglycosides are contraindicated in the presence of allergy to any aminoglycosides, renal disease, hepatic disease, preexisting hearing loss, myasthenia gravis, parkinsonism, infant botulism, lactation. Use caution in the presence of elderly patients, any patient with diminished hearing, decreased renal function, dehydration, neuromuscular disorders.

Adverse effects

- CNS: *Ototoxicity;* confusion, disorientation, depression, lethargy, nystagmus, visual disturbances, headache, fever, numbness, tingling, tremor, paresthesias, muscle twitching, convulsions, muscular weakness, neuromuscular blockade, apnea
- GI: *Nausea, vomiting, anorexia, diarrhea,* weight loss, stomatitis, increased salivation, splenomegaly
- CV: Palpitations, hypotension, hypertension
- Hematologic: Leukemoid reaction, agranulocytosis, granulocytosis, leukopenia, leukocytosis, thrombocytopenia, eosinophilia, pancytopenia, anemia, hemolytic anemia, increased or decreased reticulocyte count, electrolyte disturbances
- GU: *Nephrotoxicity*
- Hypersensitivity: Purpura, rash, urticaria, exfoliative dermatitis, itching
- Hepatic: Hepatic toxicity; hepatomegaly
- Other: *Superinfections, pain and irritation at IM injection sites*

Clinically important drug-drug interactions

- Increased ototoxic and nephrotoxic effects if taken with potent diuretics and other ototoxic and nephrotoxic drugs (eg, cephalosporins) • Increased likelihood of neuromuscular blockade if given shortly after general anesthetics, depolarizing and nondepolarizing neuromuscular junction blockers

■ Nursing Considerations

Assessment

- *History:* Allergy to any aminoglycosides, renal disease, hepatic disease, preexisting hearing loss, myasthenia gravis, parkinsonism, infant botulism, lactation, diminished hearing, decreased renal function, dehydration, neuromuscular disorders
- *Physical:* Arrange culture and sensitivity tests on infection before beginning therapy; renal function, eighth cranial nerve function, and state of hydration prior to, periodically during, and after therapy; hepatic function tests, CBC, skin—color, lesions; orientation, affect; reflexes, bilateral grip strength; body weight; bowel sounds

Implementation

- Arrange for culture and sensitivity testing of infected area before beginning treatment.
- Monitor duration of treatment: usual duration of treatment is 7–10 d. If clinical response does not occur within 3–5 d, stop therapy. Prolonged treatment leads to increased risk of toxicity. If drug is used longer than 10 d, monitor auditory and renal function daily.
- Administer IM dosage by deep IM injection.
- Ensure that patient is well hydrated before and during therapy.
- Establish safety measures if CNS, vestibular nerve effects occur (eg, use of side rails, assistance with ambulation).
- Ensure ready access to bathroom facilities in case diarrhea occurs.
- Provide small, frequent meals if nausea, anorexia occur.
- Provide comfort measures and medication for superinfections.

Drug-specific teaching points

- Take full course of oral drug; drink plenty of fluids.
- Know that the following may occur as a result of drug therapy: ringing in the ears, headache, dizziness (these effects are reversible; safety measures may need to be taken if these become severe); nausea, vomiting, loss of appetite (small, frequent meals, frequent mouth care may help).

- Report pain at injection site, severe headache, dizziness, loss of hearing, changes in urine pattern, difficulty breathing, rash or skin lesions.

Representative Drugs
amikacin sulfate
gentamicin
kanamycin
netilmicin
streptomycin
tobramycin (parenteral)
kanamycin
neomycin
paromomycin (oral)

❏ Angiotensin-Converting Enzyme (ACE) Inhibitors

Pregnancy Category C

Therapeutic actions
ACE inhibitors block ACE in the lungs from converting angiotensin I, activated when renin is released from the kidneys, to angiotensin II, a powerful vasoconstrictor. Blocking this conversion leads to decreased blood pressure, decreased aldosterone secretion, a small increase in serum potassium levels, and sodium and fluid loss; increased prostaglandin synthesis also may be involved in the antihypertensive action.

Indications
- Treatment of hypertension (alone or in combination with thiazide-type diuretics)
- Treatment of congestive heart failure in patients who do not respond adequately to conventional therapy (used with diuretics and digitalis)
- Unlabeled uses: management of hypertensive crises; treatment of rheumatoid arthritis; diabetic nephropathy, diagnosis of anatomic renal artery stenosis, hypertension related to scleroderma renal crisis; diagnosis of primary aldosteronism, idiopathic edema; Bartter's syndrome; Raynaud's syndrome; hypertension of Takayasu's disease

Contraindications/cautions
- ACE inhibitors are contraindicated in the presence of allergy to the drug, impaired renal function, CHF, salt/volume depletion, or lactation.

Adverse effects
- **GI:** *Gastric irritation, aphthous ulcers, peptic ulcers, dysgeusia*, cholestatic jaundice, hepatocellular injury, anorexia, constipation
- **CV:** *Tachycardia*, angina pectoris, **myocardial infarction**, Raynaud's syndrome, CHF, hypotension in salt/volume-depleted patients
- **Hematologic:** Neutropenia, agranulocytosis, thrombocytopenia, hemolytic anemia, **fatal pancytopenia**
- **GU:** *Proteinuria*, renal insufficiency, renal failure, polyuria, oliguria, urinary frequency
- **Dermatologic:** *Rash, pruritus,* pemphigoid-like reaction, scalded mouth sensation, exfoliative dermatitis, photosensitivity, alopecia
- **Other:** *Cough,* malaise, dry mouth, lymphadenopathy

Clinically important drug-drug interactions
- Increased risk of hypersensitivity reactions if taken concurrently with allopurinal • Decreased antihypertensive effects if taken with indomethacin

Clinically important drug-food interactions
- Decreased absorption of select agents if taken with food

Drug-lab test interferences
- False-positive test for urine acetone

■ Nursing Considerations

Assessment
- *History:* Allergy to ACE inhibitors, impaired renal function, CHF, salt/volume depletion, pregnancy, lactation
- *Physical:* Skin—color, lesions, turgor; body temperature; P, BP, peripheral perfusion; mucous membranes; bowel sounds; liver evaluation; urinalysis, renal

Adverse effects in *Italics* are most common; those in **Bold** are life-threatening.

and liver function tests, CBC and differential

Implementation
- Administer 1 h before or 2 h after meals if known to be affected by presence of food in GI tract.
- Alert surgeon and mark patient's chart with notice that ACE inhibitor is being taken; the angiotensin II formation subsequent to compensatory renin release during surgery will be blocked; hypotension may be reversed with volume expansion.
- Monitor patient closely in any situation that may lead to a fall in blood pressure secondary to reduction in fluid volume (excessive perspiration and dehydration, vomiting, diarrhea) because excessive hypotension may occur.
- Arrange for reduced dosage in patients with impaired renal function.
- Arrange for bowel program if constipation occurs.
- Provide small, frequent meals if GI upset is severe.
- Provide for frequent mouth care and oral hygiene if mouth sores, alteration in taste occur.
- Caution patient to change position slowly if orthostatic changes occur.
- Provide appropriate skin care as needed.

Drug-specific teaching points
- Take drug 1 h before or 2 h after meals; do not take with food.
- Do not stop taking the medication without consulting your physician.
- Know that the following side effects may occur: GI upset, loss of appetite, change in taste perception (these may be limited effects that will pass with time; if they persist or become a problem, consult your nurse or physician); mouth sores (frequent mouth care may help); skin rash; fast heart rate; dizziness, lightheadedness (this usually passes after the first few days of therapy; if it occurs, change position slowly, and limit your activities to those that do not require alertness and precision).
- Be careful in any situation that may lead to a drop in blood pressure (diarrhea, sweating, vomiting, dehydration); if lightheadedness or dizziness should occur, consult your nurse or physician.
- Avoid OTC medications while you are on this drug, especially cough, cold, allergy medications that may contain ingredients that will interact with this drug. If you feel that you need one of these preparations, consult your nurse or physician.
- Report mouth sores; sore throat, fever, chills; swelling of the hands, feet; irregular heartbeat, chest pains; swelling of the face, eyes, lips, tongue, difficulty in breathing.

Representative Drugs
benazepril
captopril
enalapril
enalaprilat
fosinopril
lisinopril
quinapril
ramipril
spirapril

❐ Antiarrhythmics

Pregnancy Category C

Therapeutic actions
Antiarrhythmics act at specific sites to alter the action potential of cardiac cells and interfere with the eletrical excitability of the heart. Most of these drugs may cause new or worsened arrhythmias (proarrhythmic effect) and must be used with caution and with continual cardiac monitoring and patient evaluation.

Indications
- Treatment of tachycardia when rapid but short-term control of ventricular rate is desirable (eg, patients with atrial fibrillation, flutter, in perioperative or postoperative situations)
- Treatment of noncompensatory tachycardia when heart rate requires specific intervention
- Treatment of atrial arrhythmias

Contraindications/cautions
- These drugs are reserved for emergency situations; there are no contraindications. Use caution during pregnancy or lactation.

Adverse effects
- CNS: *Lightheadedness, speech disorder, midscapular pain, weakness, rigors,* somnolence, confusion
- GI: *Taste perversion*
- CV: *Hypotension,* pallor
- GU: *Urinary retention*
- Local: *Inflammation,* induration, edema, erythema, burning at the site of infusion
- Other: Fever, rhonchi, flushing

Clinically important drug-drug interactions
- Monitor patients receiving antiarrhythmics for many drug-drug interactions; see specific drug for clinically important interactions specific to that drug.

■ Nursing Considerations

Assessment
- *History*: Cardiac disease, cerebrovascular disease
- *Physical*: P, BP, ECG; orientation, reflexes; R, adventitious sounds; urinary output

Implementation
- Ensure that more toxic drug is not used in chronic settings when transfer to another agent is anticipated.
- Monitor closely BP, heart rate, and rhythm.
- Provide appropriate comfort measures to deal with pain, rigors, fever, flushing, as appropriate and if patient is awake.
- Provide supportive measures appropriate to condition being treated.
- Provide support and encouragement to deal with drug effects, discomfort of IV lines, and so forth.

Drug-specific teaching points
- This drug is reserved for emergency use; it is best to incorporate any information about this drug into the overall teaching program for this patient. Patients maintained on oral drug will need teaching specific to that particular drug or drug type. See specific monograph for details.

Representative Drugs
Type I
  moricizine
Type IA
  disopyramide
  procainamide
  quinidine
Type B
  lidocaine
  mexilitine
  phenytoin
  tocainide
Type C
  flecainide
  propafenone
Type II
  acebutolol
  esmolol
  propranolol
Type III
  amiodarone
  bretylium
  sotalol
Type IV
  verapamil

❒ Anticoagulants

Pregnancy Category D

Therapeutic actions
Oral anticoagulants interfere with the hepatic synthesis of vitamin K-dependent clotting factors (factors II, prothrombin, VII, IX, and X), resulting in their eventual depletion and prolongation of clotting times; parenteral anticoagulants interfere with the conversion of prothrombin to thrombin, blocking the final step in clot formation but leaving the circulating levels of clotting factors unaffected.

Adverse effects in *Italics* are most common; those in **Bold** are life-threatening.

Indications

- Treatment and prevention of pulmonary embolism and venous thrombosis and its extension
- Treatment of atrial fibrillation with embolization
- Prevention of deep vein thrombosis
- Prophylaxis of systemic emobization after acute MI
- Unlabeled uses: prevention of recurrent transient ischemic attacks, prevention of recurrent myocardial infarction, and adjunt to therapy in small-cell carcinoma of the lung.

Contraindications/cautions

- Anticoagulants are contraindictated in the presence of allergy to the drug; SBE; hemorrhagic disorders; tuberculosis; hepatic diseases; GI ulcers; renal disease; indwelling catheters, spinal puncture; aneurysm; diabetes; visceral carcinoma; uncontrolled hypertension; severe trauma (including recent or contemplated CNS, eye surgery, recent placement of IUD); threatened abortion, menometrorrhagia; pregnancy (oral agents known to cause fetal damage and death); or lactation (suggest using heparin if anticoagulation is required). Use caution in the presence of CHF, diarrhea, fever; thyrotoxicosis; senile, psychotic, or depressed patients.

Adverse effects

- GI: *Nausea*, vomiting, anorexia, abdominal cramping, diarrhea, retroperitoneal hematoma, hepatitis, jaundice, mouth ulcers
- Hematologic: Granulocytosis, leukopenia, eosinophilia
- GU: Priapism, nephropathy, red-orange urine
- Dermatologic: *Alopecia, urticaria, dermatitis*
- Bleeding: *Hemorrhage*; GI or urinary tract bleeding (hematuria, dark stools; paralytic ileus; intestinal obstruction from hemorrhage into GI tract); petechiae and purpura, bleeding from mucous membranes; hemorrhagic infarction, vasculitis, skin necrosis of female breast; adrenal hemorrhage and resultant adrenal insufficiency; compressive neuropathy secondary to hemorrhage near a nerve
- Other: Fever, "purple toes" syndrome

Clinically important drug-drug interactions

- Increased bleeding tendencies if taken concurrently with salicylates, chloral hydrate, phenylbutazone, clofibrate, disulfiram, chloramphenicol, metronidazole, cimetidine, ranitidine, co-trimoxazole, sulfinpyrazone, quinidine, quinine, oxyphenbutazone, thyroid drugs, glucagon, danazol, erythromycin, androgens, amiodarone, cefamandole, cefoperazone, cefotetan, moxalactam, cefazolin, cefoxitin, ceftriaxone, meclofenamate, mefenamic acid, famotidine, nizatidine, nalidixic acid • Decreased anticoagulation effect possible if taken concurrently with barbiturates, griseofulvin, rifampin, phenytoin, glutethimide, carbamazepine, vitamin K, vitamin E, cholestyramine, aminoglutethimide, ethchlorvynol • Altered effects of warfarin if taken concurrently with methimazole, propylthiouracil • Increased activity and toxicity of phenytoin when taken with oral anticoagulants

Drug-lab test interferences

- Red-orange discoloration of alkaline urine may interfere with some lab tests.

■ Nursing Considerations

Assessment

- *History*: Allergy to the drug; SBE; hemorrhagic disorders; tuberculosis; hepatic diseases; GI ulcers; renal disease; indwelling catheters, spinal puncture; aneurysm; diabetes; visceral carcinoma; uncontrolled hypertension; severe trauma; threatened abortion, menometrorrhagia; pregnancy; lactation; CHF, diarrhea, fever; thyrotoxicosis; senile, psychotic, or depressed patients
- *Physical*: Skin—lesions, color, temperature; orientation, reflexes, affect; P, BP, peripheral perfusion, baseline ECG; R, adventitious sounds; liver evaluation,

Adverse effects in *Italics* are most common; those in **Bold** are life-threatening.

bowel sounds, normal output; CBC, urinalysis, guaiac stools, prothrombin time, renal and hepatic function tests, WBCT, APTT

Implementation
- Monitor clotting times regularly, as appropriate, to adjust dosage.
- Do not change brand names once stabilized; bioavailability problems have been documented.
- Evaluate patient regularly for signs of blood loss (eg, petechiae, bleeding gums, bruises, dark stools, dark urine).
- Establish safety measures to protect patient from injury.
- Do not give patient any IM injections. Monitor any site of invasive procedures; ensure prolonged compression of bleeding vessels.
- Double-check any other drug that is ordered for the patient for potential drug-drug interaction: dosage of both drugs may need to be adjusted.
- Use caution when discontinuing any other medication; dosage of warfarin may need to be adjusted; carefully monitor PT values.
- Maintain vitamin K on standby in case of overdose of oral agents; maintain protamine sulfate on standby for parenteral drug.
- Arrange for frequent follow-up, including blood tests to evaluate drug effects.
- Evaluate for therapeutic effects: prothrombin time, 1.5–2.5 times the control value; WBCT, 2.5–3 times control; APTT, 1.5–2 times normal.

Drug-specific teaching points
- Be aware that many factors may change your body's response to this drug—fever, change of diet, change of environment, other medications. The dosage of the drug may have to be changed on several occasions. Be sure to write down any change of dose that is prescribed.
- Do not change any medication that you are taking (adding or stopping another drug) without consulting your nurse or physician. Many other drugs affect the way that your anticoagulant works; starting or stopping another drug can cause excessive bleeding or interfere with the desired effects of the drug.
- Carry or wear a medical alert tag stating that you are on this drug. This will alert any medical personnel who might take care of you in an emergency that you are taking this drug.
- Avoid situations in which you could be easily injured, for example, contact sports, shaving with a straight razor.
- Know that the following side effects may occur: stomach bloating, cramps (this often passes with time; if it becomes too uncomfortable, contact your nurse or physician); loss of hair, skin rash (this is a frustrating and upsetting effect; if it becomes a problem, discuss it with your nurse or physician); orange-red discoloration to the urine (this may be upsetting because it can be mistaken for blood; add vinegar to your urine, and the color should disappear).
- Arrange to have periodic blood tests to check on the action of the drug. It is very important that you have these tests.
- Use contraceptive measures while taking this drug; it is important that you do not become pregnant.
- Report unusual bleeding (such as when you are brushing your teeth, excessive bleeding from injuries, excessive bruising), black or bloody stools, cloudy or dark urine, sore throat, fever, chills, severe headaches, dizziness, suspected pregnancy.

Representative Drugs
Oral
  warfarin sodium
Parenteral
  dalteparin
  enoxaparin
  heparin

☐ Antidiabetic Agents

Pregnancy Category C

Therapeutic actions
Oral antidiabetic agents are called sulfonylureas. They stimulate insulin release

from functioning beta cells in the pancreas; may improve binding between insulin and insulin receptors or increase the number of insulin receptors; second-generation sulfonylureas (glipizide and glyburide) are thought to be more potent than first-generation sulfonylureas.

Indications
- Adjuncts to diet to lower blood glucose in patients with non–insulin-dependent diabetes mellitus (type II)
- Adjuncts to insulin therapy in the stabilization of certain cases of insulin-dependent maturity-onset diabetes, reducing the insulin requirement and decreasing the chance of hypoglycemic reactions

Contraindications/cautions
- Sulfonylureas are contraindicated in the presence of allergy to sulfonylureas; diabetes complicated by fever, severe infections, severe trauma, major surgery, ketosis, acidosis, coma (insulin is indicated in these conditions); type I or juvenile diabetes, serious hepatic impairment, serious renal impairment, uremia, thyroid or endocrine impairment, glycosuria, hyperglycemia associated with primary renal disease; labor and delivery (if glipizide is used during pregnancy, discontinue drug at least 1 mo before delivery); lactation, safety not established.

Adverse effects
- **GI:** *Anorexia, nausea,* vomiting, *epigastric discomfort, heartburn, diarrhea*
- **CV:** Increased risk of cardiovascular mortality
- **Hematologic:** Leukopenia, thrombocytopenia, anemia
- **Hypersensitivity:** *Allergic skin reactions*, eczema, pruritus, erythema, urticaria, photosensitivity, fever, eosinophilia, jaundice
- **Endocrine:** *Hypoglycemia*

Clinically important drug-drug interactions
- Increased risk of hypoglycemia if taken concurrently with sulfonamides, chloramphenicol, fenfluramine, oxyphenbutazone, phenylbutazone, salicylates, clofibrate
- Decreased effectiveness of both sulfonylurea and diazoxide if taken concurrently
- Increased risk of hyperglycemia if taken with rifampin, thiazides
- Risk of hypoglycemia and hyperglycemia if taken with ethanol; "disulfiram reaction" also has been reported.

■ Nursing Considerations

Assessment
- ***History:*** Allergy to sulfonylureas; diabetes complicated by fever, severe infections, severe trauma, major surgery, ketosis, acidosis, coma (insulin is indicated in these conditions); type I or juvenile diabetes, serious hepatic impairment, serious renal impairment, uremia, thyroid or endocrine impairment, glycosuria, hyperglycemia associated with primary renal disease
- ***Physical:*** Skin—color, lesions; body temperature; orientation, reflexes, peripheral sensation; R, adventitious sounds; liver evaluation, bowel sounds; urinalysis, BUN, serum creatinine, liver function tests, blood glucose, CBC

Implementation
- Administer drug in the morning before breakfast; if severe GI upset occurs may be divided and given before meals.
- Monitor urine and serum glucose levels frequently to determine effectiveness of drug and dosage being used.
- Arrange for transfer to insulin therapy during periods of high stress (eg, infections, surgery, trauma).
- Arrange for use of IV glucose if severe hypoglycemia occurs as a result of overdose.
- Arrange for consultation with dietician to establish weight loss program and dietary control as appropriate.
- Arrange for thorough diabetic teaching program to include disease, dietary control, exercise, signs and symptoms of hypoglycemia and hyperglycemia, avoidance of infection, hygiene.
- Provide good skin care to prevent breakdown.

Adverse effects in *Italics* are most common; those in **Bold** are life-threatening.

- Ensure ready access to bathroom facilities if diarrhea occurs.
- Establish safety precautions if CNS effects occur.

Drug-specific teaching points
- Do not discontinue this medication without consulting physician.
- Monitor urine or blood for glucose and ketones as prescribed.
- Do not use this drug during pregnancy.
- Avoid alcohol while on this drug.
- Report fever, sore throat, unusual bleeding or bruising, skin rash, dark urine, light-colored stools, hypoglycemic or hyperglycemic reactions.

Representative Drugs
acetohexamide
chlorpropamide
glipizide
glyburide
metformin
tolazamide
tolbutamide

☐ Antifungals

Pregnancy Category C

Therapeutic actions
Antifungals bind to or impair sterols of fungal cell membranes, allowing increased permeability and leakage of cellular components and causing the death of the fungal cell.

Indications
- Systemic fungal infections: candidiasis, chronic mucocutaneous candidiasis, oral thrush, candiduria, blastomycosis, coccidioidomycosis, histoplasmosis, chromomycosis, paracoccidioidomycosis, dermatophytosis, ringworm infections of the skin
- Unlabeled uses: treatment of onychomycosis, pityriasis versicolor, vaginal candidiasis; CNS fungal infections (at high doses); topical treatment of tinea corporis and tinea cruris caused by *Trichophyton rubrum, Trichophyton mentagrophytes* and *Epidermophyton floccosum*; treatment of tinea versicolor caused by *Malassezia furfur* (topical administration); and reduction of scaling due to dandruff (shampoo)

Contraindications/cautions
- Antifungals are contraindicated in the presence of allergy to any antifungal, fungal meningitis, pregnancy, or lactation. Use with caution in the presence of hepatocellular failure (increased risk of hepatocellular necrosis).

Adverse effects
- **CNS**: Headache, dizziness, somnolence, photophobia
- **GI**: Hepatotoxicity, *nausea, vomiting,* abdominal pain
- **Hematologic**: Thrombocytopenia, leukopenia, hemolytic anemia
- **GU**: Impotence, oligospermia (with very high doses)
- **Hypersensitivity**: Urticaria to anaphylaxis
- **General**: *Pruritus,* fever, chills, gynecomastia
- **Local**: *Severe irritation, pruritus, stinging* with topical application

Clinically important drug-drug interactions
- Decreased blood levels if taken with rifampin • Increased blood levels of cyclosporine and risk of toxicity when taken with antifungals • Increased duration of adrenal suppression when methylprednisolone, corticosteroids are taken with antifungals

■ Nursing Considerations

Assessment
- *History*: Allergy to antifungals, fungal meningitis, hepatocellular failure, pregnancy, lactation
- *Physical*: Skin—color, lesions; orientation, reflexes, affect; bowel sounds, liver evaluation; liver function tests; CBC and differential; culture of area involved

Implementation
- Arrange for culture of fungus involved before beginning therapy; treatment

Adverse effects in Italics are most common; those in **Bold** *are life-threatening.*

should begin, however, before lab results are returned.
- Maintain epinephrine on standby in case of severe anaphylaxis after first dose.
- Administer oral drug with food to decrease GI upset.
- Continue administration for long-term therapy until infection is eradicated: candidiasis, 1–2 wk; other systemic mycoses, 6 mo; chronic mucocutaneous candidiasis, often requires maintainance therapy; tinea veriscolor, 2 wk of topical application.
- Discontinue treatment and consult physician about actual diagnosis if no improvement is seen within 2 wk of topical application.
- Discontinue topical applications if sensitivity or chemical reaction occurs.
- Administer shampoo as follows: moisten hair and scalp thoroughly with water; apply sufficient shampoo to produce a lather; gently massage for 1 min; rinse hair with warm water; repeat, leaving on hair for 3 min.
- Provide for good hygiene measures to control sources of infection or reinfection.
- Provide small, frequent meals if GI upset occurs.
- Ensure ready access to bathroom facilities if diarrhea occurs.
- Provide comfort measures appropriate to site of fungal infection.
- Arrange to monitor hepatic function tests before beginning therapy and monthly or more frequently throughout treatment.
- Establish safety precautions if CNS effects occur (eg, siderails, assistance with ambulation).

Drug-specific teaching points
- Take the full course of drug therapy. Long-term use of the drug will be needed; beneficial effects may not be seen for several weeks. Take oral drug with meals to decrease GI upset. Apply topical drug to affected area and immediate surrounding area. If using shampoo, moisten hair and scalp thoroughly with water; apply sufficient shampoo to produce a lather; gently massage for 1 min; rinse hair with warm water; repeat, leaving on hair for 3 min. Shampoo twice a week for 4 wk with at least 3 d between shampooing.
- Use appropriate hygiene measures to prevent reinfection or spread of infection.
- Know that the following side effects may occur: nausea, vomiting, diarrhea (taking the drug with food may help); sedation, dizziness, confusion (avoid driving or performing tasks that require alertness if these occur); stinging, irritation (with local application).
- Report skin rash, severe nausea, vomiting, diarrhea, fever, sore throat, unusual bleeding or bruising, yellowing of skin or eyes, dark urine or pale stools, severe irritation (local application).

Representative Drugs
amphotericin B
fluconazole
flucytosine
griseofulvin
itraconazole
ketoconazole
miconazole
nystatin

❏ Antihistamines

Pregnancy Category C

Therapeutic actions
Antihistamines competitively block the effects of histamine at peripheral H_1 receptor sites, have anticholinergic (atropine-like) and antipruritic effects.

Indications
- Symptomatic relief of symptoms associated with perennial and seasonal allergic rhinitis, vasomotor rhinitis, allergic conjunctivitis, mild, uncomplicated urticaria and angioedema
- Amelioraton of allergic reactions to blood or plasma
- Treatment of dermatographism
- Adjunctive therapy in anaphylactic reactions
- Unlabeled uses: relief of lower respiratory conditions, such as histamine-induced

bronchoconstriction in asthmatics and exercise- and hyperventilation-induced bronchospasm

Contraindications/cautions
- Antihistamines are contraindicated in the presence of allergy to any antihistamines, pregnancy, or lactation. Use with caution in the presence of narrow-angle glaucoma, stenosing peptic ulcer, symptomatic prostatic hypertrophy, asthmatic attack, bladder neck obstruction, pyloroduodenal obstruction.

Adverse effects
- CNS: *Depression, nightmares,* sedation (terfenadine is less sedating than other antihistamines)
- GI: *Dry mouth, GI upset,* anorexia, increased appetite, nausea, vomiting, diarrhea
- CV: Arrhythmia, increase in QTc intervals
- **Respiratory:** *Bronchospasm, cough, thickening of secretions*
- GU: Galactorrhea, menstrual disorders, dysuria, hesitancy
- **Dermatologic:** *Alopecia,* angioedema, skin eruption and itching
- Other: Musculoskeletal pain, mild to moderate transaminase elevations

Clinically important drug-drug interactions
- Altered antihistamine metabolism if taken concurrently with ketoconazole, troleandomycin • Increased antihistamine anticholinergic effects if taken concurrently with MAO Inhibitors • Additive CNS depressant effects if taken concurrently with alcohol, CNS depressants

■ Nursing Considerations

Assessment
- *History:* Allergy to any antihistamines, narrow-angle glaucoma, stenosing peptic ulcer, symptomatic prostatic hypertrophy, asthmatic attack, bladder neck obstruction, pyloroduodenal obstruction, pregnancy, lactation
- *Physical:* Skin—color, lesions, texture; orientation, reflexes, affect; vision exam; R, adventitious sounds; prostate palpation; serum transaminase levels

Implementation
- Administer with food if GI upset occurs.
- Provide mouth care, sugarless lozenges to suck if dry mouth is a problem.
- Arrange for use of humidifier if thickening of secretions, nasal dryness become bothersome; encourage adequate intake of fluids.
- Provide appropriate skin care if dermatologic effects occur.

Drug-specific teaching points
- Avoid excessive dosage.
- Take with food if GI upset occurs.
- Know that the following side effects may occur: dizziness, sedation, drowsiness (use caution if driving or performing tasks that require alertness if these occur); dry mouth (frequent mouth care, sucking sugarless lozenges may help); thickening of bronchial secretions, dryness of nasal mucosa (use of a humidifier may help if this becomes a problem); menstrual irregularities.
- Avoid alcohol while on this drug; serious sedation could occur.
- Report difficulty breathing, hallucinations, tremors, loss of coordination, unusual bleeding or bruising, visual disturbances, irregular heartbeat.

Representative Drugs
astemizole
azatadine
brompheniramine
chlorpheniramine
clemastine
cyproheptadine
deschlorpheniramine
diphenhydramine
loratadine
methdilazine
promethazine
terfenadine
trimeprazine
tripelennamine
triprolidine

Adverse effects in *Italics* are most common; those in **Bold** are life-threatening.

☐ Antimetabolites

Pregnancy Category D

Therapeutic actions
Antimetabolites are antineoplastic drugs that inhibit DNA polymerase. They are cell cycle phase specific to S phase (stage of DNA synthesis), causing cell death for cells in the S phase; they also block progression of cells from G_1 to S in the cell cycle.

Indications
- Induction and maintenance of remission in acute myelocytic leukemia (higher response rate in children than in adults), chronic lymphocytic leukemia
- Treatment of acute lymphocytic leukemia in adults and children, chronic myelocytic leukemia and erythroleukemia, meningeal leukemia, psoriasis and rheumatoid arthritis (methotrexate)
- Palliative treatment of GI adenocarcinoma, carcinoma of the colon, rectum, breast, stomach, pancreas
- Part of combination therapy for the treatment of non-Hodgkin's lymphoma in children

Contraindications/cautions
- Antimetabolites are contraindicated in the presence of allergy to the drug, pregnancy, lactation, and in premature infants. Use with caution in the presence of hematopoietic depression secondary to radiation or chemotherapy; impaired liver function.

Adverse effects
- CNS: Neuritis, neural toxicity
- GI: *Anorexia, nausea, vomiting, diarrhea, oral and anal inflammation or ulceration*; esophageal ulcerations, esophagitis, abdominal pain, *hepatic dysfunction* (jaundice), acute pancreatitis
- Hematologic: Bone marrow depression, hyperuricemia
- GU: Renal dysfunction, urinary retention
- Dermatologic: Fever, rash, urticaria, freckling, skin ulceration, pruritis, conjunctivitis, alopecia
- Local: Thrombophlebitis, cellulitis at injection site
- Other: *Fever, rash*

Clinically important drug-drug interactions
- Decreased therapeutic action of digoxin if taken with cytarabine • Enhanced toxicity of fluorouracil if taken with leucovorin • Potentially fatal reactions if methotrexate is taken with various NSAIDs

■ Nursing Considerations

Assessment
- *History*: Allergy to drug, hematopoietic depression, impaired liver function, lactation
- *Physical:* Weight; temperature; skin—lesions, color; hair; orientation, reflexes; R, adventitious sounds; mucous membranes, liver evaluation, abdominal exam; CBC, differential; renal and liver function tests; urinalysis

Implementation
- Arrange for tests to evaluate hematopoietic status before beginning therapy and frequently during therapy.
- Arrange for discontinuation of drug therapy if platelet count < $50,000/mm^3$, polymorphonuclear granuloctye count < $1,000/mm^3$; consult physician for dosage adjustment.
- Monitor injection site for signs of thrombophlebitis, inflammation.
- Provide frequent mouth care for mouth sores.
- Arrange for small, frequent meals and dietary consultation to maintain nutrition when GI effects are severe.
- Ensure ready access to bathroom facilities if diarrhea occurs.
- Establish safety measures if dizziness, CNS effects occur.
- Arrange for patient to obtain a wig or some other suitable head covering if alopecia occurs; ensure that head is covered in extremes of temperature.

Adverse effects in *Italics* are most common; those in **Bold** are life-threatening.

- Protect patient from exposure to infections.
- Provide appropriate skin care as needed.
- Arrange for comfort measures if anal inflammation, headache, other pain associated with cytarabine syndrome occur.
- Arrange for treatment of fever if it occurs.

Drug-specific teaching points
- Prepare a calendar of treatment days for the patient to follow.
- Know that the following side effects may occur: nausea, vomiting, loss of appetite (medication may be ordered to help; small frequent meals also may help; it is important to maintain your nutrition); malaise, weakness, lethargy (these are all effects of the drug; consult with your nurse or physician if these occur; it is advisable to avoid driving or operating dangerous machinery if these occur); mouth sores (frequent mouth care will be needed); diarrhea (ensure ready access to bathroom facilities if these occur); loss of hair (you may wish to obtain a wig or other suitable head covering; keep the head covered in extremes of temperature); anal inflammation (consult with your nurse or physician if this occurs; comfort measures can be established).
- Use birth control while on this drug; this drug may cause birth defects or miscarriages.
- Arrange to have frequent, regular medical follow-up, including frequent blood tests, to follow the effects of the drug on your body.
- Report black, tarry stools; fever, chills; sore throat; unusual bleeding or bruising; shortness of breath; chest pain; difficulty swallowing.

Representative Drugs
cytarabine
floxuridin
fluorouracil
fludarabine
mercaptopurine
methotrexate
thioguanine

❒ Antivirals

Pregnancy Category C

Therapeutic actions
Antiviral drugs inhibit viral DNA or RNA replication in the virus, preventing replication and leading to viral death.

Indications
- Initial and recurrent mucosal and cutaneous herpes simplex virus (HSV) 1 and 2 infections in immunocompromised patients, encephalitis, herpes zoster
- HIV infections (often used as combination therapy)
- CMV retinitis in patients with AIDS
- Severe initial and recurrent genital herpes infections in selected patients
- Treatment and prevention of influenza A respiratory tract illness
- Treatment of initial HSV genital infections and limited mucocutaneous HSV infections in immunocompromised patients (ointment)
- Unlabeled uses: treatment of herpes zoster, CMV and HSV infection following transplant, herpes simplex infections, infectious mononucleosis, varicella pneumonia, and varicella zoster in immunocompromised patients

Contraindications/cautions
- Antiviral drugs are contraindicated in the presence of allergy to the drug, seizures, CHF, renal disease, or lactation.

Adverse effects
Systemic Administration
- **CNS:** Headache, vertigo, depression, tremors, encephalopathic changes
- **GI:** *Nausea, vomiting,* diarrhea, anorexia
- **GU:** Crystalluria with rapid IV administration, hematuria
- **Dermatologic:** *Inflammation or phlebitis at injection sites,* rash, hair loss

Topical Administration
- **Skin:** *Transient burning at the site of application*

Adverse effects in *Italics* are most common; those in **Bold** are life-threatening.

Clinically important drug-drug interactions
• Increased drug effects if taken with probenecid • Increased nephrotoxicity with other nephrotoxic drugs

■ Nursing Considerations
Assessment
- *History*: Allergy to drug, seizures, CHF, renal disease, lactation
- *Physical*: Skin—color, lesions; orientation; BP, P, auscultation, perfusion, edema; R, adventitious sounds; urinary output; BUN, creatinine clearance

Implementation
Systemic Administration
- Ensure that the patient is well hydrated with IV fluids or PO fluids during drug use.
- Provide support and encouragement to deal with disease.
- Provide small, frequent meals if systemic therapy causes GI upset.
- Ensure ready access to bathroom facilities.
- Provide skin care, analgesics if necessary for rash.

Topical Administration
- Start treatment as soon as possible after onset of signs and symptoms.
- Wear a rubber glove or finger cot when applying drug.

Drug-specific teaching points
- Complete the full course of oral therapy, and do *not* exceed the prescribed dose.
- This drug is *not* a cure for your disease but should make you feel better.
- Know that the following side effects may occur: nausea, vomiting, loss of appetite, diarrhea, headache, dizziness.
- Avoid sexual intercourse while visible lesions are present.
- Report difficulty urinating, skin rash, increased severity or frequency of recurrences.

Topical Administration
- Wear rubber gloves or finger cots when applying the drug to prevent autoinoculation of other sites and transmission of the disease to other people.
- Know that this drug does not cure the disease; application of the drug during symptom-free periods will not prevent recurrences.
- Avoid sexual intercourse while visible lesions are present.
- Know that this drug may cause burning, stinging, itching, rash; notify your prescriber if these are pronounced.

Representative Drugs
acyclovir
acyclovir sodium
amantadine
didanosine
foscarnet
ganciclovir
ribavirin
rimantadine
stavudine
vidabarine
zalcitabine
zidovudine

❒ Barbiturates

Pregnancy Category D
C-II controlled substances

Therapeutic actions
Barbiturates act as sedatives, hypnotics, and anticonvulsants. They are general CNS depressants. Barbiturates inhibit impulse conduction in the ascending reticular activating system, depress the cerebral cortex, alter cerebellar function, depress motor output, and can produce excitation, sedation, hypnosis, anesthesia, and deep coma; at anesthetic doses, they have anticonvulsant activity.

Indications
- Sedatives or hypnotics for short-term treatment of insomnia
- Preanesthetic medications
- Anticonvulsants, in anesthetic doses, for emergency control of certain acute convulsive episodes (eg, status epilepticus, eclampsia, meningitis, tetanus, toxic reactions to strychnine or local anesthetics)

Contraindications/cautions
- Barbiturates are contraindicated in the presence of hypersensitivity to barbiturates, manifest or latent porphyria, marked liver impairment, nephritis, severe respiratory distress, respiratory disease with dyspnea, obstruction or cor pulmonale, previous addiction to sedative-hypnotic drugs, pregnancy (has caused fetal damage, neonatal withdrawal syndrome), or lactation. Use with caution in the presence of acute or chronic pain (paradoxical excitement or masking of important symptoms could result), seizure disorders (abrupt discontinuation of daily doses of drug can result in status epilepticus), fever, hyperthyroidism, diabetes mellitus, severe anemia, pulmonary or cardiac disease, status asthmaticus, shock, uremia.

Adverse effects
- CNS: *Somnolence, agitation, confusion, hyperkinesia, ataxia, vertigo, CNS depression, nightmares, lethargy, residual sedation (hangover), paradoxical excitement, nervousness, psychiatric disturbance, hallucinations, insomnia, anxiety, dizziness, thinking abnormality*
- GI: *Nausea, vomiting, constipation, diarrhea, epigastric pain*
- CV: *Bradycardia, hypotension, syncope*
- Respiratory: *Hypoventilation, apnea, respiratory depression,* laryngospasm, bronchospasm, circulatory collapse
- Hypersensitivity: Skin rashes, angioneurotic edema, serum sickness, morbiliform rash, urticaria; rarely, exfoliative dermatitis, **Stevens-Johnson syndrome**, sometimes fatal
- Local: *Pain, tissue necrosis at injection site,* gangrene; arterial spasm with inadvertent intra-arterial injection; thrombophlebitis; permanent neurologic deficit if injected near a nerve
- Other: Tolerance, psychological and physical dependence; **withdrawal syndrome** (sometimes fatal)

Clinically important drug-drug interactions
• Increased CNS depression when taken with alcohol • Increased nephrotoxicity if given concurrently with methoxyflurane • Decreased effects of the following drugs given with barbiturates: oral anticoagulants, corticosteroids, oral contraceptives and estrogens, beta-adrenergic blockers (especially propranolol, metoprolol), theophylline, metronidazole, doxycycline, griseofulvin, phenylbutazones, quinidine

■ Nursing Considerations

Assessment
- *History:* Hypersensitivity to barbiturates; manifest or latent porphyria; marked liver impairment; nephritis; severe respiratory distress; respiratory disease with dyspnea, obstruction, or cor pulmonale; previous addiction to sedative-hypnotic drugs; acute or chronic pain; seizure disorders; pregnancy; lactation; fever; hyperthyroidism; diabetes mellitus; severe anemia; pulmonary or cardiac disease; status asthmaticus; shock; uremia
- *Physical:* Body weight; body temperature; skin—color, lesions, injection site; orientation, affect, reflexes; P, BP, orthostatic BP; R, adventitious sounds; bowel sounds, normal output, liver evaluation; liver and kidney function tests, blood and urine glucose, BUN

Implementation
- Do not administer intra-arterially; may produce arteriospasm, thrombosis, gangrene.
- Administer IV doses slowly.
- Administer IM doses deep in a muscle mass.
- Do not use parenteral dosage forms if solution is discolored or contains a precipitate.
- Monitor injection sites carefully for irritation, extravasation (IV use); solutions are alkaline and very irritating to the tissues.
- Monitor P, BP, respiration carefully during IV administration.

Adverse effects in *Italics* are most common; those in **Bold** are life-threatening.

- Provide resuscitative facilities on standby in case of respiratory depression, hypersensitivity reaction.
- Ensure ready access to bathroom facilities if GI effects occur.
- Provide small, frequent meals, frequent mouth care if GI effects occur.
- Establish safety precautions if CNS changes occur (eg, side rails, accompany patient).
- Provide appropriate skin care if dermatologic effects occur.
- Provide comfort measures, reassurance for patients receiving pentobarbital for tetanus, toxic convulsions.
- Offer support and encouragement to patients receiving this drug for preanesthetic medication.
- Arrange to taper dosage gradually after repeated use, especially in epileptic patients.

Drug-specific teaching points

When giving this drug as preanesthetic medication, incorporate teaching about the drug into general teaching about the procedure. The following points should be included:
- Be aware that this drug will make you drowsy and less anxious.
- Do not try to get up after you have received this drug (request assistance if you feel you must sit up or move about for any reason).

Outpatients
- Take this drug exactly as prescribed. This drug is habit forming; its effectiveness in facilitating sleep disappears after a short time. Do not take this drug longer than 2 wk (for insomnia), and do not increase the dosage without consulting your physician. If the drug appears to be ineffective, consult your nurse or physician.
- Avoid becoming pregnant while taking this drug. The use of contraception other than oral contraceptives is recommended; these may lose their effectiveness while you are taking this drug.
- Know that the following side effects may occur: drowsiness, dizziness, "hangover," impaired thinking (these effects may become less pronounced after a few days; avoid driving a car or engaging in activities that require alertness if these occur); GI upset (taking the drug with food may help); dreams, nightmares, difficulty concentrating, fatigue, nervousness (it may help to know that these are effects of the drug that will go away when the drug is discontinued; consult your nurse or physician if these become bothersome).
- Report severe dizziness, weakness, drowsiness that persists, rash or skin lesions, pregnancy.

Representative Drugs
amobarbital
aprobarbital
butabarbital
mephobarbital
pentobarbital
pentobarbital sodium
phenobarbital
secobarbital

❒ Benzodiazepines

Pregnancy Category D
C-IV controlled substance

Therapeutic actions
Benzodiazepines are antianxiety agents, anticonvulsants, muscle relaxants, and sedative-hypnotics. Their exact mechanisms of action not understood, but it is known that benzodiazepines potentiate the effects of gamma-aminobutyrate, an inhibitory neurotransmitter.

Indications
- Management of anxiety disorders, short-term relief of symptoms of anxiety
- Short term treatment of insomnia
- Alone or as adjunct in treatment of Lennox-Gastaut syndrome (petit mal variant), akinetic and myoclonic seizures
- May be useful in patients with absence (petit mal) seizures who have not responded to succinimides; up to 30% of patients show loss of effectiveness of drug, often within 3 mo of therapy (may respond to dosage adjustment)

- Unlabeled use: treatment of panic attacks, periodic leg movements during sleep, hypokinetic dysarthria, acute manic episodes, multifocal tic disorders; adjunct treatment of schizophrenia, neuralgias; treatment of irritable bowel syndrome

Contraindications/cautions

- Benzodiazepines are contraindicated in the presence of hypersensitivity to benzodiazepines, psychoses, acute narrow-angle glaucoma, shock, coma, acute alcoholic intoxication with depression of vital signs, pregnancy (increased risk of congenital malformations, neonatal withdrawal syndrome), labor and delivery ("floppy infant" syndrome reported), or lactation (infants to become lethargic and lose weight). Use with caution in the presence of impaired liver or kidney function, debilitation.

Adverse effects

- CNS: *Transient, mild drowsiness initially; sedation, depression, lethargy, apathy, fatigue, lightheadedness, disorientation, anger, hostility,* episodes of mania and hypomania, *restlessness, confusion, crying,* delirium, *headache,* slurred speech, dysarthria, stupor, rigidity, tremor, dystonia, vertigo, euphoria, nervousness, difficulty in concentration, vivid dreams, psychomotor retardation, extrapyramidal symptoms; *mild paradoxical excitatory reactions, during first 2 wk of treatment*
- GI: *Constipation, diarrhea, dry mouth,* salivation, *nausea,* anorexia, vomiting, difficulty in swallowing, gastric disorders, hepatic dysfunction, encoporesis
- CV: Bradycardia, tachycardia, cardiovascular collapse, hypertension and hypotension, palpitations, edema
- Hematologic: Elevations of blood enzymes—LDH, alkaline phosphatase, SGOT, SGPT; blood dyscrasias—agranulocytosis, leukopenia
- GU: Incontinence, urinary retention, changes in libido, menstrual irregularities
- EENT: Visual and auditory disturbances, diplopia, nystagmus, depressed hearing, nasal congestion
- Dermatologic: Urticaria, pruritus, skin rash, dermatitis
- Other: Hiccups, fever, diaphoresis, paresthesias, muscular disturbances, gynecomastia; *drug dependence with withdrawal syndrome when drug is discontinued; more common with abrupt discontinuation of higher dosage used for longer than 4 mo*

Clinically important drug-drug interactions

• Increased CNS depression when taken with alcohol • Increased effect when given with cimetidine, disulfiram, omeprazole, oral contraceptives • Decreased effect when given with theophylline

■ Nursing Considerations

Assessment

- *History:* Hypersensitivity to benzodiazepines, psychoses, acute narrow-angle glaucoma, shock, coma, acute alcoholic intoxication with depression of vital signs, pregnancy, lactation, impaired liver or kidney function, debilitation
- *Physical:* Skin—color, lesions; body temperature; orientation, reflexes, affect, ophthalmologic exam; P, BP;R; adventitious sounds; liver evaluation, abdominal exam, bowel sounds, normal output; CBC, liver and renal function tests

Implementation

- Keep addiction-prone patients under careful surveillance because of their predisposition to habituation and drug dependence.
- Monitor liver function, blood counts periodically in patients on long-term therapy.
- Ensure ready access to bathroom facilities if GI effects occur; establish bowel program if constipation occurs.
- Provide small, frequent meals, frequent mouth care if GI effects occur.
- Provide measures appropriate to care of urinary problems (eg, protective clothing, bed changing).

Adverse effects in *Italics* are most common; those in **Bold** are life-threatening.

- Establish safety precautions if CNS changes occur (eg, side rails, accompany patient when ambulating).
- Arrange to taper dosage gradually after long-term therapy, especially in epileptic patients; arrange substitution of another antiepileptic drug, as appropriate.
- Monitor patient for therapeutic drug levels; levels vary with specific drug being used.
- Arrange for patient to wear medical alert identification indicating epilepsy and the drug therapy.

Drug-specific teaching points
- Take drug exactly as prescribed; do not to stop taking drug (long-term therapy) without consulting health care provider.
- Avoid alcohol, sleep-inducing, or OTC drugs while on this drug.
- Know that the following side effects may occur: drowsiness, dizziness (these may become less pronounced after a few days; avoid driving a car or engaging in other dangerous activities if these occur); GI upset (taking the drug with food may help); fatigue; depression; dreams; crying; nervousness; depression, emotional changes; bed wetting, urinary incontinence.
- Report severe dizziness, weakness, drowsiness that persists, rash or skin lesions, difficulty voiding, palpitations, swelling in the extremities.

Representative Drugs
alprazolam
clonazepam
clorazepate
diazepam
estazolam
flurazepam
halazepam
lorazepam
oxazepam
prazepam
quazepam
temazepam
triazolam

☐ Beta-Adrenergic Blockers

Pregnancy Category C

Therapeutic actions
Beta-adrenergic blockers are antianginals, antiarrhythmics, and antihypertensives. Beta-blockers competitively block beta-adrenergic receptors in the heart and juxtoglomerular apparatus, decreasing the influence of the sympathetic nervous system on these tissues, decreasing the excitablity of the heart, decreasing cardiac work load and oxygen consumption, decreasing the release of renin and lowering blood pressure. They have membrane-stabilizing (local anesthetic) effects that contribute to their antiarrhythmic action. They also act in the CNS to reduce sympathetic outflow and vasoconstrictor tone.

Indications
- Hypertension (alone or with other drugs, especially diuretics)
- Angina pectoris caused by coronary atherosclerosis
- Hypertrophic subaortic stenosis, to manage associated stress-induced angina, palpitations, and syncope; cardiac arrhythmias, especially supraventricular tachycardia, and ventricular tachycardias induced by digitalis or catecholamines; essential tremor, familial or hereditary
- Prevention of reinfarction in clinically stable patients 1–4 wk after MI
- Adjunctive therapy for pheochromocytoma after treatment with an alpha-adrenergic blocker, to manage tachycardia before or during surgery or if the pheochromocytoma is inoperable
- Prophylaxis for migraine headache (propranolol)
- Management of acute situational stress reaction (stage fright; (propranolol)
- Unlabeled uses: treatment of recurrent GI bleeding in cirrhotic patients, schizophrenia, essential tremors, tardive dyskinesia, acute panic symptoms, vaginal contraceptive

Contraindications/cautions
- Beta-blockers are contraindicated in the presence of allergy to beta-blocking agents, sinus bradycardia, second- or third-degree heart block, cardiogenic shock, CHF, bronchial asthma, broncho-

spasm, COPD, pregnancy (neonatal bradycardia, hypoglycemia, and apnea have occurred in human infants whose mothers received propranolol; low birth weight occurs with chronic maternal use during pregnancy), or lactation. Use with caution in the presence of hypoglycemia and diabetes, thyrotoxicosis, hepatic dysfunction.

Adverse effects
- GI: *Gastric pain, flatulence, constipation, diarrhea, nausea, vomiting,* anorexia, ischemic colitis, renal and mesenteric arterial thrombosis, retroperitoneal fibrosis, hepatomegaly, acute pancreatitis
- CV: *Bradycardia, CHF, cardiac arrhythmias, sinoartial or AV nodal block, tachycardia,* peripheral vascular insufficiency, claudication, CVA, pulmonary edema, hypotension
- Respiratory: Bronchospasm, dyspnea, cough, bronchial obstruction, nasal stuffiness, rhinitis, pharyngitis
- Neuro: Dizziness, vertigo, tinnitus, *fatigue,* emotional depression, paresthesias, sleep disturbances, hallucinations, disorientation, memory loss, slurred speech
- GU: *Impotence, decreased libido,* Peyronie's disease, dysuria, nocturia, frequency
- MS: Joint pain, arthralgia, muscle cramp
- EENT: Eye irritation, dry eyes, conjunctivitis, blurred vision
- Dermatologic: Rash, pruritus, sweating, dry skin
- Allergic reactions: Pharyngitis, erythematous rash, fever, sore throat, laryngospasm, respiratory distress
- Other: *Decreased exercise tolerance, development of antinuclear antibodies,* hyperglycemia or hypoglycemia, elevated serum transaminase, alkaline phosphatase, and LDH

Clinically important drug–drug interactions
- Increased effects of beta-blockers with verapamil • Decreased effects of beta-blockers with indomethacin, ibuprofen, piroxicam, sulindac, barbiturates • Prolonged hypoglycemic effects of insulin if taken concurrently with beta-blockers • Peripheral ishemia possible if beta-blockers combined with ergot alkaloids • Initial hypertensive episode followed by bradycardia if taken concurrently with epinephrine • Increased "first-dose response" to prazosin when taken concurrently with beta-blockers • Increased serum levels and toxic effects if taken con-currently with lidocaine, cimetidine • Increased serum levels of beta-blockers and phenothiazines, hydralazine if the two drugs are taken concurrently • Paradoxical hypertension when clonidine is given with beta-blockers; increased rebound hypertension when clonidine is discontinued in patients on beta-blockers • Decreased serum levels and therapeutic effects if beta-blocker is taken with methimazole, propylthiouracil • Decreased bronchodilator effects of theophyllines taken with beta-blockers • Decreased antihypertensive effects of beta-blockers if taken concurrently with NSAIDs (eg, ibuprofen, indomethacin, piroxicam, sulindac), rifampin

Drug-lab test interferences
- Interference with glucose or insulin tolerance tests, glaucoma screening tests

■ Nursing Considerations
Assessment
- *History:* Allergy to beta-blocking agents, sinus bradycardia, second- or third-degree heart block, cardiogenic shock, CHF, bronchial asthma, bronchospasm, COPD, hypoglycemia and diabetes, thyrotoxicosis, hepatic dysfunction, pregnancy, lactation
- *Physical:* Weight, skin—color, lesions, edema, temperature; reflexes, affect, vision, hearing, orientation; BP, P, ECG, peripheral perfusion; R, auscultation; bowel sounds, normal output, liver evaluation; bladder palpation; liver and thyroid function tests, blood and urine glucose

Implementation
- Do not discontinue drug abruptly after chronic therapy (hypersensitivity to cate-

cholamines may have developed, causing exacerbation of angina, MI, and ventricular dysrhythmias). Taper drug gradually over 2 wk with monitoring.
- Consult with physician about withdrawing drug if patient is to undergo surgery (controversial).
- Give oral drug with food to facilitate absorption.
- Provide side rails and assistance with walking if CNS, vision changes occur.
- Position patient to decrease effects of edema, respiratory obstruction.
- Space activities, and provide periodic rest periods for patient.
- Provide frequent, small meals if GI effects occur.
- Provide comfort measures to help patient cope with eye, GI, joint, CNS, dermatologic effects.

Drug-specific teaching points
- Take this drug with meals. Do not discontinue the medication abruptly; abrupt discontinuation can cause a worsening of the disorder for which you are taking the drug.
- Know that the following side effects may occur: dizziness, drowsiness, lightheadedness, blurred vision (avoid driving a car or performing hazardous tasks if these occur); nausea, loss of appetite (frequent, small meals may help); nightmares, depression (notify your health care provider who may be able to change your medication); sexual impotence (you may want to discuss this problem with your nurse or physician).
- Report difficulty breathing, night cough, swelling of extremities, slow pulse, confusion, depression, rash, fever, sore throat.
- For diabetic patients, be aware that the normal signs of hypoglycemia (sweating, tachycardia) may be blocked by this drug; monitor your blood/urine glucose carefully; be sure to eat regular meals, and take your diabetic medication regularly.

Representative Drugs
acebutolol
atenolol
betaxolol
bisoprolol
carteolol
esmolol
labetolol
metoprolol
nadolol
penbutolol
pindolol
propranolol
sotalol
timolol

☐ Calcium Channel-Blockers

Pregnancy Category C

Therapeutic actions
Calcium channel-blockers are antianginal and antihypertensive. They inhibit the movement of calcium ions across the membranes of cardiac and arterial muscle cells; this inhibition of transmembrane calcium flow results in the depression of impulse formation in specialized cardiac pacemaker cells, slowing of the velocity of conduction of the cardiac impulse, depression of myocardial contractility, and dilation of coronary arteries and arterioles and peripheral arterioles; these effects lead to decreased cardiac work, decreased cardiac energy consumption, and increased delivery of oxygen to myocardial cells.

Indications
- Treatment of angina pectoris due to coronary artery spasm (Prinzmetal's variant angina), chronic stable angina (effort-associated angina), hypertension, arrhythmias (supraventricular, those related to digoxin [verapamil]), subarachnoid hemorrhage (nimodipine)
- Orphan drug use in the treatment of interstitial cystitis, hypertensive emergencies, migraines

Contraindications/cautions
- Calcium channel-blockers are contraindicated in the presence of allergy to calcium channel-blockers, sick sinus syndrome, heart block, ventricular dys-

function, or pregnancy. Use with caution in the presence of lactation.

Adverse effects
- CNS: *Dizziness, lightheadedness, headache, asthenia,* fatigue, *nervousness,* sleep disturbances, blurred vision
- GI: *Nausea, diarrhea, constipation,* cramps, flatulence, hepatic injury
- CV: *Peripheral edema, angina,* hypotension, arrhythmias, **bradycardia, AV block,** asystole
- **Dermatologic:** *Flushing, rash,* dermatitis, pruritus, urticaria
- Other: *Nasal congestion, cough,* fever, chills, shortness of breath, muscle cramps, joint stiffnes, sexual difficulties

Clinically important drug-drug interactions
- Increased effects of calcium channel-blockers if taken concurrently with cimetidine, ranitidine

■ Nursing Considerations

Assessment
- *History:* Allergy to calcium channel-blockers, sick sinus syndrome, heart block, ventricular dysfunction; pregnancy; lactation
- *Physical:* Skin—lesions, color, edema; orientation, reflexes; P, BP, baseline ECG, peripheral perfusion, auscultation; R, adventitious sounds; liver evaluation, normal GI output; liver function tests

Implementation
- Monitor patient carefully (BP, cardiac rhythm, and output) while drug is being titrated to therapeutic dose; the dosage may be increased more rapidly in hospitalized patients under close supervision.
- Ensure that patients do not chew or divide sustained-release tablets.
- Arrange to taper dosage of beta blockers before beginning calcium channel-blocker therapy.
- Protect drug from light and moisture.
- Ensure ready access to bathroom facilities.
- Provide comfort measures for skin rash, headache, nervousness.
- Establish safety precautions if CNS changes occur.
- Position patient to alleviate peripheral edema if this occurs.
- Provide small, frequent meals if GI upset occurs.

Drug-specific teaching points
- Do not chew or divide sustained-release tablets. Swallow whole.
- Know that the following side effects may occur: nausea, vomiting (small, frequent meals may help); dizziness, light headedness, vertigo (avoid driving, operating dangerous machinery while on this drug; take special precautions to avoid falling); muscle cramps, joint stiffness, sweating, sexual difficulties (these are all uncomfortable and should disappear when the drug therapy is stopped; discuss with your nurse or physician if any of these become too uncomfortable).
- Report irregular heart beat, shortness of breath, swelling of the hands or feet, pronounced dizziness. constipation.

Representative Drugs
amlodipine
bepridil
diltiazem
felodipine
isradipine
nicardipine
nifedipine
nimodipine
verapamil

☐ Cephalosporins

Pregnancy Category B

Therapeutic actions
Cephalosporins are antibiotics. They are bactericidal, inhibiting synthesis of bacterial cell wall, causing cell death in susceptible bacteria.

Indications
- Treatment of pharyngitis, tonsillitis caused by *Streptococcus pyogenes*; otitis media caused by *Streptococcus pneu-*

Adverse effects in *Italics* are most common; those in **Bold** are life-threatening.

moniae, Haemophilus influenzae, Moraxella catarrhalis, S. pyogenes; lower respiratory tract infections caused by *S. pneumoniae, Haemophilus parainfluenxae, Staphylococcus aureus, Escherichia coli, Klebsiella, H. influenzae, S. pyogenes;* UTIs caused by *E. coli, Klebsiella pneumoniae;* dermatologic infections caused by *S. aureus, S. pyogenes, E. coli, Klebsiella, Enterobacter;* uncomplicated and disseminated gonorrhea caused by *Neisseria gonorrhoea;* septicemia caused by *S. pneumoniae, S. aureus, E. coli, Klebsiella, H. influenzae;* meningitis caused by *S. pneumoniae, H. influenzae, S. aureus, Neisseria meningitidis;* bone and joint infections caused by *S. aureus*
- Perioperative prophylaxis

Contraindications/cautions
- Cephalosporins are contraindicated in the presence of allergy to cephalosporins or penicillins, renal failure, or lactation.

Adverse effects
- CNS: Headache, dizziness, lethargy, paresthesias
- GI: *Nausea, vomiting, diarrhea, anorexia, abdominal pain, flatulence,* pseudomembranous colitis, liver toxicity
- Hematologic: Bone marrow depression: decreased WBC, decreased platelets, decreased Hct
- GU: Nephrotoxicity
- Hypersensitivity: *Ranging from rash, fever* to anaphylaxis; serum sickness reaction
- Local: *Pain,* abscess at injection site, *phlebitis,* inflammation at IV site
- Other: *Superinfections, disulfiram-like reaction with alcohol*

Clinically important drug-drug interactions
- Increased nephrotoxicity with aminoglycosides • Increased bleeding effects if taken with oral anticoagulants • Disulfiram-like reaction may occur if alcohol is taken within 72 h after cephalosporin administration

Drug-lab test interferences
- Possibility of false results on tests of urine glucose using Benedict's solution, Fehling's solution, Clinitest tablets; urinary 17-ketosteroids; direct Coombs' test

■ Nursing Considerations

Assessment
- *History:* Allergy to any cephalosporin, liver and kidney dysfunction, lactation, pregnancy
- *Physical:* Skin status, liver and kidney function test, culture of affected area, sensitivity tests

Implementation
- Culture infected area and arrange for sensitivity tests before beginning drug therapy and during therapy if expected response is not seen.
- Administer oral drug with food to decrease GI upset and enhance absorption.
- Administer oral drug to children who cannot swallow tablets; crushing the drug results in a bitter, unpleasant taste.
- Have vitamin K available in case hypoprothrombinemia occurs.
- Discontinue drug if hypersensitivy reaction occurs.
- Ensure ready access to bathroom facilities and provide small, frequent meals if GI complications occur.
- Arrange for treatment of superinfections if they occur.

Drug-specific teaching points
Oral Drug
- Take full course of therapy.
- Be aware that this drug is specific for this infection and should not be used to self-treat other problems.
- Swallow tablets whole; do not crush.
- Take the drug with food.
- Avoid drinking alcoholic beverages while on this drug and for 3 d after this drug has been stopped because severe reactions often occur (even with parenteral forms).
- Know that the following side effects may occur: stomach upset or diarrhea.
- Report severe diarrhea with blood, pus, or mucus; rash; difficulty breathing; un-

Adverse effects in *Italics* are most common; those in **Bold** are life-threatening.

usual tiredness, fatigue; unusual bleeding or bruising; unusual itching or irritation, pain at injection site.

Representative Drugs
First Generation
cefadroxil
cefazolin
cephalexin
cephalothin
cephapirin
cephradine
Second Generation
cefaclor
cefamandole
cefmetazole
cefoxitin
cefonicid
cefotetan
cefprozil
cefpodoxime
cefuroxime
loracarbef
Third Generation
cefixime
cefoperazone
cefotaxime
ceftazidime
ceftizoxime
ceftriaxone

☐ Diuretics

Pregnancy Category C

Therapeutic actions
Diuretics are divided into several subgroups. Thiazide and thiazide-related diuretics inhibit reabsorption of sodium and chloride in the distal renal tubule, increasing the excretion of sodium, chloride, and water by the kidney. Loop diuretics inhibit the reabsorption of sodium and chloride in the loop of Henle and in the distal renal tubule; because of this added effect, loop diuretics are more potent. Potassium-sparing diuretics block the effect of aldosterone on the renal tubule, leading to a loss of sodium and water and the retention of potassium; their overall effect is much weaker. Osmotic diuretics pull fluid out of the tissues with a hypertonic effect. Overall effect of diuretics is a loss of water and electrolytes from the body.

Indications
- Adjunctive therapy in edema associated with CHF, cirrhosis, corticosteroid and estrogen therapy, renal dysfunction
- Treatment of hypertension, as sole therapy or in combination with other antihypertensives
- Unlabeled uses: treatment of diabetes insipidus, especially nephrogenic diabetes insipidus, reduction of incidence of osteoporosis in postmenopausal women

Contraindications/cautions
- Diuretics are contraindicated for use in patients with fluid or electrolyte imbalances, renal or liver disease, gout, SLE, glucose tolerance abnormalities, hyperparathyroidism, manic-depressive disorders, or lactation.

Adverse effects
- CNS: *Dizziness, vertigo,* paresthesias, weakness, headache, drowsiness, fatigue
- GI: *Nausea, anorexia, vomiting, dry mouth, diarrhea, constipation*, jaundice, hepatitis, pancreatitis
- CV: Orthostatic hypotension, venous thrombosis, volume depletion, cardiac arrhythmias, chest pain
- Hematologic: Leukopenia, thrombocytopenia, agranulocytosis, aplastic anemia, neutropenia, fluid and electrolyte imbalances
- GU: *Polyuria, nocturia, impotence*, loss of libido
- Dermatologic: Photosensitivity, rash, purpura, exfoliative dermatitis
- Other: Muscle cramps and muscle spasms, fever, hives, gouty attacks, flushing, weight loss, rhinorrhea, electrolyte imbalance

Clinically important drug-drug interactions
- Increased thiazide effects and chance of acute hyperglycemia if taken with diazo-

Adverse effects in *Italics* are most common; those in **Bold** are life-threatening.

xide • Decreased absorption with cholestyramine, colestipol • Increased risk of cardiac glycoside toxicity if hypokalemia occurs • Increased risk of lithium toxicity • Increased dosage of antidiabetic agents may be needed • Risk of hyperkalemia if potassium-sparing diurectics are given with potassium preparations or ACE inhibitors • Increased risk of ototoxicity it loop diuretics are taken with aminoglycosides or cisplatin

Drug-lab test interferences
• Monitor for decreased PBI levels without clinical signs of thyroid disturbances

■ Nursing Considerations

Assessment
- *History:* Fluid or electrolyte imbalances, renal or liver disease, gout, SLE, glucose tolerance abnormalities, hyperparathyroidism, manic-depressive disorders, lactation
- *Physical:* Orientation, reflexes, muscle strength; pulses, BP, orthostatic BP, perfusion, edema, baseline ECG; respiratory rate, adventitious sounds; liver evaluation, bowel sounds; CBC, serum electrolytes, blood glucose; liver and renal function tests; serum uric acid, urinalysis

Implementation
- Administer diuretics with food or milk if GI upset occurs.
- Administer early in the day so increased urination will not disturb sleep.
- Ensure ready access to bathroom facilities when diuretic effect occurs.
- Establish safety precautions if CNS effects, orthostatic hypotension occur.
- Measure and record regular body weights to monitor fluid changes.
- Provide mouth care, small frequent meals as needed.
- Monitor IV sites for any sign of extravasation.
- Monitor electrolytes frequently with parenteral use, periodically with chronic use.

Drug-specific teaching points
- Take drug early in the day so sleep will not be disturbed by increased urination.
- Weigh yourself daily, and record weights.
- Protect skin from exposure to the sun or bright lights.
- Avoid foods high in potassium and the use of salt substitutes if taking a potassium-sparing diuretic.
- Take prescribed potassium replacement, and use foods high in potassium if taking a thiazide or loop diuretic.
- Know that increased urination will occur (stay close to bathroom facilities).
- Use caution if dizziness, drowsiness, feeling faint occur.
- Report rapid weight gain or loss, swelling in ankles or fingers, unusual bleeding or bruising, muscle cramps.

Representative Drugs
Thiazide and Related Diuretics
  bendroflumethiazide
  benzthiazide
  chlorothiazide
  chlorthalidone
  hydrochlorothiazide
  hydroflumethiazide
  indapamide
  methyclothiazide
  metolazone
  polythiazide
  quinethazone
  trichlormethiazide
Loop Diuretics
  bumetanide
  ethacrynic acid
  furosemide
  torsemide
Potassium-Sparing Diuretics
  amiloride
  spironolactone
  triamterene
Osmotic Diuretic
  mannitol

🗌 Fluoroquinolones

Pregnancy Category C

Therapeutic actions
Fluoroquinolones are antibacterial. They are bactericidal, interfering with DNA replication in susceptible gram-negative bacteria, preventing cell reproduction

and leading to death of susceptible bacteria.

Indications
- Treatment of infections caused by susceptible gram-negative bacteria, including *E. coli, Proteus mirabilis, K. pneumoniae, Enterobacter cloacae, Proteus vulgaris, Providencia rettgeri, Morganella morganii, Pseudomonas aeruginosa, Citrobacter freundii, S. aureus, S. epidermidis,* group D streptococci
- Unlabeled use: treatment of patients with cystic fibrosis who have pulmonary exacerbations

Contraindications/cautions
- Fluoroquinolones are contraindicated in presence of allergy to any fluoroquinolone, pregnancy, or lactation. Use with caution in the presence of renal dysfunction, seizures.

Adverse effects
- **CNS:** *Headache*, dizziness, insomnia, fatigue, somnolence, depression, blurred vision
- **GI:** *Nausea*, vomiting, dry mouth, *diarrhea*, abdominal pain
- **Hematologic:** Elevated BUN, SGOT, SGPT, serum creatinine and alkaline phosphatase; decreased WBC, neutrophil count, hematocrit
- **Other:** Fever, rash

Clinically important drug-drug interactions
- Decreased therapetic effect of fluoroquinolone if taken concurrently with iron salts, sucralfate • Decreased absorption of fluoroquinolone if taken with antacids • Increased effects of fluoroquinolone if taken with azlocillin • Increased serum levels and toxic effects of theophyllines if taken concurrently with fluoroquinolone

■ Nursing Considerations

Assessment
- *History:* Allergy to fluoroquinolones, renal dysfunction, seizures, lactation
- *Physical:* Skin—color, lesions; body temperature; orientation, reflexes, affect; mucous membranes, bowel sounds; renal and liver function tests

Implementation
- Arrange for culture and sensitivity tests before beginning therapy.
- Continue therapy for 2 d after the signs and symptoms of infection have disappeared.
- Administer oral drug 1 h before or 2 h after meals with a glass of water.
- Ensure that patient is well hydrated during course of drug therapy.
- Administer antacids, if needed, at least 2 h after dosing.
- Monitor clinical response; if no improvement is seen or a relapse occurs, repeat culture and sensitivity.
- Ensure ready access to bathroom facilities if diarrhea occurs.
- Arrange for appropriate bowel training program if constipation occurs.
- Provide small, frequent meals if GI upset occurs.
- Arrange for monitoring of environment (eg, noise, temperature) and analgesics, if appropriate, for headache.
- Establish safety precautions if CNS, visual changes occur.
- Encourage patient to complete full course of therapy.

Drug-specific teaching points
- Take oral drug on an empty stomach, 1 h before or 2 h after meals. If an antacid is needed, do not take it within 2 h of ciprofloxacin dose.
- Drink plenty of fluids while you are on this drug.
- Know that the following side effects may occur: nausea, vomiting, abdominal pain (small, frequent meals may help); diarrhea or constipation (consult nurse or physician if this occurs); drowsiness, blurring of vision, dizziness (observe caution if driving or using dangerous equipment).
- Report rash, visual changes, severe GI problems, weakness, tremors.

Adverse effects in *Italics* are most common; those in **Bold** are life-threatening.

Representative Drugs
ciprofloxacin
enoxacin
lomefloxacin
norfloxacin
ofloxacin

❏ Histamine$_2$ (H$_2$) Antagonist

Pregnancy Category B

Therapeutic actions
Histamine$_2$ antagonists inhibit the action of histamine at the histamine$_2$ receptors of the stomach, inhibiting gastric acid secretion and reducing total pepsin output; the resultant decrease in acid allows healing of ulcerated areas.

Indications
- Short-term treatment of active duodenal ulcer and benign gastric ulcer
- Treatment of pathologic hypersecretory conditions (eg, Zollinger-Ellison syndrome) and erosive gastroesophageal reflux
- Prophylaxis of stress-induced ulcers and acute upper GI bleed in critically ill patients

Contraindications/cautions
- H$_2$ antagonists are contraindicated in the presence of allergy to H$_2$ blockers, impaired renal or hepatic function, or lactation.

Adverse effects
- CNS: *Dizziness, somnolence, headache, confusion, hallucinations,* peripheral neuropathy, symptoms of brain stem dysfunction (dysarthria, ataxia, diplopia)
- GI: *Diarrhea*
- CV: Cardiac arrhythmias, arrest; hypotension (IV use)
- Hematologic: Increases in plasma creatinine, serum transaminase
- Other: *Impotence* (reversible with drug withdrawal), gynecomastia (in long-term treatment), rash, vasculitis, pain at IM injection site

Clinically important drug-drug interactions
- Increased risk of decreased white blood cell counts if taken with antimetabolites, alkylating agents, other drugs known to cause neutropenia • Increased serum levels and risk of toxicity of warfarin-type anticoagulants, phenytoin, beta-adrenergic blocking agents, alcohol, quinidine, lidocaine, theophylline, chloroquine, certain benzodiazepines (alprazolam, chlordiazepoxide, diazepam, flurazepam, triazolam), nifedipine, pentoxifylline, tricyclic antidepressants, procainamide, carbamazepine when taken with H$_2$ blockers

■ Nursing Considerations

Assessment
- *History:* Allergy to H$_2$ blockers, impaired renal or hepatic function, lactation
- *Physical:* Skin—lesions; orientation, affect; pulse, baseline ECG (continuous with IV use); liver evaluation, abdominal exam, normal output; CBC, liver and renal function tests

Implementation
- Administer drug with meals at bedtime.
- Arrange for decreased doses in renal dysfunction and liver dysfunction.
- Administer IM dose undiluted, deep into large muscle group.
- Ensure ready access to bathroom facilities.
- Provide comfort measures for skin rash, headache.
- Establish safety measures if CNS changes occur (eg, side rails, accompany patient).
- Arrange for regular follow-up, including blood tests to evaluate effects.

Drug-specific teaching points
- Take drug with meals and at bedtime; therapy may continue for 4–6 wk or longer.
- Take prescribed antacids exactly as prescribed, being careful of the times of administration.
- Inform your nurse or physician about your cigarette smoking habits. Cigarette

Adverse effects in *Italics* are most common; those in **Bold** are life-threatening.

smoking decreases the effectiveness of this drug.
- Have regular medical follow-up while you are on this drug to evaluate your response to it.
- Report sore throat, fever, unusual bruising or bleeding, tarry stools, confusion, hallucinations, dizziness, muscle or joint pain.

Representative Drugs
cimetidine
famotidine
nizatidine
ranitidine

☐ HMG CoA Inhibitors

Pregnancy Category X

Therapeutic actions
HMG CoA inhibitors are antihyperlipidemic. They are a fungal metabolite that inhibits the enzyme that catalyzes the first step in the cholesterol synthesis pathway in humans, resulting in a decrease in serum cholesterol, serum LDLs (associated with increased risk of coronary artery disease) and either an increase or no change in serum HDLs (associated with decreased risk of coronary artery disease).

Indications
- Adjunct to diet in the treatment of elevated total cholesterol and LDL cholesterol in patients with primary hypercholesterolemia (types IIa and IIb) whose response to dietary restriction of saturated fat and cholesterol and other nonpharmacologic measures has not been adequate.

Contraindications/cautions
- HMG CoA inhibitors are contraindicated in the presence of allergy to HMG CoA inhibitors, fungal byproducts, pregnancy, or lactation. Use with caution in the presence of impaired hepatic function, cataracts.

Adverse effects
- **CNS:** *Headache, blurred vision*, dizziness, insomnia, fatigue, muscle cramps, cataracts
- **GI:** *Flatulence, abdominal pain, cramps, constipation, nausea, vomiting*, heartburn
- **Hematologic:** Elevations of CPK, alkaline phosphatase, and transaminases

Clinically important drug-drug interactions
- Monitor patients receiving HMG CoA inhibitors for possible severe myopathy or rhabdomyolysis if taken with cyclosporine, erythromycin, gemfibrozil, niacin

■ Nursing Considerations

Assessment
- *History:* Allergy to HMG CoA inhibitors, fungal byproducts; impaired hepatic function; cataracts; pregnancy; lactation
- *Physical:* Orientation, affect, ophthalmologic exam; liver evaluation; lipid studies, liver function tests

Implementation
- Administer drug at bedtime; highest rates of cholesterol synthesis are between midnight and 5 AM.
- Consult with dietician regarding low-cholesterol diets.
- Arrange for proper consultation regarding need for diet and exercise changes.
- Arrange for regular follow-up during long-term therapy.
- Provide comfort measures to deal with headache, muscle cramps, nausea.
- Arrange for periodic ophthalmologic exam to check for cataract development.
- Offer support and encouragement to deal with disease, diet, drug therapy, and follow-up.

Drug-specific teaching points
- Take drug at bedtime.
- Institute appropriate diet changes that need to be made.
- Know that the following side effects may occur: nausea (small, frequent meals may help); headache, muscle and joint

Adverse effects in *Italics* are most common; those in **Bold** are life-threatening.

aches and pains (these may lessen with time).
- Arrange to have periodic ophthalmic exams while you are on this drug.
- Report severe GI upset, changes in vision, unusual bleeding or bruising, dark urine or light-colored stools.

Representative Drugs
fluvastatin
lovastatin
pravastatin
simvastatin

☐ Macrolide Antibiotics

Pregnancy Category B

Therapeutic actions
Macrolides are antibiotics. They are bacteriostatic or bactericidal in susceptible bacteria; they bind to cell membranes and cause changes in protein function, leading to cell death in susceptible bacteria.

Indications
- Treatment of acute infections caused by sensitive strains of *S. pneumoniae, Mycoplasma pneumoniae, Listeria monocytogenes, Legionella pneumophila;* URIs, LRIs, skin and soft-tissue infections caused by group A beta-hemolytic streptococci when oral treatment is preferred to injectable benzathine penicillin; pelvic inflammatory disease caused by *N. gonorrhoeae* in patients allergic to penicillin; intestinal amebiasis caused by *Entamoeba histolytica;* infections in the newborn and in pregnancy that are caused by *Chlamydia trachomatis* and in adult chlamydial infections when tetracycline cannot be used; primary syphilis (*Treponema pallidum*) in penicillin-allergic patients; eliminating *Bordetella pertussis* organisms from the nasopharynx of infected individuals and as prophylaxis in exposed and susceptible individuals; superficial ocular infections caused by susceptible strains of microorganisms; prophylaxis of ophthalmia neonatorum caused by *N. gonorrhoeae* or *C. trachomatis*
- Treatment of acne vulgaris and skin infections caused by sensitive microorganisms
- In conjunction with sulfonamides to treat URIs caused by *H. influenzae*
- Adjunct to antitoxin in infections caused by *Corynebacterium diphtheriae* and *Corynebacterium minutissimum*
- Prophylaxis against alpha-hemolytic streptococcal endocarditis before dental or other procedures in patients allergic to penicillin who have valvular heart disease and against infection in minor skin abrasions
- Unlabeled uses: erythromycin base is used with neomycin before colorectal surgery to reduce wound infection; treatment of severe diarrhea associated with *Campylobacter* enteritis or enterocolitis; treatment of genital, inguinal, or anorectal lymphogramuloma venereum infection; treatment of *Haemophilus ducreyi* (chancroid).

Contraindications/cautions
- Macrolides are contraindicated in the presence of allergy to any macrolide antibiotic. Use with caution in the presence of hepatic dysfunction or lactation (secreted and may be concentrated in breast milk; may modify bowel flora of nursing infant and interfere with fever workups).

Adverse effects
- **CNS:** Reversible hearing loss, confusion, uncontrollable emotions, abnormal thinking
- **GI:** *Abdominal cramping, anorexia, diarrhea, vomiting,* pseudomembranous colitis, hepatotoxicity
- **Dermatologic:** Edema, urticaria, dermatitis, angioneurotic edema
- **Hypersensitivity:** Allergic reactions ranging from rash to anaphylaxis
- **Local:** *Irritation, burning, itching* at site of application
- **Other:** *Superinfections*

Adverse effects in *Italics* are most common; those in **Bold** are life-threatening.

Pharmacologic Drug Classification ■ 37

Clinically important drug-drug interactions
- Increased serum levels of digoxin if taken with macrolide antibiotics • Increased effects of oral anticoagulants, theophyllines, carbamazepine • Increased therapeutic and toxic effects of corticosteroids • Increased levels of cyclosporine and risk of renal toxicity when taken concurrently with macrolide antibiotics • Increased irritant effects with peeling, desquamating, or abrasive agents used with dermatologic preparations

Drug-lab test interferences
- Interferes with fluorometric determination of urinary catecholamines • Decreased urinary estriol levels due to inhibition of hydrolysis of steroids in the gut

■ Nursing Considerations

Assessment
- *History:* Allergy to macrolides, hepatic dysfunction, lactation, viral, fungal, mycobacterial infections of the eye (ophthalmologic)
- *Physical:* Site of infection, skin—color, lesions; orientation, affect, hearing tests; R, adventitious sounds; GI output, bowel sounds, liver evaluation; culture and sensitivity tests of infection, urinalysis, liver function tests

Implementation
- Culture site of infection before beginning therapy.
- Administer oral erythromycin base or stearate on an empty stomach, 1 h before or 2–3 h after meals, with a full glass of water (oral erythromycin estolate, ethylsuccinate, and certain enteric-coated tablets; see manufacturer's instructions; may be given without regard to meals).
- Administer drug around the clock to maximize therapeutic effect; scheduling may have to be adjusted to minimize sleep disruption.
- Monitor liver function in patients on prolonged therapy.
- Institute appropriate hygiene measures, and arrange treatment if superinfections occur.
- If GI upset occurs with oral therapy, some preparations (see above) may be given with meals, or it may be possible to substitute one of these preparations.
- Provide small, frequent meals if GI problems occur.
- Establish safety measures (eg, accompany patient, side rails) if CNS changes occur.
- Give patient support and encouragement to continue with therapy.
- Wash affected area, rinse well, and dry before application of topical preparations.

Drug-specific teaching points
- Take oral drug on an empty stomach, 1 hour before or 2–3 h after meals, with a full glass of water, or, as appropriate, drug may be taken without regard to meals. The drug should be taken around the clock; schedule to minimize sleep disruption. It is important that you finish the *full course* of the drug therapy.
- Know that the following side effects may occur: stomach cramping, discomfort (taking the drug with meals, if appropriate, may alleviate this problem); uncontrollable emotions, crying, laughing, abnormal thinking (these will go away when the drug is stopped).
- Report severe or watery diarrhea, severe nausea or vomiting, dark urine, yellowing of the skin or eyes, loss of hearing, skin rash or itching.
- Wash and rinse area and pat it dry before applying topical solution; use fingertips or an applicator to apply; wash hands thoroughly after application.

Representative Drugs
azithromycin
clarithromycin
erythromycin
troleandomycin

❐ Narcotics

Pregnancy Category C
C-II controlled substance

Therapeutic actions

Narcotics act as agonists at specific opioid receptors in the CNS to produce analgesia, euphoria, sedation; the receptors mediating these effects are thought to be the same as those mediating the effects of endogenous opioids (enkephalins, endorphins).

Indications

- Relief of moderate to severe acute and chronic pain
- Preoperative medication to sedate and allay apprehension, facilitate induction of anesthesia, and reduce anesthetic dosage
- Analgesic adjunct during anesthesia
- A component of most preparations referred to as Brompton's Cocktail or Mixture, an oral alcoholic solution used for chronic severe pain, especially in terminal cancer patients
- Intraspinal use with microinfusion devices for the relief of intractable pain
- Unlabeled use: relief of dyspnea associated with acute left ventricular failure and pulmonary edema

Contraindications/cautions

- Narcotics are contraindicated in the presence of hypersensitivity to narcotics, diarrhea caused by poisoning until toxins are eliminated, during labor or delivery of a premature infant (may cross immature blood–brain barrier more readily), after biliary tract surgery or following surgical anastomosis, pregnancy, or labor (can cause respiratory depression of neonate; may prolong labor). Use with caution in the presence of head injury and increased intracranial pressure; acute asthma, COPD, cor pulmonale, preexisting respiratory depression, hypoxia, hypercapnia (may decrease respiratory drive and increase airway resistance); lactation (may be safer to wait 4–6 h after administration to nurse the baby); acute abdominal conditions; cardiovascular disease, supraventricular tachycardias; myxedema; convulsive disorders; acute alcoholism, delirium tremens; cerebral arteriosclerosis; ulcerative colitis; fever; kyphoscoliosis; Addison's disease; prostatic hypertrophy, urethral stricture; recent GI or GU surgery; toxic psychosis; renal or hepatic dysfunction.

Adverse effects

- **CNS:** *Lightheadedness, dizziness, sedation,* euphoria, dysphoria, delirium, insomnia, agitation, anxiety, fear, hallucinations, disorientation, drowsiness, lethargy, impaired mental and physical performance, coma, mood changes, weakness, headache, tremor, convulsions, miosis, visual disturbances, suppression of cough reflex
- **GI:** *Nausea, vomiting,* dry mouth, anorexia, constipation, biliary tract spasm; increased colonic motility in patients with chronic ulcerative colitis
- **CV:** Facial flushing, peripheral circulatory collapse, tachycardia, bradycardia, arrhythmia, palpitations, chest wall rigidity, hypertension, hypotension, orthostatic hypotension, syncope
- **GU:** Ureteral spasm, spasm of vesical sphincters, urinary retention or hesitancy, oliguria, antidiuretic effect, reduced libido or potency
- **Dermatologic:** Pruritus, urticaria, laryngospasm, bronchospasm, edema
- **Local:** Tissue irritation and induration (SC injection)
- Major hazards: **Respiratory depression, apnea, circulatory depression, respiratory arrest, shock, cardiac arrest**
- **Other:** *Sweating,* physical tolerance and dependence, psychological dependence

Clinically important drug-drug interactions

- Increased likelihood of respiratory depression, hypotension, profound sedation, or coma in patients receiving barbiturate general anesthetics

Drug-lab test interferences

- Elevated biliary tract pressure (an effect of narcotics) may cause increases in plasma

Adverse effects in *Italics* are most common; those in **Bold** are life-threatening.

Pharmacologic Drug Classification

amylase, lipase; determinations of these levels may be unreliable for 24 h

■ Nursing Considerations

Assessment
- *History:* Hypersensitivity to narcotics; diarrhea caused by poisoning; labor or delivery of a premature infant; biliary tract surgery or surgical anastomosis; head injury and increased intracranial pressure; acute asthma, COPD, cor pulmonale, preexisting respiratory depression, hypoxia, hypercapnia; acute abdominal conditions; cardiovascular disease, supraventricular tachycardias; myxedema; convulsive disorders; acute alcoholism, delirium tremens; cerebral arteriosclerosis; ulcerative colitis; fever; kyphoscoliosis; Addison's disease; prostatic hypertrophy; urethral stricture; recent GI or GU surgery; toxic psychosis; renal or hepatic dysfunction; pregnancy; lactation
- *Physical:* Body temperature; skin—color, texture, lesions; orientation, reflexes, bilateral grip strength, affect; P, auscultation, BP, orthostatic BP, perfusion; R, adventitious sounds; bowel sounds, normal output; urinary frequency, voiding pattern, normal output; ECG; EEG; thyroid, liver, kidney function tests

Implementation
- Caution patient not to chew or crush controlled-release preparations.
- Dilute and administer slowly IV to minimize likelihood of adverse effects.
- Direct patient to lie down during IV administration.
- Provide narcotic antagonist, facilities for assisted or controlled respiration on standby during IV administration.
- Use caution when injecting SC or IM into chilled areas or in patients with hypotension or in shock; impaired perfusion may delay absorption; with repeated doses, an excessive amount may be absorbed when circulation is restored.
- Monitor injection sites for irritation, extravasation.
- Instruct postoperative patients in pulmonary toilet; drug suppresses cough reflex.
- Monitor bowel function, and arrange for anthraquinone laxatives, as appropriate, for severe constipation.
- Institute safety precautions (eg, side rails, assistance with ambulation) if CNS, vision effects occur.
- Provide frequent, small meals if GI upset occurs.
- Provide environmental control if sweating, visual difficulties occur.
- Provide back rubs, positioning, and other nondrug measures to alleviate pain.
- Reassure patient about addiction liability; most patients who receive opiates for medical reasons do not develop dependence syndromes.

Drug-specific teaching points
When used as preoperative medication, teaching about the drug should be incorporated into the teaching about the procedure.
- Take this drug exactly as prescribed. Avoid alcohol, antihistamines, sedatives, tranquilizers, OTC drugs while you are taking this drug.
- Know that the following side effects may occur: nausea, loss of appetite (taking the drug with food and lying quietly should minimize these effects); constipation (notify your nurse or physician if this is severe; a laxative may help); dizziness, sedation, drowsiness, impaired visual acuity (avoid driving a car or performing other tasks that require alertness, visual acuity).
- Do not take any leftover medication for other disorders, and do not let anyone else take your prescription.
- Report severe nausea, vomiting, constipation, shortness of breath or difficulty breathing, skin rash.

Representative Drugs
codeine
fentanyl
hydrocodone
levorphanol
meperidine
methadone
morphine sulfate
oxycodone
oxymorphone

propoxyphene
sufentanil

☐ Nitrates

Pregnancy Category C

Therapeutic actions
Nitrates are antianginals. They relax vascular smooth muscle with a resultant decrease in venous return and decrease in arterial blood pressure, which reduces left ventricular workload and decreases myocardial oxygen consumption, relieving the pain of angina.

Indications
- Treatment of acute angina (sublingual, translingual, inhalant preparations)
- Prophylaxis of angina (oral sustained release, sublingual, topical, transdermal, translingual, transmucosal preparations)
- Treatment of angina unresponsive to recommended doses of organic nitrates or beta-blockers (IV preparations)
- Management of perioperative hypertension, CHF associated with acute myocardial infarction (IV preparations)
- Produce controlled hypertension during surgery (IV preparations)
- Unlabeled uses: reduction of cardiac workload in acute MI and in CHF (sublingual, topical) and adjunctive treatment of Raynaud's disease (topical)

Contraindications/cautions
- Nitrates are contraindicated in the presence of allergy to nitrates, severe anemia, early MI, head trauma, cerebral hemorrhage, hypertrophic cardiomyopathy, pregnancy, or lactation. Use with caution in the presence of hepatic or renal disease, hypotension or hypovolemia, increased intracranial pressure, constrictive pericarditis, pericardial tamponade, low ventricular filling pressure or low pulmonary capillary wedge pressure (PCWP).

Adverse effects
- CNS: Headache, apprehension, restlessness, weakness, vertigo, dizziness, faintness
- GI: Nausea, vomiting, incontinence of urine and feces, abdominal pain
- CV: Tachycardia, retrosternal discomfort, palpitations, **hypotension**, syncope, collapse, postural hypotension, angina
- Dermatologic: Rash, exfoliative dermatitis, cutaneous vasodilation with flushing, pallor, perspiration, cold sweat, contact dermatitis (transdermal preparations), topical allergic reactions (topical nitroglycerin ointment)
- Local: Local burning sensation at the point of dissolution (sublingual)
- Other: Ethanol intoxication with high dose IV use (alcohol in diluent)

Clinically important drug-drug interactions
- Increased risk of hypertension and decreased antianginal effect if taken concurrently with ergot alkaloids • Decreased pharmacologic effects of heparin if taken concurrently

Drug-lab test interferences
- False report of decreased serum cholesterol if done by the Zlatkis-Zak color reaction

■ Nursing Considerations

Assessment
- *History:* Allergy to nitrates, severe anemia, early MI, head trauma, cerebral hemorrhage, hypertrophic cardiomyopathy, hepatic or renal disease, hypotension or hypovolemia, increased intracranial pressure, constrictive pericarditis, pericardial tamponade, low ventricular filling pressure or low PCWP, pregnancy, lactation
- *Physical:* Skin—color, temperature, lesions; orientation, reflexes, affect; P, BP, orthostatic BP, baseline ECG, peripheral perfusion; R, adventitious sounds; liver evaluation, normal output; liver function tests (IV); renal function tests (IV); CBC, Hgb

Implementation
- Administer sublingual preparations under the tongue or in the buccal pouch. Encourage the patient not to swallow.

Adverse effects in *Italics* are most common; those in **Bold** are life-threatening.

Ask patient if the tablet "fizzles" or burns. Always check the expiration date on the bottle; store at room temperature, protected from light. Discard unused drug 6 mo after bottle is opened (conventional tablets); stabilized tablets (Nitrostat) are less subject to loss of potency.
- Administer sustained-release preparations with water; tell the patient not to chew the tablets or capsules; do not crush these preparations.
- Administer topical ointment by applying the ointment over a 6 × 6 in area in a thin, uniform layer using the applicator. Cover area with plastic wrap held in place by adhesive tape. Rotate sites of application to decrease the chance of inflammation and sensitization; close tube tightly when finished.
- Administer transdermal systems to skin site free of hair and not subject to much movement. Shave areas that have a lot of hair. Do not apply to distal extremities. Change sites slightly to decrease the chance of local irritation and sensitization. Remove transdermal system before attempting defibrillation or cardioversion.
- Administer transmucosal tablets by placing them between the lip and gum above the incisors or between the cheek and gum. Encourage patient not to swallow and not to chew the tablet.
- Administer the translingual spray directly onto the oral mucosa; preparation is not to be inhaled.
- Arrange to withdraw drug gradually. 4–6 wk is the recommended withdrawal period for the transdermal preparations.
- Establish safety measures if CNS effects, hypotension occur.
- Maintain control over enviroment, monitoring temperature (cool), lighting, noise.
- Provide periodic rest periods for patient.
- Provide comfort measures and arrange for analgesics if headache occurs.
- Maintain life support equipment on standby if overdose occurs or cardiac condition worsens.
- Provide support and encouragement to deal with disease, therapy, and needed lifestyle changes

Drug-specific teaching points
- Place sublingual tablets under your tongue or in your cheek; do not chew or swallow the tablet; the tablet should burn or "fizzle" under the tongue. Take the nitroglycerin before chest pain begins, when you anticipate that your activities or situation may precipitate an attack. Do not buy large quantities; this drug does not store well. Keep the drug in a dark, dry place, in a dark-colored glass bottle with a tight lid; do not combine with other drugs. You may repeat your dose every 5 min for a total of ___ tablets; if the pain is still not relieved, go to an emergency room.
- Do not chew or crush the timed-release preparations; take on an empty stomach.
- Spread a thin layer of topical ointment on the skin using the applicator. Do not rub or massage the area. Cover with plastic wrap held in place with adhesive tape. Wash your hands after application. Keep the tube tightly closed. Rotate the sites frequently to prevent local irritation.
- To use transdermal systems, you may need to shave an area for application. Apply to a slightly different area each day. Use care if changing brands; each system has a different concentration.
- Place transmucosal tablets these between the lip and gum or between the gum and cheek. Do not chew; try not to swallow.
- Spray translingual spray directly onto oral mucous membranes; do not inhale. Use 5–10 min before activities that you anticipate will precipitate an attack.
- Take drug exactly as directed; do not exceed recommended dosage.
- Know that the following side effects may occur: dizziness, lightheadedness (this may pass as you adjust to the drug; use care to change positions slowly); headache (lying down in a cool environment and resting may help; OTC preparations may not help); flushing of the neck or face (this usually passes as the drug's effects pass).

- Report blurred vision, persistent or severe headache, skin rash, more frequent or more severe angina attacks, fainting.

Representative Drugs
amyl nitrate
erythrityl tetranitrate
isosorbide
isosorbide dinitrate
nitroglycerin

☐ Nondepolarizing Neuromuscular Junction Blockers (NMJ Blockers)

Pregnancy Category C

Therapeutic actions
NMJ blockers interfere with neuromuscular transmission and cause flaccid paralysis by blocking acetylcholine receptors at the skeletal neuromuscular junction.

Indications
- Adjuncts to general anesthetics to facilitate endotracheal intubation and relax skeletal muscle, to relax skeletal muscle to facilitate mechanical ventilation.

Contraindications/cautions
- NMJ blockers are contraindicated in the presence of hypersensitivity to NMJ blockers and the bromide ion. Use with caution in the presence of myasthenia gravis; pregnancy (teratogenic in preclinical studies; may be used in cesarean section, but reversal may be difficult if patient has received magnesium sulfate to manage preeclampsia); renal or hepatic disease, respiratory depression, altered fluid/electrolyte balance; patients in whom an increase in heart rate may be dangerous.

Adverse effects
- **CV**: *Increased P*
- **Respiratory**: *Depressed respiration, apnea,* bronchospasm
- **MS**: Profound and prolonged muscle paralysis
- **Hypersensitivity**: Hypersensitivity reactions, especially rash

Clinically important drug-drug interactions
- Increased intensity and duration of neuromuscular block with some anesthetics (isoflurane, enflurane, halothane, diethyl ether, methoxyflurane), some parenteral antibiotics (aminoglycosides, clindamycin, lincomycin, bacitracin, polymyxin B, and sodium colistimethate), ketamine, quinine, quinidine, trimethaphan, calcium channel-blocking drugs (eg, verapamil), Mg^{2+} salts, and in hypokalemia (produced by K^+ depleting diuretics) • Decreased intensity of neuromuscular block with acetylcholine, cholinesterase inhibitors, K^+ salts, theophyllines, phenytoins, azathioprine, mercaptopurine, carbamazepine

■ Nursing Considerations

Assessment
- *History:* Hypersensitivity to NMJ blockers and the bromide ion, myasthenia gravis, pregnancy, renal or hepatic disease, respiratory depression, altered fluid/electrolyte balance
- *Physical:* Body weight, temperature, skin condition, hydration, reflexes, bilateral grip strength, pulse, BP, respiratory rate and adventitious sounds, liver and kidney function, serum electrolytes

Implementation
- Know that drug should be given only by trained personnel (anesthesiologists).
- Arrange to have facilities on standby to maintain airway and provide mechanical ventilation.
- Provide neostigmine, pyridostigmine, or edrophonium (cholinesterase inhibitors) on standby to overcome excessive neuromuscular block.
- Provide atropine or glycopyrrolate on standby to prevent parasympathomimetic effects of cholinesterase inhibitors.
- Provide a peripheral nerve stimulator on standby to assess degree of neuromuscular block, as needed.

Adverse effects in *Italics* are most common; those in **Bold** are life-threatening.

- Change patient's position frequently, and provide skin care to prevent decubitus ulcer formation when drug is used for other than brief periods.
- Monitor conscious patient for pain, distress that patient may not be able to communicate.
- Reassure conscious patients frequently.

Drug-specific teaching points

- Teaching points about what the drug does and how the patient will feel should be incorporated into overall teaching program about the procedure.

Representative Drugs

atracurium
doxacurium
gallamine
metocurine
mivacurium
pancuronium
pipecuronium
rocuronium
tubocurarine
vecuronium

❑ Nonsteroidal Anti-inflammatory Agents (NSAIDs)

Pregnancy Category B

Therapeutic actions

NSAIDs have anti-inflammatory, analgesic, and antipyretic activities largely related to inhibition of prostaglandins synthesis; exact mechanisms of action are not known.

Indications

- Relief of signs and symptoms of rheumatoid arthritis and osteoarthritis
- Relief of mild to moderate pain
- Treatment of primary dysmenorrhea
- Fever reduction
- Unlabeled use: treatment of juvenile rheumatoid arthritis

Contraindications/cautions

- NSAIDs are contraindicated in the presence of allergy to salicylates or other NSAIDs (more common in patients with rhinitis, asthma, chronic urticaria, nasal polyps); cardiovascular dysfunction, hypertension; peptic ulceration, GI bleeding; pregnancy; or lactation. Use with caution in the presence of impaired hepatic function; impaired renal function.

Adverse effects

- CNS: *Headache, dizziness, somnolence, insomnia,* fatigue, tiredness, dizziness, tinnitus, ophthalmologic effects
- GI: *Nausea, dyspepsia, GI pain,* diarrhea, vomiting, *constipation,* flatulence
- Respiratory: Dyspnea, hemoptysis, pharyngitis, bronchospasm, rhinitis
- Hematologic: Bleeding, platelet inhibition with higher doses, neutropenia, eosinophilia, leukopenia, pancytopenia, thrombocytopenia, agranulocytosis, granulocytopenia, aplastic anemia, decreased hemoglobin or hematocrit, bone marrow depression, menorrhagia
- GU: Dysuria, renal impairment
- Dermatologic: *Rash,* pruritus, sweating, dry mucous membranes, stomatitis
- Other: Peripheral edema, anaphylactoid reactions to fatal anaphylactic shock

Clinically important drug-drug interactions

- Increased toxic effects of lithium if taken with NSAIDs • Decreased diuretic effect if taken concurrently with loop diuretics: bumetanide, furosemide, ethacrynic acid • Potential decrease in antihypertensive effect of beta-adrenergic blocking agents

■ Nursing Considerations

Assessment

- *History:* Allergy to salicylates or other NSAIDs; cardiovascular dysfunction, hypertension; peptic ulceration, GI bleeding; impaired hepatic function; impaired renal function; pregnancy; lactation
- *Physical:* Skin—color, lesions; temperature; orientation, reflexes, ophthalmologic evaluation, audiometric evaluation, peripheral sensation; P, BP, edema; R, adventitious sounds; liver evaluation, bowel sounds; CBC, clotting times, uri-

Adverse effects in *Italics* are most common; those in **Bold** are life-threatening.

nalysis, renal and liver function tests, serum electrolytes, stool guaiac

Implementation
- Administer drug with food or after meals if GI upset occurs.
- Establish safety measures if CNS, visual disturbances occur.
- Arrange for periodic ophthalmologic examination during long-term therapy.
- Arrange for discontinuation of drug if eye changes, symptoms of liver dysfunction, renal impairment occur.
- Institute emergency procedures if overdose occurs (gastric lavage, induction of emesis, supportive therapy).
- Provide further comfort measures to reduce pain (eg, positioning, environmental control) and to reduce inflammation (eg, warmth, positioning, rest).
- Provide small, frequent meals if GI upset is severe.

Drug specific teaching points
- Use the drug only as suggested; avoid overdose. Take the drug with food or after meals if GI upset occurs. Do not exceed the prescribed dosage
- Know that the following side effects may occur: nausea, GI upset, dyspepsia (taking the drug with food may help); diarrhea or constipation (ensure ready access to bathroom facilites if diarrhea occurs); drowsiness, dizziness, vertigo, insomnia (use caution when driving or operating dangerous machinery if these occur).
- Avoid OTC drugs while you are taking this drug. Many of these drugs contain similar medications, and serious overdosage can occur. If you feel that you need one of these preparations, consult with your nurse or physician for the best possible choice.
- Report sore throat, fever, rash, itching, weight gain, swelling in ankles or fingers, changes in vision, black or tarry stools.

Representative Drugs
diclofenac
etodolac
fenoprofen
flurbiprofen
ibuprofen
indomethacin
ketoprofen
ketorolac
meclofenamate
nabumetone
naproxen
oxaprozin
piroxicam
sulindac
tolmetin

❐ Penicillins

Pregnancy Category C

Therapeutic actions
Penicillins are antibiotics. They are bactericidal, inhibiting the synthesis of cell wall of sensitive organisms, causing cell death in susceptible organisms.

Indications
- Treatment of moderate to severe infections caused by sensitive organisms: streptococci, pneumococci, staphylococci, *N. gonorrhoeae, T. pallidum,* meningococci, *Actinomyces israelii, Clostridium perfringens, Clostridium tetani, Leptotrichia buccalis* (Vincent's disease), *Spirillium minus* or *Streptobacillus moniliformis, L. monocytogenes, Pasteurella multocida, Erysipelothrix insidiosa, E. coli, Enterobacter aerogenes, Alcaligenes faecalis, Salmonella, Shigella, P. mirabilis, C. diphtheriae, Bacillus anthracis*
- Treatment of syphilis, gonococcal infections
- Unlabeled use: treatment of Lyme disease

Contraindications/cautions
- Penicillins are contraindicated in the presence of allergy to penicillins, cephalosporins, other allergens. Use with caution in the presence of renal disease, pregnancy, lactation (may cause diarrhea or candidiasis in the infant).

Adverse effects
- CNS: Lethargy, hallucinations, seizures
- GI: *Glossitis, stomatitis, gastritis, sore mouth,* furry tongue, black "hairy"

Adverse effects in *Italics* are most common; those in **Bold** are life-threatening.

tongue, *nausea, vomiting, diarrhea,* abdominal pain, bloody diarrhea, enterocolitis, pseudomembranous colitis, nonspecific hepatitis
- **Hematologic:** Anemia, thrombocytopenia, leukopenia, neutropenia, prolonged bleeding time
- **GU:** Nephritis-oliguria, proteinuria, hematuria, casts, azotemia, pyuria
- **Other:** *Superinfections,* sodium overload, leading to CHF
- **Hypersensitivity reactions:** *Rash, fever, wheezing,* anaphylaxis
- **Local:** *Pain, phlebitis,* thrombosis at injection site, Jarisch-Herxheimer reaction when used to treat syphilis

Clinically important drug-drug interactions

- Decreased effectiveness of penicillin if taken concurrently with tetracyclines
- Inactivation of parenteral aminoglycosides (amikacin, gentamicin, kanamycin, neomycin, netilmicin, streptomycin, tobramycin) if taken concurrently

Drug-lab test interferences
- False-positive Coombs' test (IV)

■ Nursing Considerations

Assessment
- *History:* Allergy to penicillins, cephalosporins, other allergens, renal disease, lactation
- *Physical:* Culture infected area; skin—rashes, lesions; R, adventitious sounds; bowel sounds, normal output; CBC, liver function tests, renal function tests, serum electrolytes, hematocrit, urinalysis; skin test with benzylpenicylloyl-polylysine if hypersensitivity reactions to penicillin have occurred

Implementation
- Culture infected area before beginning treatment; reculture area if response is not as expected.
- Use the smallest dose possible for IM injection to avoid pain and discomfort.
- Arrange to continue treatment for 48–72 h beyond the time that the patient becomes asymptomatic.
- Monitor serum electrolytes and cardiac status if penicillin G is given by IV infusion. Sodium or potassium preparations have been associated with severe electrolyte imbalances.
- Check IV site carefully for signs of thrombosis or local drug reaction.
- Do not give IM injections repeatedly in the same site; atrophy can occur. Monitor injection sites.
- Explain the reason for parenteral routes of administration; offer support and encouragement to deal with therapy.
- Provide small, frequent meals if GI upset occurs.
- Arrange for appropriate comfort and treatment measures for superinfections.
- Provide for frequent mouth care if GI effects occur.
- Ensure that bathroom facilites are readily available if diarrhea occurs.
- Maintain epinephrine, IV fluids, vasopressors, bronchodilators, oxygen, and emergency equipment on standby in case of serious hypersensitivity reaction.
- Arrange for the use of corticosteroids, antihistamines for skin reactions.

Drug-specific teaching points
- Be aware that this drug must be given by injection.
- Know that the following side effects may occur: upset stomach, nausea, vomiting (small, frequent meals may help); sore mouth (frequent mouth care may help); diarrhea (ready access to a bathroom will be necessary); pain or discomfort at the injection site (report this to your nurse if it becomes too uncomfortable).
- Report unusual bleeding, sore throat, rash, hives, fever, severe diarrhea, difficulty breathing.

Representative Drugs
amoxicillin
ampicillin
bacampicillin
carbenicillin
cloxacillin
dicloxacillin
methicillin

Adverse effects in *Italics* are most common; those in **Bold** are life-threatening.

mezlocillin
nafcillin
oxacillin
penicillin G potassium
penicillin G sodium
penicillin V
piperacillin
ticarcillin

Phenothiazines

Pregnancy Category C

Therapeutic actions
Mechanism of action of phenothiazines is not fully understood. Antipsychotic drugs block postsynaptic dopamine receptors in the brain, but this may not be necessary and sufficient for antipsychotic activity; depresses the reticular activating system, including the parts of the brain involved with wakefulness and emesis; anticholinergic, antihistaminic (H_1), and alpha-adrenergic blocking activity also may contribute to some of its therapeutic (and adverse) actions.

Indications
- Management of manifestations of psychotic disorders
- Control of severe nausea and vomiting, intractable hiccups

Contraindications/cautions
- Phenothiazines are contraindicated in the presence of coma or severe CNS depression, bone marrow depression, blood dyscrasia, circulatory collapse, subcortical brain damage, Parkinson's disease, liver damage, cerebral arteriosclerosis, coronary disease, severe hypotension or hypertension. Use with caution in the presence of respiratory disorders ("silent pneumonia" may develop); glaucoma, prostatic hypertrophy; epilepsy or history of epilepsy; breast cancer; thyrotoxicosis; peptic ulcer, decreased renal function; myelography within previous 24 h or scheduled within 48 h; exposure to heat or phosphorous insecticides; pregnancy; lactation; children younger than 12 y, especially those with chickenpox, CNS infections (children are especially susceptible to dystonias that may confound the diagnosis of Reye's syndrome).

Adverse effects
Antipsychotic Drugs
- CNS: *Drowsiness*, insomnia, vertigo, headache, weakness, tremor, ataxia, slurring, cerebral edema, seizures, exacerbation of psychotic symptoms, extrapyramidal syndromes—*pseudoparkinsonism; dystonias; akathisia*, tardive dyskinesias, potentially irreversible (no known treatment), **neuroleptic malignant syndrome**
- CV: Hypotension, orthostatic hypotension, hypertension, tachycardia, bradycardia, cardiac arrest, CHF, cardiomegaly, **refractory arrhythmias** (some fatal), pulmonary edema
- Respiratory: Bronchospasm, laryngospasm, dyspnea; suppression of cough reflex and potential for aspiration (**sudden death related to asphyxia** or cardiac arrest has been reported)
- Hematologic: Eosinophilia, leukopenia, leukocytosis, anemia; aplastic anemia; hemolytic anemia; thrombocytopenic or nonthrombocytopenic purpura; pancytopenia
- EENT: Glaucoma, *photophobia, blurred vision*, miosis, mydriasis, deposits in the cornea and lens (opacities), pigmentary retinopathy
- Hypersensitivity: Jaundice, urticaria, angioneurotic edema, laryngeal edema, photosensitivity, eczema, asthma, anaphylactoid reactions, exfoliative dermatitis
- Endocrine: Lactation, breast engorgement in females, galactorrhea; syndrome of inappropriate ADH secretion; amenorrhea, menstrual irregularities; gynecomastia in males; changes in libido; hyperglycemia or hypoglycemia; glycosuria; hyponatremia; pituitary tumor with hyperprolactinemia; inhibition of ovulation, infertility, pseudopregnancy; re-

Adverse effects in *Italics* are most common; those in **Bold** are life-threatening.

duced urinary levels of gonadotropins, estrogens, progestins
- **Autonomic:** Dry mouth, salivation, nasal congestion, nausea, vomiting, anorexia, fever, pallor, flushed facies, sweating, constipation, paralytic ileus, urinary retention, incontinence, polyuria, enuresis, priapism, ejaculation inhibition, male impotence
- **Other:** *Urine discolored pink to red-brown*

Clinically important drug-drug interactions

- Additive CNS depression with alcohol • Additive anticholinergic effects and possibly decreased antipsychotic efficacy with anticholinergic drugs • Increased likelihood of seizures with metrizamide (contrast agent used in myelography) • Increased chance of severe neuromuscular excitation and hypotension if given to patients receiving barbiturate anesthetics (methohexital, thiamylal, phenobarbital, thiopental) • Decreased antihypertensive effect of guanethidine when taken with antipsychotics

Drug-lab test interferences

- False-positive pregnancy tests (less likely if serum test is used) • Increase in protein-bound iodine, not attributable to an increase in thyroxine

■ Nursing Considerations

Assessment

- *History:* Coma or severe CNS depression; bone marrow depression; blood dyscrasia; circulatory collapse; subcortical brain damage; Parkinson's disease; liver damage; cerebral arteriosclerosis; coronary disease; severe hypotension or hypertension; respiratory disorders; glaucoma, prostatic hypertrophy; epilepsy or history of epilepsy; breast cancer; thyrotoxicosis; peptic ulcer, decreased renal function; myelography within previous 24 h or myelography scheduled within 48 h; exposure to heat or phosphorous insecticides; pregnancy; children younger than 12 y, especially those with chickenpox, CNS infections
- *Physical:* Body weight, temperature; reflexes, orientation, intraocular pressure; P, BP, orthostatic BP; R, adventitious sounds; bowel sounds and normal output, liver evaluation; urinary output, prostate size; CBC, urinalysis, thyroid, liver and kidney function tests

Implementation

- Dilute oral concentrate *only* with water, saline, 7-Up, homogenized milk, carbonated orange drink, and pineapple, apricot, prune, orange, V-8, tomato, and grapefruit juices; use 60 ml of diluent for each 16 mg (5 ml) of concentrate.
- Do *not* mix with beverages that contain caffeine (coffee, cola), tannics (tea), or pectinates (apple juice); physical incompatibility may result.
- Give IM injections only to seated or recumbent patients, and observe for adverse effects for a brief period afterward.
- Monitor pulse and BP continuously during IV administration.
- Do not change dosage in chronic therapy more often than weekly; drug requires 4–7 d to achieve steady-state plasma levels.
- Avoid skin contact with oral solution; contact dermatitis has occurred.
- Arrange for discontinuation of drug if serum creatinine, BUN become abnormal or if WBC count is depressed.
- Monitor bowel function, and arrange appropriate therapy for severe constipation; adynamic ileus with fatal complications has occurred.
- Monitor elderly patients for dehydration, and institute remedial measures promptly; sedation and decreased sensation of thirst related to CNS effects of drug can lead to severe dehydration.
- Consult physician regarding appropriate warning of patient or patient's guardian about tardive dyskinesias.
- Consult physician about dosage reduction, use of anticholinergic antiparkinsonian drugs (controversial) if extrapyramidal effects occur.
- Provide safety measures (side rails, assistance with ambulation) if sedation, ataxia, vertigo, orthostatic hypotension, vision changes occur.

Adverse effects in *Italics* are most common; those in **Bold** are life-threatening.

- Provide positioning to relieve discomfort of dystonias.
- Provide reassurance to deal with extrapyramidal effect, sexual dysfunction.

Drug-specific teaching points
- Take drug exactly as prescribed. The full effect may require 6 wk–6 mo of therapy.
- Avoid skin contact with drug solutions.
- Avoid driving a car or engaging in other dangerous activities if CNS, vision changes occur.
- Avoid prolonged exposure to sun or use a sunscreen or covering garments if exposure is necessary.
- Maintain fluid intake, and use precautions against heatstroke in hot weather.
- Report sore throat, fever, unusual bleeding or bruising, rash, weakness, tremors, impaired vision, dark urine (pink or reddish brown urine is to be expected), pale stools, yellowing of the skin or eyes.

Representative Drugs
acetophenazine
chlorpromazine
fluphenazine
mesoridazine
perphenazine
prochlorperazine
promazine
thioridazine
trifluoperazine
triflupromazine

☐ Sulfonamides

Pregnancy Category C
Pregnancy Category D (at term)

Therapeutic actions
Sulfonamides are antibiotics. They are bacteriostatic; competitively antagonize para-aminobenzoic acid, an essential component of folic acid synthesis, in susceptible gram-negative and gram-positive bacteria, causing cell death.

Indications
- Treatment of ulcerative colitis, otitis media, inclusion conjunctivitis, meningitis, nocardiosis, toxoplasmosis, trachoma, urinary tract infections
- Management of rheumatoid arthritis, collagenous colitis, Crohn's disease

Contraindications/cautions
- Sulfonamides are contraindicated in the presence of allergy to sulfonamides, sulfonylureas, thiazides; pregnancy (teratogenic in preclinical studies; at term, may bump fetal bilirubin from plasma protein binding sites and cause kernicterus); or lactation (risk of kernicterus, diarrhea, rash). Use with caution in the presence of impaired renal or hepatic function, G-6-PD deficiency, porphyria.

Adverse effects
- **CNS:** Headache, peripheral neuropathy, mental depression, convulsions, ataxia, hallucinations, tinnitus, vertigo, insomnia, hearing loss, drowsiness, transient lesions of posterior spinal column, transverse myelitis
- **GI:** Nausea, emesis, abdominal pains, diarrhea, bloody diarrhea, anorexia, pancreatitis, stomatitis, impaired folic acid absorption, hepatitis, hepatocellular necrosis
- **Hematologic:** Agranulocytosis, aplastic anemia, thrombocytopenia, leukopenia, hemolytic anemia, hypoprothrombinemia, methemoglobinemia, megaloblastic anemia
- **GU:** Crystalluria, hematuria, proteinuria, nephrotic syndrome, toxic nephrosis with oliguria and anuria, oligospermia, infertility
- **Dermatologic:** Photosensitivity, cyanosis, petechiae, alopecia
- **Hypersensitivity:** Stevens-Johnson syndrome, generalized skin eruptions, epidermal necrolysis, urticaria, serum sickness, pruritus, exfoliative dermatitis, anaphylactoid reactions, periorbital edema, conjunctival and scleral redness, photosensitization, arthralgia, allergic myocarditis, transient pulmonary changes with eosinophilia, decreased pulmonary function

Adverse effects in *Italics* are most common; those in **Bold** are life-threatening.

- **Other:** Drug fever, chills, periarteritis nodosum

Clinically important drug-drug interactions
- Increased risk of hypoglycemia when tolbutamide, tolazamide, glyburide, glipizide, acetohexamide, chlorpropamide are taken concurrently • Increased risk of folate deficiency if taking sulfonamides; monitor patients receiving folic acid carefully for signs of folate deficiency

Drug-lab test interferences
- Possible false-positive urinary glucose tests using Benedict's method

■ Nursing Considerations

Assessment
- *History:* Allergy to sulfonamides, sulfonylureas, thiazides; pregnancy; lactation; impaired renal or hepatic function; G-6-PD deficiency; porphyria
- *Physical:* Body temperature; skin—color, lesions; culture of infected site; orientation, reflexes, affect, peripheral sensation; R, adventitious sounds; mucous membranes, bowel sounds, liver evaluation; liver and renal function tests, CBC and differential, urinalysis

Implementation
- Arrange for culture and sensitivity tests of infected area before beginning therapy; repeat cultures if response is not as expected.
- Administer drug after meals or with food to prevent GI upset. Administer the drug around the clock.
- Ensure adequate fluid intake.
- Discontinue drug immediately if hypersensitivity reaction occurs.
- Establish safety precautions if CNS effects occur (eg, side rails, assistance, environmental control).
- Protect patient from exposure to light (use of sunscreen, wear protective clothing) if photosensitivity occurs.
- Provide small, frequent meals if GI upset occurs.
- Ensure ready access to bathroom facilities if diarrhea occurs.
- Provide frequent mouth care for stomatitis.
- Offer support and encouragement to deal with side effects of drug therapy, including changes in sexual function.

Drug-specific teaching points
- Complete full course of therapy.
- Take the drug with food or meals to decrease GI upset.
- Drink eight glasses of water per day.
- Be aware that this drug is specific to this disease; do not use to self-treat any other infection.
- Know that the following side effects may occur: sensitivity to sunlight (use sunscreens; wear protective clothing if exposed to the sun); dizziness, drowsiness, difficulty walking, loss of sensation (avoid driving or performing tasks that require alertness if these occur); nausea, vomiting, diarrhea (ensure ready access to bathroom facilities); loss of fertility; yellow-orange urine.
- Report blood in the urine, rash, ringing in the ears, difficulty breathing, fever, sore throat, chills.

Representative Drugs
sulfadiazine
sulfamethizole
sulfasalazine
sulfisoxazole
sulfamethoxizole

❏ Tetracyclines

Pregnancy Category D

Therapeutic actions
Tetracylines are antibiotics. They are bacteriostatic; inhibit protein synthesis of susceptible bacteria, preventing cell replication.

Indications
- Treatment of infections caused by rickettsiae; *M. pneumoniae;* agents of psittacosis, ornithosis, lymphogranuloma venereum, and granuloma inguinale; *Borrelia recurrentis, H. ducreyi, Paste-*

Adverse effects in *Italics* are most common; those in **Bold** are life-threatening.

urella pestis, Pasteurella tularensis, Bartonella bacilliformis, Bacteroides, Vibrio comma, Vibrio fetus, Brucella, E. coli, E. aerogenes, Shigella, Acinetobacter calcoaceticus, H. influenzae, Klebsiella, Diplococcus pneumoniae, S. aureus; when penicillin is contraindicated, infections caused by N. gonorrhoeae, T. pallidum, Treponema pertenue, L. monocytogenes, Clostridium, B. anthracis, Fusobacterium fusiforme, Actinomyces, N. meningitidis
- Adjunct to amebicides in acute intestinal amebiasis
- Treatment of acne
- Treatment of complicated urethral, endocervical or rectal infections in adults caused by C. trachomatis
- Treatment of superficial ocular infections due to susceptible strains of microorganisms
- Prophylaxis of ophthalmia neonatorum due to N. gonorrrhoeae or C. trachomatis

Contraindications/cautions

- Tetracyclines are contraindicated in the presence of allergy to any of the tetracyclines, allergy to tartrazine (in 250-mg tetracycline capsules marketed under brand name *Panmycin*), pregnancy (toxic to the fetus), lactation (causes damage to the teeth of infant). Use with caution in the presence of hepatic or renal dysfunction, presence of ocular viral, mycobacterial, or fungal infections.

Adverse effects

- **GI:** *Discoloring and inadequate calcification of primary teeth of fetus if used by pregnant women, discoloring and inadequate calcification of permanent teeth if used during period of dental development,* fatty liver, **liver failure,** *anorexia, nausea, vomiting, diarrhea, glossitis, dysphagia,* enterocolitis, esophageal ulcers
- **Hematologic:** Hemolytic anemia, thrombocytopenia, neutropenia, eosinophilia, leukocytosis, leukopenia
- **Dermatologic:** *Phototoxic reactions, rash,* exfoliative dermatitis
- **Hypersensitivity:** Reactions from urticaria to **anaphylaxis,** including **intracranial hypertension**
- **Local:** *Transient irritation, stinging, itching,* angioneurotic edema, urticaria, dermatitis, superinfections with ophthalmic or dermatologic use
- **Other:** *Superinfections,* local irritation at parenteral injection sites

Clinically important drug-drug interactions

• Decreased absorption of tetracyclines if used with calcium salts, magnesium salts, zinc salts, aluminum salts, bismuth salts, iron, urinary alkalinizers, food, dairy products, charcoal • Increased digoxin toxicity if taken with tetracyclines • Increased nephrotoxicity if taken with methoxyflurane • Decreased effectiveness of oral contraceptives, though rare, has been reported with a risk of breakthrough bleeding or pregnancy if taken with tetracyclines • Decreased activity of penicillins if taken with tetracyclines

■ Nursing Considerations
Assessment

- *History:* Allergy to any of the tetracyclines; allergy to tartrazine; hepatic or renal dysfunction, pregnancy, lactation; ocular viral, mycobacterial or fungal infections
- *Physical:* Site of infection, skin—color, lesions; R, adventitious sounds; bowel sounds, output, liver evaluation; urinalysis, BUN, liver function tests, renal function tests

Implementation

- Administer oral medication on an empty stomach, 1 h before or 2–3 h after meals. Do not give with antacids. If antacids must be used, give them 3 h after the dose of tetracycline.
- Culture infected area before beginning drug therapy.
- Do not use outdated drugs; degraded drug is highly nephrotoxic and should not be used.

Adverse effects in *Italics* are most common; those in **Bold** are life-threatening.

- Do not give oral drug with meals, antacids, or food.
- Ensure ready access to bathroom facilities if diarrhea occurs.
- Provide frequent hygiene measures if superinfections occur.
- Protect patient from sunlight and bright lights if photosensitivity occurs.
- Arrange for regular renal function tests if long-term therapy is used.
- Use topical preparations of this drug only when clearly indicated. Sensitization from the topical use of this drug may preclude its later use in serious infections. Topical preparations containing antibiotics that are not ordinarily given systemically are preferable.

Drug-specific teaching points

- Take the drug throughout the day for best results. The drug should be taken on an empty stomach, 1 h before or 2–3 h after meals, with a full glass of water. Do not take the drug with food, dairy products, iron preparations, or antacids.
- Finish your complete prescription; if any is left, discard it immediately. Never take an outdated product.
- Be aware that there have been reports of pregnancy occurring when taking tetracycline with oral contraceptives. To be absolutely confident of avoiding pregnancy, the use of an additional type of contraceptive is advised while on this drug.
- Know that the following side effects may occur: stomach upset, nausea (this will pass when the drug therapy is finished); superinfections in the mouth, vagina (frequent washing may help this problem; if it becomes severe, medication may be available to help); sensitivity of the skin to sunlight (use protective clothing and a sunscreen when exposed to the sun).
- Report severe cramps, watery diarrhea, rash or itching, difficulty breathing, dark urine or light-colored stools, yellowing of the skin or eyes.
- Administer eye drops as follows: lie down or tilt head backward and look at the ceiling. Drop suspension inside lower eyelid while looking up. Close eye, and apply gentle pressure to inner corner of the eye for 1 min.
- Apply ointment inside lower eyelid; close eyes, and roll eyeball in all directions.
- Be aware that this drug may cause temporary blurring of vision or stinging after application.
- Notify your nurse or physician if stinging or itching becomes severe.
- Take the full course of therapy prescribed; discard any leftover medication immediately.
- Apply dermatologic solution generously until skin is wet.
- Avoid the eyes, nose, and mouth.
- Be aware that you may experience transient stinging or burning; this will subside quickly; skin in the treated area may become yellow; this will wash off.
- Know that you may use cosmetics as you usually do.
- Wash area before applying (unless contraindicated); this drug may stain clothing.
- Report worsening of condition, rash, irritation.

Representative Drugs

demeclocycline
doxycycline
minocycline
oxytetracyline
tetracycline

❒ Tricyclic Antidepressants (TCAS)

Pregnancy Category C

Therapeutic actions

Mechanism of action of the TCAs is unknown. The TCAs are structurally related to the phenothiazine antipsychotic drugs (eg, chlorpromazine), but in contrast to the phenothiazines, TCAs inhibit the presynaptic reuptake of the neurotransmitters norepinephrine and serotonin; anticholinergic at CNS and peripheral receptors; the relation of these effects to clinical efficacy is unknown.

Indications
- Relief of symptoms of depression (endogenous depression most responsive; unlike other TCAs, protriptyline is "activating" and may be useful in withdrawn and anergic patients)
- Unlabeled use: treatment of obstructive sleep apnea

Contraindications/cautions
- TCAs are contraindicated in the presence of hypersensitivity to any tricyclic drug, concomitant therapy with an MAO inhibitor, recent MI, myelography within previous 24 h or scheduled within 48 h, pregnancy (limb reduction abnormalities reported), or lactation. Use with caution in the presence of electroshock therapy; preexisting cardiovascular disorders (eg, severe coronary heart disease, progressive heart failure, angina pectoris, paroxysmal tachycardia); angle-closure glaucoma, increased intraocular pressure, urinary retention, ureteral or urethral spasm; seizure disorders (TCAs lower the seizure threshold); hyperthyroidism (predisposes to CVS toxicity, including cardiac arrhythmias); impaired hepatic, renal function; psychiatric patients (schizophrenic or paranoid patients may exhibit a worsening of psychosis with TCA therapy); manic-depressive patients (may shift to hypomanic or manic phase); elective surgery (TCAs should be discontinued as long as possible before surgery).

Adverse effects
- CNS: *Sedation and anticholinergic (atropine-like) effects* (dry mouth, blurred vision, disturbance of accommodation for near vision, mydriasis, increased intraocular pressure), *confusion* (especially in elderly), *disturbed concentration*, hallucinations, disorientation, decreased memory, feelings of unreality, delusions, anxiety, nervousness, restlessness, agitation, panic, insomnia, nightmares, hypomania, mania, exacerbation of psychosis, drowsiness, weakness, fatigue, headache, numbness, tingling, paresthesias of extremities, incoordination, motor hyperactivity, akathisia, ataxia, tremors, peripheral neuropathy, extrapyramidal symptoms, *seizures*, speech blockage, dysarthria, tinnitus, altered EEG
- GI: *Dry mouth, constipation*, paralytic ileus, *nausea*, vomiting, anorexia, epigastric distress, diarrhea, flatulence, dysphagia, peculiar taste, increased salivation, stomatitis, glossitis, parotid swelling, abdominal cramps, black tongue
- CV: *Orthostatic hypotension*, hypertension, syncope, tachycardia, palpitations, MI, arrhythmias, heart block, precipitation of CHF, stroke
- Hematologic: Bone marrow depression, including agranulocytosis; eosinophila; purpura; thrombocytopenia; leukopenia
- GU: Urinary retention, delayed micturition, dilation of the urinary tract, gynecomastia, testicular swelling in men; breast enlargement, menstrual irregularity and galactorrhea in women; increased or decreased libido; impotence
- Hypersensitivity: Skin rash, pruritus, vasculitis, petechiae, photosensitization, edema (generalized or of face and tongue), drug fever
- Endocrine: Elevated or depressed blood sugar; elevated prolactin levels; inappropriate ADH secretion
- Withdrawal: Symptoms with abrupt discontinuation of prolonged therapy: nausea, headache, vertigo, nightmares, malaise
- Other: Nasal congestion, excessive appetite, weight gain or loss; sweating, alopecia, lacrimation, hyperthermia, flushing, chills

Clinically important drug-drug interactions
- Increased TCA levels and pharmacologic effects when given with cimetidine, fluoxetine, ranitidine • Increased half-life and therefore increased bleeding if taken with dicumarol • Altered response, including dysrhythmias and hypertension, if taken

Adverse effects in *Italics* are most common; those in **Bold** are life-threatening.

with sympathomimetics • Risk of severe hypertension when taken concurrently with clonidine • Hyperpyretic crises, severe convulsions, hypertensive episodes, and death when MAO inhibitors are given with TCAs • Decreased hypotensive activity of guanethidine if taken concurrently

■ Nursing Considerations

Assessment
- *History:* Hypersensitivity to any tricyclic drug; concomitant therapy with an MAO inhibitor; recent MI; myelography within previous 24 h or scheduled within 48 h; pregnancy; lactation; electroshock therapy; preexisting cardiovascular disorders; angle-closure glaucoma, increased intraocular pressure, urinary retention, ureteral or urethral spasm; seizure disorders; hyperthyroidism; impaired hepatic, renal function; psychiatric patients; manic-depressive patients; elective surgery
- *Physical:* Body weight; temperature; skin—color, lesions; orientation, affect, reflexes, vision and hearing; P, BP, orthostatic BP, perfusion; bowel sounds, normal output, liver evaluation; urine flow, normal output; usual sexual function, frequency of menses, breast and scrotal examination; liver function tests, urinalysis, CBC, ECG

Implementation
- Ensure that depressed and potentially suicidal patients have access to only limited quantities of drug.
- Arrange to reduce dosage if minor side effects develop; arrange to discontinue the drug if serious side effects occur.
- Arrange for CBC if patient develops fever, sore throat, or other sign of infection during therapy.
- Ensure ready access to bathroom facilities if GI effects occur; establish bowel program for constipation.
- Provide small, frequent meals, frequent mouth care if GI effects occur; provide sugarless lozenges if dry mouth becomes a problem.
- Establish safety precautions if CNS changes occur (eg, side rails, accompany patient when ambulating).

Drug-specific teaching points
- Take drug exactly as prescribed; do not stop taking this drug abruptly or without consulting the physician or nurse.
- Avoid alcohol, other sleep-inducing drugs, OTC drugs while on this drug.
- Avoid prolonged exposure to sunlight or sunlamps; use a sunscreen or protective garments if long exposure to sunlight is unavoidable.
- Know that the following side effects may occur: headache, dizziness, drowsiness, weakness, blurred vision (these effects are reversible; safety measures may need to be taken if these become severe; avoid driving or performing tasks that require alertness while these persist); nausea, vomiting, loss of appetite, dry mouth (small, frequent meals, frequent mouth care, and sucking sugarless candies may help); nightmares, inability to concentrate, confusion; changes in sexual function.
- Report dry mouth, difficulty in urination, excessive sedation.

Representative Drugs
amitriptyline
amoxapine
clomipramine
desipramine
doxepin
imipramine
nortriptyline
protriptyline
trimipramine

Part II

☐ acebutolol hydrochloride

(a se byoo' toe lole)
Monitan (CAN), Rhotral (CAN), Sectral

Pregnancy Category B

Drug classes
Beta-adrenergic blocking agent (β_1 selective)
Antiarrhythmic drug
Antihypertensive drug

Therapeutic actions
Blocks beta-adrenergic receptors of the sympathetic nervous system in the heart and juxtaglomerular apparatus (kidney), decreasing excitability of the heart, decreasing cardiac output and oxygen consumption, decreasing release of renin from the kidney, and lowering blood pressure.

Indications
- Hypertension, as a step 1 agent, alone or with other drugs, especially diuretics
- Cardiac arrhythmias, especially ventricular premature beats

Contraindications/cautions
- Contraindicated in the presence of sinus bradycardia (HR < 45 beats per minute), second- or third-degree heart block (PR interval > 0.24 sec), cardiogenic shock, CHF, asthma, COPD, lactation.
- Use caution in the presence of diabetes or thyrotoxicosis, hepatic impairment, renal failure.

Dosage
Adult
- **Hypertension:** Initially 400 mg/d in one or two doses PO; usual maintenance dosage range is 200–1,200 mg/d given in two divided doses.
- **Ventricular arrhythmias:** 200 mg bid PO; increase dosage gradually until optimum response is achieved (usually at 600–1,200 mg/d); discontinue gradually over 2 wk.

Geriatric: Because bioavailability increases twofold, lower doses may be required; do not exceed 800 mg/d maintenance dosage.
Impaired renal/hepatic function: Reduce daily dose by 50% when creatinine clearance is < 50 ml/min; reduce by 75% when creatinine clearance is < 25 ml/min; use caution with hepatic impairment.
Pediatric: Safety and efficacy not established.

Pharmacokinetics

Route	Onset	Peak	Duration
Oral	Varies	3–4 h	6–8 h

Metabolism: Hepatic, $T_{1/2}$: 3–4 h
Distribution: Crosses placenta; passes into breast milk
Excretion: Urine (30%–40%) and bile/feces (50%–60%)

Adverse effects
- **Neuro:** Dizziness, vertigo, tinnitus, fatigue, emotional depression, paresthesias, sleep disturbances, hallucinations, disorientation, memory loss, slurred speech (Because acebutolol is less lipid soluble than propranolol, it is less likely to penetrate the blood–brain barrier and cause CNS effects.)
- **GI:** *Gastric pain, flatulence, constipation, diarrhea, nausea, vomiting,* anorexia
- **CV:** **Bradycardia, CHF, cardiac arrhythmias, sinoatrial or AV nodal block, tachycardia,** peripheral vascular insufficiency, claudication, CVA, pulmonary edema, hypotension
- **Respiratory:** **Bronchospasm,** dyspnea, cough, bronchial obstruction, nasal stuffiness, rhinitis
- **GU:** *Impotence, decreased libido,* Peyronie's disease, dysuria, nocturia, frequent urination
- **MS:** Joint pain, arthralgia, muscle cramp
- **Derm:** Rash, pruritus, sweating, dry skin
- **EENT:** Eye irritation, dry eyes, conjunctivitis, blurred vision

Adverse effects in *Italics* are most common; those in **Bold** are life-threatening.

58 ■ acetaminophen

- Allergic reactions: Pharyngitis, erythematous rash, fever, sore throat, *laryngospasm, respiratory distress*
- Other: *Decreased exercise tolerance, development of antinuclear antibodies,* hyperglycemia or hypoglycemia, elevated serum transaminase

Clinically important drug-drug interactions
- Increased effects of acebutolol if taken with verapamil • Increased risk of postural hypotension if taken concurrently with prazosin • Possible increased blood pressure lowering effects if taken concurrently with aspirin, bismuth subsalicylate, magnesium salicylate, sulfinpyrazone, oral contraceptives • Decreased antihypertensive effects if taken with NSAIDs, clonidine • Possible increased hypoglycemic effect of insulin if taken with acebutol

Drug-lab test interferences
- Possible false results with glucose or insulin tolerance tests (oral)

■ Nursing Considerations

Assessment
- *History:* Sinus bradycardia, second- or third-degree heart block, cardiogenic shock, CHF, asthma, COPD, pregnancy, lactation, diabetes, or thyrotoxicosis
- *Physical:* Body weight, skin condition, neurologic status, P, BP, ECG, respiratory status, kidney and thyroid function, blood and urine glucose

Implementation
- Give with meals if needed.
- Do not discontinue drug abruptly after chronic therapy. Taper drug gradually over 2 wk with monitoring (abrupt withdrawal may cause serious beta-adrenergic rebound effects).
- Consult with physician about withdrawing drug if patient is to undergo surgery (withdrawal is controversial).
- Provide appropriate comfort measures to help patient cope with drug effects.
- Provide safety precautions if CNS effects occur.

Drug-specific teaching points
- Take drug with meals.
- Do not stop taking this drug unless instructed to do so by a health care provider.
- Avoid driving or dangerous activities if dizziness, weakness occur.
- Know that the following side effects may occur: dizziness, lightheadedness, loss of appetite, nightmares, depression, sexual impotence.
- Report difficulty breathing, night cough, swelling of extremities, slow pulse, confusion, depression, rash, fever, sore throat.

❐ acetaminophen

*(a seat a **mee'** noe fen)*
N-acetyl-P-aminophenol

Suppositories: Acephen, Neopap, Suppap

Oral: Aceta, Ace-Tabs (CAN), Atesol (CAN), Campain (CAN), Dolanex, Exdol (CAN), Genebs, Liquiprin, Oraphen (CAN), Panadol, Panex, Paraphen (CAN), Phenaphen, Robigesic (CAN), Rounox (CAN), St. Joseph's Aspirin Free, Tempra, Tylenol

Pregnancy Category B

Drug classes
Antipyretic
Analgesic (non-narcotic)

Therapeutic actions
Antipyretic: reduces fever by acting directly on the hypothalamic heat-regulating center to cause vasodilation and sweating, which helps to dissipate heat from the body
Analgesic: site and mechanism of action unclear

Indications
- Analgesic–antipyretic in patients with aspirin allergy, hemostatic disturbances, bleeding diatheses, upper GI disease, gouty arthritis

Adverse effects in *Italics* are most common; those in **Bold** are life-threatening.

- Arthritis and rheumatic disorders involving musculoskeletal pain (but lacks clinically significant antirheumatic and anti-inflammatory effects)
- Common cold, "flu," other viral and bacterial infections accompanied by pain and fever
- Unlabeled use: prophylactic for children receiving DPT vaccination to reduce incidence of fever and pain

Contraindications/cautions
- Contraindicated in the presence of allergy to acetaminophen.
- Use caution in the presence of impaired hepatic function, chronic alcoholism, pregnancy, lactation.

Dosage
Adult: By suppository, 325–650 mg q4–6h or PO, 1,000 mg three to four times per day. Do not exceed 4 g/d.
Pediatric: Doses may be repeated four to five times per day; do not exceed five doses in 24 h; give PO or by suppository.

Age	Dosage (mg)	Age	Dosage (mg)
0–3 mo	40	4–5 y	240
4–11 mo	80	6–8 y	320
1–2 y	120	9–70 y	400
2–3 y	160	11 y	480

Pharmacokinetics

Route	Onset	Peak	Duration
Oral	Varies	0.5–2 h	3–4 h

Metabolism: $T_{1/2}$: 1–3 h
Distribution: Crosses placenta; passes into breast milk
Excretion: Urine

Adverse effects
Negligible with recommended dosage.
- CNS: Headache
- GI: Hepatic toxicity and failure, jaundice
- CV: Chest pain, dyspnea, myocardial damage when doses of 5–8 g/d are ingested daily for several weeks or when doses of 4 g/d are ingested for 1 year
- Hematologic: Methemoglobinemia—cyanosis; hemolytic anemia—hematuria, anuria; neutropenia, leukopenia, pancytopenia, thrombocytopenia, hypoglycemia
- GU: Acute kidney failure, renal tubular necrosis
- Hypersensitivity reactions: Skin rash, fever
- Treatment of overdose: Monitor serum levels regularly, N-acetylcysteine should be available as a specific antidote; basic life support measures may be necessary.

Clinically important drug-drug interactions
- Increased toxicity if taken with chronic, excessive ethanol ingestion • Increased hypoprothrombinemic effect of oral anticoagulants when taken with acetaminophen • Increased risk of hepatotoxicity and possible decreased therapeutic effects if taken with barbiturates, carbamazepine, hydantoins, rifampin, sulfinpyrazone • Possible delayed or decreased effectiveness of acetaminophen when taken with anticholinergics • Possible reduced absorption of acetaminophen if taken with activated charcoal • Possible decreased effectiveness of zidovudine if taken with acetaminophen

Drug-lab test interferences
- Interference with Chemstrip G, Dextrostix, and Visidex II home blood glucose measurement systems; effects vary

■ Nursing Considerations

Assessment
- *History:* Allergy to acetaminophen, impaired hepatic function, chronic alcoholism, pregnancy, lactation
- *Physical:* Skin—color, lesions; temperature; liver evaluation; CBC, liver and renal function tests

Implementation
- Do not exceed the recommended dosage.
- Consult physician if needed for children < 3 y; if needed for longer than 10 d; if continued fever, severe or recurrent pain occurs (these may indicate serious illness).

Adverse effects in *Italics* are most common; those in **Bold** are life-threatening.

- Avoid using multiple preparations containing acetaminophen. Carefully check all OTC products.
- Administer drug with food if GI upset is noted.
- Discontinue drug if hypersensitivity reactions occur.

Drug-specific teaching points
- Do not exceed recommended dose; do not take for longer than 10 d.
- Take the drug only for complaints indicated; not an anti-inflammatory agent.
- Avoid the use of other OTC preparations while on this drug. Many of these drugs contain acetaminophen, and serious overdosage can occur. If you feel that you need one of these preparations, consult with your care provider.
- Report skin rash, unusual bleeding or bruising, yellowing of skin or eyes, changes in voiding patterns.

▢ acetazolamide

*(a set a **zole'** a mide)*

Apo-Acetazolamide (CAN), Dazamide, Diamox, Diamox Sequels

Pregnancy Category C

Drug classes
Carbonic anhydrase inhibitor
Antiglaucoma agent
Diuretic
Antiepileptic drug
Sulfonamide (nonbacteriostatic)

Therapeutic actions
Inhibits the enzyme carbonic anhydrase. This action decreases aqueous humor formation in the eye, decreases intraocular pressure, decreases hydrogen ion secretion by renal tubule cells, and increases sodium, potassium, bicarbonate, and water excretion by the kidney, causing a diuretic effect.

Indications
- Adjunctive treatment of chronic open-angle glaucoma, secondary glaucoma
- Preoperative use in acute angle-closure glaucoma when delay of surgery is desired to lower intraocular pressure
- Edema caused by congestive heart failure, drug-induced edema
- Centrencephalic epilepsy
- Prophylaxis and treatment of acute mountain sickness

Contraindications/cautions
- Contraindicated in the presence of allergy to acetazolamide, antibacterial sulfonamides, or thiazides; chronic noncongestive angle-closure glaucoma.
- Use caution in the presence of fluid or electrolyte imbalance (specifically decreased Na^+, decreased K^+, hyperchloremic acidosis), renal disease, hepatic disease (risk of hepatic coma if acetazolamide is given), adrenocortical insufficiency, respiratory acidosis, COPD, lactation.

Dosage
Adult
- ***Open-angle glaucoma:*** 250 mg–1 g/d PO, usually in divided doses. Do not exceed 1 g/d.
- ***Secondary glaucoma and preoperatively:*** 250 mg q4h or 250 mg bid PO, or 500 mg followed by 125–250 mg q4h. May be given IV for rapid relief of increased intraocular pressure.
- ***Diuresis in CHF:*** 250–375 mg (5mg/kg) qd in the morning. Most effective if given on alternate days or for 2 d alternating with a day of rest.
- ***Drug-induced edema:*** 250–375 mg qd or once daily for 1–2 d followed by a day of rest.
- ***Epilepsy:*** 8–30 mg/kg per day in divided doses. When given in combination with other antiepileptics, starting dose is 250 mg qd. Sustained-release preparation is not recommended for this use.
- ***Acute mountain sickness:*** 500–1,000 mg/d in divided doses of tablets or sustained-release capsules. For rapid ascent, the 1,000 mg dose is recommended. When possible, begin dosing 24–48 h before ascent and continue for 48 h or longer as needed while at high altitude.

acetazolamide

Pediatric
- ***Secondary glaucoma and preoperatively:*** 5–10 mg/kg IM or IV q6h, or 10–15 mg/kg per day PO in divided doses q6–8.
- ***Epilepsy:*** 8–30 mg/kg per day in divided doses. When given with other antiepileptics, starting dose is 250 mg/d.

Pharmacokinetics
Metabolism: T$_{1/2}$: 2.5–6 h

Route	Onset	Peak	Duration
Oral	1 h	2–4 h	6–12 h
Sustained release	2 h	8–12 h	18–24 h
IV	1–2 min	15–18 min	4–5 h

Distribution: Crosses placenta; passes into breast milk
Excretion: Unchanged in the urine

IV facts
Preparation: Reconstitute 500-mg vial with 5 ml of Sterile Water for Injection; stable for 1 week if refrigerated, but use within 24 h is recommended.
Infusion: Administer over 1 min for single injection; administer in solution over 4–8 h.

Adverse effects
- CNS: Weakness, fatigue, nervousness, sedation, drowsiness, dizziness, depression, tremor, ataxia, headache, paresthesias, convulsions, flaccid paralysis, transient myopia
- GI: *Anorexia, nausea, vomiting, constipation,* melena, hepatic insufficiency
- Hematologic: Bone marrow depression
- GU: Hematuria, glycosuria, *urinary frequency,* renal colic, renal calculi, crystalluria, polyuria
- Dermatologic: Urticaria, pruritis, rash, photosensitivity, erythema multiforme (Stevens-Johnson syndrome)
- Other: Weight loss, fever, acidosis

Clinically important drug-drug interactions
- Decreased renal excretion of quinidine if taken with acetazolamide • Increased excretion of salicylates, lithium when taken with acetazolamide • Increased risk of salicylate toxicity due to metabolic acidosis with acetazolamide

Drug-lab test interferences
- False-positive results of tests for urinary protein

Nursing Considerations
Assessment
- *History:* Allergy to acetazolamide, antibacterial sulfonamides, or thiazides; chronic noncongestive angle-closure glaucoma; fluid or electrolyte imbalance; renal or hepatic disease; adrenocortical insufficiency; respiratory acidosis; COPD; lactation
- *Physical:* Skin—color, lesions; edema, weight, orientation, reflexes, muscle strength, intraocular pressure; respiratory rate, pattern, adventitious sounds; liver evaluation, bowel sounds, urinary output patterns; CBC, serum electrolytes, liver and renal function tests, urinalysis

Implementation
- Administer by direct IV administration if parenteral use is necessary; IM use is painful.
- Administer with food or milk if GI upset occurs.
- Use caution if giving with other drugs with excretion inhibited by urine alkalinization.
- Make oral liquid form by crushing tablets and suspending in cherry, chocolate, raspberry, or other sweet syrup, or one tablet may be submerged in 10 ml of hot water and added to 1 ml of honey or syrup; *do not use alcohol or glycerin* as a vehicle.
- Assure ready access to bathroom facilities when diuretic effect occurs.
- Establish safety precautions if CNS effects occur; protect patient from sun or bright lights if photophobia occurs.
- Obtain regular body weights to monitor fluid changes.
- Monitor serum electrolytes and acid–base balance during course of drug therapy.

Adverse effects in *Italics* are most common; those in **Bold** are life-threatening.

Drug-specific teaching points
- Take the drug with meals if GI upset occurs.
- Arrange to have intraocular pressure checked periodically while taking this drug.
- Weigh yourself on a regular basis, at the same time of the day and in the same clothing, and record the weight on your calendar.
- Know that the following side effects may occur: increased volume and frequency of urination (have ready access to a bathroom when drug effect is greatest); dizziness, feeling faint on arising, drowsiness, fatigue (do not engage in hazardous activities like driving a car); sensitivity to sunlight (use sunglasses, wear protective clothing, or use a sunscreen when out of doors); GI upset (taking the drug with meals, having small frequent meals may help).
- Report loss or gain of more than 3 lb in 1 day, unusual bleeding or bruising, sore throat, dizziness, trembling, numbness, fatigue, muscle weakness or cramps, flank or loin pain, rash.

▢ acetohexamide

*(a set oh **hex**' a mide)*
Dimelor (CAN), Dymelor

Pregnancy Category C

Drug classes
Antidiabetic agent
Sulfonylurea—first generation

Therapeutic actions
Stimulates insulin release from functioning beta cells in the pancreas; may improve binding between insulin and insulin receptors or increase number of insulin receptors and lower blood glucose; has significant uricosuric activity.

Indications
- Adjunct to diet to lower blood glucose in patients with non–insulin-dependent diabetes mellitus (type II)
- Adjunct to insulin therapy in the stabilization of certain cases of insulin-dependent, maturity-onset diabetes, reducing the insulin requirement and decreasing the chance of hypoglycemic reactions

Contraindications/cautions
- Contraindicated in the presence of allergy to sulfonylureas; conditions in which insulin is indicated to control blood sugar—diabetes complicated by fever, severe infections, severe trauma, major surgery, ketosis, acidosis, coma; type I or juvenile diabetes; serious hepatic or serious renal impairment; uremia, thyroid, or endocrine impairment; glycosuria; hyperglycemia associated with primary renal disease; pregnancy or lactation.

Dosage
Adult: 250 mg–1.5 g/d PO. Patients on 1 g or less daily can be controlled with once-daily dosage; if patients are on 1.5 g/d twice daily dosage, before morning and evening meals is appropriate; do not exceed 1.5 g/d.
Pediatric: Safety and efficacy not established.
Geriatric: Geriatric patients tend to be more sensitive to the drug; start with a lower initial dose, monitor for 24 h, and gradually increase dose as needed.

Pharmacokinetics

Route	Onset	Peak	Duration
PO	1 h	2–4 h	12–24 h

Metabolism: Hepatic; $T_{1/2}$: 6–8 h
Distribution: Enters breast milk
Excretion: Renal

Adverse effects
- **GI:** *Anorexia, nausea, vomiting, epigastric discomfort, heartburn*
- **Hematologic:** *Hypoglycemia*, leukopenia, thrombocytopenia, anemia
- **Dermatologic:** Allergic skin reactions, eczema, pruritus, erythema, urticaria, photosensitivity
- **Hypersensitivity:** Fever, eosinophilia, jaundice

Adverse effects in *Italics* are most common; those in **Bold** are life-threatening.

- Other: Possible increased risk of cardiovascular mortality

Clinically important drug-drug interactions
• Increased risk of hypoglycemia if acetohexamide is taken concurrently with insulin, sulfonamides, chloramphenicol, fenfluramine, oxyphenbutazone, phenylbutazone, salicylates, probenecid, monoamine oxidase inhibitors, clofibrate • Decreased effect of acetohexamide if taken with beta-adrenergic blocking agents (signs of hypoglycemia also may be blocked), rifampin • Decreased effectiveness of acetohexamide and diazoxide if taken concurrently • Increased risk of hyperglycemia if acetohexamide is taken with thiazides, other diuretics, phenytoin, nicotinic acid, sympathomimetics • Risk of hypoglycemia and hyperglycemia if acetohexamide is taken with ethanol; "disulfiram reaction" also has been reported

■ Nursing Considerations

Assessment
- *History:* Renal, hepatic, endocrine disorders
- *Physical:* Skin—color, lesions; body temperature; orientation, reflexes, peripheral sensation; R, adventitious sounds; liver evaluation, bowel sounds; urinalysis, BUN, serum creatinine, liver function tests, blood glucose, CBC

Implementation
- Administer drug in the morning before breakfast. If severe GI upset occurs or if dosage is 1.5 g/d, dose may be divided with one dose before breakfast and one before the evening meal.
- Monitor serum glucose levels frequently to determine effectiveness of drug.
- Arrange for transfer to insulin therapy during periods of high stress infections, surgery, trauma, etc.
- Arrange for use of IV glucose if severe hypoglycemia occurs as a result of overdose.

Drug-specific teaching points
- Take this drug early in the morning before breakfast. If the drug is to be taken two times a day, take it before breakfast and before the evening meal.
- Do not discontinue this medication without consulting physician.
- Do not take this drug during pregnancy; if you think you are pregnant, consult your physician.
- Monitor urine or blood for glucose and ketones as prescribed.
- Avoid the use of alcohol while on this drug; serious reactions could occur.
- Report fever, sore throat, unusual bleeding or bruising, skin rash, dark urine, light-colored stools, hypoglycemic or hyperglycemic reactions.

▢ acetohydroxamic acid

(a see' toe hye drox am ik)
AHA
Lithostat

Pregnancy Category X

Drug classes
Urinary tract agent

Therapeutic actions
Inhibits the bacterial enzyme urease, inhibiting the production of ammonia in the urine and lowering the pH of urine infected with urea-splitting organisms. This enhances the effectiveness of antibiotics and increases the cure rate of these infections, which are often accompanied by kidney stone formation.

Indications
- Adjunctive therapy in chronic urea-splitting urinary tract infections

Contraindications/cautions
- Allergy to acetohydroxamic acid, physical conditions that are amenable to surgery or antimicrobial treatment, poor renal function, pregnancy (teratogenic—do not use in pregnancy and recommend

the use of birth control methods while on this drug), lactation.

Dosage
Adult: 250 mg PO tid to qid for a total dose of 10–15 mg/kg per day; recommended starting dose is 12 mg/kg per day q6–8h; do not exceed 1.5 g/d.
Pediatric: Initial dose of 10 mg/kg per day PO; dose titration may be required by hematologic response.
Geriatric or renal impaired: Serum creatinine > 1.8 mg/dl; do not exceed 1 g/d with doses at 12-h intervals; do not administer to patients with serum creatinine > 2.5 mg/dl.

Pharmacokinetics

Route	Onset	Peak
PO	1 h	15–60 min

Metabolism: Hepatic; $T_{1/2}$: 5–10 h
Distribution: Crosses placenta, may enter breast milk
Excretion: Unchanged in the urine

Adverse effects
- **CNS:** *Headache, depression, anxiety, nervousness, malaise, tremulousness*
- **GI:** *Nausea, vomiting, anorexia*
- **CV:** Superficial phlebitis of lower extremities
- **Hematologic:** Coombs' negative hemolytic anemia
- **Dermatologic:** Nonpruritic, macular skin rash in the upper extremities and face (most common after ingestion of alcohol during long-term use), alopecia

Clinically important drug-drug interactions
- Rash if taken concurrently with alcohol
- Absorption of acetohydroxamic acid and iron decreased if the two are taken concurrently

■ Nursing Considerations

Assessment
- *History:* Allergy to acetohydroxamic acid, physical conditions that are amenable to surgery or antimicrobial treatment, poor renal function, pregnancy, lactation
- *Physical:* Skin—color, lesions; orientation, affect, reflexes; peripheral perfusion, veins in lower extremities; liver evaluation; CBC, liver and renal function tests

Implementation
- Arrange for culture and sensitivity tests of urine before beginning therapy; do not administer if urine is infected with nonurease-producing organisms.
- Ensure that patient is not pregnant and is not planning on becoming pregnant while on this drug. Advise the patient to use birth control measures during the course of drug therapy.
- Administer on an empty stomach—1 h before or 2 h after meals.
- Arrange for analgesics as necessary to relieve headache.

Drug-specific teaching points
- Take the drug on an empty stomach—1 h before or 2 h after meals.
- Know that the following side effects may occur: headache (analgesics may be ordered to help); nausea, vomiting, loss of appetite (small, frequent meals may help); skin rash (this is more common when alcohol is taken with this drug; avoid alcohol while taking this drug).
- Be aware that this drug causes birth defects and should not be taken if you are, or are trying to become, pregnant; use of birth control methods is highly recommended; if you think you are pregnant, consult your physician immediately.
- Report unusual bleeding or bruising; malaise, lethargy; leg pain or swelling of the lower leg; severe nausea and vomiting.

☐ acetophenazine maleate

(a set oh fen' a zeen)
Tindal

Pregnancy Category C

Drug classes
Phenothiazine (piperazine)
Dopaminergic blocking drug
Antipsychotic drug

Therapeutic actions
Mechanism of antipsychotic action not fully understood: antipsychotic drugs block dopamine receptors in the brain, depress the reticular activating system (including those parts of the brain involved with wakefulness and emesis), and are anticholinergic and act as antihistamines.

Indications
- Management of manifestations of psychotic disorders

Contraindications/cautions
- Contraindicated in the presence of coma or severe CNS depression, bone marrow depression, blood dyscrasia, circulatory collapse, subcortical brain damage, Parkinson's disease, liver damage, cerebral arteriosclerosis, coronary disease, severe hypotension or hypertension.
- Use caution in the presence of respiratory disorders ("silent pneumonia" may develop); glaucoma, prostatic hypertrophy; epilepsy or history of epilepsy; breast cancer; thyrotoxicosis; peptic ulcer, decreased renal function; myelography within previous 24 h or myelography scheduled within 48 h; exposure to heat or phosphorous insecticides; lactation; children < 12 y, especially those with chickenpox, CNS infections (children are especially susceptible to dystonias that may confound the diagnosis of Reye's syndrome).

Dosage
Full clinical effects may require 6 wk to 6 mo of therapy.
Adult: 20 mg tid PO; total dosage range is 40–80 mg/d.
- ***Hospitalized patients:*** 80–120 mg/d PO in divided doses (doses as high as 400–600 mg/d have been used).

Pediatric: Generally not recommended for children < 12 y.
Geriatric: Use lower doses, and increase dosage more gradually than in younger patients.

Pharmacokinetics

Route	Onset	Peak	Duration
PO	2–3 h	2–4 h	36–48 h

Metabolism: Hepatic; $T_{1/2}$: 10–20 h
Distribution: Crosses the placenta; enters breast milk
Excretion: 50% renal, 50% enterohepatic

Adverse effects
- **CNS:** *Drowsiness;* insomnia; vertigo; headache; weakness; tremor; ataxia; slurring; cerebral edema; seizures; exacerbation of psychotic symptoms; extrapyramidal syndromes—*pseudoparkinsonism, dystonias; akathisia;* tardive dyskinesias; potentially irreversible (no known treatment); neuroleptic malignant syndrome (rare but 20% fatal)
- **CV:** Hypotension, orthostatic hypotension, hypertension, tachycardia, bradycardia, cardiac arrest, CHF, cardiomegaly, refractory arrhythmias (some fatal), pulmonary edema
- **Respiratory:** Bronchospasm, laryngospasm, dyspnea; suppression of cough reflex and potential for aspiration
- **Hematologic:** Eosinophilia, leukopenia, leukocytosis, anemia; aplastic anemia; hemolytic anemia; thrombocytopenic or nonthrombocytopenic purpura; pancytopenia
- **Hypersensitivity:** Jaundice, urticaria, angioneurotic edema, laryngeal edema, photosensitivity, eczema, asthma, anaphylactoid reactions, exfoliative dermatitis
- **Endocrine:** Lactation, breast engorgement in females, galactorrhea; syndrome of inappropriate ADH secretion (SIADH); amenorrhea, menstrual irregularities; gynecomastia in males; changes in libido; hyperglycemia or hypoglycemia; glycosuria; hyponatremia; pituitary tumor with hyperprolactinemia; inhibition of ovulation, infertility, pseudopregnancy; reduced urinary levels of gonadotropins, estrogens, progestins
- **Autonomic:** Dry mouth, salivation, nasal congestion, nausea, vomiting, anorexia, fever, pallor, flushed facies, sweating, constipation, paralytic ileus, urinary retention, incontinence, polyuria, enuresis,

Adverse effects in *Italics* are most common; those in **Bold** are life-threatening.

priapism, ejaculation inhibition, male impotence

Clinically important drug-drug interactions

• Additive CNS depression with barbiturates, anesthetics, ethanol • Additive anticholinergic effects and possibly decreased antipsychotic efficacy with anticholinergic drugs • Decreased absorption of oral antipsychotic drugs when given with antidiarrheal mixtures, antacids • Decreased plasma levels of antipsychotic drugs, but severe neurotoxicity with lithium • Increased neurotoxicity of phenytoin given with acetophenazine • Decreased neuromuscular block with polypeptide antibiotics (bacitracin, capreomycin, colistimethate, polymyxin B) • Increased likelihood of seizures with metrizamide (contrast agent used in myelography) • Decreased antihypertensive effect of guanethidine when taken with acetophenazine

Drug-lab test interferences

• False-positive pregnancy tests (less likely if serum test is used) • Increase in protein-bound iodine not attributable to an increase in thyroxine

■ Nursing Considerations

Assessment

- *History:* Coma or severe CNS depression; bone marrow depression; blood dyscrasia; circulatory collapse; subcortical brain damage; Parkinson's disease; liver damage; cerebral arteriosclerosis; coronary disease; severe hypotension or hypertension; respiratory disorders; glaucoma, prostatic hypertrophy; history of epilepsy; breast cancer; thyrotoxicosis; peptic ulcer, decreased renal function; myelography within previous 24 h or myelography scheduled within 48 h; exposure to heat or phosphorous insecticides; lactation
- *Physical:* Body weight, temperature; reflexes, orientation, intraocular pressure; P, BP, orthostatic BP; R, adventitious sounds; bowel sounds and normal output, liver evaluation; urinary output, prostate size; CBC, urinalysis; thyroid, liver, and kidney function tests

Implementation

- Arrange for discontinuation of drug if serum creatinine, BUN become abnormal or if WBC count is depressed.
- Monitor bowel function, and arrange appropriate therapy for severe constipation; adynamic ileus with fatal complications has occurred.
- Monitor elderly patients for dehydration, and institute remedial measures promptly; sedation and decreased sensation of thirst related to CNS effects of drug can lead to dehydration.
- Consult physician regarding appropriate warning of patient or patient's guardian about tardive dyskinesias.
- Consult physician about dosage reduction, use of anticholinergic antiparkinsonian drugs (controversial) if extrapyramidal effects occur.

Drug-specific teaching points

- Take drug exactly as prescribed.
- Know that the following side effects may occur: drowsiness (avoid driving a car or engaging in other dangerous activities), sensitivity to the sun (avoid prolonged exposure to sun or use a sunscreen or covering garments), pink or reddish brown urine.
- Maintain fluid intake, and use precautions against heatstroke in hot weather; you may not feel thirsty. Urinate before taking your drug; you may experience difficulties urinating if you have prostrate problems.
- Report sore throat, fever, unusual bleeding or bruising, rash, weakness, tremors, impaired vision, dark urine, pale stools, yellowing of the skin or eyes.

⬜ acetylcysteine

*(a se teel **sis'** tay een)*

n-acetylcysteine

Airbron (CAN), Mucomyst, Mucosal

Pregnancy Category C

Adverse effects in *Italics* are most common; those in **Bold** are life-threatening.

Drug classes
Mucolytic agent
Antidote

Therapeutic actions
Mucolytic activity: splits links in the mucoproteins contained in respiratory mucus secretions, decreasing the viscosity of the mucus

Antidote to acetaminophen hepatotoxicity: protects liver cells by maintaining cell function and detoxifying acetaminophen metabolites

Indications
- Mucolytic adjuvant therapy for abnormal, viscid, or inspissated mucus secretions in acute and chronic bronchopulmonary disease (emphysema with bronchitis, asthmatic bronchitis, tuberculosis, pneumonia), in pulmonary complications of cystic fibrosis, and in tracheostomy care; pulmonary complications associated with surgery, anesthesia, posttraumatic chest conditions; diagnostic bronchial studies
- To prevent or lessen hepatic injury that may occur after ingestion of a potentially hepatotoxic dose of acetaminophen; treatment must start as soon as possible and in any case within 24 h of ingestion
- Unlabeled uses: as ophthalmic solution to treat keratoconjunctivitis sicca (dry eye); as an enema to treat bowel obstruction due to meconium ileus or its equivalent

Contraindications/cautions
- Mucolytic use: contraindicated in the presence of hypersensitivity to acetylcysteine; use caution and discontinue immediately if bronchospasm occurs.
- Antidotal use: there are no contraindications; use caution in the presence of esophageal varices, peptic ulcer.

Dosage
Mucolytic use
- **Nebulization with face mask, mouthpiece, tracheostomy:** 1–10 ml of 20% solution or 2–20 ml of 10% solution q2–6h; the dose for most patients is 3–5 ml of the 20% solution or 6–10 ml of the 10% solution tid–qid.
- **Nebulization with tent, croupette:** Very large volumes are required, occasionally up to 300 ml, during a treatment period. The dose is the volume or solution that will maintain a very heavy mist in the tent or croupette for the desired period. Administration for intermittent or continuous prolonged periods, including overnight, may be desirable.

Instillation
- **Direct or by tracheostomy:** 1–2 ml of a 10%–20% solution q1–4h; may be introduced into a particular segment of the bronchopulmonary tree by way of a plastic catheter (inserted under local anesthesia and with direct visualization). Instill 2–5 ml of the 20% solution by a syringe connected to the catheter.
- **Percutaneous intratracheal catheter:** 1–2 ml of the 20% solution or 2–4 ml of the 10% solution q1–4h by a syringe connected to the catheter.
- **Diagnostic bronchogram:** Before the procedure, give two to three administrations of 1–2 ml of the 20% solution or 2–4 ml of the 10% solution by nebulization or intratracheal instillation.

Antidotal use: For acetaminophen overdose, administer acetylcysteine immediately if 24 h or less have elapsed from time of acetaminophen ingestion, using the following protocol:

1. Empty the stomach by lavage or by inducing emesis with syrup of ipecac; repeat dose of ipecac if emesis does not occur in 20 min.
2. If activated charcoal has been administered by lavage, charcoal may adsorb acetylcysteine and reduce its effectiveness.
3. Draw blood for acetaminophen plasma assay and for baseline SGOT, SGPT, bilirubin, prothrombin time, creatinine, BUN, blood sugar, and electrolytes; if acetaminophen assay cannot be obtained or dose is clearly in the toxic range, give full course of acetylcysteine therapy; monitor hepatic and renal function, fluid and electrolyte balance.

4. Administer acetylcysteine PO 140 mg/kg loading dose.
5. Administer 17 maintenance doses of 70 mg/kg q4h, starting 4 h after loading dose; administer full course of doses unless acetaminophen assay reveals a nontoxic level.
6. If patient vomits loading or maintenance dose within 1 h of administration, repeat that dose.
7. If patient persistently vomits the oral dose, administer by duodenal intubation.
8. Repeat blood chemistry assays in number 3 above daily if acetaminophen plasma level is in toxic range.

Pharmacokinetics

Route	Onset	Peak	Duration
Oral	30–60 min	1–2 h	
Instillation/ Inhalation	1 min	5–10 min	2–3 h

Metabolism: Hepatic, $T_{1/2}$: 6.25 h
Excretion: Urine (30%)

Adverse effects

Lytic Use
- **GI:** *Nausea*, stomatitis
- **Respiratory:** Bronchospasm, especially in asthmatics
- **Hypersensitivity:** Urticaria
- **Other:** *Rhinorrhea*

Antidotal Use
- **GI:** *Nausea, vomiting, other GI symptoms*
- **Dermatologic:** Rash

■ Nursing Considerations

Assessment
- History

Mucolytic use: Hypersensitivity to acetylcysteine, asthma
Antidotal use: Esophageal varices, peptic ulcer

- **Physical:** Body weight, body temperature, skin—color, lesions; BP; P; R, adventitious sounds, bowel sounds, liver palpation

Implementation

Mucolytic Use
- Dilute the 20% acetylcysteine solution with either Normal Saline or Sterile Water for Injection; use the 10% solution undiluted. Refrigerate unused, undiluted solution, and use within 96 h.
- Be aware that drug solution in the opened bottle may change color, but this does not alter the drug's safety or efficacy.
- Administer the following drugs separately, because they are incompatible with acetylcysteine solutions: tetracyclines, erythromycin lactobionate, amphotericin B, iodized oil, chymotrypsin, trypsin, hydrogen peroxide.
- Use water to remove residual drug solution on the patient's face after administration by face mask.
- Inform patient that nebulization may produce an initial disagreeable odor, but it will soon disappear.
- Monitor nebulizer for buildup of drug from evaporation; dilute with Sterile Water for Injection to prevent concentrate from impeding nebulization and drug delivery.
- Establish routine for pulmonary toilet to eliminate secretions as efficiently as possible; have suction equipment on standby.

Antidotal Use
- Dilute the 20% acetylcysteine solution with cola drinks or other soft drinks to a final concentration of 5%; if administered by gastric tube or Miller-Abbott tube, water may be used as diluent. Dilution minimizes the risk of vomiting.
- Prepare fresh solutions, and use within 1 h; undiluted solution in opened vials may be kept for 96 h.
- Arrange to treat fluid and electrolyte imbalance, hypoglycemia as appropriate.
- Arrange to administer vitamin K_1 if prothrombin ratio exceeds 1.5; arrange to administer fresh-frozen plasma if prothrombin time ratio exceeds 3.
- Do not administer diuretics.

Adverse effects in *Italics* are most common; those in **Bold** are life-threatening.

Drug-specific teaching points
- Know the following side effects may occur: increased productive cough, nausea, GI upset.
- Report difficulty breathing or nausea.

☐ acyclovir

(ay sye' kloe ver)
acyclovir sodium, acycloguanosine

Zovirax

Pregnancy Category C

Drug classes
Antiviral drug

Therapeutic actions
Antiviral activity; inhibits viral DNA replication

Indications
- Initial and recurrent mucosal and cutaneous herpes simplex virus (HSV) 1 and 2 infections in immunocompromised patients
- Severe initial and recurrent genital herpes infections in selected patients
- Ointment: initial HSV genital infections; limited mucocutaneous HSV infections in immunocompromised patients
- Unlabeled uses: treatment of herpes zoster, cytomegalovirus and HSV infection following transplant, herpes simplex infections, infectious mononucleosis, varicella pneumonia, varicella zoster in immunocompromised patients

Contraindications/cautions
- Allergy to acyclovir, seizures, CHF, renal disease, lactation.

Dosage
Adult
- ***Parenteral:*** 5 mg/kg infused IV over 1 h, q8h (15 mg/kg per day) for 7 d
- ***Oral***
- – *Initial genital herpes:* 200 mg q4h while awake (1,000 mg/d) for 10 d.
- – *Chronic suppressive therapy:* 400 mg bid for up to 12 mo.

Pediatric
- ***Parenteral:*** < *12 y:* 250 mg/m^2 infused IV over 1 h, every 8 h (750 mg/m^2 per day) for 7 d. > *12 y:* adult dosage.
- ***Oral:*** Safety not established.

Geriatric or renal impaired
- ***Oral:*** Creatinine clearance < 10 ml/min: 200 mg q12h
- ***IV***

Creatine clearance (ml/min)	Dosage (IV)
>50	5 mg/kg q8h
25–50	5 mg/kg q12h
10–25	5 mg/kg qd
0–10	2.5 mg/kg qd

Topical
- ***Ointment (all ages):*** Apply sufficient quantity to cover all lesions six times per day for 7 d; 1.25 cm (½ in) ribbon of ointment covers 2.5 cm^2 (4 in^2) surface area q3h.

Pharmacokinetics

Route	Onset	Peak	Duration
Oral	Varies	1.5–2 h	
IV	Immediate	1 h	8 h

Metabolism: T$_{1/2}$: 2.5–5 h
Distribution: Crosses placenta; passes into breast milk
Excretion: Unchanged in urine

IV facts
Preparation: Reconstitute drug in 10 ml Sterile Water for Injection or Bacteriostatic Water for Injection containing benzyl alcohol; concentration will be 50 mg/ml. Do *not* dilute drug with bacteriostatic water containing parabens. Use reconstituted solution within 12 h; dilute IV drug solution to concentration of 7 mg/ml or less. Do not use biologic or colloidal fluids, such as blood products or protein solutions.

Infusion: Administer by slow IV infusion of parenteral solutions; avoid bolus or rapid injection. Infuse over 1 h to avoid renal damage. Warm drug to room temperature to dissolve precipitates formed during refrigeration.

Adverse effects
Systemic Administration
- CNS: Headache, vertigo, depression, tremors, encephalopathic changes
- GI: *Nausea, vomiting,* diarrhea, anorexia
- GU: Crystalluria with rapid IV administration, hematuria
- Dermatologic: *Inflammation or phlebitis at injection sites,* rash, hair loss

Topical Administration
- Dermatologic: *Transient burning at site of application*

Clinically important drug-drug interactions
Systemic Administration
- Increased acyclovir effects if taken with probenecid • Increased nephrotoxicity with other nephrotoxic drugs • Extreme drowsiness if taken with zidovudine

■ Nursing Considerations

Assessment
- *History:* Allergy to acyclovir, seizures, CHF, renal disease, lactation
- *Physical:* Skin color, lesions; orientation; BP, P, auscultation, perfusion, edema; R, adventitious sounds; urinary output; BUN, creatinine clearance

Implementation
Systemic Administration
- Ensure that the patient is well hydrated during drug use.

Topical Administration
- Start treatment as soon as possible after onset of signs and symptoms.
- Wear a rubber glove or finger cot when applying drug.

Drug-specific teaching points
Systemic Administration
- Complete the full course of oral therapy, and do *not* exceed the prescribed dose.
- Oral acyclovir is *not* a cure for your disease but should make you feel better.
- Know that the following side effects may occur: nausea, vomiting, loss of appetite, diarrhea; headache, dizziness.
- Avoid sexual intercourse while visible lesions are present.
- Report difficulty urinating, skin rash, increased severity or frequency of recurrences.

Topical Administration
- Wear rubber gloves or finger cots when applying the drug to prevent autoinoculation of other sites and transmission of the disease to other people.
- Know that this drug does not cure the disease; application of the drug during symptom-free periods will not prevent recurrences.
- Avoid sexual intercourse while visible lesions are present.
- Know that this drug may cause burning, stinging, itching, rash; notify your physician if these are pronounced.

☐ adenosine

(a **den**' oh seen)
Adenocard

Pregnancy Category C

Drug classes
Antiarrhythmic

Therapeutic actions
Slows conduction through the AV node; can interrupt the reentry pathways through the AV node and restore sinus rhythm in patients with paroxysmal supraventricular tachycardias

Indications
- Conversion to sinus rhythm of paroxysmal supraventricular tachycardia, including that associated with accessory bypass tracts (Wolff-Parkinson-White Syndrome), after attempting vagal maneuvers when appropriate.
- Unlabeled use: assessment of patients with suspected coronary artery disease in conjuction with thallium tomography
- Orphan drug use: treatment of brain tumors in conjunction with BCNU

Adverse effects in *Italics* are most common; those in **Bold** are life-threatening.

Contraindications/cautions
- Contraindicated in the presence of hypersensitivity to adenosine; second- or third-degree AV heart block, sick sinus syndrome (unless artificial pacemake in place); atrial flutter, atrial fibrillation, ventricular tachycardia.
- Use caution in the presence of asthma (could produce bronchospasm in asthma patients).

Dosage
For rapid bolus IV use only.
Adult:
- ***Initial dose:*** 6 mg as a rapid IV bolus administered over 1–2 sec.
- ***Repeat administration:*** 12 mg as a rapid IV bolus if initial dose does not produce elimination of the supraventricular tachycardia within 1–2 min. 12-mg bolus may be repeated a second time if needed. Doses > 12 mg are not recommended.

Pediatric: Not recommended.

Pharmacokinetics

Route	Onset	Peak	Duration
IV	Immediate	10 sec	20–30 sec

Metabolism: Hepatic; $T_{1/2}$: > 10 sec
Distribution: Rapidly picked up by red blood cells

IV facts
Preparation: Store drug at room temperature; do not refrigerate. Solution must be clear at time of use; discard any unused portion of vial.
Infusion: By rapid IV bolus only, given over 1–2 sec; administer directly into a vein or as proximal as possible; follow with a rapid saline flush.

Adverse effects
- CNS: *Headache, lightheadedness,* dizziness, tingling in arms, numbness, apprehension, blurred vision, burning sensation, heaviness in arms, neck and back pain
- GI: *Nausea,* metallic taste, tightness in throat, pressure in groin
- CV: *Facial flushing, arrhythmias,* sweating, palpitations, chest pain, hypotension
- Respiratory: *Shortness of breath/dyspnea, chest pressure,* hyperventilation

Clinically important drug-drug interactions
- Increased degree of heart block if taken with carbamazepine • Increased effects of adenosine if taken with dipyridamole • Decreased effects of adenosine if taken with methylxanthines (caffeine, theophylline), which antagonize adenosine's activity

■ Nursing Considerations

Assessment
- *History:* Hypersensitivity to adenosine, second- or third-degree AV heart block, sick sinus syndrome, atrial flutter, atrial fibrillation, ventricular tachycardia, asthma (use caution), adenosine
- *Physical:* orientation, BP, P, auscultation, ECG, R, adventitious sounds

Implementation
- Assess asthma patients carefully for signs of exacerbation of asthma.
- Monitor patient's ECG continually during administration. Be alert for the possibility of arrhythmias. These usually last only a few seconds.
- Maintain emergency equipment on standby at time of administration.
- Have methylxanthines available as antagonists if problems occur.

Drug-specific teaching points
- Know that the following side effects may occur: rapid or irregular heartbeat (this usually passes quickly), facial flushing, headache, lightheadedness, dizziness, nausea, shortness of breath (tell the patient to alert the nurse or physician if he or she becomes uncomfortable, so appropriate measures can be taken).
- Report chest pain, difficulty breathing, numbness, tingling.

Adverse effects in *Italics* are most common; those in **Bold** are life-threatening.

☐ albumin, human

(al byoo' min)
normal serum albumin

5%: *Albuminar-5, Albutein 5%, Buminate 5%, Plasbumin-5*

25%: *Albuminar-25, Albutein 25%, Buminate 25%, Plasbumin-25*

Pregnancy Category C

Drug classes
Blood product
Plasma protein

Therapeutic actions
Normal blood protein; maintains plasma osmotic pressure and is important in maintaining normal blood volume

Indications
- Supportive treatment of shock due to burns, trauma, surgery, and infections
- Burns: albumin 5% used to prevent hemoconcentration and water and protein losses in conjunction with adequate infusions of crystalloid
- Hypoproteinemia in nephrotic syndrome, hepatic cirrhosis, toxemia of pregnancy, postoperative patients, tuberculous patients, premature infants
- Adult respiratory distress syndrome: albumin 25% with a diuretic may be helpful.
- Cardiopulmonary bypass: preoperative blood dilution with 25% albumin
- Acute liver failure
- Sequestration of protein-rich fluids
- Erythrocyte resuspension: albumin 25% may be added to the isotonic suspension of washed red cells immediately before transfusion.
- Acute nephrosis: albumin 25% and loop diuretic may help to control edema.
- Renal dialysis: albumin 25% may be useful in treatment of shock and hypotension
- Hyperbilirubinemia and erythroblastosis fetalis: adjunct in exchange transfusions

Contraindications/cautions
- Contraindicated in the presence of allergy to albumin; severe anemia, cardiac failure, normal or increased intravascular volume, current use of cardiopulmonary bypass.
- Use caution in the presence of hepatic or renal failure.

Dosage
Administer by IV infusion only; contains 130–160 mEq sodium/L.

Adult
- ***Hypovolemic shock:* 5% albumin**: Initial dose of 500 ml given as rapidly as possible; additional 500 ml may be given in 30 min. Base therapy on clinical response if more than 1,000 ml is required; consider the need for whole blood. In patients with low blood volume, administer at rate of 2–4 ml/min. **25% albumin:** Base therapy on clinical response. Administer as rapidly as tolerated; 1 ml/min may be given to patients with low blood volume.
- ***Hypoproteinemia:*** 5% albumin may be given for acute replacement of protein; if edema is present, use 25% albumin 50–75 g/d. Do not exceed 2 ml/min. Adjust the rate of infusion based on patient response.
- ***Burns:*** 5% or 25% albumin can be helpful in maintaining colloid osmotic pressure; suggested regimen has not been established.
- ***Hepatic cirrhosis:*** 25% may be effective in temporary restoration of plasma protein levels.
- ***Nephrosis:*** Initial dose of 100–200 ml of 25% albumin may be repeated at intervals of 1–2 d; effects are not sustained because of the underlying problem.

Pediatric
- ***Hypovolemic shock:*** 50 ml of 5% albumin; base dosage on clinical response.
- ***Hypoproteinemia:*** 25 g/d of 25% albumin.
- ***Hyperbilirubinemia and erythroblastosis fetalis:*** 1 g/kg 1–2 h before transfusion, or 50 ml of albumin may be substituted for 50 ml of plasma in the blood to be transfused.

Pharmacokinetics
Metabolism: Tissue, $T_{1/2}$: unknown
Distribution: Crosses placenta; passes into breast milk
Excretion: Urine

IV facts
Preparation: Swab stopper top immediately before removing seal with suitable antiseptic prior to entering the vial. Inspect for any particulate matter and discoloration. Store at room temperature; do not freeze. Do not dilute 5% albumin; 25% albumin may be undiluted or diluted in Normal Saline.

Infusion: Give by IV infusion; infuse slow enough to prevent rapid plasma volume expansion. Administer in combination with or through the same administration set as the usual IV solutions of saline or carbohydrates. Do not use with alcohol or protein hydrolysates—precipitates may form.

Adverse effects
- CV: Hypotension, CHF, **pulmonary edema after rapid infusion**
- Hypersensitivity reactions: Fever, chills, *changes in blood pressure*, flushing, nausea, vomiting, changes in respiration, rashes

■ Nursing Considerations
Assessment
- *History:* Allergy to albumin, severe anemia, CHF, current use of cardiopulmonary bypass, hepatic failure, renal failure
- *Physical:* Skin—color, lesions; body temperature; P, BP, peripheral perfusion; R, adventitious sounds; liver and renal function tests, hematocrit, serum electrolytes

Implementation
- Administer without regard to blood group or type.
- Consider the need for whole blood, based on the patient's clinical condition; this infusion only provides symptomatic relief of the patient's hypoproteinemia.
- Monitor blood pressure during infusion; discontinue if hypotension occurs.
- Stop infusion if headache, flushing, fever, changes in blood pressure occur; arrange to treat reaction with antihistamines. If a plasma protein is still needed, try material from a different lot number.
- Monitor patient's clinical response, and adjust infusion rate accordingly.

Drug-specific teaching points
- Report headache; nausea, vomiting; difficulty breathing; back pain.

❒ albuterol

(al byoo' ter ole)
albuterol sulfate

Salbutamol (CAN), Gen-Salbutamol Sterinebs (CAN), Novo-Salmol (CAN), Proventil, Ventodisk (CAN), Ventolin, Volmax (CAN)

Pregnancy Category C

Drug classes
Sympathomimetic drug
Beta-2 selective adrenergic agonist
Bronchodilator
Antiasthmatic drug

Therapeutic actions
In low doses, acts relatively selectively at β_2-adrenergic receptors to cause bronchodilation and vasodilation; at higher doses, β_2-selectivity is lost, and the drug acts at β_1 receptors to cause typical sympathomimetic cardiac effects.

Indications
- Relief of bronchospasm in patients with reversible obstructive airway disease
- Prevention of exercise-induced bronchospasm
- Unlabeled use: adjunct in treating serious hyperkalemia in dialysis patients; seems to lower potassium concentrations when inhaled by patients on hemodialysis

Contraindications/cautions
- Contraindicated in the presence of hypersensitivity to albuterol; tachyarrhythmias,

Adverse effects in *Italics* are most common; those in **Bold** are life-threatening.

74 ■ albuterol

tachycardia caused by digitalis intoxication; general anesthesia with halogenated hydrocarbons or cyclopropane (these sensitize the myocardium to catecholamines); unstable vasomotor system disorders; hypertension; coronary insufficiency, coronary artery disease; history of stroke; COPD patients who have developed degenerative heart disease.
- Use caution in the presence of diabetes mellitus (large IV doses can aggravate diabetes and ketoacidosis); hyperthyroidism; history of seizure disorders; psychoneurotic individuals; labor and delivery (oral use has delayed second stage of labor; parenteral use of β_2-adrenergic agonists can accelerate fetal heart beat and cause hypoglycemia, hypokalemia, pulmonary edema in the mother and hypoglycemia in the neonate); lactation.

Dosage
Adult
- ***Oral:*** Initially, 2 or 4 mg (1–2 tsp syrup) tid–qid PO; may cautiously increase dosage if necessary to 4 or 8 mg qid, not to exceed 32 mg/d.
- ***Inhalation:*** Each actuation of aerosol dispenser delivers 90 μg albuterol. 2 inhalations q4–6h; some patients may require only 1 inhalation q4h; more frequent administration or larger number of inhalations not recommended.
- ***Prevention of exercise-induced bronchospasm:*** 2 inhalations 15 min prior to exercise.

Pediatric
- **Oral, tablets**
- *12 years or older:* Same as adult.
- **Oral, syrup**
- *> 14 y:* Same as adult.
- *6–14 y:* 2 mg (1 tsp) tid–qid; if necessary, cautiously increase dosage. Do not exceed 24 mg/d in divided doses.
- *2–6 y:* Initially, 0.1 mg/kg tid, not to exceed 2 mg (1 tsp) tid; if necessary, cautiously increase dosage stepwise to 0.2 mg/kg tid. Do not exceed 4 mg (2 tsp) tid.
- *< 2 y:* Safety and efficacy not established.

- ***Inhalation***
- *12 y or older:* Same as adult.
- *< 12 y:* Safety and efficacy not established.

Geriatric and patients sensitive to β-adrenergic stimulation: Restrict initial dose to 2 mg tid–qid; individualize dosage thereafter. Patients > 60 y are more likely to develop adverse effects.

Pharmacokinetics

Route	Onset	Peak	Duration
Oral	30 min	2–2½ h	4–8 h
Inhalation	5 min	1½–2 h	3–8 h

Metabolism: Hepatic, $T_{1/2}$: 2–4 h
Distribution: Crosses placenta; passes into breast milk
Excretion: Urine

Adverse effects
- CNS: *Restlessness, apprehension, anxiety, fear, CNS stimulation*, hyperkinesia, insomnia, tremor, drowsiness, irritability, weakness, vertigo, headache
- GI: *Nausea*, vomiting, heartburn, unusual or bad taste
- CV: *Cardiac arrhythmias*, tachycardia, palpitations, PVCs (rare), anginal pain
- Respiratory: Respiratory difficulties, pulmonary edema, coughing, bronchospasm, paradoxical airway resistance with repeated, excessive use of inhalation preparations
- GU: Increased incidence of leiomyomas of uterus when given in higher than human doses in preclinical studies
- Dermatologic: *Sweating, pallor, flushing*

Clinically important drug-drug interactions
- Increased sympathomimetic effects when given with other sympathomimetic drugs
- Increased risk of toxicity, especially cardiac, when used in combination with theophylline, aminophylline, oxtriphylline
- Decreased bronchodilating effects when given with beta-adrenergic blockers (eg, propranolol)
- Decreased effectiveness of insulin, oral hypoglycemic drugs when

Adverse effects in *Italics* are most common; those in **Bold** are life-threatening.

given with albuterol • Decreased serum levels and therapeutic effects of digoxin when given with albuterol

■ Nursing Considerations

Assessment
- *History:* Hypersensitivity to albuterol; tachyarrhythmias, tachycardia caused by digitalis intoxication; general anesthesia with halogenated hydrocarbons or cyclopropane; unstable vasomotor system disorders; hypertension; coronary insufficiency, coronary artery disease; history of stroke; COPD patients who have developed degenerative heart disease; diabetes mellitus; hyperthyroidism; history of seizure disorders; psychoneurotic individuals; lactation.
- *Physical:* Body weight; skin—color, temperature, turgor; orientation, reflexes, affect; P, BP; respiratory rate, adventitious sounds; blood and urine glucose, serum electrolytes, thyroid function tests, ECG

Implementation
- Use minimal doses for minimal periods of time; drug tolerance can occur with prolonged use.
- Maintain a beta-adrenergic blocker (a cardioselective beta-blocker, such as atenolol, should be used in patients with respiratory distress) on standby in case cardiac arrhythmias occur.
- Do not exceed recommended dosage of inhalation products; administer pressurized inhalation drug forms during second half of inspiration, because the airways are open wider, and the aerosol distribution is more extensive.

Drug-specific teaching points
- Do not exceed recommended dosage; adverse effects or loss of effectiveness may result. Read the instructions that come with the product (respiratory inhalant products).
- Know that the following may occur as a result of drug therapy: dizziness, drowsiness, fatigue, headache (use caution if driving or performing tasks that require alertness if these effects occur); nausea, vomiting, change in taste (small, frequent meals may help); rapid heart rate, anxiety, sweating, flushing.
- Report chest pain, dizziness, insomnia, weakness, tremors or irregular heart beat, difficulty breathing, productive cough, failure to respond to usual dosage.

❒ aldesleukin

(al des loo' ken)
Interleukin-2, IL-2, Proleukin

Pregnancy Category C

Drug classes
Antineoplastic

Therapeutic actions
Human interleukin produced by *Escherichia coli* bacteria; activates human cellular immunity and inhibits tumor growth through increases in lymphocytes, platelets, and cytokines (tumor necrosis factor and interferon)

Indications
- Metastatic renal cell carcinoma in adults
- Unlabeled uses: treatment of Kaposi's sarcoma with zidovudine; treatment of metastatic melanoma with cyclophosphamide; treatment of non-Hodgkin's lymphoma with lymphokine-actived killer cells; treatment of phase I AIDS, advanced ARC with zidovudine

Contraindications/cautions
- Contraindicated in the presence of hypersensitivity to aldesleukin; abnormal thallium stress test; abnormal pulmonary function test; organ allografts; lactation.
- Use caution in the presence of renal, liver, or CNS impairment.

Dosage
Adult: Administer by 15 min IV infusion q8h.
- ***Metastatic renal cell carcinoma:*** Each course of treatment consists of two 5-d cycles of 600,000 IU/kg q8h IV over 15 min, separated by a rest, for a total of 14 doses, then 9 d of rest followed by

14 more doses. Treatment may be stopped because of toxicity.
Pediatric: Safety not established.

Pharmacokinetics

Route	Onset	Peak	Duration
IV	5 min	13 min	180–240 min

Metabolism: Renal, T$_{1/2}$: 85 min
Distribution: Crosses placenta; passes into breast milk
Excretion: Urine

IV facts
Preparation: Reconstitute each vial (22 million IU) with 1.2 ml Sterile Water for Injection, USP; direct the Sterile Water at the side of the vial, and swirl contents gently to avoid excess foaming; do not shake. Resultant liquid should be clear, colorless to yellow, and contain 18 million IU/ml. Use plastic, not glass, containers, and avoid in-filters while administering. Dilute in 50 ml of 5% Dextrose Injection, USP. Avoid dilution in bacteriostatic water or 0.9% Sodium Chloride Injection; aggregation can occur. Do not dilute with albumin; do not mix with any other drugs. Store vials in refrigerator before and after reconstitution; do not freeze. Administer within 48 h after reconstitution; discard any unused portions.
Infusion: Bring solution to room temperature before use; infuse over 15 min.

Adverse effects
- CNS: *Mental status changes, dizziness,* sensory dysfunction, syncope, headache, conjunctivitis
- GI: *Nausea, vomiting, diarrhea, stomatitis, anorexia,* **GI bleed**
- CV: **Capillary leak syndrome**—third spacing of fluids and severe hypotension, which may proceed to shock and death; *hypotension, sinus tachycardia, arrhythmias*
- Respiratory: *Respiratory difficulties, dyspnea,* pulmonary edema, coughing, bronchospasm
- Hematologic: *Anemia, thrombocytopenia, leukopenia,* coagulation disorders
- GU: *Oliguria/anuria,* proteinuria, hematuria
- Dermatologic: *Pruritus, erythema, rash,* dry skin, exudative dermatitis
- General: *Fever, chills, pain, fatigue, weakness, malaise, edema, infection*

Clinically important drug-drug interactions
- Increased hypotensive effects if taken with antihypertensives • Decreased effectiveness of aldesleukin if taken with corticosteroids • Increased toxicity of cardiotoxic, hepatotoxic, myelotoxic, and nephrotoxic agents: doxorubicin, methotrexate, asparaginase, aminoglycosides, indomethacin

■ Nursing Considerations
Assessment
- *History:* Hypersensitivity to aldesleukin; abnormal thallium stress test; abnormal pulmonary function test; organ allografts; lactation; renal, liver, or CNS impairment
- *Physical:* Body weight; skin—color, temperature, turgor; orientation, reflexes, affect; P, BP; rate, adventitious sounds; bowel sounds; CBC, serum electrolytes, thyroid, liver and renal function tests; ECG, stress test, pulmonary function tests

Implementation
- Aldesluekin should be given only in intensive care settings with emergency life support immediately available.
- Ensure that patient has normal thallium stress test and normal pulmonary function tests, including baseline blood gases, before giving drug.
- Monitor patient, watching vital signs, weight, cardiac monitoring (if blood pressure falls), respiratory sounds, and pulse oximetry; cardiac sounds and perfusion evaluation; orientation.
- Advise patient to use birth control methods during drug use; if nursing a baby, help patient select another method of feeding the baby.

Adverse effects in *Italics* are most common; those in **Bold** are life-threatening.

- Monitor patient for signs of infection; advise patient to avoid any situations that would involve exposure to many people or to contagious diseases.
- Arrange to hold drug dosage if patient becomes disoriented, somnolent or very lethargic; continued use could result in a coma.
- Arrange to discontinue drug if severe side effects occur; drug may often be restarted if a period of rest returns systems affected to normal.

Drug-specific teaching points

- Be aware that this drug is given in 5-d cycles with a period of rest (9 wk) to allow the body to recover. This drug can only be given IV, and you will need to be closely monitored while it is given.
- Know that you will need to have many tests to evaluate the effects of this drug and the advisability of continuing treatment.
- Avoid situations that might expose you to any infections or contagious diseases while you are on this drug (eg, crowds); you will be more susceptible to infection.
- Know that the following side effects may occur: fever, chills, rash, fluid retention, difficulty breathing, nausea, vomiting, diarrhea.
- Report chest pain, dizziness, weakness, irregular heart beat, difficulty breathing, swelling, fever, malaise, fatigue, changes in stool or urine color.

☐ alglucerase

(al gloo' sir ace)
Ceredase

Pregnancy Category C

Drug classes
Enzyme

Therapeutic actions
Modified form of a naturally occurring human enzyme that is essential for the breakdown of glucocerebroside, a breakdown product of membrane lipids.

Indications
- Long-term enzyme replacement therapy for patients with type 1 Gaucher's disease who have moderate-to-severe anemia, thrombocytopenia, bone disease, hepatomegaly, splenomegaly

Contraindications/cautions
- Contraindicated in the presence of hypersensitivity to alglucerase.
- Use caution during lactation.

Dosage
Adult: Administer by IV infusion over 1–2 h. Initial dosage of 60 U/kg per infusion, repeated every 2–4 wk depending on patient response. Dosage may be lowered every 3–6 mo.
Pediatric: Safety and efficacy not established.

Pharmacokinetics

Route	Onset	Peak	Duration
IV	3–5 min	10–15 min	60 min

Metabolism: $T_{1/2}$: 3–10 min

IV facts
Preparation: Dilute dose of alglucerase with normal saline to a final volume not to exceed 100 ml. Do not shake; shaking may render the drug inactive. Refrigerate; do not use any bottle with particulate matter or discoloration, and do not use after expiration date. Discard any unused portion.
Infusion: Infuse over 1–2 h; use an in-line particulate filter.

Adverse effects
- CNS: Fever, chills
- GI: Nausea, vomiting, abdominal discomfort
- Local: Discomfort, swelling, burning and swelling at venipuncture site

■ Nursing Considerations
Assessment
- *History:* Sensitivity to alglucerase, lactation
- *Physical:* Venipuncture site, abdominal exam, CBC, bone density evaluation

Adverse effects in *Italics* are most common; those in **Bold** are life-threatening.

allopurinol

Implementation
- Explain possible risk of viral infection when using blood products. Assure patient that side effects are usually transient.
- Monitor patient response to drug to help establish most convenient and effective treatment schedule.
- Monitor IV site for signs of irritation.

Drug-specific teaching points
- Drug must be given IV, and the schedule for receiving it will be determined by response and convenience to the patient; drug replaces an enzyme that is missing in your body and will need to be taken long-term.
- Know that the following side effects may occur: abdominal discomfort, nausea, vomiting, discomfort at injection site.
- Report swelling, burning at injection site.

☐ allopurinol

*(al oh **pure'** i nole)*

Apo-Allopurinol (CAN), Lopurin, Purinol (CAN), Zyloprim

Pregnancy Category C

Drug classes
Antigout drug

Therapeutic actions
Inhibits the enzyme responsible for the conversion of purines to uric acid, thus reducing the production of uric acid with a decrease in serum and sometimes in urinary uric acid levels, relieving the signs and symptoms of gout

Indications
- Management of the signs and symptoms of primary and secondary gout
- Management of patients with malignancies that result in elevations of serum and urinary uric acid
- Management of patients with recurrent calcium oxalate calculi whose daily uric acid excretion exceeds 800 mg/d (males) or 750 mg/d (females)
- Orphan drug use: treatment of Chagas' disease; cutaneous and visceral leishmaniasis

Contraindications/cautions
- Contraindicated in the presence of allergy to allopurinol, blood dyscrasias.
- Use caution in the presence of liver disease, renal failure, lactation.

Dosage
Adult
- ***Gout and hyperuricemia:*** 100–800 mg/d PO in divided doses, depending on the severity of the disease (200–300 mg/d is usual dose). *Maintenance:* Establish dose that maintains serum uric acid levels within normal limits.
- ***Prevention of acute gouty attacks:*** 100 mg/d PO; increase the dose by 100 mg at weekly intervals until uric acid levels are within normal limits.
- ***Prevention of uric acid nephropathy in certain malignancies:*** 600–800 mg/d for 2–3 d; maintenance dose should then be established as above.
- ***Recurrent calcium oxalate stones:*** 200–300 mg/d PO; adjust dose up or down based on 24-h urinary urate determinations.

Pediatric
- ***Secondary hyperuricemia associated with various malignancies:*** *6–10 y:* 300 mg/d PO. *< 6 y:* 150 mg/d; adjust dosage after 48 h of treatment based on serum uric acid levels.

Geriatric or renal impaired

Creatine Clearance	Dosage
10–20 ml/min	200 mg/d
<10 ml/min	100 mg/d
<3 ml/min	Intervals between doses will need to be extended, based on patient's serum uric acid levels

Adverse effects
- CNS: *Headache, drowsiness,* peripheral neuropathy, neuritis, paresthesias

Adverse effects in *Italics* are most common; those in **Bold** are life-threatening.

- **GI:** *Nausea, vomiting, diarrhea,* abdominal pain, gastritis, hepatomegaly, hyperbilirubinemia, cholestatic jaundice
- **Hematologic:** Anemia, leukopenia, agranulocytosis, thrombocytopenia, aplastic anemia, bone marrow depression
- **GU:** Exacerbation of gout and renal calculi, renal failure
- **Dermatologic: Rashes**—*maculopapular*, scaly or exfoliative—sometimes fatal

Clinically important drug-drug interactions
- Increased risk of hypersensitivity reaction if taken with ACE inhibitors • Increased toxicity if used with thiazide diuretics • Increased risk of skin rash if used with ampicillin, amoxicillin • Increased risk of bone marrow suppression if used with cyclophosphamide, other cytotoxic agents • Increased half-life of chlorpropramide, oral anticoagulants if taken with allopurinol • Increased serum levels of theophylline, 6-MP, azathioprine, dose of 6-MP (azathioprine should be reduced to one-third to one-fourth the usual dose)

Nursing Considerations
Assessment
- *History:* Allergy to allopurinol, blood dyscrasias, liver disease, renal failure, lactation
- *Physical:* Skin—lesions, color; orientation, reflexes; liver evaluation, normal output; normal output; CBC, renal and liver function tests, urinalysis

Implementation
- Administer drug following meals.
- Force fluids—2.5 to 3.0 L/d to decrease the risk of renal stone development.
- Check urine alkalinity—urates crystallize in acid urine; sodium bicarbonate or potassium citrate may be ordered to alkalinize urine.
- Arrange for regular medical follow-up and blood tests during the course of therapy.

Drug-specific teaching points
- Take the drug following meals.
- Know that the following side effects may occur: exacerbation of gouty attack or renal stones (drink plenty of fluids while on this drug, 2.5–3 L/d); nausea, vomiting, loss of appetite (taking the drug following meals or small frequent meals may help); drowsiness (use caution while driving or performing potentially hazardous tasks).
- Avoid OTC medications while you are taking this drug. Many of these preparations contain vitamin C or other agents that might increase the likelihood of kidney stone formation. If you feel you need one of these preparations, check with your nurse or physician.
- Report skin rash; unusual bleeding or bruising; fever, chills; gout attack; numbness or tingling; flank pain.

☐ alpha₁-proteinase inhibitor (human)

alpha₁-PL, Prolastin

Pregnancy Category C

Drug classes
Blood product

Therapeutic actions
A human enzyme, which inhibits neutrophil elastase, an enzyme that degrades the elastin tissue essential for maintaining lung integrity; failure to replace the enzyme in deficient patients results in slowly progressive, severe, panacinar emphysema.

Indications
- Congenital alpha₁-antitrypsin deficiency; chronic replacement in adults with early evidence of panacinar emphysema.

Contraindications/cautions
- CHF (risk of circulatory overload), hepatitis

Dosage
Adult: 60 mg/kg IV once a week to increase and maintain a level of functional alpha₁-proteinase inhibitor in the lower respiratory tract.
Pediatric: Safety and efficacy not established.

80 ■ alprazolam

IV facts
Preparation: Reconstitute with provided solution; administer within 3 h of reconstitution. Refrigerate, but avoid freezing; do not refrigerate after reconstitution. May reconstitute with Normal Saline if necessary.
Infusion: Administer alone; do not mix with other agents or diluting solutions. May be given at a rate of 0.08 ml/kg per minute or greater.

Body Weight (lb/kg)	Dosage (mg)	IV Rate (ml/min)
75/34	2,040	2.7
90/41	2,460	3.3
105/48	2,880	3.8
120/55	3,300	4.4
135/61	3,660	4.9
150/68	4,080	5.5
165/75	4,500	6.0
180/82	4,920	6.5
195/89	5,340	7.1
210/96	5,760	7.6
225/102	6,120	8.2
240/109	6,540	8.7

Adverse effects
- CNS: Lightheadedness, dizziness
- GI: Hepatitis (prepared from pools of human blood products)
- CV: *Circulatory overload*, CHF, hypertension, palpitations
- Other: Fever, usually within first 24 h of treatment

■ Nursing Considerations
Assessment
- *History:* CHF, hepatitis
- *Physical:* body temperature; P, BP, perfusion; R, adventitious sounds; liver evaluation; liver function tests, HBsAg, respiratory function tests, HIV antibody screen

Implementation
- Arrange for immunization against hepatitis B using a hepatitis B vaccine before beginning treatment with alpha$_1$-proteinase inhibitor.
- Arrange for administration of single dose of hepatitis B Immune Globulin, 0.06 ml/kg IM, at the time of administration of initial dose of hepatitis B vaccine if alpha$_1$-proteinase inhibitor is needed for treatment immediately, before the required waiting time needed for full immunization with hepatitis B vaccine.
- Monitor body temperature for first few hours of treatment; monitor patient for signs of circulatory overload: tachycardia, S$_3$, edema, rapid respirations, elevated JVP.
- Arrange for periodic screening for liver function, hepatitis B, and HIV exposure.

Drug-specific teaching points
- Know that drug must be given IV. Treatment will need to be repeated weekly to maintain lung levels of drug.
- Be aware that there is a risk of hepatitis and AIDS when receiving blood products. Blood products are carefully screened and presumed safe, but some risk remains. Immunization with hepatitis B vaccine is required to eliminate some risk.
- Know that the following side effects may occur: fever (this usually passes within a few hours); lightheadedness, dizziness
- Report shortness of breath, palpitations or irregular heart beats, fever, chills, sore throat, unusual bleeding or bruising.

❒ alprazolam

*(al **pray**' zoe lam)*
Apo-Alpraz (CAN), Novo-Alprazol (CAN), Nu-Alpraz (CAN), Xanax

Pregnancy Category D C-IV drug

Drug classes
Benzodiazepine
Antianxiety drug

Therapeutic actions
Exact mechanisms of action not understood; main sites of action may be the limbic system and reticular formation; increases the effects of gamma-aminobutyrate, an inhibitory neurotransmitter; anxiety blocking effects occur at doses

*Adverse effects in Italics are most common; those in **Bold** are life-threatening.*

alprazolam

well below those necessary to cause sedation, ataxia.

Indications
- Management of anxiety disorders or for short-term relief of symptoms of anxiety; anxiety associated with depression also is responsive.
- Treatment of panic attacks with or without agoraphobia
- Unlabeled uses: social phobia, premenstrual syndrome, depression

Contraindications/cautions
- Contraindicated in the presence of hypersensitivity to benzodiazepines, psychoses, acute narrow-angle glaucoma, shock, coma, acute alcoholic intoxication with depression of vital signs, pregnancy (crosses the placenta; increased risk of congenital malformations, neonatal withdrawal syndrome), labor and delivery ("floppy infant" syndrome reported when mothers were given benzodiazepines during labor), lactation (secreted in breast milk; has caused infants to become lethargic and lose weight).
- Use caution in the presence of impaired liver or kidney function, debilitation.

Dosage
Individualize dosage; increase dosage gradually to avoid adverse effects.

Adult
- ***Anxiety disorders:*** Initially, 0.25–0.5 mg PO tid; titrate to maximum daily dose of 4 mg/d in divided doses.
- ***Panic disorder:*** Initially 0.5 mg PO tid; increase dose at 3- to 4-d intervals in increments of no more than 1 mg/d; ranges of 1–10 mg/d have been needed.
- ***Social phobia:*** 2–8 mg/d PO.
- ***Premenstrual syndrome:*** 0.25 mg PO tid.

Geriatric patients or those with debilitating disease:
Initially 0.25 mg bid–tid; gradually increase if needed and tolerated.

Pharmacokinetics

Route	Onset	Peak	Duration
Oral	30 min	1–2 h	4–6 h

Metabolism: Hepatic, $T_{1/2}$: 12–15 h
Distribution: Crosses placenta; passes into breast milk
Excretion: Urine

Adverse effects
- **CNS:** *Transient, mild drowsiness initially; sedation, depression, lethargy, apathy, fatigue, lightheadedness, disorientation, anger, hostility,* episodes of mania and hypomania, *restlessness, confusion, crying,* delirium, *headache,* slurred speech, dysarthria, stupor, rigidity, tremor, dystonia, vertigo, euphoria, nervousness, difficulty in concentration, vivid dreams, psychomotor retardation, extrapyramidal symptoms; *mild paradoxical excitatory reactions, during first 2 weeks of treatment*
- **GI:** *Constipation, diarrhea, dry mouth,* salivation, *nausea,* anorexia, vomiting, difficulty in swallowing, gastric disorders, hepatic dysfunction
- **CV:** Bradycardia, tachycardia, cardiovascular collapse, hypertension, hypotension, palpitations, edema
- **Hematologic:** Elevations of blood enzymes—LDH, alkaline phosphatase, SGOT, SGPT; blood dyscrasias—agranulocytosis, leukopenia
- **GU:** Incontinence, urinary retention, changes in libido, menstrual irregularities
- **Dermatologic:** Urticaria, pruritus, skin rash, dermatitis
- **EENT:** Visual and auditory disturbances, diplopia, nystagmus, depressed hearing, nasal congestion
- **Other:** Hiccups, fever, diaphoresis, paresthesias, muscular disturbances, gynecomastia. *Drug dependence with withdrawal syndrome when drug is discontinued;* more common with abrupt discontinuation of higher dosage used for longer than 4 mo.

Clinically important drug-drug interactions
- Increased CNS depression when taken with alcohol, other CNS depressants, propoxyphene • Increased effect when given

Adverse effects in *Italics* are most common; those in **Bold** are life-threatening.

with cimetidine, disulfiram, omeprazole, isoniazid, oral contraceptives, valproic acid • Decreased effect when given with carbamazepine, rifampin, theophylline • Possible increased risk of digitalis toxicity if taken with digoxin • Decreased antiparkinson effectiveness of levodopa given with benzodiazepines

■ Nursing Considerations

Assessment

- *History:* Hypersensitivity to benzodiazepines; psychoses; acute narrow-angle glaucoma; shock; coma; acute alcoholic intoxication with depression of vital signs; labor and delivery; lactation; impaired liver or kidney function; debilitation.
- *Physical:* Skin—color, lesions; body temperature; orientation, reflexes, affect, ophthalmologic exam; P, BP; liver evaluation, abdominal exam, bowel sounds, normal output; CBC, liver and renal function tests

Implementation

- Arrange to taper dosage gradually after long-term therapy, especially in epileptic patients.

Drug-specific teaching points

- Take this drug exactly as prescribed.
- Do not to stop taking drug (long-term therapy) without consulting health care provider.
- Avoid the use of alcohol, sleep-inducing, or OTC drugs while on this drug.
- Know that the following side effects may occur: drowsiness, dizziness (these may become less pronounced after a few days, avoid driving a car or engaging in other dangerous activities if these occur); GI upset (taking the drug with food may help); fatigue; depression; dreams; crying; nervousness.
- Report severe dizziness, weakness, drowsiness that persists rash or skin lesions, difficulty voiding, palpitations, swelling in the extremities.

☐ alprostadil

*(al **pross'** ta dil)*
PGE1, Prostin VR Pediatric

Pregnancy Category (not applicable)

Drug classes
Prostaglandin

Therapeutic actions
Relaxes vascular smooth muscle; the smooth muscle of the ductus arteriosus is especially sensitive to this action and will relax and stay open; this is beneficial in infants who have congenital defects that restrict pulmonary or systemic blood flow and who depend on a patent ductus arteriosus for adequate blood oxygenation and lower body perfusion.

Indications

- Palliative therapy to temporarily maintain the patency of the ductus arteriosus until corrective or palliative surgery can be performed in neonates with congenital heart defects who depend on a patent ductus (eg, pulmonary atresia or stenosis, tetralogy of Fallot, coarctation of the aorta)

Contraindications/cautions

- Contraindicated in the presence of respiratory distress syndrome.
- Use caution in the presence of bleeding tendencies (drug inhibits platelet aggregation).

Dosage
Preferred administration is through a continuous IV infusion into a large vein; may be administered through an umbilical artery catheter placed at the ductal opening. Begin infusion with 0.1 μg/kg per minute. After an increase in PO_2 or in systemic blood pressure and blood pH is achieved, reduce infusion to the lowest possible dosage that maintains the response (often achieved by reducing dosage from 0.1–0.05 to 0.025–0.01 μg/kg per minute). Up to 0.4 μg/kg per minute may be used for maintenance if required; higher dosage rates are not more effective.

Pharmacokinetics

Route	Onset
IV	5–25 min

Metabolism: Lungs, $T_{1/2}$: 5–10 min
Excretion: Urine

IV facts

Preparation: Prepare solution by diluting 500 μg alprostadil with Sodium Chloride Injection or Dextrose Injection; dilute to volumes appropriate for pump delivery system being used. Discard and prepare fresh infusion solutions q24h; refrigerate drug ampules.

Infusion:

Add 500 mg Alprostadil to	Approx concentration of resulting solution	Infusion Rate
250 ml	2 mcg/ml	0.05 ml/min/kg
100 ml	5 mcg/ml	0.02 ml/min/kg
50 ml	10 mcg/ml	0.01 ml/min/kg
25 ml	20 mcg/ml	0.005 ml/min/kg

Adverse effects

- CNS: *Seizures,* cerebral bleeding, hypothermia, jitteriness, lethargy, stiffness
- GI: Diarrhea
- CV: *Bradycardia, flushing, tachycardia, hypotension,* cardiac arrest, heart block, CHF
- Respiratory: *Apnea,* respiratory distress
- Hematologic: Inhibited platelet aggregation, bleeding, anemia, disseminated intravascular coagulation, hypokalemia
- Other: Cortical proliferation of the long bones (with prolonged use, regresses after treatment is stopped), sepsis

■ Nursing Considerations

Assessment

- *History:* Respiratory distress, bleeding tendencies
- *Physical:* Body temperature; cyanosis; skeletal development, reflexes, state of agitation, arterial pressure (using auscultation or Doppler), P, auscultation, peripheral perfusion; R, adventitious sounds, bleeding times, arterial blood gases, blood pH

Implementation

- Constantly monitor arterial pressure; decrease infusion rate immediately if any fall in arterial pressure occurs.
- Regularly monitor arterial blood gases to determine efficacy of alprostadil (PO_2 in infants with restricted pulmonary flow; pH and systemic blood pressure in infants with restricted systemic flow).

Drug-specific teaching points

- Teaching about this drug should be incorporated into a total teaching program for the parent(s) of the infant with a cyanotic congential heart defect; specifics about the drug that they will need to know include:
- Your infant will be continually monitored and have frequent blood tests to follow the effects of the drug on his or her condition.
- Know that the baby may look better, breathe easier, become fussy, and so forth, but the drug treatment is only a temporary solution, and the baby will require corrective surgery.

❑ alteplase, recombinant (tissue-type plasminogen activator)

*(al ti **plaze**')*

rt-PA (recombinant tissue plasminogen activator), TPA:
Activase

Pregnancy Category C

Drug classes
Thrombolytic enzyme

Therapeutic actions
Human tissue enzyme produced by recombinant DNA techniques; converts plas-

---

Adverse effects in *Italics* are most common; those in **Bold** are life-threatening.

84 ■ alteplase, recombinant (tissue-type plasminogen activator)

minogen to the enzyme plasmin (fibrinolysin), which degrades fibrin clots; lyses thrombi and emboli; is most active at the site of the clot and causes little systemic fibrinolysis.

Indications
- Treatment of coronary artery thrombosis associated with acute MI
- Treatment of acute, massive pulmonary embolism in adults
- Unlabeled use: treatment of unstable angina

Contraindications/cautions
- Contraindicated in the presence of allergy to TPA; active internal bleeding,; recent (within 2 mo) CVA; intracranial or intraspinal surgery or neoplasm; recent major surgery, obstetric delivery, organ biopsy, or rupture of a noncompressible blood vessel; recent serious GI bleed; recent serious trauma, including CPR; SBE; hemostatic defects; cerebrovascular disease; early-onset, insulin-dependent diabetes; septic thrombosis; severe uncontrolled hypertension.
- Use caution in the presence of liver disease, old age (> 75 y—risk of bleeding may be increased).

Dosage
Careful patient assessment and evaluation are needed to determine the appropriate dose of this drug. Because experience is limited with this drug, careful monitoring is essential.

Adult

- ***Acute MI:*** Total dose of 100 mg IV given as follows: 60 mg the first hour, with an initial bolus of 6–10 mg given over 1–2 min and the rest infused slowly over the rest of the hour; then 20 mg infused slowly over the second hour and 20 mg more infused slowly over the third hour. For patients weighing less than 65 kg, decrease total dose to 1.25 mg/kg. **Do not use a total dose of 150 mg because of the increased risk of intracranial bleeding.**
- ***Pulmonary embolism:*** 100 mg administered by IV infusion over 2 h, followed immediately by heparin therapy.

Pharmacokinetics

Route	Onset	Peak	Duration
IV	Immediate	5–10 min	2½–3 h

Metabolism: $T_{1/2}$: 26 min
Distribution: Crosses placenta
Excretion: Cleared by the liver

IV facts
Preparation: Do not use if vacuum is not present; add appropriate volume of the Sterile Water for Injection provided with vial using a one large bore needle and directing stream into the cake; slight foaming may occur but will dissipate after standing undisturbed for several minutes; reconstitute immediately before use. Refrigerate reconstituted solution and use within 3 h. Do not use Bacteriostatic Water for Injection. Reconstituted solution should be colorless or pale yellow and transparent; contains 1 mg/ml with a pH of 7.3.

Infusion: Administer as reconstituted or further dilute with an equal volume of 0.9% Sodium Chloride Injection or 5% Dextrose Injection to yield 0.5 mg/ml; stable for up to 8 h in these solutions. Avoid excessive agitation; mix by gentle swirling or slow inversion. Discard unused solution.

Compatibilities: Do not add other medications to infusion solution; use 0.9% Sodium Chloride Injection or 5% Dextrose Injection and no other solutions.

Adverse effects
- **CV:** Cardiac arrhythmias with coronary reperfusion, hypotension
- **Hematologic:** *Bleeding*—particularly at venous or arterial access sites, GI bleeding, intracranial hemorrhage
- **Other:** Urticaria, nausea, vomiting, fever

Clinically important drug-drug interactions
- Increased risk of hemorrhage if used with heparin or oral anticoagulants, aspirin, dipyridamole

Adverse effects in *Italics* are most common; those in **Bold** are life-threatening.

altretamine ■ 85

■ Nursing Considerations
Assessment
- *History:* Allergy to TPA; active internal bleeding; recent (within 2 mo) obstetric delivery, organ biopsy, or rupture of a noncompressible blood vessel; recent serious GI bleed; recent serious trauma, including CPR; SBE; hemostatic defects; cerebrovascular disease; early-onset insulin-dependent diabetes; septic thrombosis; severe uncontrolled hypertension; liver disease
- *Physical:* Skin—color, temperature, lesions; orientation, reflexes; P, BP, peripheral perfusion, baseline ECG; R, adventitious sounds; liver evaluation, hematocrit, platelet count, thrombin time (TT), activated partial thromboplastin time (APTT), prothrombin time (PT)

Implementation
- Arrange to discontinue concurrent heparin and alteplase if serious bleeding occurs.
- Arrange for regular monitoring of coagulation studies.
- Apply pressure or pressure dressings to control superficial bleeding (at invaded or disturbed areas).
- Avoid any arterial invasive procedures during therapy.
- Arrange for typing and cross-matching of blood in case serious blood loss occurs and whole blood transfusions are required.
- Institute treatment within 6 h of onset of symptoms for evolving myocardial infarction.

Drug-specific teaching points
- This drug can only be given IV, and you will need to be closely monitored during drug treatment.
- Report difficulty breathing, dizziness, disorientation, headache, numbness, tingling.

☐ altretamine

(al tret' a meen)
hexamethylmelamine
Hexalen

Pregnancy Category D

Drug classes
Antineoplastic

Therapeutic actions
Cytotoxic; mechanisms by which it is able to cause cell death are not known.

Indications
- Use as a single agent in the palliative treatment of patients with persistent or recurrent ovarian cancer following first-line therapy with a cisplatin or alkylating agent-based combination

Contraindications/cautions
- Hypersensitivity to altretamine, bone marrow depression, severe neurologic toxicity, lactation.

Dosage
Adult: Dosage is determined by body surface area.
- 260 mg/m^2 per day PO given for 14 or 21 consecutive days in a 28-d cycle. Total daily dose is given as divided doses after meals and at bedtime.
- Temporarily discontinue altretamine for > 14 days if GI intolerance, WBC < 2,000/mm^3 or granuloctyes < 1,000/mm^3, platelet count < 75,000/mm^3, or progressive neuropathy occurs; restart with 200 mg/m^2 per day.

Pharmacokinetics

Route	Onset	Peak
Oral	Rapid	½–3 h

Metabolism: Hepatic, T$_{1/2}$: 4.7–10 h
Distribution: Crosses placenta; passes into breast milk
Excretion: Urine

Adverse effects
- CNS: **Peripheral sensory neuropathy** (mild to severe); fatigue; seizures
- GI: *Nausea, vomiting,* increased alkaline phosphatase, anorexia
- GU: Increased BUN
- Hematologic: **Bone marrow depression**

Adverse effects in *Italics* are most common; those in **Bold** are life-threatening.

- **Other:** Carcinogenesis, impairment of fertility, mutagenesis

Clinically important drug-drug interactions
- Increased effects of altretamine if taken concurrently with cimetidine • Increased risk of postural hypotension if taken concurrently with MAO inhibitors

■ Nursing Considerations

Assessment
- *History:* Hypersensitivity to altretamine; bone marrow depression; severe neurologic toxicity; lactation
- *Physical:* Neurologic status, body temperature, abdominal exam, kidney and liver function tests, CBC

Implementation
- Give drug with meals and at bedtime.
- Arrange to discontinue drug if GI effects are intractable; severe neuropathy occurs; bone marrow depression becomes dangerous. Reevaluate patient, and consider restarting altretamine after up to 14 d of rest.
- Arrange for blood counts before beginning therapy and at least monthly during treatment.
- Monitor patient's neurologic status frequently during treatment.
- Consider antiemetics or decreased dose if nausea and vomiting are severe.

Drug-specific teaching points
- Take drug with meals and at bedtime.
- Arrange to have regular blood tests and neurologic exams while receiving this drug.
- Know that the following side effects may occur: nausea and vomiting (this may be severe; antiemetics may be helpful and can be ordered for you; small, frequent meals also may help); weakness, lethargy (frequent rest periods will help); increased susceptibility to infection (avoid crowds and situations that might expose you to many people or diseases); numbness and tingling in the fingers or toes (use care to avoid injury to these areas; use care if trying to perform tasks that require precision).
- Report severe nausea and vomiting; fever, chills, sore throat; unusual bleeding or bruising; numbness or tingling in your fingers or toes.

❐ aluminum carbonate gel, basic

(a loo' mi num)

Basaljel

aluminum hydroxide gel

ALterna GEL, Alu-Cap, Alu-Tab, Amphojel

aluminum phosphate gel

Phosphaljel

Pregnancy Category C

Drug classes
Antacid

Therapeutic actions
Neutralizes or reduces gastric acidity, resulting in an increase in the pH of the stomach and duodenal bulb and inhibiting the proteolytic activity of pepsin, which protects the lining of the stomach and duodenum; binds with phosphate ions in the intestine to form insoluble aluminum-phosphate complexes, lowering phosphate in hyperphosphatemia and chronic renal failure but may cause hypophosphatemia in other states.

Indications
- Symptomatic relief of upset stomach associated with hyperacidity
- Hyperacidity associated with peptic ulcer, gastritis, peptic esophagitis, gastric hyperacidity, hiatal hernia
- Treatment, control, or management of hyperphosphatemia—aluminum carbonate
- Prevention of formation of phosphate urinary stones, used in conjunction with a low-phosphate diet—aluminum carbonate
- Unlabeled use for aluminum hydroxide: prophylaxis of GI bleeding, stress ulcer; reduction of phosphate absorption in

aluminum carbonate gel, basic ■ 87

hyperphosphatemia in patients with chronic renal failure

Contraindications/cautions
- Allergy to aluminum products, gastric outlet destruction, hypertension, CHF, hypophosphatemia, lactation

Dosage
Adult
Aluminum hydroxide gel: 500–1,800 mg three to six times per day PO between meals and at bedtime.
Aluminum phosphate gel: 15–30 ml undiluted PO q2h between meals and at bedtime. This preparation is no longer used as an antacid. Use is limited to reduction of fetal excretion of phosphates.
Aluminum carbonate gel
- ***Antacid:*** 2 capsules or tablets, 10 ml of regular suspension or 5 ml of extra strength suspension as often as q2h, up to 12 times per day PO
- ***Prevention of phosphate stones:*** Administer PO 1 h after meals and at bedtime.
- *Capsules or tablets:* 2 to 6;
- *suspension:* 10 to 30 ml;
- *extra strength suspension:* 5 to 15 ml in water or fruit juice.
- ***Hyperphosphatemia:*** Administer PO tid–qid with meals.
- *Capsules, tablets:* take 2;
- *suspension:* take 12 ml;
- *extra strength suspension:* take 5 ml.

Pediatric
Aluminum hydroxide gel
- ***Hyperphosphatemia:*** 50–150 mg/kg every 24 h PO in divided doses q4–6h; titrate dose to normal serum phosphorus.
- ***General guidelines:*** 5–15 ml PO q3–6h or 1–3h after meals and at bedtime.
- ***Prophylaxis of GI bleeding in critically ill infants:*** 2–5 ml/dose q1–2h PO. **For children:** 5–15 ml/dose q1–2h PO.

Pharmacokinetics

Route	Onset
Oral	Varies

Metabolism: Hepatic
Distribution: With chronic use, small amounts may be absorbed systemically and cross the placenta and enter breast milk
Excretion: GI bound in the feces

Adverse effects
- **GI:** *Constipation;* intestinal obstruction, decreased absorption of fluoride, accumulation of aluminum in serum, bone, and CNS
- **MS:** Osteomalacia and chronic phosphate deficiency with bone pain, malaise, muscular weakness

Clinically important drug-drug interactions
- Do not administer *other oral drugs* within 1–2 h of antacid administration; change in gastric pH may interfere with absorption of oral drugs. • Decreased pharmacologic effect of corticosteroids, diflunisal, digoxin, iron, isoniazid, penicillamine, phenothiazines, ranitidine, tetracyclines. • Increased pharmacologic effect of benzodiazepines if given concomitantly.

■ Nursing Considerations

Assessment
- *History:* Allergy to aluminum products; gastric outlet obstruction; hypertension, CHF; hypophosphatemia; lactation
- *Physical:* Bone strength, muscle strength; P, auscultation, BP, peripheral edema; abdominal exam, bowel sounds; serum phosphorous, serum fluoride; bone x-ray is appropriate

Implementation
- Administer drug hourly for first 2 wk when used in treatment of acute peptic ulcer; during the healing stage, administer 1–3 h after meals and at bedtime.
- Do not administer oral drugs within 1–2 h of antacid administration.
- Have patient chew tablets thoroughly before swallowing; follow with a glass of water.
- Monitor serum phosphorus levels periodically during long-term therapy.

Adverse effects in *Italics* are most common; those in **Bold** are life-threatening.

Drug-specific teaching points
- Take this drug between meals and at bedtime; ulcer patients need to strictly follow prescribed dosage pattern. If tablets are being used, chew thoroughly before swallowing, and follow with water.
- Do not take maximum dosage of antacids for more than 2 weeks except under the supervision of a physician or nurse.
- Do not take this drug with any other oral medications; absorption of those medications can be inhibited. Take other oral medications at least 1–2 h after aluminum salt.
- Know that the following side effects may occur: constipation; (appropriate measures can be taken).
- Report constipation; bone pain, muscle weakness; coffee ground vomitus, black tarry stools; no relief from symptoms being treated.

☐ amantadine HCl

(a man' ta deen)
Symadine, Symmetrel

Pregnancy Category C

Drug classes
Antiviral drug
Antiparkinsonism drug

Therapeutic actions
May inhibit penetration of influenza A virus into the host cell; may increase dopamine release in the nigostriatal pathway of parkinsonism patients, relieving their symptoms.

Indications
- Prevention and treatment of influenza A virus respiratory infection, especially in high-risk patients
- Adjunct to late vaccination against influenza A virus, to provide interim coverage; supplement to vaccination in immunodeficient patients; prophylaxis when vaccination is contraindicated
- Parkinson's disease and drug-induced extrapyramidal reactions

Contraindications/cautions
- Allergy to drug product, seizures, liver disease, eczematoid rash, psychoses, CHF, renal disease, lactation.

Dosage
Influenza A Virus
- **Adult:** *Prophylaxis:* 200 mg/d PO or 100 mg bid PO for 10 d after exposure, for up to 90 d if vaccination is impossible and exposure is repeated. *Treatment:* Same dose as above; start treatment as soon after exposure as possible, continuing for 24–48 h after symptoms are gone.
- **Patients with seizure disorders:** 100 mg/d.
- **Patients with renal disease**

Creatinine Clearance (ml/min)	Dosage
10–19	Alternate 200 mg/100 mg q7d
20–29	100 mg three/week
30–39	200 mg two/week
40–59	100 mg/d
60–79	200 mg/100 mg on alternate days
≥80	100 mg bid

- **Pediatric:** Not recommended for children < 1 y.
- *Prophylaxis:* 1–9 y: 2–4 mg/lb per d PO in two to three divided doses, not to exceed 150 mg/lb per d. 9–12 y: 100 mg PO bid.
- *Treatment:* Same dose as above; start treatment as soon after exposure as possible, continuing for 24–48 h after symptoms are gone.

Parkinsonism Treatment
- **Adult:** 100 mg bid (up to 400 mg/d) when used alone; reduce dosage in patients receiving other antiparkinsonism drugs.
- **Geriatric:** *> 65 years with no recognized renal disease:* 100 mg once daily in parkinsonism treatment; 100 mg bid (up to 400 mg/d) when used alone; reduce dosage in patients receiving other antiparkinsonian drugs.
- **Patients with renal disease**

Creatinine Clearance (ml/min)	Dosage
10–19	Alternate 200 mg/100 mg q7d

(continued)

20–29	100 mg three/week
30–39	200 mg two/week
40–59	100 mg/d
60–79	200 mg/100 mg on alternate days
≥80	100 mg bid

Drug-Induced Extrapyramidal Reactions
- **Adult:** 100 mg bid PO, up to 300 mg/d in divided doses has been used.

Pharmacokinetics

Route	Onset	Peak
Oral	36–48 h	4 h

Metabolism: $T_{1/2}$: 15–24 h
Distribution: Crosses placenta; passes into breast milk
Excretion: Unchanged in the urine

Adverse effects
- **CNS:** *Lightheadedness, dizziness, insomnia,* confusion, irritability, ataxia, psychosis, depression, hallucinations
- **GI:** *Nausea,* anorexia, constipation, dry mouth
- **CV:** CHF, orthostatic hypotension, dyspnea
- **GU:** Urinary retention

Clinically important drug-drug interactions
- Increased atropine-like side effects if taken with anticholinergic drugs • Increased amantadine effects if taken with hydrochlorothiazide, triamterene

■ Nursing Considerations

Assessment
- **History:** Allergy to drug product, seizures, liver disease, eczematoid rash, psychoses, CHF, renal disease, lactation
- **Physical:** Orientation, vision, speech, reflexes; BP, orthostatic BP, P, auscultation, perfusion, edema; R, adventitious sounds; urinary output; BUN, creatinine clearance

Implementation
- Do not discontinue this drug abruptly, when used to treat parkinsonism syndrome; parkinsonian crisis may occur.

Drug-specific teaching points
- Mark your calendar if you are on alternating dosage schedules; it is very important to take the full course of the drug.
- Know that the following may occur as a result of the drug therapy: drowsiness, blurred vision (use caution when driving or using dangerous equipment while on this drug); dizziness, light-headedness (avoid sudden position changes); irritability or mood changes (this is often an effect of the drug; if this becomes severe, the drug may need to be changed).
- Report swelling of the fingers or ankles; shortness of breath; difficulty urinating; tremors, slurred speech, difficulty walking.

☐ ambenonium chloride

*(am ne **noe'** nee um)*
Mytelase Caplets

Pregnancy Category C

Drug classes
Cholinesterase inhibitor
Parasympathomimetic drug (indirectly acting)
Antimyasthenic drug

Therapeutic actions
Increases the concentration of acetylcholine at the sites of cholinergic transmission (parasympathetic neurons and skeletal muscles) and prolongs and exaggerates the effects of acetylcholine by inhibiting the enzyme acetylcholinesterase; this causes parasympathomimetic effects and facilitates transmission at the skeletal neuromuscular junction. Also has direct stimulating effects on skeletal muscle and has a longer duration of effect and fewer side effects than other agents.

Indications
- Symptomatic control of myasthenia gravis

Contraindications/cautions
- Contraindicated in the presence of hypersensitivity to anticholinesterases; intesti-

Adverse effects in *Italics* are most common; those in **Bold** are life-threatening.

ambenonium chloride

nal or urogenital tract obstruction; peritonitis; lactation.
- Use caution in the presence of asthma, peptic ulcer, bradycardia, cardiac arrhythmias, recent coronary occlusion, vagotonia, hyperthyroidism, epilepsy.

Dosage
Adult: 5–25 mg PO tid–qid (5–75 mg per dose has been used). Start dosage with 5 mg, and gradually increase to determine optimum dosage based on optimal muscle strength and no GI disturbances; increase dose every 1–2 d. Dosage above 200 mg/d requires close supervision to avoid overdose.
Pediatric: Safety and efficacy not established.

Pharmacokinetics

Route	Onset	Peak
Oral	20–30 min	3–8 h

Metabolism: $T_{1/2}$: Unknown
Distribution: Crosses placenta; passes into breast milk
Excretion: Unknown

Adverse effects
Parasympathomimetic Effects
- **GI:** *Salivation, dysphagia, nausea, vomiting, increased peristalsis, abdominal cramps,* flatulence, diarrhea
- **CV:** *Bradycardia, cardiac arrhythmias,* AV block and nodal rhythm, **cardiac arrest;** decreased cardiac output, leading to hypotension, syncope
- **Respiratory:** *Increased pharyngeal and tracheobronchial secretions,* laryngospasm, bronchospasm, bronchiolar constriction, dyspnea
- **GU:** *Urinary frequency and incontinence,* urinary urgency
- **EENT:** *Lacrimation, miosis,* spasm of accommodation, diplopia, conjunctival hyperemia
- **Dermatologic:** Diaphoresis, flushing

Skeletal Muscle Effects
- **CNS:** Convulsions, dysarthria, dysphonia, drowsiness, dizziness, headache, loss of consciousness
- **Peripheral:** Skeletal muscle weakness, fasciculations, muscle cramps, arthralgia
- **Respiratory:** Respiratory muscle paralysis, central respiratory paralysis

Clinically important drug-drug interactions
- Decreased neuromuscular blockade of succinylcholine if taken concurrently
- Decreased effects of ambenonium and possible muscular depression if taken concurrently with corticosteroids

■ Nursing Considerations

Assessment
- *History:* Hypersensitivity to anticholinesterases, intestinal or urogenital tract obstruction, peritonitis, asthma, peptic ulcer, bradycardia, cardiac arrhythmias, recent coronary occlusion, vagotonia, hyperthyroidism, epilepsy, lactation
- *Physical:* Skin—color, texture, lesions; reflexes, bilateral grip strength; P, auscultation, BP; R, adventitious sounds; salivation, bowel sounds, normal output; frequency, voiding pattern, normal urinary output; EEG, thyroid tests

Implementation
- Be aware that overdosage with anticholinesterase drugs can cause muscle weakness (cholinergic crisis) that is difficult to differentiate from myasthenic weakness (use of edrophonium for differential diagnosis is recommended). The administration of atropine may mask the parasympathetic effects of anticholinesterase overdose and further confound the diagnosis.
- Maintain atropine sulfate on standby as an antidote and antagonist to ambenonium in case of cholinergic crisis or hypersensitivity reaction.
- Monitor patient response carefully if increasing dosage.
- Discontinue drug and consult physician if excessive salivation, emesis, frequent urination, or diarrhea occurs.
- Arrange for decreased dosage of drug if excessive sweating, nausea, or GI upset occur.

Adverse effects in *Italics* are most common; those in **Bold** are life-threatening.

Drug-specific teaching points
- Take this drug exactly as prescribed; the drug does not need to be taken during the night. Patient and significant other should receive extensive teaching about the effects of the drug, the signs and symptoms of myasthenia gravis, the fact that muscle weakness may be related to drug overdosage or to exacerbation of the disease, and that it is important to report muscle weakness promptly to the nurse or physician so that proper evaluation can be made.
- Know that the following may occur while taking this drug: blurred vision, difficulty with far vision, difficulty with dark adaptation (use caution while driving, especially at night, or performing hazardous tasks in reduced light); increased urinary frequency, abdominal cramps (these are drug effects, if these become a problem, notify your nurse or physician); sweating (avoid hot or excessively humid environments while you are taking this drug).
- Report muscle weakness, nausea, vomiting, diarrhea, severe abdominal pain, excessive sweating, excessive salivation, frequent urination, urinary urgency, irregular heartbeat, difficulty in breathing.

❏ amikacin sulfate

(am i kay' sin)
Amikacin, Amikin

Pregnancy Category C

Drug classes
Aminoglycoside antibiotic

Therapeutic actions
Bactericidal: inhibits protein synthesis in susceptible strains of gram-negative bacteria, and the functional integrity of bacterial cell membrane appears to be disrupted, causing cell death.

Indications
- Short-term treatment of serious infections caused by susceptible strains of *Pseudomonas* species, *E. coli*, indole-positive *Proteus* species, *Providencia* species, *Klebsiella*, *Enterobacter*, *Serratia* species, *Acinetobacter* species
- Suspected gram-negative infections before results of susceptibility studies are known (effective in infections caused by gentamicin- or tobramycin-resistant strains of gram-negative organisms)
- Initial treatment of staphylococcal infections when penicillin is contraindicated or infection may be caused by mixed organisms
- Neonatal sepsis when other antibiotics cannot be used (often used in combination with penicillin-type drug)
- **Unlabeled uses:** intrathecal/intraventricular administration at 8 mg/24 h; part of a multidrug regimen for treatment of *Mycobacterium avium* complex, a common infection in AIDS patients

Contraindications/cautions
- Contraindicated in the presence of allergy to any aminoglycosides, renal or hepatic disease, preexisting hearing loss, myasthenia gravis, parkinsonism, infant botulism, lactation.
- Use caution in the presence of elderly patients, any patient with diminished hearing, decreased renal function, dehydration, neuromuscular disorders.

Dosage
IM or IV (dosage is the same):
Adult and Pediatric 15 mg/kg per day divided into two to three equal doses at equal intervals, not to exceed 1.5 g/d.
- *UTIs:* 250 mg bid; treatment is usually required for 7–10 d. If treatment is required for longer, carefully monitor serum levels and renal and neurologic function.

Neonatal: Loading dose of 10 mg/kg then 7.5 mg/kg q12h.
Geriatric or renal failure patients: Reduce dosage, and carefully monitor serum drug levels and results of renal function tests throughout treatment; regulate dosage based on these values.

If Ccr is not available and patient condition is stable, calculate a dosage interval in hours for the normal dose by multiplying patient's serum creatinine by 9.

...cin sulfate

Dosage guide if Ccr is known: Maintenance dose q12h = (observed Ccr ÷ normal Ccr) × calculated loading dose (mg).

Pharmacokinetics

Route	Onset	Peak
IV	Immediate	30 min
IM	Varies	45–120 min

Metabolism: $T_{1/2}$: 2–3 hours
Distribution: Crosses placenta; passes into breast milk
Excretion: Unchanged in the urine

IV facts

Preparation: Prepare IV solution by adding the contents of a 500-mg vial to 100 or 200 ml of sterile diluent. Do not physically mix with other drugs. Administer amikacin separately. Prepared solution is stable in concentrations of 0.25 and 5 mg/ml for 24 h at room temperature.

Infusion: Administer to adults or pediatric patients over 30–60 min; infuse to infants over 1–2 h.

Compatibilities: Amikacin is stable in 5% Dextrose Injection; 5% Dextrose and 0.2%, 0.45%, or 0.9% Sodium Chloride Injection; Lactated Ringer's Injection; Normosol M in 5% Dextrose Injection; Normosol R in 5% Dextrose Injection; Plasma-Lyte 56 or 148 Injection in 5% Dextrose in Water.

Adverse effects

- CNS: *Ototoxicity*, confusion, disorientation, depression, lethargy, nystagmus, visual disturbances, headache, fever, numbness, tingling, tremor, paresthesias, muscle twitching, convulsions, muscular weakness, neuromuscular blockade, **apnea**
- GI: *Nausea, vomiting, anorexia, diarrhea*, weight loss, stomatitis, increased salivation, splenomegaly
- CV: Palpitations, hypotension, hypertension
- Hematologic: Leukemoid reaction, agranulocytosis, granulocytosis, leukopenia, leukocytosis, thrombocytopenia, eosinophilia, pancytopenia, anemia, hemolytic anemia, increased or decreased reticulocyte count, electrolyte disturbances
- GU: *Nephrotoxicity*
- Hepatic: Hepatic toxicity; hepatomegaly
- Hypersensitivity: Purpura, rash, urticaria, exfoliative dermatitis, itching
- Other: *Superinfections, pain and irritation at IM injection sites*

Clinically important drug-drug interactions

- Increased ototoxic and nephrotoxic effects if taken with potent diuretics and other ototoxic and nephrotoxic drugs (eg, cephalosporins). • Risk of inactivation of amikacin if mixed parenterally with penicillins. • Increased likelihood of neuromuscular blockade if given shortly after general anesthetics, depolarizing and nondepolarizing neuromuscular junction blockers.

■ Nursing Considerations

Assessment

- *History:* Allergy to any aminoglycosides, renal or hepatic disease, preexisting hearing loss, myasthenia gravis, parkinsonism, infant botulism, lactation, diminished hearing, decreased renal function, dehydration, neuromuscular disorders
- *Physical:* Arrange culture and sensitivity tests on infection before beginning therapy; renal function, eighth cranial nerve function and state of hydration prior to, periodically during, and after therapy; hepatic function tests, CBC, skin color and lesions, orientation and affect, reflexes, bilateral grip strength, body weight, bowel sounds.

Implementation

- Arrange for culture and sensitivity testing of infected area before beginning treatment.
- Monitor duration of treatment: usual duration of treatment is 7–10 d. If clinical response does not occur within 3-5 days, stop therapy. Prolonged treatment leads to increased risk of toxicity. If drug is used longer than 10 d, monitor auditory and renal function daily.

Adverse effects in *Italics* are most common; those in **Bold** are life-threatening.

amiloride hydrochloride ■ 93

- Administer IM dosage by deep intramuscular injection.
- Assure that patient is well hydrated before and during therapy.

Drug-specific teaching points
- Be aware that this drug is only available for IM or IV use.
- Know that the following may occur as a result of drug therapy: ringing in the ears, headache, dizziness (these effects are reversible, safety measures may need to be taken if these become severe); nausea, vomiting, loss of appetite (small frequent meals, frequent mouth care may help).
- Report pain at injection site, severe headache, dizziness, loss of hearing, changes in urine pattern, difficulty breathing, rash or skin lesions.

▢ amiloride hydrochloride

*(a **mill'** oh ride)*
Midamor

Pregnancy Category B

Drug classes
Potassium-sparing diuretic

Therapeutic actions
Inhibits sodium reabsorption in the renal distal tubule, causing loss of sodium and water and retention of potassium.

Indications
- Adjunctive therapy with thiazide or loop diuretics in edema associated with CHF and in hypertension to treat hypokalemia or to prevent hypokalemia in patients who would be at high risk if hypokalemia occurred (digitalized patients, patients with cardiac arrhythmias)
- Unlabeled uses: inhalation in the treatment of cystic fibrosis; reduction of lithium-induced polyuria without increasing lithium levels

Contraindications/cautions
- Allergy to amiloride, hyperkalemia, renal or liver disease, diabetes mellitus, metabolic or respiratory acidosis, lactation.

Dosage
Adult: Add 5 mg/d to usual antihypertensive or dosage of kaluretic diuretic; if necessary, increase dose to 10 mg/d or to 15–20 mg/d with careful monitoring of electrolytes.
- ***Single-drug therapy:*** Start with 5 mg/d; if necessary, increase to 10 mg/d or to 15–20 mg/d with careful monitoring of electrolytes.

Pediatric: Safety and efficacy not established.

Pharmacokinetics

Route	Onset	Peak	Duration
Oral	2 h	6–10 h	24 h

Metabolism: $T_{1/2}$: 6–9 h
Distribution: Crosses placenta; passes into breast milk
Excretion: Unchanged in the urine

Adverse effects
- CNS: *Headache*, dizziness, drowsiness, fatigue, paresthesias, tremors, confusion, encephalopathy
- GI: *Nausea, anorexia, vomiting, diarrhea*, dry mouth, constipation, jaundice, gas pain, GI bleeding
- Respiratory: Cough, dyspnea
- GU: *Hyperkalemia*, polyuria, dysuria, *impotence*, loss of libido
- MS: *Weakness, fatigue, muscle cramps* and muscle spasms, joint pain
- Other: Rash, pruritus, itching, alopecia

Clinically important drug-drug interactions
- Increased hyperkalemia if taken with triamterene, spironolactone, potassium supplements, diets rich in potassium, captopril, enalapril, lisinopril • Reduced effectiveness of digoxin if taken with amiloride.

■ Nursing Considerations
Assessment
- *History:* Allergy to amiloride, hyperkalemia, renal or liver disease, diabetes

---

Adverse effects in *Italics* are most common; those in **Bold** are life-threatening.

mellitus, metabolic or respiratory acidosis, lactation
- *Physical:* Skin—color, lesions, edema; orientation, reflexes, muscle strength; pulses, baseline ECG, BP; respiratory rate, pattern, adventitious sounds; liver evaluation, bowel sounds, urinary output patterns; CBC, serum electrolytes, blood sugar, liver and renal function tests, urinalysis

Implementation

- Administer with food or milk to prevent GI upset.
- Administer early in the day so increased urination does not disturb sleep.
- Measure and record regular body weights to monitor mobilization of edema fluid.
- Avoid giving patient foods rich in potassium; avoid use of salt substitutes high in potassium.
- Provide frequent mouth care, sugarless lozenges to suck.
- Arrange for regular evaluation of serum electrolytes.

Drug-specific teaching points

- Take the drug early in the day so increased urination will not disturb sleep if a single daily dose has been prescribed.
- Take the drug with food or meals to prevent GI upset.
- Avoid foods that are high in potassium, avoid using any flavoring that contains potassium (eg, salt substitute).
- Weigh yourself on a regular basis at the same time of the day and in the same clothing, and record the weight on your calendar.
- Know that the following may occur as a result of drug therapy: increased volume and frequency of urination (have ready access to a bathroom when drug effect is greatest); dizziness, feeling faint on arising, drowsiness (if these changes occur, avoid rapid position changes, hazardous activities like driving a car, and the use of alcohol which may intensify these problems); decrease in sexual function; increased thirst (sucking on sugarless lozenges may help to alleviate the thirst; frequent mouth care also may help); avoid foods that are rich in potassium (eg, fruits, Sanka).
- Report loss or gain of more than 3 lb in one day; swelling in your ankles or fingers; dizziness, trembling, numbness, fatigue; muscle weakness or cramps.

☐ amino acids

(a mee' noe)

Aminess, Aminosyn, BranchAmin, FreAmine, Hepatamine, Nephramine, Novamine, ProcalAmine, RenAmin, Travasol, Trophamine

Pregnancy Category C

Drug classes
Protein substrate
Caloric Agent

Therapeutic actions
Essential and nonessential amino acids provided in various combinations to supply calories and proteins and provide a protein-building and a protein-sparing effect for the body (a positive nitrogen balance).

Indications
- Provide nutrition to patients who are in a negative nitrogen balance when GI tract cannot absorb protein; when protein needs exceed the ability to absorb protein (burns, trauma, infections); when bowel rest is needed; when tube feeding cannot supply adequate nutrition; when health can be improved or restored by replacing lost amino acids
- Treatment of hepatic encephalopathy in patients with cirrhosis or hepatitis
- Nutritional support of uremic patients when oral nutrition is not feasible

Contraindications/cautions
- Contraindicated in the presence of hypersensitivity to any component of the solution; severe electrolyte or acid–base imbalance; inborn errors in amino acid metabolism; decreased circulating blood volume; severe kidney or liver disease;

amino acids ■ 95

hyperammonemia; bleeding abnormalities.
- Use caution in the presence of liver or renal impairment; diabetes mellitus; congestive heart failure; hypertension.

Dosage
Dosage must be individualized for each patient with careful observation of cardiac status and BUN and evaluation of metabolic needs.
Adult: 1–1.7 g/kg per day amino acid injection IV into a peripheral vein; 250–500 ml/d amino acid injection IV mixed with appropriate dextrose, vitamins, and electrolytes as part of a TPN solution.
Pediatric: 2–3 g/kg per day amino acid IV mixed with dextrose as appropriate.

Pharmacokinetics

Route	Onset
IV	Immediate

Metabolism: Part of normal anabolic processes
Distribution: Crosses placenta; passes into breast milk
Excretion: Urine as urea nitrogen

IV facts
Preparation: Strict aseptic technique is required in mixing solution; use of a laminar flow hood in the pharmacy is recommended. A 0.22-μm filter should be used to block any particulate matter and bacteria. Use mixed solution immediately. If not used within 1 h, refrigerate solution. Mixed solutions must be used within 24 h. Use strict aseptic technique when changing bottles, catheter, tubing, and so forth. Replace all IV apparatus every 24 h. Change dressing every 24 h to assess insertion site.
Infusion: Infuse using a volumetric infusion pump. Do not infuse if solution is not absolutely clear and without particulate matter. Infuse slowly, using clinical situation as a guide. If infusion falls behind, do not try to speed up infusion rate; serious overload could occur. Infusion rates of 20–30 ml/h up to a maximum of 60–100 ml/h have been used.

Compatibilities: Do not mix with amphotericin B, ampicillin, carbenicillin, cephradine, gentamicin, metronidazole, tetracycline, ticarcillin.

Adverse effects
- CNS: *Headache, dizziness,* mental confusion, **loss of consciousness**
- GI: *Nausea, vomiting,* abdominal pain, liver impairment, fatty liver
- CV: Hypertension, CHF, **pulmonary edema**, tachycardia, *generalized flushing*
- Endocrine: Hypoglycemia, hyperglycemia, fatty acid deficiency, azotemia, hyperammonemia
- Local: *Pain, infection,* phlebitis, venous thrombosis, tissue sloughing at injection site
- Hypersensitivity: Fever, chills, rash, papular eruptions

Clinically important drug-drug interactions
- Reduced protein-sparing effects of amino acids if taken with tetracyclines

■ Nursing Considerations

Assessment
- *History:* Hypersensitivity to any component of the solution; severe electrolyte or acid–base imbalance; inborn errors in amino acid metabolism; decreased circulating blood volume; kidney or liver disease; hyperammonemia; bleeding abnormalities, diabetes mellitus; congestive heart failure; hypertension
- *Physical:* Body temperature, weight, height; orientation, reflexes; P, BP, edema; R, lung auscultation; abdominal exam; urinary output; CBC, platelet count, prothrombin time, electrolytes, BUN, blood glucose, uric acid, bilirubin, creatinine, plasma proteins, renal and liver function tests; urine glucose, osmolarity

Implementation
- Assess nutritional status before and frequently during treatment; weigh patient

Adverse effects in *Italics* are most common; those in **Bold** are life-threatening.

96 ■ aminocaproic acid

daily to monitor fluid load and nutritional status.
- Monitor vital signs frequently during infusion; monitor I&O continually during treatment.
- Observe infusion site at least daily for any sign of infection, phlebitis; change dressing using strict aseptic technique at least q24h.
- Arrange to give D5W or D10W for injection by a peripheral line to avoid hypoglycemia rebound if TPN infusion needs to be stopped for any reason,
- Monitor urine glucose, acetone, and specific gravity q6h during initial infusion period, at least bid when the infusion has stabilized.
- Monitor patient for any sign of vascular overload; for any sign of hepatic impairment; arrange to decrease rate of infusion or discontinue infusion as appropriate.

Drug-specific teaching points
- Be aware that this drug can be given only through an intravenous or central line.
- Know that this drug will help you to build new proteins and regain your strength and healing power.
- Know that the following side effects could occur: headache, dizziness (medication may be ordered to help if this becomes a problem); nausea, vomiting; pain at infusion site.
- Report fever, chills, severe pain at infusion site, changes in color of urine or stool, severe headache, rash.

☐ aminocaproic acid

*(a mee noe ka **proe' ik**)*
Amicar, EACA

Pregnancy Category C

Drug classes
Systemic hemostatic agent

Therapeutic actions
Inhibits fibrinolysis by inhibiting plasminogen activator substances and by antiplasmin activity; this action prevents the breakdown of clots.

Indications
- Treatment of excessive bleeding resulting from systemic hyperfibrinolysis and urinary fibrinolysis.
- Unlabeled uses: prevention of recurrence of subarachnoid hemorrhage; management of amegakaryocytic thrombocytopenia; to decrease the need for platelet administration; to abort and treat attacks of hereditary angioneurotic edema

Contraindications/cautions
- Allergy to aminocaproic acid, active intravascular clotting (disseminated intravascular coagulation; DIC), cardiac disease, renal dysfunction, hematuria of upper urinary tract origin, hepatic dysfunction, lactation.

Dosage
Adult: Initial dose of 5 g PO or IV followed by 1–1.25 g/h to produce and sustain plasma levels of 0.13 mg/ml; do not administer more than 30 g/d.
- ***Acute bleeding:*** 4–5 g IV in 250 ml of diluent during the first hour of infusion; then continuous infusion of 1 g/h in 50 ml of diluent. Continue for 8 h or until bleeding stops.
- ***Prevention of recurrence of subarachnoid hemorrhage:*** 36 g/d in six divided doses, PO or IV.
- ***Amegakaryocytic thrombocytopenia:*** 8–24 g/d for 3 d to 13 mo.

Pediatric: 100 mg/kg PO or IV during the first hour; then 33.3 mg/kg per hour for a maximum of 18g/m^2 per day.

Pharmacokinetics

Route	Onset	Peak	Duration
Oral	Rapid	2 h	
IV	Immediate	Minutes	2–3 h

Distribution: Crosses placenta; passes into breast milk
Excretion: Unchanged in the urine

IV facts
Preparation: Dilute in compatible IV fluid. Rapid IV infusion undiluted is not recommended. Dilute 4 ml (1 g) of solution with 50 ml of diluent. For acute bleed, dilute 4–5 g in 250 ml diluent and give

over 1 h; follow with a continuous infusion of 1–1.25 g/h given in 50 ml diluent. May be stored at room temperature.
Infusion: Infuse at 4–5 g the first hour of treatment, then 1 g/h by continuous infusion; administer slowly to avoid hypotension, bradycardia, arrhythmias.
Compatibilities: Compatible with Sterile Water for Injection, Normal Saline, 5% Dextrose, Ringer's Solution.

Adverse effects
- CNS: *Dizziness, tinnitus, headache,* delirium, hallucinations, psychotic reactions, weakness, conjunctivial suffusion, nasal stuffiness
- GI: *Nausea, cramps, diarrhea*
- CV: Hypotension, cardiac myopathy
- Hematologic: *Elevated serum CPK,* aldolase, SGOT, elevated serum potassium
- GU: Intrarenal obstruction, renal failure, *fertility problems*
- MS: *Malaise,* myopathy, symptomatic weakness, fatigue
- Other: Skin rash, thrombophlebitis

Clinically important drug-drug interactions
- Risk of developing a hypercoagulable state if given concurrently with oral contraceptives, estrogens.

Drug-lab test interferences
- Elevation of serum potassium levels, especially with impaired renal function

■ Nursing Considerations

Assessment
- *History:* Allergy to aminocaproic acid, active intravascular clotting, cardiac disease, renal dysfunction; hematuria of upper urinary tract origin, hepatic dysfunction, lactation
- *Physical:* Skin—color, lesions; muscular strength; orientation, reflexes, affect; BP, P, baseine ECG, peripheral perfusion; liver evaluation, bowel sounds, output; clotting studies, CPK, urinalysis, liver and kidney function tests

Implementation
- Know that patient on oral therapy may have to take up to 10 tablets the first hour of treatment and tablets around the clock during treatment.
- Orient patient, and offer support if hallucinations, delirium, psychoses occur.
- Monitor patient for signs of clotting.

Drug-specific teaching points
- Know that the following side effects may occur: dizziness, weakness, headache, hallucinations (avoid driving or the use of dangerous machinery while you are on this drug; take special precautions to avoid injury); nausea, diarrhea, cramps (small, frequent meals may help); infertility problems (menstrual irregularities, dry ejaculation—these are drug effects and should go away when the drug is stopped); weakness, malaise (plan your day's activities, take rest periods as needed).
- Report severe headache, restlessness, muscle pain and weakness, blood in the urine.

☐ aminoglutethemide

*(a meen oh gloo **teth**' i mide)*
Cytadren

Pregnancy Category D

Drug classes
Antineoplastic
Hormone antagonist

Therapeutic actions
Inhibits the conversion of cholesterol to the steroid base necessary for producing adrenal glucocorticoids, mineralocorticoids, estrogens, and androgens.

Indications
- Suppression of adrenal function in selected patients with Cushing's syndrome—those awaiting surgery or in whom other treatment is not appropriate
- Unlabeled use: to produce medical adrenalectomy in patients with advanced

Adverse effects in *Italics* are most common; those in **Bold** are life-threatening.

breast cancer and in patients with metastatic prostate carcinoma

Contraindications/cautions
- Hypersensitivity to glutethemide or to aminoglutethemide; hypotension; hypothyroidism; pregnancy (causes fetal harm); lactation.

Dosage
Adult
- **Cushing's Disease:** 250 mg PO q6h; may be increased in increments of 250 mg/d at intervals of 1–2 wk to a total daily dose of 2 g.
- **Cancer:** 250 mg PO bid with hydrocortisone 60 mg hs, 20 mg on arising, and 20 mg at 2 PM for 2 weeks; then 250 mg PO qid and hydrocortisone 20 mg hs, 10 mg on arising, and 10 mg at 2 PM.

Pediatric: Safety and efficacy not established.

Pharmacokinetics

Route	Onset	Peak
Oral	3–5 d	36–72 h

Metabolism: $T_{1/2}$: 11–16 h
Distribution: Crosses placenta; passes into breast milk
Excretion: Urine

Adverse effects
- **CNS:** *Drowsiness*, dizziness, headache
- **GI:** *Nausea, anorexia*
- **CV:** *Hypotension*, tachycardia
- **Dermatologic:** *Morbiliform rash*, pruritus, urticaria
- **Endocrine:** Adrenal insufficiency, **hypothyroidism**, masculinization, and hirsutism
- **Other:** Myalgia, fever

Clinically important drug-drug interactions
- Decreased therapeutic effects of warfarin, anisindione, dicumarol when taken with aminoglutethemide • Possible decreased effectiveness of aminophylline, oxtriphylline, theophylline, medroxyprogesterone if taken with aminoglutethemide • Decreased effectiveness of aminoglutethemide if taken with dexamethasone, hydrocortisone

■ Nursing Considerations

Assessment
- *History:* Hypersensitivity to glutethemide or to aminoglutethemide; hypotension; hypothyroidism; pregnancy, lactation
- *Physical:* Body weight, skin condition, fever, neurologic status, reflexes, P, BP, thyroid function, renal and liver function test, cortisol levels

Implementation
- Begin therapy in a hospital setting until response has stabilized.
- Monitor patient carefully; if extreme drowsiness, severe skin rash, or excessively low cortisol levels occur, arrange to reduce dose or discontinue therapy as appropriate.
- Monitor patient for signs of hypothyroidism (slow pulse, lethargy, dry skin, thick tongue), and arrange for appropriate replacement therapy as needed.
- Arrange to discontinue drug if skin rash occurs and persists for longer than 5–8 d or if it becomes severe; it may be possible to reinstitute therapy at a lower dose once the rash has disappeared.
- Caution patient to avoid pregnancy if taking this drug; a method of birth control can be recommended.

Drug-specific teaching points
- Avoid driving or dangerous activities if dizziness, weakness occur.
- Know that the following side effects may occur: dizziness, lightheadedness (change position slowly, avoid any dangerous situations); loss of appetite, nausea your nutritional state needs to be maintained); headache (if this is severe, appropriate medication may be ordered).
- Use of a Medic-Alert system may be helpful to notify medical workers in an emergency situation that you are on this drug.
- Avoid pregnancy while taking this drug; appropriate contraceptive methods can be discussed.

Adverse effects in *Italics* are most common; those in **Bold** are life-threatening.

aminophylline

(am in off i lin)
theophylline ethylenediamine
Amoline, Phyllocontin, Truphylline

Pregnancy Category C

Drug classes
Bronchodilator
Xanthine

Therapeutic actions
Relaxes bronchial smooth muscle, causing bronchodilation and increasing vital capacity, which has been impaired by bronchospasm and air trapping; in higher concentrations, it also inhibits the release of slow-reacting substance of anaphylaxis (SRS-A) and histamine.

Indications
- Symptomatic relief or prevention of bronchial asthma and reversible bronchospasm associated with chronic bronchitis and emphysema
- Unlabeled uses: respiratory stimulant in Cheyne-Stokes respiration; treatment of apnea and bradycardia in premature babies

Contraindications/cautions
- Contraindicated in the presence of hypersensitivity to any xanthine or to ethylenediamine, peptic ulcer, active gastritis; rectal or colonic irritation or infection (use of the rectal preparations).
- Use caution in the presence of cardiac arrhythmias, acute myocardial injury, CHF, cor pulmonale, severe hypertension, severe hypoxemia, renal or hepatic disease, hyperthyroidism, alcoholism, labor, lactation.

Dosage
Individualize dosage, basing adjustments on clinical responses with monitoring of serum theophylline levels, if possible, to maintain levels in the therapeutic range of 10–20 μg/ml; base dosage on lean body mass; 127 mg aminophylline dihydrate = 100 mg theophylline anhydrous.

Adult

- ***Acute symptoms requiring rapid theophyllinization in patients not receiving theophylline:*** An initial loading dose is required, as indicated below:

Patient Group	Oral loading	Followed by	Maintenace
Young adult smokers	7.6 mg/kg	3.8 mg/kg q4h × three doses	3.8 mg/kg q6h
Nonsmoking adults who are otherwise healthy	7.6 mg/kg	3.8 mg/kg q6h × two doses	3.8 mg/kg q8h

- ***Chronic therapy:*** Usual range is 600–1,600 mg/d PO in three to four divided doses.
- ***Rectal:*** 500 mg q6–8h by rectal suppository or retention enema.

Pediatric: Use in children < 6 mo not recommended; use of timed-release products in children > 6 y not recommended. Children are very sensitive to CNS stimulant action of theophylline; use caution in younger children who cannot complain of minor side effects.

For acute symptoms requiring rapid theophyllinization in patients not receiving theophylline, to achieve a rapid effect, a loading dose is required. Dosage recommendations for oral therapy are as follows

Patient Group	Oral loading	Followed by	Maintenance
Children 6 mo–6 y	67.6 mg/kg	5.1 mg/kg q4h × three doses	5.1 mg/kg q6h
Children 9–16 y	7.6 mg/kg	3.8 mg/kg q4h × three doses	3.8 mg/kg q6h

- ***Chronic therapy:*** 12 mg/kg per 24 h PO; slow clinical titration of the oral preparations is preferred, with monitoring of clinical response and serum theophylline levels. In the absence of serum

- Report skin rash, severe drowsiness or dizziness, headache, severe nausea.

100 ■ aminophylline

levels, titrate up to the maximum dosage shown below, providing the dosage is tolerated.

Age	Maximum daily dose
<9 y	30.4 mg/kg/d
9–12 y	25.3 mg/kg/d
12–16 y	22.8 mg/kg/d
>16 y	16.5 mg/kg/d or 1,100 mg, whichever is less

Geriatric or impaired adult: Use caution, especially in elderly men and in patients with cor pulmonale, CHF, liver disease (half-life of aminophylline may be markedly prolonged in CHF, liver disease).

For acute symptoms requiring rapid theophyllinization in patients not receiving theophylline, a loading dose is necessary as follows

Patient Group	Oral loading	Followed by	Maintenance
Older patients & cor pulmonale	7.6 mg/kg	2.5 mg/kg q6h × 2 doses	2.5 mg/kg q8h
CHF	7.6 mg/kg	2.5 mg/kg q8h × 2 doses	1.3–2.5 mg/kg q12h

Pharmacokinetics

Route	Onset	Peak	Duration
Oral	1–6 h	4–6 h	6–8 h
IV	Immediate	30 min	4–8 h

Metabolism: Hepatic, $T_{1/2}$: 3–15 h
Distribution: Crosses placenta; passes into breast milk
Excretion: Urine

IV facts
Preparation: May be infused in 100–200 ml of 5% Dextrose Injection or 0.9% Sodium Chloride Injection.
Infusion: Do not exceed 25 mg/min infusion rate. Substitute oral therapy or IV therapy as soon as possible; administer maintenance infusions in a large volume to deliver the desired amount of drug each hour.

Adult: 6 mg/kg. For acute symptoms requiring rapid theophyllinization in patients receiving theophylline: a loading dose is required. Each 0.6 mg/kg IV administered as a loading dose will result in about a 1 μg/ml increase in serum theophylline. Ideally, defer loading dose until serum theophylline determination is made; otherwise, base loading dose on clinical judgment and the knowledge that 3.2 mg/kg aminophylline will increase serum theophylline levels by about 5 μg/ml and is unlikely to cause dangerous adverse effects if the patient is not experiencing theophylline toxicity before this dose. Aminophylline IV maintenance infusion rates (mg/kg per h) are given below:

Patient group	First 12 h	Beyond 12 h
Young Adult smokers	1	0.8
Nonsmoking adults, otherwise health	0.7	0.5

Pediatric: After an IV loading dose, the following maintenance rates (mg/kg per h) are recommended:

Patient group	First 12 h	Beyond 12 h
Children 6 mo–6 y	1.2	1
Children 9–16 y	1	0.8

Geriatric: After a loading dose, the following maintenance infusion rates (mg/kg per hour) are recommended:

Patient group	First 12 h	Beyond 12 h
Other patients, cor pulmonale	0.6	0.3
CHF, liver disease	0.5	0.1–0.2

Compatibility: Aminophylline is compatible with most IV solutions, but do not mix in solution with other drugs, including vitamins.

Adverse effects
- Serum theophylline levels < 20 μg/ml: adverse effects uncommon

Adverse effects in *Italics* are most common; those in **Bold** are life-threatening.

aminophylline ■ 101

- Serum theophylline levels > 20–25 μg/ml: nausea, vomiting, diarrhea, headache, insomnia, irritability (75% of patients)
- Serum theophylline levels > 30–35 μg/ml: hyperglycemia, hypotension, cardiac arrhythmias, tachycardia (> 10 μg/ml in premature newborns); **seizures, brain damage, death**
- CNS: Irritability (especially children); restlessness, dizziness, muscle twitching, convulsions, severe depression, stammering speech; abnormal behavior characterized by withdrawal, mutism and unresponsiveness alternating with hyperactive periods
- GI: Loss of appetite, hematemesis, epigastric pain, gastroesophageal reflux during sleep, increased SGOT
- CV: Palpitations, sinus tachycardia, ventricular tachycardia, life-threatening ventricular arrhythmias, circulatory failure
- Respiratory: Tachypnea, respiratory arrest
- GU: Proteinuria, increased excretion of renal tubular cells & RBCs; diuresis (dehydration), urinary retention in men with prostate enlargement
- Other: Fever, flushing, hyperglycemia, SIADH, rash

Clinically important drug-drug interactions

- Increased effects when given with cimetidine, erythromycin, troleandomycin, clindamycin, lincomycin, influenza virus vaccine, oral contraceptives • Possibly increased effects when given with thiabendazole, rifampin, allopurinol • Increased cardiac toxicity when given with halothane; increased likelihood of seizures when given with ketamine; increased likelihood of adverse GI effects when given with tetracyclines • Increased or decreased effects when given with furosemide, dextrothyroxine, leveothyroxine, liothyronine, liotrix, thyroglobulin, thyroid • Decreased effects in patients who are cigarette smokers (1–2 packs per day); theophylline dosage may need to be increased 50%–100% • Decreased effects when given with phenobarbital, aminoglutethimide • Increased effects, toxicity of sympathomimetics (especially ephedrine) when given with theophylline preparations • Decreased effects of phenytoin and theophylline preparations when given concomitantly • Decreased effects of lithium carbonate, nondepolarizing neuromuscular blockers given with theophylline preparations • Mutually antagonistic effects of beta-blockers and theophylline preparations

Clinically important drug-food interactions

- Elimination of theophylline preparations is increased by a low-carbohydrate, high-protein diet and by charcoal broiled beef • Elimination of theophylline preparations is decreased by a high-carbohydrate, low-protein diet • Food may alter bioavailability, absorption of timed-release theophylline preparations. These may rapidly release their contents in the presence of food and cause toxicity; timed-release forms should be taken on an empty stomach.

Drug-lab test interferences

- Interference with spectrophotometric determinations of serum theophylline levels by furosemide, phenylbutazone, probenecid, theobromine; coffee, tea, cola beverages, chocolate, acetaminophen cause falsely high values • Alteration in assays of uric acid, urinary catecholamines, plasma free fatty acids by theophylline preparations

■ Nursing Considerations

Assessment

- *History:* Hypersensitivity to any xanthine or to ethylenediamine, peptic ulcer, active gastritis, cardiac arrhythmias, acute myocardial injury, CHF, cor pulmonale, severe hypertension, severe hypoxemia, renal or hepatic disease, hyperthyroidism, alcoholism, labor, lactation, rectal or colonic irritation or infection (for use of aminophylline rectal preparations).
- *Physical:* Bowel sounds, normal output; P, auscultation, BP, perfusion, ECG; res-

Adverse effects in *Italics* are most common; those in **Bold** are life-threatening.

piratory rate, adventitious sounds; frequency of urination, voiding, normal output pattern, urinalysis, renal function tests; liver palpation, liver function tests; thyroid function tests; skin color, texture, lesions; reflexes, bilateral grip strength, affect, EEG

Implementation
- Administer to pregnant patients only when clearly needed — tachycardia, jitteriness, and withdrawal apnea have been observed in neonates whose mothers received xanthines up until delivery.
- Caution patient not to chew or crush enteric-coated timed-release preparations.
- Give immediate-release, liquid dosage forms with food if GI effects occur.
- Do not give timed-release preparations with food; these should be given on an empty stomach 1 h before or 2 h after meals.
- Maintain adequate hydration.
- Monitor results of serum theophylline level determinations carefully, and arrange for reduced dosage if serum levels exceed therapeutic range of 10–20 μg/ml.
- Arrange to have serum samples to determine peak theophylline concentration drawn 15–30 min after an IV loading dose.
- Monitor patient carefully for clinical signs of adverse effects, particularly if serum theophylline levels are not available.
- Maintain diazepam on standby to treat seizures.

Drug-specific teaching points
- Take this drug exactly as prescribed; if a timed-release product is prescribed, take this drug on an empty stomach, 1 h before or 2 h after meals.
- Do not to chew or crush timed-release preparations.
- Administer rectal solution or suppositories after emptying the rectum.
- Know that it may be necessary to take this drug around the clock for adequate control of asthma attacks.
- Avoid excessive intake of coffee, tea, cocoa, cola beverages, chocolate.
- Know that smoking cigarettes or other tobacco products may markedly influence the effects of theophylline; it is preferable not to smoke while taking this drug; notify the care provider if smoking habits change while taking this drug.
- Be aware that frequent blood tests may be necessary to monitor the effect of this drug and to ensure safe and effective dosage; keep all appointments for blood tests and other monitoring.
- Know that the following side effects may occur while taking this drug: nausea, loss of appetite (taking this drug with food may help if taking the immediate-release or liquid dosage forms); difficulty sleeping, depression, emotional lability (it may be reassuring to know that these are drug effects).
- Report nausea, vomiting, severe GI pain, restlessness, convulsions, irregular heartbeat.

❒ amiodarone hydrochloride

(a mee o' da rone)
Cordarone

Pregnancy Category C

Drug classes
Antiarrhythmic
Adrenergic blocker (not used as sympatholytic agent)

Therapeutic actions
Type III antiarrhythmic: acts directly on cardiac cell membrane; prolongs repolarization and refractory period; increases ventricular fibrillation threshold; acts on peripheral smooth muscle to decrease peripheral resistance

Indications
- Only for treatment of the following documented life-threatening recurrent ventricular arrhythmias that do not respond to other antiarrhythmics or when alternative agents are not tolerated: recurrent

amiodarone hydrochloride

ventricular fibrillation, recurrent hemodynamically unstable ventricular tachycardia. Serious and even fatal toxicity has been reported with this drug; use alternative agents first; very closely monitor patient receiving this drug.
- Unlabeled uses: treatment of refractory sustained or paroxysmal atrial fibrillation and paroxysmal supraventricular tachycardia; treatment of symptomatic atrial flutter; may produce benefit in left ventricular ejection fraction, exercise tolerance, and ventricular arrhythmias in patients with CHF

Contraindications/cautions
- Hypersensitivity to amiodarone, sinus node dysfunction, heart block, severe bradycardia, hypokalemia, lactation.

Dosage
Careful patient assessment and evaluation with continual monitoring of cardiac response are necessary for titrating the dosage for each patient. Therapy should begin in the hospital with continual monitoring and emergency equipment on standby. The following is a guide to usual dosage.
Adult: Loading dose: 800–1,600 mg/d PO in divided doses, for 1–3 wk; reduce dose to 600–800 mg/d in divided doses for 1 mo; if rhythm is stable, reduce dose to 400 mg/d in one to two divided doses for maintenance dose. Titrate to the lowest possible dose to limit side effects.
Pediatric: Safety and efficacy not established.

Pharmacokinetics

Route	Onset	Peak	Duration
Oral	2–3 d	3–7 h	6–8 h

Metabolism: Hepatic, $T_{1/2}$: 2.5–10 d, then 40–55 d
Distribution: Crosses placenta; passes into breast milk
Excretion: Bile and feces

Adverse effects
- CNS: *Malaise, fatigue, dizziness, tremors, ataxia,* paresthesias, lack of coordination
- GI: *Nausea, vomiting, anorexia, constipation, abnormal liver function tests,* **liver toxicity**
- CV: *Cardiac arrhythmias,* congestive heart failure, **cardiac arrest**
- Respiratory: *Pulmonary toxicity*—pneumonitis, infiltrates (shortness of breath, cough, rales, wheezes)
- Endocrine: *Hypothyroidism* or *hyperthyroidism*
- EENT: *Corneal microdeposits* (photophobia, dry eyes, halos, blurred vision)
- Other: *Photosensitivity*

Clinically important drug-drug interactions
- Increased digitalis toxicity if taken with digoxin • Increased quinidine toxicity if taken with quinidine • Increased procainamide toxicity if taken with procainamide • Increased flecainide toxicity if amiodarone is given concurrently • Increased phenytoin toxicity if taken with phenytoin, ethotoin, mephenytoin • Increased bleeding tendencies if taken with warfarin • Potential sinus arrest and heart block if taken with β-blockers, calcium channel-blockers

Drug-lab test interferences
- Increased T_4 levels, increased serum reverse T_3 levels

■ Nursing Considerations

Assessment
- *History:* Hypersensitivity to amiodarone, sinus node dysfunction, heart block, severe bradycardia, hypokalemia, lactation
- *Physical:* Skin—color, lesions; reflexes, gait, eye exam; P, BP, auscultation, continuous ECG monitoring; respiratory rate, adventitious sounds, baseline chest x-ray; liver evaluation; liver function tests, serum electrolytes, T_4 and T_3

Implementation
- Monitor patient's cardiac rhythm continuously.
- Monitor patient for an extended period when dosage adjustments are made.
- Monitor for safe and effective serum levels (0.5–2.5 μg/ml).

Adverse effects in *Italics* are most common; those in **Bold** are life-threatening.

amitriptyline hydrochloride

- Be aware that doses of digoxin, quinidine, procainamide, phenytoin, and warfarin may need to be reduced one-third to one-half when amiodarone is started.
- Administer drug with meals to decrease GI problems.
- Arrange for regular ophthalmologic exam.
- Arrange for periodic chest x-ray to evaluate pulmonary status (every 3–6 mo).
- Arrange for regular periodic blood tests for liver enzymes, thyroid hormone levels.

Drug-specific teaching points

- Be aware that your drug dosage will be changed in relation to response of arrhythmias; you will need to be hospitalized during initiation of drug therapy; you will be closely monitored when dosage is changed.
- Know that the following side effects may occur: changes in vision (halos, dry eyes, sensitivity to light; wear sunglasses, monitor light exposure); nausea, vomiting, loss of appetite (take the drug with meals; small, frequent meals may help); sensitivity to the sun (use a sunscreen or protective clothing when outdoors); constipation (a laxative may be ordered if this becomes a problem); tremors, twitching, dizziness, loss of coordination (do not drive, operate dangerous machinery, or undertake tasks that require coordination until you know your response to the drug or until your body adjusts to the drug and these side effects are lessened).
- Arrange to have regular medical follow-up, which may include monitoring of cardiac rhythm, chest x-ray, eye exam, blood tests.
- Report unusual bleeding or bruising; fever, chills; intolerance to heat or cold; shortness of breath, difficulty breathing, cough; swelling of ankles or fingers; palpitations.

☐ amitriptyline hydrochloride

(a mee trip' ti leen)

Elavil, Endep, Enovil, Levate (CAN), Meravil (CAN), Novotriptyn (CAN)

Pregnancy Category C

Drug classes
Tricyclic antidepressant (TCA; tertiary amine)

Therapeutic actions
Mechanism of action unknown; TCAs act to inhibit the reuptake of the neurotransmitters norepinephrine and serotonin, leading to an increase in their effects; anticholinergic at CNS and peripheral receptors; sedative.

Indications

- Relief of symptoms of depression (endogenous depression most responsive); sedative effects may be helpful in patients whose depression is associated with anxiety and sleep disturbance.
- Unlabeled uses: control of chronic pain (eg, intractable pain of cancer, peripheral neuropathies, postherpetic neuralgia, tic douloureux, central pain syndromes); prevention of onset of cluster and migraine headaches; treatment of pathologic weeping and laughing secondary to forebrain disease (due to multiple sclerosis)

Contraindications/cautions

- Contraindicated in the presence of hypersensitivity to any tricyclic drug; concomitant therapy with an MAO inhibitor; recent MI; myelography within previous 24 h or scheduled within 48 h; lactation.
- Use caution in the presence of electroshock therapy; preexisting cardiovascular disorders (severe coronary heart disease, progressive heart failure, angina pectoris, paroxysmal tachycardia); angle-closure glaucoma, increased intraocular pressure, urinary retention, ureteral or urethral spasm; seizure disorders; hyperthyroidism; impaired hepatic, renal function; psychiatric patients (schizophrenic or paranoid patients may exhibit a worsening of psychosis with TCA therapy); manic-depressive patients; elective surgery (TCAs should be discontinued as long as possible before surgery).

amitriptyline hydrochloride ■ 105

Dosage
Adult
- **Depression**
  - *Hospitalized patients:* Initially, 100 mg/d PO in divided doses: gradually increase to 200–300 mg/d as required. May be given IM 20–30 mg qid, initially only in patients unable or unwilling to take drug PO. Replace with oral medication as soon as possible.
  - *Outpatients:* Initially, 75 mg/d PO, in divided doses; may increase to 150 mg/d. Increases should be made in late afternoon or at bedtime. Total daily dosage may be administered at bedtime. Initiate single daily dose therapy with 50–100 mg hs; increase by 25–50 mg as necessary to a total of 150 mg/d. Maintenance dose is 40–100 mg/d, which may be given as a single bedtime dose. After satisfactory response, reduce to lowest effective dosage. Continue therapy for 3 mo or longer to lessen possibility of relapse.
- **Chronic pain:** 75–150 mg/d PO
- **Prevention of cluster/migraine headaches:** 50–150 mg/d PO.
- **Prevention of weeping in MS patients with forebrain disease:** 25–75 mg PO.

Pediatric: Not recommended in children < 12 y.

Pharmacokinetics

Route	Onset	Peak	Duration
Oral	Varies	2–4 h	20–4 wk

Metabolism: Hepatic, $T_{1/2}$: 10–50 h
Distribution: Crosses placenta; passes into breast milk
Excretion: Urine

Adverse effects
- **CNS:** *Sedation and anticholinergic (atropine-like) effects; confusion* (especially in elderly), *disturbed concentration,* hallucinations, disorientation, decreased memory, feelings of unreality, delusions, anxiety, nervousness, restlessness, agitation, panic, insomnia, nightmares, hypomania, mania, exacerbation of psychosis, drowsiness, weakness, fatigue, headache, numbness, tingling, paresthesias of extremities, incoordination, motor hyperactivity, akathisia, ataxia, tremors, peripheral neuropathy, extrapyramidal symptoms, seizures, speech blockage, dysarthria, tinnitus, altered EEG
- **GI:** *Dry mouth, constipation*, paralytic ileus, *nausea*, vomiting, anorexia, epigastric distress, diarrhea, flatulence, dysphagia, peculiar taste, increased salivation, stomatitis, glossitis, parotid swelling, abdominal cramps, black tongue, hepatitis, jaundice (rare), elevated transaminase, altered alkaline phosphatase
- **CV:** *Orthostatic hypotension*, hypertension, syncope, tachycardia, palpitations, MI, arrhythmias, **heart block**, precipitation of CHF, **stroke**
- **Hematologic:** **Bone marrow depression, including agranulocytosis**; eosinophila, purpura, thrombocytopenia, leukopenia
- **GU:** Urinary retention, delayed micturition, dilation of the urinary tract, gynecomastia, testicular swelling in men; breast enlargement, menstrual irregularity and galactorrhea in women; increased or decreased libido; impotence
- **Endocrine:** Elevated or depressed blood sugar, elevated prolactin levels, inappropriate ADH secretion
- **Hypersensitivity:** Skin rash, pruritus, vasculitis, petechiae, photosensitization, edema (generalized or of face and tongue), drug fever
- **Withdrawal:** Symptoms on abrupt discontinuation of prolonged therapy: nausea, headache, vertigo, nightmares, malaise
- **Other:** Nasal congestion, excessive appetite, weight gain or loss; sweating, alopecia, lacrimation, hyperthermia, flushing, chills

Clinically important drug-drug interactions
- Increased TCA levels and pharmacologic (especially anticholinergic) effects when given with cimetidine, fluoxetine • In-

Adverse effects in *Italics* are most common; those in **Bold** are life-threatening.

creased TCA levels when given with methylphenidate, phenothiazines, oral contraceptives, disulfiram • Hyperpyretic crises, severe convulsions, hypertensive episodes and deaths when MAO inhibitors, furazolidone are given with TCAs • Increased antidepressant response and cardiac arrhythmias when given with thyroid medication. • Increased or decreased effects of TCAs given with estrogens • Delirium when TCAs are given with disulfiram • Sympathetic hyperactivity, sinus tachycardia, hypertension, agitation when TCAs are given with levodopa • Increased biotransformation of TCAs in patients who smoke cigarettes • Increased sympathomimetic (especially α-adrenergic) effects of direct-acting sympathomimetic drugs (norepinephrine, epinephrine) when given with TCAs • Increased anticholinergic effects of anticholinergic drugs (including anticholinergic antiparkisonism drugs) when given with TCAs • Increased response (especially CNS depression) to barbiturates • Increased effects of dicumarol when given with TCAs • Decreased antihypertensive effect of guanethidine, clonidine, other antihypertensives when given with TCAs • Decreased effects of indirect-acting sympathomimetic drugs (ephedrine) when given with TCAs

■ Nursing Considerations

Assessment
- *History:* Hypersensitivity to any tricyclic drug; concomitant therapy with an MAO inhibitor; recent MI; myelography within previous 24 h or scheduled within 48 h; lactation; electroshock therapy; preexisting cardiovascular disorders; angle-closure glaucoma, increased intraocular pressure, urinary retention, ureteral or urethral spasm; seizure disorders; hyperthyroidism; impaired hepatic, renal function; psychiatric patients; manic-depressive patients; elective surgery
- *Physical:* Body weight; temperature; skin—color, lesions; orientation, affect, reflexes, vision and hearing; P, BP, orthostatic BP, perfusion; bowel sounds, normal output, liver evaluation; urine flow, normal output; usual sexual function, frequency of menses, breast and scrotal exam; liver function tests, urinalysis, CBC, ECG

Implementation
- Ensure that depressed and potentially suicidal patients have access to only limited quantities of the drug.
- Administer IM only when oral therapy is impossible.
- Do not administer IV.
- Administer major portion of dose at bedtime if drowsiness, severe anticholinergic effects occur (note that the elderly may not tolerate single daily dose therapy).
- Arrange to reduce dosage if minor side effects develop; arrange to discontinue the drug if serious side effects occur.
- Arrange for CBC if patient develops fever, sore throat, or other sign of infection during therapy.

Drug-specific teaching points
- Take drug exactly as prescribed; do not stop taking this drug abruptly or without consulting the physician or nurse.
- Avoid using alcohol, other sleep-inducing drugs, OTC drugs while on this drug.
- Avoid prolonged exposure to sunlight or sunlamps; use a sunscreen or protective garments if long exposure to sunlight is unavoidable.
- Know that the following side effects may occur: headache, dizziness, drowsiness, weakness, blurred vision (these effects are reversible; safety measures may need to be taken if these become severe, and you should avoid driving an automobile or performing tasks that require alertness while these persist); nausea, vomiting, loss of appetite, dry mouth (small frequent meals, frequent mouth care and sucking sugarless candies may help); nightmares, inability to concentrate, confusion; changes in sexual function.
- Report dry mouth, difficulty in urination, excessive sedation.

❑ amlodipine

(am loe' di peen)

Norvasc

Pregnancy Category C

amlodipine ■ 107

Drug classes
Calcium channel-blocker
Antianginal drug
Antihypertensive

Therapeutic actions
Inhibits the movement of calcium ions across the membranes of cardiac and arterial muscle cells; inhibits transmembrane calcium flow, which results in the depression of impulse formation in specialized cardiac pacemaker cells, slowing of the velocity of conduction of the cardiac impulse, depression of myocardial contractility, and dilation of coronary arteries and arterioles and peripheral arterioles; these effects lead to decreased cardiac work, decreased cardiac energy consumption, and in patients with vasospastic (Prinzmetal's) angina, increased delivery of oxygen to cardiac cells.

Indications
- Angina pectoris due to coronary artery spasm (Prinzmetal's variant angina)
- Chronic stable angina, alone or in combination with other agents
- Essential hypertension, alone or in combination with other antihypertensives

Contraindications/cautions
- Allergy to diltiazem, impaired hepatic or renal function, sick sinus syndrome, heart block (second or third degree), lactation.

Dosage
Adult: Initially 5 mg PO qd; dosage may be gradually increased over 10–14 d to a maximum dose of 10 mg PO qd.
Pediatric: Safety and efficacy not established.
Geriatric or hepatic impairment: Initially, 2.5 mg PO qd; dosage may be gradually titrated over 7–14 d based on clinical assessment

Pharmacokinetics

Route	Onset	Peak
Oral	Unknown	6–12 h

Metabolism: Hepatic, $T_{1/2}$: 30–50 h
Distribution: Crosses placenta; passes into breast milk
Excretion: Urine

Adverse effects
- **CNS:** *Dizziness, lightheadedness, headache,* asthenia, *fatigue, lethargy*
- **GI:** *Nausea,* abdominal discomfort
- **CV:** *Peripheral edema,* arrhythmias
- **Dermatologic:** *Flushing,* rash

Clinically important drug-drug interactions
- Possible increased serum levels and toxicity of cyclosporine if taken concurrently

■ Nursing Considerations

Assessment
- *History:* Allergy to diltiazem, impaired hepatic or renal function, sick sinus syndrome, heart block, lactation
- *Physical:* Skin—lesions, color, edema; P, BP, baseline ECG, peripheral perfusion, auscultation, R, adventitious sounds; liver evaluation, GI normal output; liver and renal function tests, urinalysis

Implementation
- Monitor patient carefully (BP, cardiac rhythm, and output) while drug is being titrated to therapeutic dose.
- Monitor BP very carefully if patient is also on nitrates.
- Monitor cardiac rhythm regularly during stabilization of dosage and periodically during long-term therapy.
- Administer drug without regard to meals.

Drug-specific teaching points
- Take this drug with meals if upset stomach occurs.
- Know that the following may occur as a result of drug therapy: nausea, vomiting (small, frequent meals may help); headache (monitor the lighting, noise, and temperature; medication may be ordered if this becomes severe).
- Report irregular heart beat, shortness of breath, swelling of the hands or feet, pronounced dizziness, constipation.

Adverse effects in *Italics* are most common; those in **Bold** are life-threatening.

ammonia spirit, aromatic

(ah mo' nee a)

Pregnancy Category C

Drug classes
Respiratory and circulatory stimulant

Therapeutic actions
Stimulates the respiratory and cardiovascular centers of the medulla by causing irritation of the sensory receptors in nasal membranes, esophageal mucosa, and fundus of the stomach.

Indications
- Prevention and treatment of fainting (smelling salts)

Contraindications/cautions
- Contraindicated in the presence of severe hypertension, lactation.

Dosage
Inhale vapors as required.

Pharmacokinetics
Metabolism: Lung and liver, $T_{1/2}$: unknown
Distribution: Crosses placenta; may pass into breast milk
Excretion: Unknown

Adverse effects
- **CV:** Hypertension, tachycardia
- **Local:** Nasal irritation
- **GI:** Nausea, vomiting

■ Nursing Considerations
Assessment
- *History:* Blood dyscrasias, recent infection
- *Physical:* Status of mucous membranes; BP, P

Implementation
- Wrap glass vial in gauze or cloth; break between fingers.
- Store vials out of light in tightly closed container.
- Evaluate patient if frequent fainting spells occur; refer to appropriate medical consultation.

Drug-specific teaching points
- Know that nausea, nasal irritation, headache may occur.
- Report frequent use of drug, frequent fainting spells, severe headache.

ammonium chloride

(ah mo' nee um)

Pregnancy Category C

Drug classes
Electrolyte
Urinary acidifier

Therapeutic actions
Converted to urea in the liver; liberated hydrogen and chloride ions in blood and extracellular fluid lower the pH and correct alkalosis; lowers the urinary pH, producing an acidic urine that changes the excretion rate of many metabolites and drugs.

Indications
- Treatment of hypochloremic states and metabolic alkalosis
- Acidification of urine

Contraindications/cautions
- Renal function impairment; hepatic impairment; metabolic alkalosis due to vomiting of hydrochloric acid when it is accompanied by loss of sodium

Dosage
Adult/Pediatric
- **IV:** Dosage is determined by patient's condition and tolerance; monitor dosage rate and amount by repeated serum bicarbonate determinations.

Adult
- **PO:** 4–12 g/d PO divided q4–6h for no longer than 6 d

Pediatric
- **PO:** 75 mg/kg per day PO in four divided doses for no longer than 6 d

Adverse effects in *Italics* are most common; those in **Bold** are life-threatening.

Pharmacokinetics

Route	Onset	Peak
IV	Rapid	1–3 h
PO	Varies	3–6 h

Metabolism: Hepatic
Distribution: Crosses placenta; passes into breast milk
Excretion: Urine

IV facts

Preparation: Add contents of one to two vials (100–200 mEq) to 500 or 1,000 ml isotonic (0.9%) Sodium Chloride Injection. Concentration should not exceed 1%–2% ammonium chloride. Avoid excessive heat; protect from freezing. If crystals do appear, warm the solution to room temperature in a water bath prior to use.
Infusion: Do not exceed rate of 5 ml/min in adults (1,000 ml infused over 3 h). Infuse slowly.
Compatibilities: Do not mix with codeine, levorphanol, methadone, nitrofurantoin, warfarin.

Adverse effects

- **GI:** *Nausea*, vomiting, gastric irritation (oral); **severe hepatic impairment**
- **Metabolic:** Metabolic acidosis, hypervolemia, ammonia toxicity—pallor, sweating, irregular breathing, retching, bradycarida, arrhythmias, twitching, convulsion, coma
- **Local:** *Pain or irritation at injection site*, fever, venous thrombosis, phlebitis, extravasation (IV)

Clinically important drug-drug interactions

- Decreased therapeutic levels due to increased elimination of amphetamine, methamphetamine, dextroamphetamine, ephedrine, pseudoephedrine, methadone, mexiletine when taken with ammonium chloride • Increased effects of chlorporpamide when taken with ammonium chloride

■ Nursing Considerations

Assessment

- *History:* Renal or hepatic impairment; metabolic alkalosis due to vomiting of hydrochloric acid when it is accompanied by loss of sodium
- *Physical:* P, BP; skin—color, texture; body temperature; injection site evaluation; liver evaluation; renal and liver function tests, serum bicarbonate, urinalysis

Implementation

- Infuse by IV route slowly to avoid local irritation; check infusion site frequently to monitor for local reaction.
- Monitor patient receiving IV doses for possible fluid overload.
- Monitor patient for signs of acidosis (increased R, restlessness, sweating, increased blood pH); decrease infusion as appropriate. Maintain sodium bicarbonate or sodium lactate on standby for overdose situations.

Drug-specific teaching points

- Do not take oral drug for longer than 6 d.
- Know that you will need frequent monitoring of blood tests while receiving the IV drug to determine the appropriate dosage and rate for the drug.
- Report pain or irritation at IV injection site; confusion, restlessness, sweating, headache; severe GI upset, fever, chills, changes in stool or urine color (oral drug)

☐ amobarbital

*(am oh **bar**' bi tal)*
amobarbital sodium,
amylobarbitone

Amytal Sodium, Novamobarb (CAN)

Pregnancy Category D
C-II controlled substance

Drug classes

Barbiturate (intermediate acting)
Sedative
Hypnotic
Anticonvulsant

Adverse effects in *Italics* are most common; those in **Bold** are life-threatening.

Therapeutic actions
General CNS depressant; barbiturates act on the ascending reticular activating system, depress the cerebral cortex, alter cerebellar function, depress motor output, and can produce excitation, sedation, hypnosis, anesthesia and deep coma; at anesthetic doses, has anticonvulsant activity.

Indications
- Oral: sedation and relief of anxiety; hypnotic effects; preanesthetic medication; control of convulsions
- Parenteral: management of catatonic and negativistic reactions, manic reactions and epileptiform seizures; useful in narcoanalysis and narcotherapy; diagnostic aid in schizophrenia; control of convulsive seizures, such as those due to chorea, eclampsia, meningitis, tetanus, procaine or cocaine reactions, poisoning from drugs, such as strychnine or picrotoxin.

Contraindications/cautions
- Contraindicated in the presence of hypersensitivity to barbiturates; manifest or latent porphyria; marked liver impairment; nephritis; severe respiratory distress, respiratory disease with dyspnea, obstruction, or cor pulmonale; previous addiction to sedative-hypnotic drugs; pregnancy.
- Use caution in the presence of acute or chronic pain (drug may cause paradoxical excitement or mask important symptoms); seizure disorders (abrupt discontinuation of daily doses of drug can result in status epilepticus); lactation; fever, hyperthyroidism, diabetes mellitus, severe anemia, pulmonary or cardiac disease, status asthmaticus, shock, uremia; impaired liver or kidney function, debilitation.

Dosage
Adult
- **Oral:** Usual dosage range is 15–120 mg bid–qid
- *Daytime sedation:* 30–50 mg bid–tid PO
- *Hypnotic:* 100–200 mg PO
- *Insomnia:* 65–200 mg (as sodium) at bedtime, PO
- **IM:** Usual dose is 65–500 mg; maximum dose should not exceed 500 mg: Do not give more than 5 ml of any concentration in one injection; solutions of 20% can be used to minimize volume.
- *Preanesthetic sedation:* 200 mg (as sodium) 1–2 h before surgery, IM
- *Labor:* Initial dose is 200–400 mg (as sodium); additional doses of 200–400 mg may be given at 1- to 3-h intervals for a total dose of not more than 1 g, IM
- *IV:* Same dose as IM. Do not exceed a rate of 1 ml/min. Administration of the 10% solution may cause serious respiratory depression.

Pediatric: Use caution. Barbiturates may produce irritability, excitability, inappropriate tearfulness, and aggression. Base dosage on body weight, age, and response. Because of higher metabolic rates, children tolerate comparatively higher doses; ordinarily, 65–500 mg may be given to a child 6-12 y old. Administer by slow IV injection, and monitor response carefully.

Geriatric patients or those with debilitating disease: Reduce dosage and monitor closely; may produce excitement, depression, confusion.

Pharmacokinetics

Route	Onset	Peak	Duration
Oral	45–60 min		6–8 h
IV	5 min	15 min	3–6 h

Metabolism: Hepatic, $T_{1/2}$: 16–40 h
Distribution: Crosses placenta; passes into breast milk
Excretion: Urine

IV facts
Preparation: Add Sterile Water for Injection to the vial, and rotate to facilitate solution of the powder. Do not shake the vial. Do not use a solution that is not absolutely clear after 5 min. Inject contents within 30 min of opening the vial. Amobarbital is unstable on exposure to air.

Infusion: Infuse slowly. Ensure that amobarbital is not given intra-arterially; can

cause severe spasm. Do not exceed rate of 1 ml/min. Monitor patient continually during infusion.
Compatibilities: Incompatible with many other drugs in solution; **do not mix in solution with any drugs.**

Adverse effects
- CNS: *Somnolence, agitation, confusion, hyperkinesia, ataxia, vertigo, CNS depression, nightmares, lethargy, residual sedation (hangover),* paradoxical excitement, nervousness, psychiatric disturbance, hallucinations, insomnia, anxiety, dizziness, thinking abnormality
- GI: *Nausea, vomiting, constipation, diarrhea,* epigastric pain
- CV: Bradycardia, hypotension, syncope
- Respiratory: *Hypoventilation,* **apnea, respiratory depression**, laryngospasm, bronchospasm, circulatory collapse
- Hypersensitivity: Skin rashes, angioneurotic edema, serum sickness, morbiliform rash, urticaria; rarely, exfoliative dermatitis, **Stevens-Johnson syndrome, sometimes fatal**
- Injection site: *Local pain,* tissue necrosis, gangrene; arterial spasm with inadvertent intra-arterial injection; thrombophlebitis; permanent neurologic deficit if injected near a nerve
- Other: *Tolerance, psychological and physical dependence*; withdrawal syndrome, sometimes fatal

Clinically important drug-drug interactions
- Increased CNS depression when taken with alcohol, other CNS depressants, phenothiazines, antihistamines, tranquilizers • Increased blood levels and pharmacologic effects of barbiturates when given with MAO inhibitors • Increased renal toxicity if taken with methoxyflurane • Decreased effects of the following drugs given with barbiturates: oral anticoagulants, digitoxin, tricyclic antidepressants, corticosteroids, oral contraceptives and estrogens, acetaminophen, metronidazole, phenmetrazine, carbamazepine, beta blockers, griseofulvin, phenylbutazones, theophyllines, quinidine, doxycycline • Altered effectiveness of phenytoin when given with barbiturates

■ Nursing Considerations

Assessment
- *History:* Hypersensitivity to barbiturates; manifest or latent porphyria; marked liver impairment; nephritis; severe respiratory distress, respiratory disease with dyspnea, obstruction or cor pulmonale; previous addiction to sedative-hypnotic drugs; acute or chronic pain; seizure disorders; lactation; fever, hyperthyroidism, diabetes mellitus, severe anemia, pulmonary or cardiac disease, status asthmaticus, shock, uremia; debilitation.
- *Physical:* Body weight; body temperature; skin—color, lesions; orientation, affect, reflexes; P, BP, orthostatic BP; respiratory rate, adventitious sounds; bowel sounds, normal output, liver evaluation; liver and kidney function tests, blood and urine glucose, BUN.

Implementation
- Monitor patient responses, blood levels (as appropriate) if any of the above interacting drugs are given with amobarbital; suggest alternate means of contraception to women on oral contraceptives for whom amobarbital is prescribed.
- Do not administer intra-arterially (may produce arteriospasm, thrombosis, gangrene).
- Administer IM doses deep in a muscle mass.
- Monitor injection sites carefully for irritation, extravasation with IV use (solutions are alkaline and very irritating to the tissues).
- Monitor P, BP, respiration carefully during IV administration.
- Have resuscitative facilities on standby in case of respiratory depression, hypersensitivity reaction.
- Arrange to taper dosage gradually after repeated use, especially in epileptic patients.

Adverse effects in *Italics* are most common; those in **Bold** are life-threatening.

Drug-specific teaching points

- Incorporate teaching about the drug with the general teaching about the procedure for patients receiving this drug as preanesthetic medication or during labor; include the following:
- Know that this drug will make you drowsy and less anxious.
- Do not try to get up after you have received this drug (request assistance if you feel you must sit up or move around for any reason).

Oral Use

- Know that this drug is habit forming; its effectiveness in facilitating sleep disappears after a short time.
- Do not to take this drug longer than 2 wk (for insomnia), and do not increase the dosage without consulting the physician.
- Consult care provider if the drug appears to be ineffective; do not increase the dose to get more effect.
- Avoid the use of alcohol, sleep-inducing, or OTC drugs while on this drug because these could cause dangerous effects.
- Use contraception other than oral contraceptives while on amobarbital; you should not become pregnant while taking this drug.
- Know that the following side effects may occur: drowsiness, dizziness, "hangover," impaired thinking (these effects may become less pronounced after a few days; avoid driving a car or engaging in dangerous activities if these occur); GI upset (taking the drug with food may help); dreams, nightmares, difficulty concentrating, fatigue, nervousness (it may help to know that these are effects of the drug that will go away when the drug is discontinued).
- Report severe dizziness, weakness, drowsiness that persists; rash or skin lesions; pregnancy.

☐ amoxapine

(a mox' a peen)
Asendin

Pregnancy Category C

Drug classes
Tricyclic antidepressant (TCA)
Antianxiety drug

Therapeutic actions
Mechanism of action unknown; TCAs inhibit the reuptake of the neurotransmitters norepinephrine and serotonin, leading to an increase in their effects; anticholinergic at CNS and peripheral receptors; sedative.

Indications
- Relief of symptoms of depression (endogenous depression most responsive)
- Antianxiety drug

Contraindications/cautions
- Contraindicated in the presence of hypersensitivity to any tricyclic drug; concomitant therapy with an MAO inhibitor; recent MI; myelography within previous 24 h or scheduled within 48 h; lactation.
- Use caution in the presence of electroshock therapy; preexisting cardiovascular disorders (severe coronary heart disease, progressive heart failure, angina pectoris, paroxysmal tachycardia); angle-closure glaucoma, increased intraocular pressure, urinary retention, ureteral or urethral spasm; seizure disorders; hyperthyroidism; impaired hepatic, renal function; psychiatric patients (schizophrenic or paranoid patients may exhibit a worsening of psychosis with TCA therapy); manic-depressive patients; elective surgery (TCAs should be discontinued as long as possible before surgery).

Dosage
Adult: Initially 50 mg PO bid–tid; gradually increase dosage to 100 mg bid–tid by end of first week if needed and tolerated; increase above 300 mg/d only if this dosage ineffective for at least 2 wk. Hospitalized patients refractory to antidepressant therapy and with no history of convulsive seizures may be given up to 600 mg/d in divided doses; after effective dosage is established, drug may be given in single bedtime dose (up to 300 mg).

Pediatric: Not recommended in children < 16 y.
Geriatric: Initially, 25 mg bid–tid; if tolerated, dosage may be increased by end of first week to 50 mg bid–tid. For many elderly patients, 100–150 mg/d may be adequate; some may require up to 300 mg/d.

Pharmacokinetics

Route	Onset	Peak	Duration
Oral	Varies	2–4 h	2–4 wk

Metabolism: Hepatic, $T_{1/2}$: 8–30 h
Distribution: Crosses placenta; passes into breast milk
Excretion: Urine

Adverse effects

- CNS: *Sedation and anticholinergic (atropine-like) effects*; *confusion* (especially in elderly), *disturbed concentration*, hallucinations, disorientation, decreased memory, feelings of unreality, delusions, anxiety, nervousness, restlessness, agitation, panic, insomnia, nightmares, hypomania, mania, exacerbation of psychosis, drowsiness, weakness, fatigue, headache, numbness, tingling, paresthesias of extremities, incoordination, motor hyperactivity, akathisia, ataxia, tremors, peripheral neuropathy, extrapyramidal symptoms, seizures, speech blockage, dysarthria, tinnitus, altered EEG
- GI: *Dry mouth, constipation*, paralytic ileus, *nausea*, vomiting, anorexia, epigastric distress, diarrhea, flatulence, dysphagia, peculiar taste, increased salivation, stomatitis, glossitis, parotid swelling, abdominal cramps, black tongue, hepatitis, jaundice (rare); elevated transaminase, altered alkaline phosphatase
- CV: *Orthostatic hypotension*, hypertension, syncope, tachycardia, palpitations, MI, arrhythmias, heart block, precipitation of CHF, stroke
- Hematologic:Bone marrow depression, including agranulocytosis; eosinophila, purpura, thrombocytopenia, leukopenia
- GU: Urinary retention, delayed micturition, dilation of the urinary tract, gynecomastia, testicular swelling in men; breast enlargement, menstrual irregularity, and galactorrhea in women; increased or decreased libido; impotence
- Endocrine: Elevated or depressed blood sugar, elevated prolactin levels, inappropriate ADH secretion
- **Hypersensitivity**: Skin rash, pruritus, vasculitis, petechiae, photosensitization, edema (generalized or of face and tongue), drug fever
- **Withdrawal**: Symptoms on abrupt discontinuation of prolonged therapy; nausea, headache, vertigo, nightmares, malaise
- Other: Nasal congestion, excessive appetite, weight gain or loss, sweating, alopecia, lacrimation, hyperthermia, flushing, chills

Clinically important drug-drug interactions

- Increased TCA levels and pharmacologic (especially anticholinergic) effects when given with cimetidine, fluoxetine • Increased TCA levels when given with methylphenidate, phenothiazines, oral contraceptives, disulfiram, cimetidine, ranitidine • Hyperpyretic crises, severe convulsions, hypertensive episodes, and deaths when MAO inhibitors, furazolidone are given with TCAs • Increased antidepressant response and cardiac arrhythmias when given with thyroid medication. • Increased or decreased effects of TCAs when given with estrogens • Delirium when TCAs are given with disulfiram • Sympathetic hyperactivity, sinus tachycardia, hypertension, agitation when TCAs are given with levodopa • Increased biotransformation of TCAs in patients who smoke cigarettes • Increased sympathomimetic (especially α-adrenergic) effects of direct-acting sympathomimetic drugs (norepinephrine, epinephrine) when given with TCAs • Increased anticholinergic effects of anticholinergic drugs (including anticholinergic antiparkinsonism drugs) when given

Adverse effects in *Italics* are most common; those in **Bold** are life-threatening.

with TCAs • Increased response (especially CNS depression) to barbiturates • Increased effects of dicumarol when given with TCAs • Decreased antihypertensive effect of guanethidine, clonidine, other antihypertensives when given with TCAs • Decreased effects of indirect-acting sympathomimetic drugs (ephedrine) when given with TCAs

■ Nursing Considerations

Assessment
- *History:* Hypersensitivity to any tricyclic drug; concomitant therapy with an MAO inhibitor; recent MI; myelography within previous 24 h or scheduled within 48 h; lactation; electroshock therapy; preexisting cardiovascular disorders; angle-closure glaucoma, increased intraocular pressure, urinary retention, ureteral or urethral spasm; seizure disorders; hyperthyroidism; impaired hepatic, renal function; psychiatric patients; manic-depressive patients; elective surgery
- *Physical:* Body weight; temperature; skin—color, lesions; orientation, affect, reflexes, vision and hearing; P, BP, orthostatic BP, perfusion; bowel sounds, normal output, liver evaluation; urine flow, normal output; usual sexual function, frequency of menses, breast and scrotal exam; liver function tests, urinalysis, CBC, ECG

Implementation
- Ensure that depressed and potentially suicidal patients have access to only limited quantities of drug.
- Administer major portion of dose at bedtime if drowsiness, severe anticholinergic effects occur (note that the elderly may not tolerate single daily dose therapy).
- Arrange to reduce dosage if minor side effects develop; arrange to discontinue the drug if serious side effects occur.
- Arrange for CBC if patient develops fever, sore throat, or other sign of infection during therapy.
- Encourage elderly men or men with prostate problems to void before taking drug.

Drug-specific teaching points
- Do not to stop taking this drug abruptly or without consulting the physician or nurse.
- Avoid using alcohol, other sleep-inducing drugs, OTC drugs while on this drug.
- Avoid prolonged exposure to sunlight or sunlamps, and use a sunscreen or protective garments if long exposure to sunlight is unavoidable.
- Know that the following side effects may occur: headache, dizziness, drowsiness, weakness, blurred vision (these effects are reversible; safety measures may need to be taken if these become severe; you should avoid driving an automobile or performing tasks that require alertness while these persist); nausea, vomiting, loss of appetite, dry mouth (small frequent meals, frequent mouth care and sucking sugarless candies may help); nightmares, inability to concentrate, confusion; changes in sexual function.
- Report dry mouth, difficulty in urination, excessive sedation.

❒ amoxicillin

*(a mox i **sill'** in)*

Amoxil, Apo-Amoxi (CAN), Novamoxin (CAN), Nu-Amoxi (CAN), Polymox, Trimox, Wymox

Pregnancy Category B

Drug classes
Antibiotic, penicillin–ampicillin type

Therapeutic actions
Bactericidal: inhibits synthesis of cell wall of sensitive organisms, causing cell death.

Indications
- Infections due to susceptible strains of *Haemophilus influenzae, E. coli, Proteus mirabilis, Neisseria gonorrhoeae, Streptococcus pneumoniae*, streptococci, nonpencillinase-producing staphylococci
- Unlabeled use: *Chlamydia trachomatis* in pregnancy

Contraindications/cautions
- Contraindicated in the presence of allergies to penicillins, cephalosporins, or other allergens.
- Use caution in the presence of renal disorders, lactation.

Dosage
Available in oral preparations only.

Adults and children > 20 kg
- ***URIs, GU infections, skin and soft-tissue infections:*** 250–500 mg PO q8h.
- ***Lower respiratory infections:*** 500 mg PO q8h.
- ***Uncomplicated gonococcal infections:*** 3 g amoxicillin with 1 g probenecid PO.
- ***C. trachomatis in pregnancy:*** 500 mg PO tid for 7 d.
- ***Prevention of SBE***
  - ***Dental, oral, or upper respiratory procedures:*** 3 g 1 h before procedure, then 1.5 g 6 h after initial dose.
  - ***GI or GU procedures:*** 2 g ampicillin plus 1.5 mg/kg gentamicin IM or IV one-half hour before procedure, followed by 1.5 g amoxicillin; for low-risk patients, 3 g 1 h before procedure, then 1.5 g 6 h after initial dose.

Pediatric < 20 kg
- ***URIs, GU infections, skin, and soft-tissue infections:*** 20 mg/kg per day PO in divided doses q8h.
- ***Lower respiratory infections:*** 40 mg/kg per day PO in divided doses q8h.
- ***Prevention of SBE***
  - ***Dental, oral, or upper respiratory procedures:*** 3 g 1 h before procedure, then 1.5 g 6 h after initial dose.
  - ***GI or GU procedures:*** 50 mg/kg ampicillin plus 2 mg/kg gentamicin IM or IV one-half hour before procedure followed by 25 mg/kg amoxicillin. For low-risk patients, 3 g 1 h before procedure, then 1.5 g 6 hours after initial dose

Pharmacokinetics

Route	Onset	Peak	Duration
Oral	Varies	1 h	6–8 h

Metabolism: $T_{1/2}$: 1–1.4 h
Distribution: Crosses placenta; passes into breast milk
Excretion: Unchanged in the urine

Adverse effects
- CNS: Lethargy, hallucinations, seizures
- GI: *Glossitis, stomatitis, gastritis, sore mouth,* furry tongue, black "hairy" tongue, *nausea, vomiting, diarrhea, abdominal pain,* bloody diarrhea, enterocolitis, pseudomembranous colitis, nonspecific hepatitis
- Hematologic: Anemia, thrombocytopenia, leukopenia, neutropenia, prolonged bleeding time
- GU: Nephritis
- Hypersensitivity reactions: *Rash, fever, wheezing,* **anaphylaxis**
- Other: *Superinfections*—oral and rectal moniliasis, vaginitis

Clinically important drug-drug interactions
- Increased amoxicillin effect if taken with probenecid • Decreased effectiveness if taken with tetracyclines, chloramphenicol
- Decreased efficacy of oral contraceptives if taken with amoxicillin

Clinically important drug-food interactions
- Delayed or reduced GI absorption of amoxicillin if taken with food

■ Nursing Considerations

Assessment
- *History:* Allergies to penicillins, cephalosporins, or other allergens; renal disorders; lactation
- *Physical:* Culture infected area; skin—color, lesion; R, adventitious sounds; bowel sounds; CBC, liver and renal function tests, serum electrolytes, Hct, urinalysis

Implementation
- Culture infected area before beginning treatment; reculture area if response is not as expected.
- Administer in oral preparations only; absorption may affected by presence of food;

Adverse effects in *Italics* are most common; those in **Bold** are life-threatening.

drug should be taken 1 h before or 2 h after meals.
- Arrange to continue therapy for at least 2 d after signs of infection have disappeared; continuation for 10 full days is recommended.
- Arrange for the use of corticosteroids, antihistamines for skin reactions.

Drug-specific teaching points
- Take this drug around the clock as ordered. The drug should be taken on an empty stomach, 1 h before or 2 h after meals.
- Take the full course of therapy; do not stop taking the drug just because you feel better.
- Be aware that this antibiotic is specific for this current medical problem and should not be used to self-treat other infections.
- Know that the following side effects may occur: nausea, vomiting, GI upset (small frequent meals may help); diarrhea; sore mouth (frequent mouth care may help).
- Report unusual bleeding or bruising, sore throat, fever, rash, hives, severe diarrhea, difficulty breathing.

amphotericin B

(am foe ter' i sin)

Fungizone, Fungizone Intravenous

Pregnancy Category B

Drug classes
Antifungal antibiotic

Therapeutic actions
Binds to sterols in the fungal cell membrane with a resultant change in membrane permeability, an effect that can destroy fungal cells and prevent their reproduction; fungicidal or fungistatic depending on concentration and organism.

Indications
- Reserve use for patients with progressive, potentially fatal infections: cryptococcosis; North American blastomycosis; disseminated moniliasis; coccidioidomycosis and histoplasmosis; mucormycosis caused by species of *Mucor, Rhizopus, Absidia, Entomophthora, Basidiobolus*; sporotrichosis; aspergillosis.
- Adjunct to treatment of American mucocutaneous leishmaniasis (not drug of choice in primary therapy).
- Treatment of cutaneous and mucocutaneous mycotic infections caused by *Candida* species (topical application)
- **Unlabeled use**: bladder irrigation for treatment of candiduria

Contraindications/cautions
- Allergy to amphotericin B, renal dysfunction, lactation (unless condition is life-threatening and amenable only to treatment with this drug).

Dosage
Adult and Pediatric: For test dose, give 1 mg slowly IV to determine patient tolerance. Administer by slow IV infusion over 6 h at a concentration of 0.1 mg/ml. Increase daily dose based on patient tolerance and response. Usual dose is 0.25 mg/kg per day; do not exceed 1.5 mg/kg per day.
- ***Sporotrichosis:*** 20 mg per injection; therapy may extend for 9 mo.
- ***Aspergillosis:*** Treated up to 11 mo, with a total dose of 3.6 g.
- ***Rhinocerebral phycomycosis:*** Control diabetes; amphotericin B cumulative dose of 3 g; disease is usually rapidly fatal; treatment must be aggressive.
- ***Bladder irrigation (adults):*** 50 mg/1,000 ml sterile water instilled intermittently or continously
- ***For topical application:*** Liberally apply to candidal lesions two to four times per day; treatment usually ranges from 2–4 weeks based on response.

Pharmacokinetics

Route	Onset	Peak	Duration
IV	20–30 min	1–2 h	20–24 h

Metabolism: $T_{1/2}$: 24 h initially and then 15 d
Distribution: Crosses placenta; may pass into breast milk
Excretion: Urine

amphotericin B ■ 117

IV facts

Preparation: Prepare an initial solution of 5 mg/ml concentration by rapidly injecting 10 ml Sterile Water for Injection without a bacteriostatic agent directly into the lyophilized cake using a sterile needle (minimum diameter, 20 gauge); shake vial immediately until colloidal solution is clear; 0.1 mg/ml solution is obtained by further dilution with 5% Dextrose Injection of pH above 4.2; use strict aseptic technique. Do not dilute with saline; do not use if any evidence of precipitation is found. Refrigerate vials and protect from exposure to light; concentrate may be stored in dark at room temperature for 24 h or refrigerated for 1 wk. Discard any unused material. Use solutions prepared for IV infusion promptly after preparation.

Infusion: Protect infusion from exposure to light if they will not be infused within 8 h of preparation. Infuse by slow IV infusion over 6 h.

Compatibilities: Do not mix with saline-containing solution, parenteral nutrional solutions, aminoglycosides, penicillins, phenothiazines, calcium preparations, cimetidine, metaraminol, methyldopa, polymyxin, potassium chloride, ranitidine, verapamil, clindamycin, cotrimoxazole, dopamine, dobutamine, tetracycline, vitamins, lidocaine, procaine or heparin. **If line must be flushed, do not use heparin or saline; use D5W.**

Adverse effects
Systemic Administration
- **CNS:** *Fever (often with shaking chills), headache, malaise*, generalized pain
- **GI:** *Nausea, vomiting, dyspepsia, diarrhea*, cramping, epigastric pain, anorexia
- **Hematologic:** Normochromic, normocytic anemia
- **GU:** Hypokalemia, azotemia, hyposthenuria, renal tubular acidosis, nephrocalcinosis
- **Local:** *Pain at the injection site* with phlebitis and thrombophlebitis
- **Other:** Weight loss

Topical Application
- **Skin:** *Drying effect on skin, local irritation* (cream application); *pruritus*, allergic contact dermatitis (lotion application); *local irritation* (ointment application)

Clinically important drug-drug interactions
- Do not administer with corticosteroids unless these are needed to control symptoms.
- Increased risk of nephrotoxicity if given with other nephrotoxic antibiotics, antineoplastics. • Increased effects and risk of toxicity of digitalis, skeletal muscle relaxants, flucytosine if given concurrently with amphotericin B. • Increased nephrotoxic effects if taken with cyclosporine.

■ Nursing Considerations

Assessment
- *History:* Allergy to amphotericin B, renal dysfunction, lactation
- *Physical:* Skin—color, lesions; body temperature; body weight; injection site; orientation, reflexes, affect; bowel sounds, liver evaluation; renal function tests; CBC and differential; culture of area involved

Implementation
- Arrange for appropriate culture of infection before beginning therapy; however, treatment should begin before lab results are returned.
- Monitor injection sites and veins for signs of phlebitis.
- Cleanse affected lesions before applying topical drug; apply liberally to lesions and rub in gently; do not cover with plastic wrap.
- Use soap and water to wash hands, fabrics, skin areas that may discolor as a result of topical application.
- Provide supportive measures to help patient tolerate the uncomfortable effects of the drug (aspirin, antihistamines, antiemetics, maintenance of sodium balance). IV corticosteroids may help to de-

Adverse effects in *Italics* are most common; those in **Bold** are life-threatening.

ampicillin

crease febrile reactions, but minimize use of corticosteroids. Meperidine has been used to relieve chills and fever.
- Monitor renal function tests weekly; discontinue or decrease dosage of drug at any sign of increased renal toxicity.
- Continue topical adminstration for long-term therapy until infection is eradicated, usually 2–4 wk.
- Discontinue topical application if hypersensitivity reaction occurs.

Drug-specific teaching points
- Be aware that long-term use of this drug will be needed; beneficial effects may not be seen for several weeks; the systemic form of the drug can only be given IV.
- For topical application, apply topical drug liberally to affected area after first cleansing area.
- Use hygiene measures to prevent reinfection or spread of infection.
- Know that the following side effects may occur: nausea, vomiting, diarrhea (small frequent meals may help); discoloring, drying of the skin, staining of fabric (washing with soap and water or cleaning fabric with standard cleaning fluid should remove stain; topical); stinging, irritation with local application; fever, chills, muscle aches and pains, headache (medications may be ordered to help you to deal with these discomforts of the drug).
- Report pain, irritation at injection site; GI upset, nausea, loss of appetite; difficulty breathing; local irritation, burning (topical application).

☐ ampicillin

*(am pi **sill**' in)*

Oral: Ampicin (CAN), Apo-Ampi (CAN), D-Amp, Novo-Ampicillin (CAN), Nu-Ampi (CAN), Omnipen, Penbritin (CAN), Polycillin, Principen, Totacillin

ampicillin sodium

Parenteral: Omnipen-N, Polycillin-N, Totacillin-N

Pregnancy Category B

Drug classes
Antibiotic
Penicillin

Therapeutic actions
Bactericidal action against sensitive organisms; inhibits synthesis of bacterial cell wall, causing cell death.

Indications
- Treatment of infections caused by susceptible strains of *Shigella, Salmonella, E. coli, H. influenzae, P. mirabilis, N. gonorrhoeae,* enterococci, gram-positive organisms (penicillin G-sensitive staphylococci, streptococci, pneumococci).
- Meningitis caused by *Neisseria meningitidis*.
- Unlabeled use: prophylaxis in cesarean section in certain high-risk patients

Contraindications/cautions
- Contraindicated in the presence of allergies to penicillins, cephalosporins, or other allergens.
- Use caution in the presence of renal disorders.

Dosage
Maximum recommended dosage: 8 mg/d; may be given IV, IM, or PO. Use parenteral routes for severe infections, and switch to oral route as soon as possible.

Respiratory and soft-tissue infections: Patients weighing 40 kg or more: 250–500 mg IV or IM q6h. *Patients weighing less than 40 kg:* 25–50 mg/kg per day IM or IV in equally divided doses at 6–8h intervals. *Patients weighing more than 20 kg:* 250 mg PO q6h. *Patients weighing less than 20 kg:* 50 mg/kg per day PO in equally divided doses q6–8h.

GI and GU infections, including women with N. gonorrhoeae: Patients weighing more than 40 kg: 500 mg IM or IV q6h. *Patients weighing less than 40 kg:* 50 mg/kg per day IM or IV in equally divided doses q6–8h. *Patients weighing more than 20 kg:* 500 mg PO q6h. *Patients weighing less than 20 kg:* 100 mg/kg per day PO in equallly divided doses q6–8h.

Gonococcal infections: 1 g q6h when the organism is found to be penicillin-sensitive.

ampicillin ▪ 119

Bacterial meningitis (adult and pediatric): 150–200 mg/kg per day by continuous IV drip and then IM injections in equally divided doses q3–4h.

Prevention of bacterial endocarditis for GI or GU surgery or instrumentation
- **Adult:** 2 g ampicillin IM or IV plus 1.5 mg/kg gentamicin IM or IV. First dose ½–1 h before the procedure, followed by 1.5 mg amoxicillin 6 h after initial dose, or repeat parenteral dose 8 h after initial dose.
- **Pediatric:** 50 mg/kg ampicillin plus 2 mg/kg gentamicin at the same dosage schedule as adults.

Prevention of bacterial endocarditis for dental, oral, or upper respiratory procedures
- **Adult:** 1–2 g ampicillin IM or IV plus 1.5 mg/kg gentamicin IM or IV. First dose ½–1 h before the procedure, followed by 1.5 mg amoxicillin 6 h after initial dose, or repeat parenteral dose 8 h after initial dose.
- **Pediatric:** 50 mg/kg ampicillin plus 1.5 mg/kg gentamicin at the same dosage schedule as adults.

Septicemia (adult and pediatric): 150–200 mg/kg per day IV for at least 3 days, then IM q3–4h.

Sexually transmitted diseases (adult): Rape victims: Prophylaxis against infection. *Pregnant women and patients allergic to tetracycline:* 3.5g ampicillin PO with 1 g probenecid. *Prophylaxis in cesarean section:* Single IV or IM dose of 25–100 mg/kg immediately after cord is clamped.

Pharmacokinetics

Route	Onset	Peak	Duration
Oral	30 min	2 h	6–8 h
IM	15 min	1 h	6–8 h
IV	Immediate	5 min	6–8 h

Metabolism: $T_{1/2}$: 1–2 h
Distribution: Crosses placenta; passes into breast milk
Excretion: Unchanged in the urine

IV facts

Preparation: Reconstitute with Sterile or Bacteriostatic Water for Injection; piggyback vials may be reconstituted with Sodium Chloride Injection; use reconstituted solution within 1 h. Do not mix in the same IV solution as other antibiotics. Use within 1 h after preparation because potency may decrease significantly after that.

Infusion: Direct IV administration; give slowly over 3–5 min. *Rapid administration can lead to convulsions.* **IV drip**: dilute as above before further dilution. **IV piggyback:** administer alone or further dilute with compatible solution.

Compatibility: Ampicillin is compatible with 0.9% Sodium Chloride, 5% Dextrose in Water, or 0.45% Sodium Chloride Solution, 10% Invert Sugar Water, M/6 Sodium Lactate Solution, Lactated Ringer's Solution, Sterile Water for Injection. Diluted solutions are stable for 2–8 h; check manufacturer's inserts for specifics. Discard solution after allotted time period.

Incompatibility: Do not mix with lidocaine, verapamil, other antibiotics, dextrose solutions

Adverse effects

- CNS: Lethargy, hallucinations, seizures
- GI: *Glossitis, stomatitis, gastritis, sore mouth*, furry tongue, black "hairy" tongue, *nausea, vomiting, diarrhea*, abdominal pain, bloody diarrhea, enterocolitis, pseudomembranous colitis, nonspecific hepatitis
- CV: CHF
- Hematologic: Anemia, thrombocytopenia, leukopenia, neutropenia, prolonged bleeding time
- GU: **Nephritis**
- Local: *Pain, phlebitis,* thrombosis at injection site (parenteral)
- Hypersensitivity reactions: *Rash, fever, wheezing,* **anaphylaxis**
- Other: *Superinfections*—oral and rectal moniliasis, vaginitis

Adverse effects in *Italics* are most common; those in **Bold** are life-threatening.

Clinically important drug-drug interactions

• Increased ampicillin effect if taken with probenecid • Increased risk of skin rash if taken with allopurinol • Increased bleeding effect if taken with heparin, oral anticoagulants • Decreased effectiveness if taken with tetracyclines, chloramphenicol • Decreased efficacy of oral contraceptives, atenolol if taken with ampicillin

Clinically important drug-food interactions

• Effectiveness of oral ampicillin may be reduced by the presence of food; should be taken on an empty stomach.

Drug-lab test interferences

• False-positive Coombs' test if given IV. • Decrease in plasma estrogen concentrations in pregnant women. • False-positive urine glucose tests if Clinitest, Benedict's solution, or Fehling's solution is used; enzymatic glucose oxidase methods (Clinistix, Tes-Tape) should be used to check urine glucose.

■ Nursing Considerations

Assessment
- *History:* Allergies to penicillins, cephalosporins, or other allergens; renal disorders; lactation
- *Physical:* Culture infected area; skin—color, lesion; R, adventitious sounds; bowel sounds; CBC, liver and renal function tests, serum electrolytes, hematocrit, urinalysis.

Implementation
- Culture infected area before beginning treatment; reculture area if response is not as expected.
- Check IV site carefully for signs of thrombosis or drug reaction.
- Do not give IM injections repeatedly in the same site; atrophy can occur. Monitor injection sites.
- Administer oral drug on an empty stomach, 1 h before or 2 h after meals with a full glass of water—no fruit juice or soft drinks.

Drug-specific teaching points
- Take this drug around the clock as ordered.
- Take the full course of therapy; do not stop taking the drug as soon as you feel better.
- Take the oral drug on an empty stomach, 1 h before or 2 h after meals; the oral solution is stable for 7 d at room temperature.
- Be aware that this antibiotic is specific for your medical problem and should not be used to self-treat other infections.
- Know that the following side effects may occur: nausea, vomiting, GI upset (small frequent meals may help); diarrhea may occur.
- Report pain or discomfort at injection sites, unusual bleeding or bruising, mouth sores, rash, hives, fever, itching, severe diarrhea, difficulty breathing.

❒ amrinone lactate

(am' ri none)
Inocor

Pregnancy Category C

Drug classes
Cardiotonic drug

Therapeutic actions
Increases force of contraction of ventricles (positive inotropic effect); causes vasodilation by a direct relaxant effect on vascular smooth muscle.

Indications
- CHF: short time management of patients who have not responded to digitalis, diuretics, or vasodilators

Contraindications/cautions
- Allergy to amrinone or bisulfites, severe aortic or pulmonic valvular disease, acute MI, decreased fluid volume, lactation

Dosage
Adult
- ***Initial dose:*** 0.75 mg/kg IV bolus, given over 2–3 min. A supplemental IV bolus of 0.75 mg/kg may be administered after 30 min if warranted by clinical response.

- **Maintenance infusion:** 5–10 µg/kg per minute. Do not exceed a total of 10 mg/kg per day.

Pediatric: Not recommended.

Pharmacokinetics

Route	Onset	Peak	Duration
IV	Immediate	10 min	2 h

Metabolism: Hepatic, $T_{1/2}$: 3.6–5.8 h
Distribution: Crosses placenta; may pass into breast milk
Excretion: Urine (63%) and feces (18%)

IV facts
Preparation: Administer as supplied or dilute in normal or one-half normal saline solution to a concentration of 1–3 mg/ml. Use diluted solution within 24 h. Protect ampules from exposure to light.

Infusion: Administer IV bolus slowly over 2–3 min. Maintenance infusion should not exceed 5–10 µg/kg per minute. Monitor sum of all doses; do not exceed a total daily dose of 10 mg/kg.

Compatibilities: Do not mix directly with dextrose-containing solutions; may be injected into a Y-connector or directly into tubing when a dextose solution is running. Do not mix with furosemide.

Adverse effects
- **GI:** Nausea, vomiting, abdominal pain, anorexia, hepatoxicity
- **CV:** *Arrhythmias*, hypotension
- **Hematologic:** *Thrombocytopenia*
- **Hypersensitivity:** Pericarditis, pleuritis, ascites, vasculitis
- **Other:** Fever, chest pain, burning at injection site

Clinically important drug-drug interactions
- Precipitate formation in solution if given in the same IV line with furosemide

■ Nursing Considerations
Assessment
- *History:* Allergy to amrinone or bisulfites, severe aortic or pulmonic valvular disease, acute MI, decreased fluid volume, lactation
- *Physical:* Weight, orientation, P, BP, cardiac auscultation, peripheral pulses, peripheral perfusion, R, adventitious sounds, bowel sounds, liver evaluation, urinary output, serum electrolyte levels, platelet count, liver enzymes

Implementation
- Protect drug vial from light.
- Monitor BP and P, and reduce dose if marked decreases occur.
- Monitor intake and output and electrolyte levels; record daily weights.
- Monitor platelet counts if patient is on prolonged therapy. Arrange for dose reduction if platelet levels fall.

Drug-specific teaching points
- Be aware that you will need frequent BP and P monitoring during drug therapy.
- Know that you may experience increased voiding while on this drug.
- Report pain at IV injection site; dizziness; weakness, fatigue; numbness or tingling.

❒ amyl nitrite

(am' il)
Amyl Nitrate Aspirols, Amyl Nitrate Vaporole

Pregnancy Category C

Drug classes
Antianginal drug
Nitrate

Therapeutic actions
Relaxes vascular smooth muscle, which results in a decrease in venous return and arterial blood pressure; this reduces left ventricular workload and decreases myocardial oxygen consumption.

Indications
- Relief of angina pectoris

Contraindications/cautions
- Allergy to nitrates, severe anemia, head trauma, cerebral hemorrhage, hypertrophic cardiomyopathy, lactation.

Adverse effects in *Italics* are most common; those in **Bold** are life-threatening.

amyl nitrite

Dosage
Adult: 0.18 or 0.3 ml by inhalation of vapor from crushed capsule; may repeat in 3–5 min if necessary for relief of angina. 1–6 inhalations from a capsule is usually sufficient to produce desired effect.
Pediatric: Safety and efficacy not established.

Pharmacokinetics

Route	Onset	Peak	Duration
Inhalation	30 sec	3 min	3–5 min

Metabolism: Hepatic metabolism, $T_{1/2}$: 1–4 min
Distribution: Crosses placenta; may passes into breast milk
Excretion: Urine

Adverse effects
- **CNS:** *Headache, apprehension, restlessness, weakness,* vertigo, dizziness, faintness, euphoria
- **GI:** *Nausea,* vomiting, incontinence of urine and feces, abdominal pain
- **CV:** *Tachycardia,* retrosternal discomfort, palpitations, *hypotension,* syncope, collapse, postural hypotension, angina
- **Dermatologic:** Rash, exfoliative dermatitis, *cutaneous vasodilation with flushing*
- **Drug abuse:** Abused for sexual stimulation and euphoria, effects of inhalation are instantaneous
- **Other:** Muscle twitching, pallor, perspiration, cold sweat

Clinically important drug-drug interactions
- Increased risk of severe hypotension and cardiovascular collapse if used with alcohol • Increased risk of hypotension if used with antihypertensive drugs, beta-adrenergic blockers, phenothiazines

Drug-lab test interferences
- False report of decreased serum cholesterol if done by the Zlatkis-Zak color reaction

■ Nursing Considerations

Assessment
- *History:* Allergy to nitrates, severe anemia, head trauma, cerebral hemorrhage, hypertrophic cardiomyopathy, lactation
- *Physical:* Skin—color, temperature, lesions, orientation, reflexes, affect, P, BP, orthostatic BP, baseline ECG, peripheral perfusion, respiratory rate, adventitious sounds, liver evaluation, normal output, CBC, hemoglobin

Implementation
- Administer by crushing the capsule and waving under the patient's nose; 2–6 inhalations from one capsule are usually sufficient; repeat every 3–5 min if necessary.
- Protect the drug from light; store in a cool place.
- Arrange for gradual reduction in dose if anginal treatment is being terminated; rapid discontinuation can lead to problems of withdrawal.

Drug-specific teaching points
- Crush the capsule, and inhale two to six times by waving under your nose; you can repeat in 3–5 min if necessary.
- Do not use in an environment where vapors may ignite; vapors are highly flammable.
- Protect the drug from light; store in a cool place.
- Avoid alcohol while on amyl nitrite therapy.
- Know that the following side effects may occur: dizziness, lightheadedness (this may pass as you adjust to the drug; use care to change positions slowly; lie down or sit down when you take your dose to decrease the risk of falling); headache (lying down in a cool environment and resting may help; OTC preparations may not help); flushing of the neck or face (this usually passes as the drug's effects pass).
- Report blurred vision, persistent or severe headache, skin rash, more frequent or more severe angina attacks, fainting.

Adverse effects in *Italics* are most common; those in **Bold** are life-threatening.

anistreplase

(an is tre plaze')
anisoylated plasminogen streptokinase activator complex, APSAC

Eminase

Pregnancy Category C

Drug classes
Thrombolytic enzyme

Therapeutic actions
A complex of streptokinase with human plasminogen, which is activated to plasmin in the body; plasmin lyses formed thrombi.

Indications
- Management of acute MI for the lysis of thrombi obstructing coronary arteries, the reduction of infarct size, the improvement of ventricular function following acute MI, and the reduction of mortality associated with acute MI.

Contraindications/cautions
- Known allergic reactions to anistreplase or streptokinase, active internal bleeding, recent (within 2 mo) CVA, intracranial or intraspinal surgery or neoplasm, arteriovenous malformation, aneurysm, recent major surgery, obstetric delivery, organ biopsy, rupture of a noncompressible blood vessel, recent serious GI bleed, recent serious trauma, including CPR, hemostatic defects, cerebrovascular disease, SBE, severe uncontrolled hypertension, liver disease, old age (> 75 y), lactation

Dosage
Administer as soon as possible after the onset of symptoms.
Adult: 30 U administered only by IV injection over 2–5 min into an IV line or directly into vein.

Pharmacokinetics

Route	Onset	Peak	Duration
IV	Immediate	45 min	4–6 h

Metabolism: Plasma, $T_{1/2}$: 2 h
Distribution: Crosses placenta; may pass into breast milk

IV facts
Preparation: Reconstitute by slowly adding 5 ml of Sterile Water for Injection to the vial. Gently roll the vial, mixing the dry powder and fluid; reconstituted solution should be colorless to a pale yellow transparent solution. Withdraw the entire contents of the vial. Reconstitute immediately before use. Must be used within 30 min of reconstitution. Discard any unused solution. Avoid excess agitation during dilution. Swirl gently to mix. *Do not shake.* Minimize foaming.

Infusion: Administer as soon as possible after the onset of symptoms. Administer over 2–5 min into an IV line or directly into a vein.

Compatibilities: Do not further dilute before administration; do not add to any infusion fluids. Do not add any other medications to the vial or to the syringe.

Adverse effects
- CV: **Cardiac arrhythmias with coronary reperfusion**, *hypotension*
- Hematologic: ***Bleeding***, particularly at venous or arterial access sites, gastrointestinal bleeding, intracranial hemorrhage
- Hypersensitivity: Anaphylactic and anaphylactoid reactions, bronchospasm, itching, flushing, rash
- Other: Urticaria, nausea, vomiting, fever, chills, headache

Clinically important drug-drug interactions
- Increased risk of hemorrhage if used with heparin or oral anticoagulants, aspirin, dipyridamole

Drug-lab test interferences
- Decrease in plasminogen and fibrinogen results in increases in thrombin time, APTT, prothrombin time, tests may be unreliable

Adverse effects in *Italics* are most common; those in **Bold** are life-threatening.

Nursing Considerations

Assessment
- *History:* Known allergic reactions to anistreplase or streptokinase, active internal bleeding, recent (within 2 mo) CVA, intracranial or intraspinal surgery or neoplasm, arteriovenous malformation, aneurysm, recent major surgery, obstetric delivery, organ biopsy, rupture of a noncompressible blood vessel, recent serious GI bleed, recent serious trauma, including CPR, hemostatic defects, cerebrovascular disease, SBE, severe uncontrolled hypertension, liver disease, old age (> 75 y), lactation
- *Physical:* Skin—color, temperature, lesions; orientation, reflexes; P, BP, peripheral perfusion, baseline ECG; R, adventitous sounds; liver evaluation; hematocrit, platelet count, TT, APTT, PT

Implementation
- Discontinue concurrent heparin and alteplase if serious bleeding occurs.
- Arrange for regular monitoring of coagulation studies.
- Apply pressure or pressure dressings to control superficial bleeding (at invaded or disturbed areas).
- Avoid any arterial invasive procedures during therapy.
- Arrange for typing and cross-matching of blood in case serious blood loss occurs and whole blood transfusions are required.
- Institute treatment as soon as possible after onset of symptoms for evolving MI.

Drug-specific teaching points
- Report difficulty breathing, dizziness, disorientation, headache, numbness, tingling.

☐ antihemophilic factor

*(an tee hee moe **fill'** ik)*
AHF, Factor VIII

Hemofil M, Humate-P, Koate-HS, Koate-HP, Monoclate, Profilate HP

Pregnancy Category C

Drug classes
Antihemophilic agent

Therapeutic actions
A normal plasma protein that is needed for the transformation of prothrombin to thrombin, the final step of the intrinsic clotting pathway.

Indications
- Treatment of classical hemophilia (Hemophilia A), in which there is a demonstrated deficiency of Factor VIII; provides a temporary replacement of clotting factors to correct or prevent bleeding episodes or to allow necessary surgery.

Contraindications/cautions
- Antibodies to mouse protein.

Dosage
Administer IV only using a plastic syringe; dose depends on patient weight, severity of deficiency, and severity of bleeding. Follow treatment carefully with Factor VIII level assays.
- Formulas used as a guide for dosage are:

$$\text{Expected Factor VIII increase} (\% \text{ of normal}) = \frac{\text{AHF/IU given} \times 2.0}{\text{body weight in kg}}$$

$$\text{AHF/IU required} = \text{body weight (kg)} \times \text{desired Factor VIII increase} (\% \text{ normal}) \times 0.5$$

Prophylaxis of spontaneous hemorrhage: Level of Factor VIII required to prevent spontaneous hemorrhage is 5% of normal; 30% of normal is the minimum required for hemostasis following trauma or surgery; smaller doses may be needed if treated early.

Mild hemorrhage: Do not repeat therapy unless further bleeding occurs.

Moderate hemorrhage or minor surgery: 30%–50% of normal is desired for Factor VIII levels; initial dose of 15–25 AHF/IU/kg with maintenance dose of 10–15 AHF/IU/kg is usually sufficient.

Severe hemorrhage: Factor VIII level of 80%–100% normal is desired; initial dose of 40–50 AHF/IU/kg and a maintenance dose of 20–25 AHF/IU/kg is given q8–12h.

Major surgery: Dose of AHF to achieve Factor VIII levels of 80%–100% of normal given an hour before surgery; second dose of half the size about 5 h later. Maintain Factor VIII levels at at least 30% normal for a healing period of 10–14 d.

Pharmacokinetics

Route	Onset
IV	Immediate

Metabolism: $T_{1/2}$: 12 h
Distribution: Does not readily cross placenta
Excretion: Cleared from the body by normal metabolism

IV facts

Preparation: Reconstitute using solution provided. Refrigerate unreconstituted preparations. Before reconstitution, warm diluent and dried concentrate to room temperature. Add diluent and rotate vial, or shake gently, until completely dissolved. Do not refrigerate reconstituted preparations; give within 3 h of reconstitution.

Infusion: Administer by IV route only; use a plastic syringe; solutions may stick to glass.

Administer preparations containing 34 or more U/ml at a maximum rate of 2 ml/min; give preparations containing < 34 AHF U/ml at a rate of 10–20 ml over 3 min.

Adverse effects

- **Hematologic:** Hemolysis with large or frequently repeated doses
- **Allergic reactions:** Erythema, hives, fever, backache, bronchospasm, urticaria, chills, nausea, *stinging at the infusion site*, vomiting, headache
- **Other:** Hepatitis, AIDS—risks associated with repeated use of blood products

■ Nursing Considerations

Assessment

- *History:* Antibodies to mouse protein
- *Physical:* Skin—color, lesions; P, peripheral perfusion; R, adventitious sounds; factor VIII levels, Hct, direct Coombs' test, HIV screening, hepatitis screening

Implementation

- Monitor pulse during administration; if a significant increase occurs, reduce the rate of administration, or discontinue administration and consult physician.
- Monitor patient's clinical response and factor VIII levels regularly; if no response is noted with large doses, consider the presence of factor VIII inhibitors and need for anti-inhibitor complex therapy.

Drug-specific teaching points

- Be aware that dosage varies at different times and in different situations. All known safety precautions are taken to assure that this blood product is pure and the risk of AIDS and hepatitis is as minimal as possible.
- Wear or carry a medical alert ID tag so that medical personnel who take care of you in an emergency will know that you require this treatment.
- Report headache; rash, itching; backache; difficulty breathing.

☐ antithrombin

(an' tee throm bin)
ATnativ, Kybernin, Thrombate III

Pregnancy Category C

Drug classes
Coagulation inhibitor

Therapeutic actions
A normal plasma factor identical to heparin cofactor I, necessary for heparin to exert its anticoagulant effect.

Indications
- Treatment of patients with hereditary antithrombin III (AT III) deficiency in connection with surgical or obstetric procedures or when they suffer from thromboembolism

Adverse effects in *Italics* are most common; those in **Bold** are life-threatening.

- Replacement therapy in congenital AT III deficiency

Contraindications/cautions
- Use caution in neonates of parents with AT III deficiency and in pregnancy.

Dosage
Administer IV only; dosage is based on the amount of drug needed to replace each individual patient's deficiency. Once appropriate AT III levels are achieved, maintain that level for 2–8 d depending on the situation involved.
- Formulas used as a guide for dosage are:

$$\text{Dosage Units} = \frac{[\text{desired AT-III level (\%)} - \text{baseline AT-III (\%)}] \times \text{body weight}}{1\%/(\text{IU/kg})}$$

Pediatric: Safety and efficacy not established.

Pharmacokinetics

Route	Onset
IV	Immediate

Metabolism: $T_{1/2}$: 3 d
Distribution: May cross placenta
Excretion: Cleared from the body by normal metabolism

IV facts
Preparation: Dissolve the powder in 10 ml Sterile Water for Injection, USP. Gently swirl the vial to dissolve the powder. Do not shake. Bring the solution to room temperature, and administer within 3 h following reconstitution. May be reconstituted with 0.9% Sodium Chloride Injection or 5% Dextrose Injection. After reconstitution, may be further diluted with the same diluent.
Infusion: Administer by IV route only; infuse over 5–10 min. Recommended rate is 50 IU/min (1 ml/min); do not exceed 100 IU/min (2 ml/min). Avoid rapid infusion.

Adverse effects
- **Immunologic:** Hepatitis, AIDS—risks associated with repeated use of blood products
- **Other:** Diuretic and vasodilatory effects in patients with severe DIC

Clinically important drug-drug interactions
- Increased effects of heparin if given with antithrombin III

■ Nursing Considerations

Assessment
- *History:* Clear history of AT III deficiency based on family history of venous thrombosis, decreased plasma AT III level, and exclusion of an acquired deficiency
- *Physical:* Skin—color, lesions; P, peripheral perfusion; R, adventitious sounds; AT III levels, HIV screening, hepatitis screening

Implementation
- Monitor AT III levels preceding drug therapy, 30 min after the first dose, and periodically during therapy; the first dose should increase the AT III levels to about 120% of normal. Maintenance doses, q24h, should keep that level at > 80% normal for therapeutic effect.
- Decrease heparin doses during treatment with AT III to avoid excessive bleeding.

Drug-specific teaching points
- Be aware that dosage varies at different times and in different situations. Frequent blood tests will evaluate the effectiveness of drug therapy. All known safety precautions are taken to ensure that this blood product is pure and the risk of AIDS and hepatitis is as minimal as possible.
- Wear or carry a medical alert ID tag so that medical personnel who take care of you in an emergency will know that you require this treatment in emergency situations.
- Report pain or discomfort at IV site.

Adverse effects in *Italics* are most common; those in **Bold** are life-threatening.

aprobarbital

*(a pro **bar'** bi tal)*
Alurate

Pregnancy Category D
C-III controlled substance

Drug classes
Barbiturate (short acting)
Sedative
Hypnotic

Therapeutic actions
General central nervous system depressant; barbiturates act on the ascending reticular activating system, depress the cerebral cortex, alter cerebellar function, depress motor output, and can produce excitation, sedation, hypnosis, anesthesia, and deep coma.

Indications
- Short-term sedation and sleep induction

Contraindications/cautions
- Contraindicated in the presence of hypersensitivity to barbiturates; manifest or latent porphyria; marked liver impairment; nephritis; severe respiratory distress, respiratory disease with dyspnea, obstruction or cor pulmonale; previous addiction to sedative-hypnotic drugs; pregnancy.
- Use caution in the presence of acute or chronic pain (drug may cause paradoxical excitement or mask important symptoms); seizure disorders (abrupt discontinuation of daily doses of drug can result in status epilepticus); lactation; fever, hyperthyroidism, diabetes mellitus, severe anemia, pulmonary or cardiac disease, status asthmaticus, shock, uremia; impaired liver or kidney function, debilitation.

Dosage
Adult
- **Sedation:** 40 mg tid, PO.
- **Mild insomnia:** 40–80 mg at bedtime, PO.
- **Pronounced insomnia:** 80–160 mg at bedtime, PO.

Pediatric: Safety and efficacy not established.

Geriatric patients or those with debilitating disease: Reduce dosage and monitor closely; may produce excitement, depression, confusion.

Pharmacokinetics

Route	Onset	Duration
Oral	45–60 min	6–8 h

Metabolism: Hepatic, $T_{1/2}$: 14–34 h
Distribution: Crosses placenta; passes into breast milk
Excretion: Urine

Adverse effects
- **CNS:** *Somnolence, agitation, confusion, hyperkinesia, ataxia, vertigo, CNS depression, nightmares, lethargy, residual sedation (hangover),* paradoxical excitement, nervousness, psychiatric disturbance, hallucinations, insomnia, anxiety, dizziness, thinking abnormality
- **GI:** *Nausea, vomiting, constipation, diarrhea,* epigastric pain
- **CV:** Bradycardia, hypotension, syncope
- **Respiratory:** *Hypoventilation,* **apnea, respiratory depression,** laryngospasm, bronchospasm, circulatory collapse
- **Hypersensitivity:** Skin rashes, angioneurotic edema, serum sickness, morbiliform rash, urticaria, rarely exfoliative dermatitis, **Stevens-Johnson syndrome, sometimes fatal**
- **Other:** *Tolerance, psychological and physical dependence,* withdrawal syndrome, sometimes fatal

Clinically important drug-drug interactions
- Increased CNS depression when taken with alcohol, other CNS depressants, phenothiazines, antihistamines, tranquilizers • Increased blood levels and pharmacologic effects of barbiturates when given with MAO inhibitors • Increased renal toxicity if taken with methoxyflurane • De-

Adverse effects in *Italics* are most common; those in **Bold** are life-threatening.

creased effects of the following drugs given with barbiturates: oral anticoagulants, digitoxin, tricyclic antidepressants, corticosteroids, oral contraceptives and estrogens, acetaminophen, metronidazole, phenmetrazine, carbamazepine, beta-blockers, griseofulvin, phenylbutazones, theophyllines, quinidine, doxycycline • Altered effectiveness of phenytoin given with barbiturates

■ Nursing Considerations

Assessment
- *History:* Hypersensitivity to barbiturates; manifest or latent porphyria; marked liver impairment; nephritis; severe respiratory distress, respiratory disease with dyspnea, obstruction, or cor pulmonale; previous addiction to sedative-hypnotic drugs; acute or chronic pain; seizure disorders; lactation; fever, hyperthyroidism, diabetes mellitus, severe anemia, cardiac disease, status asthmaticus, shock, uremia; debilitation.
- *Physical:* Body weight; body temperature; skin—color, lesions; orientation, affect, reflexes; P, BP, orthostatic BP; respiratory rate, adventitious sounds; bowel sounds, normal output, liver evaluation; liver and kidney function tests, blood and urine glucose, BUN.

Implementation
- Monitor patient responses, blood levels (as appropriate) if any of the above interacting drugs are given with aprobarbital; suggest alternate means of contraception to women on oral contraceptives for whom aprobarbital is prescribed.
- Arrange to taper dosage gradually after repeated use, especially in epileptic patients.

Drug-specific teaching points
- Know that this drug is habit forming; its effectiveness in facilitating sleep disappears after a short time.
- Do not to take this drug longer than 2 wk (for insomnia), and do not increase the dosage without consulting the physician.
- Consult care provider if the drug appears to be ineffective; do not increase the dose to get more effect.
- Avoid the use of alcohol, sleep-inducing, or OTC drugs while on this drug because these could cause dangerous effects.
- Use a means of contraception other than oral contraceptive preparations while on aprobarbital; you should not become pregnant while taking this drug.
- Know that the following side effects may occur: drowsiness, dizziness, "hangover," impaired thinking (these effects may become less pronounced after a few days; avoid driving a car or engaging in dangerous activities if these occur); GI upset (taking the drug with food may help); dreams, nightmares, difficulty concentrating, fatigue, nervousness (it may help to know that these are effects of the drug that will go away when the drug is discontinued).
- Report severe dizziness, weakness, drowsiness that persists; rash or skin lesions; pregnancy.

☐ aprotinin

(ah pro' tin in)
Trasylol

Pregnancy Category B

Drug classes
Systemic hemostatic

Therapeutic actions
Derived from bovine lung, aprotinin forms complexes with plasmin, kallikreins, and other factors to block activation of the kinin and fibrinolytic systems.

Indications
- Prophylactic use: to reduce blood loss and the need for transfusion in patients undergoing cardiopulmonary bypass in the course of repeat coronary artery bypass graft surgery
- Prophylactic use: to reduce blood loss in select first-time coronary bypass surgery when the patient is at special risk for bleeding

Contraindications/cautions
- Contraindictated in the presence of allergy to aprotinin, first time CABG surgery (except in special, select cases).

- Use caution in the presence of pregnancy, lactation

Dosage
Provided in a solution containing 1.4 mg/ml or 10,000 KIU/ml.
Adult: Test dose of 1 ml IV administered, followed by a loading dose of 100–200 ml administered over 20–30 min, with the patient in the supine position. Follow this with a continuous infusion of 25–50 ml/h, kept running until the surgery is over and the patient leaves the operating room.

Pharmacokinetics

Route	Peak
IV	Immediately

Metabolism: $T_{1/2}$: 150 min
Distribution: Crosses placenta; passes into breast milk
Excretion: Urine

IV facts
Preparation: No further preparation is required.
Infusion: Administer loading dose over 20–30 min and then continuous infusion of 50 ml/h.
Compatibilities: Do not administer in solution with corticosteroids, heparin, tetracyclines, fat emulsions, amino acids. Administer any other drug through a separate line.

Adverse effects
- **CV:** *Atrial fibrillation,* **MI,** CHF, atrial flutter, ventricular tachycardia, heart block, shock, hypotension
- **Respiratory:** Asthma, dyspnea, respiratory distress
- **Other:** Anaphylactic reactions

Clinically important drug-drug interactions
- Increased bleeding tendencies if taken concurrently with heparin • Blocked antihypertensive effect if taken with cimetidine

■ Nursing Considerations
Assessment
- *History:* Allergy to aprotinin, first time CABG surgery, pregnancy
- *Physical:* Skin—lesions, color, temperature; P, BP, peripheral perfusion, baseline ECG; R, adventitious sounds; prothrombin time, renal and hepatic function tests

Implementation
- Administer test dose of 10 ml before any administration.
- Administer loading dose slowly with patient in the supine position; sudden drops in blood pressure may occur.
- Evaluate patient regularly for signs of cardiovascular effects.

Drug-specific teaching points
- Patients receiving this drug will be unaware of its effects; information about this drug can be incorporated into the general teaching about coronary artery bypass surgery.

❐ asparaginase

(a **spare'** a gi nase)
colaspase
Elspar, Kidrolase (CAN)
Pregnancy Category C

Drug classes
Antineoplastic agent

Therapeutic actions
Asparaginase is an enzyme that hydrolyzes the amino acid asparagine, which is needed by some malignant cells (but not normal cells) for protein synthesis; thus, it inhibits malignant cell proliferation by interruption of protein synthesis; maximal effect in G1 phase of the cell cycle.

Indications
- Acute lymphocytic leukemia as part of combination therapy to induce remissions in children
- Unlabeled uses: other leukemias, lymphosarcoma

Contraindications/cautions
- Allergy to asparaginase, pancreatitis or history of pancreatitis, impaired hepatic

Adverse effects in *Italics* are most common; those in **Bold** are life-threatening.

function, bone marrow depression, lactation.

Dosage
Pediatric
- ***Induction regimen I:*** Prednisone 40 mg/m^2 per day PO in three divided doses for 15 d, followed by tapering of dosage as follows: 20 mg/m^2 for 2 d, 10 mg/m^2 for 2 d, 5 mg/m^2 for 2 d, 2.5 mg/m^2 for 2 d, and then discontinue. Vincristine sulfate 2 mg/m^2 IV once weekly on days 1, 8, 15; maximum dose should not exceed 2 mg. Asparaginase 1,000 IU/kg per day IV for 10 successive days beginning on day 22.
- ***Induction regimen II:*** Prednisone 40 mg/m^2 per day PO in three divided doses for 28 d, then gradually discontinue over 14 d. Vincristine sulfate 1.5 mg/m^2 IV weekly for four doses on days 1, 8, 15, 22; maximum dose should not exceed 2 mg. Asparaginase 6,000 IU/m^2 IM on days 4, 7, 10, 13, 16, 19, 22, 25, 28.
- ***Maintenance:*** When remission is obtained, institute maintenance therapy; do not use asparaginase in maintenance regimen.
- ***Single-agent induction therapy:*** Used only when combined therapy is inappropriate or when other therapies fail; 200 IU/kg per day IV for 28 d (children or adults).

Pharmacokinetics

Route	Onset
IM	Varies
IV	30–40 min

Metabolism: T$_{1/2}$: 8–30 h
Distribution: Crosses placenta; may pass into breast milk
Excretion: Urine

IV facts
Preparation: Reconstitute vial with 5 ml of Sterile Water for Injection or Sodium Chloride Injection. Ordinary shaking does not inactivate the drug. May be used for direct IV injection or further diluted with Sodium Chloride Injection or 5% Dextrose Injection. Stable for 8 h once reconstituted; do not use unless clear. Discard any cloudy solution.

Infusion: Infuse over not less than 30 min into an already running IV infusion of Sodium Chloride Injection or 5% Dextrose Injection.

Adverse effects
- Hypersensitivity: *Skin rashes, urticaria, arthralgia,* respiratory distress to anaphylaxis
- CNS: CNS depression
- GI: *Hepatotoxicity, nausea, vomiting, anorexia,* abdominal cramps, pancreatitis
- Hematologic: Bleeding problems, **bone marrow depression**
- GU: Uric acid nephropathy, **renal toxicity**
- Endocrine: Hyperglycemia—glucosuria, polyuria
- Other: Chills, fever, weight loss; **fatal hyperthermia**

Clinically important drug-drug interactions
- Increased toxicity if given IV concurrently with or immediately before vincristine or prednisone • Diminished or decreased effect of methotrexate on malignant cells if given with or immediately following asparaginase

Drug-lab test interferences
- Inaccurate interpretation of thyroid-function tests in patients taking asparaginase because of decreased serum levels of thyroxine-binding globulin; levels usually return to pretreatment levels within 4 wk of the last dose of asparaginase.

■ Nursing Considerations
Assessment
- *History:* Allergy to asparaginase, pancreatitis or history of pancreatitis, impaired hepatic function, bone marrow depression, lactation
- *Physical:* Weight; temperature; skin—color, lesions; orientation, reflexes; liver evaluation, abdominal exam; CBC, blood

Adverse effects in *Italics* are most common; those in **Bold** are life-threatening.

sugar, liver and renal function tests, serum amylase, clotting time, urinalysis, serum uric acid levels

Implementation
- Perform an intradermal skin test prior to initial administration and when it has been a week or more between doses of asparaginase because of the risk of severe hypersensitivity reactions. Prepare skin test solution as follows: reconstitute 10,000-IU vial with 5 ml of diluent; withdraw 0.1 ml (200 IU/ml), and inject it into a vial containing 9.9 ml of diluent, giving a solution of 20 IU/ml. Use 0.1 ml of this solution (2 IU) for the skin test. Observe site for 1 h for a wheal or erythema that indicates allergic reaction.
- Arrange for desensitization if hypersensitivity reaction is noted. Check manufacturer's literature for details of desensitization dosages, or arrange for patient to receive *Erwinia* asparaginase (available from the National Cancer Institute).
- Arrange for lab tests (CBC, serum amylase, blood glucose, liver function tests, uric acid) before beginning therapy and frequently during therapy.
- For IM administration, reconstitute by adding 2 ml of Sodium Chloride Injection to the 10,000-U vial. Stable for 8 h once reconstituted; use only if clear. Limit injections at each site to 2 ml; if more is required use two injection sites.
- Monitor for any sign of hypersensitivity (eg, rash, difficulty breathing). If any of these occur, discontinue drug and consult with physician.
- Monitor for pancreatitis; if serum amylase levels rise, discontinue drug and consult with physician.
- Monitor for hyperglycemia—reaction may resemble hyperosmolar, nonketotic hyperglycemia. If present, discontinue drug and be prepared for use of IV fluids and insulin if required.

Drug-specific teaching points
- Prepare a calendar for patients who will need to return for specific treatment days and additional courses of drug therapy. Drug can be given only in the hospital setting under the direct supervision of physician.
- Know that the following side effects may occur: loss of appetite, nausea, vomiting (frequent mouth care, small frequent meals may help; try to maintain good nutrition if possible; a dietician may be able to help; an antiemetic also may be ordered); fatigue, confusion, agitation, hallucinations, depression (it may help to know that these are drug effects; use special precautions to avoid injury if these occur).
- Have regular blood tests to monitor the drug's effects.
- Report fever, chills, sore throat; unusual bleeding or bruising; yellow skin or eyes; light-colored stools, dark urine; thirst, frequent urination.

▢ aspirin

(as' pir in)
Apo-ASA (CAN), Aspergum, Bayer, Easprin, Ecotrin, Empirin, Entrophen (CAN), Genprin, Norwich, Novasen (CAN), PMS-ASA (CAN), ZORprin

Buffered aspirin products:
Alka-Seltzer, Ascriptin, Buffaprin, Bufferin

Pregnancy Category D

Drug classes
Antipyretic
Analgesic (non-narcotic)
Anti-inflammatory
Antirheumatic
Antiplatelet
Salicylate
NSAID

Therapeutic actions
Analgesic and antirheumatic effects are attributable to aspirin's ability to inhibit the synthesis of prostaglandins, important mediators of inflammation. Antipyretic effects are not fully understood, but aspirin probably acts in the thermoregulatory center of the hypothalamus to

block effects of endogenous pyrogen by inhibiting synthesis of the prostaglandin intermediary. Inhibition of platelet aggregation is attributable to the inhibition of platelet synthesis of thromboxane A_2, a potent vasoconstrictor and inducer of platelet aggregation. This effect occurs at low doses and lasts for the life of the platelet (8 d). Higher doses inhibit the synthesis of prostacyclin, a potent vasodilator and inhibitor of platelet aggregation.

Indications

- Mild to moderate pain
- Fever
- Inflammatory conditions—rheumatic fever, rheumatoid arthritis, osteoarthritis
- Reduction of risk of recurrent TIAs or stroke in males with history of TIA due to fibrin platelet emboli
- Reduction of risk of death or nonfatal MI in patients with history of infarction or unstable angina pectoris
- Unlabeled use: prophylaxis against cataract formation with long-term use

Contraindications/cautions

- Allergy to salicylates or NSAIDs (more common in patients with nasal polyps, asthma, chronic urticaria); allergy to tartrazine (cross-sensitivity to aspirin is common); hemophilia, bleeding ulcers, hemmorhagic states, blood coagulation defects, hypoprothrombinemia, vitamin K deficiency (increased risk of bleeding); impaired or renal function; chickenpox, influenza (potential risk of Reye's syndrome in children and teenagers); children with fever accompanied by dehydration; surgery scheduled within 1 wk; pregnancy (maternal anemia, antepartal and postpartal hemorrhage, prolonged gestation, and prolonged labor have been reported; readily crosses the placenta; possibly teratogenic; maternal ingestion of aspirin during late pregnancy has been associated with the following adverse fetal effects: low birth weight, increased intracranial hemorrhage, stillbirths, neonatal death); lactation.

Dosage

Available in oral and suppository forms; dosage is the same. Also available as chewable tablets, gum; enteric coated, sustained release, and buffered preparations (sustained-release aspirin is not recommended for antipyresis, short-term analgesia, or children < 12 y).

Adult

- ***Minor aches and pains:*** 325–650 mg q4h.
- ***Arthritis and rheumatic conditions:*** 3.2–6.0 g/d in divided doses.
- ***Acute rheumatic fever:*** 5–8 g/d; modify to maintain serum salicylate level of 15–30 mg/dl.
- ***TIAs in men:*** 1,300 mg/d in divided doses (650 mg bid or 325 mg qid).
- ***Myocardial infarction:*** 300–325 mg/d.

Pediatric

- ***Analgesic and antipyretic:*** 65 mg/kg per 24 h in four to six divided doses, not to exceed 3.6 g/d. Dosage recommendations by age follow:

Age (years)	Dosage mg q4h
2–3	162
4–5	243
6–8	324
9–10	405
11	486
12 and older	648

- ***Juvenile rheumatoid arthritis:*** 60–110 mg/kg per 24 h in divided doses at 4- to 6-h intervals. Maintain a serum level of 200–300 μg/ml.
- ***Acute rheumatic fever:*** 100 mg/kg per day initially, then decrease to 75 mg/kg per day for 4–6 wk. Therapeutic serum salicylate level is 15–30 mg/dl.
- ***Kawasaki disease:*** 80–180 mg/kg per day; very high doses may be needed during acute febrile period; after fever resolves, dosage may be adjusted to 10 mg/kg per day.

Pharmacokinetics

Route	Onset	Peak	Duration
Oral	5–30 min	0.25–2 h	3–6 h
Rectal	1–2 h	4–5 h	6–8 h

Metabolism: Hepatic (salicylate), T$_{1/2}$: 15 min–12 h
Distribution: Crosses placenta; passes into breast milk
Excretion: Urine

Adverse effects
NSAIDs
- **GI:** *Nausea, dyspepsia, heartburn, epigastric discomfort*, anorexia, hepatotoxicity
- **Hematologic:** *Occult blood loss, hemostatic defects*
- **Hypersensitivity:** Anaphylactoid reactions to fatal anaphylactic shock
- **Aspirin intolerance:** Exacerbation of bronchospasm, rhinitis (in patients with nasal polyps, asthma, rhinitis)
- **Salicylism:** *Dizziness, tinnitus, difficulty hearing, nausea*, vomiting, diarrhea, mental confusion, lassitude (dose related)
- **Acute aspirin toxicity:** Respiratory alkalosis, hyperpnea, tachypnea, hemorrhage, excitement, confusion, asterixis, pulmonary edema, convulsions, tetany, metabolic acidosis, **fever, coma, cardiovascular collapse**, renal and respiratory failure (dose related 20–25 g in adults, 4 g in children)

Clinically important drug-drug interactions
- Increased risk of bleeding if taken with oral anticoagulants, heparin • Increased risk of GI ulceration with steroids, phenylbutazone, alcohol, NSAIDs • Increased serum salicylate levels due to decreased salicylate excretion when taken with urine acidifiers (ammonium chloride, ascorbic acid, methionine) • Increased risk of salicylate toxicity with carbonic anhydrase inhibitors, furosemide • Decreased serum salicylate levels if taken with corticosteroids • Decreased serum salicylate levels due to increased renal excretion of salicylates if taken with acetazolamide, methazolamide, certain antacids, alkalinizers • Decreased absorption of aspirin if taken with nonabsorbable antacids • Increased methotrexate levels and toxicity if taken with aspirin • Increased effects of valproic acid secondary to displacement from plasma protein sites • Greater glucose lowering effect of sulfonylureas, insulin when taken with large doses (> 2 g/d) of aspirin • Decreased antihypertensive effect of captopril, beta-adrenergic blockers if taken with salicylates; consider discontinuation of aspirin • Decreased uricosuric effect of probenecid, sulfinpyrazone • Possible decreased diuretic effects of spironolactone, furosemide (in patients with compromised renal function) • Unexpected hypotension may occur if taken with nitroglycerin

Drug-lab test interferences
- Decreased serum protein bound iodine (PBI) due to competition for binding sites • False-negative readings for urine glucose by glucose oxidase method and copper reduction method with moderate to large doses of aspirin • Interference with urine 5-HIAA determinations by fluorescent methods but not by nitrosonaphthol colorimetric method • Interference with urinary ketone determination by the ferric chloride method • Falsely elevated urine VMA levels with most tests; a false decrease in VMA using the Pisano method

■ Nursing Considerations

Assessment
- *History:* Allergy to salicylates or NSAIDs; allergy to tartrazine; hemophilia, bleeding ulcers, hemmorhagic states, blood coagulation defects, hypoprothrombinemia, vitamin K deficiency; impaired hepatic function; impaired renal function; chickenpox; influenza; children with fever accompanied by dehydration; surgery scheduled within 1 wk; pregnancy; lactation
- *Physical:* Skin—color, lesions; temperature; eighth cranial nerve function, orientation, reflexes, affect; P, BP, perfusion; R, adventitious sounds; liver evaluation, bowel sounds; CBC, clotting times, urinalysis, stool guaiac, renal and liver function tests

Adverse effects in *Italics* are most common; those in **Bold** are life-threatening.

Implementation

- Administer drug with food or after meals if GI upset occurs.
- Administer drug with full glass of water to reduce risk of tablet or capsule lodging in the esophagus.
- Do not crush, and ensure that patient does not chew sustained-release preparations.
- Do not use aspirin that has a strong vinegar-like odor.
- Institute emergency procedures if overdose occurs: gastric lavage, induction of emesis, activated charcoal, supportive therapy.

Drug-specific teaching points

- Be aware that one OTC aspirin preparation is as good as another; you do not need to pay a high price to get the desired effect.
- Use the drug only as suggested; avoid overdose. Take the drug with food or after meals if GI upset occurs.
- Know that the following side effects may occur: nausea, GI upset, heartburn (taking the drug with food may help); easy bruising, gum bleeding (these are related to aspirin's effects on blood clotting)
- Avoid the use of other OTC drugs while you are taking this drug. Many of these drugs contain aspirin, and serious overdosage can occur.
- Report ringing in the ears; dizziness, confusion; abdominal pain; rapid or difficult breathing; nausea, vomiting.
- Take extra precautions to keep this drug out of the reach of children; this drug can be very dangerous for children.

☐ astemizole

(a stem' mi zole)
Hismanal

Pregnancy Category C

Drug classes
Antihistamine (nonsedating type)

Therapeutic actions
Competitively blocks the effects of histamine at peripheral H_1 receptor sites; has anticholinergic (atropine-like) and antipruritic effects.

Indications

- Relief of symptoms associated with perennial and seasonal allergic rhinitis; vasomotor rhinitis; allergic conjunctivitis; mild, uncomplicated urticaria and angioedema
- Amelioraton of allergic reactions to blood or plasma
- Dermatographism
- Adjunctive therapy in anaphylactic reactions

Contraindications/cautions

- Allergy to any antihistamines; narrow-angle glaucoma, stenosing peptic ulcer, symptomatic prostatic hypertrophy, asthmatic attack, bladder neck obstruction, pyloroduodenal obstruction; lactation

Dosage

Adult and pediatric > 12 y: 10 mg PO bid; to achieve the optimal dose, 30 mg may be given the first day, 20 mg the second day, and 10 mg daily thereafter.
Pediatric < 12 y: Safety and efficacy not established.
Geriatric or hepatic impairment: More likely to cause dizziness, sedation, syncope, toxic confusional states, and hypotension in elderly patients; use with caution.

Pharmacokinetics

Route	Onset	Peak	Duration
Oral	1–2 h	2–4 h	4–6 h

Metabolism: Hepatic, $T_{1/2}$: 20 h first phase, 7–11 d second phase
Distribution: Crosses placenta; passes into breast milk
Excretion: Urine and feces

Adverse effects

- CNS: *Headache, nervousness, dizziness*, depression
- GI: *Appetite increase*, nausea, diarrhea, abdominal pain
- CV: Palpitation, edema

Adverse effects in *Italics* are most common; those in **Bold** are life-threatening.

- **Respiratory:** Bronchospasm, pharyngitis
- **General:** *Weight gain*
- **Other:** Fever, photosensitivity, rash, myalgia, arthralgia, angioedema

Clinically important drug-drug interactions
- Additive CNS depressant effects if taken with alcohol, other CNS depressants • Increased and prolonged anticholinergic (drying) effects if taken with MAO-inhibitors; avoid this combination

Drug-lab test interferences
- False skin testing procedures if done while patient is on antihistamines

■ Nursing Considerations

Assessment
- *History:* Allergy to any antihistamines; narrow-angle glaucoma, stenosing peptic ulcer, symptomatic prostatic hypertrophy, asthmatic attack, bladder neck obstruction, pyloroduodenal obstruction; lactation
- *Physical:* Skin—color, lesions, texture; orientation, reflexes, affect; vision exam; R, adventitious sounds; prostate palpation; serum transaminase levels.

Implementation
- Administer on an empty stomach, 1 h before or 2 h after meals.

Drug-specific teaching points
- Take this drug on an empty stomach, 1 h before or 2 h after meals or food of any kind.
- Know that the following side effects may occur: dizziness, sedation, drowsiness (use caution if driving or performing tasks that require alertness if these occur); headache (consult with your nurse or physician for appropriate treatment if this becomes a problem); thickening of bronchial secretions, dryness of nasal mucosa (a humidifier may help if this becomes a problem).
- Avoid the use of alcohol while on this drug; serious sedation could occur.
- Report difficulty breathing, hallucinations, tremors, loss of coordination, irregular heartbeat.

☐ atenolol

*(a **ten'** of lole)*

Apo-Atenol (CAN), Novo-Atenol (CAN), Tenormin

Pregnancy Category C

Drug classes
Beta-adrenergic blocking agent (β_1 selective)
Antihypertensive drug

Therapeutic actions
Blocks beta-adrenergic receptors of the sympathetic nervous system in the heart and juxtaglomerular apparatus (kidney), thus decreasing the excitability of the heart, decreasing cardiac output and oxygen consumption, decreasing the release of renin from the kidney, and lowering blood pressure.

Indications
- Treatment of angina pectoris due to coronary atherosclerosis
- Hypertension, as a step 1 agent, alone or with other drugs, especially diuretics
- Treatment of myocardial infarction
- Unlabeled uses: prevention of migraine headaches; alcohol withdrawal syndrome, treatment of ventricular arrhythmias

Contraindications/cautions
- Contraindicated in the presence of sinus bradycardia, second- or third-degree heart block, cardiogenic shock, CHF.
- Use caution in the presence of renal failure, diabetes or thyrotoxicosis (atenolol can mask the usual cardiac signs of hypoglycemia and thyrotoxicosis), lactation.

Dosage
Adult
- ***Hypertension:*** Initially 50 mg PO once a day; after 1–2 wk, dose may be increased to 100 mg
- ***Angina pectoris:*** Initially 50 mg PO qd. If optimal response is not achieved

Adverse effects in *Italics* are most common; those in **Bold** are life-threatening.

in 1 wk, increase to 100 mg qd; up to 200 mg/d may be needed.
- ***Acute myocardial infarction:*** Initially 5 mg IV given over 5 min as soon as possible after diagnosis; follow with IV injection of 5 mg 10 min later. Switch to 50 mg PO 10 min after the last IV dose; follow with 50 mg PO 12 h later. Thereafter, administer 100 mg PO qd or 50 mg PO bid for 6–9 d or until discharge from the hospital.

Geriatric or renal impaired: Dosage reduction is required because atenolol is excreted through the kidneys. The following dosage is suggested:

Creatinine Clearance (ml/min/1.73m²)	Half-Life (h)	Maximum Dosage
15–35	16–27	50 mg/d
<14	>27	50 mg qod

Hemodialysis patients: 50 mg after each dialysis; administer only under hospital administration; severe hypotension can occur.

Pediatric: Safety and efficacy not established.

Pharmacokinetics

Route	Onset	Peak	Duration
Oral	Varies	2–4 h	24 h
IV	Immediate	5 min	24 h

Metabolism: T$_{1/2}$: 6–7 h

Distribution: Crosses placenta; passes into breast milk

Excretion: Urine (40%–50%) and bile/feces (50%–60%)

IV facts

Preparation: May be diluted in Dextrose Injection, Sodium Chloride Injection, or Sodium Chloride and Dextrose Injection. Stable for 48 h after mixing.

Infusion: Initiate treatment as soon as possible after admission to the hospital; inject 5 mg over 5 min; follow with another 5-mg IV injection 10 min later.

Adverse effects
- **CNS:** Dizziness, vertigo, tinnitus, fatigue, emotional depression, paresthesias, sleep disturbances, hallucinations, disorientation, memory loss, slurred speech
- **GI:** *Gastric pain, flatulence, constipation, diarrhea, nausea, vomiting,* anorexia, ischemic colitis, renal and mesenteric arterial thrombosis, retroperitoneal fibrosis, hepatomegaly, acute pancreatitis
- **CV:** *Bradycardia, CHF, cardiac arrhythmias, sinoartial or AV nodal block, tachycardia,* peripheral vascular insufficiency, claudication, CVA, pulmonary edema, hypotension
- **Respiratory:** Bronchospasm, dyspnea, cough, bronchial obstruction, nasal stuffiness, rhinitis, pharyngitis (less likely than with propranolol)
- **GU:** *Impotence, decreased libido*, Peyronie's disease, dysuria, nocturia, frequent urination
- **MS:** Joint pain, arthralgia, muscle cramp
- **EENT:** Eye irritation, dry eyes, conjunctivitis, blurred vision
- **Dermatologic:** Rash, pruritus, sweating, dry skin
- **Allergic reactions:** Pharyngitis, erythematous rash, fever, sore throat, laryngospasm, respiratory distress
- **Other:** *Decreased exercise tolerance, development of antinuclear antibodies,* hyperglycemia or hypoglycemia, elevated serum transaminase, alkaline phosphatase, and LDH

Clinically important drug-drug interactions
- Increased effects of atenolol if taken with verapamil, anticholinergics, quinidine • Increased risk of postural hypotension if taken concurrently with prazosin • Increased risk of lidocaine toxicity if taken with atenolol • Possible increased blood pressure-lowering effects if taken concurrently with aspirin, bismuth subsalicylate, magnesium salicylate, sulfinpyrazone, oral contraceptives • Decreased antihypertensive effects if taken with NSAIDs, clonidine • Decreased antihypertensive and

antianginal effects of atenolol if taken with ampicillin, calcium salts • Possible increased hypoglycemic effect of insulin if taken with atenolol

Drug-lab test interferences
• Possible false results with glucose or insulin tolerance tests

■ Nursing Considerations
Assessment
- *History:* Sinus bradycardia, second- or third-degree heart block, cardiogenic shock, CHF, renal failure, diabetes or thyrotoxicosis, lactation
- *Physical:* Baseline body weight, skin condition, neurologic status, P, BP, ECG, respiratory status, kidney and thyroid function, blood and urine glucose

Implementation
- Do not discontinue drug abruptly after chronic therapy (hypersensitivity to catecholamines may have developed, causing exacerbation of angina, MI, and ventricular dysrhythmias). Taper drug gradually over 2 wk with monitoring.
- Consult physician about withdrawing drug if patient is to undergo surgery (withdrawal is controversial).

Drug-specific teaching points
- Take drug with meals if GI upset occurs.
- Do not stop taking this drug unless instructed to do so by a health care provider.
- Avoid driving or dangerous activities if dizziness, weakness occur.
- Know that the following side effects may occur: dizziness, lightheadedness, loss of appetite, nightmares, depression, sexual impotence.
- Report difficulty breathing, night cough, swelling of extremities, slow pulse, confusion, depression, rash, fever, sore throat.

🗌 atovaquone

(a toe' va kwon)
Mepron
Pregnancy Category C

atovaquone ■ 137

Drug classes
Antiprotozoal

Therapeutic actions
Directly inhibits enzymes required for nucleic acid and ATP synthesis in protozoa; effective against *Pneumocystis carinii*.

Indications
- Acute oral treatment of mild to moderate *P. carinii* pneumonia (PCP) in patients who are intolerant to trimethoprim-sulfamethoxazole.

Contraindications/cautions
- Contraindicated in the presence of development or history of potentially life-threatening allergic reactions to any of the components of the drug.
- Use caution in the presence of severe PCP infections, the elderly, lactation.

Dosage
Adult: 750 mg PO tid administered with food for 21 d.
Pediatric: Safety and efficacy not established.
Geriatric: Use caution, and evaluate patient response regularly.

Pharmacokinetics

Route	Onset	Peak	Duration
Oral	Varies	1–8 h	3–5 d

Metabolism: $T_{1/2}$: 2.2–2.9 d
Distribution: Crosses placenta; may pass into breast milk
Excretion: Feces

Adverse effects
- **CNS:** Dizziness, *insomnia, headache*
- **GI:** Constipation, *diarrhea, nausea, vomiting,* anorexia, abdominal pain, oral monilia infections
- **Dermatologic:** *Rash*, pruritus, sweating, dry skin
- **Other:** *Fever*, elevated liver enzymes, hyponatremia

Clinically important drug-drug interactions
- Decreased effects of other highly protein-bound drugs

Adverse effects in *Italics* are most common; those in **Bold** are life-threatening.

Clinically important drug-food interactions
- Markedly increased absorption of atovaquone when taken with food

Nursing Considerations
Assessment
- *History:* History of potentially life-threatening allergic reactions to any of the components of the drug, severe PCP infections, elderly, lactation
- *Physical:* Temperature, skin condition, neurologic status, abdominal evaluation, serum electrolytes, liver function tests

Implementation
- Give drug with meals.
- Ensure that this drug is taken for 21 d.

Drug-specific teaching points
- Take drug with food; food increases the absorption of the drug.
- Know that the following side effects may occur: dizziness, insomnia, headache (medication may be ordered to help if this occurs); nausea, vomiting (small frequent meals may help); diarrhea or constipation (consult with your health care provider for appropriate treatment); superinfections (appropriate therapy may be ordered); rash (good skin care may help).
- Report fever, mouth infection, severe headache, severe nausea or vomiting, rash.

atropine sulfate

(a' troe peen)

Parenteral and oral preparations: Minims (CAN)

ophthalmic solution:
Atropine Sulfate S.O.P., Atropisol (CAN), Dioptic's Atropine (CAN), Isopto-Atropine Ophthalmic, R.O. Atropine (CAN)

Pregnancy Category C

Drug classes
Anticholinergic
Antimuscarinic
Parasympatholytic
Antiparkinsonism drug
Antidote
Diagnostic agent (ophthalmic preparations)
Belladonna alkaloid

Therapeutic actions
Competitively blocks the effects of acetylcholine at muscarinic cholinergic receptors that mediate the effects of parasympathetic postganglionic impulses, thus depressing salivary and bronchial secretions, dilating the bronchi, inhibiting vagal influences on the heart, relaxing the GI and GU tracts, inhibiting gastric acid secretion (high doses), relaxing the pupil of the eye (mydriatic effect), and preventing accommodation for near vision (cycloplegic effect); also blocks the effects of acetylcholine in the CNS.

Indications
- Systemic administration: Antisialogogue for preanesthetic medication to prevent or reduce respiratory tract secretions
- Treatment of parkinsonism; relieves tremor and rigidity
- Restoration of cardiac rate and arterial pressure during anesthesia when vagal stimulation produced by intra-abdominal traction causes a decrease in pulse rate, lessening the degree of AV block when increased vagal tone is a factor (eg, some cases due to digitalis)
- Relief of bradycardia and syncope due to hyperactive carotid sinus reflex
- Relief of pylorospasm, hypertonicity of the small intestine, and hypermotility of the colon
- Relaxation of the spasm of biliary and ureteral colic and bronchospasm
- Relaxation of the tone of the detrusor muscle of the urinary bladder in the treatment of urinary tract disorders
- Control of crying and laughing episodes in patients with brain lesions
- Treatment of closed head injuries that cause acetylcholine release into CSF, EEG abnormalities, stupor, neurologic signs
- Relaxation of uterine hypertonicity
- Management of peptic ulcer

atropine sulfate ■ 139

- Control of rhinorrhea of acute rhinitis or hay fever
- Antidote (with external cardiac massage) for cardiovascular collapse from overdose of parasympathomimetic (cholinergic) drugs (choline esters, pilocarpine), or cholinesterase inhibitors (eg, physostigmine, isofluorphate, organophosphorus insecticides)
- Antidote for poisoning by certain species of mushroom (eg, *Amanita muscaria*)
- **Ophthalmic preparations:** diagnostically to produce mydriasis and cycloplegiapupillary dilation in acute inflammatory conditions of the iris and uveal tract

Contraindications/cautions
- Contraindicated in the presence of hypersensitivity to anticholinergic drugs.
- Systemic administration: Contraindicated in the presence of glaucoma, adhesions between iris and lens, stenosing peptic ulcer, pyloroduodenal obstruction, paralytic ileus, intestinal atony, severe ulcerative colitis, toxic megacolon, symptomatic prostatic hypertrophy, bladder neck obstruction, bronchial asthma, COPD, cardiac arrhythmias, tachycardia, myocardial ischemia, impaired metabolic, liver or kidney function, myasthenia gravis.
- Use caution in the presence of Down syndrome, brain damage, spasticity, hypertension, hyperthyroidism, lactation.
- Ophthalmic solution: Contraindicated with glaucoma or tendency to glaucoma.

Dosage
Adult
- ***Systemic administration:*** 0.4–0.6 mg IM, SC, IV
- *Hypotonic radiography:* 1 mg IM.
- *Surgery:* 0.5 mg (0.4–0.6 mg) IM (or SC, IV) prior to induction of anesthesia; during surgery, give IV; reduce dose to < 0.4 mg with cyclopropane anesthesia.
- *Bradyarrhythmias:* 0.4–1 mg (up to 2 mg) IV every 1–2 h as needed.
- *Antidote:* For poisoning due to cholinesterase inhibitor insecticides, give large doses of at least 2–3 mg parenterally, and repeat until signs of atropine intoxication appear; for "rapid" type of mushroom poisoning, give in doses sufficient to control parasympathetic signs before coma and cardiovascular collapse intervene.
- ***Ophthalmic solution:*** *For refraction:* instill 1–2 drops into eye(s) 1 h before refracting. *For uveitis:* instill 1–2 drops into eye(s) four times daily.

Pediatric
- *Systemic administration:* Refer to the following chart:

Weight		
lb	kg	Dose (mg)
7–16	3.2–7.3	0.1
16–24	7.3–10.9	0.15
24–40	10.9–18.1	0.2
40–65	18.1–29.5	0.3
65–90	29.5–40.8	0.4
>90	>40.8	0.4–0.6

- ***Surgery:*** 0.1 mg (newborn) to 0.6 mg (12 y) injected SC 30 min before surgery.

Geriatric: More likely to cause serious adverse reactions, especially CNS reactions, in elderly patients; use with caution.

Pharmacokinetics

Route	Onset	Peak	Duration
IM	10–15 min	30 min	4 h
IV	Immediate	2–4 min	4 h
SC	Varies	1–2 h	4 h
Topical	5–10 min	30–40 min	7–14 d

Metabolism: Hepatic, $T_{1/2}$: 2.5 h
Distribution: Crosses placenta; passes into breast milk
Excretion: Urine

IV facts
Preparation: Give undiluted or dilute in 10 ml sterile water.
Infusion: Give direct IV; administer 1 mg or less over 1 min

Adverse effects
Systemic Administration
- CNS: *Blurred vision, mydriasis, cycloplegia, photophobia,* increased intraocular pressure, headache, flushing, ner-

Adverse effects in *Italics* are most common; those in **Bold** are life-threatening.

vousness, weakness, dizziness, insomnia, mental confusion or excitement (after even small doses in the elderly), nasal congestion
- GI: *Dry mouth, altered taste perception, nausea,* vomiting, dysphagia, heartburn, constipation, bloated feeling, **paralytic ileus**, gastroesophageal reflux
- CV: *Palpitations, bradycardia* (low doses), *tachycardia* (higher doses)
- GU: *Urinary hesitancy and retention*; impotence
- Other: *Decreased sweating and predisposition to heat prostration,* suppression of lactation

Ophthalmic Preparations
- Local: *Transient stinging*
- Systemic: Systemic adverse effects, depending on amount absorbed

Clinically important drug-drug interactions
- Increased anticholinergic effects when given with other drugs that have anticholinergic activity: certain antihistamines, certain antiparkinson drugs, tricyclic antidepressants, MAO inhibitors. • Decreased antipsychotic effectiveness of haloperidol when given with atropine • Decreased effectiveness of phenothiazines given with atropine, but increased incidence of paralytic ileus

■ Nursing Considerations

Assessment
- *History:* Hypersensitivity to anticholinergic drugs; glaucoma; adhesions between iris and lens; stenosing peptic ulcer, pyloroduodenal obstruction, paralytic ileus, intestinal atony, severe ulcerative colitis, toxic megacolon, symptomatic prostatic hypertrophy, bladder neck obstruction, bronchial asthma, COPD, cardiac arrhythmias, myocardial ischemia, impaired metabolic, liver or kidney function, myasthenia gravis, Down syndrome, brain damage, spasticity, hypertension, hyperthyroidism, lactation
- *Physical:* Skin—color, lesions, texture; body temperature; orientation, reflexes, bilateral grip strength; affect; ophthalmic exam; P, BP; R, adventitious sounds; bowel sounds, normal GI output; normal urinary output, prostate palpation; liver and kidney function tests, ECG

Implementation
- Ensure adequate hydration; provide environmental control (temperature) to prevent hyperpyrexia.
- Encourage patient to void before taking medication if urinary retention becomes a problem.

Drug-specific teaching points
- When used preoperatively or in other acute situations, incorporate teaching about the drug with teaching about the procedure; the ophthalmic solution is used mainly acutely and will not be self-administered by the patient; the following apply to use of the oral medication for outpatients:
- Take as prescribed, 30 min before meals; avoid excessive dosage.
- Avoid hot environments while you are taking this drug; you will be heat intolerant, and dangerous reactions may occur.
- Know that the following side effects may occur: dizziness, confusion (use caution if driving or performing hazardous tasks if these occur); constipation (ensure adequate fluid intake, proper diet); dry mouth (sugarless lozenges, frequent mouth care may help; this effect sometimes lessens with time); blurred vision, sensitivity to light (it may help to know that these are drug effects that will go away when you discontinue the drug; avoid tasks that require acute vision; wear sunglasses in bright light if these occur); impotence (this is a drug effect that will go away when you discontinue the drug); difficulty in urination (it may help to empty the bladder immediately before taking each dose of drug).
- Report skin rash; flushing; eye pain; difficulty breathing; tremors, loss of coordination; irregular heartbeat, palpitations; headache; abdominal distention; hallucinations; severe or persistent dry mouth;

Adverse effects in *Italics* are most common; those in **Bold** are life-threatening.

difficulty swallowing; difficulty in urination; constipation; sensitivity to light.

☐ auranofin

(au rane' oh fin)
Ridaura

Pregnancy Category C

Drug classes
Antirheumatic agent
Gold compound

Therapeutic actions
Suppresses and prevents arthritis and synovitis—taken up by macrophages with resultant inhibition of phagocytosis and inhibition of activities of lysosomal enzymes; decreases concentrations of rheumatoid factor and immunoglobulins; exact mechanisms of action not known; no substantial evidence of remission induction.

Indications
- Management of adults with active classic or definite rheumatoid arthritis who have insufficient response or are intolerant to NSAIDs (given only orally)
- Unlabeled use: alternative or adjuvant to corticosteroids in treatment of pemphigus, SLE; for psoriatic arthritis in patients who do not tolerate or respond to NSAIDs

Contraindications/cautions
- Contraindicated in the presence of allergy to gold preparations; history of gold-induced disorders, necrotizing entercolitis, pulmonary fibrosis, exfoliative dermatitis, bone marrow aplasia, severe hematologic disorders, lactation.
- Use caution in the presence of diabetes mellitus, CHF, hypertension, compromised liver or renal function, compromised cerebral or cardiovascular circulation, inflammatory bowel disease, blood dyscrasias.

Dosage
Contains approximately 29% gold
Adult: 6 mg/d PO, either as 3 mg bid or 6 mg qd. If response is not adequate after 6 mo, dosage may be increased to 9 mg/d (3 mg tid). If response is not adequate at this dose after 3 mo, discontinue drug; do not exceed 9 mg/d.
- *Transfer from injectable gold:* Discontinue injectable agent, and start auranofin 6 mg/d PO.

Pediatric: Safety and efficacy not established.
Geriatric: Monitor patients carefully; tolerance to gold decreases with age.

Pharmacokinetics

Route	Onset	Peak
Oral	Varies	1–2 h

Metabolism: $T_{1/2}$: 26 d
Distribution: Crosses placenta; passes into breast milk
Excretion: Urine and feces

Adverse effects
- GI: *Nausea, vomiting, anorexia, abdominal cramps, diarrhea, stomatitis, glossitis,* gingivitis, metallic taste, pharyngitis, gastritis, colitis, conjunctivitis, hepatitis with jaundice
- Respiratory: Gold bronchitis, **interstitial pneumonitis and fibrosis**, cough, shortness of breath, tracheitis
- Hematologic: *Anemias,* granulocytopenia, thrombocytopenia, leukopenia, eosinophilia
- GU: Nephrotic syndrome or glomerulitis with proteinuria and hematuria; **acute tubular necrosis and renal failure,** vaginitis
- Dermatologic: *Dermatitis; pruritis, erythema,* exfoliative dermatitis, chrysiasis (gray-blue color to the skin due to gold deposition)
- **Allergic reactions:** Nitroid reactions: flushing, fainting, dizziness, sweating, nausea, vomiting, malaise, weakness

Adverse effects in *Italics* are most common; those in **Bold** are life-threatening.

Clinically important drug-drug interactions
- Do not use with penicillamine, antimalarials, cytotoxic drugs, immunosuppressive agents other than low doses of corticosteroids

■ Nursing Considerations
Assessment
- *History:* Allergy to gold preparations, history of gold-induced disorders, diabetes mellitus, CHF, hypertension, compromised liver or renal function, compromised cerebral or cardiovascular circulation, inflammatory bowel disease, blood dyscrasias, lactation
- *Physical:* Skin—color, lesions; body temperature; edema; R, adventitious sounds; GI mucous membranes, bowel sounds, liver evaluation; CBC, renal and liver function tests, chest x-ray

Implementation
- Do not administer drug to patients with history of idiosyncratic or severe reactions to gold therapy.
- Monitor hematologic status, liver and kidney function, respiratory status regularly during the course of drug therapy.
- Arrange for discontinuation of drug at first sign of toxic reaction.
- Arrange for use of low-dose systemic corticosteroids for treatment of severe stomatitis, dermatitis, renal, hematologic, pulmonary, enterocolitic complications.
- Protect patient from exposure to sunlight or ultraviolet light to decrease risk of chrysiasis.

Drug-specific teaching points
- Take this drug as prescribed; do not take more than prescribed. This drug's effects are not seen immediately; several months of therapy are needed to see results.
- Be aware that this drug does not cure the disease but does stop its effects.
- Know that the following side effects may occur: diarrhea (assure ready access to bathroom facilities); mouth sores, metallic taste (frequent mouth care will help); rash, gray-blue color to the skin (avoid exposure to the sun or ultraviolet light to help to decrease this effect); nausea, loss of appetite (small, frequent meals may help).
- Do not become pregnant while on this drug; if you decide to become pregnant, consult with physician about discontinuing drug.
- Report unusual bleeding or bruising; sore throat, fever; severe diarrhea; skin rash; mouth sores.

☐ aurothioglucose

*(aur oh thye oh **gloo**' kose)*
Solganal

Pregnancy Category C

Drug classes
Antirheumatic agent
Gold compound

Therapeutic actions
Suppresses and prevents arthritis and synovitis; taken up by macrophages with resultant inhibition of phagocytosis and inhibition of activities of lysosomal enzymes; decreases concentrations of rheumatoid factor and immunoglobulins; no substantial evidence of remission induction.

Indications
- Treatment of selected cases of adult and juvenile rheumatoid arthritis; most effective early in disease; late in disease, when damage has occurred, gold can ony prevent further damage.

Contraindications/cautions
- Allergy to gold preparations; history of gold-induced disorders—necrotizing entercolitis, pulmonary fibrosis, exfoliative dermatitis, bone marrow aplasia, severe hematologic disorders; uncontrolled diabetes mellitus; CHF; SLE; marked hypertension, compromised liver or renal function, compromised cerebral or cardiovascular circulation, inflammatory bowel disease, blood dyscrasias, recent radiation treatments; lactation.

Dosage
Contains approximately 50% gold. Administer by IM injection only, preferably intraglutteally.

aurothioglucose 143

Adult
- **Weekly injections:** First injection, 10 mg IM; second, third injections, 25 mg IM; fourth and subsequent injections, 50 mg IM until 0.8–1 g has been given. If patient has improved and has no signs of toxicity, continue 50-mg dose at 3- to 4-wk intervals many months longer.

Pediatric
- **6–12 years:** Administer one-fourth the adult dose governed by body weight; do not exceed 25 mg/dose.

Geriatric: Monitor patients carefully; tolerance to gold decreases with age.

Pharmacokinetics

Route	Onset	Peak
IM	Slow	4–6 h

Metabolism: $T_{1/2}$: 3–7 d
Distribution: Crosses placenta; passes into breast milk
Excretion: Urine and feces

Adverse effects

- GI: *Nausea, vomiting, anorexia,* abdominal cramps, diarrhea, *stomatitis, glossitis,* gingivitis, metallic taste, pharyngitis, gastritis, colitis, conjunctivitis, hepatitis with jaundice
- Respiratory: Gold bronchitis, **interstitial pneumonitis and fibrosis**, cough, shortness of breath, tracheitis
- Hematologic: *Anemias*, granulocytopenia, thromobocytopenia, leukopenia, eosinophilia
- GU: Nephrotic syndrome or glomerulitis with proteinuria and hematuria, **acute tubular necrosis** and renal failure, vaginitis
- Dermatologic: *Dermatitis; pruritis, erythema,* exfoliative dermatitis, chrysiasis (gray-blue color to the skin due to gold deposition)
- Immediate postinjection effects: **Anaphylactic shock**, syncope, bradycardia, thickening of the tongue, dysphagia, dyspnea, angioneurotic edema
- Nonvasomotor postinjection reaction: Arthralgia for 1–2 d after the injection; usually subsides after the first few injections
- Allergic reactions: Nitroid reactions: flushing, fainting, dizziness, sweating, nausea, vomiting, malaise, weakness

Clinically important drug-drug interactions

- Do not use with penicillamine, antimalarials, cytotoxic drugs, immunosuppressive agents other than low doses of corticosteroids

■ Nursing Considerations

Assessment

- *History:* Allergy to gold preparations; history of gold-induced disorders; uncontrolled diabetes mellitus; CHF; SLE; marked hypertension; compromised liver or renal function; compromised cerebral or cardiovascular circulation; inflammatory bowel disease; blood dyscrasias; recent radiation treatments; lactation
- *Physical:* Skin—color, lesions; body temperature; edema; P, BP; R, adventitious sounds; GI mucous membranes, bowel sounds, liver evaluation; CBC, renal and liver function tests, chest x-ray

Implementation

- Do not administer drug to patients with history of idosyncratic or severe reactions to gold therapy.
- Monitor hematologic status, liver and kidney function, respiratory status regularly during the course of drug therapy.
- Administer by intragluteal IM injection.
- Monitor patient carefully at time of injection for possible postinjection reaction.
- Arrange for discontinuation of drug at first sign of toxic reaction.
- Arrange for use of low-dose systemic corticosteroids for treatment of severe stomatitis, dermatitis, renal, hematologic, pulmonary, enterocolitic complications.
- Protect patient from exposure to sunlight or ultraviolet light to decrease risk of chrysiasis.

Drug-specific teaching points

- Prepare a calendar of projected injection dates. This drug's effects are not seen

Adverse effects in *Italics* are most common; those in **Bold** are life-threatening.

- immediately; several months of therapy are needed to see results.
- Know that the following side effects may occur: increased joint pain for 1–2 d after injection (this usually subsides after the first few injections); diarrhea (ensure ready access to bathroom facilities); mouth sores, metallic taste (frequent mouth care will help); rash, gray-blue color to the skin (avoid exposure to the sun or ultraviolet light to help to decrease this effect); nausea, loss of appetite (small, frequent meals may help).
- Do not become pregnant while on this drug. If you decided to become pregnant, consult with physician about discontinuing drug.
- Report unusual bleeding or bruising; sore throat; fever; severe diarrhea; skin rash; mouth sores.

☐ azatadine maleate

(a za' te deen)
Optimine

Pregnancy Category C

Drug classes
Antihistamine (piperidine type)

Therapeutic actions
Competitively blocks the effects of histamine at H_1 receptor sites; has anticholinergic (atropine-like), antiserotonin, antipruritic, sedative, and appetite-stimulating effects.

Indications
- Relief of symptoms associated with perennial and seasonal allergic rhinitis; vasomotor rhinitis; allergic conjunctivitis; mild, uncomplicated urticaria and angioedema; amelioraton of allergic reactions to blood or plasma; dermatographism; adjunctive therapy in anaphylactic reactions
- Treatment of cold urticaria
- Unlabeled uses: stimulation of appetite in underweight patients and those with anorexia nervosa; treatment of vascular cluster headaches

Contraindications/cautions
- Contraindicated in the presence of allergy to any antihistamines, lactation, third trimester of pregnancy.
- Use caution in the presence of narrow-angle glaucoma, stenosing peptic ulcer, symptomatic prostatic hypertrophy, asthmatic attack, bladder neck obstruction, pyloroduodenal obstruction.

Dosage
Adult: 1–2 mg PO bid.
Pediatric: Safety and efficacy not established in children < 12 y.
Geriatric: More likely to cause dizziness, sedation, syncope, toxic confusional states, and hypotension in elderly patients; use with caution.

Pharmacokinetics

Route	Onset	Peak
Oral	Varies	4 h

Metabolism: Hepatic, $T_{1/2}$: 12 h
Distribution: Crosses placenta; passes into breast milk
Excretion: Urine

Adverse effects
- **CNS:** *Drowsiness, sedation, dizziness, disturbed coordination,* fatigue, confusion, restlessness, excitation, nervousness, tremor, headache, blurred vision, diplopia, vertigo, tinnitus, acute labyrinthitis, hysteria, tingling, heaviness and weakness of the hands
- **GI:** *Epigastric distress,* anorexia, increased appetite and weight gain, nausea, vomiting, diarrhea or constipation
- **CV:** Hypotension, palpitations, bradycardia, tachycardia, extrasystoles
- **Respiratory:** *Thickening of bronchial secretions,* chest tightness, wheezing, nasal stuffiness, dry mouth, dry nose, dry throat, sore throat
- **Hematologic:** Hemolytic anemia, hypoplastic anemia, thrombocytopenia, leukopenia, agranulocytosis, pancytopenia

Adverse effects in *Italics* are most common; those in **Bold** are life-threatening.

- **Rheumatoid arthritis:** Usually given daily; initial dose of 1 mg/kg PO given as a single dose or bid. If necessary, dose may be increased at 6–8 wk and thereafter by steps at 4-wk intervals. Dose increments should be 0.5 mg/kg per day up to a maximum dose of 2.5 mg/kg per day. Once patient is stabilized, dose should be decreased to lowest effective dose; decrease in 0.5-mg/kg increments. Patients who do not respond in 12 wk are probably refractory.

Pediatric
- **Renal homotransplantation:** Initial dose of 3–5 mg/kg per day IV or PO followed by a maintenance dose of 1–3 mg/kg per day.

Geriatric or renal impaired: Lower doses may be required because of decreased rate of excretion and increased sensitivity to the drug.

Pharmacokinetics

Route	Onset	Peak
Oral	Varies	1–2 h
IV	Immediate	30–45 min

Metabolism: Hepatic, $T_{1/2}$: 5 h
Distribution: Crosses placenta; may pass into breast milk
Excretion: Urine

IV facts
Preparation: Add 10 ml Sterile Water for Injection and swirl until a clear solution results; use within 24 h. Further dilution into sterile saline or dextrose is usually made for infusion.
Infusion: Infuse over 30–60 min; ranges from 5 min to 8 h for the daily dose are possible.

Adverse effects
- GI: *Nausea, vomiting,* hepatotoxicity (especially in homograft patients)
- Hematologic: *Leukopenia, thrombocytopenia, macrocytic anemia*
- Other: *Serious infections* (fungal, bacterial, protozoal infections secondary to immunosuppression; may be fatal), *carcinogenesis* (increased risk of neoplasia, especially in homograft patients)

Clinically important drug-drug interactions
- Increased effects of azathioprine if taken with allopurinol; reduce the dosage of azathioprine to one-third to one-fourth the usual dose • Reversal of the neuromuscular blockade of nondepolarizing neuromuscular junction blockers (atracurium, gallamine, pancuronium, tubocurarine, vecuronium) if taken with azathioprine

■ Nursing Considerations
Assessment
- *History:* Allergy to azathioprine; rheumatoid arthritis patients previously treated with alkylating agents; pregnancy or male partners of women trying to become pregnant; lactation
- *Physical:* Body temperature; skin—color, lesions; liver evaluation, bowel sounds; renal and liver function tests, CBC

Implementation
- Administer drug by IV route only if oral administration is not possible; switch to oral route as soon as possible.
- Administer in divided daily doses or with food if GI upset occurs.
- Monitor blood counts regularly; severe hematologic effects may require the discontinuation of therapy.

Drug-specific teaching points
- Take drug in divided doses with food if GI upset occurs.
- Avoid infection while you are on this drug; avoid crowds or people who have infections. Notify your physician at once if you injure yourself.
- Notify your physician if you think you are pregnant or if you wish to become pregnant (also applies to men whose sexual partners wish to become pregnant).
- Know that the following side effects may occur: nausea, vomiting (taking the drug in divided doses or with food may help); diarrhea; skin rash.

Adverse effects in *Italics* are most common; those in **Bold** are life-threatening.

- GU: Urinary frequency, dysuria, urinary retention, early menses, decreased libido, impotence
- Other: Urticaria, rash, **anaphylactic shock**, photosensitivity, excessive perspiration

Clinically important drug-drug interactions
- Increased and prolonged anticholinergic (drying) effects if taken with MAO inhibitors

Drug-lab test interferences
- Increase in PBI not attributable to an increase in thyroxine • False-positive pregnancy test (less likely if serum test is used)

■ Nursing Considerations

Assessment
- *History:* Allergy to any antihistamines; narrow-angle glaucoma, stenosing peptic ulcer, symptomatic prostatic hypertrophy, asthmatic attack, bladder neck obstruction, pyloroduodenal obstruction; lactation
- *Physical:* Skin—color, lesions, texture; orientation, reflexes, affect; vision exam; P, BP; R, adventitious sounds; bowel sounds; prostate palpation; CBC with differential

Implementation
- Administer with food if GI upset occurs.
- Monitor patient response, and arrange for adjustment of dosage to lowest possible effective dose.

Drug-specific teaching points
- Take as prescribed; avoid excessive dosage.
- Take with food if GI upset occurs.
- Know that the following side effects may occur: dizziness, sedation, drowsiness (use caution if driving or performing tasks that require alertness if these occur); epigastric distress, diarrhea or constipation (taking the drug with meals may help; consult with nurse or physician if diarrhea or constipation becomes a problem); dry mouth (frequent mouth care, sucking sugarless lozenges may help); thickening of bronchial secretions, dryness of nasal mucosa (use of a humidifier may help if this becomes a problem).
- Avoid the use of alcohol while on this drug; serious sedation could occur.
- Report difficulty breathing, hallucinations, tremors, loss of coordination, unusual bleeding or bruising, visual disturbances, irregular heartbeat.

☐ azathioprine

*(ay za **thye'** oh preen)*
Imuran

Pregnancy Category D

Drug classes
Immunosuppressive

Therapeutic actions
Suppresses cell-mediated hypersensitivities and alters antibody production; exact mechanisms of action in increasing homograft survival and affecting autoimmune diseases not clearly understood.

Indications
- Renal homotransplantation: adjunct for prevention of rejection
- Rheumatoid arthritis: only for use in adults meeting criteria for classic rheumatoid arthritis and not responding to conventional management
- Unlabeled use: treatment of chronic ulcerative colitis, myasthenia gravis, Behçet's syndrome, Crohn's disease

Contraindications/cautions
- Allergy to azathioprine; rheumatoid arthritis patients previously treated with alkylating agents, which may greatly increase their risk for neoplasia; pregnancy.

Dosage
Adult
- ***Renal homotransplantation:*** Initial dose of 3–5 mg/kg per day PO or IV as a single dose on the day of transplant; maintenance levels are 1–3 mg/kg per day PO. Do not increase dose to decrease risk of rejection.

Adverse effects in *Italics* are most common; those in **Bold** are life-threatening.

- Report unusual bleeding or bruising; fever, sore throat, mouth sores; signs of infection; abdominal pain; severe diarrhea; darkened urine or pale stools; severe nausea and vomiting.

☐ azithromycin

*(ay zi thro **my'** sin)*
Zithromax

Pregnancy Category B

Drug classes
Macrolide antibiotic

Therapeutic actions
Bacteriostatic or bactericidal in susceptible bacteria.

Indications
- Treatment of lower respiratory tract infections: acute bacterial exacerbations of COPD due to *H. influenzae, Moraxella catarrhalis, S. pneumoniae;* community-acquired pneumonia due to *S. pneumoniae, H. influenzae*
- Treatment of lower respiratory tract infections: streptococcal pharyngitis/tonsillitis due to *Streptococcus pyogenes* in individuals who cannot take penicillins
- Treatment of uncomplicated skin infections due to *Staphylococcus aureus, S. pyogenes, Streptococcus agalactiae*
- Treatment of nongonococcal urethritis and cervicitis due to *C. trachomatis*

Contraindications/cautions
- Contraindicated in the presence of hypersensitivity to azithromycin, erythromycin, or any macrolide antibiotic.
- Use caution in the presence of gonorrhea or syphilis, pseudomembranous colitis, hepatic or renal impairment, lactation.

Dosage
Adult
- ***Mild to moderate acute bacterial exacerbations of COPD, pneumonia, pharyngitis/tonsillitis (as second-line therapy), and uncomplicated skin and skin-structure infections:*** 500 mg PO as a single dose on the first day, followed by 250 mg PO qd on days 2 through 5 for a total dose of 1.5 g
- ***Nongonococcal urethritis and cervicitis due to C. trachomatis:*** A single 1-g PO dose.

Pediatric: Safety and efficacy not established in children < 16 y.

Pharmacokinetics

Route	Onset	Peak	Duration
Oral	Varies	2.5–3.2 h	24 h

Metabolism: $T_{1/2}$: 11–48 h
Distribution: Crosses placenta; passes into breast milk
Excretion: Unchanged in biliary excretion and urine

Adverse effects
- **CNS:** Dizziness, headache, vertigo, somnolence, fatigue
- **GI:** *Diarrhea, abdominal pain, nausea,* dyspepsia, flatulence, vomiting, melena, pseudomembranous colitis
- **Other:** *Superinfections,* **angioedema**, rash, photosensitivity, vaginitis

Clinically important drug-drug interactions
- Decreased serum levels and effectiveness of azithromycin if taken with aluminum and magnesium-containing antacids
- Possible decreased effects of theophylline if taken with azithromycin
- Possible increased anticoagulant effects of warfarin if taken with azithromycin

Clinically important drug-food interactions
- Food greatly decreases the absorption of azithromycin

■ Nursing Considerations
Assessment
- *History:* Hypersensitivity to azithromycin, erythromycin, or any macrolide antibiotic; gonorrhea or syphilis, pseudomembranous colitis, hepatic or renal impairment, lactation

Adverse effects in *Italics* are most common; those in **Bold** are life-threatening.

- *Physical:* Site of infection; skin—color, lesions; orientation, GI output, bowel sounds, liver evaluation; culture and sensitivity tests of infection, urinalysis, liver and renal function tests

Implementation

- Culture site of infection before beginning therapy.
- Administer on an empty stomach—1 h before or 2–3 h after meals. Food has a marked effect on the absorption of this drug.
- Counsel patients being treated for sexually transmitted diseases about appropriate precautions and additional therapy needed.

Drug-specific teaching points

- Take this drug on an empty stomach—1 h before or 2–3 h after meals; it should never be taken with food. Take the full course of therapy prescribed.
- Know that the following side effects may occur: stomach cramping, discomfort, diarrhea; fatigue, headache (medication may be helpful); additional infections in the mouth or vagina (consult with your care provider for appropriate treatment).
- Report severe or watery diarrhea, severe nausea or vomiting, skin rash or itching, mouth sores, vaginal sores.

☐ aztreonam

(az' tree oh nam)
Azactam

Pregnancy Category B

Drug classes
Monobactam antibiotic

Therapeutic actions
Bactericidal: interferes with bacterial cell wall synthesis, causing cell death in susceptible gram-negative bacteria, ineffective against gram-positive and anaerobic bacteria.

Indications

- Treatment of urinary tract infections, lower respiratory tract infections, skin and skin-structure infections, septicemia, intra-abdominal infections and gynecologic infections caused by suseptible strains of *E. coli, Enterobacter, Serratia, Proteus, Salmonella, Providencia, Pseudomonas, Citrobacter, Haemophilus, Neisseria, Klebsiella*

Contraindications/cautions

- Contraindicated in the presence of allergy to aztreonam.
- Use caution in the presence of immediate hypersensitivity reaction to penicillins or cephalosporins, renal and hepatic disorders, lactation.

Dosage
Available for IV and IM use only; maximum recommended dose, 8 g/d.
Adult
- *UTIs:* 500 mg–1 g q8–12h.
- *Moderately severe systemic infection:* 1–2 g q8–12h.
- *Severe systemic infection:* 2 g q6–8h.

Pediatric: Safety and efficacy not established.

Geriatric or impaired renal function: Reduce dosage by one-half in patients with estimated creatinine clearances between 10 and 30 ml/min/1.73m^2 after an initial loading dose of 1 or 2 g. *Patients on hemodialysis:* give 500 mg, 1 g, or 2 g initially; maintenance dose should be one-fourth the usual initial dose at fixed intervals of 6, 8, or 12 h.

Pharmacokinetics

Route	Onset	Peak	Duration
IM	Varies	1–1.5 h	6–8 h
IV	Immediate	30 min	6–8 h

Metabolism: T$_{1/2}$: 1.5–2 h
Distribution: Crosses placenta; passes into breast milk
Excretion: Urine

IV facts
Preparation: After adding diluent to container, shake immediatley and vigorously. Constituted solutions are not for multiple-dose use; discard any unused solution. Solution should be colorless to light straw yel-

low, which may develop a slight pink tint on standing. **IV injection:** reconstitute contents of 15-ml vial with 6–10 ml Sterile Water for Injection. **IV infusion:** Reconstitute contents of 100-ml bottle to make a final concentration not > 2% w/v (add with at least 50 ml/g azetreonam of one of the following solutions per gram of aztreonam): 0.9% Sodium Chloride Injection, Ringer's Injection, Lactated Ringer's Injection, 5% or 10% Dextrose Injection, 5% Dextrose and 0.2%, 0.45%, or 0.09% Sodium Chloride, Sodium Lactate Injection, Ionosol B with 5% Dextrose, Isolyte E, Isolyte E with 5% Dextrose, Isolyte M with 5% Dextrose, Normosol-R, Normosol-R and 5% Dextrose, Normosol-M and 5% Dextrose, 5% and 10% Mannitol Injection, Lactated Ringer's and 5% Dextrose Injection, Plasma-Lyte M and 5% Dextrose, 10% Travert Injection, 10% Travert and Electrolyte no. 1, 2, or 3 Injection. Use reconstituted solutions promptly after preparation; those prepared with Sterile Water for Injection or Sodium Chloride Injection should be used within 48 h if stored at room temperature and within 7 d if refrigerated.
Infusion: IV injection: Inject slowly over 3–5 min directly into vein or into IV tubing of compatible IV infusion. **IV infusion:** Administer over 20–60 min. If giving into IV tubing that is used to administer other drugs, flush tubing with delivery solution before and after aztreonam administration.
Compatabilities: Do not mix with nafcillin sodium, cephradine, metronidazole; other admixtures are not recommended because data are not available.

Adverse effects

- GI: *Nausea, vomiting, diarrhea,* transient elevation of SGOT, SGPT, LDH
- Dermatologic: *Rash, pruritus*
- Local: *Local phlebitis/thrombophlebitis* at IV injection site, *swelling/discomfort* at IM injection site
- Hypersensitivity: **Anaphylaxis**
- Other: Superinfections

Clinically important drug-drug interactions
- Incompatible in solution with nafcillin sodium, cephradine, metronidazole

■ Nursing Considerations
Assessment
- *History:* Allergy to aztreonam, immediate hypersensitivity reaction to penicillins or cephalosporins, renal and hepatic disorders, lactation
- *Physical:* Skin—color, lesions; injection sites; body temperature; GI mucous membranes, bowel sounds, liver evaluation; GU mucous membranes; culture and sensitivity tests of infected area; liver and renal function tests

Implementation
- Arrange for culture and sensitivity tests of infected area before beginning therapy. In acutely ill patients, therapy may begin before the results of these tests are known. If therapeutic effects are not noted, reculture area.
- **IM administration:** Reconstitute contents of 15-ml vial with at least 3 ml of appropriate diluent per gram of aztreonam. Appropriate diluents are Sterile Water for Injection, Bacteriostatic Water for Injection, 0.9% Sodium Chloride Injection, Bacteriostatic Sodium Chloride Injection. Inject deeply into a large muscle mass. Do not mix with any local anesthetic.
- Discontinue drug and provide appropriate supportive measures if hypersensitivity reaction, anaphylaxis occurs.
- Monitor injection sites, and provide appropriate comfort measures.
- Arrange for appropriate treatment and comfort measures if superinfections occur.
- Monitor patient's nutritional status, and provide small, frequent meals, mouth care if GI effects, superinfections interfere with nutrition.

Drug-specific teaching points
- Be aware that this drug can only be given IM or IV.

Adverse effects in *Italics* are most common; those in **Bold** are life-threatening.

- Know that the following side effects may occur: nausea, vomiting, diarrhea.
- Report pain, soreness at injection site; difficulty breathing; mouth sores.

bacampicillin hydrochloride

(ba kam pi sill' in)
Spectrobid, Penglobe (CAN)

Pregnancy Category B

Drug classes
Antibiotic
Penicillin, ampicillin-type

Therapeutic actions
Metabolized to ampicillin during absorption; bactericidal—inhibits synthesis of cell wall of sensitive organisms, causing cell death.

Indications
- Upper and lower respiratory tract infections caused by *beta-hemolytic streptococci, Streptococcus pyogenes, Streptococcus pneumoniae, Haemophilus influenzae*, nonpenicillinase-producing staphylococci
- UTIs caused by *Escherichia coli, Proteus mirabilis, Streptococcus faecalis*
- Skin and surface-structure infections due to streptococci and susceptible staphylococci
- Gonorrhea due to *Neisseria gonorrhoeae*

Contraindications/cautions
- Contraindicated in the presence of allergies to penicillins, cephalosporins, or other allergens.
- Use caution in the presence of renal disorders, lactation.

Dosage
Available in oral preparations only.
Adult (body weight > 25 kg)
- **Upper respiratory infections, UTIs, skin and soft-structure infections:** 400 mg PO q12h.
- **Severe infections caused by less susceptible organisms:** 800 mg PO q12h.
- **Lower respiratory tract infections:** 800 mg PO q12h.
- **Gonorrhea:** 1.6 g bacampicillin plus 1 g probenecid.

Pediatric
- **Upper respiratory infections, UTIs, skin and soft-structure infections:** 25 mg/kg per day PO in two equally divided doses q12h.
- **Severe infections caused by less susceptible organisms:** 50 mg/kg per day PO in two equally divided doses q12h.
- **Lower respiratory tract infections:** 50 mg/kg per day PO in two equally divided doses q12h.

Pharmacokinetics

Route	Onset	Peak
Oral	Varies	1 h

Metabolism: Hepatic, $T_{1/2}$: 1.5 h
Distribution: Crosses placenta; passes into breast milk
Excretion: Urine

Adverse effects
- CNS: Lethargy, hallucinations, seizures
- GI: *Glossitis, stomatitis, gastritis, sore mouth,* furry tongue, black "hairy" tongue, *nausea, vomiting, diarrhea,* abdominal pain, bloody diarrhea, enterocolitis, **pseudomembranous colitis**, nonspecific hepatitis
- CV: CHF (from sodium overload with sodium preparations)
- Hematologic: Anemia, thrombocytopenia, leukopenia, neutropenia, prolonged bleeding time
- GU: Nephritis, oliguria, proteinuria, hematuria, casts, azotemia, pyuria
- Hypersensitivity reactions: *Rash, fever, wheezing,* **anaphylaxis**
- Local: *Pain, phlebitis,* thrombosis at injection site (parenteral)
- Other: *Superinfections*—oral and rectal moniliasis, vaginitis

Adverse effects in *Italics* are most common; those in **Bold** are life-threatening.

Clinically important drug-drug interactions
• Increased bacampicillin effect if taken with probenecid • Decreased effectiveness if taken with tetracyclines, chloramphenicol • Decreased efficacy of oral contraceptives if taken with bacampicillin • Do not administer to a patient who is taking disulfiram.

Clinically important drug-food interactions
• Decreased absorption and effectiveness of bacampicillin if taken with food

■ Nursing Considerations

Assessment
- *History:* Allergies to penicillins, cephalosporins, or other allergens; renal disorders; lactation
- *Physical:* Skin—color, lesion; R, adventitious sounds; bowel sounds; CBC, liver and renal function tests, serum electrolytes, hematocrit, urinalysis

Implementation
- Culture infected area before beginning treatment; reculture area if response is not as expected.
- Administer drug without regard to meals; may be given with food.
- Administer oral suspension for fasting patients; suspension should not be given with food.

Drug-specific teaching points
- Take this drug around the clock as prescribed.
- Take the full course of therapy; do not stop taking the drug when you feel better.
- Be aware that this drug can be taken with food or meals; the suspension should be taken on an empty stomach.
- Be aware that this antibiotic is specific for the current medical problem and should not be used to self-treat other infections.
- Know that the following side effects may occur: nausea, diarrhea, GI upset (small frequent meals may help); mouth sores (frequent mouth care may help).
- Report unusual bleeding or bruising; rash, hives, fever, severe diarrhea; difficulty breathing.

☐ bacitracin

*(bass i **tray**' sin)*
Powder for Injection: Baci-IM
Ophthalmic: AK-Tracin
Topical ointment: Baciguent, Bacitin (CAN)
Pregnancy Category C

Drug classes
Antibiotic

Therapeutic actions
Antibacterial: Inhibits cell wall synthesis of susceptible bacteria, primarily staphylococci, causing cell death.

Indications
- IM: Pneumonia and empyema caused by susceptible strains of staphylococci in infants
- Ophthalmic preparations: Infections of the eye caused by susceptible strains of staphylococci
- Topical ointment: Prophylaxis of minor skin abrasions; treatment of superficial infections of the skin caused by susceptible staphylococci
- Unlabeled use (oral preparation): Antibiotic-associated pseudomembranous enterocolitis

Contraindications/cautions
- Allergy to bacitracin, renal disease, lactation

Dosage
IM use
- ***Infants < 2.5 kg:*** 900 U/kg per day IM or IV in two to three divided doses.
- ***Infants > 2.5 kg:*** 1,000 U/kg per day IM or IV in two to three divided doses.

Ophthalmic use: Half-inch ribbon in the infected eye bid to q3–4h as needed.
Topical use: Apply to affected area one to five times per day; cover with sterile bandage if needed.

Pharmacokinetics

Route	Onset	Peak	Duration
IM	Rapid	1–2 h	12–14 h

Metabolism: T$_{1/2}$: 6 h
Distribution: Crosses placenta; passes into breast milk
Excretion: Urine

Adverse effects

- **GI:** Nausea, vomiting
- **GU:** *Nephrotoxicity*
- **Local:** *Pain at IM injection site* (IM); *contact dermatitis* (topical ointment); *irritation, burning, stinging, itching, blurring of vision* (ophthalmic preparations)
- **Other:** Superinfections

Clinically important drug-drug interactions

- Increased neuromuscular blockade and muscular paralysis when given with anesthetics, nondepolarizing neuromuscular blocking drugs, drugs with neuromuscular blocking activity • Increased risk of respiratory paralysis and renal failure if taken with aminoglycosides

■ Nursing Considerations

Assessment

- *History:* Allergy to bacitracin, renal disease, lactation
- *Physical:* Site of infection; skin—color, lesions; normal urinary output; urinalysis, serum creatinine, renal function tests

Implementation

- For IM use: Reconstitute 50,000-U vial with 9.8 ml Sodium Chloride Injection with 2% procaine hydrochloride; reconstitute the 10,000-U vial with 2.0 ml of diluent (this gives a concentration of 5,000 U/ml). Refrigerate unreconstituted vials. Reconstituted solutions are stable for 1 wk, refrigerated.
- For topical application: Cleanse the area before applying new ointment.
- Culture infected area before beginning therapy.
- Ensure adequate hydration to prevent renal toxicity.
- Monitor renal function tests daily during therapy (IM use).

Drug-specific teaching points

- Administer ophthalmic preparation as follows: tilt head back; place medication into eyelid and close eyes; gently hold the inner corner of the eye for 1 min. Do not touch tube to eye. For topical application, cleanse area being treated before applying new ointment; cover with sterile bandage (if appropriate).
- Know that the following side effects may occur: superinfections (frequent hygiene measures will help, but medications may be required); burning, stinging, blurring of vision with ophthalmic use (this sensation usually passes within a few minutes).
- Report rash or skin lesions; change in urinary voiding patterns; changes in vision, severe stinging, or itching (ophthalmic).

☐ baclofen

(bak' loe fen)
Alpha-Baclofen (CAN),
Lioresal

Pregnancy Category C

Drug classes
Centrally acting skeletal muscle relaxant

Therapeutic actions
Precise mechanism of action not known; GABA analog but does not appear to produce clinical effects by actions on GABA minergic systems; inhibits both monosynaptic and polysynaptic spinal reflexes; CNS depressant.

Indications

- Alleviation of signs and symptoms of spasticity resulting from multiple sclerosis, particularly for the relief of flexor spasms and concomitant pain, clonus, muscular rigidity (patients should have reversible spasticity so drug will aid in restoring residual function)
- Spinal cord injuries and other spinal cord diseases—may be of some value

baclofen ■ 153

- **Unlabeled uses**: trigeminal neuralgia (tic douloureux); may be beneficial in reducing spasticity in cerebral palsy in children (intrathecal use)

Contraindications/cautions
- Contraindicated in the presence of hypersensitivity to baclofen; skeletal muscle spasm resulting from rheumatic disorders.
- Use caution in the presence of stroke, cerebral palsy, Parkinson's disease, seizure disorders, lactation.

Dosage
Adult
- ***Oral:*** Individualize dosage; start at low dosage and increase gradually until optimum effect is achieved (usually 40–80 mg/d). The following dosage schedule is suggested: 5 mg PO tid for 3 d; 10 mg tid for 3 d; 15 mg tid for 3 d; 20 mg tid for 3 d. Thereafter, additional increases may be needed, but do not exceed 80 mg/d (20 mg qid); use lowest effective dose. If benefits are not evident after a reasonable trial period, gradually withdraw the drug.
- ***Intrathecal:*** Refer to manufacturer's instructions on pump implantation and intiation of chronic infusion. Testing is usually done with 50 μg/ml injected into intrathecal space over 1 min. Patient is observed for 24 h, then dose of 75 μg/1.5 ml is given; final screening bolus of 100 μg/2 ml is given 24 h later. Patients who do not respond to this dose are not candidates for the implant. Maintenance dose is determined by monitoring patient response and ranges from 12–1,500 μg/d. Smallest dose possible to achieve muscle tone without adverse effects is desired.

Pediatric: Safety for use in children < 12 y not established; orphan drug use to decrease spasticity in children with cerebral palsy is being studied.

Geriatric or renal impaired: Dosage reduction may be necessary; monitor closely (drug is excreted largely unchanged by the kidneys).

Pharmacokinetics

Route	Onset	Peak	Duration
Oral	1 h	2 h	4–8 h
Intrathecal	½–1 h	4 h	4–8 h

Metabolism: $T_{1/2}$: 3–4 h
Distribution: Crosses placenta; passes into breast milk
Excretion: Urine

Adverse effects
- **CNS:** *Transient drowsiness, dizziness, weakness, fatigue, confusion, headache, insomnia*
- **GI:** *Nausea, constipation*
- **CV:** *Hypotension,* palpitations
- **GU:** *Urinary frequency,* dysuria, enuresis, impotence
- **Other:** Rash, pruritus, ankle edema, excessive perspiration, weight gain, nasal congestion, increased SGOT, elevated alkaline phosphatase, elevated blood sugar

Clinically important drug-drug interactions
- Increased CNS depression when taken with alcohol, other CNS depressants

■ Nursing Considerations

Assessment
- *History:* Hypersensitivity to baclofen, skeletal muscle spasm resulting from rheumatic disorders, stroke, cerebral palsy, Parkinson's disease, seizure disorders, lactation
- *Physical:* Body weight; temperature; skin—color, lesions; orientation, affect, reflexes, bilateral grip strength, visual exam; P, BP; bowel sounds, normal GI output, liver evaluation; normal urinary output; liver and kidney function tests, blood and urine glucose

Implementation
- Patients receiving the implantable device for intrathecal delivery will need to learn about the programmable delivery system, frequent checks; needs to adjust dose and programming.
- Give with caution to patients whose spasticity contributes to upright posture or

Adverse effects in *Italics* are most common; those in **Bold** are life-threatening.

balance in locomotion or whenever spasticity is used to increase function.
- Arrange to taper dosage gradually to prevent hallucinations, possible psychosis.

Drug-specific teaching points
- Take this drug exactly as prescribed. Do not stop taking this drug without consulting the care provider; abrupt discontinuation may cause hallucinations.
- Avoid alcohol, sleep-inducing, or OTC drugs while you are on this drug because these could cause dangerous effects.
- Know that the following side effects may occur: drowsiness, dizziness, confusion (these effects may become less pronounced after a few days; avoid driving a car or engaging in activities that require alertness if these occur); nausea (frequent small meals may help); insomnia, headache, painful or frequent urination (it may help to know that these are effects of the drug that will go away when the drug is discontinued).
- Do not take this drug during pregnancy. If you decide to become pregnant or find that you are pregnant, consult your physician.
- Report frequent or painful urination, constipation, nausea, headache, insomnia, confusion that persist or are severe.

☐ beclomethasone dipropionate

(be kloe meth' a sone)

Beclodisk (CAN), Becloforte Inhaler (CAN), Beclovent, Beclovent Rotocaps (CAN), Beconase AQ Nasal Spray, Vancenase Nasal Inhaler, Vanceril

Pregnancy Category C

Drug classes
Corticosteroid
Glucocorticoid
Hormonal agent

Therapeutic actions
Anti-inflammatory effects; local administration into lower respiratory tract or nasal passages maximizes beneficial effects on these tissues while decreasing the likelihood of adverse corticosteroid effects from systemic absorption.

Indications
- Respiratory inhalant use: Control of bronchial asthma that requires corticosteroids in conjunction with other therapy
- Intranasal use: Relief of symptoms of seasonal or perennial rhinitis that respond poorly to other treatments

Contraindications/cautions
- Respiratory inhalant therapy: Acute asthmatic attack, status asthmaticus, systemic fungal infections (may cause exacerbations), allergy to any ingredient, nursing a baby
- Intranasal therapy: Untreated local infections (may cause exacerbations); nasal septal ulcers, recurrent epistaxis, nasal surgery or trauma (interferes with healing); lactation

Dosage
Respiratory inhalant use: 50 μg released at the valve delivers 42 μg to the patient.
- ***Adult:*** Two inhalations (84 μg) tid or qid. In severe asthma, start with 12 to 16 inhalations per day, and adjust dosage downward. Do not exceed 20 inhalations (840 μg/d).
- ***Pediatric (6–12 y):*** 1 or 2 inhalations tid or qid, not to exceed 10 inhalations (420 μg/d). Do not use in children < 6 y.

Intranasal Therapy: Each actuation of the inhaler delivers 42 μg. Discontinue therapy after 3 wk in the absence of significant symptomatic improvement.
- ***Adult:*** One inhalation (42 μg) in each nostril bid–qid (total dose 168–336 μg/d).
- ***Pediatric (> 12 y):*** One inhalation in each nostril bid–qid; not recommended for children < 12 y.

Pharmacokinetics

Route	Onset	Peak
Inhalation	rapid	1–2 wk

Metabolism: Lungs, GI, and liver, $T_{1/2}$: 3–15 h
Distribution: Crosses placenta; may pass into breast milk
Excretion: Feces

Adverse effects
Respiratory Inhalant Use
- Endocrine: Cushing's syndrome with overdosage, suppression of hypothalamic-pituitary-adrenal (HPA) function due to systemic absorption
- Local: *Oral, laryngeal, pharyngeal irritation,* fungal infections

Intranasal Use
- Respiratory: *Epistaxis, rebound congestion,* perforation of the nasal septum, anosmia
- Local: *Nasal irritation,* fungal infections
- Other: *Headache, nausea,* urticaria

■ Nursing Considerations

Assessment
- *History:* Acute asthmatic attack, status asthmaticus; systemic fungal infections; allergy to any ingredient; lactation; untreated local infections, nasal septal ulcers, recurrent epistaxis, nasal surgery or trauma
- *Physical:* Body weight, temperature; P, BP, auscultation; R, adventitious sounds; chest x-ray before respiratory inhalant therapy; exam of nares before intranasal therapy

Implementation
- Taper systemic steroids carefully during transfer to inhalational steroids as appropriate; deaths resulting from adrenal insufficiency have occurred during and after transfer from systemic to aerosol steroids.
- Arrange for use of decongestant nose drops to facilitate penetration of intranasal steroids if edema, excessive secretions are present.

Drug-specific teaching points
- Be aware that respiratory inhalant has been prescribed to help prevent asthmatic attacks, but it should not be used during an asthmatic attack.
- Allow at least 1 min between puffs (respiratory inhalant); if you also are using an inhalational bronchodilator (isoproterenol, metaproterenol, epinephrine), use it several minutes before using the steroid aerosol.
- Rinse your mouth after using the respiratory inhalant aerosol.
- Use a decongestant before the intranasal steroid, and clear your nose of all secretions if nasal passages are blocked; intranasal steroids may take several days to produce full benefit.
- Use this product exactly as prescribed; do not take more than prescribed, and do not stop taking the drug without consulting your health care provider. The drug must not be stopped abruptly but must be slowly tapered.
- Know that the following side effects may occur: local irritation (make sure you are using the device correctly), headache (consult your health care provider for appropriate treatment).
- Report sore throat or sore mouth.

❏ benazepril hydrochloride

(ben a' za pril)
Lotensin

Pregnancy Category C

Drug classes
Antihypertensive
Angiotensin-converting enzyme (ACE) inhibitor

Therapeutic actions
Benazepril blocks ACE from converting angiotensin I to angiotensin II, a potent vasoconstrictor, leading to decreased blood pressure, decreased aldosterone secretion, a small increase in serum potassium levels, and sodium and fluid loss; increased prostaglandin synthesis also

may be involved in the antihypertensive action.

Indications
- Treatment of hypertension alone or in combination with thiazide-type diuretics

Contraindications/cautions
- Contraindicated in the presence of allergy to benazepril or other ACE inhibitors.
- Use caution in the presence of impaired renal function, CHF, salt/volume depletion, lactation.

Dosage
Adult: Initial dose 10 mg PO qd. Maintenance dose: 20–40 mg/day PO as a single dose or two divided doses. Patients on diuretics should discontinue the diuretic 2–3 d before beginning benazepril therapy. If BP is not controlled, add diuretic slowly. If diuretic cannot be discontinued, begin benazepril therapy with 5 mg.
Pediatric: Safety and efficacy not established.
Geriatric and renal impaired: Ccr < 30 ml/min/1.73 m^2 (serum creatinine > 3 mg/dl): 5 mg PO qd. Dosage may be titrated upward until blood pressure is controlled up to a maximum of 40 mg/d.

Pharmacokinetics

Route	Onset	Peak	Duration
Oral	0.5–1 h	3–4 h	24 h

Metabolism: Hepatic, $T_{1/2}$: 10–11 h
Distribution: Crosses placenta; passes into breast milk
Excretion: Urine

Adverse effects
- **GI:** *Nausea*, abdominal pain, vomiting, constipation
- **CV:** Angina pectoris, hypotension in salt/volume depleted patients, palpitations
- **Respiratory:** *Cough*, asthma, bronchitis, dyspnea, sinusitis
- **Dermatologic:** Rash, pruritus, diaphoresis, flushing
- **Other:** Angioedema, impotence, decreased libido, asthenia, myalgia, arthralgia

Clinically important drug-drug interactions
- Increased risk of hypersensitivity reactions if taken concurrently with allopurinal • Increased coughing if taken with capsaicin • Decreased antihypertensive effects if taken with indomethacin • Increased lithium levels and neurotoxicity may occur if taken with benazepril

■ Nursing Considerations
Assessment
- *History:* Allergy to benazepril or other ACE inhibitors, impaired renal function, CHF, salt/volume depletion, lactation
- *Physical:* Skin—color, lesions, turgor; body temperature; P, BP, peripheral perfusion; mucous membranes, bowel sounds, liver evaluation; urinalysis, renal and liver function tests, CBC and differential

Implementation
- Alert surgeon, and mark patient's chart with notice that benazepril is being taken; the angiotensin II formation subsequent to compensatory renin release during surgery will be blocked; hypotension may be reversed with volume expansion.
- Monitor patient closely in any situation that may lead to a fall in blood pressure secondary to reduction in fluid volume (excessive perspiration and dehydration, vomiting, diarrhea) because excessive hypotension may occur.
- Arrange for reduced dosage in patients with impaired renal function.

Drug-specific teaching points
- Do not stop taking the medication without consulting your physician.
- Know that the following side effects may occur: GI upset, loss of appetite (these may be limited effects that will pass with time; if they persist or become a problem, consult your nurse or physician); lightheadedness (this usually passes after the first few days of therapy; if it occurs, change position slowly, and limit your activities to those that do not require

Adverse effects in *Italics* are most common; those in **Bold** are life-threatening.

alertness and precision); dry cough (this is irritating but not harmful; consult with your care provider if it becomes too bothersome).
- Be careful in any situation that may lead to a drop in blood pressure (diarrhea, sweating, vomiting, dehydration); if lightheadedness or dizziness occurs, consult your nurse or physician.
- Report mouth sores; sore throat, fever, chills; swelling of the hands, feet; irregular heartbeat, chest pains; swelling of the face, eyes, lips, tongue, difficulty in breathing, persistent cough.

☐ bendroflumethiazide

*(ben droe floo me **thye**' a zide)*
Naturetin

Pregnancy Category C

Drug classes
Thiazide diuretic

Therapeutic actions
Inhibits reabsorption of sodium and chloride in distal renal tubule, increasing the excretion of sodium, chloride, and water by the kidney.

Indications
- Adjunctive therapy in edema associated with CHF
- Hypertension, as sole therapy or in combination with other antihypertensives
- **Unlabeled uses:** calcium nephrolithiasis alone or with amiloride or allopurinal to prevent recurrences in hypercalciuric or normal calciuric patients; diabetes insipidus, especially nephrogenic diabetes insipidus

Contraindications/cautions
- Contraindicated in the presence of allergy to thiazides, sulfonamides; fluid or electrolyte imbalance; renal disease (risk of azotemia with thiazides); liver disease (thiazide-induced alterations in fluid and electrolyte balance may precipitate hepatic coma); gout (risk of precipitation of attack).
- Use caution in the presence of SLE; glucose tolerance abnormalities, diabetes mellitus; hyperparathyroidism; manic-depressive disorders aggravated by hypercalcemia; lactation.

Dosage
Adult
- ***Edema:*** 5 mg PO qd, preferably in the morning. Up to 20 mg once a day or divided into two doses. *Maintenance:* 2.5–5 mg PO qd. Intermittent therapy may be advantageous in some patients; every other day or a 3- to 5-d/wk schedule may be used.
- ***Hypertension:*** Initial: 5–20 mg/d PO. *Maintenance:* 2.5–15 mg/d PO.

Pediatric: Safety and efficacy not established.

Pharmacokinetics

Route	Onset	Peak	Duration
Oral	2 h	4 h	6–12 h

Metabolism: $T_{1/2}$: 3–4 h
Distribution: Crosses placenta; passes into breast milk
Excretion: Unchanged in the urine

Adverse effects
- **CNS:** *Dizziness, vertigo,* paresthesias, weakness, headache, blurred vision
- **GI:** *Nausea, anorexia, vomiting, dry mouth,* diarrhea, constipation, jaundice, hepatitis, pancreatitis
- **CV:** Orthostatic hypotension
- **GU:** Impotence, loss of libido
- **Dermatologic:** Photosensitivity, rash, purpura, exfoliative dermatitis, hives
- **Endocrine:** Hyperglycemia, hyperurecemia, glycosuria
- **Other:** Muscle cramps and muscle spasms, fever, gouty attacks, flushing, weight loss, rhinorrhea

Clinically important drug-drug interactions
- Increased thiazide effects if taken with diazoxide • Decreased absorption with cholestyramine, colestipol • Increased risk

of cardiac glycoside toxicity if hypokalemia occurs • Increased risk of lithium toxicity • Decreased effectiveness of antidiabetic agents when taken concurrently with bendroflumethiazide

Drug-lab test interferences
• Decreased PBI levels without clinical signs of thyroid disturbance • Increased creatinine, BUN

■ Nursing Considerations

Assessment
- *History:* Allergy to thiazides, sulfonamides; fluid or electrolyte imbalance, renal or liver disease; gout; SLE; glucose tolerance abnormalities, diabetes mellitus; hyperparathyroidism; manic-depressive disorders; lactation
- *Physical:* Skin—color, lesions, edema; orientation, reflexes, muscle strength; pulses, baseline ECG, BP, orthostatic BP, perfusion; respiratory rate, pattern, adventitious sounds; liver evaluation, bowel sounds; urinary output patterns; CBC, serum electrolytes, blood glucose, liver and renal function tests, serum uric acid, urinalysis

Implementation
- Administer with food or milk if GI upset occurs.
- Mark calendars or other reminders of drug days for outpatients if every other day or 3–5 d/wk therapy is the most advantageous for treating edema.
- Reduce dosage of other antihypertensive drugs by at least 50% if given concurrently with thiazides; readjust dosages gradually as blood pressure responds.
- Administer early in the day so increased urination will not disturb sleep; monitor body weights.

Drug-specific teaching points
- Record dates on a calendar or dated envelopes if this drug is ordered as intermittent therapy.
- Take the drug early in the day so increased urination will not disturb sleep. The drug may be taken with food or meals if GI upset occurs.
- Weigh yourself on a regular basis at the same time of the day and in the same clothing, and record the weight on your calendar.
- Know that the following side effects may occur: increased volume and frequency of urination (ensure ready access to a bathroom when drug effect is greatest); dizziness, feeling faint on arising, drowsiness (if these changes occur, avoid rapid position changes, hazardous activities, such as driving a car and alcohol, which can intensify these problems); sensitivity to sunlight (use sunglasses, wear protective clothing, or use a sunscreen when out of doors); decrease in sexual function; increased thirst (sucking on sugarless lozenges may help to alleviate the thirst, frequent mouth care also may help).
- Report loss or gain of more than 3 lb in one day, swelling in your ankles or fingers, unusual bleeding or bruising, dizziness, trembling, numbness, fatigue, muscle weakness or cramps.

❏ benzalkonium chloride

*(benz al **koe**' nee um)*
BAC, Benza, Zephiran

Pregnancy Category C

Drug classes
Antibiotic
Antiinfective
Surface active agent

Therapeutic actions
Exact mechanism of action is not known; bacteriostatic or bactericidal depending on concentration; may work by enzyme inactivation; known to have deodorant, wetting, detergent, keratolytic, and emulsifying action, possibly also due to enzyme activation.

Indications
- **Aqueous solutions:** antisepsis of skin, mucous membranes, and wounds; preoperative preparation of skin, surgeon's hands; treatment of wounds; preservation of ophthalmic solutions; irrigations of eye and body cavities, bladder, and urethra; vaginal douching

benzalkonium chloride ◾ 159

- **Tinctures and sprays:** preoperative treatment of skin; treatment of minor skin wounds and abrasions

Contraindications/cautions
- Use in occlusive dressings, casts, anal or vaginal packs (irritation and chemical burns may result)

Dosage
Adult and pediatric: Recommended dilutions for specific administration sites:
- ***Bladder retention lavage:*** 1:20,000–1:40,000 aqueous solution
- ***Bladder and urethral irrigation:*** 1:5,000–1:20,000 aqueous solution
- ***Breast/nipple hygiene:*** 1:1,000–1:2,000 aqueous solution
- ***Catheters and other adsorbent articles:*** 1:500 aqueous solution
- ***Deep infected wounds:*** 1:3,000–1:20,000 aqueous solution
- ***Denuded skin and mucous membranes:*** 1:5,000–1:10,000 aqueous solution
- ***Eye irrigation:*** 1:5,000–1:10,000 aqueous solution
- ***Hospital disinfections:*** 1:750 aqueous solution
- ***Minor wounds, lacerations:*** 1:750 tincture or spray
- ***Oozing and open infections:*** 1:2,000–1:5,000 aqueous solution
- ***Postepisiotomy care:*** 1:5,000–1:10,000 aqueous solution
- ***Preoperative disinfection of skin:*** 1:750 tincture, spray, or aqueous solution
- ***Preservation of ophthalmic solution:*** 1:5,000–1:7,500 aqueous solution
- ***Surgeon's hands and arms:*** 1:750 aqueous solution
- ***Vaginal douche/irrigation:*** 1:2,000–1:5,000 aqueous solution
- ***Wet dressings:*** 1:5,000 or less aqueous solution
- ***Preoperative prep:*** Perform preoperative periorbital skin or head prep only before the patient or eye is anesthesized

Pharmacokinetics
Not absorbed systemically.

Adverse effects
Very little systemic absorption occurs with the use of benzalkonium.
- **Allergic reactions:** Hypersensitivity reaction
- **Local:** Stinging, burning, erythema

Clinically important drug-drug interactions
- Incompatible in solution with iodine, silver nitrate, fluorescein, nitrates, peroxide, lanolin, potassium permanganate, aluminum, caramel, kaolin, pine oil, zinc sulfate, zinc oxide, yellow oxide of mercury

◾ Nursing Considerations

Assessment
- *History:* Hypersensitivity to benzalkonium
- *Physical:* Skin condition

Implementation
- Use Sterile Water for Injection as a diluent for aqueous solutions intended for deep wounds or irrigation of body cavities; otherwise, freshly distilled water may be used. Tap water contains metallic ions or organic matter that may reduce antibacterial potency.
- Do not use a cork stopper to close BAC solution container; do not store cotton, wool, rayon, or other materials in solution; use sterile gauze sponges to apply solution; dip into solution immediately before application.
- Rinse area thoroughly if soap and anionic detergents have been used; these agents may inactivate BAC.
- Avoid prolonged contact of solution with patient's skin; avoid pooling on operating table.
- Do not use tinted tincture or spray near an open flame or cautery; these contain flammable organic solvents.
- Irrigate eye immediately and repeatedly with water if solution stronger than 1:5,000 enters the eye.
- Further dilute solution if area for application is inflamed or irritated.

Adverse effects in *Italics* are most common; those in **Bold** are life-threatening.

Drug-specific teaching points
- Patient teaching should be incorporated into teaching about the procedures being performed.

☐ benzonatate

(ben zoe' na tate)
Perles, Tessalon

Pregnancy Category C

Drug classes
Antitussive (nonnarcotic)

Therapeutic actions
Related to the local anesthetic tetracaine; anesthesizes the stretch receptors in the respiratory passages, lungs, and pleura, dampering their activity and reducing the cough reflex at its source.

Indications
- Symptomatic relief of nonproductive cough

Contraindications/cautions
- Allergy to benzonatate or related compounds (tetracaine); lactation

Dosage
Adult and Pediatric (> 10 y): 100 mg PO tid; up to 600 mg/d may be used.

Pharmacokinetics

Route	Onset	Duration
Oral	15–20 min	3–8 h

Metabolism: Hepatic
Distribution: Crosses placenta; may pass into breast milk
Excretion: Urine

Adverse effects
- **CNS:** *Sedation, headache, mild dizziness*, nasal congestion, sensation of burning in the eyes
- **GI:** *Constipation, nausea*, GI upset
- **Dermatologic:** Pruritus, skin eruptions
- **Other:** Vague "chilly" feeling, numbness in the chest

■ Nursing Considerations
Assessment
- *History:* Allergy to benzonatate or related compounds (tetracaine); lactation
- *Physical:* Nasal mucous membranes; skin—color, lesions; orientation, affect; adventitious sounds

Implementation
- Adminster orally; caution patient not to chew or break capsules but to swallow them whole.

Drug-specific teaching points
- Swallow the capsules whole; do not chew or break capsules because numbness of the throat and mouth could occur, and swallowing could become difficult.
- Know that the following side effects may occur: rash, itching (skin care may help); constipation, nausea, GI upset; sedation, dizziness (avoid driving or task that require alertness if this occurs).
- Report restlessness, tremor, difficulty breathing, constipation, rash.

☐ benzquinamide hydrochloride

*(benz **kwin'** a mide)*
Emete-Con

Pregnancy Category C

Drug classes
Antiemetic

Therapeutic actions
Mechanism of action in humans is not known; antiemetic, antihistaminic, anticholinergic, and sedative activity seen in animals.

Indications
- Prevention and treatment of nausea and vomiting associated with anesthesia and surgery. Prophylactic use should be reserved for patients in whom emesis would endanger the surgical outcome or result in harm to the patient.

Adverse effects in *Italics* are most common; those in **Bold** are life-threatening.

Contraindications/cautions
- Hypersensitivity to benzquinamide; cardiovascular disease, hypertension, lactation.

Dosage
Adult
- **IM:** 50 mg (0.5–1 mg/kg). Repeat in 1 h, then q3–4 hours as necessary. Prophylactic use, give 15 min prior to emergence from anesthesia.
- **IV:** 25 mg (0.2–0.4 mg/kg) as a single dose slowly (1 ml/0.5–1 min). All subsequent doses should be IM.

Pediatric: Safety and efficacy not established.
Geriatric: Administer with caution; if given IV, give smaller dose over longer period, and monitor patient carefully.

Pharmacokinetics

Route	Onset	Peak	Duration
IM, IV	15 min	30 min	3–4 h

Metabolism: Hepatic, $T_{1/2}$: 40 min
Distribution: Crosses placenta
Excretion: Urine

IV facts
Preparation: Reconstitute initially with 2.2 ml Sterile Water or Bacteriostatic Water for Injection with benzyl alcohol or with methylparabens and propylparabens. This yields 2 ml of a solution equivalent to 25 mg benzquinamide/ml. Potent for 14 d. Store at room temperature.
Infusion: Infuse slowly; 1 ml every 30–60 sec. Do not use IV route with patients with cardiovascular disease or who are on cardiovascular drugs.

Adverse effects
- **CNS:** *Drowsiness,* dizziness, vertigo, tinnitus, fatigue, restlessness, headache, *dry mouth,* shivering, sweating, hiccoughs, fever, chills
- **GI:** Nausea, anorexia
- **CV:** *Hypertension,* hypotension, atrial arrhythmias
- **MS:** Twitching, shaking, weakness
- **Dermatologic:** Rash, pruritus, sweating

■ Nursing Considerations
Assessment
- *History:* Hypertension, hypotension, cardiovascular disease, lactation
- *Physical:* Body weight, skin condition, neurologic status, orientation, P, BP

Implementation
- Give drug to prevent postoperative nausea and vomiting 15 min prior to emergence from anesthesia.
- Do not administer IV to patients with cardiovascular disease; sudden increase or decrease in blood pressure could cause serious problems.
- Administer with caution to elderly or debilitated patients; use lower range of dose, and monitor closely.

Drug-specific teaching points
- Know that dry mouth may occur: mouth care, sugarless lozenges may help.
- Report headache, anxiety, lack of relief from nausea.

▢ benzthiazide

(benz thye' a zide)
Exna

Pregnancy Category C

Drug classes
Thiazide diuretic

Therapeutic actions
Inhibits reabsorption of sodium and chloride in distal renal tubule, increasing excretion of sodium, chloride, and water by the kidney.

Indications
- Adjunctive therapy in edema associated with CHF, cirrhosis, corticosteroid and estrogen therapy, renal dysfunction
- Hypertension as sole therapy or in combination with other antihypertensives
- **Unlabeled use:** diabetes insipidus, especially nephrogenic diabetes insipidus

Adverse effects in *Italics* are most common; those in **Bold** are life-threatening.

Contraindications/cautions
- Contraindicated in the presence of allergy to thiazides, sulfonamides; fluid or electrolyte imbalance; renal disease (risk of azotemia with thiazides); liver disease (thiazide-induced alterations in fluid and electrolyte balance may precipitate hepatic coma); gout (risk of precipitation of attack).
- Use caution in the presence of SLE; glucose tolerance abnormalities, diabetes mellitus; hyperparathyroidism; manic-depressive disorders aggravated by hypercalcemia; lactation.

Dosage
Adult
- ***Edema:*** Initially 50–200 mg PO qd for several days. Administer dosages > 100 mg/d in two divided doses. *Maintenance:* 50–150 mg qd.
- ***Hypertension:*** Initially: 50–100 mg PO qd in two doses of 25 or 50 mg each after breakfast and after lunch. *Maintenance:* individualize to patient's response; maximum dose of 200 mg/d.

Pharmacokinetics

Route	Onset	Peak	Duration
Oral	2 h	4–6 h	6–18 h

Metabolism: $T_{1/2}$: unknown
Distribution: Crosses placenta; passes into breast milk
Excretion: Urine

Adverse effects
- **CNS:** *Dizziness, vertigo,* paresthesias, weakness, headache, blurred vision
- **GI:** *Nausea, anorexia, vomiting, dry mouth,* diarrhea, constipation, jaundice, hepatitis, pancreatitis
- **CV:** Orthostatic hypotension
- **GU:** Impotence, loss of libido
- **Dermatologic:** Photosensitivity, rash, purpura, exfoliative dermatitis, hives
- **Endocrine:** Hyperglycemia, hyperuricemia, glycosuria
- **Other:** Muscle cramps and muscle spasms, fever, gouty attacks, flushing, weight loss, rhinorrhea

Clinically important drug-drug interactions
- Increased thiazide effects if taken with diazoxide • Decreased absorption with cholestyramine, colestipol • Increased risk of cardiac glycoside toxicity if hypokalemia occurs • Increased risk of lithium toxicity • Decreased effectiveness of antidiabetic agents when taken concurrently with bendroflumethiazide

Drug-lab test interferences
- Decreased PBI levels without clinical signs of thyroid disturbance • Increased creatinine, BUN

■ Nursing Considerations
Assessment
- *History:* Allergy to thiazides, sulfonamides; fluid or electrolyte imbalance, renal or liver disease; gout; SLE; glucose tolerance abnormalities, diabetes mellitus; hyperparathyroidism; manic-depressive disorders; lactation
- *Physical:* Skin—color, lesions, edema; orientation, reflexes, muscle strength; pulses, baseline ECG, BP, orthostatic BP, perfusion; respiratory rate, pattern, adventitious sounds; liver evaluation, bowel sounds; urinary output patterns; CBC, serum electrolytes, blood glucose, liver and renal function tests, serum uric acid, urinalysis

Implementation
- Administer early in the day so increased urination will not disturb sleep; administer with food or milk if GI upset occurs.

Drug-specific teaching points
- Take the drug early in the day so increased urination will not disturb sleep. The drug may be taken with food or meals if GI upset occurs.
- Weigh yourself on a regular basis, at the same time of the day and in the same clothing, and record the weight on your calendar.
- Know that the following side effects may occur: increased volume and frequency of urination (have ready access to a bathroom when drug effect is greatest);

dizziness, feeling faint on arising, drowsiness (if these changes occur, avoid rapid position changes; hazardous activities, such as driving a car; and alcohol, which can intensify these problems); sensitivity to sunlight (use sunglasses, wear protective clothing, or use a sunscreen when outdoors); decrease in sexual function; increased thirst (sucking on sugarless lozenges may help to alleviate the thirst, frequent mouth care also may help).
- Report loss or gain of more than 3 lb in one day, swelling in ankles or fingers, unusual bleeding or bruising, dizziness, trembling, numbness, fatigue, muscle weakness or cramps.

☐ benztropine mesylate

(benz' troe peen)

Apo-Benztropine (CAN), Cogentin, PMS Benztropine (CAN)

Pregnancy Category C

Drug classes
Antiparkinsonism drug (anticholinergic type)

Therapeutic actions
Has anticholinergic activity in the CNS that is believed to help normalize the hypothesized imbalance of cholinergic/dopaminergic neurotransmission in the basal ganglia of the brain of a parkinsonism patient. Reduces severity of rigidity and to a lesser extent, akinesia and tremor; less effective overall than levodopa; peripheral anticholinergic effects suppress secondary symptoms of parkinsonism, such as drooling.

Indications
- Adjunct in the therapy of parkinsonism (postencephalitic, arteriosclerotic, and idiopathic types)
- Control of extrapyramidal disorders (except tardive dyskinesia) due to neuroleptic drugs (eg, phenothiazines)

Contraindications/cautions
- Contraindicated in the presence of hypersensitivity to benztropine; glaucoma, especially angle-closure glaucoma; pyloric or duodenal obstruction, stenosing peptic ulcers, achalasia (megaesophagus); prostatic hypertrophy or bladder neck obstructions; myasthenia gravis.
- Use caution in the presence of tachycardia, cardiac arrhythmias, hypertension, hypotension, hepatic or renal dysfunction, alcoholism, chronic illness, people who work in hot environment; hot weather; lactation.

Dosage
Adult
- ***Parkinsonism:*** Initially 0.5–1 mg PO at bedtime; a total daily dose of 0.5–6 mg given at bedtime or in two to four divided doses is usual. Increase initial dose in 0.5 mg increments at 5- to 6-d intervals to the smallest amount necessary for optimal relief. Maximum daily dose is 6 mg. Also may be given parenterally (IM or IV) in same dosage as orally. When used concomitantly with other drugs, gradually substitute benztropine for all or part of the other medication, and gradually reduce dosage of the other drug.
- ***Drug-induced extrapyramidal symptoms:*** Acute dystonic reactions: Initially 1–2 mg IM (preferred) or IV to control condition; may repeat if parkinsonian effect begins to return. After that, 1–2 mg PO bid to prevent recurrences.
- ***Extrapyramidal disorders occurring early in neuroleptic treatment:*** 1–2 mg PO bid–tid. Withdraw drug after 1 or 2 wk to determine its continued need; reinstitute if disorder reappears.

Pediatric: Safety and efficacy not established.

Geriatric: Strict dosage regulation may be necessary; patients > 60 y often develop increased sensitivity to the CNS effects of anticholinergic drugs.

Pharmacokinetics

Route	Onset	Duration
Oral	1 h	6–10 h
IM/IV	15 min	6–10 h

Metabolism: Hepatic

benztropine mesylate

Distribution: Crosses placenta; passes into breast milk

IV facts
Preparation: Give undiluted. Store in tightly covered, light-resistant container. Store at room temparature.
Infusion: Administer direct IV at a rate of 1 mg over 1 min.

Adverse effects
Peripheral Anticholinergic Effects
- GI: *Dry mouth, constipation,* dilation of the colon, paralytic ileus, *nausea,* vomting, epigastric distress
- CV: Tachycardia, palpitations, hypotension, orthostatic hypotension
- GU: *Urinary retention, urinary hesitancy,* dysuria, difficulty achieving or maintaining an erection
- EENT: *Blurred vision,* mydriasis, diplopia, increased intraocular tension, angle-closure glaucoma
- Dermatologic: Skin rash, urticaria, other dermatoses
- Other: Flushing, decreased sweating, elevated temperature
- CNS effects, some of which are characteristic of centrally acting anticholinergic drugs
- CNS: *Disorientation, confusion,* memory loss, hallucinations, psychoses, agitation, nervousness, delusions, delirium, paranoia, euphoria, excitement, lightheadedness, dizziness, depression, drowsiness, weakness, giddiness, paresthesia, heaviness of the limbs
- Other: Muscular weakness, muscular cramping; inability to move certain muscle groups (high doses), numbness of fingers

Clinically important drug-drug interactions
- Paralytic ileus, sometimes fatal, when given with other anticholinergic drugs, with drugs that have anticholinergic properties (phenothiazines, tricyclic antidepressants) • Additive adverse CNS effects (toxic psychosis) with other drugs that have CNS anticholinergic properties (tricyclic antidepressants, phenothiazines) • Possible masking of the development of persistent extrapyramidal symptoms, tardive dyskinesia, in patients on long-term therapy with antipsychotic drugs (phenothiazines, haloperidol) • Decreased therapeutic efficacy of antipsychotic drugs (phenothiazines, haloperidol), possibly due to central antagonism

■ Nursing Considerations

Assessment
- *History:* Hypersensitivity to benztropine; glaucoma; pyloric or duodenal obstruction, stenosing peptic ulcers, achalasia; prostatic hypertrophy or bladder neck obstructions; myasthenia gravis; cardiac arrhythmias, hypertension, hypotension; hepatic or renal dysfunction; alcoholism, chronic illness, people who work in hot environment; lactation
- *Physical:* Body weight; temperature; skin—color, lesions; orientation, affect, reflexes, bilateral grip strength, visual exam including tonometry; P, BP, orthostatic BP; adventitious sounds; bowel sounds, normal output, liver evaluation; normal urinary output, voiding pattern, prostate palpation; liver and kidney function tests

Implementation
- Arrange to decrease dosage or discontinue drug temporarily if dry mouth is so severe that swallowing or speaking becomes difficult.
- Give with caution and arrange dosage reduction in hot weather, as appropriate to patient's lifestyle. Drug interferes with sweating and body's ability to maintain body heat equilibrium; provide sugarless lozenges, ice chips to suck if dry mouth is a problem.
- Give with meals if GI upset occurs; give before meals to patients bothered by dry mouth; give after meals if drooling is a problem or if drug causes nausea.

Adverse effects in *Italics* are most common; those in **Bold** are life-threatening.

- Ensure that patient voids just before receiving each dose of drug if urinary retention is a problem.

Drug-specific teaching points
- Take this drug exactly as prescribed.
- Avoid alcohol, sedatives, and OTC drugs while on this drug (many of these could cause dangerous effects).
- Know that the following side effects may occur: drowsiness, dizziness, confusion, blurred vision (avoid driving a car or engaging in activities that require alertness and visual acuity if these occur); nausea (frequent small meals may help); dry mouth (sucking sugarless lozenges or ice chips may help); painful or difficult urination (emptying the bladder immediately before each dose may help); constipation (if maintaining adequate fluid intake and exercising regularly do not help, consult your nurse or physician); use caution in hot weather (this drug makes you more susceptible to heat prostration).
- Report difficult or painful urination; constipation; rapid or pounding heartbeat; confusion, eye pain, or rash.

▢ bepridil hydrochloride

(be' pri dil)
Vascor

Pregnancy Category C

Drug classes
Calcium channel-blocker
Antianginal drug

Therapeutic actions
Inhibits the movement of calcium ions across the membranes of cardiac and arterial muscle cells; inhibition of transmembrane calcium flow results in the depression of impulse formation in specialized cardiac pacemaker cells, slowing of the velocity of conduction of the cardiac impulse, depression of myocardial contractility, and dilation of coronary arteries and arterioles and peripheral arterioles; these effects lead to decreased cardiac work, decreased cardiac energy consumption, and in patients with vasospastic (Prinzmetal's) angina, increased delivery of oxygen to cardiac cells.

Indications
- Chronic stable angina in patients who have failed to respond optimally to, or are intolerant of, other antianginals; can cause serious arrhythmias and agranulocytosis

Contraindications/cautions
- Allergy to bepridil, sick sinus syndrome, heart block (second or third degree), hypotension, history of serious ventricular arrhythmias, uncompensated CHF, congenital QT interval prolongation, lactation.

Dosage
Adult: Individualize dosage. Initially 200 mg/d PO. After 10 d, dosage may be adjusted upward. *Maintenance:* 300 mg/d PO. Maximum daily dose is 400 mg.
Pediatric: Safety and efficacy not established.
Geriatric: Same starting dose as adult dosage; monitor more closely for adverse effects.

Pharmacokinetics

Route	Onset	Peak
Oral	60 min	2–3 h

Metabolism: Hepatic, $T_{1/2}$: 24 h
Distribution: Crosses placenta; passes into breast milk
Excretion: Urine

Adverse effects
- **CNS:** *Dizziness, lightheadedness, nervousness, headache, asthenia,* fatigue
- **GI:** *Nausea,* hepatic injury, *constipation*
- **CV:** *Peripheral edema,* hypotension, arrhythmias, *bradycardia, AV block,* **ventricular tachycardia, asystole**
- **Hematologic: Agranulocytosis**
- **Dermatologic:** *Rash*

Adverse effects in *Italics* are most common; those in **Bold** are life-threatening.

Clinically important drug-drug interactions
- Cumulative negative chronotropic effects and decreased heart rate if bepridil taken with digoxin

■ Nursing Considerations
Assessment
- *History:* Allergy to bepridil, sick sinus syndrome, heart block, hypotension, history of serious ventricular arrhythmias, uncompensated CHF, congenital QT interval prolongation, lactation
- *Physical:* Skin—lesions, color, edema; P, BP, baseline ECG, peripheral perfusion, auscultation, R, adventitious sounds; liver evaluation, GI normal output; liver and renal function tests, CBC

Implementation
- Administer only to patients who do not respond or are intolerant to other antianginal drugs.
- Monitor patient carefully (BP, cardiac rhythm, and output) while drug is being titrated to therapeutic dose; dosage may be increased more rapidly in hospitalized patients under close supervision.
- Monitor BP carefully if patient is on concurrent doses of nitrates.
- Monitor cardiac rhythm and CBC regularly during stabilization of dosage and periodically during long-term therapy.

Drug-specific teaching points
- Take this drug exactly as prescribed.
- Know that the following side effects may occur: nausea, vomiting (small, frequent meals may help); headache (monitor the lighting, noise, and temperature; medication may be ordered if this becomes severe); dizziness, shakiness (avoid driving a car or operating dangerous machinery if these effects occur).
- Report irregular heart beat, shortness of breath, swelling of the hands or feet, pronounced dizziness, constipation, unusual bleeding or bruising.

▢ beractant

*(ber **ak'** tant)*
DDPC, natural lung surfactant
Survanta

Drug classes
Lung surfactant

Therapeutic actions
A natural bovine compound containing lipids and apoproteins that reduce surface tension and allow expansion of the alveoli; replaces the surfactant missing in the lungs of neonates suffering from respiratory distress syndrome (RDS).

Indications
- Prophylactic treatment of infants at risk of developing RDS; infants with birth weights < 1,350 g or infants with birth weights > 1,350 gm who have evidence of pulmonary immaturity
- Rescue treatment of infants who have developed RDS

Contraindications/cautions
- Because beractant is used as an emergency drug in acute respiratory situations, the benefits usually outweigh any possible risks.

Dosage
Accurate determination of birth weight is essential for determining appropriate dosage. Beractant is instilled into the trachea using a catheter inserted into the endotracheal tube.
Prophylactic treatment: Administer first dose of 100 mg phospholipids/kg birth weight (4 ml/kg) as soon as possible after birth. Four doses can be administered in the first 48 h of life. Give no more frequently than q6h.
Rescue treatment: Administer 100 mg phospholipids/kg birth weight (4 ml/kg) intratracheally. Administer the first dose as soon as possible after the diagnosis of RDS is made and when the patient is on the ventilator. Repeat doses can be given based on clinical improvement and blood gases. Administer subsequent doses no sooner than q6h.

Pharmacokinetics

Route	Onset	Peak
Intratracheal	immediate	hrs

Metabolism: Normal surfactant metabolic pathways, $T_{1/2}$: unknown
Distribution: Lung tissue

Adverse effects
- CNS: Seizures
- CV: *Patent ductus arteriosus*, **intraventricular hemorrhage**, *hypotension, bradycardia*
- Respiratory: **Pneumothorax**, *pulmonary air leak*, pulmonary hemorrhage (more often seen with infants > 700 g), *apnea*, pneumomediastinum, emphysema
- Hematologic: *Hyperbilirubinemia, thrombocytopenia*
- Other: *Sepsis, nonpulmonary infections*

■ Nursing Considerations
Assessment
- *History:* Time of birth, exact birth weight
- *Physical:* Temperature, color; R, adventitious sounds, oximeter, endotracheal tube position and patency, chest movement; ECG, P, BP, peripheral perfusion, arterial pressure (desirable); oxygen saturation, blood gases, CBC; muscular activity, facial expression, reflexes

Implementation
- Monitor ECG and transcutaneous oxygen saturation continually during administration.
- Ensure that endotracheal tube is in the correct position, with bilateral chest movement and lung sounds.
- Arrange for staff to preview teaching videotape, available from the manufacturer, before regular use to cover all the technical aspects of administration.
- Suction the infant immediately before administration, but do not suction for 2 h after administration unless clinically necessary.
- Check vial, which should appear as an off-white to brown liquid, for settling; gentle mixing should be attempted. Warm to room temperature before using—20 min or 8 min if warmed in the hand. No other warming methods should be used.
- Store drug in refrigerator. Protect from light. Enter drug vial only once. Discard remaining drug after use.
- Insert 5 French catheter into the endotracheal tube; do not instill into the mainstream bronchus.
- Instill dose slowly; inject one-fourth dose over 2–3 sec; remove catheter and reattach infant to ventilator for at least 30 sec or until stable; repeat procedure administering one-fourth dose at a time.
- Do not suction infant for 1 h after completion of full dose; do not flush catheter.
- Continually monitor patient's color, lung sounds, ECG, oximeter, and blood gas readings during administration and for at least 30 min following administration.

Drug-specific teaching points
- Details of drug effects and administration are best incorporated into parents' comprehensive teaching program.

❒ betamethasone

*(bay ta **meth**' a sone)*
Oral: Celestone

betamethasone benzoate

Topical dermatologic ointment, cream, lotion, gel: Bepen (CAN), Uticort

betamethasone dipropionate

Topical dermatologic ointment, cream, lotion, aerosol: Alphatrex, Diprolene, Diprosone, Maxivate, Occlucort (CAN), Rhoprosone (CAN), Taro-Sone (CAN)

betamethasone sodium phosphate

Systemic, including IV and local injection: Betnesol (CAN), Celestone Phosphate, Cel-U-Jec, Selestoject

betamethasone sodium phosphate and acetate

Systemic, IM, and local intraarticular, intralesional, intradermal injection: Celestone Soluspan

(continues)

Adverse effects in *Italics* are most common; those in **Bold** are life-threatening.

betamethasone valerate

Topical dermatologic ointment, cream, lotion:
Betacort (CAN), Betaderm (CAN), Betatrex, Beta-Val, Betnovate (CAN), Celestoderm (CAN), Dermabet, Prevex B (CAN), Rholosone (CAN), Valisone

Pregnancy Category C

Drug classes
Corticosteroid (long acting)
Glucocorticoid
Hormonal agent

Therapeutic actions
Binds to intracellular corticosteroid receptors, thereby initiating many natural complex reactions that are responsible for its anti-inflammatory and immunosuppressive effects.

Indications
- **Systemic administration:** Hypercalcemia associated with cancer
- Short-term management of various inflammatory and allergic disorders, such as rheumatoid arthritis, collagen diseases (eg, SLE), dermatologic diseases (eg, pemphigus), status asthmaticus, and autoimmune disorders
- *Hematologic disorders:* thrombocytopenia purpura, erythroblastopenia
- Ulcerative colitis, acute exacerbations of mutiple sclerosis, and palliation in some leukemias and lymphomas
- Trichinosis with neurologic or myocardial involvement
- *Unlabeled use:* Prevention of respiratory distress syndrome in premature neonates
- **Intra-articular or soft-tissue administration:** Arthritis, psoriatic plaques, and so forth
- **Dermatologic preparations:** Relief of inflammatory and pruritic manifestations of dermatoses that are steroid-responsive

Contraindications/cautions
- Systemic (oral and parenteral) administration: Contraindicated in the presence of infections, especially tuberculosis, fungal infections, amebiasis, vaccinia and varicella, and antibiotic-resistant infections, lactation.
- Use caution in the presence of kidney or liver disease, hypothyroidism, ulcerative colitis with impending perforation, diverticulitis, active or latent peptic ulcer, inflammatory bowel disease, CHF, hypertension, thromboembolic disorders, osteoporosis, convulsive disorders, diabetes mellitus.

Dosage
Adult
- ***Systemic administration:*** Individualize dosage, depending on the severity of the condition and the patient's response. Give daily dose before 9 AM to minimize adrenal suppression. For maintenance, reduce initial dose in small increments at intervals until the lowest dose that maintains satisfactory clinical response is reached. If long-term therapy is needed, alternate-day therapy with a short-acting corticosteroid should be considered. After long-term therapy, withdraw drug slowly to prevent adrenal insufficiency.
  - *Oral (betamethasone):* Initial dosage 0.6–7.2 mg/d
  - *IV (betamethasone sodium phosphate):* Initial dosage up to 9 mg/d.
  - *IM (betamethasone sodium phosphate; betamethasone sodium phosphate and acetate):* Initial dosage 0.5–9.0 mg/d. Usual dosage ranges are from one-third to one-half the oral dose given q12h. In life-threatening situations, dose can be in multiples of the oral dose.
  - *Intabursal, intra-articular, intradermal, intralesional (betamethasone sodium phosphate and acetate):* 0.25–2.0 ml intra-articular, depending on joint size; 0.2 ml/cm^3 intradermally, not to exceed 1 ml/wk; 0.25–1.0 ml at 3- to 7-d intervals for disorders of the foot.
  - *Topical dermatologic cream, ointment (betamethasone dipropionate):* Apply sparingly to affected area bid–qid.

betamethasone ■ 169

Pediatric: Individualize dosage on the basis of the severity of the condition and the patient's response rather than by strict adherence to formulae that correct adult doses for age or body weight. Carefully observe growth and development in infants and children on prolonged therapy.

Pharmacokinetics

Route	Onset	Duration
Systemic	Varies	3 d

Metabolism: Hepatic, $T_{1/2}$: 36–54 h
Distribution: Crosses placenta; passes into breast milk
Excretion: Unchanged in the urine

IV facts
Preparation: No further preparation needed.
Infusion: Infuse by direct IV injection over 1 min or into the tubing of running IV of dextrose or saline solutions.

Adverse effects

Effects depend on dose, route, and duration of therapy. The following are primarily associated with systemic absorption and are more likely to occur with systemically administered steroids than with locally administered preparations:

- CNS: *Vertigo, headache*, paresthesias, insomnia, convulsions, psychosis, cataracts, increased intraocular pressure, glaucoma (long-term therapy)
- GI: Peptic or esophageal ulcer, pancreatitis, abdominal distention, nausea, vomiting, *increased appetite, weight gain (long-term therapy)*
- CV: Hypotension, **shock**, hypertension, and **CHF** secondary to fluid retention, **thromboembolism**, thrombophlebitis, **fat embolism**, cardiac arrhythmias
- MS: Muscle weakness, steroid myopathy, loss of muscle mass, osteoporosis, spontaneous fractures (long-term therapy)
- Endocrine: Amenorrhea, irregular menses, growth retardation, decreased carbohydrate tolerance, diabetes mellitus, cushingoid state (long-term effect), increased blood sugar, increased serum cholesterol, decreased T_3 and T_4 levels, hypothalamic-pituitary-adrenal (HPA) suppression with systemic therapy longer than 5 d
- **Electrolyte imbalance:** *Na⁺ and fluid retention*, hypokalemia, hypocalcemia
- Other: *Immunosuppression, aggravation, or masking of infections; impaired wound healing*; thin, fragile skin; petechiae, ecchymoses, purpura, striae; subcutaneous fat atrophy

Hypersensitivity or Anaphylactoid Reactions

The following effects are related to various local routes of steroid administration:

- Intra-articular: Osteonecrosis, tendon rupture, infection
- Intralesional therapy: **Blindness**, face and head
- Topical dermatologic ointments, creams, sprays: *Local burning, irritation*, acneiform lesions, striae, skin atrophy

Systemic absorption can lead to HPA suppression (see above), growth retardation in children, and other systemic adverse effects. Children may be at special risk of systemic absorption because of their larger skin surface area to body weight ratio.

Clinically important drug-drug interactions

- Risk of severe deterioration of muscle strength when given to myasthenia gravis patients who are receiving ambenonium, edrophonium, neostigmine, pyridostigmine • Decreased steroid blood levels when taken with barbiturates, phenytoin, rifampin • Decreased effectiveness of salicylates when taken with betamethasone

Drug-lab test interferences

- False-negative nitroblue-tetrazolium test for bacterial infection • Suppression of skin test reactions.

■ Nursing Considerations

Assessment

- *History (Systemic [oral and parenteral] administration):* Infections, fun-

---

Adverse effects in *Italics* are most common; those in **Bold** are life-threatening.

gal infectons, amebiasis, vaccinia and varicella, and antibiotic-resistant infections; kidney or liver disease; hypothyroidism; ulcerative colitis with impending perforation; diverticulitis; active or latent peptic ulcer; inflammatory bowel disease; CHF; hypertension; thromboembolic disorders; osteoporosis; convulsive disorders; diabetes mellitus; lactation
- *Physical:* Baseline body weight, temperature, reflexes and grip strength, affect and orientation, P, BP, peripheral perfusion, peripheral perfusion, prominence of superficial veins, respiratory rate and adventitious sounds, serum electrolytes, blood glucose

Implementation

Systemic Use
- Administer once-a-day doses before 9 AM to mimic normal peak corticosteroid blood levels.
- Arrange for increased dosage when patient is subject to stress.
- Taper doses when discontinuing high-dose or long-term therapy.
- Do not give live virus vaccines with immunosuppressive doses of corticosteroids.

Topical Dermatologic Preparations
- Assess affected area for infections, skin integrity before application.
- Administer cautiously to pregnant patients; topical corticosteroids have caused teratogenic effects in preclinical studies and can be absorbed from systemic site.
- Use caution when occlusive dressings, tight diapers, and so forth cover affected area; these can increase systemic absorption of the drug.
- Avoid prolonged use near eyes, in genital and rectal areas, and in skin creases.

Drug-specific teaching points

Systemic Uses
- Do not to stop taking the drug (oral) without consulting health care provider.
- Take single-dose or alternate day doses before 9 AM to achieve the most effective therapy.
- Avoid exposure to infections; your ability to fight infections will be reduced.
- Wear a medial alert identification so health care providers will know that you are on this medication in an emergency.
- Know that the following side effects may occur: increase in appetite, weight gain (counting calories may be somewhat helpful); heartburn, indigestion (small, frequent meals and the use of antacids may be helpful); poor wound healing (consult with your care provider if you have a wound or injury); muscle weakness, fatigue (frequent rest periods will be helpful).
- Report unusual weight gain, swelling of the extremities, muscle weakness, black or tarry stools, fever, prolonged sore throat, colds or other infections, worsening of the disorder for which the drug is being taken.

Intrabursal, Intra-articular Therapy
- Do not overuse joint after therapy, even if pain is gone.

Topical Dermatologic Preparations
- Apply sparingly; do not cover with tight dressings.
- Avoid contact with the eyes.
- Report irritation or infection at the site of application.

▢ betaxolol hydrochloride

*(be **tax'** oh lol)*
Ophthalmic: Betoptic
Oral: Kerlone
Pregnancy Category C

Drug classes
Beta-adrenergic blocking agent (β_1 selective)
Antihypertensive
Antiglaucoma agent

Therapeutic actions
Blocks beta-adrenergic receptors of the sympathetic nervous system in the heart and juxtaglomerular apparatus (kidney), decreasing the excitability of the heart, decreasing cardiac output and oxygen consumption, decreasing the release of

betaxolol hydrochloride

renin from the kidney, and lowering blood pressure.
Decreases intraocular pressure by decreasing the secretion of aqueous humor.

Indications
- Management of hypertension, used alone or concomitantly with other antihypertensive agents, particularly thiazide-type diuretics (oral)
- Treatment of ocular hypertension and open-angle glaucoma (ophthalmic)

Contraindications/cautions
- Contraindicated in the presence of sinus bradycardia, second- or third-degree heart block, cardiogenic shock, CHF.
- Use caution in the presence of renal failure, diabetes or thyrotoxicosis (betaxolol can maks the usual cardiac signs of hypoglycemia and thyrotoxicosis), lactation.

Dosage
Adult
- ***Oral:*** Initially 10 mg PO qd, alone or added to diuretic therapy. Full antihypertensive effect is usually seen in 7–14 d. If desired response if not achieved, dose may be doubled.
- ***Ophthalmic:*** One drop bid to affected eye(s).

Pediatric: Safety and efficacy not established.

Geriatric
- ***Oral:*** Consider reducing initial dose to 5 mg PO qd.

Pharmacokinetics

Route	Onset	Peak	Duration
Oral	30–60 min	2 h	12–15 h

Metabolism: Hepatic; $T_{1/2}$: 14–22 h
Distribution: Crosses placenta; passes into breast milk
Excretion: Urine

Adverse effects
- CNS: Dizziness, vertigo, tinnitus, fatigue, emotional depression, paresthesias, sleep disturbances, hallucinations, disorientation, memory loss, slurred speech
- GI: *Gastric pain, flatulence, constipation, diarrhea, nausea, vomiting,* anorexia, ischemic colitis, renal and mesenteric arterial thrombosis, retroperitoneal fibrosis, hepatomegaly, acute pancreatitis
- CV: *Bradycardia,* **CHF,** *cardiac arrhythmias,* **sinoartial or AV nodal block,** *tachycardia,* peripheral vascular insufficiency, claudication, CVA, pulmonary edema, hypotension
- Respiratory: Bronchospasm, dyspnea, cough, bronchial obstruction, nasal stuffiness, rhinitis, pharyngitis (less likely than with propranolol)
- GU: *Impotence, decreased libido,* Peyronie's disease, dysuria, nocturia, frequent urination
- MS: Joint pain, arthralgia, muscle cramp
- EENT: Eye irritation, dry eyes, conjunctivitis, blurred vision
- Dermatologic: Rash, pruritus, sweating, dry skin
- Allergic reactions: Pharyngitis, erythematous rash, fever, sore throat, laryngospasm, respiratory distress
- Other: *Decreased exercise tolerance, development of antinuclear antibodies (ANA),* hyperglycemia or hypoglycemia, elevated serum transaminase, alkaline phosphatase, and LDH

Specifically Documented for Betaxolol Ophthalmic Solution
- CNS: Insomnia, depressive neurosis
- Local: *Brief ocular discomfort, occasional tearing, itching, decreased corneal sensitivity,* corneal staining, keratitis, photophobia

Clinically important drug-drug interactions
- Increased effects of betaxolol if taken with verapamil, anticholinergics • Increased risk of postural hypotension if taken concurrently with prazosin • Possible increased antihypertensive effects if taken concurrently with aspirin, bismuth subsalicylate, magnesium salicylate, sulfinpyrazone, oral contraceptives • Decreased antihypertensive effects if taken with NSAIDs • Possi-

Adverse effects in *Italics* are most common; those in **Bold** are life-threatening.

172 ■ bethanechol chloride

ble increased hypoglycemic effect of insulin if taken with betaxolol

Drug-lab test interferences
- Possible false results with glucose or insulin tolerance tests

■ Nursing Considerations
Assessment
- *History:* Sinus bradycardia, second- or third-degree heart block, cardiogenic shock, CHF, renal failure, diabetes or thyrotoxicosis, lactation
- *Physical:* Baseline body weight, skin condition, neurologic status, P, BP, ECG, respiratory status, kidney and thyroid function, blood and urine glucose

Implementation
- Do not discontinue drug abruptly after chronic therapy (hypersensitivity to catecholamines may have developed, causing exacerbation of angina, MI, and ventricular dysrhythmias). Taper drug gradually over 2 wk with monitoring.
- Consult with physician about withdrawing drug if patient is to undergo surgery (withdrawal is controversial).
- Protect eye from injury if corneal sensitivity is lost (ophthalmic).

Drug-specific teaching points
- Administer eye drops to minimize systemic absorption of the drug.
- Do not to stop taking this drug unless instructed to do so by a health care provider.
- Avoid driving or dangerous activities if dizziness, weakness occur.
- Know that the following side effects may occur: dizziness, lightheadedness, loss of appetite, nightmares, depression, sexual impotence.
- Report difficulty breathing, night cough, swelling of extremities, slow pulse, confusion, depression, rash, fever, sore throat, eye pain or irritation (ophthalmic).

❒ bethanechol chloride

(be than' e kole)

Duvoid, Myotonachol, PMS-Bethanechol Chloride (CAN), Urabeth, Urecholine

Pregnancy Category C

Drug classes
Parasympathomimetic drug

Therapeutic actions
Acts at cholinergic receptors in the urinary bladder (and GI tract) to mimic the effects of acetylcholine and parasympathetic stimulation; increases the tone of the detrusor muscle and causes the emptying of the urinary bladder; not destroyed by the enzyme acetylcholinesterase, so effects are more prolonged than those of acetylcholine.

Indications
- Acute postoperative and postpartum nonobstructive urinary retention and neurogenic atony of the urinary bladder with retention
- **Unlabeled use**: reflux esophagitis

Contraindications/cautions
- Contraindicated in the presence of unusual sensitivity to bethanechol, hyperthyroidism, peptic ulcer, latent or active asthma, bradycardia, vasomotor instability, coronary artery disease, epilepsy, parkinsonism, hypotension, obstructive uropathies or intestinal obstruction, recent surgery on GI tract or bladder.
- Use caution when lactating.

Dosage
Determine and use the minimum effective dose; larger doses may increase side effects.
Adult
- **Oral:** 10–50 mg bid–qid. Initial dose of 5–10 mg with gradual increases hourly until desired effect is seen; do not exceed single dose of 50 mg. Alternatively, give 10 mg initially, then 25 and 50 mg at 6-h intervals.
- **SC:** 2.5–5 mg initially; repeat this dose at 15- to 30-min intervals up to a maximum of four doses unless adverse effects intervene. Minimum effective dose may be repeated tid–qid.

Pediatric: Safety and efficacy not established for children < 8 y.

Pharmacokinetics

Route	Onset	Peak	Duration
Oral	30–90 min	60–90 min	1–6 h
SC	5–15 min	15–30 min	1–3 h

Metabolism: Unknown
Distribution: Crosses placenta; may pass into breast milk

Adverse effects

- GI: *Abdominal discomfort, salivation, nausea, vomiting,* involuntary defecation, abdominal cramps, diarrhea, belching
- CV: **Transient heart block, transient cardiac arrest**, dyspnea, orthostatic hypotension (with large doses)
- GU: Urinary urgency
- Other: Malaise, headache, *sweating, flushing*

Clinically important drug-drug interactions

- Increased cholinergic effects if taken with other cholinergic drugs, cholinesterase inhibitors

■ Nursing Considerations

Assessment

- *History:* Unusual sensitivity to bethanechol, hyperthyroidism, peptic ulcer, latent or active asthma, bradycardia, vasomotor instability, coronary artery disease, epilepsy, parkinsonism, hypotension, obstructive uropathies or intestinal obstruction, recent surgery on GI tract or bladder, lactation
- *Physical:* Skin—color, lesions; body temperature; P, rhythm, BP; bowel sounds, urinary bladder palpation; bladder tone evaluation, urinalysis

Implementation

- Administer on an empty stomach to avoid nausea and vomiting
- Do not administer IM or IV, serious reactions may occur; administer parenteral preparations by SC route only.
- Monitor patient response to establish minimum effective dose.
- Maintain atropine on standby in case needed to reverse overdosage or severe response to bethanechol.
- Monitor bowel function, especially in elderly patients who may become impacted or develop serious intestinal problems.

Drug-specific teaching points

- Take this drug on an empty stomach to avoid nausea and vomiting; if taken too soon after eating, these problems may occur.
- Know that the following side effects may occur: increased salivation, sweating, flushing, abdominal discomfort.
- Report diarrhea, headache, belching, substernal pressure or pain, dizziness.

❒ biperiden hydrochloride (oral)

*(bye **per'** i den)*

biperiden lactate (injection)
Akineton

Pregnancy Category C

Drug classes

Antiparkinsonism drug (anticholinergic type)

Therapeutic actions

Has anticholinergic activity in the CNS that is believed to help normalize the hypothesized imbalance of cholinergic/dopaminergic neurotransmission in the basal ganglia in the brain of a parkinsonism patient. Reduces severity of rigidity, and reduces to a lesser extent the akinesia and tremor that characterize parkinsonism; less effective overall than levodopa; peripheral anticholinergic effects suppress secondary symptoms of parkinsonism, such as drooling.

Indications

- Adjunct in the therapy of parkinsonism (postencephalitic, arteriosclerotic, and idiopathic types)
- Relief of symptoms of extrapyramidal disorders that accompany phenothiazine and reserpine therapy

Contraindications/cautions

- Contraindicated in the presence of hypersensitivity to benztropine; glaucoma, especially angle-closure glaucoma; pyloric

Adverse effects in *Italics* are most common; those in **Bold** are life-threatening.

or duodenal obstruction, stenosing peptic ulcers, achalasia (megaesophagus); prostatic hypertrophy or bladder neck obstructions; myasthenia gravis.
- Use caution in the presence of tachycardia, cardiac arrhythmias, hypertension, hypotension, hepatic or renal dysfunction, alcoholism, chronic illness, people who work in hot environment; hot weather; lactation.

Dosage
Adult
- ***Parkinsonism:*** 2 mg PO tid–qid; individualize dosage with a maximum dose of 16 mg/d.
- ***Drug-induced extrapyramidal disorders***
- *Oral:* 2 mg PO qid–tid.
- *Parenteral:* 2 mg IM or IV; repeat q½h until symptoms are resolved, but do not give more than four consecutive doses per 24 h.

Pediatric: Safety and efficacy not established.

Geriatric: Strict dosage regulation may be necessary; patients > 60 y often develop increased sensitivity to the CNS effects of anticholinergic drugs.

Pharmacokinetics

Route	Onset	Peak
Oral	1 h	1–1.5 h
IM	15 min	Unknown

Metabolism: Hepatic, $T_{1/2}$: 18.4–24.3 h
Distribution: Crosses placenta; passes into breast milk

IV facts
Preparation: Give undiluted. Store in tightly covered, light-resistant container. Store at room temparature.

Infusion: Administer direct IV at a rate of 1 mg over 1 min; do not give more than four consecutive doses per 24 h.

Adverse effects
- CNS: Some are characteristic of centrally acting anticholinergic drugs: *disorientation, confusion,* memory loss, hallucinations, psychoses, agitation, *nervousness,* delusions, delirium, paranoia, euphoria, excitement, *lightheadedness, dizziness,* depression, drowsiness, weakness, giddiness, paresthesia, heaviness of the limbs

Peripheral Anticholinergic Effects
- GI: *Dry mouth, constipation,* dilation of the colon, paralytic ileus, acute suppurative parotitis, nausea, vomiting, epigastric distress
- CV: Tachycardia, palpitations, hypotension, orthostatic hypotension
- GU: *Urinary retention, urinary hesitancy,* dysuria, difficulty achieving or maintaining an erection
- EENT: *Blurred vision, mydriasis,* diplopia, increased intraocular tension, angle-closure glaucoma
- Dermatologic: Skin rash, urticaria, other dermatoses
- Other: *Flushing, decreased sweating,* elevated temperature, muscular weakness, muscular cramping

Clinically important drug-drug interactions
- Paralytic ileus, sometimes fatal, when given with other anticholinergic drugs, with drugs that have anticholinergic properties (phenothiazines, tricyclic antidepressants) • Additive adverse CNS effects (toxic psychosis) with other drugs that have CNS anticholinergic properties (tricyclic antidepressants, phenothiazines) • Possible masking of the development of persistent extrapyramidal symptoms, tardive dyskinesia, in patients on long-term therapy with antipsychotic drugs (phenothiazines, haloperidol) • Decreased therapeutic efficacy of antipsychotic drugs (phenothiazines, haloperidol), possibly due to central antagonism

■ Nursing Considerations

Assessment
- *History:* Hypersensitivity to benztropine; glaucoma; pyloric or duodenal obstruction, stenosing peptic ulcers, achalasia; prostatic hypertrophy or bladder neck ob-

bismuth subsalicylate ■ 175

structions; myasthenia gravis; cardiac arrhythmias, hypertension, hypotension; hepatic or renal dysfunction; alcoholism, chronic illness, people who work in hot environment; lactation
- *Physical:* Body weight; temperature; skin—color, lesions; orientation, affect, reflexes, bilateral grip strength, visual exam, including tonometry; P, BP, orthostatic BP; adventitious sounds; bowel sounds, normal output, liver evaluation; normal urinary output, voiding pattern, prostate palpation; liver and kidney function tests

Implementation
- Arrange to decrease dosage or discontinue drug temporarily if dry mouth is so severe that swallowing or speaking becomes difficult.
- Give with caution, and arrange dosage reduction in hot weather, as appropriate to patient's lifestyle. Drug interferes with sweating and ability of body to maintain body heat equilibrium; anhidrosis and fatal hyperthermia have occurred.
- Give with meals if GI upset occurs; give before meals to patients bothered by dry mouth; give after meals if drooling is a problem or if drug causes nausea.
- Ensure that patient voids just before receiving each dose of drug if urinary retention is a problem.

Drug-specific teaching points
- Take this drug exactly as prescribed.
- Avoid the use of alcohol, sedative, and OTC drugs while you are on this drug (many of these could cause dangerous effects).
- Know that the following side effects may occur: drowsiness, dizziness, confusion, blurred vision (avoid driving a car or engaging in activities that require alertness and visual acuity if these occur); nausea (frequent small meals may help); dry mouth (sucking sugarless lozenges or ice chips may help); painful or difficult urination (emptying the bladder immediately before each dose may help); constipation (if maintaining adequate fluid intake and exercising regularly do not help, consult your nurse or physician); use caution in hot weather (this drug makes you more susceptible to heat prostration).
- Report difficult or painful urination; constipation; rapid or pounding heartbeat; confusion, eye pain, or rash.

❏ bismuth subsalicylate

(bis' mith)
Pregnancy Category C

Drug classes
Antidiarrheal agent

Therapeutic actions
Adsorbent actions remove irritants from the intestine; forms a protective coating over the mucosa and soothes the irritated bowel lining.

Indications
- Indigestion, nausea, and control of diarrhea within 24 h
- Relief of gas pains and abdominal cramps
- **Unlabeled use**: prevention and treatment of traveler's diarrhea

Contraindications/cautions
- Allergy to any components

Dosage
Adult: 2 tablets or 30 ml PO, q30 min–1 h as needed, up to eight doses/24 h.
- ***Traveler's diarrhea:*** 60 ml PO qid.

Pediatric
- ***9–12 y:*** 1 tablet or 15 ml PO.
- ***6–9 y:*** $\frac{2}{3}$ tablet or 10 ml PO.
- ***3–6 y:*** $\frac{1}{3}$ tablet or 5 ml PO.
- ***< 3 y:*** Dosage not established.

Pharmacokinetics

Route	Onset
Oral	Varies

Metabolism: Hepatic
Distribution: Crosses placenta
Excretion: Urine

Adverse effects
- GI: *Darkening of the stool,* impaction in infants, debilitated patients
- Salicylate toxicity: Ringing in the ears, rapid respirations

Clinically important drug-drug interactions
- Increased risk of salicylate toxicity if taken with other aspirin-containing products • Increased toxic effects of methotrexate, valproic acid if taken concurrently with salicylates • Use caution when taking concurrently with drugs used for diabetes • Decreased effectiveness of bismuth subsalicylate if taken concurrently with corticosteroids • Decreased absorption of oral tetracyclines if taken concomitantly • Decreased effectiveness of sulfinpyrazone if taken concurrently with salicylates

Drug-lab test interferences
- May interfere with radiologic exams of GI tract; bismuth is radiopaque

■ Nursing Considerations

Assessment
- *History:* Allergy to any components
- *Physical:* Body temperature; orientation, reflexes; R and depth of respirations; abdominal exam, bowel sounds; serum electrolytes; acid–base levels

Implementation
- Shake liquid well before administration; have patient chew tablets thoroughly or allow them to dissolve in mouth; do not swallow whole.
- Discontinue drug if any sign of salicylate toxicity occurs (eg, ringing in the ears).

Drug-specific teaching points
- Take this drug as prescribed; do not exceed prescribed dosage. Shake liquid well before using. Chew tablets thoroughly or allow them to dissolve in your mouth; do not swallow whole.
- Know that darkened stools may occur as a result of drug therapy (do not be alarmed).
- Do not take this drug with any other drug that contains aspirin or aspirin products; serious overdosage can occur.
- Report fever, diarrhea that does not stop after 2 d, ringing in the ears, rapid respirations.

❒ bisoprolol fumarate

(bis oh' pro lole)
Zebeta

Pregnancy Category C

Drug classes
Beta-adrenergic blocking agent (β1 selective)
Antihypertensive

Therapeutic actions
Blocks beta-adrenergic receptors of the sympathetic nervous system in the heart and juxtaglomerular apparatus (kidney), thus decreasing the excitability of the heart, decreasing cardiac output and oxygen consumption, decreasing the release of renin from the kidney, and lowering blood pressure.

Indications
- Management of hypertension, used alone or concomitantly with other antihypertensive agents

Contraindications/cautions
- Contraindicated in the presence of sinus bradycardia, second- or third-degree heart block, cardiogenic shock, CHF.
- Use caution in the presence of renal failure, diabetes or thyrotoxicosis (bisoprolol can mask the usual cardiac signs of hypoglycemia and thyrotoxicosis), lactation.

Dosage
Adult
- *Oral:* Initially 5 mg PO qid, alone or added to diuretic therapy; 2.5 mg may be added if appropriate; up to 20 mg PO qid has been used.

Pediatric: Safety and efficacy not established.

– *Renal or hepatic impairment:* Initially 2.5 mg PO; titrate, and use extreme caution.

Adverse effects in *Italics* are most common; those in **Bold** are life-threatening.

bisoprolol fumarate ■ 177

Pharmacokinetics

Route	Onset	Peak	Duration
Oral	30–60 min	2 h	12–15 h

Metabolism: Hepatic; $T_{1/2}$: 9–12 h
Distribution: Crosses placenta; passes into breast milk
Excretion: Urine

Adverse effects

Adverse effects are characteristic of systemic beta-blockers.
- **CNS:** Dizziness, vertigo, tinnitus, fatigue, emotional depression, paresthesias, sleep disturbances, hallucinations, disorientation, memory loss, slurred speech
- **GI:** *Gastric pain, flatulence, constipation, diarrhea, nausea, vomiting,* anorexia, ischemic colitis, renal and mesenteric arterial thrombosis, retroperitoneal fibrosis, hepatomegaly, acute pancreatitis
- **CV:** *Bradycardia, CHF, cardiac arrhythmias, sinoartial or AV nodal block, tachycardia,* peripheral vascular insufficiency, claudication, CVA, pulmonary edema, hypotension
- **Respiratory:** Bronchospasm, dyspnea, cough, bronchial obstruction, nasal stuffiness, rhinitis, pharyngitis (less likely than with propranolol)
- **GU:** *Impotence, decreased libido,* Peyronie's disease, dysuria, nocturia, frequent urination
- **MS:** Joint pain, arthralgia, muscle cramp
- **EENT:** Eye irritation, dry eyes, conjunctivitis, blurred vision
- **Dermatologic:** Rash, pruritus, sweating, dry skin
- **Allergic reactions:** Pharyngitis, erythematous rash, fever, sore throat, laryngospasm, respiratory distress
- **Other:** *Decreased exercise tolerance, development of antinuclear antibodies,* hyperglycemia or hypoglycemia, elevated serum transaminase, alkaline phosphatase, and LDH

Clinically important drug-drug interactions

- Increased effects of bisoprolol if taken with verapamil, anticholinergics • Increased risk of postural hypotension if taken concurrently with prazosin • Possible increased blood pressure-lowering effects if taken concurrently with aspirin, bismuth subsalicylate, magnesium salicylate, sulfinpyrazone, oral contraceptives • Decreased antihypertensive effects if taken with NSAIDs • Possible increased hypoglycemic effect of insulin if taken with bisoprolol

Drug-lab test interferences

- Possible false results with glucose or insulin tolerance tests

■ Nursing Considerations

Assessment

- *History:* Sinus bradycardia, cardiac arrhythmias, cardiogenic shock, CHF, renal failure, diabetes or thyrotoxicosis, lactation
- *Physical:* Baseline body weight, skin condition, neurologic status, P, BP, ECG, respiratory status, kidney and liver function, blood and urine glucose

Implementation

- Do not discontinue drug abruptly after chronic therapy (hypersensitivity to catecholamines may have developed, causing exacerbation of angina, MI, and ventricular dysrhythmias). Taper drug gradually over 2 wk with monitoring.
- Consult with physician about withdrawing drug if patient is to undergo surgery (withdrawal is controversial).

Drug-specific teaching points

- Do not to stop taking this drug unless instructed to do so by a health care provider.
- Avoid OTC medications.
- Avoid driving or dangerous activities if dizziness, weakness occur.
- Know that the following side effects may occur: dizziness, lightheadedness, loss of appetite, nightmares, depression, sexual impotence.
- Report difficulty breathing, night cough, swelling of extremities, slow pulse, confusion, depression, rash, fever, sore throat.

Adverse effects in *Italics* are most common; those in **Bold** are life-threatening.

◻ bitolterol mesylate

*(bye **tole'** ter ole)*
Tornalate

Pregnancy Category C

Drug classes
Sympathomimetic drug
β_2-selective adrenergic agonist
Bronchodilator
Antiasthmatic drug

Therapeutic actions
Prodrug that is converted by tissue and blood enzymes to active metabolite (colterol); in low doses, acts relatively selectively at β_2 adrenergic receptors to cause bronchodilation (and vasodilation); at higher doses, β_2 selectivity is lost, and the drug acts at β_1 receptors to cause typical sympathomimetic cardiac effects.

Indications
- Prophylaxis and treatment of bronchial asthma and reversible bronchospasm

Contraindications/cautions
- Hypersensitivity to bitolterol; tachyarrhythmias, tachycardia caused by digitalis intoxication; general anesthesia with halogenated hydrocarbons or cyclopropane, which sensitize the myocardium to catecholamines; unstable vasomotor system disorders; hypertension; coronary insufficiency, coronary artery disease; history of stroke; COPD patients who have developed degenerative heart disease; hyperthyroidism; history of seizure disorders; psychoneurotic individuals; labor and delivery (parenteral use of β_2-adrenergic agonists can accelerate fetal heart beat; cause hypoglycemia, hypokalemia, pulmonary edema in the mother, and hypoglycemia in the neonate; systemic absorption after inhalation use may be less than with systemic administration, but use only if potential benefit to mother justifies risk to mother and fetus); lactation

Dosage
Adult: Each actuation of aerosol dispenser delivers 0.37 mg bitolterol.
- ***Treatment of bronchospasm:*** 2 inhalations at an interval of at least 1–3 min, followed by a third inhalation if needed.
- ***Prevention of bronchospasm:*** 2 inhalations q8h; do not exceed 3 inhalations q6h or 2 inhalations q4h.

Pediatric
- **> 12 y:** Same as adult
- **< 12 y:** Safety and efficacy not established.

Geriatric: Patients > 60 y are more likely to experience adverse effects; use extreme caution.

Pharmacokinetics

Route	Onset	Peak	Duration
Inhalation	3–4 min	½–2 h	5–8 h

Metabolism: $T_{1/2}$: 3 h
Distribution: Crosses placenta; may pass into breast milk
Excretion: Lungs

Adverse effects
- **CNS:** *Restlessness, apprehension,* anxiety, fear, CNS stimulation, hyperkinesia, *insomnia,* tremor, drowsiness, *irritability,* weakness, vertigo, headache
- **CV: Cardiac arrhythmias,** tachycardia, palpitations, PVCs (rare), anginal pain (less likely with bronchodilator doses of this drug than with bronchodilator doses of a nonselective beta-agonist [ie, isoproterenol]), changes in BP (increases or decreases), sweating, pallor, flushing
- **Hypersensitivity:** Immediate hypersensitivity (allergic) reactions
- **Respiratory:** Respiratory difficulties, **pulmonary edema,** coughing, bronchospasm, paradoxical airway resistance with repeated, excessive use of inhalation preparations
- **GI:** *Nausea,* vomiting, heartburn, unusual or bad taste

Adverse effects in *Italics* are most common; those in **Bold** are life-threatening.

Clinically important drug-drug interactions
- Increased sympathomimetic effects when given with other sympathomimetic drugs
- Enhanced toxicity, especially cardiotoxicity, when taken with aminophylline, oxtriphylline, theophylline

■ Nursing Considerations
Assessment
- *History:* Hypersensitivity to bitolterol; tachyarrhythmias; general anesthesia with halogenated hydrocarbons or cyclopropane; unstable vasomotor system disorders; hypertension; coronary insufficiency; history of stroke; COPD patients who have developed degenerative heart disease; hyperthyroidism; history of seizure disorders; psychoneurotic individuals; labor or delivery; lactation
- *Physical:* Body weight, skin—color, temperature, turgor; orientation, reflexes, affect; P, BP; respiratory rate, adventitious sounds; blood and urine glucose, serum electrolytes, thyroid function tests, ECG, CBC, liver function tests (SGOT)

Implementation
- Use minimal doses for minimum time; drug tolerance can occur with prolonged use.
- Maintain a beta-adrenergic blocker (a cardioselective beta-blocker, such as atenolol should be used in patients with respiratory distress) on standby in case cardiac arrhythmias occur.
- Do not exceed recommended dosage; administer during second half of inspiration, because the airways are open wider, and the aerosol distribution is more extensive.

Drug-specific teaching points
- Do not exceed recommended dosage; adverse effects or loss of effectiveness may result. Read the instructions for use that come with the product, and ask your health care provider or pharmacist if you have any questions.
- Know that the following side effects may occur: drowsiness, dizziness, fatigue, apprehension (use caution if driving or performing tasks that require alertness if these occur); nausea, heartburn, change in taste (small, frequent meals may help, consult your nurse or physician if this is prolonged); sweating, flushing, rapid heart rate.
- Avoid OTC drugs while you are on this medication; many of them contain products that can interfere with or cause serious side effects when used with this drug. If you feel that you need one of these products, consult your nurse or physician.
- Report chest pain, dizziness, insomnia, weakness, tremor or irregular heart beat, difficulty breathing, productive cough, failure to respond to usual dosage.

▢ bleomycin sulfate

*(blee oh **mye'** sin)*
BLM, Blenoxane

Pregnancy Category D

Drug classes
Antibiotic
Antineoplastic agent

Therapeutic actions
Inhibits DNA, RNA, and protein synthesis in susceptible cells, preventing cell division; cell cycle phase-specific agent with major effects in G2 and M phases.

Indications
- Palliative treatment of squamous cell carcinoma, lymphomas, testicular carcinoma, alone or in combination with other drugs

Contraindications/cautions
- Allergy to bleomycin sulfate; lactation

Dosage
Adult: Treat lymphoma patients with 2 U or less for the first two doses; if no acute anaphylactoid reaction occurs, use the regular dosage schedule:
- ***Squamous cell carcinoma, lymphosarcoma, reticulum cell sarcoma, testicular carcinoma:*** 0.25–0.50 U/kg IV, IM, or SC, once or twice weekly.

- **Hodgkin's disease:** 0.25–0.50 U/kg IV, IM, or SC once or twice weekly. After a 50% response, give maintenance dose of 1 U/d or 5 U/wk, IV or IM. Response should be seen within 2 wk (Hodgkin's disease, testicular tumors) or 3 wk (squamous cell cancers). If no improvement is seen by then, it is unlikely to occur.

Pharmacokinetics

Route	Onset	Peak
IV	Immediate	10–20 min
IM, SC	15–20 min	30–60 min

Metabolism: $T_{1/2}$: 2 h
Distribution: May crosses placenta; may pass into breast milk
Excretion: Urine

IV facts
Preparation: Dissolve contents of vial with 5 ml physiologic saline or glucose; stable for 24 h at room temperature in NaCl, 5% Dextrose solutions, and 5% Dextrose containing heparin 100 or 1,000 U/ml; powder should be refrigerated.
Infusion: Infuse slowly over 10 min.
Compatibilities: Incompatible in solution with aminophylline, ascorbic acid, carbenicillin, diazepam, hydrocortisone, methotrexate, mitomycin, nafcillin, penicillin G, terbutaline.

Adverse effects
- **GI:** Hepatic toxicity, *stomatitis, vomiting*, anorexia, weight loss
- **Respiratory:** *Dyspnea, rales, pneumonitis,* **pulmonary fibrosis**
- **GU:** Renal toxicity
- **Dermatologic:** *Rash, striae, vesiculation, hyperpigmentation, skin tenderness, hyperkeratosis, nail changes, alopecia, pruritis*
- **Hypersensitivity:** Idiosyncratic reaction similar to anaphylaxis: hypotension, mental confusion, fever, chills, wheezing (especially in lymphoma patients, 1% occurrence)
- **Other:** *Fever, chills*

Clinically important drug-drug interactions
- Decreased serum levels and therefore effectiveness of digoxin and phenytoin if taken concurrently with bleomycin

■ Nursing Considerations

Assessment
- *History:* Allergy to bleomycin sulfate, pregnancy, lactation
- *Physical:* Temperature; skin—color, lesions; weight; R, adventitious sounds; liver evaluation, abdominal status; pulmonary function tests, urinalysis, liver and renal function tests, chest x-ray

Implementation
- Reconstitute for IM, SC use by dissolving contents of vial in 1–5 ml of Sterile Water for Injection, Sodium Chloride for Injection, 5% Dextrose Injection, Bacteriostatic Water for Injection.
- Label drug solution with date and hour of preparation; check label before use. Stable at room temperature for 24 h in Sodium Chloride, 5% Dextrose Solution, 5% Dextrose containing heparin 100 or 1,000 U/ml; discard after that time.
- Monitor pulmonary function regularly and chest x-ray weekly or biweekly to monitor onset of pulmonary toxicity; consult physician immediately if changes occur.
- Arrange for periodic monitoring of renal and liver function tests.

Drug-specific teaching points
- Be aware that this drug has to be given by injection. Prepare a calendar for dates to return for drug.
- Know that the following side effects may occur: rash, skin lesions, loss of hair, changes in nails (you may want to invest in a wig before hair loss occurs, skin care may help somewhat); loss of appetite, nausea, mouth sores (frequent mouth care, small frequent meals may help; try to maintain good nutrition).
- Report difficulty breathing, cough, yellowing of skin or eyes, severe GI upset, fever, chills.

Adverse effects in *Italics* are most common; those in **Bold** are life-threatening.

bretylium tosylate

(bre til' ee um)
Bretylate, (CAN), Bretylol

Pregnancy Category C

Drug classes
Antiarrhythmic
Adrenergic neuron blocker (not used as sympatholytic agent)

Therapeutic actions
Type III antiarrhythmic: prolongs repolarization, prolongs refractory period, and increases ventricular fibrillation threshold.

Indications
- Prevention and treatment of ventricular fibrillation
- Treatment of ventricular arrhythmias that are resistant to other antiarrhythmic agents
- **Unlabeled use**: second-line agent for advanced cardiac life support during CPR

Contraindications/cautions
- Because bretylium is used in life-threatening situations, the benefits usually outweigh any possible risks of therapy.
- Use caution in the presence of hypotension, shock; aortic stenosis; pulmonary hypertension; renal disease; lactation.

Dosage
Drug is for short-term use only. Careful patient assessment and evaluation are needed to determine the appropriate dose of this drug. Continual monitoring of cardiac response is necessary to establish the correct dosage for each patient. The following is a guide to usual dosage.

Adult
- ***Emergency use:*** Undiluted 5 mg/kg by rapid IV bolus: increase dose to 10 mg/kg, and repeat if arrhythmia persists. **Maintenance:** continuously infuse diluted solution IV at 1–2 mg/min, or infuse intermittently at 5–10 mg/kg over 10–30 min, q6h.
- ***Other arrhythmias:*** Infuse diluted solution at 5–10 mg/kg over > 8 min, and repeat q1–2h. *Maintenance:* same dose at 6-h intervals or continuous infusion of 1–2 mg/min.
- ***IM:*** 5–10 mg/kg undiluted, repeated at 1- to 2-h intervals if arrhythmia persists. *Maintenance:* same dose at 6- to 8-h intervals.

Pediatric
- ***Acute ventricular fibrillation:*** 5 mg/kg per dose IV followed by 10 mg/kg at 15- to 30-min intervals; maximum total dose 30 mg/kg. *Maintenance:* 5–10 mg/kg per dose q6h.
- ***Other ventricular arrhythmias:*** 5–10 mg/kg per dose q6h.

Pharmacokinetics

Route	Onset	Peak	Duration
IM	Varies	6–9 h	24 h
IV	Minutes	1–4 h	24 h

Metabolism: $T_{1/2}$: 6.9–8.1 h
Distribution: Crosses placenta; may pass into breast milk
Excretion: Urine

IV facts
Preparation: Dilute 1 ampule (10 ml containing 500 mg bretylium) to a minimum of 50 ml with 5% Dextrose Injection or Sodium Chloride Injection.
Infusion: Administer undiluted by rapid IV injection for emergency. Administer at a constant infusion of 1–2 mg/min using the following chart.

Amount Bretylium	Volume IV Fluid	Dose mg/min	Microdrips/min & ml/h
500 mg	50 ml	1	7
		1.5	11
		2	14
2 g	500 ml	1	16
1 g	250	1.5	24
		2	32
1 g	500	1	32
500 mg	250	1.5	47
		2	63

Compatibilities: Bretylium is compatible with 5% Dextrose Injection, 5% Dextrose in 0.45% Sodium Chloride, 5% Dextrose in 0.9% Sodium Chloride, 5% Dextrose in Lactated Ringer's, 0.9% Sodium Chloride, 5% Sodium Bicarbonate, 20% Mannitol, 1/6 M Sodium Lactate, Lactated Ringer's, Calcium

Chloride in 5% Dextrose, Potassium Chloride in 5% Dextrose.

Adverse effects
- CNS: Dizziness/lightheadedness, syncope
- GI: *Nausea, vomiting*
- CV: *Hypotension, orthostatic hypotension*, transient hypertension, cardiac arrhythmias, congestive heart failure
- Local: *Pain, burning* at injection site; tissue necrosis with extravasation

Clinically important drug-drug interactions
- Increased digitalis toxicity if taken with digitalis glycosides • Increased pressor effects of dopamine, norepinephrine, catecholamines when given with bretylium

■ Nursing Considerations

Assessment
- *History:* Hypotension, shock; aortic stenosis; pulmonary hypertension; renal disease; lactation
- *Physical:* Orientation, speech, reflexes; P, BP, auscultation, continuous ECG monitoring; R, adventitious sounds; renal function tests

Implementation
- Monitor patient's cardiac rhythm and BP continuously.
- Keep patient in supine position until tolerance of orthostatic hypotension develops.
- Increase dosage interval in patients with renal failure.
- Do not give more than 5 ml in any one IM injection site.
- Monitor for safe and effective serum drug levels (0.5–1.5 μg/ml).

Drug-specific teaching points
- Know that the drug dosage is changed frequently in relation to response of cardiac arrhythmia on monitor, and you will need frequent monitoring of cardiac rhythm and BP.
- Know that blood pressure will fall during drug therapy; because of this, it is important for you to remain lying down. Ask for assistance if you need to move or would like to sit up for any reason. You may feel lightheaded or dizzy even while lying down. Most people adjust to the blood pressure changes in a few days. It will still be important for you to change position slowly.
- Report chest pain, pain at IV site or IM injection site.

❒ bromocriptine mesylate

*(broe moe **krip'** teen)*
Parlodel

Pregnancy Category C

Drug classes
Antiparkinsonism drug
Dopamine receptor agonist
Semisynthetic ergot derivative

Therapeutic actions
Parkinsonism: Acts as an agonist directly on postsynaptic dopamine receptors of neurons in the brain, mimicking the effects of the neurotransmitter, dopamine, which is deficient in parkinsonism. Unlike levodopa, bromocriptine does not require biotransformation by the nigral neurons that are deficient in parkinsonism patients; thus, bromocriptine may be effective when levodopa has begun to lose its efficacy.
Hyperprolactinemia: Acts directly on postsynaptic dopamine receptors of the prolactin-secreting cells in the anterior pituitary, mimicking the effects of prolactin inhibitory factor, inhibiting the release of prolactin and galactorrhea. Also restores normal ovulatory menstrual cycles in patients with amenorrhea or galactorrhea, and inhibits the release of growth hormone in patients with acromegaly.

Indications
- Treatment of postencephalitic or idiopathic Parkinson's disease; may provide additional benefit in patients currently

Adverse effects in *Italics* are most common; those in **Bold** are life-threatening.

bromocriptine mesylate ■ 183

maintained on optimal dosages of levodopa with or without carbidopa, beginning to deteriorate or develop tolerance to levodopa, and experiencing "end of dose failure" on levodopa therapy; may allow reduction of levodopa dosage and decrease the dyskinesias and "on-off" phenomenon associated with long-term levodopa therapy
- Short-term treatment of amenorrhea or galactorrhea associated with hyperprolactinemia due to various etiologies, excluding demonstrable pituitary tumors
- Treatment of hyperprolactinemia associated with pituitary adenomas to reduce elevated prolactin levels, cause shrinkage of macroprolactinomas; may be used to reduce the tumor mass before surgery
- Female infertility associated with hyperprolactinemia in the absence of a demonstrable pituitary tumor
- Prevention of physiologic lactation (secretion, congestion, and engorgement) occurring after parturition when the mother does not breastfeed or after stillbirth or abortion
- *Acromegaly:* used alone or with pituitary irradiation or surgery to reduce serum growth hormone level

Contraindications/cautions
- Contraindicated in the presence of hypersensitivity to bromocriptine or any ergot alkaloid; severe ischemic heart disease or peripheral vascular disease; pregnancy, lactation.
- Use caution in the presence of history of MI with residual arrhythmias (atrial, nodal, or ventricular); renal, hepatic disease; history of peptic ulcer (fatal bleeding ulcers have occurred in patients with acromegaly treated with bromocriptine).

Dosage
Adult: Give drug with food; individualize dosage; increase dosage gradually to minimize side effects; titrate dosage carefully to optimize benefits and minimize side effects.
- **Hyperprolactinemia:** Initially, one-half to one 2.5-mg tablet PO daily; an additional 2.5-mg tablet may be added as tolerated q3–7d until optimal response is achieved; usual dosage is 5–7.5 mg/d; range is 2.5–15 mg/d. Treatment should not exceed 6 mo.
- **Physiologic lactation:** Start therapy only after vital signs have stabilized and no sooner than 4 h after delivery; 2.5 mg PO bid; usual dosage is 2.5 mg qid–tid. Continue therapy for 14 d or up to 21 d if necessary.
- **Acromegaly:** Initially, 1.25–2.5 mg PO for 3 d when going to sleep; add 1.25–2.5 mg as tolerated q3–7d until optimal response is achieved. Evaluate patient monthly, and adjust dosage based on growth hormone levels. Usual dosage range is 20–30 mg/d; do not exceed 100 mg/d; withdraw patients treated with pituitary irradiation for a yearly 4- to 8-wk reassessment period.
- **Parkinson's disease:** 1.25 mg PO bid; assess every 2 wk, and titrate dosage carefully to be sure that lowest dosage producing optimal response is not exceeded. If needed, increase dosage by increments of 2.5 mg/d q14–28d; do not exceed 100 mg/d. Efficacy for longer than 2 y not established.

Pediatric: Safety for use in children < 15 y not established.

Pharmacokinetics

Route	Onset	Peak	Duration
Oral	Varies	1–3 h	14 h

Metabolism: Hepatic; $T_{1/2}$: 3 h initial phase, 45–50 h terminal phase
Excretion: Bile

Adverse effects
Hyperprolactinemic Indications
- **CNS:** *Dizziness, fatigue, lightheadedness, nasal congestion, drowsiness,* cerebrospinal fluid rhinorrhea in patients who have had transsphenoidal surgery, pituitary radiation
- **GI:** *Nausea, vomiting, abdominal cramps, constipation, diarrhea, headache*
- **CV:** Hypotension

Adverse effects in *Italics* are most common; those in **Bold** are life-threatening.

184 ■ bromocriptine mesylate

Physiologic Lactation
- **CNS:** *Headache, dizziness, nausea, vomiting,* fatigue, syncope
- **GI:** Diarrhea, cramps
- **CV:** Hypotension

Acromegaly
- **CNS:** Nasal congestion, digital vasospasm, drowsiness
- **GI:** *Nausea, constipation, anorexia,* indigestion, dry mouth, vomiting, GI bleeding
- **CV:** Exacerbation of Raynaud's syndrome, *postural hypotension*

Parkinson's Disease
- **CNS:** *Abnormal involuntary movements, hallucinations, confusion, "on-off" phenomenon, dizziness, drowsiness, faintness, asthenia, visual disturbance, ataxia, insomnia, depression, vertigo*
- **GI:** *Nausea, vomiting, abdominal discomfort, constipation*
- **CV:** *Hypotension, shortness of breath*

Clinically important drug-drug interactions
- Increased serum bromocriptine levels and increased pharmacologic and toxic effects if taken with erythromycin • Decreased effectiveness of bromocriptine if taken concurrently with phenothiazines for treatment of prolactin-secreting tumors

■ Nursing Considerations

Assessment
- *History:* Hypersensitivity to bromocriptine or any ergot alkaloid; severe ischemic heart disease or peripheral vascular disease; pregnancy; history of MI with residual arrhythmias; renal, hepatic disease; history of peptic ulcer, lactation
- *Physical:* Skin—temperature (especially fingers), color, lesions; nasal mucous membranes; orientation, affect, reflexes, bilateral grip strength, vision exam, including visual fields; P, BP, orthostatic BP, auscultation; R, depth, adventitious sounds; bowel sounds, normal output, liver evaluation; liver and kidney function tests, CBC with differential

Implementation
- Ensure careful evaluation of patients with amenorrhea or galactorrhea before drug therapy begins; syndrome may result from pituitary adenoma that requires surgical or radiation procedures.
- Arrange to administer drug with food.
- Arrange to taper dosage in patients with Parkinson's disease if drug must be discontinued.
- Monitor blood pressure carefully for several days in patients receiving drug to inhibit postpartum lactation.
- Monitor hepatic, renal, hematopoietic function periodically during therapy.

Drug-specific teaching points
- Take this drug exactly as prescribed with food; take the first dose at bedtime while lying down.
- Do not discontinue drug without first consulting your nurse or physician (patients with macroadenoma may experience rapid growth of tumor and recurrence of original symptoms).
- Use mechanical contraceptive measures while you are taking this drug (patients receiving drug for amenorrhea or galactorrhea); pregnancy may occur before menses, and the drug is contraindicated in pregnancy (estrogen contraceptives may stimulate a prolactinoma).
- Know that the following side effects may occur: drowsiness, dizziness, confusion (avoid driving a car or engaging in activities that require alertness if these occur); nausea (taking the drug with meals, eating frequent small meals may help); dizziness or faintness when you get up (change position slowly, and exercise caution when climbing stairs); headache, nasal stuffiness (it may be possible for you to have medication for these).
- Report fainting; lightheadedness; dizziness; uncontrollable movements of the face, eyelids, mouth, tongue, neck, arms, hands, or legs; mental changes; irregular heartbeat or palpitations; severe or persistent nausea or vomiting; coffee-ground vomitus; black tarry stools; vision

Adverse effects in *Italics* are most common; those in **Bold** are life-threatening.

bromfeniramine maleate

▢ brompheniramine maleate

(brome fen ir' a meen)

parabromdylamine maleate

Bromphen, Codimal-A, Cophene-B, Dehist, Diamine T.D., Dimetane Extentabs, Dimetane-Ten, Histaject, Nasahist B, ND-Stat

Pregnancy Category C

Drug classes
Antihistamine (alkylamine type)

Therapeutic actions
Competitively blocks the effects of histamine at H_1 receptor sites; has anticholinergic (atropine-like), antipruritic, and sedative effects.

Indications
- **Oral preparations:** Symptomatic relief of symptoms associated with perennial and seasonal allergic rhinitis; vasomotor rhinitis; allergic conjunctivitis; mild, uncomplicated urticaria and angioedema; amelioraton of allergic reactions to blood or plasma; dermatographism; adjunctive therapy in anaphylactic reactions
- **Parenteral preparations:** Amelioration of allergic reactions to blood or plasma; in anaphylaxis as an adjunct to epinephrine and other measures; other uncomplicated allergic conditions when oral therapy is not possible

Contraindications/cautions
- Contraindicated in the presence of allergy to any antihistamines, third trimester of pregnancy (newborn or premature infants may have severe reactions).
- Use caution in the presence of narrow-angle glaucoma, stenosing peptic ulcer, symptomatic prostatic hypertrophy, asthmatic attack, bladder neck obstruction, pyloroduodenal obstruction, lactation.

Dosage
Adult and children > 12 y
- **Oral:** 4 mg PO q4–6h; do not exceed 24 mg in 24 h.
- **Sustained-release forms:** 8–12 mg PO q8–12h; do not exceed 24 mg in 24 h.
- **Parenteral:** 10 mg/ml injection is intended for IM, or SC administration undiluted; give IV either undiluted or 1:10 with Sterile Saline for Injection. 100 mg/ml injection is intended for IM or SC use only; use undiluted or diluted 1:10 in saline. **Usual dose:** 5–20 mg bid; maximum dose is 40 mg/24 h.

Pediatric
- **Oral**
  - *6–12 y:* 2 mg q4–6h; do not exceed 12 mg in 24 h.
  - *< 6 y:* Standard dosage not developed.
- **Sustained-release forms**
  - *6–12 y:* Use only as directed by physician.
  - *< 6 y:* Not recommended.
- **Parenteral**
  - *< 12 y:* 0.5 mg/kg per day or 15 mg/m² per day in three to four divided doses.

Geriatric: More likely to cause dizziness, sedation, syncope, toxic confusional states, and hypotension in elderly patients; use with caution.

Pharmacokinetics

Route	Onset	Peak	Duration
Oral	15–30 min	1–2 h	4–6 h
IM	20 min	1–2 h	8–12 h
IV	Immediate	30–60 min	8–12 h

Metabolism: Hepatic; $T_{1/2}$: 12–35 h
Distribution: Crosses placenta; passes into breast milk
Excretion: Urine

IV facts
Preparation: May be diluted 1:10 with Sterile Saline for Injection. May be added to Normal Saline, 5% glucose, or whole blood.

Infusion: May give IV dosage undiluted. Administer slowly.

Adverse effects

- **CNS:** *Drowsiness, sedation, dizziness, faintness, disturbed coordination,* fatigue, confusion, restlessness, excitation, nervousness, tremor, headache, blurred vision, diplopia, vertigo, tinnitus, acute labyrinthitis, hysteria, tingling, heaviness and weakness of the hands
- **GI:** *Epigastric distress,* anorexia, increased appetite and weight gain, nausea, vomiting, diarrhea or constipation
- **CV:** Hypotension, palpitations, bradycardia, tachycardia, extrasystoles
- **Respiratory:** *Thickening of bronchial secretions,* chest tightness, wheezing, nasal stuffiness, dry mouth, dry nose, dry throat, sore throat
- **Hematologic:** Hemolytic anemia, hypoplastic anemia, thrombocytopenia, leukopenia, agranulocytosis, pancytopenia
- **GU:** Urinary frequency, dysuria, urinary retention, early menses, decreased libido, impotence
- **Hypersensitivity:** Urticaria, rash, **anaphylactic shock,** photosensitivity

Clinically important drug-drug interactions

- Increased depressant effects if taken concurrently with alcohol, other CNS depressants • Increased and prolonged anticholinergic (drying) effects if taken with MAO inhibitors.

■ Nursing Considerations

Assessment

- *History:* Allergy to any antihistamines, narrow-angle glaucoma, stenosing peptic ulcer, symptomatic prostatic hypertrophy, asthmatic attack, bladder neck obstruction, pyloroduodenal obstruction, third trimester of pregnancy, lactation
- *Physical:* Skin—color, lesions, texture; orientation, reflexes, affect; vision exam; P, BP; R, adventitious sounds; bowel sounds; prostate palpation; CBC with differential

Implementation

- Administer oral preparations with food if GI upset occurs; caution patient not to crush or chew sustained-release preparations.
- Administer 10 mg/ml injection IM or SC undiluted.
- Provide appropriate supportive measures during allergic reactions that require parenteral administration.
- Maintain epinephrine 1:1,000 readily available when using parenteral preparations; hypersensitivity reactions, including anaphylaxis, have occurred.

Drug-specific teaching points

- Take as prescribed; avoid excessive dosage; take with food if GI upset occurs.
- Do not crush or chew the sustained-release preparations.
- Know that the following side effects may occur: dizziness, sedation, drowsiness (use caution if driving or performing tasks that require alertness if these occur); epigastric distress, diarrhea or constipation (taking the drug with meals may help); dry mouth (frequent mouth care, sucking sugarless lozenges may help); thickening of bronchial secretions, dryness of nasal mucosa (use of a humidifier may help if this becomes a problem).
- Avoid alcohol while on this drug; serious sedation could occur.
- Report difficulty breathing, hallucinations, tremors, loss of coordination, unusual bleeding or bruising, visual disturbances, irregular heartbeat.

❒ buclizine hydrochloride

(byoo' kli zeen)
Bucladin-S Softabs

Pregnancy Category C

Drug classes
Antiemetic
Anti-motion sickness drug

Adverse effects in *Italics* are most common; those in **Bold** are life-threatening.

buclizine hydrochloride ■ 187

Antihistamine
Anticholinergic drug

Therapeutic actions
Reduces sensitivity of the labyrinthine apparatus; probably acts at least partly by blocking cholinergic synapses in the vomiting center, which receives input from the chemoreceptor trigger zone and from peripheral nerve pathways; peripheral anticholinergic effects may contribute to efficacy; mechanism of action not totally understood.

Indications
- Control of nausea, vomiting, and dizziness of motion sickness

Contraindications/cautions
- Contraindicated in the presence of allergy to buclizine; allergy to tartrazine (more common in patients who are allergic to aspirin); lactation.
- Use caution in the presence of narrow-angle glaucoma, stenosing peptic ulcer, symptomatic prostatic hypertrophy, bronchial asthma, bladder neck obstruction, pyloroduodenal obstruction, cardiac arrhythmias (conditions that may be aggravated by anticholinergic therapy).

Dosage
Adult: 50 mg PO usually alleviates nausea. Up to 150 mg/d may be used. 50 mg PO at least ½ h before beginning to travel; for extended travel, a second tablet may be taken in 4–6 h. Usual maintenance dose is 50 mg bid; up to 150 mg/d may be given.
Pediatric: Safety and efficacy not established.
Geriatric: More likely to cause dizziness, sedation in elderly patients; use with caution.

Pharmacokinetics

Route	Onset	Duration
Oral	1 h	4–6 h

Metabolism: Hepatic
Distribution: Crosses placenta; passes into breast milk
Excretion: Urine

Adverse effects
Because this drug has anticholinergic properties, adverse effects associated with other anticholinergic drugs (atropine, scopolamine) should be kept in mind when using this drug; these include blurred vision, constipation, urinary retention, tachycardia, flushing, dryness of nose, thickening of respiratory secretions.
- CNS: *Drowsiness, dry mouth, headache, jitteriness*

■ Nursing Considerations
Assessment
- *History:* Allergy to buclizine; allergy to tartrazine; lactation; narrow-angle glaucoma, stenosing peptic ulcer, symptomatic prostatic hypertrophy, bronchial asthma, bladder neck obstruction, pyloroduodenal obstruction, cardiac arrhythmias
- *Physical:* Orientation, reflexes, affect; vision exam; P, BP; R, adventitious sounds; bowel sounds, normal GI output; prostate palpation, normal urinary output

Implementation
- Arrange for analgesics if needed for headache.

Drug-specific teaching points
- Take this drug as prescribed. Tablets can be taken without water; place tablet in mouth, and allow to dissolve or chew or swallow whole. Avoid excessive dosage.
- Use before motion sickness occurs; anti-motionsickness drugs work best if used before motion sickness occurs.
- Know that the following side effects may occur: dizziness, sedation, drowsiness (use caution if driving or performing tasks that require alertness if these occur); dry mouth (frequent mouth care, sucking sugarless lozenges may help); headache (consult your nurse or physician for recommendation of an analgesic); jitteriness (it may help to know that this is a drug effect that will go away when you discontinue the drug).
- Avoid OTC drugs when taking this drug; many of them contain ingredients that

Adverse effects in *Italics* are most common; those in **Bold** are life-threatening.

could cause serious reactions if taken with this drug.
- Avoid alcohol while taking this drug; serious sedation could occur.
- Report difficulty breathing; hallucinations, tremors, loss of coordination; visual disturbances; irregular heartbeat.

☐ budesonide

(bue des' oh nide)
Rhinocort

Pregnancy Category C

Drug classes
Corticosteroid

Therapeutic actions
Anti-inflammatory effect; local administration into nasal passages maximizes beneficial effects on these tissues, while decreasing the likelihood of adverse effects from systemic absorption.

Indications
- **Intranasal:** Management of symptoms of seasonal or perennial allergic rhinitis in adults and children; nonallergic perennial rhinitis in adults

Contraindications/cautions
- Presence of untreated local nasal infections, nasal trauma, septal ulcers, recent nasal surgery, lactation.

Dosage
Adult and children > 6 y: Initial dose 256 μg/day given as 2 sprays in each nostril morning and evening or 4 sprays in each nostril in the morning. After desired clinical effect is achieved, reduce dose to the smallest dose possible to maintain the control of symptoms. Generally takes 3–7 d to achieve maximum clinical effect.
Pediatric less than 6 y: Not recommemded.

Pharmacokinetics

Route	Onset	Peak	Duration
Intranasal	immed	rapid	8–12 h

Metabolism: Hepatic; $T_{1/2}$: unknown
Distribution: Crosses placenta; may pass into breast milk
Excretion: Urine

Adverse effects
- **GI:** Nausea, dyspepsia, dry mouth
- **Respiratory:** Epistaxis, rebound congestion, *pharyngitis, cough*
- **Dermatologic:** Rash, edema, pruritis, alopecia
- **Endocrine:** HPA suppression, Cushing's syndrome with overdosage and systemic absorption
- **Local:** *Nasal irritation,* fungal infection

■ Nursing Considerations

Assessment
- *History:* Untreated local nasal infections, nasal trauma, septal ulcers, recent nasal surgery, lactation
- *Physical:* BP, P, auscultation, R, adventitious sounds, exam of nares

Implementation
- Arrange to taper systemic steroids carefully during transfer to inhalational steroids; deaths from adrenal insufficiency have occurred.
- Arrange for use of decongestant nose drops to facilitate penetration if edema, excessive secretions are present.

Drug-specific teaching points
- Do not use this drug more often than prescribed; do not stop using this drug without consulting your health care provider.
- Be aware that it may take several days to achieve good effects; do not stop taking drug if effects are not immediate.
- Be aware that you should administer decongestant nose drops first if nasal passages are blocked.
- Know that the following side effects can occur: local irritation (make sure you are using your device correctly), dry mouth (sucking sugarless lozenges may help).
- Report sore mouth, sore throat, worsening of symptoms, severe sneezing.

Adverse effects in *Italics* are most common; those in **Bold** are life-threatening.

bumetanide

*(byoo **met'** a nide)*
Bumex

Pregnancy Category C

Drug classes
Loop (high ceiling) diuretic

Therapeutic actions
Inhibits the reabsorption of sodium and chloride from the proximal and distal renal tubules and the loop of Henle, leading to a natriuretic diuresis.

Indications
- Edema associated with CHF, cirrhosis, renal disease
- Acute pulmonary edema (IV)
- **Unlabeled use**: treatment of adult nocturia

Contraindications/cautions
- Allergy to bumetanide; electrolyte depletion; anuria, severe renal failure; hepatic coma; SLE; gout; diabetes mellitus; lactation.

Dosage
Adult: 0.5–2.0 mg/d PO in a single dose; may repeat at 4- to 5-h intervals up to a maximum daily dose of 10 mg. Intermittent dosage schedule of alternate drug and rest days or of 3–4 drug days followed by 1–2 rest days is most effective in controlling edema.
- ***Parenteral therapy:*** 0.5–1.0 mg IV or IM. Give over 1–2 min. Dose may be repeated at intervals of 2–3 h. *Do not exceed 10 mg/d.*

Pediatric: Not recommended for children < 18 y.

Geriatric or renal impaired: A continuous infusion of 12 mg over 12 h may be more effective and less toxic than intermittent bolus therapy.

Pharmacokinetics

Route	Onset	Peak	Duration
Oral	30–60 min	60–120 min	4–6 h
IV	Minutes	15–30 min	½–1 h

Metabolism: $T_{1/2}$: 60–90 min
Distribution: Crosses placenta; may pass into breast milk
Excretion: Urine

IV facts
Preparation: May be given direct IV or diluted in solution with 5% Dextrose in Water, 0.9% Sodium Chloride, Lactated Ringer's Solution. Discard unused solution after 24 h.

Infusion: Give by direct injection slowly, over 1–2 min. Further diluted in solution; give slowly.

Adverse effects
- **CNS:** *Asterixis, dizziness,* vertigo, paresthesias, confusion, fatigue, nystagmus, *weakness, headache, drowsiness,* fatigue, blurred vision, tinnitus, irreversible hearing loss
- **GI:** *Nausea, anorexia, vomiting, diarrhea,* gastric irritation and pain, dry mouth, acute pancreatitis, jaundice
- **CV:** *Orthostatic hypotension,* volume depletion, cardiac arrhythmias, thrombophlebitis
- **Hematologic:** *Hypokalemia,* leukopenia, anemia, thrombocytopenia
- **GU:** *Polyuria, nocturia,* glycosuria, renal failure
- **Local:** *Pain, phlebitis at injection site*
- **Other:** Muscle cramps and muscle spasms, weakness, arthritic pain, fatigue, hives, photosensitivity, rash, pruritus, sweating, nipple tenderness

Clinically important drug-drug interactions
- Decreased diuresis and natriuresis with NSAIDs • Increased risk of cardiac glycoside toxicity (secondary to hypokalemia) • Increased risk of ototoxicity if taken with aminoglycoside antibiotics, cisplatin

■ Nursing Considerations
Assessment
- *History:* Allergy to bumetanide, electrolyte depletion, anuria, severe renal failure, hepatic coma, SLE, gout, diabetes mellitus, lactation

Adverse effects in *Italics* are most common; those in **Bold** are life-threatening.

- *Physical:* Skin—color, lesions; edema; orientation, reflexes, hearing; pulses, baseline ECG, BP, orthostatic BP, perfusion; R, pattern, adventitious sounds; liver evaluation, bowel sounds; urinary output patterns; CBC, serum electrolytes (including calcium), blood sugar, liver and renal function tests, uric acid, urinalysis

Implementation
- Administer with food or milk to prevent GI upset.
- Mark calendars or other reminders of drug days for outpatients if intermittent therapy is the most effective for treating edema.
- Administer single daily doses early in the day so increased urination will not disturb sleep.
- Avoid IV use if oral use is possible.
- Arrange to monitor serum electrolytes, hydration, liver function during long-term therapy.
- Provide diet rich in potassium or supplemental potassium.

Drug-specific teaching points
- Record alternate day or intermittent therapy on a calendar or dated envelopes prepared for the patient.
- Take the drug early in the day so increased urination will not disturb sleep; take this drug with food or meals to prevent GI upset.
- Weigh yourself on a regular basis, at the same time of the day, and in the same clothing; record the weight on your calendar.
- Know that the following side effects may occur as a result of drug therapy: increased volume and frequency of urination (have ready access to a bathroom when drug effect is greatest); dizziness, feeling faint on arising, drowsiness (if these changes occur, avoid rapid position changes; hazardous activities, such as driving a car; and alcohol consumption, which can intensify these problems); sensitivity to sunlight (use sunglasses, wear protective clothing, or use a sunscreen when outdoors); increased thirst (sucking on sugarless lozenges may help to alleviate the thirst; frequent mouth care also may help); loss of body potassium (a potassium-rich diet, or even a potassium supplement, will be necessary).
- Report loss or gain of more than 3 lb in one day; swelling in ankles or fingers; unusual bleeding or bruising; nausea, dizziness, trembling, numbness, fatigue; muscle weakness or cramps.

buprenorphine hydrochloride

(byoo pre nor' feen)
Buprenex

Pregnancy Category C
C-V controlled substance

Drug classes
Narcotic agonist-antagonist analgesic

Therapeutic actions
Acts as an agonist at specific opioid receptors in the CNS to produce analgesia; also acts as an opioid antagonist; exact mechanism of action not understood.

Indications
- Relief of moderate-to-severe pain

Contraindications/cautions
- Contraindicated in the presence of hypersensitivity to buprenorphine.
- Use caution in the presence of physical dependence on narcotic analgesics (drug may precipitate withdrawal syndrome); compromised respiratory function; increased intracranial pressure (buprenorphine may elevate CSF pressure; may cause miosis and coma, which could interfere with patient evaluation), myxedema, Addison's disease, toxic psychosis, prostatic hypertrophy or urethral stricture, acute alcoholism, delirium tremens, kyphoscoliosis, biliary tract dysfunction (may cause spasm of the sphincter of Oddi), hepatic or renal dysfunction, lactation.

Dosage
Adult: 0.3 mg IM or by slow (over 2 min) IV injection. May repeat once, 30–60 min after first dose. If necessary, nonrisk patients

may be given up to 0.6 mg by deep IM injection.
Pediatric (< 13 y): Safety and efficacy not established.
Geriatric or debilitated: Reduce dosage to one-half usual adult dose.

Pharmacokinetics

Route	Onset	Peak	Duration
IM	15 min	1 h	6 h
IV	10 min	30–45 min	6 h

Metabolism: Hepatic; $T_{1/2}$: 2–3 h
Distribution: Crosses placenta; may pass into breast milk
Excretion: Feces

IV facts
Preparation: May be diluted with Isotonic Saline, Lactated Ringer's Solution, 5% Dextrose and 0.9% Saline, 5% Dextrose. Protect from light and excessive heat.
Infusion: Administer slowly.
Compatibilities: Compatible IV with scopolamine HBr, haloperidol, glycopyrrolate, droperidol and hydroxyzine HCl; incompatible IV with diazepam and lorazepam.

Adverse effects
- **CNS:** *Sedation, dizziness/vertigo, headache,* confusion, dreaming, psychosis, euphoria, weakness/fatigue, nervousness, slurred speech, paresthesia, depression, malaise, hallucinations, depersonalization, coma, tremor, dysphoria/agitation, convulsions, tinnitus
- **GI:** *Nausea, vomiting,* dry mouth, constipation, flatulence
- **CV:** *Hypotension,* hypertension, tachycardia, bradycardia, Wenckebach's block
- **Respiratory:** *Hypoventilation,* dyspnea, cyanosis, apnea
- **EENT:** *Miosis,* blurred vision, diplopia, conjunctivitis, visual abnormalities, amblyopia
- **Dermatologic:** *Sweating,* pruritus, rash, pallor, urticaria
- **Local:** Injection site reaction

Clinically important drug-drug interactions
- Potentiation of effects of buprenorphine when given with other narcotic analgesics, phenothiazines, tranquilizers, barbiturates, general anesthetics

Nursing Considerations
Assessment
- *History:* Hypersensitivity to buprenorphine, physical dependence on narcotic analgesics, compromised respiratory function, increased intracranial pressure, myxedema, Addison's disease, toxic psychosis, prostatic hypertrophy or urethral stricture, acute alcoholism, delirium tremens, kyphoscoliosis, biliary tract dysfunction, hepatic or renal dysfunction, lactation
- *Physical:* Skin—color, texture, lesions; orientation, reflexes, bilateral grip strength, affect; pupil size, vision; pulse, auscultation, BP; respiratory rate, adventitious sounds; bowel sounds, normal output, liver palpation; prostate palpation, normal urine output; liver, kidney, thyroid, adrenal function tests

Implementation
- Provide narcotic antagonist, facilities for assisted or controlled respiration on standby in case respiratory depression occurs.

Drug-specific teaching points
- Know that the following side effects may occur: dizziness, sedation, drowsiness, impaired visual acuity (avoid driving a car, performing other tasks that require alertness); nausea, loss of appetite (lying quietly, eating frequent small meals should minimize these effects).
- Report severe nausea, vomiting, palpitations, shortness of breath or difficulty breathing, urinary difficulty.

❒ bupropion HCl

(byoo **proe'** *pee on)*
Wellbutrin
Pregnancy Category C

Adverse effects in *Italics* are most common; those in **Bold** are life-threatening.

bupropion HCl

Drug classes
Antidepressant

Therapeutic actions
The neurochemical mechanism of the antidepressant effect of bupropion is not understood; it is chemically unrelated to other antidepressant agents; it is a weak blocker of neuronal uptake of serotonin and norepinephrine and inhibits the reuptake of dopamine to some extent.

Indications
- Treatment of depression (effectiveness if used > 6 wk is unknown)

Contraindications/cautions
- Contraindicated in the presence of hypersensitivity to bupropion; history of seizure disorder, bulimia or anorexia, head trauma, CNS tumor (increased risk of seizures); lactation.
- Use caution in the presence of treatment with MAO inhibitor; renal or liver disease; heart disease, history of MI.

Dosage
Adult: 300 mg PO given as 100 mg tid; begin treatment with 100 mg PO bid; if clinical response warrants, increase no sooner than 3 d after beginning treatment. If 4 wk after treatment, no clinical improvement is seen, dose may be increased to 150 mg PO tid (450 mg/d). Do not exceed 150 mg in any one dose. Discontinue drug if no improvement is seen within an appropriate time at the 450 mg/d level.
Pediatric: Safety and efficacy in children < 18 y not established.
Geriatric: Bupropion is excreted through the kidneys; use with caution, and monitor older patient carefully.

Pharmacokinetics

Route	Onset	Peak	Duration
Oral	Varies	2 h	8–12 h

Metabolism: Hepatic; $T_{1/2}$: 8–24 h
Distribution: May cross placenta; may pass into breast milk
Excretion: Urine and feces

Adverse effects
- **CNS:** *Agitation, insomnia, headache/migraine, tremor,* ataxia, incoordination, seizures, mania, increased libido, hallucinations, visual disturbances
- **GI:** *Dry mouth, constipation,* nausea, vomiting, stomatitis
- **CV:** *Dizziness, tachycardia,* edema, ECG abnormalities, chest pain, shortness of breath
- **GU:** Nocturia, vaginal irritation, testicular swelling
- **Dermatologic:** Rash, alopecia, dry skin
- **Other:** *Weight loss,* flulike symptoms

Clinically important drug-drug interactions
- Increased risk of adverse effects if taken concurrently with levodopa • Increased risk of bupropion toxicity if taken concurrently with MAO inhibitors • Increased risk of seizures if taken with drugs that lower seizure threshold

■ Nursing Considerations

Assessment
- *History:* Hypersensitivity to bupropion, history of seizure disorder, bulimia or anorexia, head trauma, CNS tumor, treatment with MAO inhibitor, renal or liver disease, heart disease, lactation
- *Physical:* Skin, body weight; orientation, affect, vision, coordination; P, rhythm, auscultation; R, adventitious sounds; bowel sounds, condition of mouth

Implementation
- Administer drug three times a day; do not administer more than 150 mg in any one dose.
- Increase dosage slowly to reduce the risk of seizures.
- Administer 100-mg tablets four times a day, with at least 4 h between successive doses, if patient is receiving > 300 mg/d; use combinations of 75-mg tablets to avoid giving > 150 mg in any single dose.
- Arrange for patient evaluation after 6 wk; effects of drug after 6 wk are not evaluated.

Adverse effects in *Italics* are most common; those in **Bold** are life-threatening.

- Arrange for discontinuation of MAO inhibitor therapy for at least 14 d before beginning bupropion therapy.
- Monitor liver and renal function tests in patients with a history of liver or renal impairment.
- Monitor patient's response and behavior; suicide is a potential problem in depressed patients.

Drug-specific teaching points
- Take this drug in equally divided doses three to four times a day as prescribed. Do not combine doses or make up missed doses.
- Know that the following side effects may occur: dizziness, lack of coordination, tremor (avoid driving an automobile or performing tasks that require alertness while these effects persist); dry mouth (frequent mouth care, sucking sugarless lozenges may help); headache, insomnia (consult with your nurse or physician if these become a problem; do not self-medicate); nausea, vomiting, weight loss (small, frequent meals may help).
- Avoid the use of alcohol, or limit as much as possible, while on this drug. Seizures can occur if these two drugs are combined.
- Report dark urine, light-colored stools; rapid or irregular heart beat; hallucinations; severe headache or insomnia; fever, chills, sore throat.

❒ buspirone hydrochloride

*(byoo **spye'** rone)*
BuSpar

Pregnancy Category B

Drug classes
Antianxiety agent

Therapeutic actions
Mechanism of action not known; lacks anticonvulsant, sedative, or muscle relaxant properties; binds serotonin receptors, but the clinical significance of this is not known.

Indications
- Management of anxiety disorders or short-term relief of symptoms of anxiety
- **Unlabeled use**: decreasing the symptoms (aches, pains, fatigue, cramps, irritability) of premenstrual syndrome (PMS)

Contraindications/cautions
- Hypersensitivity to buspirone; marked liver or renal impairment; lactation.

Dosage
Adult: Initially 15 mg/d PO (5 mg tid). Increase dosage 5 mg/d at intervals of 2–3 d as needed to achieve optimal therapeutic response. Do not exceed 60 mg/d. Divided doses of 20–30 mg/d have been used.
Pediatric: Safety and efficacy for children < 18 y not established.

Pharmacokinetics

Route	Onset	Peak
Oral	7–10 d	40–90 min

Metabolism: Hepatic; $T_{1/2}$: 3–11 h
Distribution: May pass into breast milk
Excretion: Urine

Adverse effects
- CNS: *Dizziness, headache, nervousness, insomnia, lightheadedness,* excitement, dream disturbances, drowsiness, decreased concentration, anger, hostility, confusion, depression, tinnitus, blurred vision, numbness, paresthesia, incoordination, tremor, depersonalization, dysphoria, noise intolerance, euphoria, akathisia, fearfulness, loss of interest, disassociative reaction, hallucinations, **suicidal ideation, seizures**, altered taste and smell, involuntary movements, slowed reaction time
- GI: *Nausea, dry mouth, vomiting, abdominal/gastric distress, diarrhea,* constipation, flatulence, anorexia, increased appetite, salivation, irritable colon and rectal bleeding

Adverse effects in *Italics* are most common; those in **Bold** are life-threatening.

- **CV:** Nonspecific chest pain, tachycardia/palpitations, syncope, hypotension, hypertension
- **Respiratory:** Hyperventilation, shortness of breath, chest congestion
- **GU:** Urinary frequency, urinary hesitancy, dysuria, increased or decreased libido, menstrual irregularity, spotting
- **Other:** Musculoskeletal aches and pains, sweating, clamminess, sore throat, nasal congestion

Clinically important drug-drug interactions
- Give with caution to patients taking alcohol, other CNS depressants • Decreased effects of buspirone if taken with fluoxetine

■ Nursing Considerations

Assessment
- *History:* Hypersensitivity to buspirone, marked liver or renal impairment, lactation
- *Physical:* Body weight; body temperature; skin—color, lesions; mucous membranes, throat—color, lesions, orientation, affect, reflexes, vision exam; P, BP; R, adventitious sounds; bowel sounds, normal GI output, liver evaluation; normal urinary output, voiding pattern; liver and kidney function tests, urinalysis, CBC and differential

Implementation
- Provide sugarless lozenges, ice chips, as appropriate, if dry mouth, altered taste occur.
- Arrange for analgesic as appropriate for patients experiencing headache, musculoskeletal aches.

Drug-specific teaching points
- Take this drug exactly as prescribed.
- Avoid the use of alcohol, sleep-inducing, or OTC drugs while on this drug; these could cause dangerous effects.
- Know that the following side effects may occur: drowsiness, dizziness, lightheadedness (avoid driving a car or operating complex machinery until you are sure that the drug does not affect you adversely); GI upset (frequent small meals may help); dry mouth (sucking ice chips or sugarless candies may help); dreams, nightmares, difficulty concentrating or sleeping, confusion, excitement (it may help to know that these are drug effects that will go away when the drug is discontinued).
- Report abnormal involuntary movements of facial or neck muscles, motor restlessness; sore or cramped muscles; abnormal posture; yellowing of the skin or eyes.

❒ busulfan

(byoo sul' fan)
Myleran

Pregnancy Category D

Drug classes
Alkylating agent
Antineoplastic drug

Therapeutic actions
Cytotoxic: interacts with cellular thiol groups causing cell death; cell cycle nonspecific.

Indications
- Palliative treatment of chronic myelogenous leukemia; less effective in patients without the Philadelphia chromosome (Ph1); ineffective in patients in the blastic stage

Contraindications/cautions
- Allergy to busulfan, history of resistance to busulfan, chronic lymphocyctic leukemia, acute leukemia, blastic phase of chronic myelogenous leukemia, hematopoietic depression, pregnancy, lactation.

Dosage
Adult
- ***Remission induction:*** 4–8 mg total dose PO daily. Continue until WBC has dropped to 15,000/mm^3; WBC may continue to fall for 1 mo after drug is discontinued. Normal WBC count is usually achieved in approximately 12–20 wk in most cases.

- *Maintenance therapy:* Resume treatment with induction dosage when WBC reaches 50,000/mm^3. If remission is shorter than 3 mo, maintenance therapy of 1–3 mg PO qid is advised to keep hematologic status under control.

Pharmacokinetics

Route	Onset	Peak	Duration
Oral	0.5–2 h	2–3 h	4 h

Metabolism: Hepatic; $T_{1/2}$: unknown
Distribution: Crosses placenta; passes into breast milk
Excretion: Urine

Adverse effects
- **GI:** Dryness of the oral mucous membranes and cheilosis
- **Respiratory: Pulmonary fibrosis,** bronchopulmonary dysplasia
- **Hematologic:** *Leukopenia, thrombocytopenia, anemia, pancytopenia* (prolonged)
- **GU:** Hyperuricemia
- **EENT:** Cataracts (with prolonged use)
- **Dermatologic:** *Hyperpigmentation*, urticaria, Stevens-Johsnson syndrome, erythema nodosum, alopecia, porphyria cutanea tarda, excessive dryness and fragility of the skin with anhidrosis
- **Endocrine:** *Amenorrhea, ovarian suppression, menopausal symptoms*; interference with spermatogenesis, testicular atrophy, syndrome resembling adrenal insufficiency (weakness, fatigue, anorexia, weight loss, nausea, vomiting, melanoderma)
- **Other:** Cancer

■ Nursing Considerations

Assessment
- *History:* Allergy to or history of resistance to busulfan, chronic lymphocytic leukemia, acute leukemia, blastic phase of chronic myelogenous leukemia, hematopoietic depression, pregnancy, lactation
- *Physical:* Weight; skin—color, lesions, turgor; earlobes—tophi; eye exam; bilateral hand grip; R, adventitious sounds; mucous membranes; CBC, differential; urinalysis; serum uric acid; pulmonary function tests; bone marrow exam if indicated

Implementation
- Arrange for blood tests to evaluate bone marrow function before beginning therapy, weekly during therapy, and for at least 3 wk after therapy has ended.
- Arrange for respiratory function tests before beginning therapy, periodically during therapy, and periodically after busulfan therapy has ended.
- Arrange for reduced dosage in cases of bone marrow depression.
- Administer medication at the same time each day.
- Suggest the use of contraceptive measures during busulfan use.
- Ensure that the patient is hydrated before beginning therapy and during therapy; alkalinization of the urine or allopurinol may be needed to prevent adverse effects of hyperuricemia.
- Monitor patient periodically for the development of cataracts.

Drug-specific teaching points
- Take the drug at the same time each day.
- Drink 10–12 glasses of fluid each day while you are on this drug.
- Know that the following side effects may occur: darkening of the skin, rash, dry and fragile skin (skin care suggestions will be outlined for you to help to prevent skin breakdown); weakness, fatigue (this can be an effect of the drug; consult with your nurse or physician if this becomes pronounced); loss of appetite, nausea, vomiting, weight loss (small frequent meals may help); amenorrhea in women, change in sperm production in men (this effect on fertility can be upsetting).
- Arrange to have regular medical follow up, including blood tests, to monitor the effects of the drug on your body.
- Consider using contraceptive measures during the course of this drug therapy. This drug has been known to cause fetal damage.

Adverse effects in *Italics* are most common; those in **Bold** are life-threatening.

- Report unusual bleeding or bruising; fever, chills, sore throat; stomach, flank, or joint pain; cough, shortness of breath.

butabarbital sodium

*(byoo ta **bar'** bi tal)*
secbutabarbital,
secbutobarbitone

Butisol Sodium, Sarisol No. 2

Pregnancy Category D
C-III controlled substance

Drug classes
Barbiturate (intermediate acting)
Sedative
Hypnotic

Therapeutic actions
General CNS depressant; barbiturates inhibit impulse conduction in the ascending reticular activating system, depress the cerebral cortex, alter cerebellar function, depress motor output, and can produce excitation (especially with subanesthetic doses in the presence of pain), sedation, hypnosis, anesthesia, deep coma.

Indications
- Short-term use as a sedative and hypnotic

Contraindications/cautions
- Contraindicated in the presence of hypersensitivity to barbiturates, tartrazine (in 30-, 50-mg tablets, and elixir marketed as *Butisol Sodium*); manifest or latent porphyria; marked liver impairment; nephritis; severe respiratory distress, respiratory disease with dyspnea, obstruction, or cor pulmonale; previous addiction to sedative-hypnotic drugs; pregnancy.
- Use caution in the presence of acute or chronic pain (drug may cause paradoxical excitement or mask important symptoms); seizure disorders (abrupt discontinuation of daily doses of drug can result in status epilepticus); lactation (has caused drowsiness in nursing infants); fever, hyperthyroidism, diabetes mellitus, severe anemia, pulmonary or cardiac disease, status asthmaticus, shock, uremia; impaired liver or kidney function, debilitation.

Dosage
Adult
- ***Daytime sedation:*** 15–30 mg PO tid–qid.
- ***Hypnotic:*** 50–100 mg PO at bedtime. Drug loses effectiveness within 2 wk and should not be used longer than that.
- ***Preanesthetic sedation:*** 50–100 mg PO 60–90 min before surgery. *Note:* It is not considered safe to administer oral medication when a patient is NPO for surgery or anesthesia.

Pediatric: Use caution: barbiturates may produce irritability, excitability, inappropriate tearfulness, and aggression.
- ***Daytime sedation:*** 7.5–30 mg PO, depending on age, weight, and sedation desired. (For methods to calculate pediatric dosage based on age and body weight, see Appendix C).
- ***Hypnotic:*** Dosage based on age and weight.
- ***Preanesthetic sedation:*** 2–6 mg/kg; maximum dose 100 mg (see note above).

Geriatric patients or those with debilitating disease: Reduce dosage and monitor closely; may produce excitement, depression, confusion.

Pharmacokinetics

Route	Onset	Peak	Duration
Oral	45–60 min	3–4 h	6–8 h

Metabolism: Hepatic; $T_{1/2}$: 50–100 h
Distribution: Crosses placenta; passes into breast milk
Excretion: Urine

Adverse effects
- CNS: *Somnolence, agitation, confusion, hyperkinesia, ataxia, vertigo, CNS depression, nightmares, lethargy, residual sedation (hangover), paradoxical excitement, nervousness, psychiatric disturbance, hallucinations, insom-*

nia, anxiety, dizziness, thinking abnormality
- GI: *Nausea, vomiting, constipation, diarrhea, epigastric pain*
- CV: *Bradycardia, hypotension, syncope*
- Respiratory: *Hypoventilation, apnea, respiratory depression,* laryngospasm, bronchospasm, **circulatory collapse**
- Hypersensitivity: Skin rashes, angioneurotic edema, serum sickness, morbiliform rash, urticaria; rarely, exfoliative dermatitis, **Stevens-Johnson syndrome, sometimes fatal**
- Other: Tolerance, psychological and physical dependence; withdrawal syndrome (sometimes fatal)

Clinically important drug-drug interactions

- Increased CNS depression when taken with alcohol • Increased risk of nephrotoxicity if taken with methoxyflurane • Decreased effects of the following drugs given with barbiturates: theophyllines, oral anticoagulants, beta-blockers, doxycycline, griseofulvin corticosteroids, oral contraceptives and estrogens, metronidazole, phenylbutazones, quinidine, carbamazepine

■ Nursing Considerations

Assessment

- *History:* Hypersensitivity to barbiturates, tartrazine, manifest or latent porphyria; marked liver impairment, nephritis, respiratory disease; previous addiction to sedative-hypnotic drugs, acute or chronic pain, seizure disorders, fever, hyperthyroidism, diabetes mellitus, severe anemia, cardiac disease, shock, uremia, debilitation, pregnancy, lactation
- *Physical:* Body weight; body temperature; skin—color, lesions; orientation, affect, reflexes; P, BP, orthostatic BP; R, adventitious sounds; bowel sounds, normal output, liver evaluation; liver and kidney function tests, blood and urine glucose, BUN

Implementation

- Monitor patient responses, blood levels (as appropriate) if any of the above interacting drugs are given with butabarbital; suggest alternate means of contraception to women on oral contraceptives for whom butabarbital is prescribed.
- Provide resuscitative facilities on standby in case of respiratory depression, hypersensitivity reaction.
- Arrange to taper dosage gradually after repeated use, especially in epileptic patients.

Drug-specific teaching points

- Know that this drug will make you drowsy and less anxious.
- Try not to get up after you have received this drug (request assistance if you feel you must sit up or move about for any reason).

Outpatients Taking This Drug

- Take this drug exactly as prescribed.
- This drug is habit-forming; its effectiveness in facilitating sleep disappears after a short time. Do not to take this drug longer than 2 wk (for insomnia), and do not increase the dosage without consulting the physician.
- Consult the care provider if the drug appears to be ineffective.
- Avoid alcohol, sleep-inducing, or OTC drugs while taking this drug because these could cause dangerous effects.
- Use a means of contraception other than oral contraceptives while on this drug (female patients); you should not become pregnant while taking this drug.
- Know that the following side effects may occur: drowsiness, dizziness, "hangover," impaired thinking (these effects may become less pronounced after a few days; avoid driving a car or engaging in dangerous activities if these occur); GI upset (taking the drug with food may help); dreams, nightmares, difficulty concentrating, fatigue, nervousness (it may help to know that these are effects of the drug that will go away when the drug is discontinued).
- Report severe dizziness, weakness, drowsiness that persists, rash or skin lesions, pregnancy.

Adverse effects in *Italics* are most common; those in **Bold** are life-threatening.

butoconazole nitrate

*(byoo toe **koe**' na zole)*
Femstat
Pregnancy Category C

Drug classes
Antifungal

Therapeutic actions
Fungicidal and fungistatic: binds to the cell membrane of the fungus with a resultant change in membrane permeability, allowing leakage of intracellular components and cell death.

Indications
- Local treatment of vulvovaginal candidiasis (moniliasis)

Contraindications/cautions
- Allergy to butoconazole or components used in preparation; lactation.

Dosage
Pregnant patients (second and third trimesters only): 1 applicator (5 g) intravaginally at bedtime for 6 d.
Nonpregnant patients: 1 applicator (5 g) intravaginally at bedtime for 3 d (may be extended to 6 d if necessary).

Pharmacokinetics

Route	Onset
Vaginal	Immediate

Metabolism: Hepatic; $T_{1/2}$: 21–24 h
Distribution: Crosses placenta; may pass into breast milk
Excretion: Urine and feces

Adverse effects
- Local: *Vulvovaginal burning,* vulvar itching; discharge, soreness, swelling, itchy fingers

■ Nursing Considerations

Assessment
- *History:* Allergy to butoconazole or components used in preparation, pregnancy, lactation
- *Physical:* Pelvic exam, exam of mucous membranes and vulvar area; culture of area involved; KOH smear to confirm diagnosis of candidiasis

Implementation
- Arrange for appropriate culture of fungus involved before beginning therapy.
- Administer vaginal cream high into vagina using the applicator supplied with the product. Administer for 3–6 consecutive nights, even during menstrual period.
- Monitor response to drug therapy; if no response is noted, arrange for further cultures to determine causative organism.
- Ensure that patient receives the full course of therapy to eradicate the fungus and prevent recurrence.
- Discontinue administration if rash or sensitivity occurs.

Drug-specific teaching points
- Take the full course of drug therapy, even if symptoms improve. Continue during menstrual period if vaginal route is being used. Vaginal cream should be inserted high into the vagina using the applicator provided.
- Use hygiene measures to prevent reinfection or spread of infection; refrain from sexual intercourse, or advise partner to use a condom to avoid reinfection.
- Be aware that this drug is specific for the fungus being treated; do not self-medicate other problems with this drug.
- Use a sanitary napkin to prevent staining of clothing.
- Know that the following side effects may occur: local irritation, burning, stinging.
- Report worsening of the condition being treated, local irritation, burning.

butorphanol tartrate

*(byoo **tor**' fa nole)*
Stadol, Stadol NS
Pregnancy Category C during pregnancy
Pregnancy Category D during labor/delivery

Adverse effects in *Italics* are most common; those in **Bold** are life-threatening.

butorphanol tartrate

Drug classes
Narcotic agonist-antagonist analgesic

Therapeutic actions
Acts as an agonist at opioid receptors in the CNS to produce analgesia, sedation (therapeutic effects), but also acts to cause hallucinations (adverse effect); has low abuse potential; not in any schedule of the Federal Controlled Substances Act.

Indications
- Relief of moderate to severe pain
- *Nasal spray:* relief of migraine headache pain
- For preoperative or preanesthetic medication, to supplement balanced anesthesia, and to relieve prepartum pain

Contraindications/cautions
- Contraindicated in the presence of hypersensitivity to butorphanol, physical dependence on a narcotic analgesic, pregnancy, lactation.
- Use caution in the presence of bronchial asthma, COPD, respiratory depression, anoxia, increased intracranial pressure, acute MI, ventricular failure, coronary insufficiency, hypertension, biliary tract surgery, renal or hepatic dysfunction.

Dosage
Adult
- *IM:* Usual single dose is 2 mg q3–4h as necessary. Dosage range is 1–4 mg q3–4h; single doses should not exceed 4 mg.
- *IV:* Usual single dose is 1 mg q3–4h as necessary. Dosage range is 0.5–2 mg q3–4h.
- *Preoperative:* 2 mg IM, 60–90 min before surgery.
- *Balanced anesthesia:* 2 mg IV shortly before induction or 0.5–1 mg IV in increments during anesthesia.
- *Labor:* 1–2 mg IV or IM at full term during early labor; repeat q4h.
- *Nasal:* 1 mg (1 spray per nostril). May repeat in 60–90 min if adequate relief is not achieved. May repeat two-dose sequence q3–4h.

Pediatric (< 18 y): Not recommended.
Geriatric or renal or hepatic impairment
- *Parenteral:* Use one-half the usual dose at twice the usual interval. Monitor patient response.
- *Nasal:* 1 mg initially. Allow 90–120 min to elapse before a second dose is given.

Pharmacokinetics

Route	Onset	Peak	Duration
IV	Rapid	0.5–1 h	3–4 h
IM	10–15 min	0.5–1 h	3–4 h
Nasal	15 min	1–2 h	4–5 h

Metabolism: Hepatic; $T_{1/2}$:2.1–9.2 h
Distribution: Crosses placenta; passes into breast milk
Excretion: Urine and feces

IV facts
Preparation: May be given undiluted. Store at room temperature. Protect from light.
Infusion: Administer direct IV at rate of 2 mg every 3–5 min.
Compatibilities: Do not mix in solution with dimenhydrinate, pentobarbital.

Adverse effects
- CNS: *Sedation, clamminess, sweating, headache, vertigo, floating feeling, dizziness, lethary, confusion, lightheadedness,* nervousness, unusual dreams, agitation, euphoria, hallucinations
- GI: *Nausea,* dry mouth
- CV: Palpitation, increase or decrease in blood pressure
- Respiratory: Slow, shallow respiration
- EENT: Diplopia, blurred vision
- Dermatologic: Rash, hives, pruritus, flushing, warmth, sensitivity to cold

Clinically important drug-drug interactions
- Potentiation of effects of butorphanol when given with barbiturate anesthetics

■ Nursing Considerations
Assessment
- *History:* Hypersensitivity to butorphanol, physical dependence on a narcotic anal-

Adverse effects in *Italics* are most common; those in **Bold** are life-threatening.

gesic, pregnancy, lactation, bronchial asthma, COPD, increased intracranial pressure, acute MI, ventricular failure, coronary insufficiency, hypertension, biliary tract surgery, renal or hepatic dysfunction
- *Physical:* Orientation, reflexes, bilateral grip strength, affect; pupil size, vision; pulse, auscultation, BP; R, adventitious sounds; bowel sounds, normal output; liver, kidney function tests

Implementation

- Provide narcotic antagonist, facilities for assisted or controlled respiration on standby during parenteral administration.

Drug-specific teaching points

- Know that the following side effects may occur: dizziness, sedation, drowsiness, impaired visual acuity (avoid driving a car, performing other tasks that require alertness); nausea, loss of appetite (lying quietly, eating frequent small meals should minimize these effects).
- Report severe nausea, vomiting, palpitations, shortness of breath or difficulty breathing, nasal lesions or discomfort (nasal spray).

☐ caffeine

(kaf een')

Caffedrine, Nodoz, Quick Pep, Tirend, Vivarin

Pregnancy Category C

Drug classes
Analeptic
Xanthine

Therapeutic actions
Increases calcium permeability in sarcoplasmic reticulum, promotes the accumulation of cAMP, and blocks adenosine receptors; stimulates the CNS, cardiac activity, gastric acid secretion, and diuresis.

Indications

- An aid in staying awake and restoring mental awareness
- Adjunct to analgesic formulations
- **IM:** possibly an analeptic in conjunction with supportive measures to treat respiratory depression associated with overdosage with CNS depressants

Contraindications/cautions

- Depression, duodenal ulcers, diabetes mellitus, lactation

Dosage
Adult: 100–200 mg PO q3–4h as needed; timed-release preparation, 200 mg PO q3–4h.
- **Respiratory depression:** 500 mg–1 g caffeine and sodium benzoate (250–500 mg caffeine) IM; do not exceed 2.5 g/d; may be given IV in severe emergency situation.

Pediatric: Safety and efficacy not established.

Pharmacokinetics

Route	Onset	Peak
Oral	15 min	15–45 min

Metabolism: Hepatic; $T_{1/2}$: 3–7.5 h
Distribution: Crosses placenta; passes into breast milk
Excretion: Urine

IV facts

Preparation: Dissolve 10 g caffeine citrate powder in 250 ml Sterile Water for Injection USP qs to 500 ml; filter and autoclave. Final concentration is 10 mg/ml caffeine base (20 mg/ml caffeine citrate). Stable for 3 mo. Or dissolve 10 mg caffeine powder and 10.94 citric acid powder in Bacteriostatic Water for Injection, USP qs to 1 L. Sterilize by filtration.
Infusion: IV single dose of 500 mg caffeine may be given slowly in emergency situations; not recommended.

Adverse effects

- CNS: *Insomnia, restlessness, excitement,* nervousness, tinnitus, muscular tremor, headaches, lightheadedness
- CV: *Tachycardia,* extrasystoles, palpitations

- **GI:** Nausea, vomiting, diarrhea, stomach pain
- **GU:** *Diuresis*
- **Other:** Withdrawal syndrome: headache, anxiety, muscle tension

Clinically important drug-drug interactions
- Increased CNS effects of caffeine if taken with cimetidine, oral contraceptives, disulfiram, ciprofloxacin, enoxacin, phenylpropanolamine • Decreased effects of caffeine if taken while smoking

Clinically important drug-food interactions
- Decreased absorption of iron if taken with or 1 h after coffee or tea

Drug-lab test interferences
- Possible false elevations of serum urate, urine VMA, resulting in false-positive diagnosis of pheochromocytoma or neuroblastoma

Nursing Considerations

Assessment
- *History:* Depression, duodenal ulcer, diabetes mellitus, lactation
- *Physical:* Neurologic status, P, BP, ECG, normal urinary output, abdominal exam, blood glucose

Implementation
- Do not stop the drug abruptly after long-term use.
- Monitor diet for presence of caffeine-containing foods that may contribute to overdose.

Drug-specific teaching points
- Do not stop taking this drug abruptly; withdrawal symptoms may occur.
- Avoid foods that are high in caffeine (coffee, tea, cola, chocolate), which may cause symptoms of overdose.
- Avoid driving or dangerous activities if dizziness, tremors, restlessness occur.
- Consult with your health care provider if fatigue continues.
- Know that the following side effects may occur: diuresis (stay near bathroom facilities if this occurs); restlessness, insomnia, muscular tremors, lightheadedness; nausea, abdominal pain.
- Report abnormal heart rate, dizziness, palpitations.

calcitonin, human

*(kal si **toe'** nin)*
Cibacalcin

calcitonin, salmon
Calcimar, Miacalcin, Miacalcin Nasal Spray

Pregnancy Category B (salmon)
Pregnancy Category C (human)

Drug classes
Hormonal agent
Calcium regulator

Therapeutic actions
The calcitonins are polypeptide hormones secreted by the thyroid; human calcitonin is a synthetic product; salmon calcitonin appears to be a chemically identical polypeptide but with greater potency per milligram and longer duration; inhibits bone resorption; lowers elevated serum calcium in children and patients with Paget's disease; increases the excretion of filtered phosphate, calcium, and sodium by the kidney.

Indications
- Paget's disease (human and salmon calcitonin)
- Postmenopausal osteoporosis in conjunction with adequate calcium and vitamin D intake to prevent loss of bone mass (salmon calcitonin)
- Hypercalcemia, emergency treatment (salmon calcitonin)

Contraindications/cautions
- Contraindicated in the presence of allergy to salmon calcitonin or fish products, lactation.

Adverse effects in Italics *are most common; those in* **Bold** *are life-threatening.*

- Use caution in the presence of renal insufficiency, osteoporosis, pernicious anemia.

Dosage
Adult
- ***Calcitonin, human:*** *Paget's disease:* starting dose of 0.5 mg/d SC; some patients may respond to 0.5 mg two to three times per week or 0.25 mg/d. Severe cases may require up to 1 mg/d for 6 mo. Discontinue therapy when symptoms are relieved.
- ***Calcitonin, salmon:*** *Skin testing:* 0.1 ml of a 10 IU/ml solution injected SC.
- *Paget's disease:* Initial dose 100 IU/d SC or IM. *Maintenance dose:* 50 IU/d or every other day. Actual dose should be determined by patient response.
- *Postmenopausal osteoporosis:* 100 IU/d SC or IM, with supplemental calcium (calcium carbonate, 1.5 g/d) and vitamin D (400 U/d).
- *Hypercalcemia: Initial dose:* 4 IU/kg q12h SC or IM. If response is not satisfactory after 1–2 d, increase to 8 IU/kg q12h; if response remains unsatisfactory after 2 more d, increase to 8 IU/kg q6h.

Pediatric: Safety and efficacy not established.

Pharmacokinetics

Route	Onset	Peak	Duration
IM, SC	15 min	3–4 h	8–24 h

Metabolism: Renal; $T_{1/2}$: 1.2 h (salmon) 1 h (human)
Distribution: May pass into breast milk
Excretion: Urine

Adverse effects
- **GI:** *Nausea, vomiting*
- **Dermatologic:** *Flushing of face or hands,* skin rash
- **GU:** *Urinary frequency* (calcitonin-human)
- **Local:** *Local inflammatory reactions at injection site* (salmon)

■ Nursing Considerations
Assessment
- *History:* Allergy to salmon calcitonin or fish products, lactation, osteoporosis, pernicious anemia, renal disease
- *Physical:* Skin—lesions, color, temperature; muscle tone; urinalysis, serum calcium, serum alkaline phosphatase and urinary hydroxyproline excretion

Implementation
- Administer skin test to patients with any history of allergies; salmon calcitonin is a protein, and the risk of allergy is significant. Prepare solution for skin test as follows: withdraw 0.05 ml of the 200 IU/ml solution or 0.1 ml of the 100 IU/ml solution into a tuberculin syringe. Fill it to 1 ml with Sodium Chloride Injection. Mix well. Discard 0.9 ml, and inject 0.1 ml (approximately 1 IU) SC into the inner aspect of the forearm. Observe after 15 min; the presence of a wheal or more than mild erythema indicates a positive response. Risk of allergy is less in patients being treated with human calcitonin.
- Use reconstituted human calcitonin within 6h.
- Maintain parenteral calcium on standby in case of development of hypocalcemic tetany.
- Monitor serum alkaline phosphatase and urinary hydroxyproline excretion prior to therapy and during the first 3 mo and q3–6 mo during long-term therapy.
- Inject doses of more than 2 ml IM, not SC; use multiple injection sites.

Drug-specific teaching points
- Be aware that this drug is given SC or IM; you, or someone who can help you, will need to learn how to do this at home. Refrigerate the drug vials.
- Know that the following side effects may occur: nausea, vomiting (this usually passes as your body adjusts to the drug); irritation at injection site (rotating injection sites will help); flushing of the face or hands, skin rash (consult with your nurse or physician if this becomes too uncomfortable).
- Report twitching, muscle spasms; dark urine; hives, skin rash; difficulty breathing.

Adverse effects in *Italics* are most common; those in **Bold** are life-threatening.

◻ calcitriol

*(kal si **trye' ole**)*
1,25-dihydroxycholecalciferol,
1,25[OH]2-D3

Calcijex, Rocaltrol

Pregnancy Category C

Drug classes
Vitamin
Calcium regulator

Therapeutic actions
Fat-soluble vitamin; helps to regulate calcium homeostasis, bone growth, and maintenance; increases serum calcium levels and decreases alkaline phosphatase, parathyroid hormone levels.

Indications
- Management of hypocalcemia in patients on chronic renal dialysis
- Reduction of elevated parathyroid hormone levels in some patients; possibly effective
- **Unlabeled use**: used orally and topically for 6 mo to decrease the severity of psoriatic lesions in patients with psoriasis vulgaris

Contraindications/cautions
- Contraindicated in the presence of allergy to vitamin D, hypercalcemia, vitamin D toxicity, hypervitaminosis D, pregnancy (teratogenic in preclinical studies).
- Use caution in the presence of renal stones, lactation.

Dosage
Adult: 0.25 µg/d PO; if satisfactory response is not observed, dosage may be increased by 0.25 µg/d at 4- to 8-wk intervals. Most patients respond to 0.5–1 µg/d. 0.5 µg IV three times per week at the end of dialysis; may need up to 3 µg IV three times per week.
Pediatric
- ***Older than 6 y:*** 0.5 – 2 µg/d PO.
- ***1–5 y:*** 0.25–0.75 µg/d.

Pharmacokinetics

Route	Onset	Peak	Duration
Oral, IV	2–6 h	10–12 h	3–5 d

Metabolism: Renal; $T_{1/2}$: 3–6 h
Distribution: May cross placenta; passes into breast milk
Excretion: Bile

IV facts
Preparation: No further preparation is needed.
Infusion: Administer undiluted, direct IV over 30–60 sec.

Adverse effects
- **CNS:** *Weakness, headache, somnolence,* irritability
- **GI:** *Nausea, vomiting, dry mouth, constipation, metallic taste,* anorexia, pancreatitis, elevated liver function tests
- **GU:** Polyuria, polydipsia, nocturia, decreased libido, elevated renal function tests
- **CV:** Hypertension, cardiac arrhythmias
- **Other:** Muscle pain, bone pain, weight loss, photophobia, rhinorrhea, pruritus, hyperthermia

Clinically important drug-drug interactions
- Risk of hypermagnesemia with magnesium-containing antacids • Reduced intestinal absorption of fat-soluble vitamins with cholestyramine, mineral oil • Possible risk of hypercalcemia if given with thiazide diuretics

■ Nursing Considerations
Assessment
- *History:* Allergy to vitamin D; hypercalcemia, vitamin D toxicity, hypervitaminosis D; renal stones; lactation
- *Physical:* Skin—color, lesions; body temperature; body weight; orientation, strength, taste; liver evaluation, mucous membranes; serum calcium, phosphorus, magnesium, alkaline phosphatase; renal and hepatic function tests; x-rays of bones

Adverse effects in *Italics* are most common; those in **Bold** are life-threatening.

Implementation
- Monitor serum calcium before beginning therapy and at least weekly during therapy; if hypercalcemia occurs, discontinue use until calcium levels return to normal.
- Provide supportive measures to help patient deal with GI, CNS effects of drug (eg, pain medication, relief of constipation, help with ADLs).
- Arrange for nutritional consultation if GI problems become severe.

Drug-specific teaching points
- Know that the following side effects may occur: weakness, bone and muscle pain, somnolence (rest often, avoid tasks that are taxing or require alertness); nausea, vomiting, constipation (consult with nurse or physician for corrective measures if this becomes a problem).
- Do not use mineral oil, antacids, or laxatives containing magnesium while on this drug.
- Arrange to have twice-weekly blood tests at first and weekly blood tests while you are on this drug to monitor your blood calcium levels.
- Report weakness, lethargy; loss of appetite, weight loss, nausea, vomiting; abdominal cramps, constipation, diarrhea; dizziness; excessive urine output, excessive thirst, dry mouth; muscle or bone pain.

☐ calcium carbonate

calcium chloride, calcium gluceptate, calcium gluconate, calcium lactate

Biocal, Calciday, Caltrate, Chooz, Dicarbosil, Equilet, Os-Cal, Oyst-Cal, Oystercal, Tums

Pregnancy Category C

Drug classes
Electrolyte
Antacid

Therapeutic actions
Essential element of the body; helps maintain the functional integrity of the nervous and muscular systems; helps maintain cardiac function, blood coagulation; is an enzyme cofactor and affects the secretory activity of endocrine and exocrine glands; neutralizes or reduces gastric acidity (oral use).

Indications
- Dietary supplement when calcium intake is inadequate
- Treatment of calcium-deficiency states that occur in tetany of the newborn, acute and chronic hypoparathyroidism, pseudohypoparathyroidism, postmenopausal and senile osteoporosis, rickets, osteomalacia
- Prevention of hypocalcemia during exchange transfusions
- Adjunctive therapy in the treatment of insect bites or stings, such as black widow spider bites; sensitivity reactions, particularly when characterized by urticaria; depression due to overdosage of magnesium sulfate; acute symptoms of lead colic
- Combats the effects of hyperkalemia as measured by ECG, pending correction of increased potassium in the extracellular fluid (calcium chloride)
- Improves weak or ineffective myocardial contractions when epinephrine fails in cardiac resuscitation, particularly after open heart surgery
- Symptomatic relief of upset stomach associated with hyperacidity; hyperacidity associated with peptic ulcer, gastritis, peptic esophagitis, gastric hyperacidity, hiatal hernia (calcium carbonate)
- Prophylaxis of GI bleeding, stress ulcers, and aspiration pneumonia; possibly useful (calcium carbonate)
- **Unlabeled use:** treatment of hypertension in some patients with indices suggesting calcium "deficiency"

Contraindications/cautions
- Allergy to calcium; renal calculi; hypercalcemia; ventricular fibrillation during cardiac resuscitation and patients with the risk of existing digitalis toxicity.

Dosage
Adult
- ***RDA:*** 800 mg.
- ***Dietary supplement:*** 500 mg–2 g PO, bid–qid.

- **Antacid:** 0.5–2.0 g PO calcium carbonate as needed.
- **Calcium chloride:** For IV use only: 1 g contains 272 mg (13.6 mEq) calcium.
  - *Hypocalcemic disorders:* 500 mg–1 g at intervals of 1–3 d.
  - *Magnesium intoxication:* 500 mg promptly. Observe patient for signs of recovery before giving another dose.
  - *Hyperkalemic ECG disturbances of cardiac function:* Adjust dose according to ECG response.
  - *Cardiac resuscitation:* 500 mg–1 g IV or 200–800 mg into the ventricular cavity.
- **Calcium gluconate:** IV infusion preferred: 1 g contains 90 mg (4.5 mEq) calcium. 0.5–2.0 g as required; daily dose 1–15 g.
- **Calcium gluceptate:** IM or IV use: 1.1 g contains 90 mg (4.5 mEq) calcium; solution for injection contains 1.1 g/5 ml. 2–5 ml IM; 5–20 ml IV.

Pediatric
- **Calcium gluconate:** 500 mg/kg per day IV given in divided doses.
- **Exchange transfusions in newborns:** 0.5 ml after every 100 ml of blood exchanged.

Pharmacokinetics

Route	Onset	Peak
Oral	3–5 min	
IV	Immediate	3–5 min

Metabolism: Hepatic; $T_{1/2}$: 1–3 h
Distribution: Crosses placenta; passes into breast milk
Excretion: Feces, urine

IV facts

Preparation: Warm solutions to body temperature; use a small needle inserted into a large vein to decrease irritation.
Infusion: Infuse slowly, 0.5–2 ml/min. Stop infusion if patient complains of discomfort; resume when symptoms disappear. Repeated injections are often necessary.

Compatibilities: Avoid mixing calcium salts with carbonates, phosphates, sulfates, tartrates.

Adverse effects

- **CV:** *Slowed heart rate, tingling, "heat waves"* (rapid IV administration); *peripheral vasodilation, local burning, fall in blood pressure* (calcium chloride injection)
- **Metabolic:** Hypercalcemia (*anorexia, nausea, vomiting, constipation*, abdominal pain, dry mouth, thirst, polyuria), *rebound hyperacidity* and milk-alkali syndrome (hypercalcemia, alkalosis, renal damage with calcium carbonate used as an antacid)
- **Local:** *Local irritation*, severe necrosis, sloughing and abscess formation (IM, SC use of calcium chloride)

Clinically important drug-drug interactions

- Decreased serum levels of oral tetracyclines, salicylates, iron salts, when taken concurrently with oral calcium salts. Administer these drugs at least 1 h apart.
- Increased serum levels of quinidine and possible toxicity if taken with calcium salts • Antagonism of effects of verapamil if given concurrently with calcium.

Clinically important drug-food interactions

- Decreased absorption of oral calcium when taken concurrently with oxalic acid (found in rhubarb and spinach), phytic acid (bran and whole cereals), phosphorus (milk and dairy products).

Drug-lab test interferences

- False-negative values for serum and urinary magnesium

■ Nursing Considerations

Assessment

- **History:** Allergy to calcium; renal calculi; hypercalcemia; ventricular fibrillation during cardiac resuscitation; digitalis toxicity
- **Physical:** Injection site; P, auscultation, BP, peripheral perfusion, ECG; abdomi-

Adverse effects in *Italics* are most common; those in **Bold** are life-threatening.

nal exam, bowel sounds, mucous membranes; serum electrolytes, urinalysis

Implementation
- Administer drug hourly for first 2 wk when used in treatement of acute peptic ulcer. During healing stage, administer 1–3 h after meals and at bedtime.
- Do not administer oral drugs within 1–2 h of antacid administration.
- Have patient chew antacid tablets thoroughly before swallowing; follow with a glass of water or milk.
- Administer calcium carbonate antacid 1 and 3 h after meals and at bedtime.
- Avoid extravasation of IV injection; it is irritating to the tissues and can cause necrosis and sloughing. Using a small needle into a large vein helps decrease the problem.
- Ensure that patient remains recumbent for a short time after IV injection.
- Administer into ventricular cavity during cardiac resuscitation, not into myocardium.
- Warm calcium gluconate if crystallization has occurred.
- Monitor serum phosphorus levels periodically during long-term oral therapy.
- Monitor cardiac response closely during parenteral treatment with calcium.

Drug-specific teaching points
Parenteral Calcium
- Report any pain or discomfort at the injection site as soon as possible.

Oral Calcium
- Take drug between meals and at bedtime. Ulcer patients need to strictly follow prescribed dosage pattern. If tablets are being used, chew thoroughly before swallowing, and follow with a glass of water or milk.
- Do not take with any other oral medications. Absorption of those medications can be blocked; take other oral medications at least 1–2 h after calcium carbonate.
- Know that the following side effects may occur: constipation (appropriate measures can be taken), nausea, GI upset, loss of appetite (special dietary consultation may be necessary).
- Report loss of appetite; nausea, vomiting, abdominal pain, constipation; dry mouth, thirst, increased voiding.

▢ capreomycin sulfate

*(kap ree oh **mye**' sin)*
Capastat Sulfate

Pregnancy Category C

Drug classes
Antituberculous drug ("third line")
Antibiotic

Therapeutic actions
Polypeptide antibiotic; mechanism of action against *Mycobacterium tuberculosis* unknown.

Indications
- Treatment of pulmonary tuberculosis that is not responsive to first-line antituberculosis agents but is sensitive to capreomycin in conjunction with other antituberculosis agents

Contraindications/cautions
- Contraindicated in the presence of allergy to capreomycin; renal insufficiency; preexisting auditory impairment.
- Use caution if lactating.

Dosage
Always give in combination with other antituberculosis drugs.
Adult: 1 g daily (not to exceed 20 mg/kg/day) IM for 60–120 d, followed by 1 g IM two to three times weekly for 18–24 mo.
Pediatric: 15 mg/kg per day (maximum 1 g) has been recommended.
Geriatric or renal impaired

Creatinine Clearance (ml/min)	Dose (mg/kg) at the Following Intervals		
	24h	48h	72h
0	1.29	2.58	3.87
10	2.43	4.87	7.3
20	3.58	7.16	10.7
30	4.72	9.45	14.2
40	5.87	11.7	
50	7.01	14	
60	8.16		
80	10.4		
100	12.7		
110	13.9		

Pharmacokinetics

Route	Onset	Peak	Duration
IM	20–30 min	1–2 h	8–12 h

Metabolism: $T_{1/2}$: 4–6 h
Distribution: Crosses placenta; may pass into breast milk
Excretion: Urine

Adverse effects
- CNS: *Ototoxicity*
- GI: Hepatic dysfunction
- Hematologic: Leukocytosis, leukopenia, eosinophilia, hypokalemia
- GU: *Nephrotoxicity*
- Hypersensitivity: Urticaria, skin rashes, fever
- Local: Pain, induration at injection sites, sterile abscesses

Clinically important drug-drug interactions
- Increased nephrotoxicity and ototoxicity if used with other nephrotoxic or ototoxic drugs • Increased risk of peripheral neuromuscular blocking action if given concurrently with nondepolarizing muscle relaxants (atracurium, gallamine, metocurine iodide, pancuronium, tubocurarine, vecuronium)

■ Nursing Considerations

Assessment
- *History:* Allergy to capreomycin; renal insufficiency; auditory impairment; lactation
- *Physical:* Skin—color, lesions; body temperature; orientation, reflexes, affect, audiometric measurement, vestibular function tests; liver evaluation; liver and renal function tests, CBC, serum K^+

Implementation
- Arrange for culture and sensitivity studies before use.
- Administer this drug only when other forms of therapy have failed.
- Administer only in conjunction with other antituberculous agents to which the mycobacteria are susceptible.
- Prepare solution by dissolving in 2 ml of 0.9% Sodium Chloride Injection or Sterile Water for Injection; allow 2–3 min for dissolution. To administer 1 g, use entire vial—if less than 1 g is needed, see the manufacturer's instructions for dilution. Reconstituted solution may be stored for 48 h at room temperature or 14 d refrigerated. Solution may acquire a straw color and darken with time; this is not associated with loss of potency.
- Administer by deep IM injection into a large muscle mass.
- Arrange for audiometric testing and assessment of vestibular function, renal function tests, and serum potassium before beginning therapy and at regular intervals during therapy.

Drug-specific teaching points
- Be aware that this drug must be given by IM injection.
- Take this drug regularly; avoid missing doses. *Do not* discontinue this drug without first consulting your physician.
- Know that the following side effects may occur: dizziness, vertigo, loss of hearing (use special precautions to avoid injury; check with your nurse or physician if these become severe).
- Arrange to have regular, periodic medical checkups, including blood.
- Report skin rash, loss of hearing, decreased urine output, palpitations.

❑ captopril

(kap' toe pril)

Apo-Capto (CAN), Capoten, Novo-Captopril (CAN), Nu-Capto (CAN), Syn-Captopril (CAN)

Pregnancy Category C

Drug classes
Antihypertensive

Adverse effects in *Italics* are most common; those in **Bold** are life-threatening.

Angiotensin-converting enzyme (ACE) inhibitor

Therapeutic actions
Blocks ACE from converting angiotensin I to angiotensin II, a powerful vasoconstrictor, leading to decreased blood pressure, decreased aldosterone secretion, a small increase in serum potassium levels, and sodium and fluid loss; increased prostaglandin synthesis also may be involved in the antihypertensive action.

Indications
- Treatment of hypertension alone or in combination with thiazide-type diuretics
- Treatment of CHF in patients who do not respond adequately to conventional therapy; used with diuretics and digitalis
- **Unlabeled uses**: management of hypertensive crises; treatment of rheumatoid arthritis; diabetic nephropathy, diagnosis of anatomic renal artery stenosis, hypertension related to scleroderma renal crisis; diagnosis of primary aldosteronism, idiopathic edema; Bartter's syndrome; Raynaud's syndrome; hypertension of Takayasu's disease

Contraindications/cautions
- Allergy to captopril; impaired renal function; CHF; salt/volume depletion, lactation.

Dosage
Adult
- ***Hypertension:*** 25 mg PO bid or tid; if satisfactory response is not noted within 1–2 wk, increase dosage to 50 mg bid–tid; usual range is 25–150 mg bid–tid PO with a mild thiazide diuretic. Do not exceed 450 mg/d.
- ***Congestive heart failure:*** 6.25–12.5 mg PO tid in patients who may be salt/volume depleted. Usual initial dose is 25 mg PO tid; maintenance dose of 50–100 mg PO tid. Do not exceed 450 mg/d. Use in conjuction with diuretic and digitalis therapy.

Pediatric: Safety and efficacy not established.
Geriatric and renal impaired: Excretion is reduced in renal failure; use smaller initial dose, and titrate at smaller doses with 1- to 2-wk intervals between increases; slowly titrate to smallest effective dose. Use of a loop diuretic is preferred with renal dysfunction.

Pharmacokinetics

Route	Onset	Peak
Oral	15 min	$\frac{1}{2}$–1$\frac{1}{2}$ h

Metabolism: $T_{1/2}$: 2 h
Distribution: Crosses placenta; passes into breast milk
Excretion: Urine

Adverse effects
- **CV:** *Tachycardia*, angina pectoris, **myocardial infarction**, Raynaud's syndrome, CHF, hypotension in salt/volume depleted patients
- **GI:** *Gastric irritation, aphthous ulcers, peptic ulcers, dysgeusia,* cholestatic jaundice, hepatocellular injury, anorexia, constipation
- **Hematologic:** Neutropenia, agranulocytosis, thrombocytopenia, hemolytic anemia, **fatal pancytopenia**
- **GU:** *Proteinuria*, renal insufficiency, renal failure, polyuria, oliguria, urinary frequency
- **Dermatologic:** *Rash, pruritus,* pemphigoid-like reaction, scalded mouth sensation, exfoliative dermatitis, photosensitivity, alopecia
- **Other:** *Cough,* malaise, dry mouth, lymphadenopathy

Clinically important drug-drug interactions
- Increased risk of hypersensitivity reactions if taken concurrently with allopurinal • Decreased antihypertensive effects if taken with indomethacin

Clinically important drug-food interactions
- Decreased absorption of captopril if taken with food

Drug-lab test interferences
- False-positive test for *urine acetone*

■ Nursing Considerations
Assessment
- *History:* Allergy to captopril, impaired renal function, CHF, salt/volume depletion, pregnancy, lactation
- *Physical:* Skin—color, lesions, turgor; body temperature; P, BP, peripheral perfusion; mucous membranes, bowel sounds, liver evaluation; urinalysis, renal and liver function tests, CBC and differential

Implementation
- Administer 1 h before or 2 h after meals.
- Alert surgeon and mark patient's chart with notice that captopril is being taken; the angiotensin II formation subsequent to compensatory renin release during surgery will be blocked; hypotension may be reversed with volume expansion.
- Monitor patient closely in any situation that may lead to a fall in blood pressure secondary to reduction in fluid volume (excessive perspiration and dehydration, vomiting, diarrhea) because excessive hypotension may occur.
- Arrange for reduced dosage in patients with impaired renal function.

Drug-specific teaching points
- Take drug 1 h before or 2 h after meals; do not take with food. Do not stop taking the medication without consulting your physician.
- Know that the following side effects may occur: GI upset, loss of appetite, change in taste perception (these may be limited effects that will pass with time); mouth sores (frequent mouth care may help); skin rash; fast heart rate; dizziness, lightheadedness (this usually passes after the first few days of therapy; if it occurs, change position slowly, and limit your activities to those that do not require alertness and precision).
- Be careful in any situation that may lead to a drop in blood pressure (diarrhea, sweating, vomiting, dehydration); if lightheadedness or dizziness occurs, consult your care provider.
- Avoid OTC medications while you are on this drug, especially cough, cold, allergy medications that may contain ingredients that will interact with it.
- Report mouth sores; sore throat, fever, chills; swelling of the hands, feet; irregular heartbeat, chest pains; swelling of the face, eyes, lips, tongue, difficulty breathing.

▢ carbamazepine

*(kar ba **maz**' e peen)*

Apo-Carbamazepine (CAN), Novo-Carbamaz (CAN), Tegretol

Pregnancy Category C

Drug classes
Antiepileptic

Therapeutic actions
Mechanism of action not understood; antiepileptic activity may be related to its ability to inhibit polysynaptic responses and block post-tetanic potentiation. Drug is chemically related to the tricyclic antidepressants (TCAs).

Indications
- Refractory seizure disorders: partial seizures with complex symptoms (psychomotor, temporal lobe epilepsy), generalized tonic-clonic (grand mal) seizures, mixed seizure patterns or other partial or generalized seizures (carbamazepine should be reserved for patients who have not responded satisfactorily to other agents, whose seizures are difficult to control, or who are experiencing marked side effects, such as excessive sedation)
- Trigeminal neuralgia (tic douloureux): treatment of pain associated with true trigeminal neuralgia; also beneficial in glossopharyngeal neuralgia
- **Unlabeled uses**: neurogenic diabetes insipidus; certain psychiatric disorders, including bipolar disorders, schizoaffective illness, resistant schizophrenia, and dyscontrol syndrome associated with limbic system dysfunction; alcohol withdrawal

carbamazepine

Contraindications/cautions
- Contraindicated in the presence of hypersensitivity to carbamazepine or tricyclic antidepressants; history of bone marrow depression; concomitant use of monoamine oxidase inhibitors (MAOIs), lactation.
- Use caution with history of adverse hematologic reaction to any drug (may be at increased risk of severe hematologic toxicity); glaucoma or increased intraocular pressure; history of cardiac, hepatic, or renal damage; psychiatric patients (may activate latent psychosis).

Dosage
Individualize dosage; a low initial dosage with gradual increase is advised.

Adult
- ***Epilepsy:*** Initial dose of 200 mg PO bid on the first day; increase gradually by up to 200 mg/d in divided doses q6–8h, until the best response is obtained. Do not exceed 1200 mg/d in patients older than 15 y; in rare instances, doses up to 1600 mg/d have been used in adults. *Maintenance:* adjust to minimum effective level, usually 800–1200 mg/d.
- ***Trigeminal neuralgia:*** Initial dose of 100 mg PO bid on the first day; may increase by up to 200 mg/d, using 100-mg increments q12h as needed. Do not exceed 1200 mg/d. *Maintenance:* control of pain can usually be maintained with 400–800 mg/d (range 200–1200 mg/d). Attempt to reduce the dose to the minimum effective level or to discontinue the drug at least once every 3 mo.
- ***Combination therapy:*** When added to existing antiepileptic therapy, do so gradually while other antiepileptics are maintained or discontinued.

Pediatric
- ***Children older than 12 y:*** Use adult dosage. Do not exceed 1000 mg/d in patients 12–15 y; 1200 mg/d in patients older than 15 y.
- ***Children 6–12 y:*** Initial dose is 100 mg PO bid on the first day. Increase gradually by adding 100 mg/d at 6- to 8-h intervals until the best response is obtained. Do not exceed 1000 mg/d. Dosage also may be calculated on the basis of 20–30 mg/kg per day in divided doses tid–qid.
- ***Children younger than 6 y:*** Safety and efficacy not established.

Geriatric: Use caution; drug may cause confusion, agitation.

Pharmacokinetics

Route	Onset	Peak
Oral	Slow	4–5 h

Metabolism: Hepatic; $T_{1/2}$: 25–65 h, then 12–17 h
Distribution: Crosses placenta; passes into breast milk
Excretion: Urine and feces

Adverse effects
- CNS: *Dizziness, drowsiness, unsteadiness,* disturbance of coordination, confusion, headache, fatigue, visual hallucinations, depression with agitation, behavioral changes in children, talkativeness, speech disturbances, abnormal involuntary movements, paralysis and other symptoms of cerebral arterial insufficiency, peripheral neuritis and paresthesias, tinnitus, hyperacusis, blurred vision, transient diplopia and oculomotor disturbances, nystagmus, scattered punctate cortical lens opacities, conjunctivitis, ophthalmoplegia, fever, chills; syndrome of inappropriate antidiuretic hormone (SIADH)
- GI: *Nausea, vomiting,* gastric distress, abdominal pain, diarrhea, constipation, anorexia, dryness of mouth or pharynx, glossitis, stomatitis; abnormal liver function tests, cholestatic and hepatocellular jaundice, **fatal hepatitis, fatal massive hepatic cellular necrosis with total loss of intact liver tissue**
- CV: Congestive heart faliure, aggravation of hypertension, hypotension, syncope and collapse, edema, primary thrombophlebitis, recurrence of thrombophlebitis, aggravation of coronary artery disease,

Adverse effects in *Italics* are most common; those in **Bold** are life-threatening.

arrhythmias and AV block; **fatal cardiovascular complications**
- Respiratory: Pulmonary hypersensitivity characterized by fever, dyspnea, pneumonitis or pneumonia
- Hematologic: **Potentially fatal hematologic disorders**
- GU: Urinary frequency, acute urinary retention, oliguria with hypertension, renal failure, azotemia, impotence, proteinuria, glueyosuria, elevated BUN, microscopic deposits in urine
- Dermatologic: Pruritic and erythematous rashes, urticaria, Stevens-Johnson syndrome, photosensitivity reactions, alterations in pigmentation, exfoliative dermatitis, alopecia, diaphoresis, erythema multiforme and nodosum, purpura, aggravation of lupus erythematosus

Clinically important drug-drug interactions

- Increased serum levels and manifestations of toxicity if given with erythromycin, troleandomycin, cimetidine, danazol, isoniazid, propoxyphene, verapamil; dosage of carbamazepine may need to be reduced (reductions of about 50% are recommended when given with erythromycin) • Increased CNS toxicity when given with lithium • Increased risk of hepatotoxicity when given with isoniazid (MAOI); because of the chemical similarity of carbamazepine to the tricyclic antidepressants and because of the serious adverse interaction documented for the TCAs and MAOIs, discontinue MAOIs for a minimum of 14 d before carbamazepine administration • Decreased absorption when given with charcoal • Decreased serum levels and decreased effects of carbamazepine when taken with barbiturates • Increased metabolism but no loss of seizure control when given with phenytoin, primidone • Increased metabolism of phenytoin, valproic acid given with carbamazepine • Decreased anticoagulant effect of warfarin, oral antyicoagulants given with carbamazepine; dosage of warfarin may need to be increased during concomitant therapy but decreased if carbamazepine is withdrawn • Decreased effects of nondepolarizing muscle relaxants, haloperidol if taken concurrently • Decreased antimicrobial effects of doxycycline given with carbamazepine

■ Nursing Considerations

Assessment

- *History:* Hypersensitivity to carbamazepine or tricyclic antidepressants; history of bone marrow depression; concomitant use of MAOIs; history of adverse hematologic reaction to any drug; glaucoma or increased intraocular pressure; history of cardiac, hepatic, or renal damage; psychiatric history; lactation
- *Physical:* Body weight; body temperature; skin—color, lesions; palpation of lymph glands; orientation, affect, reflexes; ophthalmologic exam (including tonometry, funduscopy, slit lamp exam); P, BP, perfusion; auscultation; peripheral vascular exam; R, adventitious sounds; bowel sounds, normal output; oral mucous membranes; normal urinary output, voiding pattern; CBC including platelet, reticulocyte counts and serum iron; hepatic function tests, urinalysis, BUN, thyroid function tests, EEG

Implementation

- Use this drug only for classifications listed in indications. Although it may relieve the pain of trigeminal neuralgia, it is not a general analgesic. It should be used only for epileptic seizures that are refractory to other safer agents.
- Give drug with food to prevent GI upset.
- Arrange to reduce dosage, discontinue carbamazepine, or substitute other antiepileptic medication gradually. Abrupt discontinuation of all antiepileptic medication may precipitate status epilepticus.
- Arrange for frequent liver function tests; arrange to discontinue drug immediately if hepatic dysfunction occurs.
- Arrange for patient to have CBC, including platelet, reticulocyte counts, and serum iron determination, before initiating

Adverse effects in *Italics* are most common; those in **Bold** are life-threatening.

therapy; this is done weekly for the first 3 mo of therapy and monthly thereafter for at least 2–3 y. Arrange to discontinue drug if there is evidence of marrow suppression, as follows:

Erythrocytes	<4 million/mm³
Hematocrit	<32%
Hemoglobin	<11g/100 ml
Leukocytes	<4000/mm³
Platelets	<100,000/mm³
Reticulocytes	<0.3% (20,000/mm³)
Serum iron	>150 g/100 ml

- Arrange for frequent eye exams, urinalysis, and BUN determinations.
- Arrange for frequent monitoring of serum levels of carbamazepine and other antiepileptic drugs given concomitantly, especially during the first few weeks of therapy. Arrange to adjust dosage as appropriate on the basis of these data and clinical response.
- Arrange for appropriate counseling for women of childbearing age who wish to become pregnant.
- Evaluate for therapeutic serum levels (usually 4–12 μg/ml).

Drug-specific teaching points
- Take this drug with food exactly as prescribed.
- Do not discontinue this drug abruptly or change dosage, except on the advice of your physician.
- Avoid alcohol, sleep-inducing, or OTC drugs while you are on this drug; these could cause dangerous effects.
- Arrange for frequent checkups, including blood tests, to monitor your response to this drug. It is important that you keep all appointments for checkups.
- Use contraceptive techniques at all times; if you wish to become pregnant while you are taking this drug, you should consult your physician.
- Know that the following side effects may occur: drowsiness, dizziness, blurred vision (avoid driving a car or performing other tasks requiring alertness or visual acuity if this occurs); GI upset (taking the drug with food or milk and eating frequent small meals may help).
- Wear a medical alert tag at all times so that any emergency medical personnel taking care of you will know that you are an epileptic taking antiepileptic medication.
- Report bruising, unusual bleeding, abdominal pain, yellowing of the skin or eyes, pale feces, darkened urine, impotence, CNS disturbances, edema, fever, chills, sore throat, mouth ulcers, skin rash, pregnancy.

carbenicillin indanyl sodium

(kar ben i sill' in)
Geocillin, Geopen Oral (CAN)

Pregnancy Category B

Drug classes
Antibiotic
Penicillin with extended spectrum

Therapeutic actions
Bactericidal: inhibits synthesis of cell wall of sensitive organisms, causing cell death.

Indications
- UTIs caused by susceptible strains of *Escherichia coli, Proteus mirabilis, Morganella morganii, Providencia rettgeri, Proteus vulgaris, Pseudomonas, Enterobacter*, and enterococci
- Treatment of prostatitis due to susceptible strains of *E. coli, Streptococcus faecalis, P. mirabilis, Clostridium Enterobacter*

Contraindications/cautions
- Contraindicated in the presence of allergies to penicillins, cephalosporins, or other allergens.
- Use caution in the presence of renal disorders, lactation (may cause diarrhea or candidiasis in the infant).

Dosage
Adult
- ***UTIs caused by E. coli, Proteus, Enterobacter:*** 382–764 mg PO qid.
- ***UTIs caused by Pseudomonas, Enterococci:*** 764 mg qid PO.

Pediatric: Safety and efficacy not established.

Pharmacokinetics

Route	Onset	Peak
Oral	Varies	1 h

Metabolism: $T_{1/2}$: 60–70 min
Distribution: Crosses placenta; passes into breast milk
Excretion: Urine

Adverse effects

- **CNS:** Lethargy, hallucinations, seizures, decreased reflexes
- **GI:** *Glossitis, stomatitis, gastritis, sore mouth,* furry tongue, black "hairy" tongue, *nausea, vomiting, diarrhea,* abdominal pain, bloody diarrhea, enterocolitis, pseudomembranous colitis, nonspecific hepatitis
- **Hematologic:** Anemia, thrombocytopenia, leukopenia, neutropenia, prolonged bleeding time, hemorrhagic episodes at high doses
- **GU:** Nephritis: oliguria, proteinuria, hematuria, casts, azotemia, pyuria
- **Hypersensitivity reactions:** *Rash, fever, wheezing,* **anaphylaxis**
- **Other:** *Superinfections:* oral and rectal moniliasis, vaginitis

Clinically important drug-drug interactions

• Increased bleeding effects if taken in high doses with heparin, oral anticoagulants • Decreased effectiveness if taken with tetracyclines • Decreased activity of gentamicin, tobramycin, kanamycin, neomycin, amikacin, netilimicin, streptomycin if given with carbenicillin • Decreased efficacy of oral contraceptives is possible if taken with carbenicillin.

Clinically important drug-food interactions

• Decreased absorption and decreased serum levels if taken with food

■ Nursing Considerations

Assessment

- *History:* Allergies to penicillins, cephalosporins, or other allergens; renal disorders; lactation
- *Physical:* Culture infected area; skin—color, lesion; R, adventitious sounds; bowel sounds; CBC, liver and renal function tests, serum electrolytes, hematocrit, urinalysis

Implementation

- Administer on an empty stomach, 1 h before or 2 h after meals, with a full glass of water. Do not give with fruit juice or soft drinks.
- Arrange to continue treatment for 10 d.

Drug-specific teaching points

- Take drug around the clock as prescribed; take the full course of therapy, usually 10 d.
- Take the drug on an empty stomach, 1 h before or 2 h after meals, with a full glass of water.
- Be aware that this antibiotic is specific for this infection and should not be used to self-treat other infections.
- Know that the following side effects may occur: stomach upset, nausea, diarrhea, mouth sores (if these become severe, consult with nurse or physician for appropriate treatment).
- Report unusual bleeding or bruising, fever, chills, sore throat, hives, rash, severe diarrhea, difficulty breathing.

carboplatin

(kar' boe pla tin)
Paraplatin

Pregnancy Category D

Drug classes
Alkylating agent
Antineoplastic agent

Therapeutic actions

Cytotoxic: heavy metal that produces cross-links within and between strands of DNA, thus preventing cell replication; cell cycle nonspecific.

Indications

- Palliative treatment of patients with ovarian carcinoma recurrent after prior che-

Adverse effects in *Italics* are most common; those in **Bold** are life-threatening.

motherapy, including patients who have been treated with cisplatin
- **Unlabeled uses**: alone or in combination with other agents in the treatment of small-cell lung cancer, squamous cell cancer of the head and neck, endometrial cancer, relapsed or refractory acute leukemia, seminoma of testicular cancer

Contraindications/cautions
- Contraindicated with a history of severe allergic reactions to carboplatin, cisplatin, platinum compounds, mannitol; severe bone marrow depression; pregnancy, lactation.
- Use caution in renal impairment.

Dosage
Adult
- ***As a single agent:*** 360 mg/m² IV on day 1 every 4 wk. Do not repeat single doses of carboplatin until the neutrophil count is at least 2,000/mm³ and the platelet count is at least 100,000/mm³. The following adjustment of dosage can be used: platelets > 100,00 and neutrophils > 2,000—dosage 125% prior course; platelets 100,000 and neutrophils 2,000—no adjustment in dosage; platelets < 50,000 and neutophils < 500—dosage 75% of previous course. Doses > 125% are not recommended.

Pediatric: Safety and efficacy not established.

Geriatric and renal impaired: Increased risk of bone marrow depression in patients with renal impairment. Use caution.

Creatinine Clearance (ml/min)	Dose (mg/m² on day 1)
41–59	250
16–40	200
≤14	No data available

Pharmacokinetics

Route	Onset	Duration
IV	Rapid	48–96 h

Metabolism: T$_{1/2}$: 1.2–2 h, then 2.6–5.9 h

Distribution: Crosses placenta; may pass into breast milk
Excretion: Urine

IV facts
Preparation: Immediately before use, reconstitute the content of each vial with Sterile Water for Injection, 5% Dextrose in Water, or Sodium Chloride Injection. For a concentration of 10 mg/ml, combine 50-mg vial with 5 ml of diluent, 150-mg vial with 15 ml of diluent, or 450-mg vial with 45 ml of diluent. Carboplatin can be further diluted using 5% Dextrose in Water or Sodium Chloride Injection. Store unopened vials at room temperature. Protect from exposure to light. Reconstituted solution is stable for 8 h at room temperature. Discard after 8 h. Do not use needles of IV administration sets that contain aluminum; carboplatin cam precipitate and lose effectiveness when in contact with aluminum.
Infusion: Administer by slow infusion lasting >15 min.

Adverse effects
- CNS: *Peripheral neuropathies*, ototoxicity, visual disturbances, change in taste perception
- GI: *Vomiting, nausea, abdominal pain, diarrhea, constipation*
- Hematologic: **Bone marrow depression**, *decreased serum sodium, magnesium, calcium, potassium*
- GU: *Increased BUN or serum creatinine*
- Hypersensitivity: *Anaphylactic-like reaction*, rash, urticaria, erythema, pruritis, brochospasm
- Other: *Pain, alopecia, asthenia,* cancer

Clinically important drug-drug interactions
- Decreased potency of carboplatin and precipitate formation in solution if given using needles or administration sets containing aluminum

■ Nursing Considerations
Assessment
- *History:* Severe allergic reactions to carboplatin, cisplatin, platinum com-

pounds, mannitol; severe bone marrow depression; renal impairment; pregnancy, lactation
- *Physical:* Weight, skin, and hair evaluation; eighth cranial nerve evaluation; reflexes; sensation; CBC, differential; renal function tests; serum electrolytes; serum uric acid; audiogram

Implementation
- Arrange for tests to evaluate bone marrow function before beginning therapy and periodically during therapy. Do not administer next dose if bone marrow depression is marked. Consult physician for dosage.
- Maintain epinephrine, corticosteroids, and antihistamines on standby in case of anaphylatic-like reactions, which may occur with minutes of administration.
- Arrange for an antiemetic if nausea and vomiting are severe.

Drug-specific teaching points
- Be aware that this drug can only be given IV. Prepare a calendar of treatment days.
- Know that the following side effects may occur: nausea, vomiting (medication may be ordered to help; small, frequent meals also may help); numbness, tingling, loss of taste, ringing in the ears, dizziness, loss of hearing (these are all effects of the drug); rash, loss of hair (you may want to purchase a wig if hair loss occurs).
- Use birth control while on this drug. This drug may cause birth defects or miscarriages.
- Arrange to have frequent, regular medical follow-up, including blood tests to follow the effects of the drug on your body.
- Report loss of hearing, dizziness; unusual bleeding or bruising; fever, chills, sore throat; leg cramps, muscle twitching; changes in voiding patterns; difficulty breathing.

❏ carboprost tromethamine

(kar' boe prost)
Hemabate

Pregnancy Category C

carboprost tromethamine ■ 215

Drug classes
Prostaglandin
Abortifacient

Therapeutic actions
Stimulates the myometrium of the gravid uterus to contract in a manner that is similar to the contractions of the uterus during labor, thus evacuating the contents of the gravid uterus.

Indications
- Termination of pregnancy 13–20 wk from the first day of the last menstrual period
- Evacuation of the uterus in the management of missed abortion or intrauterine fetal death in the second trimester
- Postpartum hemmorhage due to uterine atony, which has not responded to conventional methods

Contraindications/cautions
- Contraindicated in the presence of allergy to prostaglandin preparations; acute pelvic inflammatory disease; active cardiac, hepatic, pulmonary, renal disease.
- Use caution with history of asthma; hypotension; hypertension; cardiovascular, adrenal, renal, or hepatic disease; anemia; jaundice; diabetes; epilepsy; scarred uterus; cervicitis, infected endocervical lesions; acute vaginitis.

Dosage
Adult
- ***Abortion:*** 250 μg (1 ml) IM; give 250 μg IM at 1½- to 3½-h intervals, depending on uterine response; may be increased to 500 μg if uterine contractility is inadequate after several 250-μg doses; do not exceed 12 mg total dose or continuous administration over 2 d.
- ***Refractory postpartum uterine bleeding:*** 250 μg IM as one dose; in some cases, multiple doses at 15- to 90-min intervals may be used; do not exceed a total dose of 2 mg (8 doses)

Pharmacokinetics

Route	Onset	Peak
IM	15 min	2 h

Metabolism: Hepatic and lung; $T_{1/2}$: 8 h

216 ■ carisoprodol

Distribution: Crosses placenta; passes into breast milk
Excretion: Urine

Adverse effects
- **CNS:** Headache, paresthesias, *flushing,* anxiety, weakness, syncope, dizziness
- **GI:** Vomiting, diarrhea, *nausea*
- **CV:** *Hypotension*, arrhythmias, chest pain
- **Respiratory:** Coughing, dyspnea
- **GU:** Endometritis, perforated uterus, uterine rupture, uterine/vaginal pain, incomplete abortion
- **Other:** Chills, diaphoresis, backache, breast tenderness, eye pain, skin rash, pyrexia

■ Nursing Considerations

Assessment
- *History:* Allergy to prostaglandin preparations; acute pelvic inflammatory disease; active cardiac, hepatic, pulmonary, renal disease; history of asthma; hypotension; hypertension; anemia; jaundice; diabetes; epilepsy; scarred uterus; cervicitis, infected endocervical lesions; acute vaginitis
- *Physical:* Body temperature; BP, P, auscultation; R, adventitious sounds; bowel sounds, liver evaluation; vaginal discharge, pelvic exam, uterine tone; liver and renal function tests, WBC, urinalysis, CBC

Implementation
- Refrigerate unopened vials. Stable at room temperature for 9 d.
- Administer a test dose of 100 μg (0.4 ml) prior to abortion if indicated.
- Administer by deep IM injection.
- Arrange for pretreatment or concurrent treatment with antiemetic and antidiarrheal drugs to decrease the incidence of GI side effects.
- Ensure that abortion is complete or that other measures are used to complete the abortion if drug effects are not sufficient.
- Monitor body temperature, using care to differentiate prostaglandin-induced pyrexia from postabortion endometritis pyrexia.
- Monitor uterine tone and vaginal discharge throughout procedure and several days after the procedure to assess drug effects and recovery.
- Ensure adequate hydration throughout procedure.

Drug-specific teaching points
- Be aware that several IM injections may be required to achieve desired effect.
- Know that the following side effects may occur: nausea, vomiting, diarrhea, uterine/vaginal pain, fever, headache, weakness, dizziness.
- Report severe pain, difficulty breathing, palpitations, eye pain, rash.

☐ carisoprodol

*(kar eye soe **proe'** dol)*
isomeprobamate
Soma

Pregnancy Category C

Drug classes
Centrally acting skeletal muscle relaxant

Therapeutic actions
Precise mechanism of action not known; chemically related to meprobamate, an antianxiety drug; has sedative properties; also found in animal studies to inhibit interneuronal activity in descending reticular formation and spinal cord; does not directly relax tense skeletal muscles.

Indications
- Relief of discomfort associated with acute, painful musculoskeletal conditions as an adjunct to rest, physical therapy, and other measures

Contraindications/cautions
- Allergic or idiosyncratic reactions to carisoprodol, meprobamate (cross-reactions with meprobamate have been reported); acute intermittent porphyria, suspected porphyria, lactation.

Adverse effects in *Italics* are most common; those in **Bold** are life-threatening.

Dosage

Adult: 350 mg PO tid–qid; take the last dose at bedtime.
Pediatric: Not recommended for children younger than 12 y.
Geriatric patients or those with hepatic or renal impairment: Dosage reduction may be necessary; monitor closely.

Pharmacokinetics

Route	Onset	Peak	Duration
Oral	30 min	1–2 h	4–6 h

Metabolism: Hepatic; $T_{1/2}$: 8 h
Distribution: Crosses placenta; passes into breast milk
Excretion: Urine

Adverse effects

- **CNS:** *Dizziness, drowsiness, vertigo, ataxia, tremor, agitation, irritability*
- **GI:** Nausea, vomiting, hiccups, epigastric distress
- **CV:** Tachycardia, postural hypotension, facial flushing
- Hypersensitivity: **Allergic or idiosyncratic reactions** (usually seen with first to fourth dose in patients without previous contact with drug): skin rash, erythema multiforme, pruritus, eosinophila, fixed drug eruption; asthmatic episodes, fever, weakness, dizziness, angioneurotic edema, smarting eyes, hypotension, anaphylactoid shock

■ Nursing Considerations

Assessment

- *History:* Allergic or idiosyncratic reactions to carisoprodol, meprobamate; acute intermittent porphyria, suspected porphyria; lactation
- *Physical:* Body temperature; Skin—color, lesions; orientation, affect; P, BP, orthostatic BP; bowel sounds, liver evaluation; liver and kidney function tests, CBC

Implementation

- Arrange to reduce dosage in patients with liver dysfunction.

Drug-specific teaching points

- Take this drug exactly as prescribed; do not take a higher dosage than that prescribed for you.
- Avoid alcohol, sleep-inducing, or OTC drugs while on this drug; these could cause dangerous effects; if you feel you need one of these preparations, consult your nurse or physician.
- Know that the following side effects may occur: drowsiness, dizziness, vertigo (avoid driving a car or engaging in activities that require alertness if these occur); dizziness when you get up or climb stairs (avoid sudden changes in position, and use caution when climbing stairs); nausea (taking drug with food and eating frequent small meals may help); insomnia, headache, depression (it may help to know that these are effects of the drug that will go away when the drug is discontinued; consult your nurse or physician if these are bothersome or persistent).
- Report skin rash, severe nausea, dizziness, insomnia, fever, difficulty breathing.

❑ carmustine

*(car **mus'** teen)*
BCNU, Bicnu

Pregnancy Category D

Drug classes

Alkylating agent, nitrosourea
Antineoplastic drug

Therapeutic actions

Cytotoxic: alkylates DNA and RNA and inhibits several enzymatic processes, leading to cell death.

Indications

Palliative therapy alone or in combination with other agents for the following:

- Brain tumors: glioblastomas, brainstem glioma, medullablastoma, astrocytoma, ependymoma, metastatic brain tumors

Adverse effects in *Italics* are most common; those in **Bold** are life-threatening.

218 ■ carmustine

- Hodgkin's disease and non-Hodgkin's lymphomas (as secondary therapy)
- Multiple myeloma (in combination with prednisolone)

Contraindications/cautions
- Allergy to carmustine; radiation therapy; chemotherapy; hematopoietic depression; impaired renal or hepatic function; pregnancy (teratogenic, and embryotoxic in preclinical studies); lactation.

Dosage
Do not give repeat doses more frequently than every 6 wk because of delayed bone marrow toxicity.

Adult and pediatric: As single agent in untreated patients: 150–200 mg/m^2 IV every 6 wk as a single dose or in divided daily injections (75–100 mg/m^2 on 2 successive d). Do not give a repeat dose until platelets > 100,000/mm^3, leukocytes > 4,000/mm^3, adjust dosage after initial dose based on hematologic response, as follows:

Leukocytes	Platelets	Percentage of Prior Dose to Give
>4,000	>100,000	100%
3,000–3,999	75,000–99,999	100%
2,000–2,999	25,000–74,999	70%
<2,000	<25,000	50%

Pharmacokinetics

Route	Onset	Peak
IV	Immediate	15 min

Metabolism: Hepatic; T$_{1/2}$: 15–30 min
Distribution: Crosses placenta; passes into breast milk
Excretion: Urine and lungs (10%)

IV facts
Preparation: Reconstitute with 3 ml of the supplied sterile diluent, then add 27 ml of Sterile Water for Injection to the alcohol solution; resulting solution contains 3.3 mg/ml of carmustine in 10% ethanol, pH is 5.6–6.0; may be further diluted with Sodium Chloride Injection or 5% Dextrose Injection. Refrigerate unopened vials. Protect reconstituted solution from light; no preservatives are added, and the solution decomposes with time. Check vials before use to ensure that no oil film residue is present; if so, discard the vial.

Infusion: Administer reconstituted solution by IV drip over 1–2 h; shorter infusion time may cause intense pain and burning.

Adverse effects
- CNS: Ocular toxicity: nerve fiber-layer infarcts, retinal hemorrhage
- GI: *Nausea, vomiting, stomatitis,* hepatotoxicity
- Respiratory: *Pulmonary infiltrates,* fibrosis
- Hematologic: *Myelosuppression, leukopenia, thrombocytopenia, anemia;* delayed for 4–6 wk
- GU: Renal toxicity: decreased renal size, azotemia, renal failure
- Other: *Local burning at site of injection;* intense flushing of the skin, suffusion of the conjunctiva with rapid IV infusion; cancer

Clinically important drug-drug interactions
- Increased toxicity and myelosuppression if taken concurrently with cimetidine • Decreased serum levels of digoxin, phenytoin if taken concurrently with carmustine

■ Nursing Considerations
Assessment
- *History:* Allergy to carmustine; radiation therapy; chemotherapy; hematopoietic depression; impaired renal or hepatic function; pregnancy; lactation
- *Physical:* Temperature; weight; ophthalmologic exam; R, adventitious sounds; mucous membranes, liver evaluation; CBC, differential; urinalysis, liver and renal function tests; pulmonary function tests

Implementation
- Arrange for blood tests to evaluate hematopoietic function before beginning ther-

Adverse effects in *Italics* are most common; those in **Bold** are life-threatening.

apy and weekly during and for at least 6 wk after therapy.
- Do not give full dosage within 2–3 wk after a full course of radiation therapy or chemotherapy because of the risk of severe bone marrow depression; reduced dosage may be needed.
- Arrange for reduced dosage in patients with depressed bone marrow function.
- Arrange for pretherapy medicating with antiemetic to decrease the severity of nausea and vomiting.
- Monitor injection site for any adverse reaction; accidental contact of carmustine with the skin can cause burning and hyperpigmentation of the area.
- Arrange for monitoring of ophthalmologic status during therapy.
- Monitor urine output for volume and any sign of renal failure.
- Arrange for monitoring of liver, renal, and pulmonary function tests during course of therapy.

Drug-specific teaching points

- Be aware that this drug can only be given IV.
- Know that the following side effects may occur: nausea, vomiting, loss of appetite (an antiemetic may be ordered for you; small frequent meals also may help); increased susceptibility to infection (avoid exposure to infection by avoiding crowded places, and take precautions to avoid injury).
- Try to maintain your fluid intake and nutrition while on this drug.
- Use birth control methods while on this drug; this drug can cause severe birth defects.
- Report unusual bleeding or bruising; fever, chills, sore throat; stomach or flank pain; changes in vision; difficulty breathing, shortness of breath; burning or pain at IV injection site.

▢ carteolol hydrochloride

(*kar' tee oh lole*)
Cartrol

Pregnancy Category C

Drug classes
Beta-adrenergic blocking agent
Antihypertensive drug

Therapeutic actions
Blocks beta-adrenergic receptors of the sympathetic nervous system in the heart and juxtaglomerular apparatus (kidney), thus decreasing the excitability of the heart, decreasing cardiac output and oxygen consumption, decreasing the release of renin from the kidney, and lowering blood pressure.

Indications
- Management of hypertension, used alone as a Step 1 agent, or in combination with other drugs, particularly a thiazide diuretic.
- **Unlabeled use**: prophylaxis for angina attacks

Contraindications/cautions
- Contraindicated in the presence of sinus bradycardia (HR < 45 beats per minute), second- or third-degree heart block (PR interval > 0.24 sec), cardiogenic shock, CHF, asthma, COPD, lactation.
- Use with caution in the presence of diabetes or thyrotoxicosis, hepatic impairment, renal failure.

Dosage
Adult: Initially 2.5 mg as a single daily oral dose, either alone or with a diuretic. If adequate response is not seen, gradually increase to 5–10 mg as a single daily dose. Doses > 10 mg are not likely to produce further benefit and may actually decrease response. *Maintenance:* 2.5–5 mg PO qd.
Pediatric: Safety and efficacy not established.
Geriatric or impaired renal function: Because bioavailability increases twofold, lower doses may be required. Creatinine clearance of > 60 ml/min, administer q24h; creatinine clearance of 20–60 ml/min, administer q48h; creatinine clearance of < 30 ml/min, administer q72h.

Pharmacokinetics

Route	Onset	Peak	Duration
Oral	Varies	1–3 h	24–48 h

Metabolism: Hepatic; $T_{1/2}$: 6 h
Distribution: Crosses placenta; passes into breast milk
Excretion: Urine

Adverse effects

- CNS: Dizziness, vertigo, tinnitus, fatigue, emotional depression, paresthesias, sleep disturbances, hallucinations, disorientation, memory loss, slurred speech (carteolol is less lipid-soluble than propranolol; it is less likely to penetrate the blood–brain barrier and cause CNS effects)
- GI: *Gastric pain, flatulence, constipation, diarrhea, nausea, vomiting,* anorexia,
- CV: *Bradycardia, CHF, cardiac arrhythmias, sinoartial or AV nodal block, tachycardia,* peripheral vascular insufficiency, claudication, CVA, pulmonary edema, hypotension
- Respiratory: **Bronchospasm,** dyspnea, cough, bronchial obstruction, nasal stuffiness, rhinitis
- GU: *Impotence, decreased libido,* Peyronie's disease, dysuria, nocturia, frequent urination
- MS: Joint pain, arthralgia, muscle cramp
- EENT: Eye irritation, dry eyes, conjunctivitis, blurred vision
- Dermatologic: Rash, pruritus, sweating, dry skin
- Allergic: Pharyngitis, erythematous rash, fever, sore throat, **laryngospasm, respiratory distress**
- Other: *Decreased exercise tolerance, development of antinuclear antibodies,* hyperglycemia or hypoglycemia, elevated serum transaminase

Clinically important drug-drug interactions

- Increased effects of carteolol if taken with verapamil • Decreased effects of theophyllines and carteolol if taken concurrently • Increased risk of postural hypotension if taken concurrently with prazosin • Possible increased blood pressure-lowering effects if taken concurrently with aspirin, bismuth subsalicylate, magnesium salicylate, sulfinpyrazone • Decreased antihypertensive effects if taken with NSAIDs, clonidine • Possible increased hypoglycemic effect of insulin if taken with carteolol • Initial hypertensive episode followed by bradycardia if combined with epinephrine • Peripheral ischemia and possible gangrene if combined with ergot alkaloids

Drug-lab test interferences

- Monitor for possible false results with glucose or insulin tolerance tests.

■ Nursing Considerations

Assessment

- *History:* Arrhythmias, cardiogenic shock, CHF, asthma, COPD, pregnancy, lactation, diabetes or thyrotoxicosis
- *Physical:* Body weight, skin condition, neurologic status, P, BP, ECG, respiratory status, kidney and thyroid function, blood and urine glucose

Implementation

- Administer carteolol once a day. Monitor response and maintain at lowest possible dose.
- Do not discontinue drug abruptly after chronic therapy (hypersensitivity to catecholamines may have developed, causing exacerbation of angina, MI, and ventricular dysrhythmias; taper drug gradually over 2 wk with monitoring).
- Consult with physician about withdrawing drug if patient is to undergo surgery (withdrawal is controversial).

Drug-specific teaching points

- Take drug with meals.
- Do not stop taking this drug unless instructed to do so by a health care provider.
- Avoid driving or dangerous activities if dizziness, weakness occur.
- Know that the following side effects may occur: dizziness, lightheadedness, loss of appetite, nightmares, depression, sexual impotence.
- Report difficulty breathing, night cough, swelling of extremities, slow pulse, confusion, depression, rash, fever, sore throat

Adverse effects in *Italics* are most common; those in **Bold** are life-threatening.

cefaclor

(sef' a klor)
Ceclor

Pregnancy Category B

Drug classes
Antibiotic
Cephalosporin (first generation)

Therapeutic actions
Bactericidal: inhibits synthesis of bacterial cell wall, causing cell death.

Indications
- Lower respiratory tract infections caused by *Streptococcus pneumoniae, Haemophilus influenzae, S. pyogenes*
- Upper respiratory infections caused by *S. pyogenes*
- Dermatologic infections caused by *Staphylococcus aureus, S. pyogenes*
- UTIs caused by *E. coli, P. mirabilis, Klebsiella*, coagulase-negative staphylococci
- Otitis media caused by *S. pneumoniae, H. influenzae, S. pyogenes,* staphylococci
- **Unlabeled use**: acute uncomplicated UTI in select patients, single 2-g dose

Contraindications/cautions
- Allergy to cephalosporins or penicillins; renal failure; lactation

Dosage
Adult: 250 mg PO q8h; dosage may be doubled in severe cases. **Do not exceed 4 g/d.**
Pediatric: 20 mg/kg per day PO in divided doses q8h; in severe cases 40 mg/kg per day may be given. **Do not exceed 1 mg/d.**
- *Otitis media and pharyngitis:* Total daily dosage may be divided and administered q12h.

Pharmacokinetics

Route	Peak	Duration
PO	30–60 min	8–10 h

Metabolism: $T_{1/2}$: 30–60 min
Distribution: Crosses the placenta; enters breast milk
Excretion: Renal, unchanged

Adverse effects
- **CNS:** Headache, dizziness, lethargy, paresthesias
- **GI:** *Nausea, vomiting, diarrhea, anorexia, abdominal pain, flatulence, pseudomembranous colitis,* liver toxicity
- **Hematologic:** Bone marrow depression
- **GU:** Nephrotoxicity
- **Hypersensitivity:** *Ranging from rash, fever* to *anaphylaxis*; serum sickness reaction
- **Other:** *Superinfections*

Clinically important drug-drug interactions
- Increased nephrotoxicity with aminoglycosides • Increased bleeding effects if taken with oral anticoagulants • Disulfiram-like reaction may occur if alcohol is taken within 72 h after cefaclor administration.

Drug-lab test interferences
- Possibility of false results on tests of urine glucose using Benedict's solution, Fehling's solution, Clinitest tablets; urinary 17-ketosteroids; direct Coombs' test.

■ Nursing Considerations

Assessment
- *History:* Penicillin or cephalosporin allergy, pregnancy or lactation
- *Physical:* Kidney function, respiratory status, skin status, culture and sensitivity tests of infected area

Implementation
- Culture infected area before beginning drug therapy.
- Give drug with meals or food to decrease GI discomfort.
- Refrigerate suspension after reconstitution, and discard after 14 d.
- Discontinue drug if hypersensitivy reaction occurs.
- Give patient yogurt or buttermilk in case of diarrhea.

Adverse effects in *Italics* are most common; those in **Bold** are life-threatening.

- Arrange for oral vancomycin for serious colitis that fails to respond to discontinuation of drug.

Drug-specific teaching points
- Take this drug with meals or food.
- Complete the full course of this drug, even if you feel better before the course of treatment is over.
- Be aware that this drug is prescribed for this particular infection; do not self-treat any other infection with this drug.
- Know that the following side effects may occur: stomach upset, loss of appetite, nausea (taking the drug with food may help); diarrhea (stay near bathroom facilities); headache, dizziness.
- Report severe diarrhea with blood, pus, or mucus; rash or hives; difficulty breathing; unusual tiredness, fatigue; unusual bleeding or bruising.

cefadroxil

*(sef a **drox'** ill)*
Duricef, Ultracef

Pregnancy Category B

Drug classes
Antibiotic
Cephalosporin (first generation)

Therapeutic actions
Bacteridical: inhibits the formation of bacterial cell wall, causing the cell's death.

Indications
- UTIs caused by *E. coli, P. mirabilis, Klebsiella*
- Pharyngitis, tonsillitis caused by group A β-hemolytic streptococci
- Dermatologic infections caused by staphylococci, streptococci

Contraindications/cautions
- Allergy to cephalosporins or penicillins, renal failure, lactation

Dosage
Adult
- ***UTIs:*** 1–2 g/d PO in single or two divided doses for uncomplicated lower UTIs. For all other UTIs, 2 g/d in two divided doses.
- ***Dermatologic infections:*** 1 g/d PO in single or two divided doses.
- ***Pharyngitis, tonsillitis caused by group A β-hemolytic streptococci:*** 1 g/d PO in single or two divided doses for 10 d.

Pediatric
- ***UTIs, dematologic infections:*** 30 mg/kg per day PO in divided doses q12h.
- ***Pharyngitis, tonsillitis caused by group A β-hemolytic streptococci:*** 30 mg/kg per day in single or two divided doses, continue for 10 d.

Geriatric or impaired renal function: 1 g PO loading dose, followed by 500 mg PO at the following intervals:

Creatinine Clearance (ml/min)	Interval (hours)
0–10	36
10–25	24
25–50	12
>50	Usual adult dosage

Pharmacokinetics

Route	Peak	Duration
PO	1.5–2 h	20–22 h

Metabolism: $T_{1/2}$: 78–96 min
Distribution: Crosses the placenta; enters breast milk
Excretion: Renal

Adverse effects
- CNS: Headache, dizziness, lethargy, paresthesias
- GI: *Nausea, vomiting, diarrhea, anorexia, abdominal pain, flatulence,* **pseudomembranous colitis**, liver toxicity
- Hematologic: Bone marrow depression
- GU: Nephrotoxicity

Adverse effects in *Italics* are most common; those in **Bold** are life-threatening.

- **Hypersensitivity:** *Ranging from rash to fever to* **anaphylaxis**; serum sickness reaction
- **Other:** *Superinfections*

Clinically important drug-drug interactions
- Decreased bactericidal activity if used with bacteriostatic agents • Increased serum levels of cephalosporins if used with probenecid

Drug-lab test interferences
- False-positive urine glucose using Benedict's solution, Fehling's solution, Clinitest tablets • False-positive direct Coombs' test • Falsely elevated urinary 17-ketosteroids

Nursing Considerations

Assessment
- *History:* Penicillin or cephalosporin allergy, pregnancy or lactation
- *Physical:* Kidney function, respiratory status, skin status, culture and sensitivity tests of infected area

Implementation
- Culture infected area before beginning drug therapy.
- Give drug with meals or food to decrease GI discomfort.
- Refrigerate suspension after reconstitution, and discard after 14 d; shake refrigerated suspension well before using.
- Discontinue drug if hypersensitivy reaction occurs.
- Give the patient yogurt or buttermilk in case of diarrhea.
- Arrange for oral vancomycin for serious colitis that fails to respond to discontinuation of drug.

Drug-specific teaching points
- Take this drug only for this specific infection, and do not use to self-treat other problems.
- Refrigerate the suspension, and discard unused portion after 14 d; shake suspension well before each use.
- Know that the following side effects may occur: stomach upset, loss of appetite, nausea (taking the drug with food may help), diarrhea (stay near bathroom facilities), headache, dizziness.
- Report severe diarrhea with blood, pus, or mucus; skin rash; difficulty breathing; unusual tiredness, fatigue; unusual bleeding or bruising.

❏ cefamandole nafate

*(sef a **man'** dole)*
Mandole

Pregnancy Category B

Drug classes
Antibiotic
Cephalosporin (second generation)

Therapeutic actions
Bactericidal: inhibits synthesis of bacterial cell wall and causes cell death.

Indications
- Lower respiratory tract infections caused by *S. pneumoniae, S. aureus,* group A β-hemolytic streptococci, *Klebsiella, H. influenzae, P. mirabilis*
- Dermatologic infections caused by *S. aureus, S. pyogenes, E. coli, P. mirabilis, H. influenzae, Enterobacter* species
- UTIs caused by *E. coli, Proteus* species, *Klebsiella, Enterobacter* species, *S. epidermidis,* group D streptococci
- Septicemia caused by *S. pneumoniae, S. aureus,* group A β-hemolytic streptocci, *E. coli, H. infuenzae*
- Peritonitis caused by *E. coli, Enterobacter* species
- Bone and joint infections caused by *S. aureus*
- Mixed infections with many organisms isolated
- Perioperative prophylaxis

Contraindications/cautions
- Allergy to cephalosporins or penicillins, renal failure, pregnancy, lactation.

Dosage
Adult: 500 mg–1 g IM or IV q4–8h, depending on severity of infection.
- *Acute UTI:* 500 mg q8h to 1 g q8h.

Adverse effects in *Italics* are most common; those in **Bold** are life-threatening.

- **Severe infections:** 1 g q4–6h, up to 2 g q4h.
- **Perioperative prophylaxis:** 1–2 g IM or IV ½–1 h prior to initial incision; 1–2 g q6h for 24 h after surgery.
- **Prosthetic arthroplasty:** Continue above doses for 72 h.
- **Cesarean section:** Administer first dose just prior to clamping or after cord is clamped.

Pediatric: 50–100 mg/kg per day IM or IV in equally divided doses q4–8h. Up to 150 mg/kg per day in severe infections.
- **Perioperative prophylaxis:** 50–100 mg/kg per day in equally divided doses, starting ½–1 h before initial incision and continuing for 24 h after surgery.

Geriatric (or impaired renal function): IM loading dose of 1–2 g. Maintenance dosages are as follows:

Creatinine Clearance (ml/min)	Severe Infection	Less Severe Infection
>80	2 g q4h	1.2 g q6h
50–80	1.4 g q4h or 2 g q6h	0.75–1.5 g q6h
25–50	1.5 g q6h or 2 g q8h	0.75–1.5 g q8h
10–25	1 g q6h or 1.25 g q8h	0.5–1 g q8h
2–10	0.67 g q8h or 1 g q12h	0.5–0.75 g q12h
<2	0.5 g q8h or 0.75 g q12h	0.25–0.5 g q12h

Pharmacokinetics

Route	Peak	Duration
IM	30–120 min	6–8 h
IV	10 min	6–8 h

Metabolism: $T_{1/2}$: 30–60 min
Distribution: Crosses the placenta; enters breast milk
Excretion: Renal

IV facts

Preparation: Dilute each gram of drug with 10 ml of Sterile Water for Injection, 5% Dextrose Injection, or 0.9% Sodium Chloride Injection, or add drug to IV solutions of 5% Dextrose Injection; 5% or 10% Dextrose and 0.2%, 0.45%, or 0.9% Sodium Chloride Injection; or Sodium Lactate Injection (M/6). To give by continuous IV infusion, dilute each gram with 10 ml Sterile Water for Injection; may be added to IV container of any of the above solutions. Stable for 96 h if refrigerated, 24 h at room temperature.

Infusion: By intermittent IV injections, inject slowly over 3–5 min. If using a piggy-back IV setup, discontinue the other solution while cefamandole is being given. If given as part of combination therapy with aminoglycosides, give each antibiotic at a different site.

Incompatibilities: Do not mix aminoglycosides and cefamandole in the same IV solution.

Adverse effects

- CNS: Headache, dizziness, lethargy, paresthesias
- GI: *Nausea, vomiting, diarrhea, anorexia, abdominal pain, flatulence,* **pseudomembranous colitis**, liver toxicity
- Hematologic: Bone marrow depression
- GU: Nephrotoxicity
- Hypersensitivity: *Ranging from rash* to *fever* to **anaphylaxis;** serum sickness reaction
- Other: *Superinfections, pain,* abscess (redness, tenderness, heat, tissue sloughing), inflammation at injection site, *phlebitis, disulfiram-like reaction with alcohol*

Clinically important drug-drug interactions

- Increased nephrotoxicity with aminoglycosides • Increased bleeding effects if taken with oral anticoagulants • Disulfiram-like reaction may occur if alcohol is taken within 72 h after cefamandole administration.

Adverse effects in *Italics* are most common; those in **Bold** are life-threatening.

Drug-lab test interferences

- False results of urine glucose using Benedict's solution, Fehling's solution, Clinitest tablets; urinary 17-ketosteroids; direct Coombs' test.

■ Nursing Considerations

Assessment
- *History:* Penicillin or cephalosporin allergy, pregnancy or lactation
- *Physical:* Kidney function, respiratory status, skin status, culture and sensitivity tests of infected area, injection site

Implementation
- Culture infected area, and arrange for sensitivity tests before beginning drug therapy.
- Dilute each gram with 3 ml Sterile Water for Injection, Bacteriostatic Water for Injection, 0.9% Sodium Chloride Injection, or Bacteriostatic Sodium Chloride Injection for IM use. Shake well until dissolved.
- Reconstituted solution is stable for 24 h at room temperature or 4 d if refrigerated.
- Discontinue drug if hypersensitivy reaction occurs.
- Have vitamin K available in case hypoprothrombinemia occurs.

Drug-specific teaching points
- Do not use alcoholic beverages while on this drug and for 3 d after this drug has been stopped, because severe reactions often occur.
- Know that the following side effects may occur: stomach upset, loss of appetite, nausea (taking the drug with food may help); diarrhea (stay near bathroom facilities); headache, dizziness.
- Report severe diarrhea, difficulty breathing, unusual tiredness or fatigue, pain at injection site.

❏ cefazolin sodium

(sef a' zoe lin)
Ancef (CAN), Gen-Cefazolin (CAN), Kefzol, Zolicef

Pregnancy Category B

Drug classes
Antibiotic
Cephalosporin (first generation)

Therapeutic actions
Bactericidal: inhibits synthesis of bacterial cell wall and causes cell death.

Indications
- Respiratory tract infections caused by *S. pneumoniae, S. aureus,* group A β-hemolytic streptococci, *Klebsiella, H. influenzae*
- Dermatologic infections caused by *S. aureus,* group A β-hemolytic streptococci, other strains of streptococci
- GU infections caused by *E. coli, P. mirabilis, Klebsiella,* sensitive strains of *Enterobacter,* and enterococci
- Biliary tract infections caused by *E. coli,* streptococci, *P. mirabilis, Klebsiella, S. aureus*
- Septicemia caused by *S. pneumoniae, S. aureus, E. coli, P. mirabilis, Klebsiella*
- Bone and joint infections caused by *S. aureus*
- Endocarditis caused by *S. aureus,* group A β-hemolytic streptococci
- Perioperative prophylaxis

Contraindications/cautions
- Allergy to cephalosporins or penicillins, renal failure, lactation

Dosage
Adult: 250–500 mg IM or IV q4–8h.
- ***Moderate to severe infection:*** 500 mg–1 g IM or IV q6–8h.
- ***Life-threatening infections:*** 1–1.5 g IM or IV q6h.
- ***Acute UTI:*** 1 g IM or IV q12h.
- ***Perioperative prophylaxis:*** 1 g IV ½–1 h prior to initial incision; 0.5–1 g IV or IM during surgery at appropriate intervals; 0.5–1 g IV or IM q6–8h for 24 h after surgery. Prophylactic treatment may be continued for 3–5 d.

Pediatric
- ***Mild infections:*** 25–50 mg/kg per day IM or IV in three to four equally divided doses.
- ***Severe infections:*** Increase total daily dose to 100 mg/kg. Adjust dosage

cefazolin sodium

for impaired renal function (see package insert for details).

Premature infants and infants younger than 1 mo: Safety and efficacy not established.

- *Perioperative prophylaxis:* Dosage adjustment is made according to body weight or age (see Appendix III for formulas).

Geriatric or impaired renal function: IV or IM loading dose of 500 mg; maximum maintenance dosages are as follows:

CCr (ml/min)	Mild to Moderate Infection	Severe Infection
≥55	250–500 mg q6–8h	500–1,000 mg q6–8h
35–54	250–500 mg q8h	500–1,000 mg q12
11–34	125–250 mg q12h	250–500 mg q12h
≤10	125–250 mg q18–24h	250–800 mg q18–24h

Pharmacokinetics

Route	Onset	Peak	Duration
IM	30 min	1.5–2 h	6–8 h
IV	Immediate	5 min	6–8 h

Metabolism: T$_{1/2}$: 90–120 min
Distribution: Crosses the placenta; enters breast milk
Excretion: Renal, unchanged

IV facts

Preparation: Use a volume control set or separate piggy-back container. Dilute reconstituted 500 mg–1 g of cefazolin in 50–100 ml of 0.9% Sodium Chloride Injection; 5% or 10% Dextrose Injection; 5% Dextrose in Lactated Ringer's Injection; 5% Dextrose and 0.2%, 0.45%, or 0.9% Sodium Chloride Injection; Lactated Ringer's Injection; 5% or 10% Invert Sugar in Sterile Water for Injection; 5% Sodium Bicarbonate in Sterile Water for Injection; Ringer's Injection; Normosol-M in D5-W; Ionosol B with Dextrose 5%; Plasma-Lyte with 5% Dextrose. For direct IV injection as follows: dilute reconstituted 500 mg–1 g cefazolin with at least 10 ml of Sterile Water for Injection. Shake well until dissolved. Stable for 24 h at room temperature.

Infusion: By direct IV injection, inject slowly over 3–5 min.

Incompatibilities: If given as part of combination therapy with aminoglycosides, give each antibiotic at a different site. **Do not mix aminoglycosides and cefazolin in the same IV solution.**

Adverse effects

- CNS: Headache, dizziness, lethargy, paresthesias
- GI: *Nausea, vomiting, diarrhea, anorexia, abdominal pain, flatulence,* **pseudomembranous colitis,** liver toxicity
- Hematologic: Bone marrow depression
- GU: Nephrotoxicity
- Hypersensitivity: *Ranging from rash* to *fever* to **anaphylaxis;** serum sickness reaction
- Other: *Superinfections, pain,* abscess (redness, tenderness, heat, tissue sloughing), inflammation at injection site, *phlebitis, disulfiram-like reaction with alcohol*

Clinically important drug-drug interactions

- Increased nephrotoxicity with aminoglycosides • Increased bleeding effects if taken with oral anticoagulants • Disulfiram-like reaction may occur if alcohol is taken within 72 h after cefazolin administration.

Drug-lab test interferences

- False results of urine glucose using Benedict's solution, Fehling's solution, Clinitest tablets; urinary 17-ketosteroids; direct Coombs' test.

■ Nursing Considerations

Assessment

- *History:* Penicillin or cephalosporin allergy, pregnancy or lactation

Adverse effects in *Italics* are most common; those in **Bold** are life-threatening.

- *Physical:* Kidney function, respiratory status, skin status; culture and sensitivity tests of infected area, injection site

Implementation
- Culture infected area, and arrange for sensitivity tests before beginning drug therapy.
- Reconstitute for IM use using Sterile Water for Injection or Bacteriostatic Water for Injection or 0.9% Sodium Chloride Injection as follows:

Vial Size	Diluent to Add	Available Volume	Concentration
250 mg	2 ml	2 ml	125 mg/ml
500 mg	2 ml	2.2 ml	225 mg/ml
1 g	2.5 ml	3 ml	330 mg/ml

- Inject IM doses deeply into large muscle group.
- Be aware that solution is stable for 24 h at room temperature or 4 d if refrigerated; redissolve by warming to room temperature and agitating slightly.
- Have vitamin K available in case hypoprothrombinemia occurs.

Drug-specific teaching points
- Do not use alcoholic beverages while on this drug and for 3 d after this drug has been stopped because severe reactions often occur.
- Know that the following side effects may occur: stomach upset, loss of appetite, nausea (taking the drug with food may help); diarrhea (stay near bathroom facilities); headache, dizziness.
- Report severe diarrhea, difficulty breathing, unusual tiredness or fatigue, pain at injection site.

❒ cefixime

*(sef **icks'** ime)*
Suprax

Pregnancy Category B

Drug classes
Antibiotic
Cephalosporin (third generation)

Therapeutic actions
Bactericidal: inhibits synthesis of bacterial cell wall, causing cell death.

Indications
- Uncomplicated UTIs caused by *E. coli, P. mirabilis*
- Otitis media caused by *H. influenzae* (beta-lactamase positive and negative strains), *Moraxella catarrhalis, S. pyogenes*
- Pharyngitis, tonsillitis caused by *S. pyogenes*
- Acute bronchitis and acute exacerbations of chronic bronchitis caused by *S. pneumoniae, H. influenzae* (beta-lactamase positive and negative strains)
- Uncomplicated gonorrhea caused by *Neisseria gonorrhoeae*

Contraindications/cautions
- Allergy to cephalosporins or penicillins; renal failure; lactation

Dosage
Adult and children more than 50 kg or younger than 12 y: 400 mg/d PO as a single 400-mg tablet or as 200 mg q12h. For *S. pyogenes* infections, administer cefixime for at least 10 d.
Pediatric: 8 mg/kg per day suspension as a single daily dose or as 4 mg/kg q12h. Treat otitis media with suspension; in clinical studies, the suspension resulted in higher blood levels than tablets.
Geriatric or impaired renal function:

Creatine Clearance (ml/min)	Dosage
>60	Standard
21–60, or on hemodialysis	75% of standard
≤20 or continuous peritoneal dialysis	50% of standard

Pharmacokinetics

Route	Peak
PO	2–6 h

Metabolism: $T_{1/2}$: 3–4 h
Distribution: Crosses the placenta; enters breast milk
Excretion: Renal and bile

Adverse effects
- CNS: Headache, dizziness, lethargy, paresthesias
- GI: *Nausea, vomiting, diarrhea, anorexia, abdominal pain, flatulence*, **pseudomembranous colitis**, liver toxicity
- Hematologic: Bone marrow depression
- GU: Nephrotoxicity
- Hypersensitivity: *Ranging from rash to fever* to **anaphylaxis**; serum sickness reaction
- Other: *Superinfections*

Clinically important drug-drug interactions
- Decreased bactericidal activity if used with bacteriostatic agents • Increased serum levels of cephalosporins if used with probenecid

Drug-lab test interferences
- False-positive urine glucose using Benedict's solution, Fehling's solution, Clinitest tablets • False-positive direct Coombs' test • Falsely elevated urinary 17-ketosteroids

■ Nursing Considerations

Assessment
- *History:* Penicillin or cephalosporin allergy, pregnancy or lactation
- *Physical:* Kidney function, respiratory status, skin status, culture and sensitivity tests of infected area

Implementation
- Culture infected area before beginning drug therapy.
- Shake refrigerated suspension well before using.
- Give drug with meals or food to decrease GI discomfort.
- Refrigerate suspension after reconstitution, and discard after 14 d.
- Discontinue drug if hypersensitivy reaction occurs.
- Give the patient yogurt or buttermilk in case of diarrhea.
- Arrange for oral vancomycin for serious colitis that fails to respond to discontinuation of drug.

Drug-specific teaching points
- Take this drug only for this specific infection, and do not use to self-treat other problems.
- Refrigerate suspension, and discard unused portion after 14 d; shake suspension well before each use.
- Know that the following side effects may occur: stomach upset, loss of appetite, nausea (taking the drug with food may help); diarrhea (stay near bathroom facilities); headache, dizziness.
- Report severe diarrhea with blood, pus, or mucus; skin rash; difficulty breathing; unusual tiredness, fatigue; unusual bleeding or bruising.

❒ cefmetazole sodium

*(sef **met**' a zol)*
Zefazone

Pregnancy Category B

Drug classes
Antibiotic
Cephalosporin (second generation)

Therapeutic actions
Bactericidal: inhibits the formation of bacterial cell wall, causing cell death.

Indications
- UTIs caused by *E. coli*
- Lower respiratory tract infections caused by *S. aureus, S. pneumoniae, E. coli, H. influenzae*
- Dermatologic infections caused by *S. aureus, S. epidermidis, S. pyogenes, Streptococcus agalactiae, E. coli, P. mirabilis, P. vulgaris, M. morganii, Proteus stuartii, Klebsiella pneumoniae, Klebsiella oxytoca, Bacteroides fragilis, Bacteroides melaninogenicus*
- Intra-abdominal infections caused by *E. coli, K. pneumoniae, K. oxytoca, B. fragilis, Clostridium perfringens*
- Perioperative prophylaxis for cesarean section, abdominal or vaginal hysterectomy, cholecystectomy, colorectal surgery

Adverse effects in *Italics* are most common; those in **Bold** are life-threatening.

Contraindications/cautions
- Allergy to cephalosporins or penicillins, renal failure, lactation

Dosage
Adult: 2 g IV q6–12h for 5–14 d.
- **Perioperative prophylaxis:** *Vaginal hysterectomy:* 2-g single dose 30–90 min before surgery or 1-g doses 30–90 min before surgery and repeated 8 and 16 h later. *Abdominal hysterectomy:* 1 g-doses 30–90 min before surgery and repeated 8 and 16 h later. *Cesarean section:* 2-g single dose after clamping cord or 1-g doses after clamping cord; repeated at 8 and 16 h later. *Colorectal surgery:* 2-g single dose 30–90 min before surgery or 2-g doses 30–90 min before surgery and repeated 8 and 16 h later. *Cholecystectomy (high risk):* 1-g doses 30–90 min before surgery and repeated 8 and 16 h later.

Pediatric: Safety and efficacy not established.

Geriatric or impaired renal function:

Creatinine Clearance (ml/min)	Dose (g)	Frequency
50–90	1–2	q12h
30–49	1–2	q16h
10–29	1–2	q24h
<10	1–2	q48h

Pharmacokinetics

Route	Onset	Peak
IV	Rapid	End of infusion

Metabolism: $T_{1/2}$: 1.2 h
Distribution: Enters breast milk
Excretion: Urine

IV facts
Preparation: Use Sterile Water for Injection, Bacteriostatic Water for Injection, or 0.9% Sodium Chloride Injection. Dilute 1 g with 3.7 ml to yield 250 mg/ml or 1 g with 10 ml to yield 100 mg/ml; 2 g diluted with 7 ml will yield 250 mg/ml, or 2 g with 15 ml yields 125 mg/ml. Primary solutions may be further diluted to concentrations of 1–20 mg/ml in 0.9% Sodium Chloride Injection, 5% Dextrose Injection, or Lactated Ringer's Injection. Stable for 24 h at room temperature, 7 d if refrigerated, or 6 wk if frozen. Do not refreeze thawed solutions; discard any unused solution.

Infusion: If using a piggy-back IV setup, discontinue the other solution while cefmetazole is being given. If given as part of combination therapy with aminoglycosides, give each antibiotic at a different site. Do not mix aminoglycosides and cefmetazole in the same IV solution. Direct IV infusion over 3–5 min; slow infusion over 10–60 min.

Incompatabilites: Do not mix in solution with aminoglycosides.

Adverse effects
- CNS: Headache, dizziness, lethargy, paresthesias
- GI: *Nausea, vomiting, diarrhea, anorexia, abdominal pain, flatulence,* pseudomembranous colitis, liver toxicity
- Hematologic: bone marrow depression: decreased WBC, decreased platelets, decreased Hct
- GU: Nephrotoxicity
- Hypersensitivity: *Ranging from rash* to *fever* to anaphylaxis, serum sickness reaction
- Local: *Pain,* abscess at injection site, *phlebitis,* inflammation at IV site
- Other: *Superinfections, disulfiram-like reaction with alcohol*

Clinically important drug-drug interactions
- Increased nephrotoxicity with aminoglycosides • Increased bleeding effects if taken with oral anticoagulants • Disulfiram-like reaction may occur if alcohol is taken within 72 h after cefmetazole administration.

Drug-lab test interferences
- Possibility of false results on tests of urine glucose using Benedict's solution, Fehling's

solution, Clinitest tablets; urinary 17-ketosteroids; direct Coombs' test.

■ Nursing Considerations
Assessment
- *History:* Liver and kidney dysfunction, lactation, pregnancy
- *Physical:* Skin status, liver and kidney function test, culture of affected area, sensitivity tests

Implementation
- Have vitamin K available in case hypoprothrombinemia occurs.
- Discontinue drug if hypersensitivy reaction occurs.

Drug-specific teaching points
- Be aware that side effects may include stomach upset or diarrhea.
- Avoid drinking alcoholic beverages while on this drug and for 3 d after this drug has been stopped because severe reactions often occur.
- Report severe diarrhea, difficulty breathing, unusual tiredness or fatigue, pain at injection site.

☐ cefonicid

(se fon' i sid)
Monocid

Pregnancy Category B

Drug classes
Antibiotic
Cephalosporin (second generation)

Therapeutic actions
Bactericidal: inhibits synthesis of bacterial cell wall, causing cell death.

Indications
- Lower respiratory tract infections caused by *S. pneumoniae, K. pneumoniae, H. influenzae, E. coli*
- UTIs caused by *E. coli, Proteus* species, *K. pneumoniae*
- Dermatologic infections caused by *S. aureus, S. pyogenes, S. epidermidis, S. agalactiae*
- Septicemia caused by *S. pneumoniae, E. coli*
- Bone and joint infections caused by *S. aureus*
- Perioperative prophylaxis

Contraindications/cautions
- Allergy to cephalosporins or penicillins, renal failure, lactation.

Dosage
Adult: 1 g/d IM or IV. Up to 2 g/d may be tolerated.
- *Perioperative prophylaxis:* 1 g IV 1 h prior to initial incision; 1 g/d for 24 h after surgery.
- *Cesarean section:* Give *after* the cord is clamped.

Geriatric (or impaired renal function): Initial dose of 7.5 mg/kg IV or IM followed by:

Creatinine Clearance (ml/min)	Dosage Moderate Infections	Dosage Severe Infections
60–79	10 mg/kg q24h	25 mg/kg q24h
40–59	8 mg/kg q24h	20 mg/kg q24h
20–39	4 mg/kg q24h	15 mg/kg q24h
10–19	4 mg/kg q48h	15 mg/kg q48h
5–9	4 mg/kg q 3–5 d	15 mg/kg q 3–5 d
<5	3 mg/kg q 3–5 d	4 mg/kg q 3–5 d

Pharmacokinetics

Route	Onset	Peak	Duration
IV	Immediate	5 min	24 h
IM	1 h	1 h	24 h

Metabolism: $T_{1/2}$: 4.5–5.8 h
Distribution: Enters breast milk
Excretion: Urine

IV facts
Preparation: Reconstitute single-dose vials as follows: 500-mg vial, add 2 ml Sterile Water for Injection (220 mg/ml concentration); 1-g vial, add 2.5 ml Sterile Water for Injection (325 mg/ml concentration). For IV infusion, add reconstituted solution to 50–100 ml of one of the follow-

ing: 0.9% Sodium Chloride; 5% or 10% Dextrose Injection; 5% Dextrose and 0.2%, 0.45%, or 0.9% Sodium Chloride Injection; Ringer's Injection; Lactated Ringer's Injection; 5% Dextrose and Lactated Ringer's Injection; 10% Invert Sugar in Sterile Water for Injection; 5% Dextrose and 0.15% Potassium Chloride Injection; Sodium Lactate Injection. Reconstituted or diluted solution is stable for up to 24 h at room temperature, 72 h if refrigerated; discard unused solutions within the allotted time period.

Infusion: Give bolus injections slowly over 3–5 min into vein or IV tubing. If given as part of combination therapy with aminoglycosides, give each antibiotic at a different site: do not mix aminoglycosides and cefonicid in the same IV solution.

Incompatibilities: Incompatible in solution with aminoglycosides.

Adverse effects

- CNS: Headache, dizziness, lethargy, paresthesias
- GI: *Nausea, vomiting, diarrhea, anorexia, abdominal pain, flatulence,* pseudomembranous colitis, liver toxicity
- Hematologic: Bone marrow depression: decreased WBC, decreased platelets, decreased Hct
- GU: Nephrotoxicity
- Hypersensitivity: *Ranging from rash* to *fever* to anaphylaxis; serum sickness reaction
- Local: *Pain,* abscess at injection site, *phlebitis,* inflammation at IV site
- Other: *Superinfections, disulfiram-like reaction with alcohol*

Clinically important drug-drug interactions

- Increased nephrotoxicity with aminoglycosides • Increased bleeding effects if taken with oral anticoagulants • Disulfiram-like reaction may occur if alcohol is taken within 72 h after cefonicid administration.

Drug-lab test interferences

- Possibility of false results on tests of urine glucose using Benedict's solution, Fehling's solution, Clinitest tablets; urinary 17-ketosteroids; direct Coombs' test.

■ Nursing Considerations

Assessment

- *History:* Liver and kidney dysfunction, lactation, pregnancy
- *Physical:* Skin status, liver and kidney function test, culture of affected area, sensitivity tests

Implementation

- Culture infected area, and arrange for sensitivity tests before beginning drug therapy and during therapy if expected response is not seen.
- Divide IM doses of 2 g once daily and give as two equal doses deeply into two different large muscles.
- Have vitamin K available in case hypoprothrombinemia occurs.
- Discontinue drug if hypersensitivy reaction occurs.

Drug-specific teaching points

- Be aware that side effects may include stomach upset or diarrhea.
- Avoid drinking alcoholic beverages while on this drug and for 3 d after this drug has been stopped, because severe reactions often occur.
- Report severe diarrhea, difficulty breathing, unusual tiredness or fatigue, pain at injection site.

⬜ cefoperazone sodium

*(sef ob **per'** a zone)*
Cefobid

Pregnancy Category B

Drug classes
Antibiotic
Cephalosporin (third generation)

Therapeutic actions
Bactericidal: inhibits synthesis of bacterial cell wall, causing cell death.

Indications

- Respiratory tract infections caused by *S. pneumoniae, S. aureus, S. pyogenes,*

Adverse effects in *Italics* are most common; those in **Bold** are life-threatening.

Pseudomonas aeruginosa, K. pneumoniae, H. influenzae, E. coli, Proteus, Enterobacter
- Dermatologic infections caused by *S. aureus, S. pyogenes, P. aeruginosa*
- UTIs caused by *E. coli, P. aeruginosa*
- Septicemia caused by *S. pneumoniae, S. aureus, S. agalactiae,* enterococci, *H. influenzae, P. aeruginosa, E. coli, Klebsiella, Proteus, Clostridium,* anaerobic gram-positive cocci
- Peritonitis and intra-abdominal infections caused by *E. coli, P. aeruginosa,* anaerobic gram-positive cocci, anaerobic gram-positive and gram-negative bacilli
- Pelvic inflammatory disease, endometritis caused by *N. gonorrhoeae, S. epidermidis, S. agalactiae, E. coli, Clostridium, Bacteroides,* and anaerobic gram-positive cocci

Contraindications/cautions
- Allergy to cephalosporins or penicillins, hepatic failure, lactation.

Dosage
Adult: 2–4 g/d IM or IV in equal divided doses q12h; up to 6–12 g/d have been used in severe cases.
Pediatric: Safety and efficacy not established.
Hepatic impaired: Total daily dose of 4 g. Monitor patient carefully.

Pharmacokinetics

Route	Onset	Peak	Duration
IV	5–10 min	15–20 min	6–12 h
IM	1 h	1–2 h	6–12 h

Metabolism: $T_{1/2}$: 1.75–2.5 h
Distribution: Enters breast milk
Excretion: Bile

IV facts
Preparation: For administration by IV infusion; concentrations of 2–50 mg/ml are recommended. Reconstitute powder for IV use in 5% or 10% Dextrose Injection; 5% Dextrose and 0.2% or 0.9% Sodium Chloride Injection; 5% Dextrose and Lactated Ringer's Injection; Lactated Ringer's Injection; 0.9% Sodium Chloride Injection; Normosol M and 5% Dextrose Injection; Normosol R. After reconstituting solutions, allow to stand until any sign of foaming is gone; vigorous agitation may be necessary. Reconstituted solution is stable for 24 h at room temperature or up to 5 d if refrigerated.

Vial Dose	Desired Concentration	Diluent to Add	Resulting Volume
1 g	333 mg/ml	2.6 ml	3 ml
	250 mg/ml	3.8 ml	4 ml
2 g	333 mg/ml	5 ml	6 ml
	250 mg/ml	7.2 ml	8 ml

Infusion: If using a piggy-back IV setup, discontinue the other solution while cefoperazone is being given. If given as part of combination therapy with aminoglycosides, give each antibiotic at a different site.
Incompatibilities: Do not mix aminoglycosides and cefoperazone in the same IV solution.

Adverse effects
- CNS: Headache, dizziness, lethargy, paresthesias
- GI: *Nausea, vomiting, diarrhea, anorexia, abdominal pain, flatulence,* pseudomembranous colitis, liver toxicity
- Hematologic: **Bone marrow depression:** decreased WBC, decreased platelets, decreased Hct
- GU: Nephrotoxicity
- Hypersensitivity: *Ranging from rash* to *fever* to anaphylaxis; serum sickness reaction
- Local: *Pain,* abscess at injection site; *phlebitis,* inflammation at IV site
- Other: *superinfections, disulfiram-like reaction with alcohol*

Clinically important drug-drug interactions
- Increased nephrotoxicity with aminoglycosides • Increased bleeding effects if taken with oral anticoagulants • Disulfiram-like reaction may occur if alcohol is taken within 72 h after cefoperazone administration.

cefotaxime sodium ■ 233

Drug-lab test interferences
- Possibility of false results on tests of urine glucose using Benedict's solution, Fehling's solution, Clinitest tablets; urinary 17-ketosteroids; direct Coombs' test.

■ Nursing Considerations

Assessment
- *History:* Liver and kidney dysfunction, lactation, pregnancy
- *Physical:* Skin status, liver and kidney function test, culture of affected area, sensitivity tests

Implementation
- Culture infected area, and arrange for sensitivity tests before beginning drug therapy and during therapy if expected response is not seen.
- Keep dosage under 4 g/d, or monitor serum concentrations in patients with liver disease or biliary obstruction.
- To prepare drug for IM use: reconstitute powder in Bacteriostatic Water for Injection; Sterile Water for Injection; or 0.5% Lidocaine HCl Injection (when concentrations greater than 250 mg/ml are to be used).
- Maintain vitamin K on standby in case hypoprothrombinemia occurs.
- Discontinue drug if hypersensitivy reaction occurs.

Drug-specific teaching points
- Be aware that side effects may include stomach upset or diarrhea.
- Avoid drinking alcoholic beverages while on this drug and for 3 d after this drug has been stopped because severe reactions often occur.
- Report severe diarrhea, difficulty breathing, unusual tiredness or fatigue, pain at injection site.

❒ cefotaxime sodium

*(sef oh **taks**' eem)*
Claforan

Pregnancy Category B

Drug classes
Antibiotic
Cephalosporin (third generation)

Therapeutic actions
Bactericidal: inhibits synthesis of bacterial cell wall, causing cell death.

Indications
- Lower respiratory tract infections caused by *S. pneumoniae, S. aureus, Klebsiella, H. influenzae, E. coli, P. mirabilis, Enterobacter, Serratia marcescens, S. pyogenes*
- UTIs caused by *Enterococcus, S. epidermidis, S. aureus, Citrobacter, Enterobacter, E. coli, Klebsiella, P. mirabilis, Proteus, S. marcescens*
- Gyn infections caused by *S. epidermidis, Enterococcus, E. coli, P. mirabilis, Bacteroides, Clostridium, Peptococcus, Peptostreptococcus,* streptococci; and uncomplicated gonorrhea caused by *N. gonorrhoeae*
- Dermatologic infections caused by *S. aureus, E. coli, Serratia, Proteus, Klebsiella, Enterobacter, Pseudomonas, S. marcescens, Bacteroides, Peptococcus, Peptostreptococcus, P. mirabilis, S. epidermidis, S. pyogenes, Enterococcus*
- Septicemia caused by *E. coli, Klebsiella, S. marcescens*
- Peritonitis and intra-abdominal infections caused by *E. coli, Peptostreptococcus, Bacteroides, Peptococcus, Klebsiella*
- CNS infections caused by *E. coli, H. influenzae, Neisseria meningitidis, S. pneumoniae, K. pneumoniae*
- Bone and joint infections caused by *S. aureus*
- Perioperative prophylaxis

Contraindications/cautions
- Allergy to cephalosporins or penicillins, renal failure, lactation.

Dosage
Adult: 2–8 g/d IM or IV in equally divided doses q6–8h. Do not exceed 12 g/d.
- ***Gonorrhea:*** 1 g IM in a single injection.
- ***Disseminated infection:*** 500 mg IV qid for 7 d.

cefotaxime sodium

- **Gonococcal ophthalmia:** 500 mg IV qid.
- **Perioperative prophylaxis:** 1 g IV or IM 30–90 min before surgery.
- **Cesarean section:** 1 g IV after cord is clamped and then 1 g IV or IM at 6 and 12 h.

Pediatric
- **0–1 wk:** 50 mg/kg IV q12h.
- **1–4 wk:** 50 mg/kg IV q8h.
- **1 mo–12 y (<50 kg):** 50–180 mg/kg per day IV or IM in four to six divided doses.

Geriatric (or reduced renal function): If creatinine clearance is < 20 ml/min, reduce dosage by half.

Pharmacokinetics

Route	Onset	Peak	Duration
IV	Immediate	5 min	18–24 h
IM	5–10 min	30 min	18–24 h

Metabolism: $T_{1/2}$: 1 h
Distribution: Crosses the placenta; enters breast milk
Excretion: Urine

IV facts

Preparation: Reconstitute for intermittent IV injection with 1 or 2 g with 10 ml Sterile Water for Injection. Reconstitute vials for IV infusion with 10 ml of Sterile Water for Injection. Reconstitute infusion bottles with 50 or 100 ml of 0.9% Sodium Chloride Injection or 5% Dextrose Injection. Drug solution may be further diluted with 50–100 ml of 5% or 10% Dextrose Injection; 5% Dextrose and 0.2%, 0.45%, or 0.9% Sodium Chloride Injection; Lactated Ringer's Solution; 0.9% Sodium Chloride Injection; Sodium Lactate Injection (M/6); 10% Invert Sugar. Reconstituted solution is stable for 24 h at room temperature or 5 d if refrigerated. Powder and reconstituted solution darken with storage.

Infusion: Inject slowly into vein over 3–5 min or over a longer time through IV tubing. If administered with aminoglycosides, administer at different sites.

Incompatibilities: Do not mix in solutions with aminoglycoside solutions.

Adverse effects

- **CNS:** Headache, dizziness, lethargy, paresthesias
- **GI:** *Nausea, vomiting, diarrhea, anorexia, abdominal pain, flatulence,* pseudomembranous colitis, liver toxicity
- **Hematologic:** Bone marrow depression: decreased WBC, decreased platelets, decreased Hct
- **GU:** Nephrotoxicity
- **Hypersensitivity:** *Ranging from rash* to *fever* to anaphylaxis; serum sickness reaction
- **Local:** *Pain,* abscess at injection site, *phlebitis,* inflammation at IV site
- **Other:** *Superinfections, disulfiram-like reaction with alcohol*

Clinically important drug-drug interactions

- Increased nephrotoxicity with aminoglycosides • Increased bleeding effects if taken with oral anticoagulants • Disulfiram-like reaction may occur if alcohol is taken within 72 h after cefotaxime administration.

Drug-lab test interferences

- Possibility of false results on tests of urine glucose using Benedict's solution, Fehling's solution, Clinitest tablets; urinary 17-ketosteroids; direct Coombs' test.

■ Nursing Considerations

Assessment

- *History:* Liver and kidney dysfunction, lactation, pregnancy
- *Physical:* Skin status, liver and kidney function test, culture of affected area, sensitivity tests

Implementation

- Culture infected area, and arrange for sensitivity tests before beginning drug therapy and during therapy if expected response is not seen.

Adverse effects in *Italics* are most common; those in **Bold** are life-threatening.

is 182–195 mg/ml. Reconstituted solution is stable for 24 h at room temperature or 4 d if refrigerated. Protect drug from light.
Infusion: Inject slowly over 3–5 min into vein or over a longer time into IV tubing. Discontinue infusion of other solutions temporarily while cefotetan is running. If given as part of combination therapy with aminoglycosides, give each antibiotic at a different site.

Incompatibilities: Do not mix aminoglycosides and cefotetan in the same IV solution.

Adverse effects

- CNS: Headache, dizziness, lethargy, paresthesias
- GI: *Nausea, vomiting, diarrhea, anorexia, abdominal pain, flatulence*, pseudomembranous colitis, liver toxicity
- Hematologic: Bone marrow depression: decreased WBC, decreased platelets, decreased Hct
- GU: Nephrotoxicity
- Hypersensitivity: *Ranging from rash* to *fever* to anaphylaxis, serum sickness reaction
- Local: *Pain,* abscess at injection site; *phlebitis,* inflammation at IV site
- Other: *Superinfection, disulfiram-like reaction with alcohol*

Clinically important drug-drug interactions

- Increased nephrotoxicity with aminoglycosides • Increased bleeding effects if taken with oral anticoagulants • Disulfiram-like reaction may occur if alcohol is taken within 72 h after cefotetan administration.

Drug-lab test interferences

- Possibility of false results on tests of urine glucose using Benedict's solution, Fehling's solution, Clinitest tablets; urinary 17-ketosteroids; direct Coombs' test.

■ Nursing Considerations

Assessment

- *History:* Liver and kidney dysfunction, lactation, pregnancy
- *Physical:* Skin status, liver and kidney function test, culture of affected area, sensitivity tests

Implementation

- Culture infected area, and arrange sensitivity tests before beginning therapy and during therapy if expected response is not seen.
- Reconstitute for IM use with Sterile Water for Injection, 0.9% Sodium Chloride solution, Bacteriostatic Water for Injection, 0.5% or 1% lidocaine HCl; inject deep into large muscle group.
- Protect drug from light.
- Have vitamin K available in case hypoprothrombinemia occurs.
- Discontinue drug if hypersensitivy reaction occurs.

Drug-specific teaching points

- Be aware that side effects may include stomach upset or diarrhea.
- Avoid drinking alcoholic beverages while on this drug and for 3 d after this drug has been stopped because severe reactions often occur.
- Report severe diarrhea, difficulty breathing, unusual tiredness or fatigue, pain at injection site.

☐ cefoxitin sodium

*(se **fox**' i tin)*

Mefoxin

Pregnancy Category B

Drug classes
Antibiotic
Cephalosporin (second generation)

Therapeutic actions
Bactericidal: inhibits synthesis of bacterial cell wall, causing cell death.

Indications

- Lower respiratory tract infections caused by *S. pneumoniae, S. aureus,* streptococci, *E. coli, Klebsiella, H. influenzae, Bacteroides*

Adverse effects in *Italics* are most common; those in **Bold** are life-threatening.

cefoxitin sodium ■ 237

- Dermatologic infections caused by *S. aureus, S. epidermidis*, streptococci, *E. coli, P. mirabilis, Klebsiella, Bacteroides, Clostridium, Peptococcus, Peptostreptococcus*
- UTIs caused by *E. coli, P. mirabilis, Klebsiella, M. morganii, P. rettgeri, P. vulgaris, Providencia*, uncomplicated gonorrhea caused by *N. gonorrhoeae*
- Intra-abdominal infections caused by *E. coli, Klebsiella, Bacteroides, Clostridium*
- Gynecologic infections caused by *E. coli, N. gonorrhoeae, Bacteroides, Clostridium, Peptococcus, Peptostreptococcus*, group B streptococci
- Septicemia caused by *S. pneumoniae, S. aureus, E. coli, Klebsiella, Bacteroides*
- Bone and joint infections caused by *S. aureus*
- Perioperative prophylaxis

Contraindications/cautions
- Allergy to cephalosporins or penicillins, renal failure, lactation.

Dosage
Adult: 1–2 g IM or IV q6–8h, depending on the severity of the infection.
- ***Uncomplicated gonorrhea:*** 2 g IM with 1 g oral probenecid.
- ***Perioperative prophylaxis:*** 2 g IV or IM ½–1 h prior to initial incision and q6h for 24 h after surgery.
- ***Cesarean section:*** 2 g IV as soon as the umbilical cord is clamped, followed by 2 g IM or IV at 4 and 8 h, then q6h for up to 24 h.
- ***Transurethral prostatectomy:*** 1 g prior to surgery and then 1 g q8h for up to 5 d.

Pediatric
- ***Older than 3 mo:*** 80–160 mg/kg per day IM or IV in divided doses q4–6h. Do not exceed 12 g/d.
- ***Prophylactic use:*** 30–40 mg/kg per dose IV or IM q6h.

Geriatric (or impaired renal function): IV loading dose of 1–2 g;. Maintenance dosages are as follows:

Creatinine Clearance (ml/min)	Maintenance Dosage
30–50	1–2 g q8–12h
10–29	1–2 g q12–24h
5–9	0.5–1 g q12–24h
<5	0.5–1 g q24–48h

Pharmacokinetics

Route	Onset	Peak	Duration
IV	Immediate	5 min	6–8 h
IM	5–10 min	20–30 min	6–8 h

Metabolism: $T_{1/2}$: 45–60 min
Distribution: Crosses the placenta; enters breast milk
Excretion: Urine

IV facts
Preparation: For IV intermittent administration, reconstitute 1 or 2 g with 10–20 ml Sterile Water for Injection. For continuous IV infusion, add reconstituted solution to 5% Dextrose Injection, 0.9% Sodium Chloride Injection, 5% Dextrose and 0.9% Sodium Chloride Injection, or 5% Dextrose Injection with 0.02% Sodium Bicarbonate Solution. Store dry powder in cool, dry area. Powder and reconstituted solution darkens with storage. Stable for 24 h at room temperature.

Infusion: *Intermittent administration:* slowly inject over 3–5 min, or give over longer time through IV tubing; discontinue other solutions temporarily. If given as part of combination therapy with aminoglycosides, give each antibiotic at a different site.

Incompatibilities: Do not mix aminoglycosides and cefoxitin in the same IV solution.

Adverse effects
- CNS: Headache, dizziness, lethargy, paresthesias
- GI: *Nausea, vomiting, diarrhea, anorexia, abdominal pain, flatulence,* pseudomembranous colitis, liver toxicity
- Hematologic: Bone marrow depression: decreased WBC, decreased platelets, decreased Hct

Adverse effects in *Italics* are most common; those in **Bold** are life-threatening.

- **GU:** Nephrotoxicity
- **Hypersensitivity:** *Ranging from rash to fever* to anaphylaxis, serum sickness reaction
- **Local:** *Pain,* abscess at injection site, *phlebitis,* inflammation at IV site
- **Other:** *Superinfections, disulfiram-like reaction with alcohol*

Clinically important drug-drug interactions
- Increased nephrotoxicity with aminoglycosides • Increased bleeding effects if taken with oral anticoagulants • Disulfiram-like reaction may occur if alcohol is taken within 72 h after cefoxitin administration

Drug-lab test interferences
- Possibility of false results on tests of urine glucose using Benedict's solution, Fehling's solution, Clinitest tablets; urinary 17-ketosteroids; direct Coombs' test.

■ Nursing Considerations
Assessment
- *History:* Liver and kidney dysfunction, lactation, pregnancy
- *Physical:* Skin status, liver and kidney function test, culture of affected area, sensitivity tests

Implementation
- Culture infected area, and arrange for sensitivity tests before beginning drug therapy and during therapy if expected response is not seen.
- Reconstitute each gram for IM use with 2 ml Sterile Water for Injection or with 2 ml of 0.5% Lidocaine HCl Solution (without epinephrine) to decrease pain at injection site. Inject deeply into large muscle group.
- Know that the dry powder and reconstituted solutions darken slightly at room temperature.
- Have vitamin K available in case hypoprothrombinemia occurs.
- Discontinue drug if hypersensitivity reaction occurs.

Drug-specific teaching points
- Know that the following side effects may occur: stomach upset or diarrhea.
- Avoid drinking alcoholic beverages while on this drug and for 3 d after this drug has been stopped because severe reactions often occur.
- Report severe diarrhea, difficulty breathing, unusual tiredness or fatigue, pain at injection site.

▢ cefpodoxime proxetil

*(sef poe **docks'** eem)*
Vantin

Pregnancy Category B

Drug classes
Antibiotic
Cephalosporin (second generation)

Therapeutic actions
Bactericidal: inhibits synthesis of bacterial cell wall, causing cell death.

Indications
- Lower respiratory tract infections caused by *S. pneumoniae, H. influenzae*
- Upper respiratory infections caused by *S. pyogenes, H. influenzae, Moraxella catharrhalis*
- Dermatologic infections caused by *S. aureus, S. pyogenes*
- UTIs caused by *E. coli, P. mirabilis, Klebsiella, Staphylococcus saprophyticus*
- Otitis media caused by *S. pneumoniae, H. influenzae, M. catarrhalis*
- Sexually transmitted disease caused by *N. gonorrhoeae*

Contraindications/cautions
- Allergy to cephalosporins or penicillins, renal failure, lactation.

Dosage
Adult: 100–400 mg q12h PO depending on severity of infection; continue for 7–14 d
Pediatric: 5 mg/kg per dose PO q12h; do not exceed 100–200 mg per dose; continue for 10 d
Geriatric or renal impaired: Creatinine clearance < 30 ml/min: increase dosing interval to q24h.

Adverse effects in *Italics* are most common; those in **Bold** are life-threatening.

Pharmacokinetics

Route	Peak	Duration
PO	30–60 min	16–18 h

Metabolism: $T_{1/2}$: 120–180 min
Distribution: Crosses the placenta; enters breast milk;
Excretion: Renal, unchanged

Adverse effects
- CNS: Headache, dizziness, lethargy, paresthesias
- GI: *Nausea, vomiting, diarrhea, anorexia, abdominal pain, flatulence, pseudomembranous colitis,* liver toxicity
- Hematologic: Bone marrow depression
- GU: Nephrotoxicity
- Hypersensitivity: *Ranging from rash to fever to anaphylaxis*; serum sickness reaction
- Other: *Superinfections*

Clinically important drug-drug interactions
- Increased nephrotoxicity with aminoglycosides • Increased bleeding effects if taken with oral anticoagulants • Disulfiram-like reaction if alcohol is taken within 72 h after cefpodoxime administration

Clinically important drug-food interactions
- Increased absorption and increased effects of cefpodoxime if taken with food

Drug-lab test interferences
- Possibility of false results on tests of urine glucose using Benedict's solution, Fehling's solution, Clinitest tablets; urinary 17-ketosteroids; direct Coombs' test.

■ Nursing Considerations

Assessment
- *History:* Penicillin or cephalosporin allergy, pregnancy or lactation
- *Physical:* Kidney function, respiratory status, skin status; culture and sensitivity tests of infected area

Implementation
- Culture infected area before beginning drug therapy.
- Give drug with meals or food to enhance absorption.
- Prepare suspension as follows: suspend 50 mg/5 ml strength in a total of 58 ml distilled water. Gently tap the bottle to loosen the powder. Add 25 ml distilled water and shake vigorously for 15 seconds. Add 33 ml distilled water, and shake vigorously for 3 min or until all particles are suspended. Suspend 100 mg/5 ml strength in a total of 57 ml distilled water. Proceed as above, adding 25 ml distilled water and 32 ml distilled water, respectively.
- Refrigerate suspension after reconstitution; shake vigorously before use, and discard after 14 d.
- Discontinue drug if hypersensitivity reaction occurs.
- Give the patient yogurt or buttermilk in case of diarrhea.
- Arrange for oral vancomycin for serious colitis that fails to respond to discontinuation

Drug-specific teaching points
- Take this drug with meals or food.
- Complete the full course of this drug, even if you feel better before the course of treatment is over.
- Be aware that this drug is prescribed for this particular infection; do not self-treat any other infection with this drug.
- Know that the following side effects may occur: stomach upset, loss of appetite, nausea (taking the drug with food may help); diarrhea (stay near bathroom facilities); headache, dizziness.
- Report severe diarrhea with blood, pus, or mucus; rash or hives; difficulty breathing; unusual tiredness, fatigue; unusual bleeding or bruising.

❑ cefprozil monohydrate

(sef pro' zil)
Cefzil

Pregnancy Category B

Adverse effects in *Italics* are most common; those in **Bold** are life-threatening.

cefprozil monohydrate

Drug classes
Antibiotic
Cephalosporin (second generation)

Therapeutic actions
Bactericidal: inhibits synthesis of bacterial cell wall, causing cell death.

Indications
- Pharyngitis/tonsillitis caused by *S. pyogenes*
- Secondary bacterial infection of acute bronchitis and exacerbation of chronic bronchitis caused by *S. pneumoniae, H. influenzae, M. catarrhalis*
- Dermatologic infections caused by *S. aureus, S. pyogenes*
- UTIs caused by *E. coli, P. mirabilis, Klebsiella,* coagulase-negative staphylococci
- Otitis media caused by *S. pneumoniae, H. influenzae, M. catarrhalis*

Contraindications/cautions
- Allergy to cephalosporins or penicillins, renal failure, lactation.

Dosage
Adult: 250–500 mg PO q12h. Continue treatment for 10 d.
Pediatric: 7.5–15 mg/kg PO q12h. Continue treatment for 10 d.
Geriatric or renal impaired: Creatinine clearance 30–120 ml/min, use standard dose; creatinine clearance 0–30 ml/min, use 50% of standard dose.

Pharmacokinetics

Route	Peak	Duration
PO	6–10 h	24–28 h

Metabolism: $T_{1/2}$: 78 min
Distribution: Crosses the placenta, enters breast milk
Excretion: Renal, unchanged

Adverse effects
- CNS: Headache, dizziness, lethargy, paresthesias
- GI: *Nausea, vomiting, diarrhea, anorexia, abdominal pain, flatulence,* **pseudomembranous colitis,** liver toxicity
- Hematologic: Bone marrow depression
- GU: Nephrotoxicity
- **Hypersensitivity:** *Ranging from rash* to *fever* to *anaphylaxis;* serum sickness reaction
- Other: *Superinfections*

Clinically important drug-drug interactions
- Increased nephrotoxicity with aminoglycosides • Increased bleeding effects if taken with oral anticoagulants • Disulfiram-like reaction if alcohol is taken within 72 h after cefprozil administration

Drug-lab test interferences
- Possibility of false results on tests of urine glucose using Benedict's solution, Fehling's solution, Clinitest tablets; urinary 17-ketosteroids; direct Coombs' test.

■ Nursing Considerations

Assessment
- *History:* Penicillin or cephalosporin allergy, pregnancy or lactation
- *Physical:* Kidney function, respiratory status, skin status, culture and sensitivity tests of infected area

Implementation
- Culture infected area before beginning drug therapy.
- Give drug with meals or food to decrease GI discomfort.
- Refrigerate suspension after reconstitution, and discard after 14 d.
- Discontinue drug if hypersensitivy reaction occurs.
- Give the patient yogurt or buttermilk in case of diarrhea.
- Arrange for oral vancomycin for serious colitis that fails to respond to discontinuation

Drug-specific teaching points
- Take this drug with meals or food.
- Complete the full course of this drug, even if you feel better before the course of treatment is over.
- Be aware that this drug is prescribed for this particular infection; do not self-treat any other infection with this drug.

Adverse effects in *Italics* are most common; those in **Bold** are life-threatening.

- Know that the following side effects may occur: stomach upset, loss of appetite, nausea (taking the drug with food may help); diarrhea (stay near bathroom facilities); headache, dizziness.
- Report severe diarrhea with blood, pus, or mucus; rash or hives; difficulty breathing; unusual tiredness, fatigue; unusual bleeding or bruising.

ceftazidime

(sef tay zi deem)
Fortaz, Tazicef, Tazidime

Pregnancy Category B

Drug classes
Antibiotic
Cephalosporin (third generation)

Therapeutic actions
Bactericidal: inhibits synthesis of bacterial cell wall, causing cell death.

Indications
- Lower respiratory tract infections caused by *P. aeruginosa*, other *Pseudomonas*, *S. pneumoniae*, *S. aureus*, *Klebsiella*, *H. influenzae*, *P. mirabilis*, *E. coli*, *Enterobacter*, *Serratia*, *Citrobacter*
- UTIs caused by *P. aeruginosa*, *Enterobacter*, *E. coli*, *Klebsiella*, *P. mirabilis*, *Proteus*
- Gynecologic infections caused by *E. coli*
- Dermatologic infections caused by *P. aeruginosa*, *S. aureus*, *E. coli*, *Serratia*, *Proteus*, *Klebsiella*, *Enterobacter*, *S. pyogenes*
- Septicemia caused by *P. aeruginosa*, *E. coli*, *Klebsiella*, *H. influenzae*, *Serratia*, *S. pneumoniae*, *S. aureus*
- Intra-abdominal infections caused by *E. coli*, *S. aureus*, *Bacteroides*, *Klebsiella*
- CNS infections caused by *H. influenzae*, *N. meningitidis*
- Bone and joint infections caused by *P. aeruginosa*, *Klebsiella*, *Enterobacter*, *S. aureus*

Contraindications/cautions
- Allergy to cephalosporins or penicillins, renal failure, lactation.

Dosage
Adult: Usual dose: 1 g (range 250 mg–2 g) q8–12h IM or IV. Do not exceed 6 g/d. Dosage will vary with infection.
- **UTI:** 250–500 mg IV or IM q8–12h.
- **Pneumonia, dermatologic infections:** 500 mg–1 g IV or IM q8h.
- **Bone and joint infections:** 2 g IV q12h.
- **Gynecologic, intra-abdominal, life-threatening infections, meningitis:** 2 g IV q8h.

Pediatric
- **0–4 wk:** 30 mg/kg IV q12h.
- **1 mo–12 y:** 30–50 mg/kg IV q8h. Do not exceed 6 g/d.

Geriatric or reduced renal function: Loading dose of 1 g, followed by:

Creatinine Clearance (ml/min)	Dosage
50–31	1 g q12h
30–16	1 g q24h
15–6	500 mg q24h
<5	500 mg q48h

Pharmacokinetics

Route	Onset	Peak	Duration
IV	Rapid	1 h	24–28 h
IM	30 min	1 h	24–28 h

Metabolism: $T_{1/2}$: 114–120 min
Distribution: Crosses the placenta; enters breast milk
Excretion: Urine

IV facts
Preparation: Reconstitute drug for direct IV injection with Sterile Water for Injection. Reconstituted solution is stable for 18 h at room temperature or 7 d if refrigerated. **500-mg vial:** mix with 5 ml diluent; resulting concentration, 11 mg/ml. **1-g vial:** mix with 5 (10) ml diluent; resulting concentration, 180 (100) mg/ml. **2-g vial** mix with 10 ml diluent; resulting concentration, 170–180 mg/ml.

Infusion: For IV, reconstitute 1- or 2-g infusion pack with 100 ml Sterile Water for Injection; infuse slowly. Direct injection: slowly over 3–5 min. Infusion: slow infusion. If patient is also receiving aminoglycosides, administer at seperate sites.

ceftizoxime sodium

Incompatibilities: Sodium Bicarbonate Injection and aminoglycoside solutions.

Adverse effects
- CNS: Headache, dizziness, lethargy, paresthesias
- GI: *Nausea, vomiting, diarrhea, anorexia, abdominal pain, flatulence,* pseudomembranous colitis, liver toxicity
- Hematologic: Bone marrow depression: decreased WBC, decreased platelets, decreased Hct
- GU: Nephrotoxicity
- Hypersensitivity: *Ranging from rash* to *fever* to anaphylaxis; serum sickness reaction
- Local: *Pain,* abscess at injection site; *phlebitis,* inflammation at IV site
- Other: Superinfections, *disulfiram-like reaction with alcohol*

Clinically important drug-drug interactions
- Increased nephrotoxicity with aminoglycosides • Increased bleeding effects if taken with oral anticoagulants • Disulfiram-like reaction may occur if alcohol is taken within 72 h after ceftazidime administration.

Drug-lab test interferences
- Possibility of false results on tests of urine glucose using Benedict's solution, Fehling's solution, Clinitest tablets; urinary 17-ketosteroids; direct Coombs' test.

■ Nursing Considerations

Assessment
- *History:* Liver and kidney dysfunction, lactation, pregnancy
- *Physical:* Skin status, liver and kidney function test, culture of affected area, sensitivity tests

Implementation
- Culture infected area, and arrange for sensitivity tests before beginning drug therapy and during therapy if expected response is not seen.
- Reconstitute drug for IM use with Sterile Water or Bacteriostatic Water for Injection or with 0.5% or 1% Lidocaine HCl Injection to reduce pain; inject deep into large muscle group.
- Do *not* mix with aminoglycoside solutions. Administer these drugs seperately.
- Know that powder and reconstituted solution darken with storage.
- Have vitamin K available in case hypoprothrombinemia occurs.
- Discontinue drug if hypersensitivity reaction occurs.

Drug-specific teaching points
- Know that the following side effects may occur stomach upset or diarrhea.
- Avoid drinking alcoholic beverages while on this drug and for 3 d after this drug has been stopped because severe reactions often occur.
- Report severe diarrhea, difficulty breathing, unusual tiredness or fatigue, pain at injection site.

☐ ceftizoxime sodium

*(sef ti **zox**' eem)*
Cefizox

Pregnancy Category B

Drug classes
Antibiotic
Cephalosporin (third generation)

Therapeutic actions
Bactericidal: inhibits synthesis of bacterial cell wall, causing cell death.

Indications
- Lower respiratory tract infections caused by *S. pneumoniae, S. aureus, Klebsiella, H. influenzae, E. coli, P. mirabilis, Enterobacter, Serratia, Bacteroides*
- UTIs caused by *S. aureus, Citrobacter, Enterobacter, E. coli, Klebsiella, P. aeruginosa, P. vulgaris, P. rettgeri, P. mirabilis, M. morganii, S. marcescens, Enterobacter*
- Uncomplicated cervical and urethral gonorrhea caused by *N. gonorrhoeae*

Adverse effects in *Italics* are most common; those in **Bold** are life-threatening.

ceftizoxime sodium

- Pelvic inflammatory disease caused by *N. gonnorrhoeae, E. coli, S. agalactiae*
- Intra-abdominal infections caused by *E. coli, S. epidermidis, Streptococcus* (except enterococci), *Enterobacter, Klebsiella, Bacteroides, Peptococcus, Peptostreptococcus*
- Dermatologic infections caused by *S. aureus, E. coli, Klebsiella, Enterobacter, Bacteroides, Peptococcus, Peptostreptococcus, P. mirabilis, S. epidermidis, S. pyogenes*
- Septicemia caused by *E. coli, Klebsiella, S. pneumoniae, S. aureus, Bacteroides, Serratia*
- Bone and joint infections caused by *S. aureus, Streptococci* (excluding enterococci), *P. mirabilis, Bacteroides, Peptococcus, Peptostreptococcus*
- Meningitis caused by *H. influenzae*, some cases caused by *S. pneumoniae*

Contraindications/cautions
- Allergy to cephalosporins or penicillins, renal failure, lactation

Dosage
Adult: Usual dose: 1–2 g (range 1–4 g) IM or IV q8–12h. Do not exceed 12 g/d. Dosage will vary with infection.
- ***Gonorrhea:*** Single 1-gm IM dose.
- ***Uncomplicated UTIs:*** 500 mg q12h IM or IV
- ***PID:*** 2 g q8h IV

Pediatric
- ***Older than 6 mo:*** 50 mg/kg q6–8h; up to 200 mg/kg per day in severe infections

Geriatric or reduced renal function: Initial dose of 500 mg–1 g IM or IV followed by:

CCr (ml/min)	Usual Dosage	Maximum Dosage
79–80	500 mg q8h	0.75–1.5 g q8h
49–5	250–500 mg q12h	0.5–1 g q12h
4–0	500 mg q48h or 250 mg q24h	0.5–1 g q48h or 0.5 g q24h

Pharmacokinetics

Route	Onset	Peak	Duration
IV	Rapid	1 h	18–24 h
IM	30 min	1 h	18–24 h

Metabolism: $T_{1/2}$: 84–114 min
Distribution: Crosses the placenta; enters breast milk
Excretion: Urine

IV facts
Preparation: Dilute reconstituted solution for IV infusion with 50–100 ml of 5% or 10% Dextrose Injection; 5% Dextrose and 0.2%, 0.45%, or 0.9% Sodium Chloride Injection; Lactated Ringer's Injection; Ringer's Injection; 0.9% Sodium Chloride Injection; Invert Sugar 10% in Sterile Water for Injection; 5% Sodium Bicarbonate in Sterile Water for Injection; or 5% Dextrose in Lactated Ringer's Injection if reconstituted with 4% Sodium Bicarbonate Injection.

Package Size	Diluent to Add	Volumes	Resulting Concentration
1-g vial	10 ml	10.7 ml	95 mg/ml
2-g vial	20 ml	21.4 ml	95 mg/ml
10-g vial	30 ml	37 ml	1 g/3.5 ml
	45 ml	51 ml	1 g/5 ml

Piggy-back vials should be reconstituted with 50–100 ml of any of the above solutions. Shake well, and administer as a single dose with primary IV fluids. Reconstituted solution is stable for 24 h at room temperature or 4 d if refrigerated; discard solution after allotted time.

Infusion: If given as part of combination therapy with aminoglycosides, give each antibiotic at a different site. Direct injection: administer slowly over 3–5 min directly or through tubing.

Incompatibilities: Do not mix aminoglycosides and ceftizoxime in the same IV solution.

Adverse effects
- CNS: Headache, dizziness, lethargy, paresthesias

Adverse effects in *Italics* are most common; those in **Bold** are life-threatening.

- **GI:** *Nausea, vomiting, diarrhea, anorexia, abdominal pain, flatulence,* pseudomembranous colitis, liver toxicity
- **Hematologic:** Bone marrow depression: decreased WBC, decreased platelets, decreased Hct
- **GU:** Nephrotoxicity
- **Hypersensitivity:** *Ranging from rash to fever* to anaphylaxis; serum sickness reaction
- **Local:** *Pain,* abscess at injection site; *phlebitis,* inflammation at IV site
- **Other:** *Superinfections, disulfiram-like reaction with alcohol*

Clinically important drug-drug interactions

• Increased nephrotoxicity with aminoglycosides • Increased bleeding effects if taken with oral anticoagulants • Disulfiram-like reaction may occur if alcohol is taken within 72 h after ceftizoxime administration.

Drug-lab test interferences

• Possibility of false results on tests of urine glucose using Benedict's solution, Fehling's solution, Clinitest tablets; urinary 17-ketosteroids; direct Coombs' test.

■ Nursing Considerations

Assessment
- *History:* Liver and kidney dysfunction, lactation, pregnancy
- *Physical:* Skin status, liver and kidney function test, culture of affected area, sensitivity tests

Implementation
- Culture infected area, and arrange for sensitivity tests before beginning drug therapy and during therapy if expected response is not seen.
- Divide and administer IM doses of 2 g at two different sites by deep IM injection.
- Give each antibiotic at a different site, if given as part of combination therapy with aminoglycosides.
- Discontinue drug if hypersensitivy reaction occurs.
- Have vitamin K available in case hypoprothrombinemia occurs.

Drug-specific teaching points
- Know that the following side effects may occur: stomach upset or diarrhea.
- Avoid drinking alcoholic beverages while on this drug and for 3 d after this drug has been stopped because severe reactions often occur.
- Report severe diarrhea, difficulty breathing, unusual tiredness or fatigue, pain at injection site.

☐ ceftriaxone sodium

*(sef try **ax'** one)*
Rocephin

Pregnancy Category B

Drug classes
Antibiotic
Cephalosporin (third generation)

Therapeutic actions
Bactericidal: inhibits synthesis of bacterial cell wall, causing cell death.

Indications
- Lower respiratory tract infections caused by *S. pneumoniae, S. aureus, Klebsiella, H. influenzae, E. coli, P. mirabilis, E. aerogens, Serratia maecescens, Haemophilus parainfluenzae,* Streptococcus (excluding enterococci)
- UTIs caused by *E. coli, Klebsiella, P. vulgaris, P. mirabilis, M. morganii*
- Gonorrhea caused by *N. gonorrhoeae*
- Intra-abdominal infections caused by *E. coli, K. pneumoniae*
- Pelvic inflammatory disease caused by *N. gonorrhoeae*
- Dermatologic infections caused by *S. aureus, Klebsiella, Enterobacter cloacae, P. mirabilis, S. epidermidis, P. aeruginosa, Streptococcus* (excluding enterococci)
- Septicemia caused by *E. coli, S. pneumoniae, H. influenzae, S. aureus, K. pneumoniae*
- Bone and joint infections caused by *S. aureus, Streptococci* (excluding entero-

cocci), *P. mirabilis, S. pneumoniae, E. coli, K. pneumoniae, Enterobacter*
- Meningitis caused by *H. influenzae, S. pneumoniae, N. meningitidis*
- Perioperative prophylaxis for patients undergoing coronary artery bypass surgery
- **Unlabeled use**: treatment of Lyme disease in doses of 2 g IV bid for 14 d

Contraindications/cautions
- Allergy to cephalosporins or penicillins, renal failure, lactation

Dosage
Adult: 1–2 g/d IM or IV qid or in equal divided doses bid. Do not exceed 4 g/d.
- ***Gonorrhea:*** Single 250 mg IM dose.
- ***Meningitis:*** 100 mg/kg per day in divided doses q12h. Do not exceed 4 g/d.
- ***Perioperative prophylaxis:*** 1 g $\frac{1}{2}$–1 h before surgery.

Pediatric: 50–75 mg/kg per day in divided doses q12h. Do not exceed 2 g/d.
- ***Meningitis:*** 100 mg/kg per day in divided doses q12h, with or without a loading dose of 75 mg/kg

Pharmacokinetics

Route	Onset	Peak	Duration
IV	Rapid	Immediate	15–18 h
IM	30 min	1.5–4 h	15–18 h

Metabolism: $T_{1/2}$: 5–10 h
Distribution: Crosses the placenta; enters breast milk
Excretion: Urine and bile

IV facts
Preparation: Dilute reconstituted solution for IV infusion with 50–100 ml of 5% or 10% Dextrose Injection, 5% Dextrose and 0.45% or 0.9% Sodium Chloride Injection, 0.9% Sodium Chloride Injection, 10% Invert Sugar, 5% Sodium Bicarbonate, FreAmine 111, Normosol-M in 5% Dextrose, Ionosol-B in 5% Dextrose, 5% or 10% Mannitol, Sodium Lactate. Stability of reconstituted and diluted solution depends on diluent, concentration and type of container (eg, glass, PVC); check manufacturer's inserts for specific details. Protect drug from light.

Package Size	Diluent to Add	Resulting Concentration
250-mg vial	2.4 ml	100 mg/ml
500-g vial	4.8 ml	100 mg/ml
1-g vial	9.6 ml	100 mg/ml
2-g vial	19.2 ml	100 mg/ml
Piggyback 1 g	10 ml	
Piggyback 2 g	20 ml	

Infusion: Administer by intermittent infusion. Do not mix ceftriaxone with any other antimicrobial drug.
Incompatibilities: Do not mix aminoglycosides and ceftriaxone in the same IV solution.

Adverse effects
- CNS: Headache, dizziness, lethargy, paresthesias
- GI: *Nausea, vomiting, diarrhea, anorexia, abdominal pain, flatulence*, pseudomembranous colitis, liver toxicity
- Hematologic: Bone marrow depression: decreased WBC, decreased platelets, decreased Hct
- GU: Nephrotoxicity
- Hypersensitivity: *Ranging from rash* to *fever* to anaphylaxis; serum sickness reaction
- Local: *Pain,* abscess at injection site; *phlebitis,* inflammation at IV site
- Other: *Superinfections, disulfiram-like reaction with alcohol*

Clinically important drug-drug interactions
- Increased nephrotoxicity with aminoglycosides • Increased bleeding effects if taken with oral anticoagulants • Disulfiram-like reaction may occur if alcohol is taken within 72 h after ceftriaxone administration.

Drug-lab test interferences
- Possibility of false results on tests of urine glucose using Benedict's solution, Fehling's solution, Clinitest tablets; urinary 17-ketosteroids; direct Coombs' test.

■ Nursing Considerations
Assessment
- *History:* Liver and kidney dysfunction, lactation, pregnancy

- *Physical:* Skin status, liver and kidney function test, culture of affected area, sensitivity tests

Implementation
- Culture infected area, and arrange for sensitivity tests before beginning drug therapy and during therapy if expected response is not seen.
- Reconstitute for IM use with Sterile Water for Injection, 0.9% Sodium Chloride Solution, 5% Dextrose Solution, Bacteriostatic Water with 0.9% Benzyl Alcohol, or 1% Lidocaine Solution (without epinephrine); inject deeply into a large muscle group.
- Check manufacturer's inserts for specific details. Stability of reconstituted and diluted solution depends on diluent, concentration and type of container (eg, glass, PVC).
- Protect drug from light.
- Do not mix ceftriaxone with any other antimicrobial drug.
- Monitor ceftriaxone blood levels in patients with severe renal impairment and in patients with renal and hepatic impairment.
- Have vitamin K available in case hypoprothrombinemia occurs.
- Discontinue drug if hypersensitivy reaction occurs.

Drug-specific teaching points
- Know that the following side effects may occur: stomach upset or diarrhea.
- Avoid drinking alcoholic beverages while on this drug and for 3 d after this drug has been stopped because severe reactions often occur.
- Report severe diarrhea, difficulty breathing, unusual tiredness or fatigue, pain at injection site.

☐ cefuroxime axetil

(se fyoor ox' em)
Ceftin

cefuroxime sodium
Kefurox, Zinacef

Pregnancy Category B

Drug classes
Antibiotic
Cephalosporin (second generation)

Therapeutic actions
Bactericidal: inhibits synthesis of bacterial cell wall, causing cell death.

Indications
Oral (Cefuroxime Axetil)
- Pharyngitis, tonsilitis caused by *S. pyogenes*
- Otitis media caused by *S. pneumoniae, H. influenzae, M. catarrhalis, S. pyogenes*
- Lower respiratory tract infections caused by *S. pneumoniae, H. parainfluenxae, H. influenzae*
- UTIs caused by *E. coli, K. pneumoniae*
- Dermatologic infections, including impetigo caused by *S. aureus, S. pyogenes*

Parenteral (Cefuroxime Sodium)
- Lower respiratory tract infections caused by *S. pneumoniae, S. aureus, E. coli, Klebsiella, H. influenzae, S. pyogenes*
- Dermatologic infections caused by *S. aureus, S. pyogenes, E. coli, Klebsiella, Enterobacter*
- UTIs caused by *E. coli, Klebsiella*
- Uncomplicated and disseminated gonorrhea caused by *N. gonorrhoea*
- Septicemia caused by *S. pneumoniae, S. aureus, E. coli, Klebsiella, H. influenzae*
- Meningitis caused by *S. pneumoniae, H. influenzae, S. aureus, N. meningitidis*
- Bone and joint infections caused by *S. aureus*
- Perioperative prophylaxis

Contraindications/cautions
- Allergy to cephalosporins or penicillins, renal failure, lactation

Dosage
Oral
- ***Adult and children older than 12 y:*** 250 mg bid. For severe infections, may be increased to 500 mg bid.
  - *Uncomplicated UTIs:* 125 mg bid. May be increased to 250 mg bid in severe cases.
- ***Pediatric***
  - *Younger than 12 y:* 125 mg bid.

– *Otitis media: younger than 2 y:* 125 mg bid. *Older than 2 y*: 250 mg bid.
Parenteral
- **Adult:** 750 mg–1.5 g IM or IV q8h, depending on severity of infection.
– *Uncomplicated gonorrhea:* 1.5 g IM (at two different sites) with 1 g of oral probenecid.
– *Perioperative prophylaxis:* 1.5 g IV ½–1 h prior to initial incision; then 750 mg IV or IM q8h for 24 h after surgery.
- **Pediatric**
– *Older than 3 mo:* 50–100 mg/kg per day IM or IV in divided doses q6–8h.
– *Bacterial meningitis:* 200–240 mg/kg per day IV in divided doses q6–8h.
– *Impaired renal function:* Adjust adult dosage for renal impairment by weight or age of child
- **Geriatric or adult impaired renal function**

Creatinine Clearance (ml/min)	Dosage
>20	750 mg–1.5 g q8h
10–20	750 mg q12h
<10	750 mg q24h

Pharmacokinetics

Route	Onset	Peak	Duration
IV	Rapid	Immediate	18–24 h
IM	20 min	30 min	18–24 h
PO	Varies	2 h	18–24 h

Metabolism: $T_{1/2}$: 1–2 h
Distribution: Crosses the placenta; enters breast milk
Excretion: Urine

IV facts
Preparation: Preparation of parenteral drug solutions and suspensions differs for different starting preparations and different brand names; check the manufacturer's directions carefully. Reconstitute parenteral drug with Sterile Water for Injection, 5% Dextrose in Water, 0.9% Sodium Chloride, or any of the following, which also may be used for further dilution: 0.9% Sodium Chloride, 5% or 10% Dextrose Injection, 5% Dextrose and 0.45% or 0.9% Sodium Chloride Injection, or M/6 Sodium Lactate Injection. Stability of solutions depends on diluent and concentration: Check manufacturer's specifications. **Do not mix** with IV solutions containing aminoglycosides. Powder form, solutions, and suspensions darken during storage.

Infusion: Inject slowly over 3–5 minutes directly into vein for IV administration, or infuse. Administer aminoglycosides and cefuroxime at different sites.

Incompatibilities: Do not mix aminoglycosides and cefuroxime in the same IV solution.

Adverse effects
- CNS: Headache, dizziness, lethargy, paresthesias
- GI: *Nausea, vomiting, diarrhea, anorexia, abdominal pain, flatulence*, pseudomembranous colitis, liver toxicity
- Hematologic: Bone marrow depression: decreased WBC, decreased platelets, decreased Hct
- GU: Nephrotoxicity
- Hypersensitivity: *Ranging from rash* to *fever* to anaphylaxis, serum sickness reaction
- Local: *Pain*, abscess at injection site; *phlebitis*, inflammation at IV site
- Other: *Superinfections, disulfiram-like reaction with alcohol*

Clinically important drug-drug interactions
- Increased nephrotoxicity with aminoglycosides • Increased bleeding effects if taken with oral anticoagulants • Disulfiram-like reaction may occur if alcohol is taken within 72 h after cefuroxime administration.

Drug-lab test interferences
- Possibility of false results on tests of urine glucose using Benedict's solution, Fehling's solution, Clinitest tablets; urinary 17-ketosteroids; direct Coombs' test.

■ Nursing Considerations
Assessment
- *History:* Liver and kidney dysfunction, lactation, pregnancy

248 ■ cellulose sodium phosphate

- *Physical:* Skin status, liver and kidney function test, culture of affected area, sensitivity tests

Implementation
- Culture infected area, and arrange for sensitivity tests before beginning drug therapy and during therapy if expected response is not seen.
- Administer oral drug with food to decrease GI upset and enhance absorption.
- Administer oral drug to children who can swallow tablets; crushing the drug results in a bitter, unpleasant taste.
- Have vitamin K available in case hypoprothrombinemia occurs.
- Discontinue drug if hypersensitivy reaction occurs.

Drug-specific teaching points for parenteral drug
- Know that the following side effects may occur: stomach upset or diarrhea.
- Avoid drinking alcoholic beverages while on this drug and for 3 d after this drug has been stopped because severe reactions often occur.
- Report severe diarrhea, difficulty breathing, unusual tiredness or fatigue, pain at injection site.

Drug-specific teaching points for oral drug
- Take full course of therapy.
- Be aware that this drug is specific for this infection and should not be used to self-treat other problems.
- Swallow tablets whole; do not crush. Take the drug with food.
- Know that the following side effects may occur: stomach upset or diarrhea.
- Report severe diarrhea with blood, pus, or mucus; rash; difficulty breathing; unusual tiredness, fatigue; unusual bleeding or bruising; unusual itching or irritation.

❒ cellulose sodium phosphate

(sell' u loos)
CSP, Calcibind, Calcisorb (CAN)

Pregnancy Category C

Drug classes
Antilithic
Resin exchange agent
Cation

Therapeutic actions
Binds calcium and magnesium in the bowel; promotes the excretion of calcium and reduces serum calcium levels, decreasing the formation of renal calculi.

Indications
- Absorptive hypercalciuria Type I (recurrent passage or formation of calcium oxalate or calcium phosphate renal stones not eliminated by diet)
- **Unlabeled uses**: adjunct in the treatment of hypercalcemia, management of calcinosis cutis

Contraindications/cautions
- Contraindicated in the presence of primary or secondary hyperparathyroidism; high fasting urinary calcium or hypophosphatemia; pregnancy; children.
- Use with caution in the presence of CHF, ascites, nephrotic syndrome.

Dosage
Adult: Initial dose of 15 g/d PO (5 g with each meal) in patients with urinary calcium > 300 mg/d; when urinary calcium declines to < 150 mg/d, reduce to 10 g/d (5 g with supper and 2.5 g with two other meals). Patients with urinary calcium < 300 mg/d but > 200 mg/d, 10 g/d.
Pediatric: Safety and efficacy not established.

Pharmacokinetics
Not absorbed systemically.

Adverse effects
- GI: *Bad taste, loose stools, diarrhea, dyspepsia*
- Other: *Decreased magnesium levels*

■ Nursing Considerations
Assessment
- *History:* Primary or secondary hyperparathyroidism; high fasting urinary calcium or hypophosphatemia; lactation; CHF, ascites, nephrotic syndrome

Adverse effects in *Italics* are most common; those in **Bold** are life-threatening.

- *Physical:* Body weight, skin condition, neurologic status, abdominal exam, urinary calcium, serum electrolytes

Implementation
- Administer drug with meals.
- Arrange for supplemental magnesium gluconate while receiving this drug. Those receiving 15 g CSP/d should receive 1.5 g magnesium gluconate before breakfast and again at bedtime. Those receiving 10 g CSP/d should receive 1 g magnesium gluconate twice a day. Administer magnesium 1 h before or 2 h after CSP to prevent binding.
- Suspend each dose of CSP powder in a glass of water, soft drink, or fruit juice. Administer 1 h before meal.
- Monitor 24-h urinary calcium levels periodically during therapy; arrange for dosage adjustment accordingly.
- Arrange for dietary consultation to help patient moderate calcium intake and dietary oxalate intake.
- Encourage patient to increase fluid intake each day.

Drug-specific teaching points
- Take drug 1 h before meals as ordered. Take the magnesium supplement 1 h before the CSP; suspend each dose of the drug in a glass of water, soft drink, or fruit juice.
- Avoid the use of vitamin C supplements while on this drug.
- Try to drink as much fluid per day as tolerable while on this drug.
- Moderate your calcium intake (dairy products), oxalate intake (spinach, rhubarb, chocolate, brewed tea), salt intake while on this drug.
- Know that the following side effects may occur: bad taste, loose stools, diarrhea, indigestion.
- Report swelling of extremities, tremors, palpitations

☐ cephalexin

*(sef a **lex**' in)*

Apo-Cephalex (CAN), Keflex, Novo-Lexin (CAN), Nu-Cephalex (CAN)

cephalexin hydrochloride monohydrate

Biocef, Cefanex, Keftab, Zartan

Pregnancy Category B

Drug classes
Antibiotic
Cephalosporin (first generation)

Therapeutic actions
Bactericidal: inhibits synthesis of bacterial cell wall, causing cell death.

Indications
- Respiratory tract infections caused by *S. pneumoniae,* group A β-hemolytic streptococci
- Dermatologic infections caused by staphylococci, streptococci
- Otitis media caused by *S. pneumoniae, H. influenzae,* streptococci, staphylococci, *M. catarrhalis*
- Bone infections caused by staphylococci, *P. mirabilis*
- GU infections caused by *E. coli, P. mirabilis, Klebsiella*

Contraindications/cautions
- Allergy to cephalosporins or penicillins; renal failure; lactation

Dosage
Adult: 1–4 g/d in divided dose; 250 mg PO q6h usual dose.
- ***Skin and skin-structure infections:*** 500 mg PO q12h. Larger doses may be needed in severe cases; *do not exceed* 4 g/d.

Pediatric: 25–50 mg/kg per day PO in divided doses.
- ***Skin and skin-structure infections:*** Divide total daily dose, and give q12h. Dosage may be doubled in severe cases.
- ***Otitis media:*** 75–100 mg/kg per day PO in four divided doses. Safety and efficacy of cephalexin hydrochloride monohydrate not established for children.

Pharmacokinetics

Route	Peak	Duration
PO	60 min	8–10 h

Metabolism: $T_{1/2}$: 50–80 min
Distribution: Crosses the placenta, enters breast milk
Excretion: Renal

Adverse effects

- **CNS:** Headache, dizziness, lethargy, paresthesias
- **GI:** *Nausea, vomiting, diarrhea, anorexia, abdominal pain, flatulence,* **pseudomembranous colitis,** liver toxicity
- **Hematologic:** Bone marrow depression
- **GU:** Nephrotoxicity
- **Hypersensitivity:** *Ranging from rash to fever* to **anaphylaxis;** serum sickness reaction
- **Other:** *Superinfections*

Clinically important drug-drug interactions

- Increased nephrotoxicity with aminoglycosides • Increased bleeding effects if taken with oral anticoagulants • Disulfiram-like reaction may occur if alcohol is taken within 72 h after cephalexin administration.

Drug-lab test interferences

- Possibility of false results on tests of urine glucose using Benedict's solution, Fehling's solution, Clinitest tablets; urinary 17-ketosteroids; direct Coombs' test.

■ Nursing Considerations

Assessment

- *History:* Penicillin or cephalosporin allergy, pregnancy or lactation
- *Physical:* Kidney function, respiratory status, skin status; culture and sensitivity tests of infected area

Implementation

- Arrange for culture and sensitivity tests of infected area before beginning drug therapy and during therapy if infection does not resolve.
- Give drug with meals; arrange for small, frequent meals if GI complications occur.
- Refrigerate suspension, and discard after 14 d.

Drug-specific teaching points

- Take this drug with meals or food. Refrigerate suspension; discard any drug after 14 d.
- Complete the full course of this drug, even if you feel better before the course of treatment is over.
- Be aware that this drug is prescribed for this particular infection; do not self-treat any other infection with this drug.
- Know that the following side effects may occur: stomach upset, loss of appetite, nausea (taking the drug with food may help); diarrhea (stay near bathroom facilities); headache, dizziness.
- Report severe diarrhea with blood, pus, or mucus; rash or hives; difficulty breathing; unusual tiredness, fatigue; unusual bleeding or bruising.

▢ cephalothin sodium

(sef a' loe thin)
Keflin

Pregnancy Category B

Drug classes
Antibiotic
Cephalosporin (first generation)

Therapeutic actions
Bactericidal: inhibits synthesis of bacterial cell wall, causing cell death.

Indications

- Respiratory tract infections caused by *S. pneumoniae,* staphylococci, group A β-hemolytic streptococci, *Klebsiella, H. influenzae*
- Dermatologic infections caused by staphylococci, group A β-hemolytic streptococci, *E. coli, P. mirabilis,, Klebsiella*
- GU infections caused by *E. coli, P. mirabilis, Klebsiella*

cephalothin sodium ■ 251

- Septicemia caused by *S. pneumoniae*, staphylococci, group A β-hemolytic streptocci, *S. viridans, E. coli, P. mirabilis, Klebsiella*
- GI infections caused by *Salmonella, Shigella*
- Meningitis caused by *S. pneumoniae*, group A β-hemolytic streptococci, staphylococci
- Bone and joint infections caused by staphylococci
- Perioperative prophylaxis

Contraindications/cautions
- Allergy to cephalosporins or penicillins, renal failure, lactation

Dosage
Adult: 500 mg–1 g IM or IV q4–6h, depending on severity of infection (up to 2 g q4h in life-threatening infections).
- ***Perioperative prophylaxis:*** 1–2 g $\frac{1}{2}$–1 h before initial incision; 1–2 g during surgery; 1–2 g q6h for 24 h after surgery.

Pediatric: Usual dose 100 mg/kg per day (range 80–160 mg/kg per day) IM or IV in divided doses.
- ***Perioperative prophylaxis:*** 20–30 mg/kg $\frac{1}{2}$–1 h before initial incision; 20–30 mg/kg during surgery; 20–30 mg/kg q6h for 24 h after surgery.

Geriatric or impaired renal function: IV loading dose of 1–2 g. Maximum maintenance dosages are:

Creatinine Clearance (ml/min)	Maximum Dosage
50–80	2 g q6h
25–50	1.5 g q6h
10–25	1 g q6h
2–10	0.5 g q6h
<2	0.5 g q8h

Pharmacokinetics

Route	Onset	Peak	Duration
IV	Rapid	15 min	18–24 h
IM	20 min	30 min	18–24 h

Metabolism: $T_{1/2}$: 30–50 min

Distribution: Crosses the placenta; enters breast milk
Excretion: Urine

IV facts
Preparation: Dilute 1–2 g with at least 10 ml of Sterile Water for Injection and add to Acetated Ringer's Injection, 5% Dextrose Injection, 5% Dextrose in Lactated Ringer's Injection, Ionosol B in D5W, Isolyte M with 5% Dextrose, Lactated Ringer's Injection, Normosol-M in D5-W, Plasma-Lyte Injection, Plasma-Lyte-M in 5% Dextrose, Ringer's Injection, or 0.9% Sodium Chloride Injection. Concentrated solutions darken slightly at room temperature. Use IV infusions within 12 h, and complete use within 24 h. Discard solution after 24 h; solution is stable for 4 d if refrigerated. Redissolve prepared solution by warming to room temperature and agitating slightly.

Infusion: Administer intermittent IV injection by slowly injecting a solution of 1 g in 10 ml diluent directly into the vein over 3–5 min or inject into IV tubing.

Incompatibilities: Do not mix aminoglycosides and cephalothin in the same IV solution.

Adverse effects
- CNS: Headache, dizziness, lethargy, paresthesias
- GI: *Nausea, vomiting, diarrhea, anorexia, abdominal pain, flatulence*, pseudomembranous colitis, liver toxicity
- Hematologic: Bone marrow depression: decreased WBC, decreased platelets, decreased Hct
- GU: Nephrotoxicity
- Hypersensitivity: *Ranging from rash* to *fever* to anaphylaxis; serum sickness reaction
- Local: *Pain,* abscess at injection site; *phlebitis,* inflammation at IV site
- Other: *Superinfections, disulfiram-like reaction with alcohol*

Clinically important drug-drug interactions
- Increased nephrotoxicity with aminoglycosides • Increased bleeding effects if taken

Adverse effects in *Italics* are most common; those in **Bold** are life-threatening.

252 ■ cephapirin sodium

with oral anticoagulants • Disulfiram-like reaction may occur if alcohol is taken within 72 h after cephalothin administration.

Drug-lab test interferences
- Possibility of false results on tests of urine glucose using Benedict's solution, Fehling's solution, Clinitest tablets; urinary 17-ketosteroids; direct Coombs' test, creatinine levels.

■ **Nursing Considerations**

Assessment
- *History:* Liver and kidney dysfunction, lactation, pregnancy
- *Physical:* Skin status, liver and kidney function test, culture of affected area, sensitivity tests

Implementation
- Culture infected area, and arrange for sensitivity tests before beginning drug therapy and during therapy if expected response is not seen.
- Add 6 mg/100 ml cephalothin to peritoneal dialysis solution, and instill into the peritoneum if necessary.
- Prepare for IM injection as follows: Reconstitute each gram with 4 ml Sterile Water; if contents do not dissolve, add 0.2–0.4 ml diluent, and warm gently; use within 12 h.
- Administer IM injections deeply into large muscle mass.
- Arrange for patient to have yogurt or buttermilk if diarrhea occurs.
- Arrange for oral vancomycin for severe colitis that does not respond to discontinuation of drug.
- Arrange for continuation of prophylactic dose for 3–5 d if postoperative site shows signs of infection; do culture and sensitivity tests on site and arrange for change of antibiotic as appropriate.

Drug-specific teaching points
- Know that the following side effects may occur: stomach upset or diarrhea, headache, dizziness.
- Avoid drinking alcoholic beverages while on this drug and for 3 d after this drug has been stopped because severe reactions often occur.

- Report severe diarrhea, difficulty breathing, unusual tiredness or fatigue, pain at injection site.

❒ cephapirin sodium

(sef a pye' rin)
Cefadyl

Pregnancy Category B

Drug classes
Antibiotic
Cephalosporin (first generation)

Therapeutic actions
Bactericidal: inhibits synthesis of bacterial cell wall, causing cell death.

Indications
- Respiratory tract infections caused by *S. pneumoniae, S. aureus,* group A β-hemolytic streptococci, *Klebsiella, H. influenzae*
- Dermatologic infections caused by *S. aureus,* group A β-hemolytic streptococci, *E. coli, P. mirabilis, Klebsiella, S. epidermidis*
- GU infections caused by *S. aureus, E. coli, P. mirabilis, Klebsiella*
- Septicemia caused by *S. aureus,* group A β-hemolytic streptococci, *S. viridans, E. coli, Klebsiella*
- Endocarditis caused by *S. viridans, S. aureus*
- Osteomyelitis caused by *S. aureus, Klebsiella, P. mirabilis,* group A β-hemolytic streptococci
- Perioperative prophylaxis

Contraindications/cautions
- Allergy to cephalosporins or penicillins, renal failure, lactation.

Dosage
Adult: 500 mg–1 g IM or IV q4–6h, depending on severity of infection; up to 12 g daily in severe cases.
- *Perioperative prophylaxis:* 1–2 g ½–1 h before initial incision; 1–2 g during surgery; 1–2 g q6h for 24 h after surgery or up to 3–5 d.

cephapirin sodium ■ 253

Pediatric: 40–80 mg/kg per day IM or IV in four divided doses. **Do not use in infants younger than 3 mo.**

- ***Perioperative prophylaxis:*** Reduce adult dose according to body weight or age (see Appendix III for formulas).

Geriatric or renal impaired: Serum creatinine > 5 mg/100 ml, 7.5–15 mg/kg q12h.

Pharmacokinetics

Route	Onset	Peak	Duration
IV	Rapid	5 min	6–8 h
IM	10 min	30 min	6–8 h

Metabolism: $T_{1/2}$: 24–36 min
Distribution: Crosses the placenta; enters breast milk
Excretion: Urine

IV facts

Preparation: Prepare IV intermittent doses, reconstituting 500 mg or 1- to 2-g vial with 10 ml diluent. Stability of diluted IV solutions varies: See manufacturer's inserts. Prepare IV doses with compatible solutions: Sodium Chloride Injection; 5% Sodium Chloride in Water; 5%, 10%, 20% Dextrose in Water; Sodium Lactate Injection; 10% Invert Sugar in Normal Saline or Water; 5% Lactated Ringer's Injection; Lactated Ringer's with 5% Dextrose; Ringer's Injection; Sterile Water for Injection; 5% Dextrose in Ringer's Injection; Normosol R; Normosol R in 5% Dextrose Injection; Ionosol D-CM; Ionosol G in 10% Dextrose Injection.

Infusion: Inject intermittent dose slowly over 3–5 min. If giving cephapirin IV piggyback, stop the other infusion while the cephapirin is being infused. Administer aminoglycosides and cefuroxime at different sites.

Incompatibilities: Do not mix aminoglycosides and cephapirin in the same IV solution.

Adverse effects

- CNS: Headache, dizziness, lethargy, paresthesias
- GI: *Nausea, vomiting, diarrhea, anorexia, abdominal pain, flatulence,* pseudomembranous colitis, liver toxicity
- Hematologic: Bone marrow depression: decreased WBC, decreased platelets, decreased Hct
- GU: Nephrotoxicity
- Hypersensitivity: *Ranging from rash* to *fever* to anaphylaxis; serum sickness reaction
- Local: *Pain,* abscess at injection site; *phlebitis,* inflammation at IV site
- Other: *Superinfections, disulfiram-like reaction with alcohol*

Clinically important drug-drug interactions

- Increased nephrotoxicity with aminoglycosides • Increased bleeding effects if taken with oral anticoagulants • Disulfiram-like reaction if alcohol is taken within 72 h after cephapirin administration

Drug-lab test interferences

- Possibility of false results on tests of urine glucose using Benedict's solution, Fehling's solution, Clinitest tablets; urinary 17-ketosteroids; direct Coombs' test.

■ Nursing Considerations

Assessment

- *History:* Liver and kidney dysfunction, lactation, pregnancy
- *Physical:* Skin status, liver and kidney function test, culture of affected area, sensitivity tests

Implementation

- Culture infected area, and arrange for sensitivity tests before beginning drug therapy and during therapy if expected response is not seen.
- Prepare IM solution as follows: reconstitute 500-mg vials with 1 ml of Sterile Water for Injection or Bacteriostatic Water for Injection; reconstitute 1-g vials with 2 ml of diluent; each 1.2 ml contains 500 mg cephapirin.
- Administer IM injections deeply into large muscle mass.
- Have vitamin K available in case hypoprothrombinemia occurs.

Adverse effects in *Italics* are most common; those in **Bold** are life-threatening.

- Discontinue drug if hypersensitivy reaction occurs.

Drug-specific teaching points
- Know that the following side effects may occur: stomach upset or diarrhea.
- Avoid drinking alcoholic beverages while on this drug and for 3 d after this drug has been stopped because severe reactions often occur.
- Report severe diarrhea, difficulty breathing, unusual tiredness or fatigue, pain at injection site.

cephradine

(sef ra deen)
Velosef

Pregnancy Category B

Drug classes
Antibiotic
Cephalosporin (first generation)

Therapeutic actions
Bactericidal: inhibits synthesis of bacterial cell wall, causing cell death.

Indications
Oral Use
- Respiratory tract infections caused by group A β-hemolytic streptococci, *S. pneumoniae*
- Otitis media caused by group A β-hemolytic streptococci, *S. pneumoniae, H. influenzae,* and staphylococci
- Dermatologic infections caused by staphylococci and β-hemolytic streptococci
- UTIs caused by *E. coli, P. mirabilis, Klebsiella,* enterococci

Parenteral Use
- Respiratory tract infections caused by *S. pneumoniae, Klebsiella, H. influenzae, S. aureus,* and group A β-hemolytic streptococci
- UTIs caused by *E. coli, P. mirabilis, Klebsiella*
- Dermatologic infections caused by *S. aureus,* group A β-hemolytic streptococci
- Bone infections caused by *S. aureus*
- Septicemia caused by *S. pneumoniae, S. aureus, P. mirabilis, E. coli*
- Perioperative prophylaxis

Contraindications/cautions
- Allergy to cephalosporins or penicillins, renal failure, lactation

Dosage
Adult: 250–500 mg PO q6–12h (dose depends on the severity of infection); 2–4 g/d IV or IM in equal divided doses qid.
- ***Perioperative prophylaxis:*** 1 g IV or IM 30–90 min before surgery; then 1 g q4–6h for up to 24 h.
- ***Cesarean section:*** 1 g IV as soon as cord is clamped; then 1 g IM or IV at 6 and 12 h.

Pediatric
- ***Older than 9 mo:*** 25–50 mg/kg per day in equally divided doses PO q6–12h.
- ***Otitis media:*** 75–100 mg/kg per day PO in equal divided doses q6–12h. **Do not exceed 4 g/d.** 50–100 mg/kg per day IV or IM in four equally divided doses.

Geriatric or reduced renal function: Loading dose of 1 g and then maintenance dosage as follows:

CCr (ml/min)	Dosage
>20	500 mg q6h
5–20	250 mg q6h
<5	250 mg q12h

Pharmacokinetics

Route	Onset	Peak	Duration
IV	Rapid	5 min	6–8 h
IM	20 min	1–2 h	6–8 h
PO	Varies	1 h	6–8 h

Metabolism: $T_{1/2}$: 48–80 min
Distribution: Crosses the placenta; enters breast milk
Excretion: Urine

IV facts
Preparation: Prepare for direct IV injections by diluting drug with Sterile Water for Injection, 5% Dextrose Injection, or Sodium Chloride Injection using 5 ml with the 250- to 500-mg vials, 10 ml with the 1-g vial, or 20 ml with the 2-g vial. Prepare for IV

cephradine ■ 255

infusion as follows: add 10, 20, or 40 ml Sterile Water for Injection to 1-, 2-, or 4-g preparations; withdraw and dilute further with 5% or 10% Dextrose Injection, Sodium Chloride Injection, M/6 Sodium Lactate, Dextrose and Sodium Chloride Injection, 10% Invert Sugar in Water, Normosol-R, or Ionosol B with 5% Dextrose. Use direct IV solutions within 2 h at room temperature. IV infusion solution is stable for 10 h at room temperature or 48 h if refrigerated; for prolonged infusions replace solution every 10 h. Protect solutions from light or direct sunlight.

Infusion: Inject direct IV slowly over 3–5 min, or give through IV tubing.

Incompatibilities: Do not mix cephradine with any other antibiotic. Do not use with Lactated Ringer's Injection.

Adverse effects

- CNS: Headache, dizziness, lethargy, paresthesias
- GI: *Nausea, vomiting, diarrhea, anorexia, abdominal pain, flatulence,* pseudomembranous colitis, liver toxicity
- Hematologic: Bone marrow depression: decreased WBC, decreased platelets, decreased Hct
- GU: Nephrotoxicity
- Hypersensitivity: *Ranging from rash* to *fever* to anaphylaxis; serum sickness reaction
- Local: *Pain,* abscess at injection site; *phlebitis,* inflammation at IV site
- Other: *Superinfections, disulfiram-like reaction with alcohol*

Clinically important drug-drug interactions

- Increased nephrotoxicity with aminoglycosides • Increased bleeding effects if taken with oral anticoagulants • Disulfiram-like reaction may occur if alcohol is taken within 72 h after cephradine administration.

Drug-lab test interferences

- Possibility of false results on tests of urine glucose using Benedict's solution, Fehling's solution, Clinitest tablets; urinary 17-ketosteroids; direct Coombs' test.

■ Nursing Considerations

Assessment
- *History:* Liver and kidney dysfunction, lactation, pregnancy
- *Physical:* Skin status, liver and kidney function test, culture of affected area, sensitivity tests

Implementation
- Culture infected area, and arrange for sensitivity tests before beginning drug therapy and during therapy if expected response is not seen.
- Prepare for IM use by reconstituting drug with Sterile Water or Bacteriostatic Water for Injection; inject deeply into large muscle group.
- Use IM solution within 2 h if stored at room temperature.
- Protect solutions from light or direct sunlight.
- Do not mix cephradine with any other antibiotic.
- Give oral drug with meals.
- Have vitamin K available in case hypoprothrombinemia occurs.
- Discontinue drug if hypersensitivy reaction occurs.

Drug-specific teaching points for parenteral drug
- Know that the following side effects may occur stomach upset or diarrhea.
- Avoid drinking alcoholic beverages while on this drug and for 3 d after this drug has been stopped because severe reactions often occur.
- Report severe diarrhea, difficulty breathing, unusual tiredness or fatigue, pain at injection site.

Drug-specific teaching points for oral drug
- Take full course of therapy.
- Be aware that this drug is specific for this infection and should not be used to self-treat other problems.
- Swallow tablets whole; do not crush. Take the drug with food.

Adverse effects in *Italics* are most common; those in **Bold** are life-threatening.

- Avoid drinking alcoholic beverages while on this drug and for 3 d after this drug has been stopped because severe reactions often occur.
- Know that the following side effects may occur: stomach upset or diarrhea.
- Report severe diarrhea with blood, pus, or mucus; rash; difficulty breathing; unusual tiredness, fatigue; unusual bleeding or bruising; unusual itching or irritation.

charcoal, activated

(char' kole)

Actidose-Aqua, Actidose with Sorbitol, Activated Charcoal, Charcoaid, Charcodote (Can), Liqui-Char

Pregnancy Category C

Drug classes
Antidote

Therapeutic actions
Adsorbs toxic substances swallowed into the GI tract, inhibiting GI absorption; maximum amount of toxin absorbed is 100–1,000 mg/g charcoal.

Indications
- Emergency treatment in poisoning by most drugs and chemicals

Contraindications/cautions
- Poisoning or overdosage of cyanide, mineral acids, alkalies, ethanol, methanol, and iron salts

Dosage
Adult: 30–100 g or 1 g/kg or approximately 5–10 times the amount of poison ingested, as an oral suspension; administer as soon as possible after poisoning.
- *Gastric dialysis:* 20–40 g q6h for 1–2 d may be used for severe poisonings; for optimum effect, administer within 30 min of poisoning.

Pharmacokinetics
Not absorbed systemically. Excreted in the feces.

Adverse effects
- **GI:** *Vomiting* (related to rapid ingestion of high doses), *constipation, diarrhea,* black stools

Clinically important drug-drug interactions
- Adsorption and inactivation of syrup of ipecac, laxatives if taken with activated charcoal • Decreased effectiveness of other medications when used with charcoal because of the adsorption by activated charcoal

■ Nursing Considerations
Assessment
- *History:* Poisoning or overdosage of cyanide, mineral acids, alkalies, ethanol, methanol, and iron salts
- *Physical:* Stools, bowel sounds

Implementation
- Induce emesis before administering activated charcoal.
- Administer drug to conscious patients only.
- Administer drug as soon after poisoning as possible; most effective results are seen if administered within 30 min.
- Prepare suspension of powder in 6–8 oz of water; taste may be gritty and disagreeable. Sorbitol is added to some preparations to improve taste; diarrhea more likely with these preparations.
- Store in closed containers; activated charcoal adsorbs gases from the air and will lose its effectiveness with prolonged exposure to air.
- Maintain life-support equipment on standby for poisoning and overdose.

Drug-specific teaching points
- Know that the following side effects may occur: black stools, diarrhea or constipation.

chenodiol

*(kee noe **dye'** ole)*
chenodeoxycholic acid

Pregnancy Category X

Adverse effects in *Italics* are most common; those in **Bold** are life-threatening.

Drug classes
Gallstone-solubilizing agent

Therapeutic actions
Suppresses hepatic synthesis of cholesterol and cholic acid, leading to cholesterol in the bile and dissolution of cholesterol gallstones.

Indications
- Treatment of selected patients with radiolucent gallstones in well-opacifying gallbladders when elective surgery is contraindicated

Contraindications/cautions
- Allergy to chenodiol, hepatic dysfunction, bile ductal abnormalities, pregnancy, lactation

Dosage
Adult: 13–16 mg/kg per day PO in two divided doses, morning and night. Start with 250 mg bid for 2 wk, and increase by 250 mg/d each week thereafter until the recommended dose is reached.
Pediatric: Safety and efficacy not established.

Pharmacokinetics

Route	Onset	Peak	Duration
Oral	Varies	15–14 min	2–4 h

Metabolism: Hepatic; $T_{1/2}$: 3.1 min, then 16½ min
Distribution: Crosses placenta; may pass into breast milk
Excretion: Feces

Adverse effects
- **GI:** Increased incidence of intrahepatic cholestasis; *hepatitis; elevated SGPT, diarrhea, cramps,* heartburn, constipation, nausea, vomiting, anorexia, epigastric distress, dyspepsia, flatulence, abdominal pain
- **Hematologic:** *Elevated serum total cholesterol, LDL;* decreased serum triglycerides; decreased WBC count
- Other: **Colon cancer**

Clinically important drug-drug interactions
- Decreased absorption of chenodiol if taken with bile acid sequestering agents (cholestyramine, colestipol) • Reduced absorption of acetaminophen, barbiturates, carbamazepine, digitoxin, digoxin, furosemide, glutethimide, hydantoins, methotrexate, nizatidine, phenothiazines, phenylbutazones, propoxyphene, salicylates, sulfones, sulfonylureas, tetracyclines, theophyllines, tricyclic antidepressants, valproic acid

■ Nursing Considerations
Assessment
- *History:* Allergy to chenodiol, hepatic dysfunction, bile ductal abnormalities, pregnancy, lactation
- *Physical:* Liver evaluation, abdominal exam; liver function tests, serum lipids, WBC, serum aminotransferase, serum cholesterol; hepatic and biliary radiologic studies

Implementation
- Administer drug twice a day, in the morning and at night.
- Arrange for periodic, regular monitoring of serum aminotransferase levels, serum cholesterol.
- Arrange for patient to be scheduled for periodic oral cholecystograms or ultrasonograms to evaluate drug effectiveness.
- Caution patient to use birth control while taking this drug; the drug can cause serious problems for the fetus.

Drug-specific teaching points
- Take this drug twice a day in the morning and at night. Continue to take the drug as long as prescribed.
- Be aware that this drug may dissolve the gallstones that you have now; it does not "cure" the problem that caused the stones in the first place, and in many cases the stones can recur; medical follow-up is important.
- Use birth control methods while on this drug; this drug must not be taken by pregnant women. If you think that you have become pregnant, consult with your physician immediately.
- Arrange to receive periodic x-rays or ultrasound tests of your gallbladder; you also will need periodic blood tests to

Adverse effects in *Italics* are most common; those in **Bold** are life-threatening.

evaluate your response to this drug. These tests are important, and you should make every effort to keep follow-up appointments.
- Know that the following side effects may occur: diarrhea (if this becomes a serious problem, consult with your nurse or physician about changing your dose); nausea, GI upset, flatulence (small, frequent meals may help).
- Report gallstone attacks (abdominal pain, nausea, vomiting); yellowing of the skin or eyes.

chloral hydrate

(klor' al hye' drate)
Aquachloral Supprettes

Pregnancy Category C
C-IV controlled substance

Drug classes
Sedative/hypnotic (nonbarbiturate)

Therapeutic actions
Mechanism by which CNS is affected is not known; hypnotic dosage produces mild cerebral depression and quiet, deep sleep; does not depress REM sleep, produces less "hangover" than most barbiturates and benzodiazepines.

Indications
- Nocturnal sedation
- Preoperative sedation to lessen anxiety and induce sleep without depressing respiration or cough reflex
- Adjunct to opiates and analgesics in postoperative care and control of pain

Contraindications/cautions
- Contraindicated in the presence of hypersensitivity to chloral derivatives; allergy to tartrazine (in 324-mg suppositories marketed as *Aquachloral Supprettes*); severe cardiac disease, gastritis; hepatic or renal impairment; lactation.
- Use caution in the presence of acute intermittent porphyria (may precipitate attacks).

Dosage
Adult: Single doses or daily dosage should not exceed 2 g.
- ***Hypnotic:*** 500 mg–1 g PO or rectally 15–30 min before bedtime or 30 min before surgery (*Note:* it is not usually considered safe practice to administer oral medication to patients who are NPO for anesthesia or surgery).
- ***Sedative:*** 250 mg PO or rectally tid after meals.

Pediatric
- ***Hypnotic:*** 50 mg/kg per day PO up to 1 g per single dose; may be given in divided doses.
- ***Sedative:*** 25 mg/kg per day PO up to 500 mg per single dose; may be given in divided doses.

Pharmacokinetics

Route	Onset	Peak	Duration
Oral/PR	30–60 min	1–3 h	4–8 h

Metabolism: Hepatic; $T_{1/2}$: 7–10 h
Distribution: Crosses placenta; passes into breast milk
Excretion: Urine and bile

Adverse effects
- CNS: *Somnambulism, disorientation, incoherence, paranoid behavior,* excitement, delirium, drowsiness, staggering gait, ataxia, lightheadedness, vertigo, nightmares, malaise, mental confusion, headache, hallucinations
- GI: *Gastric irritation, nausea, vomiting,* **gastric necrosis** (following intoxicating doses), flatulence, diarrhea, unpleasant taste
- Hematologic: *Leukopenia, eosinophilia*
- Dermatologic: *Skin irritation*; allergic skin rashes including hives, erythema, eczematoid dermatitis, urticaria
- Other: Physical, psychological dependence; tolerance; withdrawal reaction

Clinically important drug-drug interactions
- Additive CNS depression when given with **alcohol,** other CNS depressants • Mutual inhibition of metabolism with alcohol (may

Adverse effects in *Italics* are most common; those in **Bold** are life-threatening.

develop a vasodilation reaction charaterized by tachycardia, palpitations, and facial flushing) • Complex effects on oral (coumarin) anticoagulants given with chloral hydrate (monitor prothrombin levels and adjust coumarin dosage accordingly whenever chloral hydrate is instituted or withdrawn from the drug regimen)

Drug-lab test interferences
• Interference with the copper sulfate test for glycosuria, fluorometric tests for urine catecholamines, and urinary 17-hydroxycorticosteroid determinations (when using the Reddy, Jenkins, and Thorn procedure)

■ Nursing Considerations

Assessment
- *History:* Hypersensitivity to chloral derivatives, allergy to tartrazine, severe cardiac disease, gastritis, hepatic or renal impairment, acute intermittent porphyria, lactation
- *Physical:* Skin—color, lesions; orientation, affect, reflexes; P, BP, perfusion; bowel sounds, normal output, liver evaluation; liver and kidney function tests, CBC and differential, stool guaiac test

Implementation
- Give capsules with a full glass of liquid; ensure that patient swallows capsules whole; give syrup in half glass of water, fruit juice, or ginger ale.
- Supervise carefully dose and amount of drug prescribed for patients who are addiction prone or alcoholic; dispense least amount of drug feasible to patients who are depressed or suicidal.
- Withdraw gradually over 2 wk if patient has been maintained on high doses for weeks or months; if patient has built up high tolerance, withdrawal should be undertaken in a hospital, using supportive therapy similar to that for withdrawal from barbiturates; fatal withdrawal reactions have occurred.
- Arrange for reevaluation of patients with prolonged insomnia; therapy of the underlying cause of insomnia (eg, pain, depression) is preferable to prolonged therapy with sedative–hypnotic drugs.

Drug-specific teaching points
- Take this drug exactly as prescribed: Swallow capsules whole with a full glass of liquid (take syrup in half glass of water, fruit juice, or ginger ale).
- Do not discontinue the drug abruptly. Consult your care provider if you wish to discontinue the drug before you are instructed to do so.
- Avoid alcohol, sleep-inducing, or OTC drugs while you are on this drug; these could cause dangerous effects.
- Know that the following side effects may occur: drowsiness, dizziness, lightheadedness (avoid driving a car or performing other tasks requiring alertness if these occur); GI upset (frequent small meals may help); sleep-walking, nightmares, confusion (use caution if these occur, eg, close doors, keep medications out of reach so inadvertent overdose does not occur while confused).
- Report skin rash, coffee ground vomitus, black or tarry stools, severe GI upset, fever, sore throat.

☐ chlorambucil

*(klor **am**' byoo sil)*
Leukeran

Pregnancy Category D

Drug classes
Alkylating agent, nitrogen mustard
Antineoplastic drug

Therapeutic actions
Cytotoxic: alkylates cellular DNA, interfering with the replication of susceptible cells.

Indications
- Palliative treatment of chronic lymphocytic leukemia; malignant lymphomas, including lymphosarcoma; giant follicular lymphoma; and Hodgkin's disease
- **Unlabeled uses:** treatment of uveitis and meningoencephalitis associated with Behçet's disease; treatment of idiopathic membranous nephropathy; treatment of rheumatoid arthritis

Contraindications/cautions
- Allergy to chlorambucil; cross-sensitization with melphalen; radiation therapy, chemotherapy; hematopoietic depression; pregnancy, lactation.

Dosage
Individualize dosage based on hematologic profile and response.
Adult
- ***Initial dose and short course therapy:*** 0.1–0.2 mg/kg per day PO for 3–6 wk; daily dose may be given as a single dose.
- ***Chronic lymphocytic leukemia (alternate regimen):*** 0.4 mg/kg q2 wk, increasing by 0.1 mg/kg with each dose until therapeutic or toxic effect occurs.
- ***Maintenance dose:*** 0.03–0.1 mg/kg per day. Do not exceed 0.1 mg/kg per day. Short courses of therapy are safer than continuous maintenance therapy; base dosage and duration on patient response and bone marrow status.

Pediatric: Safety and efficacy not established.

Pharmacokinetics

Route	Onset	Peak	Duration
Oral	Varies	1 h	15–20

Metabolism: Hepatic; $T_{1/2}$: 60 min
Distribution: Crosses placenta; passes into breast milk
Excretion: Urine

Adverse effects
- **CNS:** *Tremors, muscular twitching, confusion,* agitation, ataxia, flaccid paresis, hallucinations, seizures
- **GI:** Nausea, vomiting, anorexia, **hepatotoxicity**, jaundice (rare)
- **Respiratory:** Bronchopulmonary dysplasia, pulmonary fibrosis
- **Hematologic:** *Bone marrow depression,* hyperuricemia
- **GU:** *Sterility* (especially if given to prepubertal or pubertal males and adult men); amenorrhea can occur in females)
- **Dermatologic:** Skin rash, urticaria, alopecia, keratitis
- **Other:** *Cancer, acute leukemia*

■ Nursing Considerations
Assessment
- *History:* Allergy to chlorambucil, cross-sensitization with melphalen (skin rash), radiation therapy, chemotherapy, hematopoietic depression, pregnancy, lactation
- *Physical:* Temperature; weight; Skin—color, lesions; R, adventitious sounds; liver evaluation; CBC, differential, hemoglobin, uric acid, liver function tests

Implementation
- Arrange for blood tests to evaluate hematopoietic function before beginning therapy and weekly during therapy.
- Do not give full dosage within 4 wk after a full course of radiation therapy or chemotherapy because of the risk of severe bone marrow depression.
- Ensure that patient is well hydrated before treatment.
- Monitor uric acid levels; ensure adequate fluid intake, and prepare for appropriate treatment of hyperuricemia if it occurs.
- Arrange to divide single daily dose if nausea and vomiting occur with large single dose.

Drug-specific teaching points
- Take this drug once a day. If nausea and vomiting occur, consult with nurse or physician about dividing the dose.
- Know that the following side effects may occur: nausea, vomiting, loss of appetite (dividing the dose may help; small frequent meals also may help; it is important that you try to maintain your fluid intake and nutrition while on this drug; drink at least 10–12 glassses of fluid each day); infertility (from irregular menses to complete amenorrhea; men may stop producing sperm; this may be an irreversible problem; discuss your feelings with your nurse or physician); severe birth defects—advisable to use birth control methods while on this drug.

Adverse effects in *Italics* are most common; those in **Bold** are life-threatening.

chloramphenicol

- Report unusual bleeding or bruising; fever, chills, sore throat; cough, shortness of breath; yellow color of the skin or eyes; flank or stomach pain.

☐ chloramphenicol

(klor am fen' i kole)
Oral: Chloromycetin Kapseals
Ophthalmic solution: Chloromycetin Ophthalmic, Chloroptic Ophthalmic
Otic solution: Chloromycetin Otic
Topical dermatologic cream: Diochloram (CAN), Minims (CAN), Sopamycetin (CAN)

chloramphenical palmitate
Oral: Chloromycetin Palmitate

chloramphenical sodium succinate
Parenteral, IV: Chloromycetin Succinate

Pregnancy Category C

Drug classes
Antibiotic

Therapeutic actions
Bacteriostatic effect against susceptible bacteria; prevents cell replication.

Indications
- **Systemic:** Serious infections for which no other antibiotic is effective
- Acute infections caused by *Salmonella typhi*
- Serious infections caused by *Salmonella, H. influenzae*, rickettsiae, lymphogranuloma—psittacosis group
- Cystic fibrosis regimen
- **Ophthalmic preparations:** Treatment of superficial ocular infections caused by susceptible microorganisms
- **Otic solution:** Treatment of superficial infections of the external auditory canal (inner ear infections should be treated with systemic antibiotics)
- **Topical dermatologic cream:** Treatment of superficial infections of the skin caused by susceptible organisms.

Contraindications/cautions
- Allergy to chloramphenical, renal failure, hepatic failure, G-6-PD deficiency, intermittent porphyria, pregnancy (may cause gray syndrome), lactation

Dosage
Systemic
Severe and sometimes fatal blood dyscrasias (adults) and severe and sometimes fatal gray syndromes (in newborns and premature infants) may occur. Use should be restricted to situations in which no other antibiotic is effective. Serum levels should be monitored at least weekly to minimize risk of toxicity (therapeutic concentrations: peak, 10–20 µg/ml; trough, 5–10 µg/ml).
Adult and pediatric: 50 mg/kg per day in divided doses q6h up to 100 mg/kg per day in severe cases.
- ***Newborns:*** 25 mg/kg per day in four doses q6h; after 2 weeks of age, full-term infants usually tolerate 50 mg/kg per day in four doses q6h (dosage should be monitored using serum concentrations of the drug as a guide).
- ***Infants and children with immature metabolic processes:*** 25 mg/kg per day (monitor serum concentration carefully).

Geriatric or renal or hepatic failure: Use serum concentration of the drug to adjust dosage.
– *Otic:* Instill 2–3 drops into the ear tid.
– *Ophthalmic:* Instill ointment or solution as prescribed.
– *Topical:* Apply tid–qid to infected area.

Pharmacokinetics

Route	Onset	Peak	Duration
Oral	Varies	1–3 h	48–72 h
IV	20–30 min	1 h	48–72 h

Metabolism: Hepatic; $T_{1/2}$: 1.5–4 h
Distribution: Crosses placenta; passes into breast milk
Excretion: Urine

IV facts
Preparation: Dilute with 10 ml of Water for Injection, or 5% Dextrose Injection.

chloramphenicol

Infusion: Administer as a 10% solution over at least 1 min. Substitute oral dosage as soon as possible.

Adverse effects
Systemic
- CNS: *Headache,* mild depression, mental confusion, delirium
- GI: *Nausea, vomiting, glossitis, stomatitis, diarrhea*
- Hematologic: *Blood dyscrasias*
- Other: Fever, macular rashes, urticaria, anaphylaxis; *gray syndrome* (see in neonates and premature babies: abdominal distension, pallid cyanosis, vasomotor collapse, irregular respirations; may lead to death), superinfections

Ophthalmic Solution, Otic Solution, Dermatologic Cream
- Hematologic: **Bone marrow hypoplasia, aplastic anemia**, and **death** with prolonged or frequent intermittent ocular use
- Hypersensitivity: *Irritation, burning, itching,* angioneurotic edema, urticaria, dermatitis
- Other: Superinfections

Clinically important drug-drug interactions
- Increased serum levels and drug effects of dicumarol, anisindione, warfarin, phenytoins, tolbutamide, acetohexamide, glipizide, glyburide, tolazamide if taken with chloramphenicol • Decreased hematologic response to iron salts, vitamin B_{12} when taken with chloramphenicol

■ Nursing Considerations
Assessment
- *History:* Allergy to chloramphenicol, renal or hepatic failure, G-6-PD deficiency, intermittent porphyria, lactation
- *Physical:* Culture site of infection; orientation, reflexes, sensation; respiratory rate, adventitious sounds; bowel sounds, output, liver function; urinalysis, BUN, CBC, liver function tests, renal function tests

Implementation
Systemic Administration
- Culture infected area before beginning therapy.
- Give drug on an empty stomach, 1 h before or 2 h after meals. If severe GI upset occurs; drug may be given with meals.
- **Do not** give this drug IM because it is ineffective by that route.
- Monitor hematologic data carefully, especially with long-term therapy by any route of administration.
- Arrange for dosage reduction in patients with renal or hepatic disease.
- Monitor serum levels periodically as indicated in dosage section.

Ophthalmic and Otic Solution, Topical Dermatologic Cream
- Topical preparations of the drug should be used only when necessary. Sensitization from the topical use of this drug dmay preclude its later use in serious infections. Topical preparations that contain antibiotics that are not ordinarily given systemically are preferable.

Drug-specific teaching points
- **Never** use any leftover medication to self-treat any other infection.

Oral Therapy
- Take this drug q6h around the clock; schedule doses to minimize sleep disruption. The drug should be taken on an empty stomach, 1 h before or 2 h after meals. Take the full course of this medication.
- Know that the following side effects may occur: nausea, vomiting (if this becomes severe, the drug can be taken with food); diarrhea (this will stop when the drug is stopped); headache (medication to help the pain may be available); confusion (avoid driving a car or operating delicate machinery if this occurs); superinfections (frequent hygiene measures may help; medications are available if superinfections become severe).
- Report sore throat, tiredness; unusual bleeding or bruising (even if these occur several weeks after you finish the drug); numbness, tingling, pain in the extremities; pregnancy.

Adverse effects in *Italics* are most common; those in **Bold** are life-threatening.

Ophthalmic Solution
- Administer eye drops as follows: lie down or tilt head backward, and look at ceiling. Drop solution inside lower eyelid while looking up. After instilling eye drops, close eyes, and apply gentle pressure to the inside corner of the eye for 1 min.
- Know that the following side effects may occur: temporary stinging or blurring of vision after administration (notify your nurse or physician if these become pronounced).

Otic Solution
- Administer as follows: lie on side or tilt head so that ear to be treated is uppermost. Grasp ear and gently pull up and back (adults) or down and back (children); drop medication into the ear canal. Stay in this position for 2–3 min. Solution should be warmed to near body temperature before use; **do not** use cold or hot solutions.

Topical Dermatologic Cream
- Cleanse affected area of skin before application (unless otherwise indicated).

☐ chlordiazepoxide hydrochloride

*(klor dye az e **pox**' ide)*
metaminodiazepoxide hydrochloride

Apo-Chlorodiazepoxide (CAN), Librium, Libritabs, Mitran, Reposans-10, Solium (CAN)

Pregnancy Category D
C-IV controlled substance

Drug classes
Benzodiazepine
Antianxiety drug

Therapeutic actions
Exact mechanisms of action not understood; acts mainly at subcortical levels of the CNS; main sites of action may be the limbic system and reticular formation; potentiates the effects of gamma-aminobutyric acid (GABA).

Indications
- Management of anxiety disorders or for short-term relief of symptoms of anxiety
- Acute alcohol withdrawal; may be useful in symptomatic relief of acute agitation, tremor, delirium tremens, hallucinosis
- Preoperative relief of anxiety and tension

Contraindications/cautions
- Contraindicated in the presence of hypersensitivity to benzodiazepines, psychoses, acute narrow-angle glaucoma, shock, coma, acute alcoholic intoxication with depression of vital signs, pregnancy (increased risk of congenital malformations, neonatal withdrawal syndrome), labor and delivery ("floppy infant" syndrome reported), lactation (infants to become lethargic and lose weight).
- Use caution in the presence of impaired liver or kidney function, debilitation.

Dosage
Individualize dosage; increase dosage cautiously to avoid adverse effects.

Adult
- ***Oral:*** *Anxiety disorders:* 5 or 10 mg, up to 20 or 25 mg, tid–qid, depending on severity of symptoms. *Preoperative apprehension:* 5–10 mg tid–qid on days preceding surgery. *Alcohol withdrawal:* Parenteral form usually used initially. If given orally, initial dose is 50–100 mg, followed by repeated doses as needed, up to 300 mg/d; then reduce to maintenance levels.
- ***Parenteral:*** *Severe anxiety:* 50–100 mg IM or IV initially; then 25–50 mg tid–qid if necessary, or switch to oral dosage form. *Preoperative apprehension:* 50–100 mg IM 1 h prior to surgery. *Alcohol withdrawal:* 50–100 mg IM or IV initially; repeat in 2–4 h if necessary. Up to 300 mg may be given in 6 h; do not exceed 300 mg/24 h.

Pediatric
- ***Oral:*** *Older than 6 y:* 5 mg bid–qid initially; may be increased in some children to 10 mg bid–tid. *Younger than 6 y:* Not recommended.
- ***Parenteral, older children:*** 25–50 mg IM or IV.

chlordiazepoxide hydrochloride

Geriatric patients or those with debilitating disease: 5 mg PO bid–qid; 25–50 mg IM or IV.

Pharmacokinetics

Route	Onset	Peak	Duration
Oral	Varies	1–4 h	48–72 h
IM	10–15 min	15–30 min	48–72 h
IV	Immediate	3–30 min	48–72 h

Metabolism: Hepatic; $T_{1/2}$: 5–30 h
Distribution: Crosses placenta; passes into breast milk
Excretion: Urine

IV facts
Preparation: Add 5 ml sterile physiologic saline or Sterile Water for Injection to contents of ampule; agitate gently until drug is dissolved.

Infusion: Administer IV doses slowly over 1 min. Arrange to change patients on IV therapy to oral therapy as soon as possible.

Adverse effects
- CNS: *Transient, mild drowsiness initially; sedation, depression, lethargy, apathy, fatigue, lightheadedness, disorientation, restlessness, confusion,* crying, delirium, headache, slurred speech, dysarthria, stupor, rigidity, tremor, psychomotor retardation, extrapyramidal symptoms; *mild paradoxical excitatory reactions, during first 2 wk of treatment* (especially in psychiatric patients, aggressive children, and with high dosage), visual and auditory disturbances, diplopia, nystagmus, depressed hearing, nasal congestion
- GI: *Constipation, diarrhea,* dry mouth, salivation, nausea, anorexia, vomiting, difficulty in swallowing, gastric disorders, hepatic dysfunction, jaundice
- CV: *Bradycardia, tachycardia,* cardiovascular collapse, hypertension and hypotension, palpitations, edema
- Hematologic: Decreased hematocrit, blood dyscrasias
- GU: *Incontinence, urinary retention, changes in libido,* menstrual irregularities
- **Dermatologic:** Urticaria, pruritus, skin rash, dermatitis
- **Dependence:** *Drug dependence with withdrawal syndrome* when drug is discontinued (more common with abrupt discontinuation of higher dosage used for longer than 4 mo)
- **Other:** Phlebitis and thrombosis at IV injection sites, hiccups, fever, diaphoresis, paresthesias, muscular disturbances, gynecomastia, pain, burning, and redness after IM injection

Clinically important drug-drug interactions
- Increased CNS depression when taken with alcohol, omeprazole • Increased pharmacologic effects of chlordiazepoxide when given with cimetidine, disulfiram, oral contraceptives • Decreased sedative effects of chlordiazepoxide if taken concurrently with theophylline, aminophylline, dyphylline, oxitriphylline

■ Nursing Considerations

Assessment
- *History:* Hypersensitivity to benzodiazepines; psychoses; acute narrow-angle glaucoma; shock; coma; acute alcoholic intoxication; pregnancy; lactation; impaired liver or kidney function, debilitation.
- *Physical:* Skin—color, lesions; body temperature; orientation, reflexes, affect, ophthalmologic exam; P, BP; R, adventitious sounds; liver evaluation, abdominal exam, bowel sounds, normal output; CBC, liver and renal function tests.

Implementation
- Do not administer intra-arterially; arteriospasm, gangrene may result.
- Reconstitute solutions for IM injection only with special diluent provided; do not use diluent if it is opalescent or hazy; prepare injection immediately before use, and discard any unused solution.

Adverse effects in *Italics* are most common; those in **Bold** are life-threatening.

chloroquine hydrochloride ■ 265

- Do not use drug solutions made with physiologic saline or Sterile Water for Injection for IM injections because of pain.
- Give IM injection slowly into upper outer quadrant of the gluteus muscle; monitor injection sites.
- Do not use small veins (dorsum of hand or wrist) for IV injection.
- Monitor P, BP, respiration carefully during IV administration.
- Maintain patients receiving parenteral benzodiazepines in bed for 3 h; do not permit ambulatory patients to operate a vehicle following an injection.
- Arrange to reduce dosage of narcotic analgesics in patients receiving IV benzodiazepines; doses should be reduced by at least one-third or totally eliminated.
- Arrange to monitor liver and kidney function, CBC at intervals during long-term therapy.
- Arrange to taper dosage gradually after long-term therapy, especially in epileptic patients.

Drug-specific teaching points
- Take drug exactly as prescribed.
- Do not to stop taking this drug (long-term therapy) without consulting the health care provider. Avoid alcohol, sleep-inducing, or OTC drugs while on this drug.
- Know that the following side effects may occur: drowsiness, dizziness (these may become less pronounced after a few days; avoid driving a car or engaging in other dangerous activities if these occur); GI upset (taking the drug with water may help); depression, dreams, emotional upset, crying.
- Report severe dizziness, weakness, drowsiness that persists, rash or skin lesions, palpitations, swelling of the extremities, visual changes, difficulty voiding.

❒ chloroquine hydrochloride

(klo' ro kwin)
IM: Aralen HCl

chloroquine phosphate
Oral: Aralen Phosphate
Pregnancy Category C

Drug classes
Amebicide
Antimalarial
4-aminoquinoline

Therapeutic actions
Inhibits protozoal reproduction and protein synthesis. Mechanism of anti-inflammatory action in rheumatoid arthritis is not known.

Indications
- Treatment of extraintestinal amebiasis
- Prophylaxis and treatment of acute attacks of malaria caused by susceptible strains of *Plasmodia*
- **Unlabeled use**: treatment of rheumatoid arthritis and discoid lupus erythematosus

Contraindications/cautions
- Allergy to chloroquine and other 4-aminoquinolines, porphyria, psoriasis, retinal disease, hepatic disease, G-6-PD deficiency, alcoholism, lactation.

Dosage
Adult
- ***Amebicide:*** *Oral*: 1 g (600 mg base)/d for 2 d; then 500 mg (300 mg base)/d for 2–3 wk. *IM*: 200–250 mg (160–200 mg base)/d for 10–12 d.
- ***Antimalarial:*** *Suppression:* 300 mg base PO once a week on the same day for 2 wk before exposure and continuing until 6–8 wk after exposure. *Acute attack:* 600 mg base PO initially; then 300 mg 6 h later and on days 2 and 3; or 160–200 mg base IM initially and 6 h later if needed. Do not exceed 800 mg base/day. *Antirheumatoid:* 200 mg (160 mg base) PO qid or bid.

Pediatric
- ***Amebicide:*** Not recommended.
- ***Antimalarial:*** *Suppression:* 5 mg base/kg PO once a week on the same day for 2 wk before exposure and continuing until 6–8 wk after exposure. *Acute attack:* 10 mg base/kg PO initially; then 5 mg base/kg 6 h later and on days 2 and 3; or 5 mg base/kg IM initially and 6 h later if needed. Do not exceed 10 mg base/kg per day.

Pharmacokinetics

Route	Onset	Peak	Duration
Oral	Varies	1–2 h	wk
IM	Rapid	45–60 min	wk

Metabolism: Hepatic; $T_{1/2}$: 70–120 h
Distribution: Crosses placenta; passes into breast milk
Excretion: Urine

Adverse effects

- CNS: *Visual disturbances*, retinal changes (may be manifested by blurring of vision, difficulty in focusing), ototoxicity, muscle weakness
- GI: *Nausea, vomiting, diarrhea*, loss of appetite, abdominal pain
- CV: *Hypotension, ECG changes*
- Hematologic: Blood dyscrasias, hemolysis in patients with G-6-PD deficiency

Clinically important drug-drug interactions

- Increased effects of chloroquine if taken concurrently with cimetidine • Decreased GI absorption of both drugs if taken with magnesium trisilicate

■ Nursing Considerations

Assessment

- *History:* Allergy to chloroquine and other 4-aminoquinolines, porphyria, psoriasis, retinal disease, hepatic disease, G-6-PD deficiency, alcoholism, lactation
- *Physical:* Reflexes, muscle strength, auditory and ophthalmologic screening; BP, ECG; liver palpation; CBC, G-6-PD in deficient patients, liver function tests

Implementation

- Administer with meals if GI upset occurs.
- Schedule dosages for weekly, same-day therapy on a calendar.
- Double check pediatric doses; children are very susceptible to overdosage.
- Arrange for ophthalmologic exams during long-term therapy.

Drug-specific teaching points

- Take full course of drug therapy. Take drug with meals if GI upset occurs. Mark your calendar with the drug days for malarial prophylaxis.
- Know that the following side effects may occur: stomach pain, loss of appetite, nausea, vomiting, or diarrhea.
- Arrange to have regular ophthalmologic exams if long-term use is indicated.
- Report blurring of vision, loss of hearing, ringing in the ears, muscle weakness, fever.

☐ chlorothiazide

(klor oh *thye'* a zide)
Diurigen, Diuril

chlorothiazide sodium
Diuril Sodium

Pregnancy Category C

Drug classes
Thiazide diuretic

Therapeutic actions
Inhibits reabsorption of sodium and chloride in distal renal tubule, increasing the excretion of sodium, chloride, and water by the kidney.

Indications

- Adjunctive therapy in edema associated with CHF, cirrhosis, corticosteroid, and estrogen therapy, renal dysfunction
- Treatment of hypertension, as sole therapy or in combination with other antihypertensives
- **Unlabeled uses**: treatment of diabetes insipidus, especially nephrogenic diabetes insipidus; reduction of incidence of osteoporosis in postmenopausal women

Contraindications/cautions

- Fluid or electrolyte imbalances, renal or liver disease, gout, SLE, glucose tolerance abnormalities, hyperparathyroidism, manic-depressive disorders, lactation

Dosage
Adult

- ***Edema:*** 0.5–2 g PO or IV (if patient unable to take PO) qid or bid.

Adverse effects in *Italics* are most common; those in **Bold** are life-threatening.

- **Hypertension:** 0.5–2 g/d PO as a single or divided dose; adjust dose to BP response, giving up to 2 g/d in divided doses. IV use is not recommended.
Pediatric: 22 mg/kg per day PO in two doses.
- **Infants younger than 6 mo:** Up to 33 mg/kg per day in two doses. IV use not recommended.

Pharmacokinetics

Route	Onset	Peak	Duration
Oral	2 h	3–6 h	6–12 h
IV	15 min	30 min	2 h

Metabolism: $T_{1/2}$: 45–120 min
Distribution: Crosses placenta; passes into breast milk
Excretion: Urine

IV facts
Preparation: Dilute vial for parenteral solution with 18 ml Sterile Water for Injection. Never add less than 18 ml. Discard diluted solution after 24 h.
Infusion: Administer slowly. Switch to oral drug as soon as possible.
Incompatibilities: Compatible with dextrose and sodium chloride solutions. Do not give parenteral solution with whole blood or blood products.

Adverse effects
- **CNS:** *Dizziness, vertigo,* paresthesias, weakness, headache, drowsiness, fatigue
- **GI:** *Nausea, anorexia, vomiting, dry mouth, diarrhea, constipation,* jaundice, hepatitis, pancreatitis
- **CV:** Orthostatic hypotension, venous thrombosis, volume depletion, cardiac arrhythmias, chest pain
- **Hematologic:** Leukopenia, thrombocytopenia, agranulocytosis, aplastic anemia, neutropenia, fluid and electrolyte imbalances
- **GU:** *Polyuria, nocturia, impotence,* loss of libido
- **Dermatologic:** Photosensitivity, rash, purpura, exfoliative dermatitis
- **Other:** Muscle cramps and muscle spasms, fever, hives, gouty attacks, flushing, weight loss, rhinorrhea

Clinically important drug-drug interactions
- Increased thiazide effects and chance of acute hyperglycemia if taken with diazoxide • Decreased absorption with cholestyramine • Increased risk of cardiac glycoside toxicity if hypokalemia occurs • Increased risk of lithium toxicity • Increased dosage of antidiabetic agents may needed

Drug-lab test interferences
- Monitor for decreased PBI levels without clinical signs of thyroid disturbances.

■ Nursing Considerations
Assessment
- *History:* Fluid or electrolyte imbalances, renal or liver disease, gout, SLE, glucose tolerance abnormalities, hyperparathyroidism, manic-depressive disorders, lactation
- *Physical:* Orientation, reflexes, muscle strength; pulses, BP, orthostatic BP, perfusion, edema, baseline ECG; R, adventitious sounds; liver evaluation, bowel sounds; CBC, serum electrolytes, blood glucose, liver and renal function tests, serum uric acid, urinalysis

Implementation
- Administer with food or milk if GI upset occurs.
- Administer early in the day, so increased urination will not disturb sleep.
- Measure and record regular body weights to monitor fluid changes.

Drug-specific teaching points
- Take drug early in the day, so sleep will not be disturbed by increased urination.
- Weigh yourself daily, and record weights.
- Protect skin from exposure to the sun or bright lights.
- Know that increased urination will occur (stay close to bathroom facilities).
- Use caution if dizziness, drowsiness, feeling faint occur.

Adverse effects in *Italics* are most common; those in **Bold** are life-threatening.

chlorotrianisene

(klor oh trye an' i seen)
TACE

Pregnancy Category X

Drug classes
Hormone
Estrogen

Therapeutic actions
Estrogens are endogenous female sex hormones; important in the development of the female reproductive system and secondary sex characteristics; cause capillary dilatation, fluid retention, protein anabolism, and thin cervical mucus; conserve calcium and phosphorus and encourage bone formation; inhibit ovulation and prevent postpartum breast discomfort.

Indications
- Palliation of moderate to severe vasomotor symptoms, atrophic vaginitis, kraurosis vulvae associated with menopause
- Treatment of female hypogonadism
- Treatment of postpartum breast engorgement
- Palliation in prostatic carcinoma (inoperable and progressing)

Contraindications/cautions
- Contraindicated in the presence of allergy to estrogens, breast cancer, estrogen-dependent neoplasm; undiagnosed abnormal genital bleeding, active thrombophlebitis or thromboembolic disorders or history of such from previous estrogen use, pregnancy, lactation.
- Use with caution in the presence of metabolic bone disease, renal insufficiency, CHF.

Dosage
Administer PO; give cyclically (3 wk of estrogen therapy followed by 1 wk of rest), and use for short term unless otherwise indicated.

Adult
- ***Postpartum breast engorgement:*** 12 mg PO qid for 7 d or 50 mg PO q6h for six doses. Administer first dose within 8 h of delivery.
- ***Moderate to severe vasomotor symptoms associated with menopause:*** 12–25 mg/d PO given cyclically for 30 d; one or more courses may be used.
- ***Atrophic vaginitis and kraurosis vulvae:*** 12–25 mg/d PO given cyclically for 30–60 d.
- ***Female hypogonadism:*** 12–25 mg/d PO given cyclically for 21 d; may be followed immediately by 100 mg progesterone IM or by an oral progestin during the last 5 d of therapy. Next course may begin on the fifth day of induced uterine bleeding.
- ***Prostatic carcinoma:*** 12–25 mg/d PO given chronically.

Pediatric: Not recommended due to effect on the growth of the long bones.

Pharmacokinetics

Route	Onset
Oral	14 d

Metabolism: Hepatic
Distribution: Crosses placenta; passes into breast milk

Adverse effects
- CNS: *Steepening of the corneal curvature with a resultant change in visual acuity and intolerance to contact lenses, headache,* migraine, dizziness, mental depression, chorea, convulsions
- GI: *Gallbladder disease, nausea, vomiting, abdominal cramps, bloating,* cholestatic jaundice, colitis, acute pancreatitis, **hepatic adenoma**
- CV: *Increased blood pressure,* **thromboembolic and thrombotic disease**, peripheral edema
- GU: *Increased risk of endometrial cancer* in postmenopausal women, *breakthrough bleeding, change in menstrual*

- Report rapid weight gain or loss, swelling in ankles or fingers, unusual bleeding or bruising, muscle cramps.

chlorotrianisene

flow, *dysmenorrhea, premenstrual-like syndrome, amenorrhea,* vaginal candidiasis, cystitis-like syndrome, endometrial cystic hyperplasia, changes in libido
- **Dermatologic:** Photosensitivity, chloasma, erythema nodosum or multiforme, hemorrhagic eruption, loss of scalp hair, hirsutism, urticaria, dermatitis
- **Other:** Decreased glucose tolerance, *weight changes,* aggravation of porphyria, *breast tenderness*

Clinically important drug-drug interactions

- Increased therapeutic and toxic effects of corticosteroids if given with chlorotrianisene
- Risk of breakthrough bleeding, pregnancy, spotting if taken concurrently with barbiturates, hydantoins, rifampin

Drug-lab test interferences

- Increased sulfobromophthalein retention • Increased prothrombin and factors VII, VIII, IX, and X • Decreased antithrombin III • Increased thyroid binding globulin with increased PBI, T_4, increased uptake of free T_3 resin (free T_4 is unaltered) • Impaired glucose tolerance • Decreased pregnanediol excretion • Reduced response to metyrapone test • Reduced serum folate concentration • Increased serum triglycerides and phospholipid concentration

■ Nursing Considerations

Assessment

- *History:* Allergy to estrogens, breast cancer, estrogen-dependent neoplasm, undiagnosed abnormal genital bleeding, active thrombophlebitis or thromboembolic disorders or history of such from previous estrogen use, metabolic bone disease, renal insufficiency, CHF, pregnancy, lactation
- *Physical:* Skin—color, lesions, edema; breast exam; orientation, affect, reflexes; P, auscultation, BP, peripheral perfusion; R, adventitious sounds; bowel sounds, liver evaluation, abdominal exam; pelvic exam; serum calcium, phosphorus; liver and renal function tests; Pap smear; glucose tolerance test

Implementation

- Arrange for pretreatment and periodic (at least annual) history and physical, which should include BP, breasts, abdomen, pelvic organs, and a Pap smear.
- Caution patient before beginning therapy of the risks involved with estrogen use, the need to prevent pregnancy during treatment, the need for frequent medical followup, the need for periodic rests from drug treatment, as appropriate.
- Administer cyclically for short-term or cyclic use only when treating postmenopausal conditions because of the risk of endometrial neoplasm; taper to the lowest effective dose, and provide a drug-free week each month if at all possible.
- Arrange for the concomitant use of progestin therapy during chronic estrogen therapy in women; this will mimic normal physiologic cycling and allow for a cyclic uterine bleeding, which may decrease the risk of endometrial cancer.
- Protect patient from exposure to sun or ultraviolet light if photosensitivity occurs.

Drug-specific teaching points

- Use this drug in cycles or for short periods.
- Prepare a calendar of drug days, rest days, and drug-free period.
- Know that many potentially serious problems have occurred with the use of this drug, including development of cancers, blood clots, liver problems; this drug cannot be given to pregnant women because of serious toxic effects to the baby.
- Arrange for periodic medical exams throughout therapy.
- Know that the following side effects may occur: nausea, vomiting, bloating; headache, dizziness, mental depression (use caution if driving or performing tasks that require alertness if this occurs); sensitivity to sunlight (use a sunscreen and wear protective clothing until your tolerance to this effect of the drug is known); skin rash, loss of scalp hair, darkening of the skin on the face; changes in menstrual patterns.

Adverse effects in *Italics* are most common; those in **Bold** are life-threatening.

- Report pain in the groin or calves, chest pain or sudden shortness of breath, abnormal vaginal bleeding, lumps in the breast, sudden severe headache, dizziness or fainting, changes in vision or speech, weakness or numbness in the arm or leg, severe abdominal pain, yellowing of the skin or eyes, severe mental depression.

☐ chlorphenesin carbamate

(klor fen' e sin)
Maolate

Pregnancy Category C

Drug classes
Centrally acting skeletal muscle relaxant

Therapeutic actions
Precise mechanism of action not known; has sedative properties; does not directly relax tense skeletal muscles; does not directly affect the motor endplate or motor nerves.

Indications
- Relief of discomfort associated with acute, painful musculoskeletal conditions
- Adjunct to rest, physical therapy, and other measures

Contraindications/cautions
- Allergic or idiosyncratic reactions to chlorphenesin, tartrazine; lactation.

Dosage
Adult: Initially, 800 mg PO tid until the desired effect is obtained; reduce dosage for maintenance to 400 mg qid or less as required. Safety for use longer than 8 wk not established.
Pediatric: Safety and efficacy not established for children younger than 12 y.
Geriatric patients or those with hepatic impairment: Dosage reduction may be necessary; monitor closely.

Pharmacokinetics

Route	Onset	Peak	Duration
Oral	Varies	1–3 h	8–12 h

Metabolism: Hepatic; $T_{1/2}$: 3.5 h
Distribution: Crosses placenta; may pass into breast milk
Excretion: Urine

Adverse effects
- CNS: *Dizziness, drowsiness, confusion,* paradoxical stimulation, insomnia, headache
- GI: *Nausea, epigastric distress*
- Hematologic: Leukopenia, thrombocytopenia, agranulocytosis, pancytopenia
- Hypersensitivity: **Anaphylactoid reactions,** drug fever

■ Nursing Considerations

Assessment
- *History:* Allergic or idiosyncratic reactions to chlorphenesin, tartrazine, lactation
- *Physical:* Skin—color, lesions; orientation, affect; liver evaluation; liver function tests, CBC with differential

Implementation
- Arrange to reduce dosage in patients with liver dysfunction.

Drug-specific teaching points
- Take this drug exactly as prescribed; do not take a higher dosage than that prescribed for you.
- Avoid the use of alcohol, sleep-inducing, or OTC drugs while you are on this drug; these could cause dangerous effects.
- Know that the following side effects may occur: drowsiness, dizziness, confusion (avoid driving a car or engaging in activities that require alertness if these occur); nausea (taking drug with food and eating frequent small meals may help); insomnia, headache (it may help to know that these are effects of the drug that will go away when the drug is discontinued).
- Report skin rash, severe nausea, dizziness, insomnia, fever, difficulty breathing.

Adverse effects in *Italics* are most common; those in **Bold** are life-threatening.

☐ chlorpheniramine maleate

(klor fen ir' a meen)

Chlorphen (CAN), Chlor-Pro, Chlorspan, Chlortab, Chlor-Trimeton, Chlor-Tripolon (CAN), Novopheniram (CAN), Phenetron, Telachlor

Pregnancy Category B

Drug classes
Antihistamine (alkylamine type)

Therapeutic actions
Competitively blocks the effects of histamine at H_1 receptor sites; has atropine-like, antipruritic, and sedative effects.

Indications
- Oral preparations: symptomatic relief of symptoms associated with perennial and seasonal allergic rhinitis; vasomotor rhinitis; allergic conjunctivitis; mild, uncomplicated urticaria and angioedema; amelioraton of allergic reactions to blood or plasma; dermatographism; adjunctive therapy in anaphylactic reactions.
- Parenteral preparations: amelioration of allergic reactions to blood or plasma; in anaphylaxis as an adjunct to epinephrine and other measures; other uncomplicated allergic conditions when oral therapy is not possible.

Contraindications/cautions
- Contraindicated in the presence of allergy to any antihistamines, narrow-angle glaucoma, stenosing peptic ulcer, symptomatic prostatic hypertrophy, asthmatic attack, bladder neck obstruction, pyloroduodenal obstruction, third trimester of pregnancy, lactation.
- Use caution in pregnancy.

Dosage
Adult and children older than 12 y
- **Tablets or syrup:** 4 mg PO q4–6h; do not exceed 24 mg in 24 h.
- **Sustained-release forms:** 8–12 mg PO at bedtime or q8–12h during the day; do not exceed 24 mg in 24 h.
- *Parenteral:* 10 mg/ml injection is intended for IV, IM, or SC administration; 100 mg/ml injection is intended for IM or SC use only.
- *Allergic reactions to blood or plasma:* 10–20 mg IM, IV, or SC, as a single dose; maximum recommended dose is 40 mg in 24 h.
- *Anaphylaxis:* 10–20 mg IV as a single dose.
- *Uncomplicated allergic conditions:* 5–20 mg IM, IV, or SC, as a single dose.

Pediatric
- **Tablets or syrup:** *6–12 y:* 2 mg q4–6h PO; do not exceed 12 mg in 24 h. *2–5 y:* 1 mg q4–6h PO; do not exceed 4 mg in 24 h.
- **Sustained-release forms:** *6–12 y:* 8 mg PO at bedtime or during the day as indicated. *Younger than 6 y:* Not recommended.

Geriatric: More likely to cause dizziness, sedation, syncope, toxic confusional states, and hypotension in elderly patients; use with caution.

Pharmacokinetics

Route	Onset	Peak
Oral	½–6 h	2–6 h

Metabolism: Hepatic, $T_{1/2}$: 12–15 h
Distribution: Crosses placenta; enters breast milk
Excretion: Urine

IV facts
Preparation: No preparation necessary.
Infusion: Administer slowly by direct injection or into tubing of running line.

Adverse effects
- CNS: *Drowsiness, sedation, dizziness, disturbed coordination*, fatigue, confusion, restlessness, excitation, nervousness, tremor, headache, blurred vision, diplopia, vertigo, tinnitus, acute labryinthitis, hysteria, tingling, heaviness and weakness of the hands

Adverse effects in *Italics* are most common; those in **Bold** are life-threatening.

- **GI:** *Epigastric distress,* anorexia, increased appetite and weight gain, nausea, vomiting, diarrhea or constipation
- **CV:** Hypotension, palpitations, bradycardia, tachycardia, extrasystoles
- **Respiratory:** *Thickening of bronchial secretions,* chest tightness, wheezing, nasal stuffiness, dry mouth, dry nose, dry throat, sore throat
- **Hematologic:** Hemolytic anemia, hypoplastic anemia, thrombocytopenia, leukopenia, agranulocytosis, pancytopenia
- **GU:** Urinary frequency, dysuria, urinary retention, early menses, decreased libido, impotence
- **Other:** Urticaria, rash, anaphylactic shock, photosensitivity, excessive perspiration, chills

Clinically important drug-drug interactions
- Increased depressant effects if taken concurrently with alcohol, other CNS depressants

■ Nursing Considerations

Assessment
- *History:* Allergy to any antihistamines; narrow-angle glaucoma, stenosing peptic ulcer, symptomatic prostatic hypertrophy, asthmatic attack, bladder neck obstruction, pyloroduodenal obstruction, pregnancy, lactation
- *Physical:* Skin—color, lesions, texture; orientation, reflexes, affect; vision exam; P, BP ; R, adventitious sounds; bowel sounds; prostate palpation; CBC with differential

Implementation
- Administer oral preparations with food if GI upset occurs.
- Caution patient not to crush or chew sustained-release preparations.
- Administer 10 mg/ml injection IV, IM, or SC; administer 100 mg/ml injection only IM or SC.
- Maintain epinephrine 1:1000 readily available when using parenteral preparations; hypersensitivity reactions, including anaphylaxis, have occurred.
- Arrange for periodic blood tests during prolonged therapy.

Drug-specific teaching points
- Take as prescribed; avoid excessive dosage. Take with food if GI upset occurs; do not crush or chew the sustained-release preparations.
- Know that the following side effects may occur: dizziness, sedation, drowsiness (use caution if driving or performing tasks that require alertness if these occur); epigastric distress, diarrhea, or constipation (taking the drug with meals may help; consult care provider if diarrhea or constipation becomes a problem); dry mouth (frequent mouth care, sucking sugarless lozenges may help); thickening of bronchial secretions, dryness of nasal mucosa (use of a humidifier may help if this becomes a problem).
- Avoid OTC drugs while you are on this drug; many contain ingredients that could cause serious reactions if taken with this antihistamine.
- Avoid alcohol while on this drug; serious sedation could occur.
- Report difficulty breathing; hallucinations, tremors, loss of coordination; unusual bleeding or bruising; visual disturbances; irregular heartbeat.

▢ chlorpromazine hydrochloride

*(klor **proe'** ma zeen)*
Largactil (CAN), Ormazine, Thorazine

Pregnancy Category C

Drug classes
Phenothiazine
Dopaminergic blocking drug
Antipsychotic drug
Antiemetic drug
Antianxiety drug

Therapeutic actions
Mechanism of action not fully understood; antipsychotic drugs block postsynaptic

chlorpromazine hydrochloride

dopamine receptors in the brain; depresses those parts of the brain involved with wakefulness and emesis; anticholinergic, antihistaminic (H_1), and alpha-adrenergic blocking.

Indications
- Management of manifestations of psychotic disorders; control of manic type of manic-depressive illness
- Relief of preoperative restlessness and apprehension
- Adjunct in treatment of tetanus
- Treatment of acute intermittent porphyria
- Treatment of severe behavioral problems in children marked by combativeness, hyperactivity
- Control of nausea and vomiting and intractable hiccups
- Possibly effective in the treatment of nonpsychotic anxiety (not drug of choice)

Contraindications/cautions
- Allergy to chlorpromazine; comatose or severely depressed states; bone marrow depression; circulatory collapse; subcortical brain damage, Parkinson's disease; liver damage; cerebral or coronary arteriosclerosis; severe hypotension or hypertension; respiratory disorders; glaucoma; epilepsy or history of epilepsy; peptic ulcer or history of peptic ulcer; decreased renal function; prostate hypertrophy; breast cancer; thyrotoxicosis; myelography within 24 h or scheduled within 48 h; lactation; exposure to heat, phosphorous insecticides; children with chickenpox, CNS infections (such children are more susceptible to dystonias, which may confound the diagnosis of Reye's syndrome or other encephalopathy; antiemetic effects of drug may mask symptoms of Reye's syndrome, encephalopathies)

Dosage
Full clinical antipsychotic effects may require 6 wk to 6 mo of therapy.
Adult
- **Excessive anxiety, agitation in psychiatric patients:** 25 mg IM; may repeat in 1 h. Increase dosage gradually in inpatients, up to 400 mg q4–6h. Switch to oral dosage as soon as possible: 25–50 mg PO tid for outpatients; up to 2,000 mg/d PO for inpatients. Usual initial oral dosage: 10 mg tid–qid PO or 25 mg PO bid–tid; increase daily dosage by 20–50 mg semiweekly until optimum dosage is reached (maximum response may require months); doses of 200–800 mg/d PO are not uncommon in discharged mental patients.
- **Surgery:** Preoperatively, 25–50 mg PO 2–3 h before surgery or 12.5–25.0 mg IM 1–2 h before surgery; intraoperatively, 12.5 mg IM, repeated in ½ h or 2 mg IV repeated q 2 min up to 25 mg total to control vomiting (if no hypotension occurs); postoperatively, 10–25 mg PO q4–6h or 12.5–25.0 mg IM repeated in 1 h (if not, hypotension occurs).
- **Acute intermittent porphyria:** 25–50 mg PO or 25 mg IM tid–qid.
- **Tetanus:** 25–50 mg IM tid–qid, usually with barbiturates, or 25–50 mg IV diluted and infused at rate of 1 mg/min.
- **Antiemetic:** 10–25 mg PO q4–6h; 50–100 mg rectally q6–8h; 25 mg IM. If no hypotension, give 25–50 mg q3–4h. Switch to oral dosage as soon as vomiting stops.
- **Intractable hiccups:** 25–50 mg PO tid–qid. If symptoms persist for 2–3 d, give 25–50 mg IM; if inadequate response, give 25–50 mg IV in 500–1,000 ml of saline with BP monitoring.

Pediatric: Generally not used in children younger than 6 mo.
- **Psychiatric outpatients:** 0.5 mg/kg PO q4–6h; 1 mg/kg rectally q6–8h; 0.5 mg/kg IM q6–8h, not to exceed 40 mg/d (up to 5 y) or 75 mg/d (5–12 y).
- **Surgery:** Preoperatively, 0.5 mg/kg PO 2–3 h before surgery or 0.5 mg/kg IM 1–2 h before surgery; intraoperatively, 0.25 mg/kg IM or 1 mg (diluted) IV, repeated at 2-min intervals up to total IM dose; postoperatively, 0.5 mg/kg PO q4–6h or 0.5 mg/kg IM, repeated in 1 h if no hypotension.
- **Psychiatric inpatients:** 50–100 mg/d PO; maximum of 40 mg/d IM for children up to 5 y; maximum of 75 mg/d IM for children 5–12 y.

274 ■ chlorpromazine hydrochloride

- ***Tetanus:*** 0.5 mg/kg IM q6–8h or 0.5 mg/min IV, not to exceed 40 mg/d for children up to 23 kg; 75 mg/d for children 23–45 kg.
- ***Antiemetic:*** 0.55 mg/kg PO q4–6h; 1.1 mg/kg rectally q6–8h or 0.55 mg/kg IM q6–8h. Maximum IM dosage 40 mg/d for children up to 5 y or 75 mg/d for children 5–12 y.

Geriatric: Institute dosage at one-fourth to one-third that recommended for younger adults and increase more gradually.

Pharmacokinetics

Route	Onset	Peak	Duration
Oral	30–60 min	2–4 h	4–6 h
IM	10–15 min	15–20 min	4–6 h

Metabolism: Hepatic, $T_{1/2}$: 2 h, then 30 h
Distribution: Crosses placenta; enters breast milk
Excretion: Urine

IV facts
Preparation: Dilute drug for IV injection to a concentration of 1 mg/ml or less.
Infusion: Reserve IV injections for hiccups, tetanus, or use during surgery. Administer at a rate of 1 mg/2 min.
Incompatibilities: Precipitate or discoloration may occur when mixed with morphine, meperidine, products containing cresols.

Adverse effects

- CNS: *Drowsiness, insomnia, vertigo,* headache, weakness, tremors, ataxia, slurring, cerebral edema, seizures, exacerbation of psychotic symptoms, *extrapyramidal syndromes,* neuroleptic malignant syndrome
- GI: *Dry mouth, salivation, nausea, vomiting, anorexia, constipation,* paralytic ileus, incontinence
- CV: *Hypotension, orthostatic hypotension,* hypertension, tachycardia, bradycardia, cardiac arrest, CHF, cardiomegaly, refractory arrhythmias, pulmonary edema
- Respiratory: Bronchospasm, laryngospasm, dyspnea, suppression of cough reflex and potential aspiration
- Hematologic: **Eosinophilia, leukopenia, leukocytosis**, *anemia*, aplastic anemia, hemolytic anemia, thrombocytopenic or nonthrombocytopenic purpura, pancytopenia, elevated serum cholesterol
- GU: *Urinary retention,* polyuria, incontinence, priapism, ejaculation inhibition, male impotence, urine discolored pink to red-brown
- EENT: Nasal congestion, glaucoma, *photophobia, blurred vision,* miosis, mydriasis, deposits in the cornea and lens, pigmentary retinopathy
- Hypersensitivity: Jaundice, *urticaria*, angioneurotic edema, laryngeal edema, photosensitivity, eczema, asthma, anaphylactoid reactions, exfoliative dermatitis, contact dermatitis with drug solutions
- Endocrine: Lactation, breast engorgement in females, galactorrhea, syndrome of inappropriate ADH secretion, amenorrhea, menstrual irregularities, gynecomastia in males, changes in libido, hyperglycemia, inhibition of ovulation, infertility, pseudopregnancy, reduced urinary levels of gonadotropins, estrogens and progestins
- Other: Fever, heat stroke, pallor, flushed facies, sweating, *photosensitivity*

Clinically important drug-drug interactions

• Additive anticholinergic effects and possibly decreased antipsychotic efficacy if taken concurrently with anticholinergic drugs • Additive CNS depression, hypotension if given preoperatively with barbiturate anesthetics, alcohol, meperidine • Additive effects of both drugs if concurrently with beta-blockers • Increased risk of tachycardia, hypotension if given concurrently with epinephrine, norepinephrine • Increased risk of seizure if taken with metrizamide • Decreased hypotension effect if taken concurrently with guanethidine

Adverse effects in *Italics* are most common; those in **Bold** are life-threatening.

chlorpromazine hydrochloride ■ 275

Drug-lab test interferences
• False-positive pregnancy tests (less likely if serum test is used) • Increase in protein-bound iodine, not attributable to an increase in thyroxine

■ Nursing Considerations
Assessment
- *History:* Allergy to chlorpromazine; comatose or severely depressed states; bone marrow depression; circulatory collapse; subcortical brain damage, Parkinson's disease; liver damage; cerebral or coronary arteriosclerosis; severe hypotension or hypertension; respiratory disorders; glaucoma; epilepsy or history of epilepsy; peptic ulcer or history of peptic ulcer; decreased renal function; prostate hypertrophy; breast cancer; thyrotoxicosis; myelography within 24 h or scheduled within 48 h; lactation; exposure to heat, phosphorous insecticides; children with chickenpox; CNS infections
- *Physical:* Body temperature, body weight; skin—color, turgor; reflexes, orientation, intraocular pressure, ophthalmologic exam; P, BP, orthostatic BP, ECG; R, adventitious sounds; bowel sounds, normal output, liver evaluation; prostate palpation, normal urine output; CBC; urinalysis; thyroid, liver, and kidney function tests; EEG (as appropriate)

Implementation
- Do not change brand names of oral dosage forms or rectal suppositories; bioavailability differences have been documented for different brands.
- Dilute the oral concentrate just before administration in 60 ml or more of tomato or fruit juice, milk, simple syrup, orange syrup, carbonated beverage, coffee, tea, or water, or in semisolid foods (soup, puddings).
- Protect oral concentrate from light.
- Do not allow the patient to crush or chew the sustained-release capsules.
- Do not give by SC injection; give slowly by deep IM injection into upper outer quadrant of buttock.
- Keep the patient recumbent for ½ h after injection to avoid orthostatic hypotension.
- Avoid skin contact with oral concentrates and parenteral drug solutions because of the possibility of contact dermatitis.
- Consult with physician regarding warning patient or the patient's guardian about the possibility of tardive dyskinesias developing with continued use.
- Be alert to potential for aspiration because of suppressed cough reflex.
- Monitor renal function tests, and arrange for discontinuation of drug if serum creatinine, BUN become abnormal.
- Monitor CBC, and arrange for discontinuation of drug if WBC count is depressed.
- Consult with physician about dosage reduction or use of anticholinergic antiparkinsonian drugs (controversial) if extrapyramidal effects occur.
- Arrange to withdraw drug gradually after high-dose therapy; gastritis, nausea, dizziness, headache, tachycardia, insomnia have occurred after abrupt withdrawal.
- Monitor elderly patients for dehydration; sedation and decreased sensation of thirst owing to CNS effects can lead to dehydration, hemoconcentration, and reduced pulmonary ventilation; promptly institute remedial measures.
- Avoid epinephrine as vasopressor if drug-induced hypotension occurs.

Drug-specific teaching points
- Take drug exactly as prescribed. Avoid OTC medications and alcohol unless you have first consulted your health care provider.
- Do not change brand names of your drug without consulting your health care provider.
- Learn how to dilute oral drug concentrate; how to administer rectal suppository as appropriate.
- Do not get oral concentrate on your skin or clothes; contact dermatitis can occur.
- Know that the following side effects may occur: drowsiness (avoid driving a car or operating dangerous machinery if this occurs; avoid the use of alcohol, which will increase the drowsiness); sensitivity to the sun (avoid prolonged sun exposure, and wear garments that cover you or use a sunscreen if you must be out

in the sun); pink or reddish-brown urine (this is an expected drug effect that does not indicate blood is in your urine or that anything is wrong); faintness, dizziness (change position slowly; use caution climbing stairs; this effect usually goes away after several weeks of therapy).
- Use caution in hot weather; you may be prone to heat stroke while on this drug; keep up fluid intake, and do not exercise unduly in a hot climate.
- Report sore throat, fever, unusual bleeding or bruising, rash, weakness, tremors, impaired vision, dark urine, pale stools, yellowing of the skin and eyes.

☐ chlorpropamide

*(klor **proe'** pa mide)*
Apo-Chlorpropamide (CAN), Diabinese

Pregnancy Category C

Drug classes
Antidiabetic agent
Sulfonylurea, first generation

Therapeutic actions
Stimulates insulin release from functioning beta cells in the pancreas; may improve binding between insulin and insulin receptors or increase the number of insulin receptors; can increase the effect of ADH (antidiuretic hormone).

Indications
- Adjunct to diet to lower blood glucose in patients with non–insulin-dependent diabetes mellitus (type II)
- **Unlabeled uses**: treatment of neurogenic diabetes insipidus at doses of 200–500 mg/d; temporary adjunct to insulin therapy in type II diabetes to improve diabetic control

Contraindications/cautions
- Allergy to sulfonylureas; diabetes complicated by fever, severe infections, severe trauma, major surgery, ketosis, acidosis, coma; type I or juvenile diabetes, serious hepatic impairment, serious renal impairment, uremia, thyroid or endocrine impairment, glycosuria, hyperglycemia associated with primary renal disease; pregnancy, lactation

Dosage
Adult
- ***Initial therapy:*** 250 mg/d PO. *Maintenance therapy:* 100–250 mg/d PO. Up to 500 mg/d may be needed; do not exceed 750 mg/d.

Pediatric: Safety and efficacy not established.

Geriatric: Geriatric patients tend to be more sensitive to the drug; start with initial dose of 100–125 mg/d PO; monitor for 24 h, and gradually increase dose as needed.

Pharmacokinetics

Route	Onset	Peak	Duration
Oral	1 h	3–4 h	60 h

Metabolism: Hepatic, $T_{1/2}$: 36 h
Distribution: Crosses placenta; enters breast milk
Excretion: Urine and bile

Adverse effects
- **GI**: *Anorexia, nausea, vomiting, epigastric discomfort, heartburn*
- **CV**: Possible increased risk of cardiovascular mortality
- **Hematologic**: *Hypoglycemia*, leukopenia, thrombocytopenia, anemia
- **Hypersensitivity**: Allergic skin reactions, eczema, pruritus, erythema, urticaria, photosensitivity, fever, jaundice
- **Endocrine**: SIADH

Clinically important drug-drug interactions
- Increased risk of hypoglycemia if chlorpropamide is taken concurrently with sulfonamides, urine acidifiers, chloramphenicol, fenfluramine, oxyphenbutazone, phenylbutazone, salicylates, monoamine oxidase inhibitors, clofibrate, dicumarol, rifampin • Decreased effectiveness of chlorpropamide and diazoxide if taken concurrently • Increased risk of hyperglycemia if chlorpropamide is taken with urine alkalin-

Adverse effects in *Italics* are most common; those in **Bold** are life-threatening.

izers, thiazides, other diuretics • Risk of hypoglycemia and hyperglycemia if chlorpropamide is taken with ethanol; "disulfiram reaction" also has been reported

■ Nursing Considerations

Assessment
- *History:* Allergy to sulfonylureas; diabetes complicated by fever, severe infections, severe trauma, major surgery, ketosis, acidosis, coma; type I or juvenile diabetes, serious hepatic or renal impairment, uremia, thyroid or endocrine impairment, glycosuria, hyperglycemia associated with primary renal disease; pregnancy, lactation
- *Physical:* Skin—color, lesions; body temperature; orientation, reflexes, peripheral sensation; R, adventitious sounds; liver evaluation, bowel sounds; urinalysis, BUN, serum creatinine, liver function tests, blood glucose, CBC

Implementation
- Administer drug in the morning before breakfast; if severe GI upset occurs, dose may be divided with one dose before breakfast and one before evening meal.
- Monitor urine and serum glucose levels frequently to determine effectiveness of drug and dosage being used.
- Arrange for transfer to insulin therapy during periods of high stress (eg, infections, surgery, trauma).
- Arrange for use of IV glucose if severe hypoglycemia occurs as a result of overdose; support and monitoring of patient may be prolonged for 3–5 d because of the long half-life of chlorpropamide.

Drug-specific teaching points
- Do not to discontinue this medication without consulting physician.
- Monitor urine or blood for glucose and ketones as prescribed.
- Do not use this drug during pregnancy.
- Avoid the use of OTC drugs and alcohol while taking this drug.
- Report fever, sore throat, unusual bleeding or bruising, skin rash, dark urine, light-colored stools, hypoglycemic or hyperglycemic reactions.

☐ chlorprothixene hydrochloride and lactate

*(klor proe **thix**' een)*

Pregnancy Category C

Drug classes
Dopaminergic blocking agent
Antipsychotic drug
Thioxanthene

Therapeutic actions
Mechanism of action not understood; antipsychotic drugs block postsynaptic dopamine receptors in the brain.

Indications
- Management of manifestations of psychotic disorders.

Contraindications/cautions
- Contraindicated in the presence of coma or severe CNS depression; bone marrow depression; blood dyscrasia; circulatory collapse; subcortical brain damage; Parkinson's disease; liver damage; cerebral arteriosclerosis; coronary disease; severe hypotension or hypertension; children younger than 12 y, especially those with chickenpox, CNS infections (children are especially susceptible to dystonias that may confound the diagnosis of Reye's syndrome).
- Use caution in cases of respiratory disorders; glaucoma, prostatic hypertrophy; epilepsy or history of epilepsy; breast cancer; thyrotoxicosis; peptic ulcer, decreased renal function; myelography within previous 24 h or scheduled within 48 h; exposure to heat or phosphorous insecticides; pregnancy, lactation.

Dosage
Full clinical effects may require 6 wk–6 mo of therapy.
Adult
- ***Oral:*** Initially 25–50 mg tid–qid; increase as needed. Doses exceeding 600 mg/d are rarely required.
- ***IM:*** 25–50 mg tid–qid. Institute oral medication as soon as feasible.

Pediatric: Not recommended for oral use in children younger than 6 y; not recommended for parenteral use in children younger than 12 y.
- *Oral:* 10–25 mg tid–qid.
- *IM:* 25–50 mg tid–qid.

Geriatric and debilitated patients: Initiate treatment with 10–25 mg tid–qid. Increase dosage more gradually than in younger patients.

Pharmacokinetics

Route	Onset	Peak	Duration
Oral	Varies	2–4 h	weeks
IM	10–30 min	1–2 h	weeks

Metabolism: Hepatic, $T_{1/2}$: 10–20 h
Distribution: Crosses placenta; enters breast milk
Excretion: Urine and bile

Adverse effects

- CNS: *Drowsiness, insomnia, vertigo,* headache, weakness, tremors, ataxia, slurring, cerebral edema, seizures, exacerbation of psychotic symptoms, *extrapyramidal syndromes, tardive dyskinesias,* NMS
- GI: *Dry mouth, salivation, nausea, vomiting, anorexia, constipation,* paralytic ileus, incontinence
- CV: *Hypotension, orthostatic hypotension,* hypertension, tachycardia, bradycardia, cardiac arrest, CHF, cardiomegaly, refractory arrhythmias, pulmonary edema
- Respiratory: Bronchospasm, **laryngospasm**, dyspnea, suppression of cough reflex and potential aspiration
- Hematologic: *Eosinophilia, leukopenia, leukocytosis, anemia,* aplastic anemia, hemolytic anemia, thrombocytopenic or nonthrombocytopenic purpura, pancytopenia, elevated serum cholesterol
- GU: *Urinary retention,* polyuria, incontinence, priapism, ejaculation inhibition, male impotence, urine discolored pink to red-brown
- EENT: Nasal congestion, glaucoma, *photophobia, blurred vision,* miosis, mydriasis
- **Hypersensitivity**: Jaundice, *urticaria,* angioneurotic edema, laryngeal edema, *photosensitivity,* eczema, asthma, anaphylactoid reactions, exfoliative dermatitis, contact dermatitis with drug solutions
- Endocrine: Lactation, breast engorgement in females, galactorrhea, SIADH secretion, amenorrhea, menstrual irregularities, gynecomastia in males, changes in libido, hyperglycemia, inhibition of ovulation, infertility, pseudopregnancy, reduced urinary levels of gonadotropins, estrogens and progestins
- Other: Fever, heatstroke, pallor, flushed facies, sweating

Drug-lab test interferences

- False-positive pregnancy tests (less likely if serum test is used) • Increase in *protein-bound iodine,* not attributable to an increase in thyroxine

■ Nursing Considerations

Assessment

- *History:* Allergy to aspirin, tartrazine, coma, or severe CNS depression; bone marrow depression; blood dyscrasia; circulatory collapse; subcortical brain damage; Parkinson's disease; liver damage; cerebral arteriosclerosis; coronary disease; severe hypotension or hypertension; respiratory disorder; glaucoma; prostatic hypertrophy; epilepsy or history of epilepsy; breast cancer; thyrotoxicosis; peptic ulcer, decreased renal function; myelography within previous 24 h or scheduled within 48 h; exposure to heat or phosphorous insecticides; pregnancy, lactation; children younger than 12 y, especially those with chickenpox, CNS infections
- *Physical:* Body weight, temperature; reflexes, orientation, intraocular pressure; P, BP, orthostatic BP; R, adventitious sounds; bowel sounds and normal output, liver evaluation; urinary output, prostate size; CBC, urinalysis, thyroid, liver and kidney function tests

Adverse effects in *Italics* are most common; those in **Bold** are life-threatening.

Implementation
- Arrange for discontinuation of drug if serum creatinine, BUN become abnormal or if WBC count is depressed.
- Administer oral concentrate undiluted or in milk, water, fruit juice, coffee, or carbonated beverages.
- Administer IM doses with patient seated or recumbent to prevent orthostatic hypotension.
- Change from IM to oral administration by giving oral and parenteral doses alternately on the same day and then oral doses only, adjusted to the required maintenance level.
- Avoid skin contact with drug solution; contact dermatitis may occur.
- Monitor elderly patients for dehydration, and institute remedial measures promptly; sedation and decreased sensation of thirst related to CNS effects of drug can lead to dehydration.
- Consult physician regarding appropriate warning of patient or patient's guardian about tardive dyskinesias.
- Consult physician about dosage reduction, use of anticholinergic antiparkinsonian drugs (controversial) if extrapyramidal effects occur.

Drug-specific teaching points
- Take drug exactly as prescribed.
- Avoid driving a car or engaging in other dangerous activities if CNS, vision changes occur.
- Avoid prolonged exposure to sun, or use a sunscreen or covering garments if this is necessary.
- Maintain fluid intake, and use precautions against heat stroke in hot weather.
- Report sore throat, fever, unusual bleeding or bruising, rash, weakness, tremors, impaired vision, dark urine (pink or reddish-brown urine is to be expected), pale stools, yellow of the skin or eyes.

◻ chlorthalidone

(klor thal' i done)
Apo-Chlorthalidone (CAN), Hygroton, Thalitone
Pregnancy Category C

Drug classes
Thiazide-like diuretic

Therapeutic actions
Inhibits reabsorption of sodium and chloride in distal renal tubule, increasing excretion of sodium, chloride, and water by the kidney.

Indications
- Adjunctive therapy in edema associated with CHF, cirrhosis, corticosteroid and estrogen therapy, renal dysfunction
- Hypertension, as sole therapy or in combination with other antihypertensives
- **Unlabeled uses**: calcium nephrolithiasis alone or in combination with amiloride or allopurinol to prevent recurrences in hypercalciuric or normal calciuric patients; diabetes insipidus, especially nephrogenic diabetes insipidus

Contraindications/cautions
- Fluid or electrolyte imbalances, renal or liver disease, gout, SLE, glucose tolerance abnormalities, hyperparathyroidism, manic-depressive disorders, lactation

Dosage
Adult
- ***Edema:*** 50–100 mg/d PO or 100 mg every other day: up to 200 mg/d.
- ***Hypertension:*** 25–100 mg/d PO based on patient response (doses > 25 mg/d are likely to increase K^+ excretion, but provide no further increase in Na^+ excretion or decrease in BP).
- ***Calcium nephrolithiasis:*** 50 mg/d PO.

Pediatric: Safety and efficacy not established.

Pharmacokinetics

Route	Onset	Peak	Duration
Oral	2 h	3–6 h	24–72 h

Metabolism: Hepatic, $T_{1/2}$: 54 h
Distribution: Crosses placenta; enters breast milk
Excretion: Urine

Adverse effects
- **CNS:** *Dizziness, vertigo,* paresthesias, weakness, headache, drowsiness, fatigue
- **GI:** *Nausea, anorexia, vomiting, dry mouth, diarrhea, constipation,* jaundice, hepatitis, pancreatitis
- **GU:** *Polyuria, nocturia, impotence,* loss of libido
- **Hematologic:** Leukopenia, thrombocytopenia, agranulocytosis, aplastic anemia, neutropenia, fluid and electrolyte imbalances
- **CV:** Orthostatic hypotension, venous thrombosis, volume depletion, cardiac arrhythmias, chest pain
- **Dermatologic:** Photosensitivity, rash, purpura, exfoliative dermatitis
- **Other:** Muscle cramps and muscle spasms, fever, hives, gouty attacks, flushing, weight loss

Clinically important drug-drug interactions
- Increased thiazide effects and chance of acute hyperglycemia if taken with diazoxide • Decreased absorption with cholestyramine, colestipol • Increased risk of cardiac glycoside toxicity if hypokalemia occurs • Increased risk of lithium toxicity • Increased dosage of antidiabetic agents may be needed

Drug-lab test interferences
- Decreased PBI levels without clinical signs of thyroid disturbances.

■ Nursing Considerations

Assessment
- *History:* Fluid or electrolyte imbalances, renal or liver disease, gout, SLE, glucose tolerance abnormalities, hyperparathyroidism, manic-depressive disorders, lactation
- *Physical:* Skin—color and lesions; orientation, reflexes, muscle strength; pulses, BP, orthostatic BP, perfusion, edema, baseline ECG; R, adventitious sounds; liver evaluation, bowel sounds; CBC, serum electrolytes, blood glucose, liver and renal function tests, serum uric acid, urinalysis

Implementation
- Administer with food or milk if GI upset occurs.
- Administer early in the day, so increased urination will not disturb sleep.
- Mark calendars or other reminders of drug days for outpatients on every other day or 3- to 5-d/wk therapy.
- Measure and record regular body weights to monitor fluid changes.

Drug-specific teaching points
- Take drug early in the day, so sleep will not be disturbed by increased urination.
- Weigh yourself daily, and record weights.
- Protect skin from exposure to the sun or bright lights.
- Be aware that increased urination will occur (stay close to bathroom facilities).
- Use caution if dizziness, drowsiness, feeling faint occur.
- Report rapid weight gain or loss, swelling in ankles or fingers, unusual bleeding or bruising, muscle cramps.

☐ chlorzoxazone

(klor zox' a zone)
Paraflex, Parafon Forte DSC, Remular-S

Pregnancy Category C

Drug classes
Centrally acting skeletal muscle relaxant

Therapeutic actions
Precise mechanism of action not known; has sedative properties; acts at spinal and supraspinal levels of the CNS to depress reflex arcs involved in producing and maintaining skeletal muscle spasm.

Indications
- Relief of discomfort associated with acute, painful musculoskeletal conditions, as an adjunct to rest, physical therapy, and other measures

Contraindications/cautions
- Contraindicated with allergic or idiosyncratic reactions to chlorzoxazone.

Adverse effects in *Italics* are most common; those in **Bold** are life-threatening.

- Use caution in the presence of history of allergies or allergic drug reactions, lactation.

Dosage
Adult: Initially, 500 mg PO tid–qid; may increase to 750 mg tid–qid; reduce dosage as improvement occurs.
Pediatric: Safety and efficacy not established.

Pharmacokinetics

Route	Onset	Peak	Duration
Oral	30–60 min	1–2 h	3–4 h

Metabolism: Hepatic, $T_{1/2}$: 60 min
Distribution: Crosses placenta; may enter breast milk
Excretion: Urine

Adverse effects
- CNS: *Dizziness, drowsiness, lightheadedness,* malaise, overstimulation
- GI: *GI disturbances*; GI bleeding (rare)
- GU: Urine discoloration—orange to purple-red
- Hypersensitivity: skin rashes, petechiae, ecchymoses, angioneurotic edema, **anaphylaxis** (rare)

Clinically important drug-drug interactions
- Additive CNS effects with alcohol, other CNS depressants

■ Nursing Considerations
Assessment
- *History:* Allergic or idiosyncratic reactions to chlorzoxazone; history of allergies or allergic drug reactions; lactation
- *Physical:* Skin—color, lesions; orientation; liver evaluation; liver function tests

Implementation
- Arrange to discontinue drug if signs or symptoms of liver dysfunction or allergic reaction (urticaria, redness, or itching) occur.

Drug-specific teaching points
- Take this drug exactly as prescribed; do not take a higher dosage than that prescribed for you.
- Avoid alcohol, sleep-inducing, or OTC drugs while you are on this drug; these could cause dangerous effects.
- Know that the following side effects may occur: drowsiness, dizziness, lightheadedness (avoid driving a car or engaging in activities that require alertness if these occur); nausea (taking drug with food and eating frequent small meals may help); discolored urine (this is an expected effect of the drug that you should not worry about).
- Report skin rash, severe nausea, coffee-ground vomitus, black or tarry stools, pale stools, yellow skin or eyes, difficulty breathing.

☐ cholestyramine

(koe **less'** tir a meen)
Cholybar, Questran

Pregnancy Category C

Drug classes
Antihyperlipidemic agent
Bile acid sequestrant

Therapeutic actions
Binds bile acids in the intestine, allowing excretion in the feces; as a result, cholesterol is oxidized in the liver to replace the bile acids lost; serum cholesterol and LDL are lowered.

Indications
- Adjunctive therapy: reduction of elevated serum cholesterol in patients with primary hypercholesterolemia (elevated LDL)
- Pruritus associated with partial biliary obstruction
- **Unlabeled uses**: antibiotic-induced pseudomembranous colitis; bile salt-mediated diarrhea, postvagotomy diarrhea; chlordecone (*Kepone*) pesticide poisoning to bind the poison in the intestine

Contraindications/cautions
- Allergy to bile acid sequestrants, tartrazine (tartrazine sensitivity is seen more

*Adverse effects in Italics are most common; those in **Bold** are life-threatening.*

282 ■ choline magnesium trisalicylate

often in patients allergic to aspirin); complete biliary obstruction; abnormal intestinal function; pregnancy; lactation.

Dosage
Adult: 4 g one to six times per day PO. Individualize dose according to patient's response.
Pediatric: Safety and efficacy not established.

Pharmacokinetics
Not absorbed systemically; excreted in the feces.

Adverse effects
- CNS: Headache, anxiety, vertigo, dizziness, fatigue, syncope, drowsiness
- GI: *Constipation to fecal impaction, exacerbation of hemorrhoids,* abdominal cramps, pain, flatulence, anorexia, heartburn, nausea, vomiting, steatorrhea
- Hematologic: *Increased bleeding tendencies related to vitamin K malabsorption,* vitamins A and D deficiencies, reduced serum and red cell folate, hyperchloremic acidosis
- GU: Hematuria, dysuria, diuresis
- Dermatologic: Rash and irritation of skin, tongue, perianal area
- Other: Osteoporosis, backache, muscle and joint pain, arthritis, fever

Clinically important drug-drug interactions
- Decreased or delayed absorption if taken concurrently with warfarin, dicumarol, thiazide diuretics, digitalis preparations, thyroid, corticosteroids • Malabsorption of fat-soluble vitamins if taken concurrently with cholestyramine

■ Nursing Considerations
Assessment
- *History:* allergy to bile acid sequestrants, tartrazine; complete biliary obstruction; abnormal intestinal function; lactation
- *Physical:* Skin—lesions, color, temperature; orientation, affect, reflexes; P, auscultation, baseline ECG, peripheral perfusion; liver evaluation, bowel sounds; lipid studies, liver function tests, clotting profile

Implementation
- Mix the contents of one packet or one level scoopful of powder with 4–6 fluid oz of beverage (water, milk, fruit juices, other noncarbonated beverage), highly fluid soup, pulpy fruits (applesauce, pineapple); do not administer drug in dry form.
- Administer drug before meals.
- Monitor administration of other oral medications; because of the risk of binding in the intestine and delayed or decreased absorption of other oral medications, give them 1 h before or 4–6 h after the cholestyramine.
- Consult with patient and appropriate sources to cope with the high cost of the drug.

Drug-specific teaching points
- Take drug before meals; do not take the powder in the dry form; mix one packet or one scoopful with 4–6 oz of fluid—water, milk, fruit juice, noncarbonated beverages, highly fluid soups, cereals, pulpy fruits.
- Take other medications 1 h before or 4–6 h after cholestyramine.
- Know that the following side effects may occur: constipation (this may resolve; or other measures may need to be taken to alleviate this problem); nausea, heartburn, loss of appetite (small, frequent meals may help); dizziness, drowsiness, vertigo, fainting (avoid driving and operating dangerous machinery until you know how this drug affects you); headache, muscle and joint aches and pains (this may lessen with time).
- Report unusual bleeding or bruising, severe constipation, severe GI upset, chest pain, difficulty breathing, rash, fever.

❐ choline magnesium trisalicylate

(ko' leen mag nee' see um tri sal' i ci late)

Tricosal, Trilisate

Pregnancy Category C

Adverse effects in *Italics* are most common; those in **Bold** are life-threatening.

Drug classes
NSAID
Salicylate
Analgesic–antipyretic

Therapeutic actions
Inhibits prostaglandin synthesis; this action lowers fever, decreases inflammation.

Indications
- Treatment of osteoarthritis, rheumatoid arthritis
- Relief of moderate pain, fever

Contraindications/cautions
- Contraindicated in the presence of allergy to salicylates, NSAIDs.
- Use caution in the presence of chronic renal failure, peptic ulcer, hepatic failure, children with chickenpox or CNS symptoms, lactation.

Dosage
Adult
- **Arthritis:** 1.5–2.5 g/d PO in one to three divided doses. Do not exceed 4.5 g/d.
- **Pain, fever:** 2–3 g/d PO in two divided doses.

Pediatric
- **Pain, fever:** 50 mg/kg per day PO in two divided doses.

Pharmacokinetics

Route	Onset	Peak
Oral	30 min	1–3 h

Metabolism: Hepatic, $T_{1/2}$: 2–3 h
Distribution: Crosses placenta; passes into breast milk
Excretion: Urine

Adverse effects
- CNS: Dizziness, vertigo, confusion, drowsiness, headache, tinnitus
- GI: *Diarrhea, nausea,* GI lesion, GI bleed

Clinically important drug-drug interactions
- Increased risk of salicylate toxicity if taken with aminosalicylic acid, ammonium chloride, acidifying agents, carbonic anhydrase inhibitors • Increased risk of bleeding if taken with oral anticoagulants • Increased risk of toxicity of methotrexate if taken with choline magnesium trisalicylate • Decreased effectiveness of probenecid, sulfinpyrazone

■ Nursing Considerations

Assessment
- *History:* Allergy to salicylates or NSAIDs, peptic ulcer disease, hepatic failure, chronic renal failure, lactation
- *Physical:* Skin condition, T, neurologic status, abdominal exam, kidney and liver function tests, urinalysis, bleeding times

Implementation
- Give with meals to decrease GI effects.

Drug-specific teaching points
- Take drug with meals; use the drug only as prescribed.
- Know that the following side effects may occur: dizziness, lightheadedness, drowsiness (avoid driving or operating dangerous machinery it this occurs); nausea, diarrhea.
- Report sore throat, fever, rash, itching, black or tarry stools.

☐ choline salicylate

(ko' leen sal' i ci late)
Arthropan

Pregnancy Category C

Drug classes
NSAID
Salicylate
Analgesic–antipyretic

Therapeutic actions
Inhibits prostaglandin synthesis, which lowers fever, decreases inflammation.

Indications
- Treatment of osteoarthritis, rheumatoid arthritis
- Relief of moderate pain, fever

Adverse effects in *Italics* are most common; those in **Bold** are life-threatening.

Contraindications/cautions
- Contraindicated in the presence of allergy to salicylates, NSAIDs.
- Use caution in the presence of chronic renal failure, peptic ulcer, hepatic failure, children with chickenpox or CNS symptoms, lactation.

Dosage
Adult and children older than 12 y: 870 mg PO q3–4h; do not exceed six doses per day. Patients with rheumatoid arthritis may start with 5–10 ml, up to qid.
Pediatric: 2 g/m^2 per day PO in four to six divided doses.

Pharmacokinetics

Route	Onset	Peak
Oral	5–10 min	10–30 min

Metabolism: Hepatic, T$_{1/2}$: 2–3 h
Distribution: Crosses placenta; enters breast milk
Excretion: Urine

Adverse effects
- CNS: Dizziness, vertigo, confusion, drowsiness, headache, tinnitus, sweating
- GI: *Diarrhea, nausea,* hepatotoxicity

Clinically important drug-drug interactions
- Increased risk of salicylate toxicity if taken with aminosalicylic acid, ammonium chloride, acidifying agents, carbonic anhydrase inhibitors • Increased risk of bleeding if taken with oral anticoagulants • Increased risk of toxicity of methotrexate if taken with choline magnesium trisalicylate • Decreased effectiveness of probenecid, sulfinpyrazone

■ Nursing Considerations

Assessment
- *History:* Allergy to salicylates or NSAIDs, peptic ulcer disease, hepatic or chronic renal failure, lactation
- *Physical:* Skin condition, T, neurologic status, abdominal exam, kidney and liver function tests, urinalysis, bleeding times

Implementation
- Give with meals to decrease GI effects; may be mixed with fruit juice or carbonated beverage to improve taste.

Drug-specific teaching points
- Take drug with meals; use drug only as prescribed. May take with fruit juice, carbonated beverages to improve taste. Store drug at room temperature.
- Know that the following side effects may occur: dizziness, lightheadedness, drowsiness (avoid driving or operating dangerous machinery it this occurs); nausea, diarrhea.
- Report sore throat, fever, rash, itching, black or tarry stools.

☐ chorionic gonadotropin

(goe nad' oh troe pin)

human chorionic gonadotropin (HCG)

A.P.L., Chorex, Chorigon, Choron 10, Follutein, Glukor, Gonic, Pregnyl, Profasi HP

Pregnancy Category C

Drug classes
Hormone

Therapeutic actions
A human placental hormone with actions identical to pituitary leutenizing hormone (LH); stimulates production of testosterone and progesterone.

Indications
- Prepubertal cryptorchidism not due to anatomic obstruction
- Treatment of selected cases of hypogonadotropic hypogonadism in males
- Induction of ovulation in the anovulatory, infertile woman in whom the cause of anovulation is secondary and not due to primary ovarian failure and who has been pretreated with human menotropins

Contraindications/cautions
- Contraindicated in presence of known sensitivity to chorionic gonadotropin,

Adverse effects in *Italics* are most common; those in **Bold** are life-threatening.

Dosage

For IM use only; individualize dosage; the following dosage regimens are suggested:

Prepubertal cryptorchidism not due to anatomic obstruction: 4,000 USP U IM, three times per week for 3 wk; 5,000 USP U IM, every second day for four injections; 15 injections of 500–1,000 USP U over 6 wk; 500 USP U three times per week for 4–6 wk; if not successful, start another course 1 mo later, giving 1,000 USP U/injection.

Hypogonadotropic hypogonadism in males: 500–1,000 USP U, IM three times per week for 3 wk; followed by the same dose twice a week for 3 wk; 1,000–2,000 USP U IM three times per week; 4,000 USP U three times per week for 6–9 mo; reduce dosage to 2,000 USP Units three times per week for an additional 3 mo.

Use with menotropins to stimulate spermatogenesis: 5,000 IU IM three times per week for 4–6 mo; with the beginning of menotropins therapy, HCG dose is continued at 2,000 IU twice a week.

Induction of ovulation and pregnancy: 5,000–10,000 IU IM, 1 d following the last dose of menotropins.

Pharmacokinetics

Route	Onset	Peak
IM	2 h	6 h

Metabolism: Hepatic, $T_{1/2}$: 23 h
Distribution: Crosses placenta; may enter breast milk
Excretion: Urine

Adverse effects

- CNS: *Headache, irritablilty, restlessness,* depression, fatigue
- CV: Edema, arterial thromboembolism
- Endocrine: *Precocious puberty, gynecomastia,* ovarian hyperstimulation (sudden ovarian enlargement, ascites, rupture of ovarian cysts, multiple births)
- **Other:** *Pain at injection site*

■ Nursing Considerations

Assessment

- *History:* Sensitivity to chorionic gonadotropin, precocious puberty, prostatic carcinoma or androgen-dependent neoplasm, epilepsy, migraine, asthma, cardiac or renal disease, lactation
- *Physical:* Skin—texture, edema; prostate exam; injection site; sexual development; orientation, affect, reflexes; R, adventitious sounds; P, auscultation, BP, peripheral edema; liver evaluation; renal function tests

Implementation

- Prepare solution for injection using manufacturers' instructions; each brand and concentration varies.
- Discontinue drug at any sign of ovarian overstimulation, and arrange to have patient admitted to the hospital for observation and supportive measures.
- Provide appropriate comfort measures to help patient deal with CNS effects, pain at injection site.

Drug-specific teaching points

- Know that this drug can only be given IM. Prepare a calendar showing the treatment schedule.
- Know that the following side effects may occur: headache, irritability, restlessness, depression, fatigue (it may help to know that these are drug effects; if they become too uncomfortable, consult physician or nurse).
- Report pain at injection site, severe headache, restlessness, swelling of ankles or fingers, difficulty breathing, severe abdominal pain.

☐ chymopapain

(kye' moe pa pane)
Chymodiactin

Pregnancy Category C

Adverse effects in *Italics* are most common; those in **Bold** are life-threatening.

Drug classes
Enzyme

Therapeutic actions
A protein-dissolving enzyme, which hydrolyzes the polypeptides and proteins that maintain the structure of the chondromucoproteins when injected into the lumbar intervertebral disk. This decreases the pressure and relieves compression symptoms in that area.

Indications
- Treatment of herniated lumbar intervertebral disks when symptoms have not responded to conservative therapy.

Contraindications/cautions
- Allergy to chymopapain, papaya; severe spondyloisthesis; spinal stenosis; paralysis; spinal cord tumor; previous injection of chymopapain; use in any spinal region other than the lumbar area

Dosage
Adult: 2–4 nKat U/disk injected; usually 3 nKat U/disk, or a volume of injection of 1–2 ml. Maximum dose in patient with multiple herniations is 8 nKat U injected.
Pediatric: Safety and efficacy not established.

Pharmacokinetics

Route	Onset	Duration
Intradiscal	30 min	24 h

Metabolism: Plasma, $T_{1/2}$: 18–20 h
Distribution: May cross placenta
Excretion: Urine

Adverse effects
- **CNS:** Paraplegia, paralysis, CNS hemorrhage, myelopathy, paraparesis, headache, dizziness, hypalegesia, leg weakness, calf cramping, foot drop, tingling and numbness in toes and legs
- **GI:** Nausea, paralytic ileus
- **GU:** Urinary retention
- **MS:** *Back pain, stiffness, soreness; back spasm;* **discitis**
- **Allergic:** Erythema, pilomotor erection, rash, pruritic urticaria, conjunctivitis, vasomotor rhinitis, angioedema, **anaphylaxis**

■ Nursing Considerations
Assessment
- *History:* Lumbar spine lesion, allergy to papaya or chymopapain, previous injection with chymopapain, spinal tumor, paralysis, spinal stenosis
- *Physical:* Body weight, neurologic status, skin evaluation, abdominal exam, normal urinary output

Implementation
- Pretreat patient with histamine receptor agonists to lessen severity of allergic reaction. Cimetidine 300 mg PO q6h and diphenhydramine 50 mg PO q6h for 24 h before procedure.
- Prepare solution as follows: cleanse vial stopper with alcohol; allow to air dry before inserting needle (alcohol deactives the enzyme); reconstitute with 5 ml Sterile Water for Injection. Do not use Bacteriostatic Water for Injection. Store refrigerated. Use within 2 h of reconstitution. Discard drug after that time.
- Provide appropriate comfort measures to help patient cope with pain of injection, back spasm, and back pain (which may persist for several weeks).

Drug-specific teaching points
- Be aware that this drug will be injected directly into the lumbar spine.
- Know that the following side effects may occur: back spasm, back pain, back soreness, numbness and tingling.
- Report difficulty breathing, rash, itchy or runny eyes, running nose, swelling, vomiting, loss of movement and feeling in the extremities.

❒ cimetidine

*(sye **met'** i deen)*

Novo-Cimetine (CAN), Nu-Cimet (CAN), Peptol (CAN), Tagamet

Pregnancy Category B

Adverse effects in *Italics* are most common; those in **Bold** are life-threatening.

cimetidine ■ 287

Drug classes
H$_2$ antagonist

Therapeutic actions
Inhibits the action of histamine at the histamine$_2$ (H$_2$) receptors of the stomach, inhibiting gastric acid secretion and reducing total pepsin output.

Indications
- Short-term treatment of active duodenal ulcer
- Short-term treatment of benign gastric ulcer
- Treatment of pathologic hypersecretory conditions (eg, Zollinger-Ellison syndrome)
- Prophylaxis of stress-induced ulcers and acute upper GI bleed in critically ill patients
- Treatment of erosive gastroesophageal reflux

Contraindications/cautions
- Allergy to cimetidine, impaired renal or hepatic function, lactation.

Dosage
Adult
- ***Active duodenal ulcer:*** 800 mg PO at bedtime or 300 mg PO qid at meals and bedtime or 400 mg PO bid; continue for 4–6 wk. For intractable ulcers, 300 mg IM or IV q6–8h.
- ***Maintenance therapy for duodenal ulcer:*** 400 mg PO at bedtime.
- ***Active gastric ulcer:*** 300 mg PO qid at meals and at bedtime.
- ***Pathologic hypersecretory syndrome:*** 300 mg PO qid at meals and at bedtime, or 300 mg IV or IM q6h. Individualize doses as needed; **do not exceed 2,400 mg/d**.
- ***Erosive gastroesophageal reflux disease:*** 1,600 mg PO qd for 12 wk.
- ***Prevention of upper GI bleeding:*** Continuous IV infusion of 50 mg/h. Do not treat beyond 7 d.

Pediatric: Not recommended for children younger than 16 y.

Geriatric or impaired renal function: Accumulation may occur. Use lowest dose possible: 300 mg PO or IV q12h; may be increased to q8h if patient tolerates it, and levels are monitored.

Pharmacokinetics

Route	Onset	Peak
Oral	Varies	1–1.5 h
IV/IM	Rapid	1–1.5 h

Metabolism: Hepatic, T$_{1/2}$: 2 h
Distribution: Crosses placenta; enters breast milk
Excretion: Urine

IV facts
Preparation: IV injections: dilute in 0.9% Sodium Chloride Injection, 5% or 10% Dextrose Injection, Lactated Ringer's Solution, 5% Sodium Bicarbonate Injection to a volume of 20 ml. Solution is stable for 48 h at room temperature. **IV infusions**: dilute 300 mg in 100 ml of 5% Dextrose Injection or one of above listed solutions.
Infusion: Inject by direct injection over not less than 2 min; by infusion, slowly over 15–20 min.
Incompatibilities: Incompatible with aminophylline, barbiturate in IV solutions; pentobarbital sodium and pentobarbital sodium/atropine in the same syringe.

Adverse effects
- CNS: *Dizziness, somnolence, headache, confusion, hallucinations*, peripheral neuropathy; symptoms of brain stem dysfunction (dysarthria, ataxia, diplopia)
- GI: *Diarrhea*
- CV: Cardiac arrhythmias, arrest; hypotension (IV use)
- Hematologic: Increases in plasma creatinine, serum transaminase
- Other: *Impotence* (reversible with drug withdrawal), gynecomastia (in long-term treatment), rash, vasculitis, pain at IM injection site

Clinically important drug-drug interactions
- Increased risk of decreased white blood cell counts if taken with antimetabolites, alkylating agents, other drugs known to cause neutropenia • Increased serum levels

Adverse effects in *Italics* are most common; those in **Bold** are life-threatening.

cinoxacin

and risk of toxicity of warfarin-type anticoagulants, phenytoin, beta-adrenergic blocking agents, alcohol, quinidine, lidocaine, theophylline, chloroquine, certain benzodiazepines (alprazolam, chlordiazepoxide, diazepam, flurazepam, triazolam), nifedipine, pentoxifylline, **tricyclic antidepressants, procainamide**, carbamazepine when taken with cimetidine

■ Nursing Considerations

Assessment
- *History:* Allergy to cimetidine, impaired renal or hepatic function, lactation
- *Physical:* Skin—lesions; orientation, affect; pulse, baseline ECG (continuous with IV use); liver evaluation, abdominal exam, normal output; CBC, liver and renal function tests

Implementation
- Administer drug with meals and at bedtime.
- Arrange for decreased doses in renal dysfunction and liver dysfunction.
- Administer IM dose undiluted deep into large muscle group.
- Arrange for regular followup, including blood tests to evaluate effects.

Drug-specific teaching points
- Take drug with meals and at bedtime; therapy may continue for 4–6 wk or longer.
- Take prescribed antacids exactly as prescribed, being careful of the times of administration.
- Inform your nurse or physician about your cigarette smoking habits. Cigarette smoking decreases the effectiveness of this drug.
- Have regular medical followup while you are on this drug to evaluate your response to it.
- Report sore throat, fever, unusual bruising or bleeding, tarry stools, confusion, hallucinations, dizziness, muscle or joint pain.

◻ cinoxacin

(sin ox' a sin)
Cinobac Pulvules
Pregnancy Category B

Drug classes
Urinary tract anti-infective
Antibacterial drug

Therapeutic actions
Bactericidal; interferes with DNA replication in susceptible gram-negative bacteria, preventing cell division.

Indications
- Urinary tract infections caused by susceptible gram-negative bacteria, including *E. coli, P. mirabilis, P. vulgaris, K. pneumoniae, Klebsiella* species, *Enterobacter* species

Contraindications/cautions
- Allergy to cinoxacin; renal dysfunction (do not use with anuric patients); liver dysfunction; pregnancy, lactation

Dosage
Adult: 1 g/d in two to four divided doses PO for 7–14 d.
Pediatric: Not recommended for younger than 12 y.
Geriatric or impaired renal function: Initial dose of 500 mg PO, then the following maintenance schedule is suggested:

Creatinine Clearance (ml/min)	Dosage
>80	500 mg bid
80–50	250 mg tid
50–20	250 mg bid
<20	250 mg/d

Pharmacokinetics

Route	Onset	Peak	Duration
Oral	2 h	2–4 h	10–12 h

Metabolism: Hepatic, $T_{1/2}$: 1–1.5 h
Distribution: Crosses placenta; enters breast milk
Excretion: Urine

Adverse effects
- CNS: *Headache, dizziness,* insomnia, nervousness, confusion

Adverse effects in *Italics* are most common; those in **Bold** are life-threatening.

- **GI:** *Nausea*, abdominal cramps, vomiting, diarrhea, anorexia, perineal burning
- **Hematologic:** Elevated BUN, SGOT, SGPT, serum creatinine, alkaline phosphatase
- **Hypersensitivity:** *Rash, urticaria, pruritis,* edema

Clinically important drug-drug interactions
- Lowered urine concentrations of cinoxacin if pretreated with probenecid

Nursing Considerations

Assessment
- *History:* Allergy to cinoxacin, renal or liver dysfunction, pregnancy, lactation
- *Physical:* Skin—color, lesions; orientation, reflexes; liver and renal function tests

Implementation
- Arrange for culture and sensitivity tests.
- Administer drug with food if GI upset occurs.
- Arrange for periodic renal and liver function tests during prolonged therapy.
- Monitor clinical response; if no improvement is seen or a relapse occurs, send urine for repeat culture and sensitivity.
- Encourage patient to complete full course of therapy.

Drug-specific teaching points
- Take drug with food. Complete full course of drug therapy to ensure a resolution of the infection.
- Know that the following side effects may occur: nausea, vomiting, abdominal pain (small, frequent meals may help); diarrhea (ensure ready access to a bathroom if this occurs); drowsiness, blurring of vision, dizziness (observe caution if driving or using dangerous equipment).
- Report rash, visual changes, severe GI problems, weakness, tremors.

ciprofloxacin hydrochloride

*(si proe **flox'** a sin)*
Ciloxin (CAN), Cipro

Pregnancy Category C

Drug classes
Antibacterial drug

Therapeutic actions
Bactericidal; interferes with DNA replication in susceptible gram-negative bacteria preventing cell reproduction.

Indications
- For the treatment of infections caused by susceptible gram-negative bacteria, including *E. coli, P. mirabilis, K. pneumoniae,* Enterobacter cloacae, *P. vulgaris, P. rettgeri, M. morganii, P. aeruginosa, Citrobacter freundii, S. aureus, S. epidermidis,* group D streptococci
- **Unlabeled use:** effective in patients with cystic fibrosis who have pulmonary exacerbations

Contraindications/cautions
- Contraindicated in the presence of allergy to ciprofloxacin, norfloxacin, pregnancy, lactation.
- Use caution in the presence of renal dysfunction, seizures.

Dosage
Adult
- ***Uncomplicated urinary tract infections:*** 250 mg q12h PO for 7–14 d or 200 mg IV q12h.
- ***Complicated urinary tract infections:*** 500 mg bid PO for 10–21 d or 400 mg IV.
- ***Respiratory, bone, joint infections:*** 500 mg q12h PO for 4–6 wk or 400 mg IV.
- ***Severe skin infections:*** 750 mg q12h PO for 4–6 wk.
- ***Infectious diarrhea:*** 500 mg q12h PO for 5–7 d.

Adverse effects in *Italics* are most common; those in **Bold** are life-threatening.

ciprofloxacin hydrochloride

Pediatric: Not recommended; produced lesions of joint cartilage in immature experimental animals.

Geriatric or impaired renal function
- **Creatinine clearance > 50 (oral), > 30 (IV):** *Usual dosage (30–50)*: 250–500 mg q12h; *5–29*: 250–500 mg q18h (oral), 200–400 mg q18–24h (IV); *hemodialysis*: 250–500 mg q24h, after dialysis.

Pharmacokinetics

Route	Onset	Peak	Duration
Oral	Varies	1–1½ h	4–5 h
IV	10 min	30 min	4–5 h

Metabolism: Hepatic, $T_{1/2}$: 3½–4 h
Distribution: Crosses placenta; enters breast milk
Excretion: Urine and bile

IV facts

Preparation: Dilute to a final concentration of 1–2 mg/ml with 0.9% NaCl Injection or 5% Dextrose Injection. Stable up to 14 d refrigerated or at room temperature.
Infusion: Administer slowly over 60 min.
Incompatibilities: Discontinue the administration of any other solutions during ciprofloxacin infusion.

Adverse effects

- CNS: *Headache*, dizziness, insomnia, fatigue, somnolence, depression, blurred vision
- GI: *Nausea*, vomiting, dry mouth, *diarrhea*, abdominal pain
- Hematologic: Elevated BUN, SGOT, SGPT, serum creatinine and alkaline phosphatase; decreased WBC, neutrophil count, hematocrit
- Other: Fever, rash

Clinically important drug-drug interactions

- Decreased therapeutic effect of ciprofloxacin if taken concurrently with iron salts, sulcrafate • Decreased absorption of ciprofloxacin if taken with antacids • Increased effects of ciprofloxacin if taken with azlocillin • Increased serum levels and toxic effects of theophyllines if taken concurrently with ciprofloxacin

■ Nursing Considerations

Assessment
- *History:* Allergy to ciprofloxacin, norfloxacin; renal dysfunction; seizures; lactation
- *Physical:* Skin—color, lesions; body temperature; orientation, reflexes, affect; mucous membranes, bowel sounds; renal and liver function tests

Implementation
- Arrange for culture and sensitivity tests before beginning therapy.
- Continue therapy for 2 d after the signs and symptoms of infection have disappeared.
- Administer oral drug 1 h before or 2 h after meals with a glass of water.
- Ensure that patient is well hydrated during course of drug therapy.
- Administer antacids if needed at least 2 h after dosing.
- Monitor clinical response; if no improvement is seen or a relapse occurs, repeat culture and sensitivity.
- Encourage patient to complete full course of therapy.

Drug-specific teaching points
- Take oral drug on an empty stomach— 1 h before or 2 h after meals. If an antacid is needed, do not take it within 2 h of ciprofloxacin dose.
- Drink plenty of fluids while you are on this drug.
- Know that the following side effects may occur: nausea, vomiting, abdominal pain (small, frequent meals may help); diarrhea or constipation; drowsiness, blurring of vision, dizziness (observe caution if driving or using dangerous equipment).
- Report rash, visual changes, severe GI problems, weakness, tremors.

Adverse effects in *Italics* are most common; those in **Bold** are life-threatening.

cisapride

(sis' a pride)
Propulsid

Pregnancy Category C

Drug classes
Prokinetic agent
GI drug

Therapeutic actions
Increases the release of acetylcholine in the myenteric plexus; thus, improves GI motility with little to no dopaminergic action.

Indications
- Symptomatic treatment of nocturnal heartburn due to gastroesophageal reflux disease

Contraindications/cautions
- Allergy to cisapride, gallbladder disease, GI hemorrhage, GI obstruction, pregnancy, lactation, prolonged Q-T interval.

Dosage
Adult: 5–20 mg PO tid; usual dose, 10 mg qid. Administer drug at least 15 min before meals and at HS.
Pediatric: Safety and efficacy not established.

Pharmacokinetics

Route	Onset	Peak	Duration
Oral	Rapid	1–1½ h	8–10 h

Metabolism: Hepatic, $T_{1/2}$: 6–12 h
Distribution: Crosses placenta; enters breast milk
Excretion: Urine and feces

Adverse effects
- CNS: *Headache,* fatigue, somnolence
- GI: *Abdominal pain, diarrhea, constipation, nausea, vomiting,* borborygamus, bloating
- CV: **Serious cardiac arrhythmias** when used in combination drug regimens
- Respiratory: *Rhinitis,* sinusitis, coughing, upper respiratory infections

Clinically important drug-drug interactions
- Increased sedative effects if taken with alcohol, benzodiazepines • Increased coagulation times if taken with oral anticoagulants • Risk of serious ventricular arrhythmias if taken with ketoconazole, itraconazol, miconazole IV, troleandomycin

■ Nursing Considerations

Assessment
- *History:* Severe gallbladder disease, GI bleeding, GI obstruction, pregnancy, lactation
- *Physical:* Neurologic status, abdominal exam, R, adventitious sounds, ECG including Q-T interval

Implementation
- Administer at least 15 min before each meal and at bedtime.

Drug-specific teaching points
- Take drug at least 15 min before meals and at bedtime.
- Avoid alcohol while on this drug; serious sedation could occur.
- Know that the following side effects may occur: headache (consult with your nurse or physician if this becomes a problem; appropriate medication may be ordered), stomach rumbling, diarrhea, abdominal pain, nausea, vomiting, constipation.
- Report severe abdominal pain, prolonged diarrhea, weight loss, extreme fatigue.

cisplatin

(sis' pla tin)
CDDP, Platinol, Platinol-AQ

Pregnancy Category D

Drug classes
Alkylating agent
Antineoplastic drug

Therapeutic actions
Cytotoxic: heavy metal that inhibits cell replication; cell cycle nonspecific.

Adverse effects in *Italics* are most common; those in **Bold** are life-threatening.

Indications
- *Metastatic testicular tumors:* combination therapy with bleomycin sulfate and vinblastine sulfate after surgery or radiotherapy
- *Metastatic ovarian tumors:* as single therapy in resistant patients or in combination therapy with doxorubicin after surgery or radiotherapy
- *Advanced bladder cancer:* single agent for transitional cell bladder cancer no longer amenable to surgery or radiotherapy

Contraindications/cautions
- Allergy to cisplatin, platinum-containing products; hematopoietic depression; impaired renal function; hearing impairment; pregnancy; lactation

Dosage
Adult
- **Metastatic testicular tumors**
  - *Remission induction:* Cisplatin: 20 mg/m² per day IV for 5 consecutive d (days 1–5) every 3 wk for three courses of therapy. Bleomycin: 30 U IV weekly (day 2 of each week) for 12 consecutive doses. Vinblastine: 0.15–0.2 mg/kg IV twice weekly (days 1 and 2) every 3 wk for four courses.
  - *Maintenance:* Vinblastine: 0.3 mg/kg IV every 4 wk for 2 y.
- **Metastatic ovarian tumors:** Combination therapy: administer cisplatin and doxorubicin sequentially. *Cisplatin:* 50 mg/m² IV once every 3 wk (day 1). *Doxorubicin:* 50 mg/m² IV once every 3 wk (day 1). As a single agent: 100 mg/m² IV every 4 wk.
- **Advanced bladder cancer:** 50–70 mg/m² IV once every 3–4 wk; in heavily pretreated (radiotherapy or chemotherapy) patients, give an initial dose of 50 mg/m² repeated every 4 wk. Do not give repeated courses until serum creatinine is < 1.5 mg/100 ml or BUN is > 25 mg/100 ml or until platelets > 100,000/mm³ and WBC > 4,000/mm³. Do not give subsequent doses until audiometry indicates hearing is within normal range.

Pharmacokinetics

Route	Onset	Peak	Duration
IV	8–10 h	18–23 d	30–35 d

Metabolism: Hepatic, $T_{1/2}$: 25–49 min, then 58–73 h
Distribution: Crosses placenta; enters breast milk
Excretion: Urine

IV facts
Preparation: Dissolve the powder in the 10-mg and 50-mg vials with 10 or 50 ml of Sterile Water for Injection respectively; resulting solution contains 1 mg/ml cisplatin; stable for 20 h at room temperature—do not refrigerate. Dilute reconstituted drug in 1–2 L of 5% Dextrose in One-Half or One-Third Normal Saline containing 37.5 g mannitol.
Infusion: Hydrate patient with 1–2 L of fluid infused for 8–12 h before drug therapy; infuse dilute drug over 6–8 h.

Adverse effects
- CNS: *Ototoxicity*, peripheral neuropathies, seizures, loss of taste
- GI: *Nausea, vomiting, anorexia*
- Hematologic: *Leukopenia, thrombocytopenia, anemia*, hypomagnesemia, hypocalcemia, hypokalemia, hypophosphatemia, hyperuricemia
- GU: *Nephrotoxicity*, dose limiting
- Hypersensitivity: **Anaphylactic-like reactions**, facial edema, bronchoconstriction, tachycardia, hypotension (treat with epinephrine, corticosteroids, antihistamines)

Clinically important drug-drug interactions
- Additive ototoxicity if taken concurrently with furosemide, bumetanide, ethacrynic acid • Decreased serum levels of phenytoins if taken with cisplatin

■ Nursing Considerations
Assessment
- *History:* Allergy to cisplatin, platinum-containing products; hematopoietic de-

---
Adverse effects in *Italics* are most common; those in **Bold** are life-threatening.

pression; impaired renal function; hearing impairment; pregnancy, lactation
- *Physical:* Weight; eighth cranial nerve evaluation; reflexes; sensation; CBC, differential; renal function tests; serum electrolytes; serum uric acid; audiogram

Implementation
- Arrange for tests to evaluate serum creatinine, BUN, creatinine clearance, magnesium, calcium, potassium levels before initiating therapy and before each subsequent course of therapy. Do not administer if there is evidence of nephrotoxicity; consult with physician.
- Arrange for audiometric testing before beginning therapy and prior to subsequent doses. Do not administer dose if audiometric acuity is not within normal limits; consult with physician.
- Do not use needles of IV sets containing aluminum parts; can cause precipitate and loss of drug potency. Use gloves while preparing drug to prevent contact with the skin or mucosa; contact can cause skin reactions. If contact should occur, wash area immediately with soap and water.
- Maintain adequate hydration and urinary output for the 24 h following drug therapy.
- Arrange for an antiemetic if nausea and vomiting are severe; metoclopramide has been successful.
- Arrange for monitoring of uric acid levels; if markedly increased, allopurinol may be ordered.
- Arrange for monitoring of electrolytes and appropriate supplementation if necessary.

Drug-specific teaching points
- Know that this drug can only be given IV. Prepare a calendar of treatment days.
- Know that the following side effects may occur: nausea, vomiting (medication may be ordered to help; small frequent meals also may help); numbness, tingling, loss of taste, ringing in the ears, dizziness, loss of hearing (these are all effects of the drug).
- Use birth control while taking this drug; this drug may cause birth defects or miscarriages.
- Arrange to have frequent, regular medical follow-up, including frequent blood tests to follow the effects of the drug on your body.
- Report loss of hearing, dizziness; unusual bleeding or bruising, fever, chills, sore throat, leg cramps, muscle twitching, changes in voiding patterns.

cladribine

(kla' dri been)
CdA, 2-chlorodeoxyadenosine

Leustatin

Pregnancy Category D

Drug classes
Antineoplastic

Therapeutic actions
Blocks DNA synthesis and repair, causing cell death in active and resting lymphocytes and monocytes.

Indications
- Treatment of active hairy cell leukemia
- **Unlabeled uses**: advanced cutaneous T-cell lymphomas, chronic lymphocytic leukemia, non-Hodgkin's lymphomas, acute myeloid leukemia, autoimmune hemolytic anemia, mycosis fungoides, Sezary syndrome

Contraindications/cautions
- Contraindicated in the presence of hypersensitivity to cladribine or any components, pregnancy, lactation.
- Use caution in the presence of active infection, myelosuppression, debilitating illness, renal or hepatic impairment.

Dosage
Adult: Single course given by continuous IV infusion of 0.09 mg/kg per day for 7 d.
Pediatric: Safety and efficacy not established.

Pharmacokinetics

Route	Onset	Duration
IV	Rapid	8–10 h

Metabolism: Hepatic, $T_{1/2}$: 5.4 h
Distribution: Crosses placenta; may enter breast milk
Excretion: Urine

IV facts

Preparation: Prepare daily dose by adding calculated dose to 500-ml bag of 0.9% Sodium Chloride Injection. Stable for 24 h at room temperature. Prepare 7-d infusion using aseptic technique, and add calculated dose to 100 ml Bacteriostatic, 0.9% Sodium Chloride Injection (0.9% benzyl alcohol preserved) through a sterile 0.22-μm filter. Store unopened vials in refrigerator, and protect from light. Vials are single-use only and should be discarded after use.

Infusion: Infuse daily dose slowly over 24 h. 7-d dose should be infused continuously over the 7-d period.

Incompatibilities: Do not mix with any other solutions, drugs, or additives. Do not infuse through IV line with any other drug or additive.

Adverse effects

- **GI:** *Nausea, anorexia, vomiting, diarrhea,* constipation, abdominal pain
- **CNS:** *Fatigue, headache,* dizziness, insomnia, **neurotoxicity**
- **CV:** Tachycardia, edema
- **Respiratory:** *Cough, abnormal breath sounds,* shortness of breath
- **Hematologic:** *Neutropenia,* **myelosuppression**
- **Dermatologic:** *Rash,* pruritus, pain, erythema, petechiae, purpura
- **Local:** *Injection site redness, swelling, pain;* thrombosis, phlebitis
- **Other:** *Fever, chills,* asthenia, diaphoresis, myalgia, arthralgia, **infection**, cancer

■ Nursing Considerations

Assessment

- *History:* Allergy to cladribine or any component, renal or hepatic impairment, myelosuppression, infection, pregnancy, lactation
- *Physical:* Body weight, skin condition, neurologic status, abdominal exam, P, respiratory status, kidney and liver function tests, CBC, uric acid levels

Implementation

- Use disposable gloves and protective garments when handling cladribine. If drug contacts skin or mucous membranes, wash immediately with copious amounts of water.
- Ensure continuous infusion of drug over 7 d.
- Caution patients of childbearing age of the severe effects of drug on the fetus; advise the use of birth control measures during and for several weeks after treatment.
- Monitor complete hematologic profile, renal and liver function tests before and frequently during treatment. Consult with physician at first sign of toxicity; consider delaying or discontinuing dose if neurotoxicity or renal toxicity occur.

Drug-specific teaching points

- Be aware that this drug must be given continuously for 7 d and must be given IV.
- Be aware that frequent monitoring of blood tests will be needed during the treatment and for several weeks after treatment to assess the drug's effects on your body.
- Know that the following side effects may occur: fever, headache, rash, nausea, vomiting, fatigue, pain at injection site.
- Report numbness or tingling, severe headache, nausea, rash, extreme fatigue, edema, pain or swelling at injection site.

❒ clarithromycin

*(klar **ith'** ro my sin)*
Biaxin Filmtabs

Pregnancy Category C

clarithromycin ■ 295

Drug classes
Macrolide antibiotic

Therapeutic actions
Inhibits protein synthesis in susceptible bacteria, causing cell death.

Indications
- Treatment of upper respiratory infections caused by *S. pyogenes, S. pneumoniae*
- Treatment of lower respiratory infections caused by *Mycoplasma pneumoniae, S. pneumoniae, H. influenzae, M. catarrhalis*
- Treatment of skin and structure infections caused by *S. aureus, S. pyogenes*

Contraindications/cautions
- Contraindicated in the presences of hypersensitivity to clarithromycin, erythromycin, or any macrolide antibiotic.
- Use caution in the presence of colitis, hepatic or renal impairment, pregnancy, lactation.

Dosage
Adult
- ***Pharyngitis, tonsilitis; pneumonia due to S. pneumoniae, M. pneumoniae; skin or skin-structure infections; lower respiratory tract infections due to S. pneumonie, M. catarrhalis:*** 250 mg PO q12h for 7–14 d.
- ***Acute maxillary sinusitis, lower respiratory infection caused by H. influenzae:*** 500 mg PO q12h for 7–14 d.

Pediatric: Safety and efficacy not established in children younger than 12 y.
Geriatric or impaired renal function: Decrease dosage or prolong dosing intervals as appropriate.

Pharmacokinetics

Route	Onset	Peak
Oral	Varies	2 h

Metabolism: Hepatic, $T_{1/2}$: 3–7 h
Distribution: Crosses placenta; enters breast milk
Excretion: Urine

Adverse effects
- CNS: Dizziness, headache, vertigo, somnolence, fatigue
- GI: *Diarrhea, abdominal pain, nausea,* dyspepsia, flatulence, vomiting, melena, **pseudomembranous colitis**
- Other: *Superinfections*

Clinically important drug-drug interactions
- Increased serum levels and effects of carbamazepine, theophylline when taken with clarithromycin

Clinically important drug-food interactions
- Food decreases the rate of absorption of clarithromycin but does not alter effectiveness

■ **Nursing Considerations**

Assessment
- *History:* Hypersensitivity to clarithromycin, erythromycin, or any macrolide antibiotic; pseudomembranous colitis, hepatic or renal impairment, lactation
- *Physical:* Site of infection, Skin—color, lesions; orientation, GI output, bowel sounds, liver evaluation; culture and sensitivity tests of infection, urinalysis, liver and renal function tests

Implementation
- Culture site of infection before beginning therapy.
- Monitor patient for anticipated response during treatment.
- Administer without regard to meals; administer with food if GI effects occur.

Drug-specific teaching points
- Take this drug with food if GI effects occur. Take the full course of therapy prescribed.
- Know that the following side effects may occur: stomach cramping, discomfort, diarrhea (ensure ready access to bathroom facilities); fatigue, headache (medication may be helpful); additional infections in the mouth or vagina (consult with your care provider for appropriate treatment).

Adverse effects in *Italics* are most common; those in **Bold** are life-threatening.

- Report severe or watery diarrhea, severe nausea or vomiting, skin rash or itching, mouth sores, vaginal sores.

☐ clemastine fumarate

(klem' as teen)
Tavist, Tavist-1

Pregnancy Category B

Drug classes
Antihistamine

Therapeutic actions
Blocks the effects of histamine at H_1 receptor sites; has atropine-like, antipruritic, and sedative effects.

Indications
- Symptomatic relief of symptoms associated with perennial and seasonal allergic rhinitis; vasomotor rhinitis; allergic conjunctivitis; mild, uncomplicated urticaria and angioedema; amelioraton of allergic reactions to blood or plasma; dermatographism; adjunctive therapy in anaphylactic reactions.

Contraindications/cautions
- Contraindicated in the presence of allergy to any antihistamines, third trimester of pregnancy, lactation.
- Use caution in the presence of narrow-angle glaucoma, stenosing peptic ulcer, symptomatic prostatic hypertrophy, asthmatic attack, bladder neck obstruction, pyloroduodenal obstruction.

Dosage
Adult and pediatric older than 12 y: 1.34 mg PO bid to 2.68 mg PO tid. Do not exceed 8.04 mg/d. For dermatologic conditions, use 2.68 mg tid only.
Pediatric younger than 12 y: Safety and efficacy not established.
Geriatric: More likely to cause dizziness, sedation, syncope, toxic confusional states, and hypotension in elderly patients; use with caution.

Pharmacokinetics

Route	Onset	Peak	Duration
Oral	15–30 min	1–2 h	4–6 h

Metabolism: Hepatic, $T_{1/2}$: 3–4 h
Distribution: Crosses placenta; enters breast milk
Excretion: Urine

Adverse effects
- **CNS:** *Drowsiness, sedation, dizziness, disturbed coordination,* fatigue, confusion, restlessness, excitation, nervousness, tremor, headache, blurred vision, diplopia, vertigo, tinnitus, acute labyrinthitis, hysteria, tingling, heaviness and weakness of the hands
- **GI:** *Epigastric distress,* anorexia, increased appetite and weight gain, nausea, vomiting, diarrhea or constipation
- **CV:** Hypotension, palpitations, bradycardia, tachycardia, extrasystoles
- **Respiratory:** *Thickening of bronchial secretions,* chest tightness, wheezing, nasal stuffiness, dry mouth, dry nose, dry throat, sore throat
- **Hematologic:** Hemolytic anemia, hypoplastic anemia, thrombocytopenia, leukopenia, agranulocytosis, pancytopenia
- **GU:** Urinary frequency, dysuria, urinary retention, early menses, decreased libido, impotence
- **Other:** Urticaria, rash, anaphylactic shock, photosensitivity, excessive perspiration, chills

Clinically important drug-drug interactions
- Increased depressant effects if taken concurrently with alcohol, other CNS depressants • Increased and prolonged anticholinergic (drying) effects if taken with MAO inhibitors.

■ Nursing Considerations

Assessment
- *History:* Allergy to any antihistamines; narrow-angle glaucoma, stenosing peptic ulcer, symptomatic prostatic hypertrophy, asthmatic attack, bladder neck obstruction, pyloroduodenal obstruction; lactation
- *Physical:* Skin—color, lesions, texture; orientation, reflexes, affect; vision exam; P, BP; R, adventitious sounds; bowel

sounds; prostate palpation; CBC with differential

Implementation
- Administer with food if GI upset occurs.
- Administer syrup form if patient is unable to take tablets.
- Monitor patient response, and arrange for adjustment of dosage to lowest possible effective dose.

Drug-specific teaching points
- Take this drug as prescribed; avoid excessive dosage.
- Take with food if GI upset occurs.
- Know that the following side effects may occur: dizziness, sedation, drowsiness (use caution if driving or performing tasks that require alertness if these occur); epigastric distress, diarrhea, or constipation (taking the drug with meals may help; consult with care provider if diarrhea or constipation becomes a problem); dry mouth (frequent mouth care, sucking sugarless lozenges may help); thickening of bronchial secretions, dryness of nasal mucosa (a humidifier may help).
- Avoid alcohol while on this drug; serious sedation could occur.
- Report difficulty breathing, hallucinations, tremors, loss of coordination, unusual bleeding or bruising, visual disturbances, irregular heartbeat.

❒ clindamycin hydrochloride

(klin da mye' sin)
Oral: Cleocin

clindamycin palmitate hydrochloride
Oral: Cleocin Pediatric

clindamycin phosphate
Oral, parenteral, topical dermatologic solution for acne, vaginal preparation:
Cleocin Phosphate, Cleocin T, Dalacin C (CAN)

Pregnancy Category B

Drug classes
Lincosamide antibiotic

Therapeutic actions
Inhibits protein synthesis in susceptible bacteria, causing cell death.

Indications
- *Systemic administration:* serious infections caused by susceptible strains of anaerobes, streptococci, staphylococci, pneumococci; reserve use for penicillin-allergic patients or when penicillin is inappropriate; less toxic antibiotics (erythromycin) should be considered
- *Parenteral form:* treatment of speticemia caused by staphylococci, streptococci; acute hematogenous osteomyelitis; adjunct to surgical treatment of chronic bone and joint infections due to susceptible organisms
- *Topical dermatologic solution:* Treatment of acne vulgaris
- *Vaginal preparation:* Treatment of bacterial vaginosis; do not use to treat meningitis; does not cross the blood–brain barrier.

Contraindications/cautions
- *Systemic administration:* allergy to clindamycin, history of asthma or other allergies, tartrazine (in 75- and 150-mg capsules); hepatic or renal dysfunction; lactation.
- *Topical dermatologic solution, vaginal preparation:* allergy to clindamycin or lincomycin; history of regional enteritis or ulcerative colitis; history of antibiotic-associated colitis.

Dosage
Adult
- **Oral:** 150–300 mg q6h, up to 300–450 mg q6h in more severe infections.
- **Parenteral:** 600–2,700 mg/d in two to four equal doses; up to 4.8 g/d IV or IM may be used for life-threatening situations.
- **Vaginal preparation:** One applicator (100 mg clindamycin phosphate) intravaginally, preferably at bedtime, for 7 consecutive d.

Pediatric
- **Oral:** *Clindamycin HCl:* 8–20 mg/kg per day in three to four equal doses; *Clin-*

298 ■ clindamycin hydrochloride

damycin palmitate HCl: 8–25 mg/kg per day in three to four equal doses; children weighing < 10 kg—37.5 mg tid as the minimum dose.
- ***Parenteral (older than 1 mo):*** 15–40 mg/kg per day in three to four equal doses; in severe infections, give 300 mg/d regardless of weight.

Geriatric or renal failure patients: Reduce dose, and monitor patient's serum levels carefully.

Topical dermatologic solution: Apply a thin film to affected area bid.

Pharmacokinetics

Route	Onset	Peak	Duration
Oral	Varies	1–2 h	8–12 h
IM	20–30 min	1–3 h	8–12 h
IV	Immediate	Minutes	8–12 h
Topical	Minimally absorbed systemically		

Metabolism: Hepatic, $T_{1/2}$: 2–3 h
Distribution: Crosses placenta; enters breast milk
Excretion: Urine and feces

IV facts
Preparation: Store unreconstituted product at room temperature. Reconstitute by adding 75 ml of water to 100-ml bottle of palmitate in two portions. Shake well; do *not* refrigerate reconstituted solution. Reconstituted solution is stable for 2 wk at room temperature. Dilute reconstituted solution to a concentration of 300 mg/50 ml or more of diluent using 0.9% Sodium Chloride Injection, 5% Dextrose Injection, or Lactated Ringer's solution. Solution is stable for 16 d at room temperature.

Infusion: Do not administer more than 1,200 mg in a single 1-h infusion. Infusion rates: 300 mg in 50 ml diluent, 10 min; 600 mg in 50 ml diluent, 20 min; 900 mg in 50–100 ml diluent, 30 min; 1,200 mg in 100 ml diluent, 40 min.

Incompatibilities: Calcium gluconate, ampicillin, phenytoin, barbiturates, aminophylline, and magnesium sulfate. May be mixed with sodium chloride, dextrose, calcium, potassium, vitamin B complex, cephalothin, kanamycin, gentamicin, penicillin, carbencillin.

Adverse effects
Systemic Administration
- **GI:** Severe colitis, including **pseudomembranous colitis**, *nausea, vomiting, diarrhea, abdominal pain, esophagitis, anorexia,* jaundice, liver function changes
- **Hematologic:** Neutropenia, leukopenia, agranulocytosis, eosinophilia
- **Hypersensitivity:** *Skin rashes,* urticaria to anaphylactoid reactions
- **Local:** *Pain following injection,* induration and sterile abscess after IM injection, thrombophlebitis after IV use

Topical Dermatologic Solution
- **CNS:** *Fatigue, headache*
- **GI:** Pseudomembranous colitis, diarrhea, bloody diarrhea; abdominal pain, sore throat
- **GU:** Urinary frequency
- **Dermatologic:** *Contact dermatitis, dryness,* gram-negative folliculitis

Vaginal Preparation
- **GU:** *Cervicitis, vaginitis,* vulvar irritation

Clinically important drug-drug interactions
Systemic Administration
- Increased neuromuscular blockade if taken with neuromuscular blocking agents
- Decreased GI absorption if taken with **kaolin, aluminum salts**

■ Nursing Considerations
Assessment
- *History:* Allergy to clindamycin, history of asthma or other allergies, allergy to tartrazine (in 75- and 150-mg capsules); hepatic or renal dysfunction; lactation; history of regional enteritis or ulcerative colitis; history of antibiotic associated colitis
- *Physical:* Site of infection or acne, as appropriate; Skin—color, lesions; BP; respiratory rate, adventitious sounds; bowel sounds, output, liver evaluation; complete blood count, renal and liver function tests

Adverse effects in *Italics* are most common; those in **Bold** are life-threatening.

Implementation

Systemic Administration
- Administer oral drug with a full glass of water or with food to prevent esophageal irritation.
- Do not give IM injections of more than 600 mg; inject deep into large muscle to avoid serious problems.
- Culture site of infection before beginning therapy.
- Do not use for minor bacterial or viral infections.
- Monitor renal and liver function tests, and blood counts with prolonged therapy.

Topical Dermatologic Administration
- Keep solution out of the eyes, mouth and away from abraded skin or mucous membranes; alcohol base will cause stinging.
- Keep cool tap water available to bathe eye, mucous membranes, abraded skin inadvertently contacted by drug solution.

Vaginal Preparation
- Administer intravaginally, preferably at bedtime.

Drug-specific teaching points
- Take oral drug with a full glass of water or with food. Apply thin film of acne solution to affected area twice daily, being careful to avoid eyes, mucous membranes, abraded skin; if solution contacts one of these areas, flush with copious amounts of cool water. Use vaginal prepartion for 7 consecutive d, preferably at betime.
- Take the full prescribed course of this drug (oral). Do not stop taking this drug without notifying your nurse or physician.

Vaginal Preparation
- Refrain from sexual intercourse during treatment with this product.
- Know that the following side effects may occur: nausea, vomiting (small frequent meals may help); superinfections in the mouth, vagina (frequent hygiene measures will help, ask your health care provider for appropriate treatment if it becomes severe).
- Report with oral therapy, severe or watery diarrhea, abdominal pain, inflamed mouth or vagina, skin rash or lesions. With acne solution, abdominal pain, diarrhea. With vaginal preparation: vaginal irritation, itching; diarrhea, no improvement in complaint being treated.

❒ clofazimine

(kloe fa' zi meen)
Lamprene

Pregnancy Category C

Drug classes
Leprostatic

Therapeutic actions
Inhibits growth of *Mycobacterium leprae*, leading to cell death; has anti-inflammatory effects in controlling erythema nodosum leprosum reactions.

Indications
- Treatment of lepromatous leprosy, including dapsone-resistant lepromatous leprosy and lepromatous leprosy complicated by erythema nodosum leprosum
- Part of combination drug therapy in the initial treatment of multibacillary leprosy to prevent the development of drug resistance

Contraindications/cautions
- Contraindicated in the presence of allergy to clofazimine.
- Use caution in the presence of GI problems, diarrhea, pregnancy (infant may be born with pigmented skin), lactation.

Dosage
Adult
- ***Dapsone-resistant leprosy:*** 100 mg/d PO with one or more other antileprosy drugs for 3 y, then 100 mg/d as single agent.
- ***Dapsone-sensitive multibacillary leprosy:*** Give triple-drug regimen for at least 2 y, and continue until negative skin smears are obtained; then monotherapy with the appropriate agent.
- ***Erythema nodosum leprosum:*** 100 mg/d PO. If nerve injury or skin

ulceration is threatened, give corticosteroids. If prolonged corticosteroid therapy is needed, give 100–200 mg clofazimine/d for up to 3 mo; do not exceed 200 mg/d, and taper to 100 mg/d a soon as possible. Keep patient under medical surveillance.

Pediatric: Safety and efficacy not established.

Pharmacokinetics

Route	Onset	Duration
Oral	Varies	Months

Metabolism: Hepatic, $T_{1/2}$: 70 d
Distribution: Crosses placenta; enters breast milk
Excretion: Urine, bile, sputum, sweat

Adverse effects

- CNS: Depression, suicidal tendencies
- GI: *Abdominal, epigastric pain; diarrhea; nausea; vomiting; GI intolerance*; splenic infarction
- Hematologic: Elevated blood sugar, elevated sedimentation rate
- GU: *Discolored urine or feces, sputum, sweat*
- EENT: Conjunctival and corneal pigmentation due to crystal deposits, dryness, burning, itching, irritation
- Dermatologic: *Pink to brownish-black pigmentation of skin; ichthyosis and dryness; rash and pruritus*

■ Nursing Considerations

Assessment

- *History:* Allergy to clofazimine, GI problems, diarrhea, lactation
- *Physical:* Skin—lesions, color, turgor texture; ocular exam; bowel sounds, feces color; culture of lesions

Implementation

- Assess patient, and consult with physician if leprosy reactional episodes occur (worsening of leprosy activity related to therapy). Use of other leprostatics, analgesics, corticosteroids, or surgery may be necessary.
- Protect drug from exposure to moisture, heat.
- Administer drug with meals.
- Provide appropriate skin care for dermatologic reactions. Apply oil if dryness and ichthyosis occur.
- Arrange for treatment with corticosteroids if needed with erythema nodosum leprosum; monitor closely.
- Arrange to reduce dosage if abdominal pain, diarrhea, colic occur. Monitor patient for possible severe abdominal symptoms.
- Caution patient that tears, sweat, sputum, urine, feces may be discolored as a result of therapy.
- Offer support and encouragement to deal with skin pigmentation; assure patient that it is usually reversible but may take several months to years to disappear. Suicides have been reported due to severe depression due to pigmentation effects.
- Contact support groups to help the patient to cope with disease and drug therapy: National Hansen's Disease Center; Carville, LA, 70721; telephone: (504) 642-7771.

Drug-specific teaching points

- Follow the prescription carefully, do not exceed the prescribed dose. Take the drug with meals. To be effective, this drug will be needed for a prolonged period.
- Arrange for regular medical followup while you are on this drug.
- Know that the following side effects may occur: nausea, loss of appetite, vomiting, diarrhea (taking the drug with meals may help); discoloring of the tears, sweat, sputum, urine, feces, whites of the eyes, pigmentation of the skin from pink to brownish-black (these effects are reversible when the drug is discontinued; return of the skin to normal color make take several months or years); dryness of the skin (apply oil as needed).
- Report worsening of Hansen's disease symptoms, severe GI upset, colicky pain, severe depression.

Adverse effects in *Italics* are most common; those in **Bold** are life-threatening.

clofibrate

(kloe fye' brate)
Atromid S

Pregnancy Category C

Drug classes
Antihyperlipidemic agent

Therapeutic actions
Stimulates the liver to increase breakdown of VLDL to LDL; decreases liver synthesis of VLDL; inhibits cholesterol formation, lowering serum lipid levels; has antiplatelet effect.

Indications
- Primary dysbetalipoproteinemia (type III hyperlipidemia) that does not respond to diet
- Very high serum triglycerides (type IV and V hyperlipidemia) with abdominal pain and pancreatitis that does not respond to diet

Contraindications/cautions
- Allergy to clofibrate, hepatic or renal dysfunction, primary biliary cirrhosis, peptic ulcer, pregnancy, lactation.

Dosage
Adult: 2 g/d PO in divided doses. **Caution:** use this drug only if strongly indicated, and lipid studies show a definite response; hepatic tumorigenicity occurs in lab animals.
Pediatric: Safety and efficacy not established.

Pharmacokinetics

Route	Onset	Peak	Duration
Oral	Varies	3–6 h	Weeks

Metabolism: Hepatic, $T_{1/2}$: 15 h
Distribution: Crosses placenta; enters breast milk
Excretion: Urine

Adverse effects
- **GI:** *Nausea*, vomiting, diarrhea, dyspepsia, flatulence, bloating, stomatitis, gastritis, gallstones (with long-term therapy), peptic ulcer, GI hemorrhage
- **CV:** Angina, arrhythmias, swelling, phlebitis, thrombophlebitis, pulmonary emboli
- **Hematologic:** Leukopenia, anemia, eosinophilia, increased SGOT and SGPT, increased thymol turbidity, increased CPK, BSP retention
- **GU:** *Impotence, decreased libido*, dysuria, hematuria, proteinuria, decreased urine output
- **Dermatologic:** *Skin rash*, alopecia, dry skin, dry and brittle hair, pruritus, urticaria
- **Other:** *Myalgia, "flu-like" syndromes,* arthralgia, weight gain, polyphagia, increased perspiration, systemic lupus erythematosus, blurred vision, gynecomastia

Clinically important drug-drug interactions
- Increased bleeding tendencies if oral anticoagulants are given with clofibrate; reduce dosage of anticoagulant, usually by 50% • Increased pharmacologic effects of sulfonylureas, insulin, with resultant increased risk of hypoglycemia if given concurrently with clofibrate

■ Nursing Considerations

Assessment
- *History:* Allergy to clofibrate, hepatic or renal dysfunction, primary biliary cirrhosis, peptic ulcer, lactation
- *Physical:* Skin—lesions, color, temperature; P, BP, auscultation, baseline ECG, peripheral perfusion, edema; bowel sounds, normal output, liver evaluation; normal output; lipid studies, CBC, clotting profile, liver and renal function tests, urinalysis

Implementation
- Administer drug with meals or milk if GI upset occurs.
- Arrange for regular follow-up including blood tests for lipids, liver function, CBC during long-term therapy.
- Monitor urine output.

Adverse effects in *Italics* are most common; those in **Bold** are life-threatening.

Drug-specific teaching points

- Take the drug with meals or with milk if GI upset occurs.
- Know that the following side effects may occur: diarrhea, loss of appetite (ensure ready access to the bathroom if this occurs; small frequent meals may help); dry skin, dry and brittle hair, excessive sweating (frequent skin care, use of nonabrasive lotion may help); loss of libido, impotence (this can be very upsetting).
- Arrange to have regular follow-up visits to your doctor for blood tests.
- Report chest pain, shortness of breath, palpitations, severe stomach pain with nausea and vomiting, fever and chills or sore throat, blood in the urine, little urine output, swelling of the ankles or legs, unusual weight gain.

☐ clomiphene citrate

(kloe' mi feen)

Clomid, Milophene, Serophene

Pregnancy Category X

Drug classes
Hormonal agent
Fertility drug

Therapeutic actions
Binds to estrogen receptors, decreasing the number of available estrogen receptors, which gives the hypothalamus the false signal to increase in FSH and LH secretion, resulting in ovarian stimulation.

Indications
- Treatment of ovarian failure in patients with normal liver function and normal endogenous estrogen levels, whose partners are fertile and potent
- **Unlabeled use:** treatment of male infertility

Contraindications/cautions
- Known sensitivity to clomiphene, liver disease, abnormal bleeding of undetermined origin, ovarian cyst, lactation.

Dosage
Treatment of ovarian failure
- ***Initial therapy:*** 50 mg/day PO for 5 d started anytime there has been no recent uterine bleeding or about the fifth day of the cycle if uterine bleeding does occur.
- ***Second course:*** If ovulation does not occur after the first course, administer 100 mg/d PO for 5 d; start this course as early as 30 d after the previous one.
- ***Third course:*** Repeat second course regimen; if patient does not respond to three courses of treatment, further treatment is not recommended.

Male sterility: 25 mg/d PO for 25 d with a 5-d rest; or 100 mg PO every Monday, Wednesday, and Friday.

Pharmacokinetics

Route	Onset	Duration
Oral	5–8 d	6 wk

Metabolism: Hepatic, $T_{1/2}$: 5 d
Distribution: Crosses placenta
Excretion: Feces

Adverse effects
- **CNS:** Visual symptoms (blurring, spots, flashes), nervousness, insomnia, dizziness, light headedness
- **GI:** *Abdominal discomfort, distention, bloating, nausea, vomiting*
- **CV:** *Vasomotor flushing*
- **GU:** Uterine bleeding, *ovarian enlargement*, ovarian overstimulation, birth defects in resulting pregnancies
- **Other:** *Breast tenderness*

Drug-lab test interferences
- Increased levels of serum thyroxine, thyroxine-binding globulin

■ Nursing Considerations

Assessment
- *History:* Sensitivity to clomiphene, liver disease, abnormal bleeding of undetermined origin, ovarian cyst, pregnancy
- *Physical:* Skin—color, temperature; affect, orientation, ophthalmologic exam; abdominal exam, pelvic exam, liver eval-

Adverse effects in *Italics* are most common; those in **Bold** are life-threatening.

uation; urinary estrogens and estriol levels (women); liver function tests

Implementation
- Arrange for a complete pelvic exam before each course of treatment to rule out ovarian enlargement, pregnancy, other uterine difficulties.
- Arrange for check of urine estrogen and estriol levels before beginning therapy; normal levels indicate appropriate patient selection for this drug.
- Refer patient for complete ophthalmic exam; if visual symptoms occur, discontinue drug.
- Discontinue drug at any sign of ovarian overstimulation, and arrange to have patient admitted to the hospital for observation and supportive measures.
- Provide women with calendar of treatment days and explanations about signs of estrogen and progesterone activity; caution patient that 24-h urine collections will be needed periodically; timing of intercourse is important for achieving pregnancy.
- Caution patient about the risks and hazards of multiple births.
- Explain to patient that if no response has occurred after three courses of therapy, this drug will probably not help, and treatment will be discontinued.

Drug-specific teaching points
- Prepare a calendar showing the treatment schedule, plotting ovulation, and so forth.
- Know that the following side effects may occur: abdominal distention; flushing; breast tenderness; dizziness, drowsiness, lightheadedness, visual disturbances (use caution if driving or performing tasks that require alertness if these occur).
- Be aware that there is an increased incidence of multiple births in women using this drug.
- Report bloating, stomach pain, blurred vision, yellow skin or eyes, unusual bleeding or bruising, fever, chills, visual changes or blurring.

☐ clomipramine hydrochloride

*(kloe **mi**' pra meen)*
Anafranil

Pregnancy Cateogory C

Drug classes
Tricyclic antidepressant (TCA; tertiary amine)

Therapeutic actions
Mechanism of action unknown; inhibits the presynaptic reuptake of the neurotransmitters norepinephrine and serotonin; anticholinergic at CNS and peripheral receptors; sedative.

Indications
- Treatment of obsessions and compulsions in patients with obsessive-compulsive disorder (OCD), whose obsessions or compulsions cause marked distress, are time-consuming, or interfere with social or occupational functioning.

Contraindications/cautions
- Contraindicated in the presence of hypersensitivity to any tricyclic drug, concomitant therapy with an MAO inhibitor, recent MI, myelography within previous 24 h or scheduled within 48 h, lactation.
- Use caution in the presence of electroshock therapy, preexisting cardiovascular disorders (eg, severe coronary heart disease, progressive heart failure, angina pectoris, paroxysmal tachycardia); angle-closure glaucoma, increased intraocular pressure, urinary retention, ureteral or urethral spasm; seizure disorders; hyperthyroidism; impaired hepatic, renal function; psychiatric patients (schizophrenic or paranoid patients may exhibit a worsening of psychosis with TCA therapy); manic-depressive patients; elective surgery.

Dosage
Adult
- ***Initial:*** 25 mg PO qid; gradually increase as tolerated to approximately 100 mg during the first 2 wk. Then increase gradually over the next several weeks to

a maximum dose of 250 mg/d. After reaching the maximum dose, administer once a day at bedtime to minimize sedation.
- **Maintenance:** Adjust the dosage to maintain the lowest effective dosage, and periodically assess patient to determine the need for treatment. Effectiveness after 10 wk has not been documented.

Pediatric
- **Initial:** 25 mg PO qid; gradually increase as tolerated during the first 2 wk to a maximum of 3 mg/kg or 100 mg, whichever is smaller. Then increase dosage to a daily maximum of 3 mg/kg or 200 mg, whichever is smaller. After reaching the maximum dose, administer once a day at bedtime to minimize sedation.
- **Maintenance:** Adjust dosage to maintain lowest effective dosage, and periodically assess patient to determine the need for treatment. Effectiveness after 10 wk has not been documented.

Pharmacokinetics

Route	Onset	Duration
Oral	slow	1–6 wk

Metabolism: Hepatic, $T_{1/2}$: 21–31 h
Distribution: Crosses placenta; enters breast milk
Excretion: Bile/feces

Adverse effects

- CNS: *Sedation and anticholinergic (atropine-like) effects; confusion* (especially in elderly), *disturbed concentration*, hallucinations, disorientation, decreased memory, feelings of unreality, delusions, anxiety, nervousness, restlessness, agitation, panic, insomnia, nightmares, hypomania, mania, *asthenia, aggressive reaction*
- GI: *Dry mouth, constipation,* paralytic ileus, *nausea*, vomiting, anorexia, epigastric distress, diarrhea, flatulence, dysphagia, peculiar taste, increased salivation, stomatitis, parotid swelling, abdominal cramps, black tongue, *eructation*
- CV: *Orthostatic hypotension,* hypertension, syncope, tachycardia, palpitations, MI, arrhythmias, heart block, precipitation of CHF, stroke
- Hematologic: Bone marrow depression, including agranulocytosis; eosinophila, purpura, thrombocytopenia, leukopenia, *anemia*
- GU: Urinary retention, delayed micturition, dilation of the urinary tract, gynecomastia, testicular swelling in men; breast enlargement, *menstrual irregularity* and galactorrhea in women; increased or decreased libido; *impotence*
- Endocrine: Elevated or depressed blood sugar; elevated prolactin levels; SIADH secretion
- Hypersensitivity: Skin rash, pruritus, vasculitis, petechiae, photosensitization, edema (generalized or of face and tongue), drug fever
- Withdrawal: Symptoms on abrupt discontinuation of prolonged therapy: nausea, headache, vertigo, nightmares, malaise
- Other: *Nasal congestion, laryngitis,* excessive appetite, weight gain or loss; sweating hyperthermia, flushing, chills

Clinically important drug-drug interactions

- Increased TCA levels and pharmacologic effects when given with cimetidine. • Increased TCA levels when given with fluoxetine, methylphenidate, phenothiazines, oral contraceptives, disulfiram • Hyperpyretic crises, severe convulsions, hypertensive episodes and deaths when MAO inhibitors, furazolidone are given with TCAs • Increased antidepressant response and cardiac arrhythmias when given with thyroid medication • Increased anticholinergic effects of anticholinergic drugs when given with TCAs • Increased response to alcohol, barbiturates, benzodiazepines, other CNS depressants when given with TCAs • Decreased effects of indirect-acting sympathomimetic drugs (ephedrine) when given with TCAs

Adverse effects in *Italics* are most common; those in **Bold** are life-threatening.

Nursing Considerations

Assessment
- *History:* Hypersensitivity to any tricyclic drug; concomitant therapy with an MAO inhibitor; recent MI; myelography within previous 24 h or scheduled within 48 h; lactation; electroshock therapy; preexisting cardiovascular disorders; angle-closure glaucoma, increased intraocular pressure, urinary retention, ureteral or urethral spasm; seizure disorders; hyperthyroidism, impaired hepatic, renal function; psychiatric patients; elective surgery.
- *Physical:* Body weight; temperature; skin—color, lesions; orientation, affect, reflexes, vision and hearing; P, BP, orthostatic BP, perfusion; bowel sounds, normal output; liver evaluation; urine flow, normal output; usual sexual function, frequency of menses, breast and scrotal exam; liver function tests, urinalysis, CBC, ECG.

Implementation
- Ensure that depressed and potentially suicidal patients have access to only limited quantities of the drug.
- Administer in divided doses with meals to reduce GI side effects while increasing dosage to therapeutic levels.
- Administer maintenance dosage as a once-daily dose at bedtime to decrease daytime sedation.
- Arrange to reduce dosage if minor side effects develop; arrange to discontinue the drug if serious side effects occur.
- Arrange for CBC if patient develops fever, sore throat, or other sign of infection during therapy.

Drug-specific teaching points
- Take this drug exactly as prescribed; do not to stop taking this drug abruptly or without consulting the physician or nurse.
- Avoid alcohol, other sleep-inducing drugs, OTC drugs while on this drug.
- Avoid prolonged exposure to sunlight or sunlamps; use a sunscreen or protective garments if long exposure to sunlight is unavoidable.
- Know that the following side effects may occur: headache, dizziness, drowsiness, weakness, blurred vision (these effects are reversible; safety measures may need to be taken if these become severe; you should avoid driving an automobile or performing tasks that require alertness while these persist); nausea, vomiting, loss of appetite, dry mouth (small, frequent meals; frequent mouth care; and sucking sugarless candies may help); nightmares, inability to concentrate, confusion; changes in sexual function.
- Report dry mouth, difficulty urinating, excessive sedation.

clonazepam

(kloe na' ze pam)
Klonopin, Rivotril (CAN)

C-IV controlled substance
Pregnancy Category D

Drug classes
Benzodiazepine
Antiepileptic drug

Therapeutic actions
Exact mechanisms of action not understood; benzodiazepines potentiate the effects of GABA, an inhibitory neurotransmitter.

Indications
- Used alone or as adjunct in treatment of Lennox-Gastaut syndrome (petit mal variant), akinetic and myoclonic seizures; may be useful in patients with absence (petit mal) seizures who have not responded to succinimides; up to 30% of patients show loss of effectiveness of drug, often within 3 mo of therapy (may respond to dosage adjustment).
- **Unlabeled uses**: treatment of panic attacks, periodic leg movements during sleep, hypokinetic dysarthria, acute manic episodes, multifocal tic disorders, adjunct treatment of schizophrenia, neuralgias

Contraindications/cautions
- Contraindicated in the presence of hypersensitivity to benzodiazepines, psychoses, acute narrow-angle glaucoma, shock,

coma, acute alcoholic intoxication with depression of vital signs; pregnancy (increased risk of congenital malformations, neonatal withdrawal syndrome), labor and delivery ("floppy infant" syndrome reported), lactation (infants become lethargic and lose weight).
- Use caution in the presence of impaired liver or kidney function, debilitation.

Dosage

Individualize dosage; increase dosage gradually to avoid adverse effects; drug is available only in oral dosage forms.

Adult: Initial dose should not exceed 1.5 mg/d PO divided into three doses; increase in increment of 0.5–1 mg PO every 3 days until seizures are adequately controlled or until side effects preclude further dosage increases. Maximum recommended dosage is 20 mg/d.

Pediatric: Infants and children up to 10 y or 30 kg: 0.01–0.03 mg/kg per day PO initially; do not exceed 0.05 mg/kg per day PO, given in two to three doses. Increase dosage by not more than 0.25–0.5 mg every third day until a daily maintenance dose of 0.1–0.2 mg/kg has been reached, unless seizures are controlled by lower dosage or side effects preclude dosage increases. Whenever possible, divide daily dose into three equal doses, or give largest dose at bedtime.

Pharmacokinetics

Route	Onset	Peak	Duration
Oral	Varies	1–2 h	weeks

Metabolism: Hepatic, $T_{1/2}$: 18–50 h
Distribution: Crosses placenta; enters breast milk
Excretion: Urine

Adverse effects

- CNS: *Transient, mild drowsiness initially; sedation, depression, lethargy, apathy, fatigue, lightheadedness, disorientation, anger, hostility,* episodes of mania and hypomania, *restlessness, confusion, crying,* delirium, *headache,* slurred speech, dysarthria, stupor, rigidity, tremor, dystonia, vertigo, euphoria, nervousness, difficulty in concentration, vivid dreams, psychomotor retardation, extrapyramidal symptoms; *mild paradoxical excitatory reactions, during first two weeks of treatment*
- GI: *Constipation, diarrhea, dry mouth,* salivation, *nausea,* anorexia, vomiting, difficulty in swallowing, gastric disorders, hepatic dysfunction, encoporesis
- CV: Bradycardia, tachycardia, cardiovascular collapse, hypertension and hypotension, palpitations, edema
- Hematologic: Elevations of blood enzymes: LDH, alkaline phosphatase, SGOT, SGPT; blood dyscrasias: agranulocytosis, leukopenia
- GU: Incontinence, urinary retention, changes in libido, menstrual irregularities
- EENT: Visual and auditory disturbances, diplopia, nystagmus, depressed hearing, nasal congestion
- Dermatologic: Urticaria, pruritus, skin rash, dermatitis
- Other: Hiccups, fever, diaphoresis, paresthesias, muscular disturbances, gynecomastia. Drug dependence with withdrawal syndrome when drug is discontinued more common with abrupt discontinuation of higher dosage used for longer than 4 mo.

Clinically important drug-drug interactions

- Increased CNS depression when taken with alcohol • Increased effect when given with cimetidine, disulfiram, omeprazole, oral contraceptives • Decreased effect when given with theophylline

■ Nursing Considerations

Assessment

- *History:* Hypersensitivity to benzodiazepines; psychoses; acute narrow-angle glaucoma; shock; coma; acute alcoholic intoxication; pregnancy; lactation; impaired liver or kidney function, debilitation.
- *Physical:* Skin—color, lesions; body temperature; orientation, reflexes, affect,

ophthalmologic exam; P, BP; R, adventitious sounds; liver evaluation, abdominal exam, bowel sounds, normal output; CBC, liver and renal function tests.

Implementation
- Keep addiction-prone patients under careful surveillance because of their predisposition to habituation and drug dependence.
- Monitor liver function, blood counts periodically in patients on long-term therapy.
- Arrange to taper dosage gradually after long-term therapy, especially in epileptic patients; arrange substitution of another antielipetic drug as appropriate.
- Monitor patient for therapeutic drug levels: 20–80 ng/ml.
- Arrange for patient to wear medical alert identification indicating epilepsy and drug therapy.

Drug-specific teaching points
- Take drug exactly as prescribed; do not to stop taking drug (long-term therapy) without consulting health care provider.
- Avoid alcohol, sleep-inducing, or OTC drugs while on this drug.
- Know that the following side effects may occur: drowsiness, dizziness (these may become less pronounced after a few days; avoid driving a car or engaging in other dangerous activities if these occur); GI upset (taking the drug with food may help); fatigue; dreams; crying; nervousness; depression, emotional changes; bed-wetting, urinary incontinence.
- Report severe dizziness, weakness, drowsiness that persists, rash or skin lesions, difficulty voiding, palpitations, swelling in the extremities.

☐ clonidine hydrochloride

(kloe' ni deen)

Apo-Clonidine (CAN), Catapres, Catapres-TTS (transdermal preparation), Dixarit (CAN), Nu-Clonidine (CAN)

Pregnancy Category C

Drug classes
Antihypertensive drug
Centrally acting sympatholytic drug

Therapeutic actions
Stimulates CNS alpha$_2$-adrenergic receptors, inhibits sympathetic cardioaccelerator and vasoconstrictor centers, and decreases sympathetic outflow from the CNS.

Indications
- Hypertension (in the stepped-care approach, clonidine is a step 2 drug)
- **Unlabeled uses**: Gilles de la Tourette's syndrome; migraine, to decrease the severity and frequency of attacks; menopausal flushing, to decrease the severity and frequency of episodes; detoxification of patients from chronic methadone administration; rapid opiate detoxification (in doses up to 17 μg/kg per day); treatment of alcohol and benzodiazepine withdrawal; management of hypertensive "urgencies" (oral clonidine "loading" is used; initial dose of 0.2 mg then 0.1 mg every hour until a dose of 0.7 mg is reached or until blood pressure is controlled)

Contraindications/cautions
- Contraindicated in the presence of hypersensitivity to clonidine or any component of the adhesive layer of the transdermal system.
- Use caution in the presence of severe coronary insufficiency, recent myocardial infarction, cerebrovascular disease; chronic renal failure; pregnancy, lactation.

Dosage
Adult
- **Oral therapy:** Individualize dosage. *Initial dose*: 0.1 mg bid; maintenance dose: increments of 0.1 or 0.2 mg/d may be made until desired response is achieved. Most common range is 0.2–0.8 mg/d given in divided doses; maximum dose is 2.4 mg/d. Minimize sedative effects by slowly increasing the daily dosage and giving the majority of the daily dose at bedtime.

- **Transdermal system:** Apply to a hairless area of intact skin of upper arm or torso once every 7 d. Use a different skin site from the previous application. If system loosens during the 7-d wearing, apply the adhesive overlay directly over the system to ensure good adhesion. Start with the 0.1-mg system (releases 0.1 mg/24 h); if, after 1–2 wk, desired BP reduction is not achieved, add another 0.1-mg system, or use a larger system. Dosage of more than two 0.3-mg systems usually does not improve efficacy. Antihypertensive effect may not commence until 2–3 d after application; therefore, when substituting the transdermal system in patients on previous antihypertensive medication, a gradual reduction of prior dosage is advised. Previous antihypertensive medication may have to be continued, particularly in patients with severe hypertension.

Pediatric: Safety and efficacy not established.

Pharmacokinetics

Route	Onset	Peak	Duration
Oral	30–60 min	3–5 h	24 h
Transdermal	Slow	2–3 d	7 d

Metabolism: Hepatic, $T_{1/2}$: 12–16 h, 19 h (transdermal system)
Distribution: Crosses placenta; enters breast milk
Excretion: Urine

Adverse effects

- CNS: *Drowsiness, sedation, dizziness,* headache, fatigue that tend to diminish within 4–6 wk, dreams, nightmares, insomnia, hallucinations, delirium, nervousness, restlessness, anxiety, depression, retinal degeneration
- GI: *Dry mouth, constipation,* anorexia, malaise, nausea, vomiting, parotid pain, parotitis, mild transient abnormalitities in liver function tests
- CV: Congestive heart failure, orhtostatic hypotension, palpitations, tachycardia, bradycardia, Raynaud's phenomenon, ECG abnormalities manifested as Wenckebach period or ventricular trigeminy
- GU: Impotence, decreased sexual activity, loss of libido, nocturia, difficulty in micturition, urinary retention
- Dermatologic: Rash, angioneurotic edema, hives, urticaria, hair thinning and alopecia, pruritus, dryness, itching or burning of the eyes, pallor
- Other: Weight gain, transient elevation of blood glucose or serum creatine phosphokinase, gynecomastia, weakness, muscle or joint pain, cramps of the lower limbs, dryness of the nasal mucosa, fever

Transdermal System
- CNS: *Drowsiness,* fatigue, headache, lethargy, sedation, insomnia, nervousness
- GI: *Dry mouth,* constipation, nausea, change in taste, dry throat
- GU: Impotence, sexual dysfunction
- Local: *Transient localized skin reactions,* pruritus, erythema, allergic contact sensitization and contact dermatitis, localized vesiculation, hyperpigmentation, edema, excoriation, burning, papules, throbbing, blanching, generalized macular rash

Clinically important drug-drug interactions

- Decreased antihypertensive effects when given with tricyclic antidepressants (eg, imipramine) • Paradoxical hypertension when given with propranolol; also greater withdrawal hypertension when clonidine is abruptly discontinued and patient is taking beta-adrenergic blocking agents

■ Nursing Considerations

Assessment

- *History:* Hypersensitivity to clonidine or any component of the adhesive layer of the transdermal system; severe coronary insufficiency, recent myocardial infarction, cerebrovascular disease; chronic renal failure; lactation
- *Physical:* Body weight; body temperature; Skin—color, lesions, temperature; mucous membranes—color, lesion; breast exam; orientation, affect, reflexes;

Adverse effects in *Italics* are most common; those in **Bold** are life-threatening.

ophthalmologic exam; P, BP, orthostatic BP, perfusion, edema, auscultation; bowel sounds, normal output, liver evaluation, palpation of salivary glands; normal urinary output, voiding pattern; liver function tests, ECG

Implementation

- Do not discontinue drug abruptly; discontinue therapy by reducing the dosage gradually over 2–4 d to avoid rebound hypertension, tachycardia, flushing, nausea, vomiting, cardiac arrhythmias (hypertensive encephlopathy and death have occurred after abrupt cessation of clonidine).
- Do not discontinue clonidine if patient needs surgery; arrange to monitor BP carefully during surgery; have other blood pressure-controlling drugs on standby.
- Arrange to reevaluate the therapy if clonidine tolerance occurs; the concomitant administration of a diuretic increases the antihypertensive efficacy of clonidine.
- Monitor blood pressure carefully when discontinuing clonidine; hypertension usually returns within 48 h.
- Assess compliance with drug regimen in a nonthreatening, supportive manner; pill counts, other methods of evaluation may be needed.

Drug-specific teaching points

- Take this drug exactly as prescribed. It is important that you not miss doses. Do not discontinue the drug unless instructed to do so. Do not discontinue abruptly; life-threatening adverse effects may occur. If you are going out of town, be sure that you have an adequate supply of the drug with you.
- Use the transdermal system exactly as prescribed; refer to directions in package insert, or contact your nurse or physician if you have questions.
- Attempt lifestyle changes (as appropriate) that will contribute to BP reduction: discontinue smoking and the use of alcohol; lose weight; restrict your intake of sodium (salt); exercise regularly.
- Use caution if you ingest alcohol. You may become very sensitive to the effects of alcohol while you are taking this drug.
- Know that the following side effects may occur: drowsiness, dizziness, lightheadedness, headache, weakness (these are often transient symptoms that go away after 4–6 wk of treatment; observe caution while driving or performing other tasks that require alertness or physical dexterity while you are experiencing these symptoms); dry mouth (sucking on sugarless lozenges or ice chips may help); GI upset (frequent small meals may help); dreams, nightmares (it may help to know that these are drug effects); dizziness, lightheadedness when you change position (get up slowly; use caution when climbing stairs); impotence, other sexual dysfunction, decreased libido (you may wish to discuss these with your nurse or physician); breast enlargement, sore breasts; palpitations.
- Report urinary retention, changes in vision, blanching of fingers, skin rash.

▢ clorazepate dipotassium

(klor az' e pate)

Apo-Clorazepate (CAN), Gen-Xene, Novo-Clopate (CAN), Tranxene

Pregnancy Category D
C-IV Controlled Substance

Drug classes
Benzodiazepine
Antianxiety drug
Antiepileptic drug

Therapeutic actions
Exact mechanisms of action not understood; benzodiazepines potentiate the effects of GABA, an inhibitory neurotransmitter; anxiolytic effects occur at doses well below those necessary to cause sedation, ataxia.

Indications
- Management of anxiety disorders or for short-term relief of symptoms of anxiety

310 ■ clorazepate dipotassium

- Symptomatic relief of acute alcohol withdrawal
- Adjunctive therapy in the management of partial seizures

Contraindications/cautions
- Contraindicated in the presence of hypersensitivity to benzodiazepines; psychoses; acute narrow-angle glaucoma; shock; coma; acute alcoholic intoxication with depression of vital signs; pregnancy (increased risk of congenital malformations, neonatal withdrawal syndrome); labor and delivery ("floppy infant" syndrome reported); lactation (infants tend to become lethargic and lose weight).
- Use caution in the presence of impaired liver or kidney function, debilitation.

Dosage
Individualize dosage; increase dosage gradually to avoid adverse effects. Drug is available only in oral forms.

Adult
- **Anxiety:** Usual dose is 30 mg/d PO in divided doses tid; adjust gradually within the range of 15–60 mg/d; also may be administered as a single daily dose at bedtime; start with a dose of 15 mg. *Maintenance:* give the 22.5-mg PO tablet in a single daily dose as an alternate dosage form for patients stabilized on 7.5 mg PO tid; do not use to initiate therapy; the 11.5-mg tablet may be given as a single daily dose.
- **Adjunct to antiepileptic medication:** Maximum initial dose is 7.5 mg PO tid. Increase dosage by no more than 7.5 mg every week, and do not exceed 90 mg/d.
- **Acute alcohol withdrawal:** *Day 1:* 30 mg PO initially, then 30–60 mg in divided doses. *Day 2:* 45–90 mg PO in divided doses. *Day 3:* 22.5–45 mg PO in divided doses. *Day 4:* 15–30 mg PO in divided doses. Thereafter, gradually reduce dose to 7.5–15 mg/d PO, and discontinue as soon as patient's condition is stable.

Pediatric
- **Adjunct to antiepileptic medication:** *Older than 12 y:* Same as adult. *9–12 y:* maximum initial dose is 7.5 mg PO bid; increase dosage by no more than 7.5 mg every week, and do not exceed 60 mg/d. *Younger than 9 y:* Not recommended.

Geriatric patients or those with debilitating disease
- **Anxiety:** Initially, 7.5–15 mg/d PO in divided doses. Adjust as needed and tolerated.

Pharmacokinetics

Route	Onset	Peak	Duration
Oral	Fast	1–2 h	Days

Metabolism: Hepatic, $T_{1/2}$: 30–100 h
Distribution: Crosses placenta; enters breast milk
Excretion: Urine

Adverse effects
- CNS: *Transient, mild drowsiness initially; sedation, depression, lethargy, apathy, fatigue, lightheadedness, disorientation, anger, hostility,* episodes of mania and hypomania, *restlessness, confusion, crying,* delirium, *headache,* slurred speech, dysarthria, stupor, rigidity, tremor, dystonia, vertigo, euphoria, nervousness, difficulty in concentration, vivid dreams, psychomotor retardation, extrapyramidal symptoms; *mild paradoxical excitatory reactions, during first 2 wk of treatment*
- GI: *Constipation, diarrhea, dry mouth,* salivation, *nausea,* anorexia, vomiting, difficulty in swallowing, gastric disorders, hepatic dysfunction, encoporesis
- CV: Bradycardia, tachycardia, cardiovascular collapse, hypertension and hypotension, palpitations, edema
- Hematologic: Elevations of blood enzymes—LDH, alkaline phosphatase, SGOT, SGPT; blood dyscrasias—agranulocytosis, leukopenia
- GU: Incontinence, urinary retention, changes in libido, menstrual irregularities

Adverse effects in *Italics* are most common; those in **Bold** are life-threatening.

- **EENT:** Visual and auditory disturbances, diplopia, nystagmus, depressed hearing, nasal congestion
- **Dermatologic:** Urticaria, pruritus, skin rash, dermatitis
- **Other:** Hiccups, fever, diaphoresis, paresthesias, muscular disturbances, gynecomastia. Drug dependence with withdrawal syndrome when drug is discontinued more common with abrupt discontinuation of higher dosage used for longer than 4 mo.

Clinically important drug-drug interactions

• Increased CNS depression when taken with alcohol • Increased effect when given with cimetidine, disulfiram, omeprazole, oral contraceptives • Decreased effect when given with theophylline

Nursing Considerations

Assessment

- *History:* Hypersensitivity to benzodiazepines; psychoses; acute narrow-angle glaucoma; shock; coma; acute alcoholic intoxication; pregnancy; lactation; impaired liver or kidney function; debilitation
- *Physical:* Skin—color, lesions; body temperature; orientation, reflexes, affect, ophthalmologic exam; P, BP; R, adventitious sounds; liver evaluation, abdominal exam, bowel sounds, normal output; CBC, liver and renal function tests

Implementation

- Arrange to taper dosage gradually after long-term therapy, especially in epileptic patients.
- Arrange for epileptic patients to wear medical alert identification, indicating medication usage and epilepsy.

Drug-specific teaching points

- Take drug exactly as prescribed; do not stop taking drug (long-term therapy) without consulting health care provider.
- Avoid alcohol, sleep-inducing, or OTC drugs while on this drug.
- Know that the following side effects may occur: drowsiness, dizziness (these may become less pronounced after a few days; avoid driving a car or engaging in other dangerous activities if these occur); GI upset (taking the drug with food may help); fatigue; depression; dreams; crying; nervousness; depression, emotional changes; bed-wetting, urinary incontinence.
- Report severe dizziness, weakness, drowsiness that persists, rash or skin lesions, difficulty voiding, palpitations, swelling in the extremities.

clotrimazole

*(kloe **trim'** a zole)*

Troche preparation: Canesten (CAN), Mycelex

Vaginal preparations: Gyne-Lotrimin, Mycelex-G, Myclo (CAN)

Topical preparations: Clotrimaderm (CAN), Lotrimin, Mycelex

Pregnancy Category C (troche)
Pregnancy Category B (topical, vaginal)

Drug classes
Antifungal

Therapeutic actions
Fungicidal and fungistatic: binds to fungal cell membrane with a resultant change in membrane permeability, allowing leakage of intracellular components, causing cell death.

Indications

- Treatment of oropharyngeal candidiasis (troche)
- Local treatment of vulvovaginal candidiasis (moniliasis; vaginal preparations)
- Topical treatment of tinea pedia, tinea cruris, tinea corporis due to *Trichophyton rubrum, Trichophyton mentagrophytes, Epidermophyton floccosum, Microsporum canis*; candidiasis due to *Candida albicans*; tinea versicolor due

Adverse effects in *Italics* are most common; those in **Bold** are life-threatening.

to *Microsporum furfur* (topical preparations)

Contraindications/cautions
- Allergy to clotrimazole or components used in preparation

Dosage
Troche: Administer 1 troche five times a day for 14 consecutive d.
Vaginal preparation, tablet: Insert one 100-mg tablet intravaginally at bedtime for 7 nights or two 100-mg tablets intravaginally at bedtime for 3 nights, or insert one 500-mg tablet intravaginally one time only.
Vaginal preparation, cream: One applicator (5 g/d), preferably at bedtime for 7–14 consecutive d; 14-d treatments have a higher success rate.
Topical: Gently massage into affected and surrounding skin areas bid in the morning and evening for 1–4 wk. With no improvement in 4 wk, reevaluate diagnosis.

Pharmacokinetics
Action is primarily local; pharmacokinetics are not known.

Adverse effects
Troche
- GI: *Nausea, vomiting, abnormal liver function tests*

Vaginal
- GI: *Lower abdominal cramps,* bloating
- GU: *Slight urinary frequency; burning or irritation in the sexual partner*
- Dermatologic: Skin rash

Topical
- Local: *Erythema, stinging,* blistering, peeling, edema, pruritus, urticaria, general skin irritation

■ Nursing Considerations

Assessment
- *History:* Allergy to clotrimazole or components used in preparation
- *Physical:* Skin—color, lesions, area around lesions; bowel sounds; culture of area involved, liver function tests

Implementation
- Arrange for appropriate culture of fungus involved before beginning therapy.
- Have patient dissolve troche slowly in mouth.
- Insert vaginal tablets high into the vagina; administer preferably at bedtime; if this is not possible, have patient remain recumbent for 10–15 min after insertion. Provide sanitary napkin to protect clothing from stains.
- Administer vaginal cream high into vagina using the applicator supplied with the product. Administer for 7–14 consecutive nights, even during menstrual period.
- Cleanse affected area before topical application, unless otherwise indicated. Do not apply to eyes or eye areas.
- Monitor response to drug therapy. If no response is noted, arrange for more cultures to determine causative organism.
- Ensure that patient receives full course of therapy to eradicate the fungus and prevent recurrence.
- Discontinue topical or vaginal administration if rash or sensitivity occurs.

Drug-specific teaching points
- Take the full course of drug therapy, even if symptoms improve. Continue during menstrual period if vaginal route is being used. Long-term use of the drug may be needed; beneficial effects may not be seen for several weeks. Vaginal tablets and creams should be inserted high into the vagina. Troche preparation should be allowed to dissolve slowly in the mouth. Apply topical preparation with a gently massage into the affected area.
- Use hygiene measures to prevent reinfection or spread of infection.
- **Vaginal use:** Refrain from sexual intercourse, or advise partner to use a condom to avoid reinfection. Use a sanitary napkin to prevent staining of clothing.
- Know that the following side effects may occur: nausea, vomiting, diarrhea (oral use); irritation, burning, stinging (local use).
- Report worsening of the condition being treated, local irritation, burning (topical application), rash, irritation, pelvic pain

cloxacillin sodium ■ 313

(vaginal use), nausea, GI distress (oral administration).

☐ cloxacillin sodium

(klox a sill' in)
Apo-Cloxi (CAN), Cloxapen, Novo-Cloxin (CAN), Nu-Cloxi (CAN), Orbenin (CAN), Tegopen

Pregnancy Category B

Drug classes
Antibiotic
Penicillinase-resistant pencillin

Therapeutic actions
Bactericidal: inhibits cell wall synthesis of sensitive organisms, causing cell death.

Indications
- Infections due to penicillinase-producing staphylococci

Contraindications/cautions
- Contraindicated in the presence of allergies to penicillins, cephalosporins, or other allergens.
- Use caution in the presence of renal disorders, lactation (may cause diarrhea or candidiasis in the infant).

Dosage
Adult: 250 mg q6h PO; up to 500 mg q6h PO in severe infections.
Pediatric: < 20 kg: 50 mg/kg/day PO in equally divided doses q6h; up to 100 mg/kg per day PO in equally divided doses q6h in severe infections.

Pharmacokinetics

Route	Onset	Peak
Oral	Varies	1 h

Metabolism: $T_{1/2}$: 30–90 min
Distribution: Crosses placenta; enters breast milk
Excretion: Urine

Adverse effects
- **CNS:** Lethargy, hallucinations, seizures, decreased reflexes
- **GI:** *Glossitis, stomatitis, gastritis, sore mouth,* furry tongue, black "hairy" tongue, *nausea, vomiting, diarrhea,* abdominal pain, bloody diarrhea, enterocolitis, pseudomembranous colitis, nonspecific hepatitis
- **Hematologic:** Anemia, thrombocytopenia, leukopenia, neutropenia, prolonged bleeding time, hemorrhagic episodes at high doses
- **GU:** Nephritis—oliguria, proteinuria, hematuria, casts, azotemia, pyuria
- **Hypersensitivity:** *Rash, fever, wheezing,* **anaphylaxis**
- **Other:** *Superinfections*—oral and rectal moniliasis, vaginitis

Clinically important drug-drug interactions
- Decreased effectiveness if taken with tetracyclines • Decreased efficacy of oral contraceptives is possible if taken with cloxacillin

Clinically important drug-food interactions
- Decreased absorption and decreased serum levels if taken with food

■ Nursing Considerations

Assessment
- *History:* Allergies to penicillins, cephalosporins, or other allergens; renal disorders, lactation
- *Physical:* Culture infected area; skin—color, lesion; R, adventitious sounds; bowel sounds; CBC, liver and renal function tests, serum electrolytes, Hct, urinalysis

Implementation
- Administer on an empty stomach, 1 h before or 2 h after meals, with a full glass of water. Do not give with fruit juice or soft drinks.
- Arrange to continue treatment for 10 full d.

Adverse effects in *Italics* are most common; those in **Bold** are life-threatening.

Drug-specific teaching points

- Take drug around the clock as prescribed; take the full course of therapy, usually 10 d. Take the drug on an empty stomach, 1 h before or 2 h after meals, with a full glass of water.
- Be aware that this antibiotic is specific for this infection and should not be used to self-treat other infections.
- Know that the following side effects may occur: stomach upset, nausea, diarrhea, mouth sores (if these become severe, consult with nurse or physician for appropriate treatment).
- Report unusual bleeding or bruising, fever, chills, sore throat, hives, rash, severe diarrhea, difficulty breathing.

☐ clozapine

(kloe ' za peen)

Clozaril

Pregnancy Category B

Drug classes
Antipsychotic drug
Dopaminergic blocking drug

Therapeutic actions
Mechanism of action not fully understod: blocks dopamine receptors in the brain, depresses the reticular activating system; anticholinergic, antihistaminic (H_1), and alpha-adrenergic blocking activity may contribute to some of its therapeutic (and adverse) actions. Clozapine produces fewer extrapyramidal effects than other antipsychotics.

Indications
- Management of severely ill schizophrenic patients who fail to respond adequately to standard antipsychotic drug treatment.

Contraindications/cautions
- Contraindicated in the presence of allergy to clozapine, myeloproliferative disorders, history of clozapine-induced agranulocytosis or severe granulocytopenia, severe CNS depression, comatose states, history or seizure disorders, lactation.
- Use caution in the presence of cardiovascular disease, prostate enlargement, narrow-angle glaucoma, pregnancy.

Dosage
Adult
- ***Initial:*** 25 mg PO qid or bid; then gradually continue to increase with daily dosage increments of 25–50 mg/d, if tolerated, to a dose of 300–450 mg/d by the end of second week. Make subsequent dosage increments no more than once or twice weekly in increments not to exceed 100 mg. Do not exceed 900 mg/d.
- ***Maintenance:*** Maintain at the lowest effective dose needed to maintain remission of symptoms.
- ***Discontinuation:*** Gradual reduction of dose over a 2-wk period is preferred. If abrupt discontinuation is required, carefully monitor patient for signs of acute psychotic symptoms.
- ***Reinitiation of treatment:*** Follow initial dosage guidelines, using extreme care due to increased risk of severe adverse effects with reexposure.

Pediatric: Safety and efficacy in children younger than 16 y not established.

Pharmacokinetics

Route	Onset	Peak	Duration
Oral	Varies	1–6 h	Weeks

Metabolism: Hepatic, $T_{1/2}$: 4–12 h
Distribution: Crosses placenta; enters breast milk
Excretion: Urine and feces

Adverse effects
- **CNS:** *Drowsiness, sedation, seizures, dizziness, syncope, headache,* tremor, distubed sleep, nightmares, restlessness, agitation, increased salivation, sweating
- **GI:** *Nausea, vomiting, constipation,* abdominal discomfort, dry mouth
- **CV:** *Tachycardia, hypotension,* ECG changes, hypertension

Adverse effects in *Italics* are most common; those in **Bold** are life-threatening.

- Hematologic: Leukopenia, granulocytopenia, agranulocytopenia
- GU: Urinary abnormalities
- Other: *Fever,* weight gain, rash

Clinically important drug-drug interactions

- Increased therapeutic and toxic effects of clozapine if taken with cimetidine • Decreased therapeutic effect of clozapine if taken with phenytoin, mephenytoin, ethotoin

■ Nursing Considerations

Assessment

- *History:* Allergy to clozapine, myeloproliferative disorders, history of clozapine-induced agranulocytosis or severe granulocytopenia, severe CNS depression, comatose states, history or seizure disorders, cardiovascular disease, prostate enlargement, narrow-angle glaucoma, lactation
- *Physical:* Body temperature, weight; reflexes, orientation, intraocular pressure, ophthalmologic exam; P, BP, orthostatic BP, ECG; R, adventitious sounds; bowel sounds, normal output, liver evaluation; prostate palpation, normal urine output; CBC, urinalysis, liver and kidney function tests, EEG as appropriate

Implementation

- Administer only after patient has been tried on conventional antipsychotic drugs and found to be unresponsive to that drug therapy.
- Arrange to obtain clozapine through the *Clozaril Patient Management System.*
- Do not dispense more than 1 wk supply at a time.
- Monitor WBC carefully before administering first dose.
- Arrange for periodic monitoring of WBC weekly during treatment and for the 4 wk following the discontinuation of clozapine.
- Monitor body temperature. If fever occurs, determine that no underlying infection is present, and consult physician for appropriate comfort measures.
- Monitor elderly patients for dehydration, and institute remedial measures promptly; sedation and decreased sensation of thirst related to CNS effects of drug can lead to dehydration.
- Encourage voiding before taking the drug to help decrease anticholinergic effects of urinary retention.
- Follow guidelines for discontinuation or reinstitution of the drug carefully.

Drug-specific teaching points

- Be aware that weekly blood tests will be taken to determine safe dosage; dosage will be increased gradually to achieve most effective dose. Only 1 wk of medication can be dispensed at a time. Do not take more than your prescribed dosage. Do not make up missed doses, contact your nurse of physician if this occurs. Do not stop taking this drug suddenly; gradual reduction of dosage is needed to prevent side effects.
- Know that the following effects may occur as a result of drug therapy: drowsiness, dizziness, sedation, seizures (avoid driving a car, operating machinery, or performing tasks that require concentration); dizziness, faintness on arising (change positions slowly; use caution if this occurs); increased salivation (it might help to know that this is a drug effect); constipation (consult with your care provider for appropriate relief measures); fast heart rate (rest, take your time if this occurs).
- Know that this drug cannot be taken during pregnancy. If you think you are pregnant or wish to become pregnant, contact your nurse or physician.
- Report lethargy, weakness, fever, sore throat, malaise, mouth ulcers, and "flu-like" symptoms.

❒ codeine phosphate

(koe' deen)
codeine sulfate

Pregnancy Category C during pregnancy
Pregnancy Category D during labor
C-II Controlled Substance

Adverse effects in *Italics* are most common; those in **Bold** are life-threatening.

codeine phosphate

Drug classes
Narcotic agonist analgesic
Antitussive

Therapeutic actions
Acts at opioid receptors in the CNS to produce analgesia, euphoria, sedation; acts in medullary cough center to depress cough reflex.

Indications
- Relief of mild to moderate pain in adults and children
- Coughing induced by chemical or mechanical irritation of the respiratory system

Contraindications/cautions
- Contraindicated in the presence of hypersensitivity to narcotics, physical dependence on a narcotic analgesic (drug may precipitate withdrawal).
- Use caution in the presence of pregnancy, labor, lactation, bronchial asthma, COPD, respiratory depression, anoxia, increased intracranial pressure, acute myocardial infarction, ventricular failure, coronary insufficiency, hypertension, biliary tract surgery, renal or hepatic dysfunction.

Dosage
Adult
- ***Analgesic:*** 15–60 mg PO, IM, IV or SC q4–6h; do not exceed 120 mg/24 h.
- ***Antitussive:*** 10–20 mg PO q4–6h; do not exceed 120 mg/24 h.

Pediatric: Contraindicated in premature infants.
- ***Analgesic:*** *1 y or older*: 0.5 mg/kg SC, IM or PO q4–6h.
- ***Antitussive:*** *6–12 y*: 5–10 mg PO q4–6h; do not exceed 60 mg/24 h. *2–6 y*: 2.5–5 mg PO q4–6h; do not exceed 30 mg/24 h.

Geriatric or impaired adult: Use caution; respiratory depression may occur in elderly, the very ill, those with respiratory problems. Reduced dosage may be necessary.

Pharmacokinetics

Route	Onset	Peak	Duration
Oral/IM/IV	10–30 min	30–60 min	4–6 h

Metabolism: Hepatic, $T_{1/2}$: 2.5–4 h
Distribution: Crosses placenta; enters breast milk
Excretion: Urine

IV facts
Preparation: Protect vials from light.
Infusion: Administer slowly by direct injection or into running IV tubing.

Adverse effects
- **CNS:** *Sedation, clamminess, sweating, headache, vertigo, floating feeling, dizziness, lethargy, confusion, lightheadedness,* nervousness, unusual dreams, agitation, euphoria, hallucinations, delirium, insomnia, anxiety, fear, disorientation, impaired mental and physical performance, coma, mood changes, weakness, headache, tremor, convulsions
- **GI:** *Nausea, vomiting,* dry mouth, anorexia, constipation, biliary tract spasm
- **CV:** Palpitation, increase or decrease in blood pressure, circulatory depression, **cardiac arrest, shock,** tachycardia, bradycardia, arrhythmia, palpitations
- **Respiratory:** Slow, shallow respiration; apnea; suppression of cough reflex; laryngospasm; bronchospasm
- **GU:** Ureteral spasm, spasm of vesical sphincters, urinary retention or hesitancy, oliguria, antidiuretic effect, reduced libido or potency
- **EENT:** Diplopia, blurred vision
- **Dermatologic:** Rash, hives, pruritus, flushing, warmth, sensitivity to cold
- **Local:** Phlebitis following IV injection, pain at injection site; tissue irritation and induration (SC injection)
- **Other:** Physical tolerance and dependence, psychological dependence

Clinically important drug-drug interactions
- Potentiation of effects of codeine when given with barbiturate anesthetics; decrease dose of codeine when coadministering.

Drug-lab test interferences
- Elevated biliary tract pressure may cause increases in plasma amylase, lipase; determinations of these levels may be unreliable for 24 h after administration of narcotics.

■ Nursing Considerations
Assessment
- *History:* Hypersensitivity to butorphanol, physical dependence on a narcotic analgesic, pregnancy, labor, lactation, bronchial asthma, COPD, increased intracranial pressure, acute myocardial infarction, ventricular failure, coronary insufficiency, hypertension, biliary tract surgery, renal or hepatic dysfunction
- *Physical:* Orientation, reflexes, bilateral grip strength, affect; pupil size, vision; pulse, auscultation, BP; respiratory rate, adventitious sounds; bowel sounds, normal output; liver and kidney function tests

Implementation
- Administer to women who are nursing a baby 4–6 h before the next scheduled feeding to minimize the amount in milk.
- Provide narcotic antagonist, facilities for assisted or controlled respiration on standby during parenteral administration.
- Use caution when injecting SC into chilled body areas or in patients with hypotension or in shock; impaired perfusion may delay absorption; with repeated doses, an excessive amount may be absorbed when circulation is restored.
- Instruct postoperative patients in pulmonary toilet; drug suppresses cough reflex.
- Monitor bowel function, and arrange for laxatives (especially senna compounds—approximate dose of 187 mg senna concentrate per 120 mg codeine equivalent), bowel training program, as appropriate, if severe constipation occurs.

Drug-specific teaching points
- Take drug exactly as prescribed.
- Know that the following side effects may occur: dizziness, sedation, drowsiness, impaired visual acuity (avoid driving a car, performing other tasks that require alertness); nausea, loss of appetite (lying quietly, eating frequent small meals should minimize these effects); constipation (a laxative may help).
- Do not to take any leftover medication for other disorders, and do not to let anyone else take the prescription.
- Report severe nausea, vomiting, palpitations, shortness of breath or difficulty breathing.

☐ colchicine

(kol chi seen)

Pregnancy Category C
Pregnancy Category D (parenteral)

Drug classes
Antigout drug

Therapeutic actions
Exact mechanism of action unknown; decreases deposition of uric acid; inhibits kinin formation and phagocytosis, and decreases inflammatory reaction to urate crystal deposition.

Indications
- Pain relief of acute gout attack; also used between attacks as prophylaxis
- *Orphan drug use:* arrest progression of neurologic disability caused by chronic progressive multiple sclerosis
- **Unlabeled uses**: hepatic cirrhosis, familial Mediterranean fever, skin manifestations of scleroderma, psoriasis, dermatitis herpetiformis, treatment of Behçet's disease

Contraindications/cautions
- Allergy to colchicine, blood dyscrasias, serious GI disorders, liver, renal or cardiac disorders, pregnancy, lactation

Dosage
Adult
- ***Acute gouty arthritis:*** 0.5–1.2 mg PO followed by 0.5–1.2 mg q1–2h until pain is relieved or nausea, vomiting, or diarrhea occurs. *IV dose:* 2 mg IV followed by 0.5 mg q6h until desired effect is achieved; *do not exceed 4 g/24 h.*

318 ■ colchicine

- ***Prophylaxis in intercritical periods:*** *Less than one attack per year:* 0.5–0.6 mg/d PO for 3–4 d/wk. More frequent attacks (> 1/y): 0.5–0.6 mg/d; up to 1.8 mg/d PO may be needed in severe cases. *IV dose:* 0.5–1 mg qid or bid; change to oral therapy as soon as possible.
- ***Prophylaxis for patients undergoing surgery:*** 0.5–0.6 mg tid PO for 3 d before and 3 d after the procedure.

Pediatric: Safety and efficacy not established.

Geriatric or renal impaired: Use with caution; reduce dosage if weakness, anorexia, nausea, vomiting, or diarrhea occurs.

Pharmacokinetics

Route	Onset	Peak
Oral	0.5–2 h	12 h
IV	30–50 min	6–12 h

Metabolism: Hepatic, $T_{1/2}$: 20–60 min
Distribution: Crosses placenta; enters breast milk
Excretion: Urine and bile

IV facts
Preparation: Use undiluted or diluted in 0.9% Sodium Chloride Injection, which does not have a bacteriostatic agent. Do not dilute with 5% Dextrose in Water. Do not use solutions that have become turbid.

Infusion: Infuse slowly over 2–5 min by direct injection or into tubing of running IV.

Adverse effects
- **CNS:** Peripheral neuritis, purpura, myopathy
- **GI:** *Diarrhea, vomiting,* abdominal pain, nausea
- **Hematologic:** Bone marrow depression, elevated alkaline phosphatase, SGOT levels
- **GU:** Azoospermia (reversible)
- **Dermatologic:** Dermatoses, loss of hair
- **Local:** Thrombophlebitis at IV sites

Clinically important drug-drug interactions
- Decreased absorption of vitamin B_{12} when taken with colchicine

Drug-lab test interferences
- False-positive results for urine RBC, urine hemoglobin

■ Nursing Considerations
Assessment
- *History:* Allergy to colchicine, blood dyscrasias, serious GI, liver, renal or cardiac disorders, pregnancy, lactation
- *Physical:* Skin—lesions, color; orientation, reflexes; P, cardiac auscultation, BP; liver evaluation, normal bowel output; normal urinary output; CBC, renal and liver function tests, urinalysis

Implementation
- Monitor for relief of pain and signs and symptoms of gout attack; usually abate within 12 h and are gone within 24–48 h.
- Know that parenteral drug is to be used IV only; SC or IM use will cause severe irritation.
- Arrange for opiate antidiarrheal medication if diarrhea is severe.
- Discuss the dosage regimen with patients who have been using colchicine; these patients know when to stop the medication before GI side effects occur.
- Administration of colchicine should begin at the first warning of an acute attack; delay can decrease the effectiveness of the drug in alleviating the signs and symptoms of gout.
- Arrange for regular medical follow-up and blood tests during the course of therapy.

Drug-specific teaching points
- Take this drug at the first warning of an acute attack; delay will impair the drug's effectiveness in relieving your symptoms. Stop the drug at the first sign of nausea, vomiting, stomach pain, or diarrhea.
- Know that the following side effects may occur: nausea, vomiting, loss of appetite

Adverse effects in *Italics* are most common; those in **Bold** are life-threatening.

(taking the drug following meals or small, frequent meals may help); loss of fertility (this is reversible and should resolve when the drug is stopped); loss of hair (this is reversible and should resolve when the drug is stopped).
- Report severe diarrhea, skin rash, sore throat, fever, unusual bleeding or bruising, fever, chills, sore throat, persistence of gout attack, numbness or tingling, tiredness, weakness.

colestipol hydrochloride

(koe les' ti pole)
Colestid
Pregnancy Category C

Drug classes
Antihyperlipidemic agent
Bile acid sequestrant

Therapeutic actions
Binds bile acids in the intestine to form a complex that is excreted in the feces; as a result, cholesterol is lost, oxidized in the liver, and serum cholesterol and LDL are lowered.

Indications
- Reduction of elevated serum cholesterol in patients with primary hypercholesterolemia (elevated LDL) (adjunctive therapy)

Contraindications/cautions
- Allergy to bile acid sequestrants, complete biliary obstruction, abnormal intestinal function, pregnancy, lactation

Dosage
Adult: 5–30 g/d PO in divided doses two to four times per day. Start with 5 g qid or bid PO, and increase in 5-g/d increments at 1- to 2-mo intervals.
Pediatric: Safety and efficacy not established.

Pharmacokinetics
Not absorbed systemically. Eliminated in the feces.

Adverse effects
- **CNS:** *Headache*, anxiety, vertigo, dizziness, fatigue, syncope, drowsiness
- **GI:** *Constipation* to fecal impaction, *exacerbation of hemorrhoids*, abdominal cramps, *abdominal pain*, flatulence, anorexia, heartburn, nausea, vomiting, steatorrhea
- **Hematologic:** Increased bleeding tendencies related to vitamin K malabsorption, vitamin A and D deficiencies, hyperchloremic acidosis
- **GU:** Hematuria, dysuria, diuresis
- **Dermatologic:** Rash and irritation of skin, tongue, perianal area
- **Other:** Osteoporosis, chest pain, backache, muscle and joint pain, arthritis, fever

Clinically important drug-drug interactions
- Decreased serum levels or delayed absorption of thiazide diuretics, digitalis preparations taken with colestipol • Malabsorption of fat-soluble vitamins if taken concurrently with colestipol

■ Nursing Considerations

Assessment
- *History:* Allergy to bile acid sequestrant, complete biliary obstruction, abnormal intestinal function, pregnancy, lactation
- *Physical:* Skin—lesions, color, temperature; orientation, affect, reflexes; P, auscultation, baseline ECG, peripheral perfusion; liver evaluation, bowel sounds; lipid studies, liver function tests, clotting profile

Implementation
- Do not administer drug in dry form. Mix in liquids, soups, cereals, or pulpy fruits; add the prescribed amount to a glassful (90 ml) of liquid; stir until completely mixed. The granules will not dissolve. May be mixed with carbonated beverages, slowly stirred in a large glass. Rinse the glass with a small amount of additional beverage to ensure all of the dose has been taken.
- Administer drug before meals.

Adverse effects in *Italics* are most common; those in **Bold** are life-threatening.

- Monitor administration of other oral medications because of the risk of binding in the intestine and delayed or decreased absorption of the other medications. Give them 1 h before or 4–6 h after the colestipol.
- Arrange for regular follow-up during long-term therapy.
- Consult with patient and appropriate sources to cope with the high cost of the drug.

Drug-specific teaching points

- Take drug before meals. Do not take the powder in the dry form. Mix in liquids, soups, cereals, or pulpy fruit; add the prescribed amount to a glassful of the liquid; stir until completely mixed. The granules will not dissolve; rinse the glass with a small amount of additional liquid to ensure that you receive the entire dose of the drug; carbonated beverages may be used; mix by slowly stirring in a large glass.
- Be aware that this drug may interfere with the absorption of other oral medications. If you take other oral medications, take them 1 h before or 4–6 h after colestipol.
- Know that the following side effects may occur: constipation (this may resolve, or other measures may need to be taken to alleviate this problem); nausea, heartburn, loss of appetite (small, frequent meals may help); dizziness, drowsiness, vertigo, fainting (avoid driving and operating dangerous machinery until you know how this drug affects you); headache, muscle and joint aches and pains (these may lessen with time).
- Report unusual bleeding or bruising, severe constipation, severe GI upset, chest pain, difficulty breathing, rash, fever.

☐ colfosceril palmitate

(kole fos' seer el)
synthetic lung surfactant, dipalmitoylphosphatidylcholine, DPPC

Exosurf Neonatal

Drug classes
Lung surfactant

Therapeutic actions
A natural compound that reduces surface tension in the alveoli, allowing expansion of the alveoli; replaces the surfactant missing in the lungs of neonates suffering from RDS.

Indications
- Prophylactic treatment of infants at risk of developing RDS; infants with birth weights < 1,350 g or infants with birth weights > 1,350 g who have evidence of pulmonary immaturity
- Rescue treatment of infants who have developed RDS

Contraindications/cautions
- Colfosceril is used as an emergency drug in acute respiratory situations; benefits outweigh any potential risks of therapy.

Dosage
Accurate determination of birth weight is essential for determining appropriate dosage. Colfosceril is instilled into the trachea using the endotracheal tube adapter that comes with the product.

Prophylactic treatment: Administer first dose as a single 5-ml/kg intratracheal dose as soon as possible after birth. Administer second and third dose at 12 h and 24 h, respectively to all infants who remain on mechanical ventilation.

Rescue treatment: Administer in two 5-ml/kg doses. Administer first dose as soon after the diagnosis of RDS is made as possible. The second dose should be given in 12 h, if the infant remains on mechanical ventilation. Data on safety and efficacy of rescue treatment with more than two doses are not available.

Pharmacokinetics

Route	Onset	Duration
Intratracheal	Rapid	12 h

Metabolism: Lung, $T_{1/2}$: 12 h
Excretion: Respiratory

Adverse effects
- CNS: **Seizures**
- CV: *Patent ductus arteriosus, intraventricular hemorrhage, hypotension*
- Respiratory: *Pneumothorax, pulmonary air leak,* **pulmonary hemorrhage**, *apnea,* pneumomediastinum, emphysema
- Hematologic: *Hyperbilirubinemia, thrombocytopenia*
- Other: *Sepsis, nonpulmonary infections*

■ Nursing Considerations
Assessment
- *History:* Time of birth, history of gestation
- *Physical:* Temperature, color; R, adventitious sounds, oximeter, endotracheal tube position and patency, chest movement; ECG, P, BP, peripheral perfusion, arterial pressure (desirable); oxygen saturation, blood gases, CBC; motor activity, facial expression, reflexes

Implementation
- Monitor ECG and transcutaneous oxygen saturation continually during administration.
- Ensure that endotracheal tube is in the correct position, with bilateral chest movement and lung sounds.
- Arrange for staff to preview teaching videotape, available from the manufacturer, before regular use to cover all the technical aspects of administration.
- Suction the infant immediately before administration; do not suction for 2 h after administration unless clinically necessary.
- Reconstitute immediately before use with the 8 ml of diluent that comes with the product; **do not use** Bacteriostatic Water for Injection. Reconstitute using the manufacturer's directions to ensure proper mixing and dilution.
- Check reconstituted vial, which should appear as a milky liquid, for flakes or precipitates; gentle mixing should be attempted. If precipitate remains, do not use.
- Insert endotracheal adapter of the correct size into the endotracheal tube; attach the breathing circuit to the adapter; remove cap from the sideport of the adapter; attach syringe containing the drug into the sideport and administer correct dose.
- Instill dose slowly over 1–2 min, 30–50 ventilations, moving infant after each half dose to ensure adequate instillation into both lungs.
- Continually monitor patient's color, lung sounds, ECG, oximeter, and blood gas readings during administration and for at least 30 min following administration.

Drug-specific teaching points
- Parents of the critically ill infant will need a comprehensive teaching and support program, including details of drug effects.

❒ corticotropin injection

*(kor ti koe **troe'** pin)*
ACTH, adenocorticotropin, corticotrophin

Acthar

corticotropin repository injection

H.P. Acthar Gel

Pregnancy Category C

Drug classes
Anterior pituitary hormone
Diagnostic agent

Therapeutic actions
Stimulates the adrenal cortex to synthesize and secrete adrenocortical hormones.

Indications
- Diagnostic tests of adrenal function
- Therapy of some glucocorticoid-sensitive disorders
- Nonsuppurative thyroiditis
- Hypercalcemia associated with cancer
- Acute exacerbations of multiple sclerosis

Adverse effects in *Italics* are most common; those in **Bold** are life-threatening.

- Tuberculous meningitis with subarachnoid block
- Trichinosis with neurologic or myocardial involvement
- Rheumatic, collagen, dermatologic, allergic, ophthalmologic, respiratory, hematologic, edematous, and GI diseases
- **Unlabeled use**: treatment of infantile spasms

Contraindications/cautions
- Adrenocortical insufficiency or hyperfunction; infections, especially systemic fungal infections, ocular herpes simplex; scleroderma, osteoporosis; recent surgery; CHF, hypertension; allergy to pork or pork products (corticotropin is isolated from porcine pituitaries); liver disease; ulcerative colitis with impending perforation; diverticulitis; recent GI surgery; active or latent peptic ulcer; inflammatory bowel disease; diabetes mellitus; hypothyroidism; pregnancy, lactation

Dosage
Adult
- ***Diagnostic tests:*** 10–25 U dissolved in 500 ml of 5% dextrose injection infused IV over 8 h.
- ***Therapy:*** 20 U IM or SC qid; when indicated, gradually reduce dosage by increasing intervals between injections or decreasing the dose injected, or both.
- ***Acute exacerbations of multiple sclerosis:*** 80–120 U/d IM for 2–3 wk.
- ***Repository injection:*** 40–80 U IM or SC q24–72h.

Pediatric: Use only if necessary, and then only intermittently and with careful observation. Prolonged use will inhibit skeletal growth.
- ***Infantile spasms:*** 20–40 U/d or 80 U every other day IM for 3 mo or 1 mo after cessation of seizures.

Pharmacokinetics

Route	Onset	Peak	Duration
IM/IV	Rapid	1 h	2–4 h

Metabolism: $T_{1/2}$: 15 min

Distribution: Does not cross placenta; may enter breast milk

IV facts
Preparation: Reconstitute powder by dissolving in Sterile Water for Injection or Sodium Chloride Injection. Refrigerate reconstituted solution. Stable for 24 h.
Infusion: 10–25 U dissolved in 500 ml of 5% Dextrose Injection infused over 8 h.

Adverse effects
- **CNS:** Convulsions, vertigo, *headaches*, pseudotumor cerebri, *euphoria, insomnia, mood swings, depression,* psychosis, intracerebral hemorrhage, reversible cerebral atrophy in infants, cataracts, increased intraocular pressure, glaucoma
- **GI:** Peptic or esophageal ulcer, pancreatitis, abdominal distention
- **CV:** *Hypertension,* CHF, necrotizing angiitis
- **Hematologic:** *Fluid and electrolyte disturbances,* negative nitrogen balance
- **GU:** *Amenorrhea, irregular menses*
- **MS:** *Muscle weakness,* steroid myopathy, loss of muscle mass, osteoporosis, spontaneous fractures
- **Endocrine:** Growth retardation, decreased carbohydrate tolerance, diabetes mellitus, cushingoid state, *secondary adrenocortical and pituitary unresponsiveness*
- **Hypersensitivity: Anaphylactoid** or hypersensitivity reactions
- **Other:** *Impaired wound healing, petechiae, ecchymoses, increased sweating, thin and fragile skin, acne, immunosuppression and masking of signs of infection,* activation of latent infections, including tuberculosis, fungal, and viral eye infections, pneumonia, abscess, septic infection, GI and GU infections

Clinically important drug-drug interactions
- Decreased effects of corticotropin if taken with barbiturates • Decreased effects of anticholinesterases if taken concurrently with

corticotropin; profound muscular depression is possible

Drug-lab test interferences
- Suppression of skin test reactions

■ Nursing Considerations

Assessment
- *History:* Adrenocortical insufficiency or hyperfunction; infections, ocular herpes simplex; scleroderma, osteoporosis; recent surgery; CHF, hypertension; allergy to pork or pork products; liver disease: cirrhosis; ulcerative colitis; diverticulitis; active or latent peptic ulcer; inflammatory bowel disease, lactation; diabetes mellitus; hypothyroidism
- *Physical:* Body weight, temperature; skin—color, integrity; reflexes, bilateral grip strength, ophthalmologic exam, affect, orientation; P, BP, auscultation, peripheral perfusion, status of veins; R, adventitious sounds, chest x-ray; upper GI x-ray (if symptoms of peptic ulcer), liver palpation; CBC, serum electrolytes, 2-h postprandial blood glucose, thyroid function tests, urinalysis

Implementation
- Verify adrenal responsiveness (ie, increase in urinary and plasma corticosteroid levels) to corticotropin before beginning therapy, using the route of administration proposed for treatment.
- Administer corticotropin repository injection only by IM or SC injection.
- Administer IV injections only for diagnostic purposes or to treat thrombocytopenic purpura.
- Prepare solutions for IM and SC injections as follows: Reconstitute powder by dissolving in Sterile Water for Injection or Sodium Chloride Injection so that the individual dose will be contained in 1–2 ml of solution. Refrigerate reconstituted solutions, and use within 24 h.
- Use minimal doses for minimal duration of time to minimize adverse effects.
- Taper doses when discontinuing high-dose or long-term therapy.
- Administer a rapidly acting corticosteroid before, during, and after stress when patients are on long-term corticotropin therapy.
- Do not give patients live virus vaccines while they are on this drug.

Drug-specific teaching points
- Avoid immunizations with live vaccines.
- Be aware that if you are a diabetic, you may require an increased dosage of insulin or oral hypoglycemic drug; your health care provider will give you details.
- Take antacids between meals (if appropriate) to reduce "heartburn."
- Avoid unnecessary exposure to people and contagious diseases. This drug may mask signs of infection and decrease your resistance to infection; wash your hands carefully after touching contaminated surfaces.
- Report unusual weight gain, swelling of lower extremities, muscle weakness, abdominal pain, seizures, headache, fever, prolonged sore throat, cold or other infection, worsening of symptoms for which drug is being taken.

❐ cortisone acetate

(kor' ti sone)
Cortone Acetate

Pregnancy Category C

Drug classes
Adrenal cortical hormone
Corticosteroid, short acting
Hormonal agent

Therapeutic actions
Enters target cells where it has anti-inflammatory and immunosuppressive (glucocorticoid) and salt-retaining (mineralocorticoid) effects.

Indications
- Replacement therapy in adrenal cortical insufficiency
- Hypercalcemia associated with cancer
- Short-term management of various inflammatory and allergic disorders, such as rheumatoid arthritis, collagen diseases (eg, SLE), dermatologic diseases (eg,

pemphigus), status asthmaticus, and autoimmune disorders
- Hematologic disorders: thrombocytopenic purpura, erythroblastopenia
- Trichinosis with neurologic or myocardial involvement
- Ulcerative colitis, acute exacerbations of multiple sclerosis, and palliation in some leukemias and lymphomas

Contraindications/cautions
- Contraindicated in the presence of infections, especially tuberculosis, fungal infections, amebiasis, vaccinia and varicella, and antibiotic-resistant infections, pregnancy, lactation.
- Use caution in the presence of renal or hepatic disease; hypothyroidism, ulcerative colitis with impending perforation; diverticulitis; active or latent peptic ulcer; inflammatory bowel disease; CHF, hypertension, thromboembolic disorders; osteoporosis; convulsive disorders; diabetes mellitus.

Dosage
Physiologic replacement: 0.5–0.75 mg/kg per day PO or 25 mg/m^2 per day PO divided into equal doses q8h; 0.25–0.35 mg/kg per day or 12–15 mg/m^2 per day IM.
Adult: Individualize dosage, depending on the severity of the condition and the patient's response. If long-term therapy is needed, alternate-day therapy should be considered. After long-term therapy, withdraw drug slowly to avoid adrenal insufficiency.
- ***Initial:*** 25–300 mg/d PO; 20–330 mg/d IM.
- ***Maintenance:*** Reduce dose in small increments at intervals until the lowest dose that maintains satisfactory clinical response is reached.

Pediatric: Individualize dosage on the basis of severity of the condition and the patient's response, rather than by strict adherence to formulas that correct adult doses for age or body weight. Carefully observe growth and development in infants and children on prolonged therapy.

Pharmacokinetics

Route	Onset	Peak	Duration
Oral	Rapid	2 h	1–1.5 d
IM	Slow	20–40 h	1–1.5 d

Metabolism: Hepatic, T$_{1/2}$: 30 min
Distribution: Crosses placenta; enters breast milk
Excretion: Urine

Adverse effects
- **CNS:** Convulsions, *vertigo, headaches,* pseudotumor cerebri, *euphoria, insomnia, mood swings, depression,* psychosis, **intracerebral hemorrhage**, reversible cerebral atrophy in infants, cataracts, increased intraocular pressure, glaucoma
- **GI:** Peptic or esophageal ulcer, pancreatitis, abdominal distention
- **CV:** *Hypertension,* CHF, necrotizing angiitis
- **Hematologic:** *Fluid and electrolyte disturbances,* negative nitrogen balance, increased blood sugar, glycosuria, increased serum cholesterol, decreased serum T$_3$ and T$_4$ levels
- **GU:** *Amenorrhea, irregular menses*
- **MS:** *Muscle weakness,* steroid myopathy, loss of muscle mass, osteoporosis, spontaneous fractures
- **Endocrine:** Growth retardation, decreased carbohydrate tolerance, diabetes mellitus, cushingoid state, *secondary adrenocortical and pituitary unresponsiveness*
- **Hypersensitivity:** Anaphylactoid or hypersensitivity reactions
- **Other:** *Impaired wound healing, petechiae, ecchymoses, increased sweating, thin and fragile skin,* acne, *immunosuppression and masking of signs of infection,* activation of latent infections including tuberculosis, fungal and viral eye infections, pneumonia, abscess, septic infection, GI and GU infections

Clinically important drug-drug interactions
- Increased therapeutic and toxic effects of cortisone if taken concurrently with trolean-

domycin • Decreased effects of anticholinesterases if taken concurrently with corticotropin; profound muscular depression is possible • Decreased steroid blood levels if taken concurrently with phenytoin, phenobarbital, rifampin • Decreased serum levels of salicylates if taken concurrently with cortisone.

Drug-lab test interferences
• False-negative nitroblue-tetrazolium test for bacterial infection • Suppression of skin test reactions

Nursing Considerations

Assessment
- *History:* Infections, hypothyroidism, ulcerative colitis; diverticulitis; active or latent peptic ulcer; inflammatory bowel disease; CHF, hypertension, thromboembolic disorders; osteoporosis; convulsive disorders; diabetes mellitus, lactation
- *Physical:* Baseline body weight, temperature; reflexes, and grip strength, affect, and orientation; P, BP, peripheral perfusion, prominence of superficial veins; R and adventitious sounds; serum electrolytes, blood glucose

Implementation
- Administer once-a-day doses before 9 AM to mimic normal peak corticosteroid blood levels.
- Arrange for increased dosage when patient is subject to stress.
- Taper doses when discontinuing high-dose or long-term therapy.
- Do not give live virus vaccines with immunosuppressive doses of corticosteroids.

Drug-specific teaching points
- Do not to stop taking the drug (oral) without consulting health care provider.
- Avoid exposure to infection.
- Report unusual weight gain, swelling of the extremities, muscle weakness, black or tarry stools, fever, prolonged sore throat, colds or other infections, worsening of the disorder for which the drug is being taken.

cosyntropin

(koe sin troe' pin)
Cortrosyn, Synacthen Depot (CAN)

Pregnancy Category C

Drug classes
Diagnostic agent

Therapeutic actions
Stimulates the adrenal cortex to synthesize and secrete adrenocortical hormones.

Indications
• Diagnostic tests of adrenal function

Contraindications/cautions
• Adrenocortical insufficiency or hyperfunction; infections, especially systemic fungal infections, ocular herpes simplex; scleroderma, osteoporosis; recent surgery; CHF, hypertension; liver disease; ulcerative colitis with impending perforation; diverticulitis; recent GI surgery; active or latent peptic ulcer; inflammatory bowel disease; diabetes mellitus; hypothyroidism; pregnancy, lactation.

Dosage
Adult: 0.25–0.075 mg IM or IV; 0.25 mg IM is suggested starting point.
Pediatric: Younger than 2 y: 0.125 mg IM or IV.

Pharmacokinetics

Route	Onset	Peak	Duration
IM/IV	Rapid	1 h	2–4 h

Metabolism: $T_{1/2}$: 15 min
Distribution: Does not cross placenta; may enter breast milk

IV facts
Preparation : Add 0.25 mg to dextrose or saline solution.
Infusion: Infuse at a rate of 0.04 mg/h over 4–8 h.

Adverse effects
- CNS: **Convulsions**, vertigo, *headaches*, pseudotumor cerebri, *euphoria, insomnia, mood swings, depression,* psychosis, intracerebral hemorrhage, reversible cerebral atrophy in infants
- GI: Peptic or esophageal ulcer, pancreatitis, abdominal distention
- CV: *Hypertension,* CHF, necrotizing angiitis
- Hematologic: *Fluid and electrolyte disturbances,* negative nitrogen balance
- GU: *Amenorrhea, irregular menses*
- MS: *Muscle weakness,* steroid myopathy, loss of muscle mass, osteoporosis, spontaneous fractures
- Endocrine: *Secondary adrenocortical and pituitary unresponsiveness*
- Hypersensitivity: **Anaphylactoid** or hypersensitivity reactions
- Other: *Impaired wound healing, petechiae, ecchymoses, increased sweating, thin and fragile skin, acne, immunosuppression and masking of signs of infection,* activation of latent infections including tuberculosis, fungal and viral eye infections, pneumonia, abscess, septic infection, GI and GU infections

Clinically important drug-drug interactions
- Decreased effects of corticotropin if taken with barbiturates • Decreased effects of anticholinesterases if taken concurrently with corticotropin, profound muscular depression is possible

Drug-lab test interferences
- Suppression of skin test reactions

■ Nursing Considerations

Assessment
- *History:* Adrenocortical insufficiency or hyperfunction; infections; scleroderma, osteoporosis; recent surgery; CHF, hypertension; liver disease; ulcerative colitis; diverticulitis; active or latent peptic ulcer; inflammatory bowel disease; lactation; diabetes mellitus; hypothyroidism
- *Physical:* Body weight, temperature; skin—color, integrity; reflexes, bilateral grip strength, ophthalmologic exam, affect, orientation; P, BP, auscultation, peripheral perfusion, status of veins; R, adventitious sounds, chest x-ray; upper GI x-ray (if symptoms of peptic ulcer), liver palpation; CBC, serum electrolytes, 2-h postprandial blood glucose, thyroid function tests, urinalysis

Implementation
- Verify adrenal responsiveness (ie, increase in urinary and plasma corticosteroid levels) to corticotropin before beginning therapy, using the route of administration proposed for treatment.
- Prepare solutions for IM injections as follows: dissolve suggested dose in Sterile Saline.
- Do not give patients live virus vaccines while they are on this drug.

Drug-specific teaching points
- Be aware that if you are a diabetic, you may require an increased dosage of insulin or oral hypoglycemic drug; your health care provider will give you details.
- Know that this drug may mask signs of infection and decrease your resistance to infection; wash your hands carefully after touching contaminated surfaces. Avoid unnecessary exposure to people and contagious diseases.
- Report unusual weight gain, swelling of lower extremities, muscle weakness, abdominal pain, seizures, headache, fever, prolonged sore throat, cold or other infection, pain at injection site.

❐ cromolyn sodium

(kroe' moe lin)

disodium cromoglycate, cromoglicic acid, cromoglycic acid

Gastrocrom

Respiratory inhalant, nasal solution, ophthalmic solution: Intal, Nasalcrom, Opticrom 4%, Rynacrom (CAN)

Pregnancy Category B

Adverse effects in *Italics* are most common; those in **Bold** are life-threatening.

cromolyn sodium ■ 327

Drug classes
Antiasthmatic drug (prophylactic)
Antiallergic drug

Therapeutic actions
Inhibits the allergen-triggered release of histamine and slow-releasing substance of anaphylaxis, leukotriene, from mast cells; decreases the overall allergic response.

Indications
- *Respiratory inhalant:* Prophylaxis of severe bronchial asthma; prevention of exercise-induced bronchospasm
- *Nasal preparations:* Prevention and treatment of allergic rhinitis
- *Ophthalmic solution:* Treatment of allergic disorders (vernal keratoconjunctivitis and conjunctivitis, giant papillary conjunctivitis, vernal keratitis, allergic keratoconjunctivitis)
- *Oral use:* orphan drug use—mastocytosis
- *Unlabeled uses*: prevention of GI and systemic reactions in patients with food allergies; treatment of eczema, dermatitis, ulcerations, urticaria pigmentosa, chronic urticaria, hay fever, postexercise bronchospasm

Contraindications/cautions
- Allergy to cromolyn, pregnancy, lactation.
- **Respiratory inhalant and nasal products:** Impaired renal or hepatic function.

Dosage
Respiratory Inhalant Product Used in Spinhaler
- *Adult and children older than 5 y:* Initially 20 mg (contents of 1 capsule) inhaled qid at regular intervals.
- *Children younger than 5 y:* Safety and efficacy not established; use of capsule product not recommended.

Nebulizer Solution for Oral Inhalation
- *Adults and children older than 2 y:* Initially 20 mg qid at regular intervals, administered from a power-operated nebulizer with an adequate flow rate and equipped with a suitable face mask; do not use a hand-operated nebulizer.
- *Children younger than 2 y:* Safety and efficacy not established.
- *Prevention of exercise-induced bronchospasm:* Inhale 20 mg no more than 1 h before anticipated exercise; during prolonged exercise, repeat as needed for protection.

Nasal Solution Used With Nasalmatic Metered-Spray Device
- *Adults and children older than 6 y:* 1 spray in each nostril three to six times per day at regular intervals.
- *Children younger than 6 y:* Safety and efficacy not established.
- *Seasonal (pollenotic) rhinitis and prevention of rhinitis caused by exposure to other specific inhalant allergens:* Begin treatment before expected exposure, and continue during exposure period.

Ophthalmic Solution
- *Adults and children older than 4 y:* 1–2 drops in each eye from four to six times per day at regular intervals.
- *Children younger than 4 y:* Safety and efficacy not established.

Oral
- *Adults:* 2 capsules qid PO, ½ h before meals and at bedtime.
- *Pediatric*
  - *Premature to term infants:* Not recommended.
  - *Term to 2 y:* 20 mg/kg PO per day in four divided doses.
  - *2–12 y:* One capsule PO qid ½ h before meals and at bedtime. Dosage may be increased if satisfactory results are seen within 2–3 wk. Do not exceed 40 mg/kg per day (30 mg/kg per day in children 6 mo–2 y).

Pharmacokinetics

Route	Onset	Peak	Duration
All	1 wk	15 min	6–8 h

Metabolism: Hepatic, $T_{1/2}$: 80 min
Distribution: Crosses placenta; may enter breast milk

Excretion: Urine and bile; respiratory (inhalation)

Adverse effects
Respiratory Inhalant Product
- CNS: *Dizziness, headache,* lacrimation
- GI: *Nausea, dry and irritated throat,* swollen parotid glands
- GU: Dysuria, frequency
- Dermatologic: Urticaria, rash, angioedema, joint swelling and pain

Nebulizer Solution
- GI: Abdominal pain
- Respiratory: *Cough, nasal congestion, wheezing, sneezing,* nasal itching, epistaxis, nose burning

Nasal Solution
- CNS: *Headaches*
- GI: Bad taste in mouth
- Respiratory: *Sneezing, nasal stinging or burning, nasal irritation,* epistaxis, postnasal drip
- Dermatologic: Rash

Ophthalmic Solution
- Local: *Transient ocular stinging or burning on instillation*

Oral
- CNS: *Dizziness, fatigue, paresthesia, headache,* migraine, psychosis, anxiety, depression, insomnia, behavior change, hallucinations, lethargy
- GI: *Taste perversion, diarrhea,* esophagospasm, flatulence, dysphagia, hepatic function tests abnormality, burning in the mouth and throat
- Dermatologic: *Flushing,* urticaria, angioedema, skin erythema and burning

■ Nursing Considerations

Assessment
- *History:* Allergy to cromolyn, impaired renal or hepatic function, lactation
- *Physical:* Skin—color, lesions; palpation of parotid glands; joint size, overlying color and temperature; orientation; R, auscultation, patency of nasal passages (patients using respiratory inhalant and nasal products); liver evaluation; normal output; renal and liver function tests, urinalysis

Implementation

Respiratory Inhalant Products
- Do not use during acute asthma attack; begin therapy when acute episode has been controlled and patient can inhale adequately.
- Arrange for continuation of treatment with bronchodilators and corticosteroids, as appropriate, during initial cromolyn therapy, tapering corticosteroids and reinstituting when patient is subject to stress.
- Use caution if cough or bronchospasm occurs after inhalation; this may (rarely) preclude continuation of treatment.
- Arrange for discontinuation of therapy if eosinophilic pneumonia occurs.
- Taper cromolyn when withdrawal is desirable.
- Mix cromolyn solution only with compatible solutions: compatible with metaproterenol sulfate, isoproterenol HCl, 0.25% isoetharine HCl, epinephrine HCl, terbutaline sulfate, and 20% acetylcysterine solution for at least 1 h after their admixture.
- Store nebulizer solution below 30°C; protect from light.

Nasal Solution
- Have patient clear nasal passages before use.
- Have patient inhale through nose during administration.
- Be aware that response to treatment may become apparent only after 2–4 wk of therapy (perennial allergic rhinitis); concomitant use of antihistamines and nasal decongestants may be necessary initially.
- Replace *Nasalmatic* pump device every 6 mo.

Ophthalmic Solution
- Instruct patients not to wear soft contact lenses during treatment.
- Be aware that symptomatic response is usually evident within a few days, but treatment for up to 6 wk may be necessary.

Adverse effects in *Italics* are most common; those in **Bold** are life-threatening.

All
- Administer corticosteroids concomitantly if indicated.
- Carefully teach patients how to use the specialized *Spinhaler*, *Nasalmatic*, or power nebulizer devices.

Oral
- Administer drug ½ h before meals and at bedtime.
- Prepare solution for patients who cannot take capsules as follows: open capsule, and pour contents into half glass of hot water; stir until completely dissolved; add equal quantity of cold water. Do not mix with fruit juice, milk, or foods. Drink all of the liquid.
- Do not administer oral capsules for inhalation.

Drug-specific teaching points
- Take drug at regular intervals. If drug is being used to prevent reactions after specific allergen exposure or to prevent exercise-induced bronchospasm, patient should be instructed as to optimal time to administer drug.
- Administer the drug as follows: *Respiratory inhalant and nasal solution:* See manufacturer's insert; do not swallow capsule used in Spinhaler. *Ophthalmic solution:* Lie down or tilt head back, and look at ceiling; drop solution inside lower eyelid while looking up. After instilling eye drops, close eyes; apply gentle pressure to inside corner of eye for 1 min.
- Do not discontinue drug abruptly except on advice of your health care provider (respiratory inhalant and nasal products).
- Do not wear soft contact lenses while using cromolyn eye drops.
- Be aware that you may experience transient stinging or burning in your eyes on instillation of the eye drops.
- Know that you may experience dizziness, drowsiness, fatigue while you are taking the oral drug. If this occurs, avoid driving or operating dangerous machinery.
- Report coughing, wheezing (respiratory products); change in vision (ophthalmic products); swelling, difficulty swallowing, depression (oral product).

cyclizine hydrochloride

(sye' kli zeen)
Marezine

Pregnancy Category B

Drug classes
Antiemetic
Antimotion sickness drug
Antihistamine
Anticholinergic drug

Therapeutic actions
Reduces sensitivity of the labyrinthine apparatus; peripheral anticholinergic effects may contribute to efficacy.

Indications
- Prevention and treatment of nausea, vomiting, motion sickness

Contraindications/cautions
- Contraindicated in presence of allergy to cyclizine.
- Use caution in the presence of pregnancy, lactation, narrow-angle glaucoma, stenosing peptic ulcer, symptomatic prostatic hypertrophy, bronchial asthma, bladder neck obstruction, pyloroduodenal obstruction, cardiac arrhythmias; postoperative patients (hypotensive effects of drug may be confusing and dangerous).

Dosage
Adult: 50 mg PO ½ h before exposure to motion; repeat q4–6h. Do not exceed 200 mg in 24 h.
Pediatric (6–12 y): 25 mg PO up to three times a day.
Geriatric: More likely to cause dizziness, sedation, syncope, toxic confusional states, and hypotension in elderly patients; use with caution.

Pharmacokinetics

Route	Onset	Peak	Duration
Oral	30–60 min	1–1½ h	4–6 h

Metabolism: Hepatic, $T_{1/2}$: 2–3 h

cyclobenzaprine hydrochloride

Distribution: Crosses placenta; enters breast milk
Excretion: Unknown

Adverse effects
- **CNS:** *Drowsiness, confusion,* euphoria, nervousness, restlessness, insomnia and excitement, convulsions, vertigo, tinnitus, blurred vision, diplopia, auditory and visual hallucinations
- **GI:** *Dry mouth, anorexia, nausea,* vomiting, diarrhea or constipation, cholestatic jaundice
- **CV:** Hypotension, palpitations, tachycardia
- **Respiratory:** Respiratory depression, **death**, dry nose and throat
- **GU:** *Urinary frequency, difficult urination,* urinary retention
- **Dermatologic:** Urticaria, drug rash

Clinically important drug-drug interactions
- Increased depressant effects if taken concurrently with alcohol, other CNS depressants

■ Nursing Considerations

Assessment
- *History:* Allergy to cyclizine, narrow-angle glaucoma, stenosing peptic ulcer, symptomatic prostatic hypertrophy, bronchial asthma, bladder neck obstruction, pyloroduodenal obstruction, cardiac arrhythmias, recent surgery, lactation
- *Physical:* Skin—color, lesions, texture; orientation, reflexes, affect; vision exam; P, BP; R, adventitious sounds; bowel sounds; prostate palpation; CBC

Implementation
- Maintain epinephrine 1:1,000 readily available when using parenteral preparations; hypersensitivity reactions, including anaphylaxis, have occurred.

Drug-specific teaching points
- Take drug as prescribed; avoid excessive dosage.
- Use before motion sickness occurs; antimotion sickness drugs work best if used prophylactically.
- Know that the following side effects may occur: dizziness, sedation, drowsiness (use caution if driving or performing tasks that require alertness if these occur); epigastric distress, diarrhea or constipation (taking the drug with food may help); dry mouth (frequent mouth care, sucking sugarless lozenges may help); thickening of bronchial secretions, dryness of nasal mucosa (if this is a problem, another type of motion sickness remedy may be preferable).
- Avoid alcohol while taking this drug; serious sedation could occur.
- Report difficulty breathing, hallucinations, tremors, loss of coordination, unusual bleeding or bruising, visual disturbances, irregular heartbeat.

☐ cyclobenzaprine hydrochloride

(sye kloe ben' za preen)
Flexeril

Pregnancy Category B

Drug classes
Centrally acting skeletal muscle relaxant

Therapeutic actions
Precise mechanism of action not known; does not directly relax tense skeletal muscles but appears to act mainly at brain stem levels or in the spinal cord.

Indications
- Relief of discomfort associated with acute, painful musculoskeletal conditions, as an adjunct to rest, physical therapy
- **Unlabeled use:** adjunct in the management of fibrositis syndrome

Contraindications/cautions
- Contraindicated in the presence of hypersensitivity to cyclobenzaprine, acute recovery phase of myocardial infarction, arrhythmias, heart block or conduction disturbances, CHF, hyperthyroidism.

Adverse effects in *Italics* are most common; those in **Bold** are life-threatening.

- Use with caution in the presence of urinary retention, angle-closure glaucoma, increased intraocular pressure, lactation.

Dosage
Adult: 10 mg PO tid (range 20–40 mg/d in divided doses); do not exceed 60 mg/d; do not use longer than 2 or 3 wk.
Pediatric: Safety and efficacy in children younger than 15 y not established.

Pharmacokinetics

Route	Onset	Peak	Duration
Oral	1 h	4–6 h	12–24 h

Metabolism: Hepatic, $T_{1/2}$: 1–3 d
Distribution: Crosses placenta; may enter breast milk
Excretion: Urine

Adverse effects
- CNS: *Drowsiness, dizziness,* fatigue, tiredness, asthenia, blurred vision, headache, nervousness, confusion
- GI: *Dry mouth*, nausea, constipation, dyspepsia, unpleasant taste, liver toxicity in preclinical studies

Clinically important drug-drug interactions
- Additive CNS effects with **alcohol, barbiturates,** other CNS depressants

■ Nursing Considerations
Assessment
- *History:* Hypersensitivity to cyclobenzaprine, acute recovery phase of myocardial infarction, arrhythmias, CHF, hyperthyroidism, urinary retention, angle-closure glaucoma, increased intraocular pressure, lactation
- *Physical:* Orientation, affect, ophthalmic exam (tonometry); bowel sounds, normal GI output; prostate palpation, normal voiding pattern; thyroid function tests

Implementation
- Arrange for analgesics if headache occurs (and possibly as adjunct to cyclobenzaprine for relief of discomfort of muscle spasm).

Drug-specific teaching points
- Take this drug exactly as prescribed. Do not take a higher dosage than that prescribed for you.
- Avoid alcohol, sleep-inducing, or OTC drugs while you are on this drug; these could cause dangerous effects.
- Know that the following side effects may occur: drowsiness, dizziness, blurred vision (avoid driving a car or engaging in activities that require alertness if these occur); dyspepsia (taking drug with food and eating frequent small meals may help); dry mouth (sucking sugarless lozenges or ice chips may help).
- Report urinary retention or difficulty voiding, pale stools, yellow skin or eyes.

☐ cyclophosphamide

(sye kloe foss' fa mide)
Cytoxan, Neosar, Procytox (CAN)

Pregnancy Category D

Drug classes
Alkylating agent
Nitrogen mustard
Antineoplastic drug

Therapeutic actions
Cytotoxic: interferes with the replication of susceptible cells. *Immunosuppressive:* lymphocytes are especially sensitive to drug effects.

Indications
- Treatment of malignant lymphomas, multiple myeloma, leukemias, mycosis fungoides, neuroblastoma, adenocarcinoma of the ovary, retinoblastoma, carcinoma of the breast; used concurrently or sequentially with other antineoplastic drugs
- **Unlabeled uses**: severe rheumatologic conditions, Wegener's granulomatosis, steroid-resistant vasculidites, SLE

Contraindications/cautions
- Contraindicated in presence of allergy to cyclophosphamide, allergy to tartrazine

Adverse effects in *Italics* are most common; those in **Bold** are life-threatening.

cyclophosphamide

(in tablets marketed as *Cytoxan*), pregnancy, lactation.
- Use caution in the presence of radiation therapy; chemotherapy; tumor cell infiltration of the bone marrow; adrenalectomy with steroid therapy; infections, especially varicella-zoster; hematopoietic depression, impaired hepatic or renal function.

Dosage
Individualize dosage based on hematologic profile and response.

Adult
- ***Induction therapy:*** 40–50 mg/kg IV given in divided doses over 2–5 d or 1–5 mg/kg per day PO.
- ***Maintenance therapy:*** 1–5 mg/kg per day PO, 10–15 mg/kg IV every 7–10 d, or 3–5 mg/kg IV twice weekly.
- ***Hepatic dysfunction:*** Bilirubin of 3.1–5.0 mg% or SGOT > 180: reduce dose by 25%. Bilirubin > 5 mg%: omit dose.
- ***Renal dysfunction:*** Glomerular filtration rate < 10 ml/min: decrease dose by 50%.

Pharmacokinetics

Route	Onset	Peak
Oral	Varies	1 h
IV	Rapid	15–30 min

Metabolism: Hepatic, $T_{1/2}$: 4–6 h
Distribution: Crosses placenta; enters breast milk
Excretion: Urine

IV facts
Preparation: Add Sterile Water for Injection or Bacteriostatic Water for Injection to the vial, and shake gently. Use 5 ml for 100-mg vial, 10 ml for 200-mg vial, 25 ml for 500-mg vial, 50 ml for 1-g vial. Prepared solutions may be injected IV, IM, intraperitoneally, intrapleurally. Use within 24 h if stored at room temperature or within 6 d if refrigerated.

Infusion: Infuse in 5% Dextrose Injection, 5% Dextrose and 0.9% Sodium Chloride Injection.

Adverse effects
- **GI:** *Anorexia, nausea, vomiting, diarrhea,* stomatitis
- **CV:** Cardiotoxicity
- **Respiratory:** Interstitial pulmonary fibrosis
- **Hematologic:** *Leukopenia,* thrombocytopenia, anemia (rare), increased serum uric acid levels
- **GU:** *Hemorrhagic cystitis,* bladder fibrosis, hematuria to potentially fatal **hemorrhagic cystitis,** increased urine uric acid levels, gonadal suppression
- **Dermatologic:** *Alopecia,* darkening of skin and fingernails
- **Other:** SIADH, immunosuppression secondary neoplasia

Clinically important drug-drug interactions
- Prolonged apnea with succinylcholine: metabolism is inhibited by cyclophosphamide • Decreased serum levels and therapeutic acitivity of digoxin taken concurrently with cyclophosphamide

■ Nursing Considerations

Assessment
- *History:* Allergy to cyclophosphamide, allergy to tartrazine, radiation therapy, chemotherapy, tumor cell infiltration of the bone marrow, adrenalectomy with steroid therapy, infections, hematopoietic depression, impaired hepatic or renal function, pregnancy, lactation
- *Physical:* Temperature; weight; skin—color, lesions; hair; P, auscultation, baseline ECG; R, adventitious sounds; mucous membranes, liver evaluation; CBC, differential; urinalysis; liver and renal function tests

Implementation
- Arrange for blood tests to evaluate hematopoietic function before beginning therapy and weekly during therapy.
- Do not give full dosage within 4 wk after a full course of radiation therapy or chemotherapy because of the risk of severe bone marrow depression; reduced dosage may be needed.

Adverse effects in *Italics* are most common; those in **Bold** are life-threatening.

- Arrange for reduced dosage in patients with impaired renal or hepatic function.
- Ensure that patient is well hydrated before treatment to decrease risk of cystitis.
- Prepare oral solution by dissolving injectable cyclophosphamide in aromatic elixir. Refrigerate and use within 14 d.
- Administer tablets on an empty stomach. If severe GI upset occurs, tablet may be given with food.
- Counsel male patients not to father a child during or immediately after therapy; infant cardiac and limb abnormalities have occurred.

Drug-specific teaching points
- Take drug on an empty stomach. If severe GI upset occurs, the tablet may be taken with food.
- Know that the following side effects may occur: nausea, vomiting, loss of appetite (taking the drug with food, small frequent meals also may help); darkening of the skin and fingernails; loss of hair (you may wish to obtain a wig or arrange for some other head covering before the loss of hair occurs; it is important to keep the head covered in extremes of temperature).
- Try to maintain your fluid intake and nutrition while on this drug (drink at least 10–12 glassses of fluid each day).
- Use birth control methods while on this drug and for a time afterwards (male and female patients); this drug can cause severe birth defects.
- Report unusual bleeding or bruising, fever, chills, sore throat, cough, shortness of breath, blood in the urine, painful urination, rapid heart beat, swelling of the feet or hands, stomach or flank pain.

cycloserine

(sye kloe ser' een)
Seromycin Pulvules
Pregnancy Category C

Drug classes
Antituberculous drug ("third line")
Antibiotic

Therapeutic actions
Inhibits cell wall synthesis in susceptible strains of gram-positive and gram-negative bacteria and in *Mycobacterium tuberculosis*, causing cell death.

Indications
- Treatment of active pulmonary and extrapulmonary (including renal) tuberculosis that is not responsive to first-line antituberculous drugs in conjunction with other antituberculous drugs
- UTIs caused by susceptible bacteria

Contraindications/cautions
- Allergy to cycloserine, epilepsy, depression, severe anxiety or psychosis, severe renal insufficiency, excessive concurrent use of alcohol, lactation.

Dosage
Adult
- ***Initial dose:*** 250 mg bid PO at 12-h intervals for first 2 wk; monitor serum levels (above 30 μg/ml is generally toxic).
- ***Maintenance dose:*** 500 mg–1 g/d PO in divided doses.

Pediatric: Safety and dosage not established.

Pharmacokinetics

Route	Onset	Peak	Duration
Oral	Varies	3–4 h	48–72 h

Metabolism: $T_{1/2}$: 10 h
Distribution: Crosses placenta; enters breast milk
Excretion: Urine and feces

Adverse effects
- CNS: *Convulsions, drowsiness, somnolence, headache, tremor, vertigo, confusion*, disorientation, loss of memory, **psychoses** (possibly with suicidal tendencies), hyperirritability, aggression, paresis, hyperreflexia, paresthesias, seizures, coma

Adverse effects in *Italics* are most common; those in **Bold** are life-threatening.

- Hematologic: Elevated serum transaminase levels
- Dermatologic: Skin rash

■ Nursing Considerations
Assessment
- *History:* Allergy to cycloserine, epilepsy, depression, severe anxiety or psychosis, severe renal insufficiency, excessive concurrent use of alcohol, nursing a baby
- *Physical:* Skin—color, lesions; orientation, reflexes, affect, EEG if appropriate; liver evaluation; liver function tests

Implementation
- Arrange for culture and sensitivity studies before use.
- Administer this drug only when other forms of therapy have failed, and only in conjunction with other antituberculosis agents when being used to treat tuberculosis.
- Arrange for follow-up of liver and renal function tests, hematologic tests, and serum drug levels.
- Consult with physician regarding the possible use of anticonvulsant drugs, sedatives, or pyridoxine if CNS effects become too severe.
- Discontinue drug, and notify physician if skin rash, severe CNS reactions occur.

Drug-specific teaching points
- Avoid excessive alcohol consumption while on this drug.
- Take this drug regularly; avoid missing doses. *Do not* discontinue this drug without first consulting your physician.
- Know that the following side effects may occur: drowsiness, tremor, disorientation (use caution if operating a car or dangerous machinery); take special precautions to avoid injury); depression, personality change, numbness and tingling (it might help to know that these are related to the drug therapy).
- Arrange for regular, periodic medical checkups, which will include blood tests to evaluate the drug effects.
- Report skin rash, headache, tremors, shaking, confusion, dizziness.

❐ cyclosporine

(sye' kloe spor een)
cyclosporin A, Sandimmune

Pregnancy Category C

Drug classes
Immunosuppressive agent

Therapeutic actions
Exact mechanism of immunosuppressant action is not known; specifically and reversibly inhibits immunocompetent lymphocytes in the G_0 or G_1 phase of the cell cycle; inhibits T-helper and T-suppressor cells, lymphokine production, and release of interleukin-2 and T-cell growth factor.

Indications
- Prophylaxis for organ rejection in kidney, liver, and heart transplants in conjunction with adrenal corticosteroids
- Treatment of chronic rejection in patients previously treated with other immunosuppressive agents
- **Unlabeled use**: limited but successful use in other procedures, including pancreas, bone marrow, heart and lung transplants

Contraindications/cautions
- Contraindicated in the presence of allergy to cyclosporine or polyoxyethylated castor oil (in oral preparation), pregnancy, lactation.
- Use caution in the presence of impaired renal function, malabsorption.

Dosage
Adult, pediatric
- ***Oral:*** 15 mg/kg per day PO initially given 4–12 h prior to transplantation; continue dose postoperatively for 1–2 wk, then taper by 5%/wk to a maintainence level of 5–10 mg/kg per day.
- ***Parenteral:*** Patients unable to take oral solution preoperatively or postoperatively may be given IV infusion at one-third the oral dose (ie, 5–6 mg/kg per day given 4–12 h prior to transplantation,

Adverse effects in *Italics* are most common; those in **Bold** are life-threatening.

cyclosporine ■ 335

administered as a slow infusion over 2–6 h). Continue this daily dose postoperatively. Switch to oral drug as soon as possible.

Pharmacokinetics

Route	Onset	Peak
Oral	Varies	3½ h
IV	Rapid	1–2 h

Metabolism: Hepatic, $T_{1/2}$: 19–27 h
Distribution: Crosses placenta; enters breast milk
Excretion: Bile and urine

IV facts
Preparation: Dilute IV solution immediately before use. Dilute 1 ml concentrate in 20–100 ml of 0.9% Sodium Chloride Injection or 5% Dextrose Injection. Protect from exposure to light.
Infusion: Give in a slow IV infusion over 2–6 h.

Adverse effects
- CNS: *Tremor*, convulsions, headache, paresthesias
- GI: **Hepatotoxicity**, *gum hyperplasia*, *diarrhea*, nausea, vomiting
- CV: *Hypertension*
- Hematologic: Leukopenia
- GU: *Renal dysfunction*, nephrotoxicity
- Other: *Hirsuitism*, *acne*, lymphomas, infections

Clinically important drug-drug interactions
- Increased risk of nephrotoxicity if taken with other nephrotoxic agents (erythromycin) • Increased risk of digoxin toxicity if taken concurrently with cyclosporine • Risk of severe myopathy or rhabdomyolysis if taken with lovastatin • Increased risk of toxicity if taken with diltiazem, metoclopramide, nicardipine • Increased plasma concentration of cyclosporine if taken with ketoconazole • Decreased therapeutic effect of cyclosporine if taken with hydantoins, rifampin, sulfonamides

■ Nursing Considerations
Assessment
- *History:* Allergy to cyclosporine or polyoxyethylated castor oil, impaired renal function, malabsorption, lactation
- *Physical:* Body temperature; Skin—color, lesions; BP, peripheral perfusion; liver evaluation, bowel sounds, gum evaluation; renal and liver function tests, CBC

Implementation
- Mix oral solution with milk, chocolate milk, or orange juice at room temperature. Stir well, and administer at once. Do not allow mixture to stand before drinking. Use a glass container, and rinse with more diluent to ensure that the total dose is taken.
- Use parenteral administration only if patient is unable to take the oral solution; transfer to oral solution as soon as possible.
- Do not refrigerate oral solution; store at room temperature and use within 2 mo after opening.
- Monitor renal and liver function tests before and periodically during therapy; marked decreases in function could require changes in dosage or discontinuation of the drug.
- Monitor blood pressure; some heart transplant patients have required concomitant antihypertensive therapy.

Drug-specific teaching points
- Dilute solution with milk, chocolate milk, or orange juice at room temperature; drink immediately after mixing. Rinse the glass with the solution to ensure that all the dose is taken. Store solution at room temperature. Use solution within 2 mo of opening the bottle.
- Avoid infection while you are on this drug; avoid crowds or people who have infections. Notify your physician at once if you injure yourself.

Adverse effects in *Italics* are most common; those in **Bold** are life-threatening.

- Know that the following side effects may occur: nausea, vomiting (taking the drug with food may help); diarrhea (ensure ready access to bathroom facilities if this occurs); skin rash; mouth sores (frequent mouth care will help).
- Be aware that this drug should not be taken during pregnancy. If you think that you are pregnant or you want to become pregnant, discuss this with your physician.
- Arrange to have periodic blood tests to monitor your response to this drug and its effects on your body.
- Do not discontinue this medication without your physician's advice.
- Report unusual bleeding or bruising, fever, sore throat, mouth sores, tiredness.

cyproheptadine hydrochloride

(si proe hep' ta deen)
Periactin, PMS-Cyproheptadine (CAN)

Pregnancy Category B

Drug classes
Antihistamine (piperidine type)

Therapeutic actions
Blocks the effects of histamine at H_1 receptor sites; has atropine-like, antiserotonin, antipruritic, sedative, and appetite-stimulating effects.

Indications
- Relief of symptoms associated with perennial and seasonal allergic rhinitis; vasomotor rhinitis; allergic conjunctivitis; mild, uncomplicated urticaria and angioedema; amelioraton of allergic reactions to blood or plasma; dermatographism; adjunctive therapy in anaphylactic reactions
- Treatment of cold urticaria
- **Unlabeled uses**: stimulation of appetite in underweight patients and those with anorexia nervosa; treatment of vascular cluster headaches

Contraindications/cautions
- Contraindicated in the presence of allergy to any antihistamines, third trimester of pregnancy.
- Use caution in the presence of narrow-angle glaucoma, stenosing peptic ulcer, symptomatic prostatic hypertrophy, asthmatic attack, bladder neck obstruction, pyloroduodenal obstruction, lactation.

Dosage
Adult
- ***Initial therapy:*** 4 mg tid PO.
- ***Maintenance therapy:*** 4–20 mg/d PO; do not exceed 0.5 mg/kg per day.

Pediatric: 0.25 mg/kg per day PO or 8 mg/m^2
- ***7–14 y:*** 4 mg PO bid or tid; do not exceed 16 mg/d.
- ***2–6 y:*** 2 mg PO bid or tid; do not exceed 12 mg/d.

Geriatric: More likely to cause dizziness, sedation, syncope, toxic confusional states, and hypotension in elderly patients; use with caution.

Pharmacokinetics

Route	Onset	Peak	Duration
Oral	15–30 min	1–2 h	4–6 h

Metabolism: Hepatic, $T_{1/2}$: 3–4 h
Distribution: Crosses placenta; enters breast milk
Excretion: Urine

Adverse effects
- **CNS**: *Drowsiness, sedation, dizziness, disturbed coordination,* fatigue, confusion, restlessness, excitation, nervousness, tremor, headache, blurred vision, diplopia, vertigo, tinnitus, acute labyrinthitis, hysteria, tingling, heaviness and weakness of the hands
- **GI**: *Epigastric distress,* anorexia, increased appetite and weight gain, nausea, vomiting, diarrhea or constipation
- **CV**: Hypotension, palpitations, bradycardia, tachycardia, extrasystoles
- **Respiratory**: *Thickening of bronchial secretions,* chest tightness, wheezing, nasal stuffiness, dry mouth, dry nose, dry throat, sore throat

Adverse effects in *Italics* are most common; those in **Bold** are life-threatening.

- **Hematologic:** Hemolytic anemia, hypoplastic anemia, thrombocytopenia, leukopenia, agranulocytosis, pancytopenia
- **GU:** Urinary frequency, dysuria, urinary retention, early menses, decreased libido, impotence
- **Other:** Urticaria, rash, anaphylactic shock, photosensitivity, excessive perspiration, chills

Clinically important drug-drug interactions

- Subnormal pituitary-adrenal response to metyrapone if taken with cyproheptadine • Decreased effects of fluoxetine taken with cyproheptadine • Increased and prolonged anticholinergic (drying) effects if taken with MAO inhibitors

Nursing Considerations

Assessment

- *History:* Allergy to any antihistamines; narrow-angle glaucoma, stenosing peptic ulcer, symptomatic prostatic hypertrophy, asthmatic attack, bladder neck obstruction, pyloroduodenal obstruction; lactation
- *Physical:* Skin—color, lesions, texture; orientation, reflexes, affect; vision exam; P, BP; R, adventitious sounds; bowel sounds; prostate palpation; CBC with differential

Implementation

- Administer with food if GI upset occurs.
- Administer syrup form if patient is unable to take tablets.
- Monitor patient response, and arrange for adjustment of dosage to lowest possible effective dose.

Drug-specific teaching points

- Take as prescribed; avoid excessive dosage.
- Take this drug with food if GI upset occurs.
- Know that the following side effects may occur: dizziness, sedation, drowsiness (use caution if driving or performing tasks that require alertness if these occur); epigastric distress, diarrhea, or constipation (taking the drug with meals may help; dry mouth (frequent mouth care, sucking sugarless lozenges may help); thickening of bronchial secretions, dryness of nasal mucosa (use of a humidifier may help if this becomes a problem).
- Avoid the use of alcohol while on this drug; serious sedation could occur.
- Report difficulty breathing, hallucinations, tremors, loss of coordination, unusual bleeding or bruising, visual disturbances, irregular heartbeat.

cysteamine bitartrate

(sis tee' ah meen)
Cystagon

Pregnancy Category C

Drug classes
Urinary tract agent

Therapeutic actions
Depletes cystine in the cells of patients with cystinosis, an inherited defect of lysosomal transport by participating with the lysosomes in an interchange reaction which allows cystine byproducts to exit the lysosome.

Indications
- Management of adults and children with nephropathic cystinosis

Contraindications/cautions
- Allergy to cysteamine or penicillamine, pregnancy, lactation.

Dosage
Maintenance dosage should be reached over a 5–6 wk period with slow incrementation based on leukocyte cystine measurement.
Adult and children >12 yr: 2 g/d PO divided into 4 doses.
Pediatric up to age 12 yr: 1.3 g/m^2/d of free base divided into 4 doses. Do not give intact capsules to children >6 y; open capsule and sprinkle over food.

Pharmacokinetics

Route	Onset	Peak
Oral	Slow	5–6 h

Adverse effects in *Italics* are most common; those in **Bold** are life-threatening.

Metabolism: T$_{1/2}$: unknown
Distribution: Crosses placenta; may pass into breast milk
Excretion: Urine

Adverse effects

- CNS: Nervousness, abnormal thinking, depression, emotional lability, hallucinations, nightmares, *headache*, ataxia, confusion, **seizures**
- GI: *Nausea, vomiting, bad breath, abdominal pain,* dyspepsia, constipation, gastroenteritis, duodenitis, duodenal ulcer
- Hematologic: Abnormal liver function tests, leukopenia, anemia
- Other: *Rash, fever*

■ Nursing Considerations

Assessment

- *History:* Allergy to cysteamine or penicillamine, pregnancy, lactation.
- *Physical:* Skin—color, lesions, turgor; body temperature; mucous membranes, bowel sounds, liver evaluation; urinalysis, renal and liver function tests, CBC and differential; leukocyte cystine measurement

Implementation

- Obtain leukocyte cystine measurements 5–6 h after dose administration for new patients; at 3 wk intervals with any dosage change; every 3 mo during maintenance treatment.
- Arrange to temporarily discontinue drug if initial therapy is poorly tolerated due to GI symptoms or rash; drug may be reinstituted at a lower dose with gradual increases.

Drug-specific teaching points

- Do not stop taking the medication without consulting your physician.
- Arrange to have regular blood tests during treatment with this drug.
- Know that the following side effects may occur: GI upset, loss of appetite (these may be limited effects that will pass with time), skin rash, dizziness, loss of sleep, abnormal thinking (avoid driving or performing tasks that require alertness if these occur).
- Report fever, rash, severe GI complaints, changes in gait, concentration

☐ cytarabine

(sye **tare'** a been)
cytosine arabinoside
Ara-C, Cytosar-U
Pregnancy Category D

Drug classes
Antimetabolite
Antineoplastic drug

Therapeutic actions
Inhibits DNA polymerase; cell cycle phase specific—S phase (stage of DNA synthesis); also blocks progression of cells from G_1 to S.

Indications

- Induction and maintenance of remission in acute myelocytic leukemia (higher response rate in children than in adults)
- Treatment of acute lymphocytic leukemia in adults and children; treatment of chronic myelocytic leukemia and erythroleukemia
- Treatment of meningeal leukemia (intrathecal use)
- Treatment of non-Hodgkin's lymphoma in children (part of combination therapy)

Contraindications/cautions

- Contraindicated in presence of allergy to cytarabine, pregnancy, lactation, premature infants.
- Use caution in the presence of hematopoietic depression secondary to radiation or chemotherapy; impaired liver function.

Dosage
Given by IV infusion or injection or SC.
Adult

- ***Acute myelocytic leukemia (AML) induction of remission:*** 200 mg/m^2 per day by continuous infu-

sion for 5 d for a total dose of 1000 mg/m²; repeat every 2 wk. Individualize dosage based on hematologic response.
- **Maintenance of AML:** Use same dosage and schedule as induction; often a longer rest period is allowed.
- **Acute lymphocytic leukemia (ALL):** Dosage similar to AML.
- **Intrathecal use for meningeal leukemia:** 5 mg/m² to 75 mg/m² once daily for 4 d or once every 4 d. Most common dose is 30 mg/m² every 4 d until CSF is normal, followed by one more treatment.

Pediatric
- **Remission induction and maintenance of AML:** Calculate dose by body weight or surface area. (See Appendix C).
- **ALL:** Same dosage as AML.
- **Intrathecal use (has been used as treatment of meningeal leukemia and prophylaxis in newly diagnosed children with ALL):** Cytarabine, 30 mg/m²; hydrocortisone sodium succinate, 15 mg/m²; methotrexate, 15 mg/m²
- **Combination therapies: For persistent leukemias—give at 2- to 4-wk intervals: Cytarabine:** 100 mg/m² per day by continous IV infusion, days 1–10. **Doxorubicin:** 30 mg/m² per day by IV infusion over 30 min, days 1–3.
- **Cytarabine:** 100 mg/m² per day by IV infusion over 30 min q12h, days 1–7. *Thioguanine:* 100 mg/m² PO q12h, days 1–7. *Daunorubicin:* 60 mg/m² per day by IV infusion, days 5–7.
- **Cytarabine:** 100 mg/m² per day by contiuous infusion, days 1–7. *Doxorubicin:* 30 mg/m² per day by IV infusion, days 1–3. *Vincristine:* 1.5 mg/m² per day by IV infusion, days 1 and 5. *Prednisone:* 40 mg/m² per day by IV infusion q12h, days 1–5.
- **Cytarabine:** 100 mg/m² per day IV q12h, days 1–7. *Daunorubicin:* 70 mg/m² per day by infusion, days 1–3. *Thioguanine:* 100 mg/m² per day PO q12h, days 1–7. *Prednisone:* 40 mg/m² per day PO, days 1–7. *Vincristine:* 1 mg/m² per day by IV infusion, days 1 and 7.
- **Cytarabine:** 100 mg/m² per day by continous infusion, days 1–7. *Daunorubicin:* 45 mg/m² per day by IV push, days 1–3.

Pharmacokinetics

Route	Onset	Peak	Duration
IV	Rapid	20–60 min	12–18 h

Metabolism: Hepatic, $T_{1/2}$: 1–3 h
Distribution: Crosses placenta; enters breast milk
Excretion: Urine

IV facts
Preparation: Reconstitute 100-mg vial with 5 ml of Bacteriostatic Water for Injection with benzyl alcohol 0.9%; resultant solution contains 20 mg/ml cytarabine. Reconstitute 500-mg vial with 10 ml of the above; resultant solution contains 50 mg/ml cytarabine. Store at room temperature for up to 48 h. Discard solution if a slight haze appears. Can be further diluted with Water for Injection, 5% Dextrose in Water, or Sodium Chloride Injection; stable for 8 d.

Infusion: Administer by IV infusion, IV injection, or SC; patients can usually tolerate higher doses when given by rapid IV injection. There is no clinical advantage to any particular route.

Adverse effects
- CNS: Neuritis, neural toxicity
- GI: *Anorexia, nausea, vomiting, diarrhea, oral and anal inflammation or ulceration*; esophageal ulcerations, esophagitis, abdominal pain, *hepatic dysfunction* (jaundice), acute pancreatitis
- Hematologic: **Bone marrow depression,** hyperuricemia
- GU: Renal dysfunction, urinary retention
- Dermatologic: Fever, rash, urticaria, freckling, skin ulceration, pruritus, conjunctivitis, alopecia

Adverse effects in *Italics* are most common; those in **Bold** are life-threatening.

- **Local:** Thrombophlebitis, cellulitis at injection site
- **Other:** Cytarabine syndrome (fever, myalgia, bone pain, occasional chest pain, maculopapular rash, conjunctivitis, malaise, which is sometimes responsive to corticosteroids), *fever, rash*

Clinically important drug-drug interactions
- Decreased therapeutic action of digoxin if taken with cytarabine

■ Nursing Considerations
Assessment
- *History:* Allergy to cytarabine, hematopoietic depression, impaired liver function, lactation
- *Physical:* Weight; temperature; skin—lesions, color; hair; orientation, reflexes; R, adventitious sounds; mucous membranes, liver evaluation, abdominal exam; CBC, differential; renal and liver function tests; urinalysis

Implementation
- Arrange for tests to evaluate hematopoietic status before beginning therapy and frequently during therapy.
- Arrange for discontinuation of drug therapy if platelet count < 50,000/mm^3, polymorphonuclear granuloctye count < 1,000/mm^3; consult physician for dosage adjustment.
- Use a special diluent (Elliott's B solution), similar to CSF, for intrathecal use.
- Arrange for comfort measures if anal inflammation, headache, other pain associated with cytarabine syndrome occur.

Drug-specific teaching points
- Prepare a calendar of treatment days to follow. Drug must be given IV or SC.
- Know that the following side effects may occur: nausea, vomiting, loss of appetite (medication may be ordered to help; small frequent meals may also help; it is important to maintain your nutrition); malaise, weakness, lethargy (these are all effects of the drug; it is advisable to avoid driving or operating dangerous machinery if these occur); mouth sores (frequent mouth care will be needed); diarrhea (ensure yourself ready access to bathroom facilities if these occur); loss of hair (you may wish to obtain a wig or other suitable head covering; it is important to keep the head covered at extremes of temperature); anal inflammation (comfort measures can be established).
- Use birth control while on this drug; this drug may cause birth defects or miscarriages.
- Arrange to have frequent, regular medical follow-up, including frequent blood tests to follow the effects of the drug on your body.
- Report black, tarry stools, fever, chills, sore throat, unusual bleeding or bruising, shortness of breath, chest pain, difficulty swallowing.

❐ dacarbazine

(da kar' ba zeen)
DTIC, imidazole carboxamide

DTIC-Dome

Pregnancy Category C

Drug classes
Antineoplastic agent

Therapeutic actions
Cytotoxic: exact mechanism of action unknown; inhibits DNA and RNA synthesis, causing cell death; cell cycle nonspecific.

Indications
- Metastatic malignant melanoma
- Hodgkin's disease—second-line therapy in combination with other drugs

Contraindications/cautions
- Contraindicated in the presence of allergy to dacarbazine, pregnancy, lactation.
- Use caution in the presence of impaired hepatic function, bone marrow depression.

Dosage
Malignant melanoma: 2–4.5 mg/kg per day IV for 10 d, repeated at 4-wk intervals or 250 mg/m^2 per day IV for 5 d, repeated every 3 wk.

Adverse effects in *Italics* are most common; those in **Bold** are life-threatening.

Hodgkin's disease: 150 mg/m^2 per day for 5 d in combination with other drugs, repeated every 4 wk or 375 mg/m^2 on day 1 in combination with other drugs, repeated every 15 d.

Pharmacokinetics

Route	Onset	Duration
IV	15–20 min	6–8 h

Metabolism: Hepatic; T$_{1/2}$: 19 min then 5 h
Distribution: Crosses placenta; enters breast milk
Excretion: Urine

IV facts

Preparation: Reconstitute 100-mg vials with 9.9 ml and the 200-mg vials with 19.7 ml of Sterile Water for Injection; the resulting solution contains 10 mg/ml of dacarbazine. Reconstituted solution may be further diluted with 5% Dextrose Injection or Sodium Chloride Injection and administered as an IV infusion. Reconstituted solution is stable for 72 h if refrigerated, 8 h at room temperature. If further diluted, solution is stable for 24 h if refrigerated or 8 h at room temperature.

Infusion: Infuse slowly; use care to avoid extravasation.

Adverse effects

- **GI:** *Anorexia, nausea, vomiting,* hepatotoxicity, **hepatic necrosis**
- **Hematologic:** *Hemopoietic depression*
- **Dermatologic:** *Photosensitivity,* erythematous and urticarial rashes, alopecia
- **Hypersensitivity:** Anaphylaxis
- **Local:** *Local tissue damage and pain if extravasation occurs*
- **Other:** Facial paresthesias, flulike syndrome, cancer

■ Nursing Considerations

Assessment

- *History:* Allergy to dacarbazine, impaired hepatic function, bone marrow depression, lactation

- *Physical:* Weight; temperature; skin—color, lesions; hair; mucous membranes, liver evaluation; CBC, liver function tests

Implementation

- Arrange for lab tests (WBC, RBC, platelets) before beginning therapy and frequently during therapy.
- Administer IV only; use care to prevent extravasation into the subcutaneous tissues during administration because tissue damage and severe pain may occur.
- Apply hot packs to relieve pain locally if extravasation occurs.
- Restrict the patient's oral intake of fluid and foods for 4–6 h before therapy to alleviate nausea and vomiting.
- Consult with physician for antiemetic if severe nausea and vomiting occur. Phenobarbital and prochloperazine have been found useful. Assure patient that nausea usually subsides after 1–2 d.

Drug-specific teaching points

- Prepare a calendar for specific treatment days and additional courses of drug therapy.
- Know that the following side effects may occur: loss of appetite, nausea, vomiting (frequent mouth care, small frequent meals may help; try to maintain good nutrition if at all possible; a dietician may be able to help; an antiemetic may also be ordered); rash, loss of hair (these are effects of the drug; they should pass when the drug is discontinued; you may want to arrange for a wig or other suitable head covering before hair loss occurs; it is important to keep head covered in extremes of temperature); sensitivity to ultraviolet light (use a sunscreen and protective clothing if exposed to sunlight or ultrviolet lights).
- Arrange to have regular blood tests to monitor the drug's effects.
- Report fever, chills, sore throat, unusual bleeding or bruising, yellow skin or eyes, light-colored stools, dark urine, pain or burning at IV injection site.

Adverse effects in *Italics* are most common; those in **Bold** are life-threatening.

◻ dactinomycin

*(dak ti noe **mye'** sin)*

actinomycin D, ACT

Cosmegan

Pregnancy Category C

Drug classes
Antibiotic
Antineoplastic agent

Therapeutic actions
Cytotoxic: inhibits synthesis of messenger RNA, causing cell death; cell cycle nonspecific.

Indications
- Wilms' tumor, rhabdomyosarcoma, metastatic and nonmetastatic choriocarcinoma, Ewing's sarcoma, sarcoma botryoides, as part of a combination therapy regimen
- Nonseminomatous testicular carcinoma
- Potentiation of effects of radiation therapy

Contraindications/cautions
- Contraindicated in the presence of allergy to dactinomycin; chickenpox, herpes zoster (severe, generalized disease and death could result); pregnancy; lactation.
- Use caution in the presence of bone marrow suppression, radiation therapy.

Dosage
Individualize dosage. Toxic reactions are frequent and limit the amount of the drug that can be given. Administer drug in short courses.
Adult
- **IV:** 0.5 mg/d for up to 5 d. Administer a second course after at least 3 wk. Do not exceed 15 µg/kg per day for 5 d. Calculate dosage for obese or edematous patients on the basis of surface area as an attempt to relate dosage to lean body mass. Do not exceed 400–600 µg/m^2 per day.
- ***Isolation-perfusion technique:*** 0.05 mg/kg for lower extremity or pelvis; 0.035 mg/kg for upper extremity. Use lower dose for obese patients or when previous therapy has been used.

Pediatric: Do not give to children younger than 6–12 mo.
- **IV:** 0.015 mg/kg per day for 5 d or a total dose of 2.5 mg/m^2 over 1 wk; administer a second course after at least 3 wk.

Pharmacokinetics

Route	Onset	Duration
IV	Rapid	9 d

Metabolism: Hepatic; T$_{1/2}$: 36 h
Distribution: Crosses placenta; enters breast milk
Excretion: Urine and bile

IV facts
Preparation: Reconstitute by adding 1.1 ml of Sterile Water for Injection (*without preservatives*) to vial, which gives a solution with concentration of 0.5 mg/ml. Discard any unused portion.

Infusion: Add to IV infusions of 5% Dextrose or to Sodium Chloride, or inject into IV tubing of a running IV infusion. If drug is given directly into a vein without an infusion, use two needles, one sterile needle to remove drug from vial and another for the direct IV injection. Do not inject into IV lines with cellulose ester membrane filters; drug may be partially removed by filter.

Adverse effects
- **GI:** *Cheilitis, dysphagia, esophagitis,* ulcerative stomatitis, pharyngitis, *anorexia, abdominal pain, diarrhea,* GI ulceration, proctitis, nausea, vomiting, hepatic abnormalities
- **Hematologic:** *Anemia, aplastic anemia, agranulocytosis, leukopenia, thrombocytopenia, pancytopenia, reticulopenia*
- **Dermatologic:** *Alopecia, skin eruptions,* acne, erythema, increased pigmentation of GU renal abnormalities
- **Local:** *Tissue necrosis at sites of extravasation*
- **Other:** *Malaise, fever, fatigue, lethargy, myalgia,* hypocalcemia, death, increased

Adverse effects in *Italics* are most common; those in **Bold** are life-threatening.

incidence of second primary tumors when used with radiation

Drug-lab test interferences
- Inaccurate bioassay procedure results for determination of antibacterial drug levels

■ Nursing Considerations

Assessment
- *History:* Allergy to dactinomycin; chickenpox, herpes zoster; bone marrow suppression, radiation therapy; pregnancy, lactation
- *Physical:* Temperature; skin—color, lesions; weight; hair; local injection site; mucous membranes, abdominal exam; CBC, hepatic and renal function tests, urinalysis

Implementation
- Do not administer IM or SC because severe local reaction and tissue necrosis occur; for IV use only.
- Monitor injection site for extravasation, reports of burning, or stinging. Discontinue infusion immediately, and restart in another vein; apply cold compresses to the area. Local infiltration with injectable corticosteroid and flushing of the area with saline may lessen the local reaction.
- Monitor patient's response, including CBC, frequently at beginning of therapy; adverse effects may require a decrease in drug dose or discontinuation of the drug; consult physician.
- Warn patient that adverse effects may not occur immediately, may be maximal 1–2 wk after therapy.

Drug-specific teaching points
- Prepare a calendar for return days for drug therapy.
- Know that the following side effects may occur: rash, skin lesions, loss of hair (you may want to invest in a wig before hair loss occurs; skin care may help somewhat); loss of appetite, nausea, mouth sores (frequent mouth care, small frequent meals may help; you will need to try to maintain good nutrition if at all possible; a dietician may be able to help; an antiemetic also may be ordered).
- Know that adverse effects of the drug may not occur immediately; it may take up to 1–2 wk following administration for the maximal effects.
- Arrange for regular medical followup, which will include blood tests to monitor the drug's effects.
- Report severe GI upset, diarrhea, vomiting, burning or pain at injection site, unusual bleeding or bruising, severe mouth sores, GI lesions.

❒ dalteparin

(dahl' ta pear in)
Fragmin

Pregnancy Category B

Drug classes
Anticoagulant

Therapeutic actions
Low molecular weight heparin that inhibits thrombus and clot formation by blocking factor Xa, factor IIa, preventing the formation of clots.

Indications
- Prevention of deep vein thrombosis, which may lead to pulmonary embolism, following abdominal surgery.

Contraindications/cautions
- Contraindicated in the presence of hypersensitivity to dalteparin, heparin, pork products; severe thrombocytopenia; uncontrolled bleeding.
- Use caution in the presence of pregnancy or lactation, history of GI bleed.

Dosage
Adult: Not yet available
Pediatric: Safety and efficacy not established

Pharmacokinetics

Route	Onset	Peak	Duration
SC	20–60 min	3–5 h	12 h

Adverse effects in *Italics* are most common; those in **Bold** are life-threatening.

Metabolism: T$_{1/2}$: 4.5 h; distribution: may cross placenta, may enter breast milk
Excretion: Urine

Adverse effects
- Hematologic: **Hemorrhage**; *bruising*; thrombocytopenia; elevated SGOT, SGPT levels; hyperkalemia
- Hypersensitivity: Chills, fever, urticaria, asthma
- Treatment of overdose: Protamine sulfate (1% solution). Each mg of protamine neutralizes 1 mg dalteparin. Give very slowly IV over 10 min.
- Other: Fever; pain; local irritation, hematoma, erythema at site of injection

Clinically important drug-drug interactions
- Increased bleeding tendencies with oral anticoagulants, salicylates, penicillins, cephalosporins

Drug-lab test interferences
- Increased AST, ALT levels

■ Nursing Considerations

Assessment
- *History*: Recent surgery or injury; sensitivity to heparin, pork products, enoxaparin; lactation; history of GI bleed.
- *Physical*: Peripheral perfusion, R, stool guaiac test, partial thromboplastin time (PTT) or other tests of blood coagulation, platelet count, kidney function tests

Implementation
- Arrange to give drug as soon as possible after abdominal surgery.
- Give deep subcutaneous injections; **do not** give dalteparin by IM injection.
- Administer by deep SC injection; patient should be lying down; alternate administration between the left and right anterolateral and left and right posterolateral abdominal wall. Introduce the whole length of the needle into a skin fold held between the thumb and forefinger; hold the skin fold througout the injection.
- Apply pressure to all injection sites after needle is withdrawn; inspect injection sites for signs of hematoma.
- Do not massage injection sites.
- Do not mix with other injections or infusions.
- Store at room temperature; fluid should be clear, colorless to pale yellow.
- Alert all health care providers that patient is on dalteparin.
- If thromboembolic episode should occur despite therapy, discontinue and initiate appropriate therapy.
- Have protamine sulfate (dalteparin antidote) on standby in case of overdose.

Drug-specific teaching points
- Know that this drug must be given by a parenteral route (cannot be taken orally).
- Periodic blood tests will be needed to monitor your response to this drug.
- Be careful to avoid injury while you are on this drug: use an electric razor, avoid activities that might lead to injury.
- Report nose bleed, bleeding of the gums, unusual bruising, black or tarry stools, cloudy or dark urine, abdominal or lower back pain, severe headache.

❐ danazol

(da na zole)
Cyclomen (CAN), Danocrine

Pregnancy Category C

Drug classes
Androgen
Hormonal agent

Therapeutic actions
Synthetic androgen that suppresses the release of the pituitary gonadotropins FSH and LH, which inhibits ovulation and decreases estrogen and progesterone levels; inhibits sex steroid synthesis and binds to steroid receptors in cells of target tissues. Therapeutic effects in hereditary angioedema are probably due to effects of the drug in the liver; danazol partially or completely corrects the primary defect in this disorder.

Adverse effects in *Italics* are most common; those in **Bold** are life-threatening.

Indications
- Treatment of endometriosis amenable to hormonal management
- Treatment of fibrocystic breast disease; decreases nodularity, pain, and tenderness; symptoms return after cessation of therapy
- Prevention of attacks of hereditary angioedema
- **Unlabeled uses**: treatment of precocious puberty, gynecomastia, menorrhagia

Contraindications/cautions
- Known sensitivity to danazol; undiagnosed abnormal genital bleeding; impaired hepatic, renal, or cardiac function; pregnancy; lactation.

Dosage
Adult
- ***Endometriosis:*** Begin therapy during menstruation, or ensure that patient is not pregnant; 800 mg/d PO, in two divided doses; downward titration to a dose sufficient to maintain amenorrhea may be considered. For mild cases, give 200–400 mg PO, in two divided doses. Continue therapy for 3–6 mo or up to 9 mo. Reinstitute therapy if symptoms recur after termination of therapy.
- ***Fibrocystic breast disease:*** Begin therapy during menstruation, or ensure that patient is not pregnant; 100–400 mg/d PO in two divided doses; 2–6 mo of therapy may be required to alleviate all signs and symptoms.
- ***Hereditary angioedema:*** Individualize dosage; starting dose of 200 mg PO bid or tid. After favorable response, decrease dose by 50% or less at 1- to 3-mo intervals. If an attack occurs, increase dose to 200 mg/d; monitor response closely during adjustment of dose.

Pharmacokinetics

Route	Peak	Duration
Oral	6–8 wk	3–6 mo

Metabolism: Hepatic; $T_{1/2}$: 4½ h

Distribution: Crosses placenta; enters breast milk
Excretion: Unknown

Adverse effects
- CNS: Dizziness, headache, sleep disorders, fatigue, tremor
- GI: Hepatic dysfunction
- GU: Fluid retention
- Endocrine: *Androgenic effects* (acne, edema, mild hirsutism, decrease in breast size, deepening of the voice, oily skin or hair, weight gain, clitoral hypertrophy or testicular atrophy), *hypoestrogenic effects* (flushing, sweating, vaginitis, nervousness, emotional lability)

Clinically important drug-drug interactions
- Prolongation of prothrombin time in patients stabilized on oral anticoagulants • Increased carbamazepine toxicity if taken concurrently with danazol

■ Nursing Considerations

Assessment
- *History:* Known sensitivity to danazol; undiagnosed abnormal genital bleeding; impaired hepatic, renal or cardiac function; pregnancy; lactation
- *Physical:* Body weight; hair distribution pattern; skin—color, texture, lesions; breast exam; orientation, affect, reflexes; P, auscultation, BP, peripheral edema; liver evaluation; liver and renal function tests, semen and sperm evaluation

Implementation
- Ensure that patient is not pregnant before beginning therapy; begin therapy for endometriosis and fibrocystic breast disease during menstrual period.
- Ensure that patient does not have carcinoma of the breast before beginning therapy for fibrocystic breast disease; rule out carcinoma during therapy if nodule persists or enlarges.
- Caution patient that androgenic effects may not be reversible when the drug is withdrawn.

Adverse effects in *Italics* are most common; those in **Bold** are life-threatening.

- Arrange for periodic liver function tests during therapy; heptic dysfunction has been reported with long-term use.
- Arrange for periodic tests of semen and sperm, especially in adolescents; marked changes may indicate need to discontinue therapy.

Drug-specific teaching points
- Know that the following side effects may occur: masculinizing effects (acne, hair growth, deepening of voice, oily skin or hair; these effects may not be reversible when the drug is withdrawn), low-estrogen effects (flushing, sweating, vaginal irritation, mood changes, nervousness).
- Use a nonhormonal form of birth control during drug therapy. If you become pregnant, discontinue the drug, and consult with your physician immediately. This drug is contraindicated during pregnancy.
- Report abnormal growth of facial hair, deepening of the voice, unusual bleeding or bruising, fever, chills, sore throat, vaginal itching or irritation.

☐ dantrolene sodium

(dan' troe leen)

Dantrium

Pregnancy Category C

Drug classes
Direct-acting skeletal muscle relaxant

Therapeutic actions
Relaxes skeletal muscle within the skeletal muscle fiber, probably by interfering with the release of calcium from the sarcoplasmic reticulum; does not interfere with neuromuscular transmission or affect the surface membrane of skeletal muscle.

Indications
- **Oral:** Control of clinical spasticity resulting from upper motor neuron disorders, such as spinal cord injury, stroke, cerebral palsy, or multiple sclerosis; not indicated for relief of skeletal muscle spasm resulting from rheumatic disorders; continued long-term administration is justified if use of the drug: significantly reduces painful or disabling spasticity, such as clonus; significantly reduces the intensity or degree of nursing care required; rids the patient of any annoying manifestation of spasticity considered important by the patient.
- Preoperatively to prevent or attenuate the development of malignant hyperthermia in susceptible patients who must undergo surgery or anesthesia; after a malignant hyperthermia crisis to prevent recurrence
- **Unlabeled use**: exercise-induced muscle pain
- **Parenteral (IV):** management of the fulminant hypermetabolism of skeletal muscle characteristic of malignant hyperthermia crisis

Contraindications/cautions
Refer to the chronic use of oral dantrolene to treat spasticity; malignant hyperthermia is a medical emergency that would override contraindications and cautions.
- Contraindicated in the presence of active hepatic disease; spasticity used to sustain upright posture and balance in locomotion or to obtain or maintain increased function; lactation.
- Use caution in the presence of female patients and patients > 35 y (greater likelihood of drug-induced, potentially fatal, hepatocellular disease in these populations); impaired pulmonary function; severely impaired cardiac function due to myocardial disease; history of previous liver disease or dysfunction.

Dosage
Adult
- *Oral*
  - *Chronic spasticity:* Titrate and individualize dosage; establish a therapeutic goal before therapy, and increase dosage until maximum performance compatible with the dysfunction is achieved. Initially, 25 mg qd; increase to 25 mg bid–qid; then increase in increments of 25 mg up to as high as 100 mg bid–qid if necessary. Most patients will respond to 400 mg/d or less; maintain each dosage

dantrolene sodium ■ 347

level for 4–7 d to evaluate response. Discontinue drug after 45 d if benefits are not evident.
- *Preoperative prophylaxis of malignant hyperthermia:* 4–8 mg/kg per d PO in three to four divided doses for 1–2 d prior to surgery, with the last dose given approximately 3–4 h before scheduled surgery with a minimum of water. Adjust dosage to within the recommended range to prevent incapacitation due to drowsiness and to prevent excessive GI irritation.
- *Postcrisis follow-up:* 4–8 mg/kg per d PO in four divided doses for 1–3 d to prevent recurrence.
• **Parenteral (treatment of malignant hyperthermia):** Discontinue all anesthetic agents as soon as problem is recognized. Give dantrolene by continuous rapid IV push beginning at a minimum dose of 1 mg/kg and continuing until symptoms subside or a maximum cumulative dose of 10 mg/kg has been given. If physiologic and metabolic abnormalities reappear, repeat regimen. Administration should be continuous until symptoms subside.

Pediatric: Safety for use in children < 5 y not established. Because adverse effects could become apparent only after many years, weigh benefits and risks of long-term use carefully.
• **Oral**
- *Chronic spasticity:* Use an approach similar to that described above for the adult. Initially, 0.5 mg/kg bid PO. Increase to 0.5 mg/kg tid–qid; then increase by increments of 0.5 mg/kg up to 3 mg/kg, bid–qid if necessary;. Do not exceed dosage of 100 mg qid.
- *Malignant hyperthermia:* Dosage orally and IV is same as adult.

Pharmacokinetics

Route	Onset	Peak	Duration
Oral	Slow	4–6 h	8–10 h
IV	Rapid	5 h	6–8 h

Metabolism: Hepatic; $T_{1/2}$: 9 h (oral) 4–8 h (IV)
Distribution: Crosses placenta; enters breast milk
Excretion: Urine

IV facts
Preparation: Add 60 ml of Sterile Water for Injection (without bacteriostatic agents); shake until solution is clear. Protect from light, and use within 6 h. Store at room temperature, protected from light.
Infusion: Administer by rapid continuous IV push. Administer continuously until symptoms subside.

Adverse effects
Oral
- CNS: *Drowsiness, dizziness, weakness, general malaise, fatigue,* speech disturbance, seizure, headache, lightheadedness, visual disturbance, diplopia, alteration of taste, insomnia, mental depression, mental confusion, increased nervousness
- GI: *Diarrhea,* constipation, GI bleeding, anorexia, dysphagia, gastric irritation, abdominal cramps, **hepatitis**
- CV: Tachycardia, erratic blood pressure, phlebitis, effusion with pericarditis
- GU: Increased urinary frequency, hematuria, crystalluria, difficult erection, urinary incontinence, nocturia, dysuria, urinary retention
- Dermatologic: Abnormal hair growth, acnelike rash, pruritus, urticaria, eczematoid eruption, sweating, photosensitivity
- Other: Myalgia, backache, chills and fever, feeling of suffocation
- Parenteral: None of the above reactions with short-term IV therapy for malignant hyperthermia

■ Nursing Considerations
Assessment
- *History:* Active hepatic disease; spasticity used to sustain upright posture and balance in locomotion or to obtain or maintain increased function; female patient

Adverse effects in *Italics* are most common; those in **Bold** are life-threatening.

and patients > 35 y; impaired pulmonary function; severely impaired cardiac function; history of previous liver disease; lactation
- *Physical:* Body temperature; skin—color, lesions; orientation, affect, reflexes, bilateral grip strength, vision; P, BP, auscultation; adventitious sounds; bowel sounds, normal GI output; prostate palpation, normal output, voiding pattern; urinalysis, liver function tests (SGOT, SGPT, alkaline phosphatase, total bilirubin)

Implementation

- Monitor IV injection sites, and ensure that extravasation does not occur—drug is very alkaline and irritating to tissues.
- Ensure that other measures are used to treat malignant hyperthermia: discontinuation of triggering agents, monitoring and providing for increased oxygen requirements, managing metabolic acidosis and electrolyte imbalance, cooling if necessary.
- Establish a therapeutic goal before beginning chronic oral therapy (eg, regaining and maintaining a specific function, such as therapeutic exercise program, use of braces, transfer maneuvers).
- Arrange to withdraw drug for 2–4 d if needed to reinforce a clinical impression of benefit of continued drug therapy; exacerbation of spasticity would indicate continued need for this potentially dangerous drug.
- Arrange to discontinue drug if diarrhea is severe; it may be possible to reinstitute it at a lower dose.
- Monitor liver function tests periodically during treatment, and arrange to discontinue drug at first sign of abnormality; early detection of liver abnormalities may permit reversion to normal function.

Drug-specific teaching points

Preoperative Prophylaxis of Malignant Hyperthermia
- Call for assistance when you wish to get up; you should not move about unaccompanied; this drug may cause you to be drowsy.
- Report GI upset; a change in dosage may be possible, and small frequent meals may help.

Chronic Oral Therapy for Spasticity
- Take this drug exactly as prescribed; do not take a higher dosage than that prescribed for you.
- Avoid alcohol, sleep-inducing, or OTC drugs while you are on this drug; these could cause dangerous effects.
- Know that the following side effects may occur: drowsiness, dizziness, blurred vision (avoid driving a car or engaging in activities that require alertness if these occur); diarrhea (ensure ready access to bathroom facilities); nausea (taking drug with food and eating frequent small meals may help); difficulty urinating, increased urinary frequency, urinary incontinence (be sure that you empty the bladder just before taking the medication); headache, malaise (it may be possible for you to use an analgesic); photosensitivity (use sunscreens, protective clothing if you cannot avoid exposure to sunlight or ultraviolet light).
- Report skin rash, itching, bloody or black tarry stools, pale stools, yellowish discoloration of the skin or eyes, severe diarrhea.

☐ dapsone

(dap' sone)
DDS, diaphenylsulfone
Avlosulfan (CAN)

Pregnancy Category A

Drug classes
Leprostatic

Therapeutic actions
Bactericidal and bacteriostatic against *Mycobacterium leprae*; mechanism of action in dermatitis herpetiformis is not established.

Indications
- Hansen's disease (leprosy—all forms)
- Dermatitis herpetiformis

dapsone

- **Orphan drug use**: alone or in combination with trimethoprim for treatment of *Pneumocystis carinii* pneumonia
- **Unlabeled uses:** Relapsing polychondritis, prophylaxis of malaria

Contraindications/cautions
- Contraindicated in the presence of allergy to dapsone or its derivatives, lactation.
- Use caution in the presence of anemia, severe cardiopulmonary disease, G-6-PD deficiency, methemoglobin reductase deficiency, hemoglobin M, hepatic dysfunction, pregnancy.

Dosage
Adult
- **Dermatitis herpetiformis:** 50 mg daily PO; individualize dosage to 50–300 mg daily. Maintenance dosage may be reduced after 6 mo on a gluten-free diet.
- **Leprosy:** 6–10 mg/kg per week PO (50–100 mg daily).
- **Bacteriologically negative tuberculoid and indeterminate type leprosy:** 50 mg/d PO. Continue therapy for at least 3 y after clinical control is established.
- **Lepromatous and borderline patients:** 50 mg/d PO for *at least 10 y* after patient is bacteriologically negative, usually for life.

Pediatric: Use correspondingly smaller doses than with adults.

Pharmacokinetics

Route	Onset	Peak	Duration
Oral	8 d	4–8 h	3 wk

Metabolism: Hepatic; $T_{1/2}$: 28 h
Distribution: May cross placenta; enters breast milk
Excretion: Urine

Adverse effects
- CNS: Peripheral neuropathy in nonleprosy patients, headache, psychosis, insomnia, vertigo, paresthesias, blurred vision, tinnitus
- GI: *Nausea, vomiting,* abdominal pain, anorexia, toxic hepatitis, cholestatic jaundice
- Hematologic: *Hemolysis, including hemolytic anemia,* aplastic anemia, agranulocytosis; methemoglobinemia, hypoalbuminemia
- GU: Albuminuria, nephrotic syndrome, renal papillary necrosis, male infertility
- Dermatologic: Hyperpigmented macules, drug-induced lupus erythematosus, phototoxicity
- Other: Fever, carcinogenic in small animals

■ Nursing Considerations

Assessment
- *History:* Allergy to dapsone or its derivatives, anemia, severe cardiopulmonary disease, G-6-PD deficiency, methemoglobin reductase deficiency, hemoglobin M, hepatic dysfunction, lactation
- *Physical:* Skin—lesions, color; temperature; orientation, affect, reflexes, vision; P, auscultation, BP, edema; R, auscultation; bowel sounds, liver evaluation; CBC, liver and renal function tests

Implementation
- Monitor patient closely during administration; fatalities have been reported from agranulocytosis, aplastic anemia, and other blood dyscrasias.
- Arrange for regular blood counts during therapy: weekly for first month, monthly for 6 mo, and then every 6 mo is recommended. Arrange for discontinuation of drug, and consult with physician if significant leukopenia, thrombocytopenia, or decreased hematopoiesis occurs.
- Arrange for discontinuation of drug, and consult with physician if any sign of hypersensitivity occurs (dermatologic reactions).
- Arrange for monitoring of liver function tests during therapy; arrange to discontinue drug and consult with physician if any abnormality occurs.
- Assess patient and consult with physician if leprosy reactional episodes occur (worsening of leprosy activity related to therapy); use of other leprostatics, analgesics, steroids, or surgery may be necessary.

Adverse effects in *Italics* are most common; those in **Bold** are life-threatening.

- Administer drug with meals if GI upset occurs.
- Suspect secondary dapsone resistance when a lepromatous or borderline lepromatous patient relapses clinically and bacteriologically. Arrange for clinical confirmation of dapsone resistance, and change drugs as ordered.
- Contact support groups to help the patient to cope with disease and drug therapy: National Hansen's Disease Center; Carville, LA, 70721; telephone, (504) 642-7771.

Drug-specific teaching points
- Take the drug with food if GI upset occurs. Follow the prescription carefully: to be effective, this drug will be needed for a prolonged period.
- Arrange regular medical followup while you are on this drug, including blood tests.
- Know that the following side effects may occur: nausea, loss of appetite, vomiting (taking the drug with meals may help); sensitivity to sunlight (wear protective clothing; use a sunscreen); numbness, tingling, weakness (use caution to avoid injury).
- Report worsening of Hansen's disease symptoms, severe GI upset, unusual bleeding or bruising, sore throat, fever, chills, yellowing of skin or eyes.

▢ daunorubicin hydrochloride

*(daw noe **roo'** bi sin)*
daunomycin, DNR
Cerubidine

Pregnancy Category D

Drug classes
Antibiotic
Antineoplastic agent

Therapeutic actions
Cytotoxic, antimiotic, immunosuppressive: binds to DNA and inhibits DNA synthesis, causing cell death.

Indications
- Remission induction in acute non-lymphocytic leukemia of adults, alone and in combination with cytarabine
- Remission induction in childhood acute lymphocytic leukemia in combination with vincristine and prednisone (addition of daunorubicin gives longer remission than use of only vincristine and prednisone)

Contraindications/cautions
- Contraindicated in the presence of allergy to daunorubicin; systemic infections; myelosuppression; cardiac disease; previous therapy with doxorubicin or cumulative doses of daunorubicin > 550 mg/mm^2 (adults), 300 mg/mm^2 (children > 2y), or 10 mg/kg (children < 2 y) leads to increased risk of cardiotoxicity; pregnancy; lactation.
- Use caution in the presence of impaired hepatic or renal function, previous cumulative doses of doxorubicin or daunorubicin.

Dosage
Adult
- ***As a single agent:*** 60 mg/m^2 per day IV on days 1, 2, and 3, every 3–4 wk.
- ***In combination:*** 45 mg/m^2 per day IV on days 1, 2, and 3 of the first course and on days 1 and 2 of subsequent courses with 100 mg/m^2 per day cytarabine by IV infusion daily for 7 d for the first course and for 5 d for subsequent courses. Up to three courses may be needed to attain a normal-appearing bone marrow.

Pediatric
- ***Acute lymphocytic leukemia:*** 25 mg/m^2 IV on day 1 every week, vincristine 1.5 mg/m^2 IV on day 1 every week, prednisone 40 mg/m^2 orally daily. Four to six courses are usually sufficient to achieve complete remission.

Children < 2 y or less than 0.5 m^2: Calculate dose based on body weight rather than surface area. Maintenance therapy and CNS prophylaxis must be instituted after complete remission is induced.

daunorubicin hydrochloride

Impaired hepatic or renal function

Serum Bilirubin (mg/dl)	Serum Creatinine (mg/dl)	Dose
1.2–3.0		3/4 normal dose
>3	>3	1/2 normal dose

Pharmacokinetics

Route	Onset	Duration
IV	slow	8 d

Metabolism: Hepatic; $T_{1/2}$: 22 h
Distribution: Crosses placenta; enters breast milk
Excretion: Bile and urine

IV facts

Preparation: Reconstitute vial contents with 4 ml of Sterile Water for Injection to prepare a solution of 5 mg/ml; withdraw the desired dose into a syringe containing 10–15 ml of normal saline. Reconstituted solution is stable for 24 h at room temperature and 48 h if refrigerated. Protect from sunlight.

Infusion: Inject into the tubing of a free-flowing IV infusion of 5% glucose or normal saline solution.

Incompatibilities: Do not mix with other drugs or heparin.

Adverse effects

- **GI:** *Nausea, vomiting,* mucositis, diarrhea
- **CV:** Cardiac toxicity, **CHF**
- **Hematologic:** *Myelosuppression*
- **GU:** *Hyperuricemia* due to cell lysis, *red urine*
- **Dermatologic:** *Complete but reversible alopecia*, skin rash
- **Local:** *Local tissue necrosis if extravasation occurs*
- **Other:** Fever, chills, cancer

■ Nursing Considerations

Assessment

- *History:* Allergy to daunorubicin; systemic infections; myelosuppression; cardiac disease; previous therapy with doxorubicin; impaired hepatic or renal function; lactation.
- *Physical:* Temperature; skin—color, lesions; weight; hair; local injection site; auscultation, peripheral perfusion, pulses, ECG; R, adventitious sounds; liver evaluation, mucus membranes; CBC, liver and renal function tests, serum uric acid

Implementation

- Do not administer IM or SC because severe local reaction and tissue necrosis occurs.
- Monitor injection site for extravasation: reports of burning or stinging. Discontinue infusion immediately, and restart in another vein. Local SC extravasation: local infiltration with corticosteroid may be ordered, flood area with normal saline; apply cold compress to area. If ulceration begins, arrange consultation with plastic surgeon.
- Monitor patient's response to therapy, frequently at beginning of therapy: serum uric acid level, cardiac output (listen for S_3), ECG, CBC. Changes may require a decrease in the dose; consult physician. Drug therapy for hyperuricemia, CHF may be advisable.
- Record doses received to monitor total dosage—toxic effects are often dose related.

Drug-specific teaching points

- Prepare a calendar for dates to return for drug therapy.
- Know that the following side effects may occur: rash, skin lesions, loss of hair, changes in nails (you may want to invest in a wig before hair loss occurs; skin care may help somewhat); loss of appetite, nausea, mouth sores (frequent mouth care, small frequent meals may help; you will need to try to maintain good nutrition if possible; a dietician may be able to help; an antiemetic also may be ordered); red urine (this is a result of drug therapy and will pass after a few days).
- Arrange for regular medical followup, which will include blood tests to monitor the drug's effects.

Adverse effects in *Italics* are most common; those in **Bold** are life-threatening.

- Report difficulty breathing, sudden weight gain, swelling, burning or pain at injection site, unusual bleeding or bruising.

☐ deferoxamine mesylate

(de fer ox' a meen)
Desferal

Pregnancy Category C

Drug classes
Chelating agent
Antidote

Therapeutic actions
Binds with iron and prevents it from entering into chemical reactions.

Indications
- Acute iron toxicity
- Treatment of chronic iron overload
- **Unlabeled use**: management of aluminum accumulation in bone in renal failure and aluminum-induced dialysis encephalopathy

Contraindications/cautions
- Severe renal disease, anuria, primary hemochromatosis, lactation.

Dosage
Adult
- ***Acute iron toxicity:*** 1 g IM, then 0.5 g IM q4h. Subsequently give 0.5 g q4–12h based on response. Do not exceed 6 g/d. Or 15 mg/kg per hour IV; switch to IM as soon as possible.
- ***Chronic overload:*** 0.5–1 g IM qid. Give 2 g IV with each unit of blood. Do not exceed 15 mg/kg per day. Or 1–2 g/d (20–40 mg/kg per day) SC over 8–24 h with a continuous infusion pump.

Pediatric: 50 mg/kg per dose IM or IV q6h or up to 15 mg/kg per hour by continuous IV infusion. Do not exceed 6 g/24 h or 2 g/dose.

Pharmacokinetics

Route	Onset
IV, IM	Rapid

Metabolism: Plasma; $T_{1/2}$: 1 h
Distribution: Crosses placenta; enters breast milk
Excretion: Urine

IV facts
Preparation: Add 2 ml Sterile Water for Injection to each vial. Add to saline, glucose in water, or Ringer's Lactate Solution for infusion. Protect from light. Do not store reconstituted solution longer than 1 wk.
Infusion: Infuse slowly; use of an unfusion pump is preferable.

Adverse effects
- **GI:** Diarrhea, abdominal discomfort
- **CNS:** Blurred vision, cataracts (long-term use), auditory disturbances, loss of hearing
- **Local:** *Pain, induration at injection site*, skin irritation and swelling
- **Hypersensitivity:** Generalized itching, rash, anaphylactic reaction
- **Other:** Tachycardia, fever

■ Nursing Considerations

Assessment
- *History:* Severe renal disease, anuria, primary hemochromatosis, lactation
- *Physical:* Skin condition, neurologic exam, including vision and hearing, eye exam, abdominal exam, CBC, serum iron levels

Implementation
- Administer IM, by continuous SC infusion, or by slow IV infusion.
- Monitor patient response to drug, including evaluation for cataracts, skin reaction, local injection site.

Drug-specific teaching points
- Be aware that this drug is given IM, SC, or IV. Its effects will be monitored carefully.
- Know that the following side effects may occur: discomfort at injection site, skin

Adverse effects in *Italics* are most common; those in **Bold** are life-threatening.

rash, vision changes (use caution if vision becomes impaired).
- Report loss of hearing, vision changes, skin rash with itching, difficulty breathing, fever, pain at injection site.

☐ demeclocycline hydrochloride

(dem e kloe sye' kleen)
demethylchlortetracycline hydrochloride

Declomycin

Pregnancy Category D

Drug classes
Antibiotic
Tetracycline

Therapeutic actions
Bacteriostatic: inhibits protein synthesis of susceptible bacteria, preventing cell reproduction.

Indications
- Infections caused by rickettsiae; *Mycoplasma pneumoniae*; agents of psittacosis, ornithosis, lymphogranuloma venereum, and granuloma inguinale; *Borrelia recurrentis; Haemophilus ducreyi; Pasteurellia pestis; Pasteurellia tularensis; Bartonella bacilliformis; Bacteroides; Vibrio comma; Vibrio fetus; Brucella; Escherichia coli; Enterobacter aerogenes; Shigella; Acinetobacter calcoaceticus; Haemophilus influenzae; Klebsiella; Diplococcus pneumoniae; Staphylococcus aureus*
- When penicillin is contraindicated, infections caused by *Neisseria gonorrhoeae, Treponema pallidum, Treponema pertenue, Listeria monocytogenes, Clostridium, Bacillus anthracis, Fusobacterium fusiforme, Actinomyces, Neisseria meningitidis*
- As an adjunct to amebicides in acute intestinal amebiasis
- Treatment of acne, uncomplicated urethral, endocervical or rectal infections in adults caused by *Chlamydia trachomatis*
- **Unlabeled use**: management of the chronic form of the syndrome of inappropriate antidiuretic hormone secretion (SIADH)

Contraindications/cautions
- Allergy to tetracyclines, renal or hepatic dysfunction, pregnancy, lactation.

Dosage
Adult: 150 mg qid PO or 300 mg bid PO
- *Gonococcal infection:* 600 mg PO then 300 mg q12h for 4 d to a total of 3 g.

Pediatric (> 8 y): 6–12 mg/kg per day PO in two to four divided doses. Not recommended for children < 8 y.

Pharmacokinetics

Route	Onset	Peak	Duration
Oral	Varies	3–4 h	18–20 h

Metabolism: Hepatic; $T_{1/2}$: 12–16 h
Distribution: Crosses placenta; enters breast milk
Excretion: Urine and feces

Adverse effects
- **GI**: Fatty liver, **liver failure**, *anorexia, nausea, vomiting, diarrhea, glossitis,* dysphagia, enterocolitis, esophageal ulcer
- **Hematologic**: Hemolytic anemia, thrombocytopenia, neutropenia, eosinophilia, leukocytosis, leukopenia
- **Dermatologic**: *Phototoxic reactions, rash,* exfoliative dermatitis (more frequent and more severe with this tetracycline than with any others)
- **Dental**: *Discoloring and inadequate calcification of primary teeth of fetus if used by pregnant women, discoloring and inadequate calcification of permanent teeth if used during period of dental development*
- **Other**: Superinfections, nephrogenic diabetes insipidus syndrome (polyuria, polydipsia, weakness) in patients being treated for SIADH

Adverse effects in *Italics* are most common; those in **Bold** are life-threatening.

Clinically important drug-drug interactions
- Decreased absorption of demeclocycline if taken with antacids, iron, alkali • Increased digoxin toxicity if taken with demeclocycline • Increased nephrotoxicity if taken with methoxyflurane • Decreased activity of penicillin if taken with demeclocycline.

Clinically important drug-food interactions
- Decreased effectiveness of demeclocycline if taken with food, dairy products

Drug-lab test interferences
- Interference with culture studies for several days following therapy

■ Nursing Considerations

Assessment
- *History:* Allergy to tetracyclines, renal or hepatic dysfunction, pregnancy, lactation.
- *Physical:* Skin status, R and sounds, GI function and liver evaluation, urinary output and concentration, urinalysis and BUN, liver and renal function tests; culture infected area before beginning therapy.

Implementation
- Administer in oral form only on an empty stomach; if severe GI upset occurs, administer with food.
- Arrange for discontinuation of drug if diabetes insipidus occurs in SIADH patients.

Drug-specific teaching points
- Take drug throughout the day for best results; take on an empty stomach, 1 h before or 1 h after meals, unless GI upset occurs; then it can be taken with food.
- Know that the following side effects may occur: sensitivity to sunlight (wear protective clothing, and use a sunscreen), diarrhea.
- Report rash, itching; difficulty breathing; dark urine or light-colored stools; severe cramps; increased thirst, increased urination, weakness (SIADH patients).

❒ desipramine hydrochloride

*(dess **ip'** ra meen)*
Norpramin, Pertofrane

Pregnancy Category C

Drug classes
Tricyclic antidepressant (TCA; secondary amine)

Therapeutic actions
Mechanism of action unknown; inhibits the presynaptic reuptake of the neurotransmitters norepinephrine and serotonin; anticholinergic at CNS and peripheral receptors; sedating.

Indications
- Relief of symptoms of depression (endogenous depression most responsive)
- **Unlabeled uses**: facilitation of cocaine withdrawal (50–200 mg/d), treatment of eating disorders

Contraindications/cautions
- Contraindicated in the presence of hypersensitivity to any tricyclic drug, concomitant therapy with an MAO inhibitor, recent MI, myelography within previous 24 h or scheduled within 48 h, lactation.
- Use caution in the presence of electroshock therapy; preexisting cardiovascular disorders (eg, severe coronary heart disease, progressive heart failure, angina pectoris, paroxysmal tachycardia; possibly increased risk of serious CVS toxicity with TCAs); angle-closure glaucoma, increased intraocular pressure, urinary retention, ureteral or urethral spasm (anticholinergic effects of TCAs may exacerbate these conditions); seizure disorders (TCAs lower the seizure threshold); hyperthyroidism (predisposes to CVS toxicity, including cardiac arrhythmias); impaired hepatic, renal function; psychiatric patients (schizophrenic or paranoid patients may exhibit a worsening of psychosis with TCA therapy); manic-depressive patients (may shift to hypomanic or manic phase); elective surgery (TCAs should be discontinued as long as possible before surgery).

desipramine hydrochloride ■ 355

Dosage
Adult
- **Depression:** 100–200 mg/d PO as single dose or in divided doses initially. May gradually increase to 300 mg/d if necessary. Do not exceed 300 mg/d. Patients requiring 300 mg/d should generally have treatment initiated in a hospital. Continue a reduced maintenance dosage for at least 2 mo after a satisfactory response has been achieved.

Pediatric: Not recommended in children < 12 y.

Geriatric: Initially 25–100 mg/d PO; dosages more than 150 mg are not recommended.

Pharmacokinetics

Route	Onset	Peak	Duration
Oral	Varies	2–4 h	3–4 d

Metabolism: Hepatic; $T_{1/2}$: 12–24 h
Distribution: Crosses placenta; enters breast milk
Excretion: Urine

Adverse effects
- **CNS:** *Sedation and anticholinergic effects, confusion* (especially in elderly), *disturbed concentration*, hallucinations, disorientation, decreased memory, feelings of unreality, delusions, anxiety, nervousness, restlessness, agitation, panic, insomnia, nightmares, hypomania, mania, exacerbation of psychosis, drowsiness, weakness, fatigue, headache, numbness, tingling, paresthesias of extremities, incoordination, motor hyperactivity, akathisia, ataxia, tremors, peripheral neuropathy, extrapyramidal symptoms, *seizures*, speech blockage, dysarthria, tinnitus, altered EEG
- **GI:** *Dry mouth, constipation*, paralytic ileus, *nausea*, vomiting, anorexia, epigastric distress, diarrhea, flatulence, dysphagia, peculiar taste, increased salivation, stomatitis, glossitis, parotid swelling, abdominal cramps, black tongue
- **CV:** *Orthostatic hypotension*, hypertension, syncope, tachycardia, palpitations, MI, arrhythmias, heart block, precipitation of CHF, stroke
- **Hematologic:** Bone marrow depression
- **GU:** Urinary retention, delayed micturition, dilation of the urinary tract, gynecomastia, testicular swelling in men; breast enlargement, menstrual irregularity and galactorrhea in women; increased or decreased libido; impotence
- **Endocrine:** Elevated or depressed blood sugar; elevated prolactin levels; SIADH secretion
- **Hypersensitivity:** Skin rash, pruritus, vasculitis, petechiae, photosensitization, edema (generalized or of face and tongue), drug fever
- **Withdrawal:** Symptoms on abrupt discontinuation of prolonged therapy: nausea, headache, vertigo, nightmares, malaise
- **Other:** Nasal congestion, excessive appetite, weight gain or loss; sweating (paradoxical effect in a drug with prominent anticholinergic effects), alopecia, lacrimation, hyperthermia, flushing, chills

Clinically important drug-drug interactions
- Increased TCA levels and pharmacologic (especially anticholinergic) effects when given with cimetidine, fluoxetine, ranitidine • Increased serum levels and risk of bleeding if taken concurrently with oral anticoagulants. • Altered response, including dysrhythmias and hypertension if taken with sympathomimetics • Risk of severe hypertension when taken concurrently with clonidine • Hyperpyretic crises, severe convulsions, hypertensive episodes, and deaths when MAO inhibitors are given with TCAs • Decreased hypotensive activity of guanethidine if taken concurrently with desipramine.

■ Nursing Considerations

Assessment
- *History:* Hypersensitivity to any tricyclic drug; concomitant therapy with an MAO

Adverse effects in *Italics* are most common; those in **Bold** are life-threatening.

inhibitor; recent MI; myelography within previous 24 h or scheduled within 48 h; lactation; electroshock therapy; preexisting cardiovascular disorders; angle-closure glaucoma, increased intraocular pressure, urinary retention, ureteral or urethral spasm; seizure disorders; hyperthyroidism; impaired hepatic, renal function; psychiatric patients; elective surgery.
- *Physical:* Body weight; temperature; skin—color, lesions; orientation, affect, reflexes, vision and hearing; P, BP, orthostatic BP, perfusion; bowel sounds, normal output, liver evaluation; urine flow, normal output; usual sexual function, frequency of menses, breast and scrotal exam; liver function tests, urinalysis, CBC, ECG.

Implementation
- Ensure that depressed and potentially suicidal patients have access to only limited quantities of the drug.
- Administer major portion of dose at bedtime if drowsiness, severe anticholinergic effects occur.
- Arrange to reduce dosage if minor side effects develop; arrange to discontinue the drug if serious side effects occur.
- Arrange for CBC if patient develops fever, sore throat, or other sign of infection during therapy.

Drug-specific teaching points
- Take drug exactly as prescribed; do not to stop taking this drug abruptly or without consulting the physician or nurse.
- Avoid alcohol, other sleep-inducing drugs, OTC drugs while on this drug.
- Avoid prolonged exposure to sunlight or sunlamps; use a sunscreen or protective garments if long exposure to sunlight is unavoidable.
- Know that the following side effects may occur: headache, dizziness, drowsiness, weakness, blurred vision (these effects are reversible; safety measures may need to be taken if these become severe; avoid driving an automobile or performing tasks that require alertness while these persist); nausea, vomiting, loss of appetite, dry mouth (small frequent meals, frequent mouth care, and sucking sugarless candies may help); nightmares, inability to concentrate, confusion; changes in sexual function.
- Report dry mouth, difficulty in urination, excessive sedation.

◻ desmopressin acetate

*(des moe **press'** in)*
1-deamino-8-D-arginine vasopressin
DDAVP, Concentraid, Stimate

Pregnancy Category B

Drug classes
Hormonal agent

Therapeutic actions
Synthetic analog of human ADH; promotes resorption of water in the renal tubule; increases levels of clotting factor VIII.

Indications
- **DDAVP:** neurogenic diabetes insipidus (not nephrogenic in origin; intranasal and parenteral)
- Hemophilia A (with factor VIII levels > 5%) (parenteral)
- Von Willebrand's disease (type I; parenteral)
- **Orphan drug uses**: treatment of hemophilia A, certain types of von Willebrand's disease
- **Concentraid:** Diagnosis of renal concentrating ability

Contraindications/cautions
- Contraindicated in the presence of allergy to desmopressin acetate; type II von Willebrand's disease.
- Use caution in the presence of vascular disease or hypertension, lactation.

Dosage
Adult
- *Diabetes insipidus:* 0.1–0.4 ml/d intranasally as a single dose or divided into two to three doses; 1 spray/nostril for total of 300 mg. 0.5–1.0 ml/d SC or IV, divided into two doses, adjusted to achieve a diurnal water turnover pattern.

desmopressin acetate ■ 357

- **Hemophilia A or von Willebrand's disease:** 0.3 μg/kg diluted in 50 ml sterile physiologic saline; infuse IV slowly over 15–30 min. If needed preoperatively, infuse 30 min before the procedure. Determine need for repeated administration based on patient reponse.
- **Renal concentration testing:** 40 μg of Concentraid intranasally (20 μg in each nostril). Discard the urine voided within 1 h of administration; test two urines voided within 8 h of administration. Patient should drink only small amounts of fluid during that time.

Pediatric
- **Diabetes insipidus (3 mo–12 y):** 0.05–0.3 ml/d intranasally as a single dose or divided into two doses; 1 spray per nostril for total of 300 mg.
- **Hemophilia A or von Willebrand's disease (10 kg or less):** 0.3 μg/kg diluted in 10 ml of sterile physiologic saline. Infuse IV slowly over 15–30 min.
- **Renal concentration testing (12 mo–12 y):** Restrict fluid intake; administer 20 μg intranasally in the morning. Measure osmolality and specific gravity in urine voided over next 3–5 h. Safety and efficacy not established in children < 12 y (parenteral) or 3 mo (intranasal).

Pharmacokinetics

Route	Onset	Peak	Duration
IV/SC	30 min		90–120 min
Nasal	15–60 min	1–5 h	5–21 h

Metabolism: $T_{1/2}$: 7.8 min then 75.5 min
Distribution: Crosses placenta; enters breast milk

IV facts
Preparation: Use drug as provided; refrigerate vial.
Infusion: Administer by direct IV injection.

Adverse effects
- CNS: Transient headache
- GI: Nausea, mild abdominal cramps
- CV: Slight elevation of BP, facial flushing (with high doses)
- GU: Vulval pain, fluid retention, water intoxication, hyponatremia (high doses)
- Local: *Local erythema, swelling, burning pain* (parenteral injection)

■ Nursing Considerations

Assessment
- *History:* Allergy to desmopressin acetate; type II von Willebrand's disease; vascular disease or hypertension; lactation
- *Physical:* Nasal mucous membranes; skin—color; P, BP, edema; R, adventitous sounds; bowel sounds, abdominal exam; urine volume and osmolality, plasma osmolality; factor VIII coagulant activity, skin bleeding times, factor VIII coagulant levels, factor VIII antigen and ristocetin cofactor levels (as appropriate)

Implementation
- Store nasal solution and injection in the refrigerator.
- Administer intranasally by drawing solution into the rhinyle or flexible calibrated plastic tube supplied with preparation. Insert one end of tube into nostril; blow on the other end to deposit solution deep into nasal cavity. Administer to infants, young children, or obtunded adults by using an air-filled syringe attached to the plastic tube. Spray form also available (1 spray/nostril).
- Arrange for appropriate collection and analysis of urine when administering renal concentration test.
- Monitor condition of nasal passages during long-term therapy; inappropriate administration can lead to nasal ulcerations.
- Monitor patients with cardiovascular diseases very carefully for cardiac reactions.
- Arrange to individualize dosage to establish a diurnal pattern of water turnover; estimate response by adequate duration of sleep and adequate, not excessive, water turnover.
- Monitor pulse and blood pressure during infusion for hemophilia A or von Wille-

Adverse effects in *Italics* are most common; those in **Bold** are life-threatening.

brand's disease. Monitor clinical response and lab reports to determine effectiveness of therapy and need for more desmopression or use of blood products.

Drug-specific teaching points
- Administer intranasally by drawing solution into the rhinyle or flexible calibrated plastic tube supplied with preparation. Insert one end of tube into nostril; blow on the other end to deposit soluton deep into nasal cavity. Review proper administration technique for nasal use.
- Know that the following side effects may occur: GI cramping, facial flushing, headache, nasal irritation (proper administration may decrease these problems).
- Limit fluids as much as possible during the testing period if undergoing the renal concentration testing; it is important to maintain accurate urine collection.
- Report any of the following to your nurse or physician: drowsiness, listlessness, headache, shortness of breath, heartburn, abdominal cramps, vulval pain, severe nasal congestion or irritation.

▢ dexamethasone

(dex a meth' a sone)

Oral, topical dermatologic aerosol and gel, ophthalmic suspension: Aeroseb-Dex, Decaderm, Decadron, Decaspray, Dexasone (CAN), Dexone, Hexadrol, Maxidex Ophthalmic

dexamethasone acetate

IM, intra-articular, or soft-tissue injection: Dalalone, Decadron-LA, Decaject-L.A., Decameth L.A., Desxasone-L.A., Dexone L.A., Solurex L.A.

dexamethasone sodium phosphate

IV, IM, intra-articular, interlesional injection; respiratory inhalant; intranasal steroid; ophthalmic solution and ointment; topical dermatologic cream: AK-Dex, AK-Dex Ophthalmic, Dalalone, Decadrol, Decadron Phosphate, Decadron Phosphate Ophthalmic, Decadron Phosphate Respihaler, Decaject, Dexacen-4, Dexasone, Dexone, Hexadrol Phosphate, Maxidex Ophthalmic, Solurex, Turbinaire Decadron Phosphate

Pregnancy Category C

Drug classes
Corticosteroid, long acting
Glucocorticoid
Hormonal agent

Therapeutic actions
Enters target cells and binds to specific receptors, initiating many complex reactions that are responsible for its anti-inflammatory and immunosuppressive effects.

Indications
- Hypercalcemia associated with cancer
- Short-term management of various inflammatory and allergic disorders, such as rheumatoid arthritis, collagen diseases (eg, SLE), dermatologic diseases (eg, pemphigus), status asthmaticus, and autoimmune disorders
- **Hematologic disorders**: thrombocytopenic purpura, erythroblastopenia
- Trichinosis with neurologic or myocardial involvement
- Ulcerative colitis, acute exacerbations of multiple sclerosis, and palliation in some leukemias and lymphomas
- Cerebral edema associated with brain tumor, craniotomy, or head injury
- Testing adrenocortical hyperfunction
- **Unlabeled uses:** Antiemetic for cisplatin-induced vomiting, diagnosis of depression
- **Intra-articular or soft-tissue administration:** Arthritis, psoriatic plaques

dexamethasone ■ 359

- **Respiratory inhalant:** Control of bronchial asthma requiring corticosteroids in conjunction with other therapy
- **Intranasal:** Relief of symptoms of seasonal or perennial rhinitis that responds poorly to other treatments
- **Dermatologic preparations:** Relief of inflammatory and pruritic manifestations of dermatoses that are steroid-responsive
- **Ophthalmic preparations:** Inflammation of the lid, conjunctiva, cornea, and globe

Contraindications/cautions
- Contraindicated in the presence of infections, especially tuberculosis, fungal infections, amebiasis, vaccinia and varicella, and antibiotic-resistant infections.
- Use caution in the presence of renal or hepatic disease; hypothyroidism, ulcerative colitis with impending perforation; diverticulitis; active or latent peptic ulcer; inflammatory bowel disease; CHF, hypertension, thromboembolic disorders; osteoporosis; convulsive disorders; diabetes mellitus; lactation.

Dosage
Systemic Administration
- **Adult:** Individualize dosage, depending on the severity of the condition and the patient's response. Give daily dose before 9 AM to minimize adrenal suppression. If long-term therapy is needed, alternate-day therapy with a short-acting steroid should be considered. After long-term therapy, withdraw drug slowly to avoid adrenal insufficiency. For maintenance therapy, reduce initial dose in small increments at intervals until the lowest dose that maintains satisfactory clinical response is reached.
- **Pediatric:** Individualize dosage, depending on the severity of the condition and the patient's response, rather than by strict adherence to formulas that correct adult doses for age or body weight. Carefully observe growth and development in infants and children on long-term therapy.

Initial adult dosage
- **Oral (dexamethasone, oral):** 0.75–9.0 mg/d.
  - *Suppression tests: For Cushing's syndrome:* 1 mg at 11 PM; assay plasma cortisol at 8 PM the next day. For greater accuracy, give 0.5 mg q6h for 48 h, and collect 24-h urine to determine 17-OH-corticosteroid excretion. *Test to distinguish Cushing's syndrome due to ACTH excess from that resulting from other causes:* 2 mg q6h for 48 h. Collect 24-h urine to determine 17-OH-corticosteroid excretion.
- **IM (dexamethasone acetate):** 8–16 mg; may repeat in 1–3 wk. Dexamethasone phosphate: 0.5–0.9 mg/d; usual dose range is one-third to one-half the oral dose.
- **IV (dexamethasone sodium phosphate):** 0.5–9.0 mg/d.
  - *Cerebral edema:* 10 mg IV and then 4 mg IM q6h; change to oral therapy, 1–3 mg tid, as soon as possible and taper over 5–7 d. *Pediatric:* Oral therapy preferred (0.2 mg/kg per day in divided doses).
  - *Unresponsive shock:* 1–6 mg/kg as a single IV injection (as much as 40 mg initially followed by repeated injections q2–6h has been reported).
  - *Dexamethasone acetate:* 4–16 mg intra-articular, soft tissue; 0.8–1.6 mg intralesional.
  - *Dexamethasone sodium phosphate:* 0.4–6.0 mg (depending on joint or soft-tissue injection site).

Respiratory Inhalant (Dexamethasone Sodium Phosphate) (84 μg released with each actuation).
- **Adult:** 3 inhalations tid–qid, not to exceed 12 inhalations/d.
- **Pediatric:** 2 inhalations tid–qid, not to exceed 8 inhalations/d.

Intranasal (Dexamethasone Sodium Phosphate) (Each spray delivers 84 μg dexamethasone).
- **Adult:** 2 sprays (168 μg) into each nostril bid–tid, not to exceed 12 sprays (1,008 μg)/d.
- **Pediatric:** 1 or 2 sprays (84–168 μg) into each nostril bid, depending on age,

360 ■ dexamethasone

not to exceed 8 sprays (672 μg). Arrange to reduce dose and discontinue therapy as soon as possible.

Topical Dermatologic Preparations: Apply sparingly to affected area bid–qid.

Ophthalmic Solutions / Suspensions: Instill 1–2 drops into the conjunctival sac q1h during the day and q2h during the night; after a favorable response, reduce dose to 1 drop q4h and then 1 drop tid–qid.

Ophthalmic Ointment: Apply a thin coating in the lower conjunctival sac tid–qid; reduce dosage to bid and then qid after improvement.

Pharmacokinetics

Route	Onset	Peak	Duration
Oral	Slow	1–2 h	2–3 d
IM	Rapid	30–60 min	2–3 d
IV	Rapid	30–60 min	2–3 d

Metabolism: Hepatic; $T_{1/2}$: 110–210 min
Distribution: Crosses placenta; enters breast milk
Excretion: Urine

IV facts

Preparation: No preparation required.
Infusion: Administer by slow, direct IV injection.

Adverse effects

Adverse effects depend on dose, route, and duration of therapy. The first list is primarily associated with systemic absorption; the list following is related to specific routes of administration.

- **CNS:** Convulsions, *vertigo, headaches,* pseudotumor cerebri, *euphoria, insomnia, mood swings, depression,* psychosis, intracerebral hemorrhage, reversible cerebral atrophy in infants, cataracts, increased intraocular pressure, glaucoma
- **GI:** Peptic or esophageal ulcer, pancreatitis, abdominal distention
- **CV:** *Hypertension,* CHF, necrotizing angiitis
- **Hematologic:** *Fluid and electrolyte disturbances,* negative nitrogen balance, increased blood sugar, glycosuria, increased serum cholesterol, decreased serum T_3 and T_4 levels
- **GU:** *Amenorrhea, irregular menses*
- **MS:** *Muscle weakness,* steroid myopathy, loss of muscle mass, osteoporosis, spontaneous fractures
- **Endocrine:** Growth retardation, decreased carbohydrate tolerance, diabetes mellitus, cushingoid state, *secondary adrenocortical and pituitary unresponsiveness*
- **Hypersensitivity:** Anaphylactoid or hypersensitivity reactions
- **Other:** *Impaired wound healing; petechiae; ecchymoses; increased sweating; thin and fragile skin; acne; immunosuppression and masking of signs of infection;* activation of latent infections, including tuberculosis, fungal, and viral eye infections; pneumonia; abscess; septic infection; GI and GU infections

Intra-articular

- **Musculoskeletal:** Osteonecrosis, tendon rupture, infection

Intralesional Therapy

- **CNS:** Blindness (when used on face and head—rare)

Respiratory Inhalant

- **Respiratory:** Oral, laryngeal, pahryngeal irritation
- **Endocrine:** Suppression of HPA function due to systemic absorption
- **Other:** Fungal infections

Intranasal

- **CNS:** Headache
- **GI:** Nausea
- **Respiratory:** Nasal irritation, fungal infections, epistaxis, rebound congestion, perforation of the nasal septum, anosmia
- **Dermatologic:** Urticaria
- **Endocrine:** suppression of HPA function due to systemic absorption

Topical Dermatologic Ointments, Creams, Sprays

- **Local:** Local burning, irritation, acneiform lesions, striae, skin atrophy
- **Endocrine:** Suppression of HPA function due to systemic absorption, growth retar-

Adverse effects in *Italics* are most common; those in **Bold** are life-threatening.

dation in children (children may be at special risk for systemic absorption because of their large skin surface area to body weight ratio)

Ophthalmic Preparations
- **Local:** Infections, especially fungal; glaucoma, cataracts with long-term use
- **Endocrine:** Suppression of HPA function due to systemic absorption; more common with long-term use

Clinically important drug-drug interactions
- Increased therapeutic and toxic effects of cortisone if taken concurrently with troleandomycin • Decreased effects of anticholinesterases if taken concurrently with corticotropin; profound muscular depression is possible • Decreased steroid blood levels if taken concurrently with phenytoin, phenobarbital, rifampin • Decreased serum levels of salicylates if taken concurrently with cortisone.

Drug-lab test interferences
- False-negative nitroblue-tetrazolium test for bacterial infection • Suppression of skin test reactions

■ Nursing Considerations

Assessment
- *History (for systemic administration):* Active infections; renal or hepatic disease; hypothyroidism, ulcerative colitis; diverticulitis; active or latent peptic ulcer; inflammatory bowel disease; CHF, hypertension, thromboembolic disorders; osteoporosis; convulsive disorders; diabetes mellitus; lactation. *For ophthalmic preparations:* Acute superficial herpes simplex keratitis, fungal infections of ocular structures; vaccinia, varicella, and other viral diseases of the cornea and conjunctiva; ocular tuberculosis.
- *Physical (for systemic administration):* Baseline body weight, temperature; reflexes, and grip strength, affect, and orientation; P, BP, peripheral perfusion, prominence of superficial veins; R and adventitious sounds; serum electrolytes, blood glucose. *For topical dermatologic preparations:* Affected area for infections, skin injury

Implementation
- *For systemic administration:* Do not give drug to nursing mothers; drug is secreted in breast milk.
- Administer once-a-day doses before 9 AM to mimic normal peak corticosteroid blood levels.
- Arrange for increased dosage when patient is subject to stress.
- Taper doses when discontinuing high-dose or long-term therapy.
- Do not give live virus vaccines with immunosuppressive doses of corticosteroids.
- *For respiratory inhalant, intranasal preparation:* Do not use respiratory inhalant product during an acute asthmatic attack or to manage status asthmaticus.
- Do not use intranasal product in patients with untreated local nasal infections, epistaxis, nasal trauma, septal ulcers, or recent nasal surgery.
- Arrange to taper systemic steroids carefully during transfer to inhalational steriods; deaths caused by adrenal insufficiency have occurred.
- *For topical dermatologic preparations:* Use caution when occlusive dressings, tight diapers, and so forth cover affected area; these can increase systemic absorption of the drug.
- Avoid prolonged use near the eyes, in genital and rectal areas, and in skin creases.

Drug-specific teaching points
- *For systemic administration:* Do not stop taking the drug (oral) without consulting health-care provider.
- Avoid exposure to infection.
- Report unusual weight gain, swelling of the extremities, muscle weakness, black or tarry stools, fever, prolonged sore throat, colds or other infections, worsening of the disorder for which the drug is being taken.

Adverse effects in *Italics* are most common; those in **Bold** are life-threatening.

- *For intra-articular administration:* Do not overuse joint after therapy, even if pain is gone.
- *For respiratory inhalant, intranasal preparation:* Do not use this drug more often than prescribed.
- Do not stop using this drug without consulting health care provider.
- Use the inhalational bronchodilator drug first if using the oral inhalant product concomitantly with bronchodilator therapy.
- Administer decongestant nose drops first if nasal passages are blocked.
- *For topical dermatologic preparations:* Apply the drug sparingly.
- Avoid contact with eyes.
- Report any irritation or infection at the site of application.
- *For ophthalmic preparations:* Administer as follows: Lie down or tilt head backward and look at ceiling. Warm tube of ointment in hand for several minutes. Apply ¼–½ inch of ointment, or drop suspension inside lower eyelid while looking up. After applying ointment, close eyelids and roll eyeball in all directions. After instilling eye drops, release lower lid, but do not blink for at least 30 sec; apply gentle pressure to the inside corner of the eye for 1 min. Do not close eyes tightly, and try not to blink more often than usual; do not touch ointment tube or dropper to eye, fingers, or any surface.
- Wait at least 10 min before using any other eye preparations.
- Know that the eyes become more sensitive to light (sunglasses will help).
- Report worsening of the condition, pain, itching, swelling of the eye, failure of the condition to improve after 1 wk.

☐ dexchlorpheniramine maleate

(dex klor fen ir' a meen)
Dexchlor, Poladex, Polaramine
Pregnancy Category B

Drug classes
Antihistamine (alkylamine type)

Therapeutic actions
Blocks the effects of histamine at H_1 receptor sites, has atropine-like, antipruritic, and sedative effects.

Indications
- Relief of symptoms associated with perennial and seasonal allergic rhinitis; vasomotor rhinitis; allergic conjunctivitis; mild, uncomplicated urticaria and angioedema; amelioraton of allergic reactions to blood or plasma; dermatographism; adjunctive therapy in anaphylactic reactions

Contraindications/cautions
- Contraindicated in the presence of allergy to any antihistamines, narrow-angle glaucoma, stenosing peptic ulcer, symptomatic prostatic hypertrophy, asthmatic attack, bladder neck obstruction, pyloroduodenal obstruction, third trimester of pregnancy, lactation.
- Use caution in pregnancy.

Dosage
Adult and pediatric > 12 y: 2 mg q4–6h PO, or 4–6 mg repeat-action tablets at bedtime PO or q8–10h PO during the day.
Pediatric
- *6–11 y:* 1 mg q4–6h PO or 4 mg repeat-action tablet once daily at bedtime.
- *2–5 y:* 0.5 mg q4–6h PO; do not use repeat-action tablets.

Geriatric: More likely to cause dizziness, sedation, syncope, toxic confusional states, and hypotension in elderly patients; use with caution.

Pharmacokinetics

Route	Onset	Peak
Oral	15–30 min	3 h

Metabolism: Hepatic; $T_{1/2}$: 12–15 h
Distribution: Crosses placenta; enters breast milk
Excretion: Urine

Adverse effects
- **CNS:** *Drowsiness, sedation, dizziness, disturbed coordination,* fatigue, confusion, restlessness, excitation, nervousness, tremor, headache, blurred vision, diplopia, vertigo, tinnitus, acute labyrinthitis, hysteria, tingling, heaviness and weakness of the hands
- **GI:** *Epigastric distress,* anorexia, increased appetite and weight gain, nausea, vomiting, diarrhea or constipation
- **CV:** Hypotension, palpitations, bradycardia, tachycardia, extrasystoles
- **Respiratory:** *Thickening of bronchial secretions,* chest tightness, wheezing, nasal stuffiness, dry mouth, dry nose, dry throat, sore throat
- **Hematologic:** Hemolytic anemia, hypoplastic anemia, thrombocytopenia, leukopenia, agranulocytosis, pancytopenia
- **GU:** Urinary frequency, dysuria, urinary retention, early menses, decreased libido
- **Other:** Urticaria, rash, anaphylactic shock, photosensitivity, excessive perspiration

Clinically important drug-drug interactions
- Increased depressant effects if taken concurrently with alcohol, other CNS depressants

■ Nursing Considerations

Assessment
- *History:* Allergy to any antihistamines; narrow-angle glaucoma, stenosing peptic ulcer, symptomatic prostatic hypertrophy, asthmatic attack, bladder neck obstruction, pyloroduodenal obstruction, pregnancy, lactation
- *Physical:* Skin—color, lesions, texture; orientation, reflexes, affect; vision exam; P, BP ; R, adventitious sounds; bowel sounds; prostate palpation; CBC with differential

Implementation
- Administer with food if GI upset occurs.
- Administer syrup form if patient is unable to take tablets.
- Monitor patient response, and arrange for adjustment of dosage to lowest possible effective dose.

Drug-specific teaching points
- Take as prescribed; avoid excessive dosage. Take with food if GI upset occurs; do not crush or chew the sustained-release preparations.
- Know that the following side effects may occur: dizziness, sedation, drowsiness (use caution if driving or performing tasks that require alertness if these occur); epigastric distress, diarrhea, or constipation (taking the drug with meals may help); dry mouth (frequent mouth care, sucking sugarless lozenges may help); thickening of bronchial secretions, dryness of nasal mucosa (use of a humidifier may help if this becomes a problem).
- Avoid alcohol while on this drug; serious sedation could occur.
- Report difficulty breathing; hallucinations, tremors, loss of coordination; unusual bleeding or bruising; visual disturbances; irregular heartbeat.

◻ dexpanthenol

*(dex **pan**' the nole)*
dextropantothenyl alcohol
Ilopan

Pregnancy Category C

Drug classes
GI stimulant

Therapeutic actions
Mechanism of action is unknown; is the alcohol analog of pantothenic acid, a cofactor in the synthesis of the neurotransmitter acetylcholine; acetylcholine is the transmitter released by parasympathetic postganglionic nerves; the parasympathetic nervous system provides stimulation to maintain intestinal function.

Indications
- Prophylactic use immediately after major abdominal surgery to minimize paralytic

Adverse effects in *Italics* are most common; those in **Bold** are life-threatening.

ileus, intestinal atony causing abdominal distention.
- Treatment of intestinal atony causing abdominal distention; postoperative or postpartum retention of flatus; postoperative delay in resumption of intestinal motility; paralytic ileus

Contraindications/cautions
- Allergy to dexpanthenol, hemophilia, ileus due to mechanical obstruction, lactation.

Dosage
Adult
- ***Prevention of postoperative adynamic ileus:*** 250–500 mg IM; repeat in 2 h, then q6h until danger of adynamic ileus has passed.
- ***Treatment of adynamic ileus:*** 500 mg IM; repeat in 2 h, then q6h as needed.
- ***IV administration:*** 500 mg diluted in IV solutions.

Pediatric: Safety and efficacy not established.

Pharmacokinetics

Route	Onset	Peak
IM	Rapid	4 h

Metabolism: Hepatic; $T_{1/2}$: unknown
Distribution: Crosses placenta; enters breast milk
Excretion: Urine and feces

IV facts
Preparation: Dilute with bulk solutions of glucose or Lactated Ringer's.
Infusion: Infuse slowly. Do not administer by direct IV injection.

Adverse effects
- GI: *Intestinal colic ($\frac{1}{2}$ h after administration), nausea, vomiting; diarrhea*
- CV: *slight drop in blood pressure*
- Respiratory: Dyspnea
- Dermatologic: Itching, tingling, red patches of skin, generalized dermatitis, urticaria

■ Nursing Considerations
Assessment
- *History:* Allergy to dexpanthenol, hemophilia, ileus due to mechanical obstruction, lactation.
- *Physical:* Skin—color, lesions, texture; P, BP; bowel sounds, normal output

Implementation
- Monitor BP carefully during IV administration.

Drug-specific teaching points
- Teaching about this drug should be incorporated into the overall postoperative or postpartum teaching, as appropriate. Specific point to include is to know that intestinal colic may occur within $\frac{1}{2}$ h of administration.
- Know that the following side effects may occur: nausea, vomiting, diarrhea, itching, skin rash.
- Report difficulty breathing, severe itching, or rash.

☐ dextran, high molecular weight

(dex' tran)

Dextran 70, Dextran 75, Gentran 75, Macrodex

Pregnancy Category C

Drug classes
Plasma expander

Therapeutic actions
Synthetic polysaccharide used to approximate the colloidal properties of albumin.

Indications
- Adjunctive therapy for treatment of shock or impending shock due to hemorrhage, burns, surgery, or trauma; to be used only in emergency situations when blood or blood products are not available

Contraindications/cautions
- Allergy to dextran (dextran 1 can be used prophylactically in patients known to be allergic to clinical dextran); marked hemostatic defects (risk for increased bleeding effects); severe cardiac congestion; renal failure or anuria.

Dosage
Adult: 500 ml, given at a rate of 24–40 ml/min IV as an emergency procedure. Do not exceed 20 ml/kg the first 24 h of treatment.
Pediatric: Determine dosage by body weight or surface area of the patient. Do not exceed 20 ml/kg IV.

Pharmacokinetics

Route	Onset	Peak	Duration
IV	Minutes	Minutes	12 h

Metabolism: Hepatic; $T_{1/2}$: 24 h
Distribution: Crosses placenta; enters breast milk
Excretion: Urine

IV facts
Preparation: Administer in unit provided. Discard any partially used containers. Do not use unless the solution is clear.
Infusion: Infuse at rate of 20–40 ml/min.

Adverse effects
- **GI:** Nausea, vomiting
- **Hematologic:** *Hypervolemia, coagulation problems*
- **Hypersensitivity:** Urticaria, nasal congestion, wheezing, tightness of chest, mild hypotension (antihistamines may be helpful in relieving these symptoms)
- **Local:** Infection at injection site, extravasation
- **Other:** Fever, joint pains

Drug-lab test interferences
- Falsely elevated blood glucose assays
- Interference with bilirubin assays in which alcohol is used, with total protein assays using biuret reagent • Blood typing and cross-matching procedures using enzyme techniques may give unreliable readings; draw blood samples before giving infusion of dextran

■ Nursing Considerations
Assessment
- *History:* Allergy to dextran; marked hemostatic defects; severe cardiac congestion; renal failure or anuria
- *Physical:* Body temperature; skin—color, lesions; P, BP, adventitious sounds, peripheral edema; R, adventitious sounds; urinalysis, renal and liver function tests, clotting times, PT, PTT, hemoglobin, hematocrit, urine output

Implementation
- Administer by IV infusion only; monitor rates based on patient response.
- Do not administer more than recommended dose.
- Use only clear solutions. Discard partially used containers; solution contains no bacteriostat.
- Monitor patients carefully for any sign of hypervolemia or the development of CHF; supportive measures may be needed.

Drug-specific teaching points
- Report difficulty breathing, skin rash, unusual bleeding or bruising, pain at IV site.

☐ dextran, low molecular weight

(dex' tran)

Dextran 40, Gentran 40, 10% LMD, Rheomacrodex

Pregnancy Category C

Drug classes
Plasma expander

Therapeutic actions
Synthetic polysaccharide used to approximate the colloidal properties of albumin.

Indications
- Adjunctive therapy for treatment of shock or impending shock due to hemorrhage, burns, surgery or trauma

Adverse effects in *Italics* are most common; those in **Bold** are life-threatening.

- Priming fluid in pump oxygenators during extracorporeal circulation
- Prophylaxis against deep vein thrombosis (DVT) and pulmonary emboli (PE) in patients undergoing procedures known to be associated with a high incidence of thromboembolic complications, such as hip surgery

Contraindications/cautions
- Allergy to dextran (dextran 1 can be used prophylactically in patients known to be allergic to clinical dextran); marked hemostatic defects; severe cardiac congestion; renal failure or anuria.

Dosage
Adult
- ***Adjunctive therapy in shock:*** Total dosage of 20 ml/kg IV in the first 24 h. The first 10 ml/kg should be infused rapidly, the remaining dose being administered slowly. Beyond 24 h, total daily dosage should not exceed 10 ml/kg. Do not continue therapy for more than 5 d.
- ***Hemodiluent in extracorporeal circulation:*** Generally 10–20 ml/kg are added to perfusion circuit. Do not exceed a total dosage of 20 ml/kg.
- ***Prophylaxis therapy for DVT, PE:*** 500–1,000 ml IV on the day of surgery, continue treatment at a dose of 500 ml/d for an additional 2–3 d. Thereafter, depending on procedure and risk involved, 500 ml may be administered every second to third day for up to 2 wk.

Pharmacokinetics

Route	Onset	Peak	Duration
IV	Immediate	Minutes	12 h

Metabolism: Hepatic; $T_{1/2}$: 3 h
Distribution: Crosses placenta; enters breast milk
Excretion: Urine

IV facts
Preparation: Protect from freezing. Use in bottles provided, no further preparation necessary.

Infusion: Administer first 10 ml rapidly, remainder of solution slowly, monitoring patient response.

Adverse effects
- **GI:** Nausea, vomiting
- **CV:** Hypotension, **anaphylactoid shock**, *hypervolemia*
- **Hypersensitivity:** Ranging from mild cutaneous eruptions to generalized urticaria
- **Local:** Infection at site of injection, extravasation, venous thrombosis or phlebitis
- **Other:** Headache, fever, wheezing

Drug-lab test interferences
- Falsely elevated blood glucose assays
- Interference with bilirubin assays in which alcohol is used, with total protein assays using biuret reagent • Blood typing and cross-matching procedures using enzyme techniques may give unreliable readings; draw blood samples before giving infusion of dextran

■ Nursing Considerations
Assessment
- *History:* Allergy to dextran; marked hemostatic defects; severe cardiac congestion; renal failure or anuria; lactation
- *Physical:* Body temperature; skin—color, lesions; P, BP, adventitious sounds, peripheral edema; R, adventitious sounds; urinalysis, renal and liver function tests, clotting times, PT, PTT, hemoglobin, hematocrit, urine output

Implementation
- Administer by IV infusion only; monitor rates based on patient response.
- Do not administer more than recommended dose.
- Monitor urinary output carefully; if no increase in output is noted after 500 ml of dextran, discontinue drug until diuresis can be induced by other means.
- Monitor patients carefully for any sign of hypervolemia or the development of CHF.

Adverse effects in *Italics* are most common; those in **Bold** are life-threatening.

Drug-specific teaching points
- Report difficulty breathing, skin rash, unusual bleeding or bruising, pain at IV site.

dextroamphetamine sulfate

(dex troe am fet' a meen)
Dexedrine

Pregnancy Category C
C-II controlled substance

Drug classes
Amphetamine
Anorexiant
CNS stimulant

Therapeutic actions
Acts in the CNS to release norepinephrine from nerve terminals; in higher doses also releases dopamine; suppressess appetite; increases alertness, elevates mood; often improves physical performance, especially when fatigue and sleep-deprivation have caused impairment; efficacy in hyperkinetic syndrome, attention-deficit disorders in children appears paradoxical and is not understood.

Indications
- Narcolepsy
- Abnormal behavioral syndrome in children (attention-deficit disorder, hyperkinetic syndrome) as part of treatment program that includes psychological, social, educational measures
- Exogenous obesity as short-term adjunct to caloric restriction in patients refractory to alternative therapy

Contraindications/cautions
- Hypersensitivity to sympathomimetic amines, tartrazine (in preparations marketed as *Dexedrine*); advanced arteriosclerosis, symptomatic cardiovascular disease, moderate to severe hypertension, hyperthyroidism, glaucoma, agitated states, history of drug abuse; pregnancy; lactation.

Dosage
Adult
- ***Narcolepsy:*** Start with 10 mg/d PO in divided doses; increase in increments of 10 mg/d at weekly intervals. If adverse reactions (insomnia, anorexia) occur, reduce dose. Usual dosage is 5–60 mg/d PO in divided doses. Give first dose on awakening, additional doses (1 or 2) q4–6h; long-acting forms can be given once a day.
- ***Exogenous obesity:*** 5–30 mg/d PO in divided doses of 5–10 mg, 30–60 min before meals. *Long-acting form:* 10–15 mg in the morning.

Pediatric
- ***Narcolepsy:*** *6–12 y:* Condition is rare in children < 12 y; when it does occur, initial dose is 5 mg/d PO. Increase in increments of 5 mg at weekly intervals until optimal response is obtained. *12 y or older:* Use adult dosage.
- ***Attention-deficit disorder:*** *< 3 y:* Not recommended. *3–5 y:* 2.5 mg/d PO. Increase in increments of 2.5 mg/d at weekly intervals until optimal response is obtained. *6 y or older:* 5 mg PO qd–bid. Increase in increments of 5 mg/d at weekly intervals until optimal respnse is obtained. Dosage will rarely exceed 40 mg/d. Give first dose on awakening, additional doses (1 or 2) q4–6h. Long-acting forms may be used once a day.
- ***Obesity:*** Not recommended for children < 12 y.

Pharmacokinetics

Route	Onset	Peak	Duration
Oral	Rapid	1–5 h	8–10 h

Metabolism: Hepatic; $T_{1/2}$: 10–30 h
Distribution: Crosses placenta; enters breast milk
Excretion: Urine

Adverse effects
- CNS: *Overstimulation, restlessness, dizziness, insomnia*, dyskinesia, euphoria, dysphoria, tremor, headache, psychotic episodes

Adverse effects in *Italics* are most common; those in **Bold** are life-threatening.

- **GI:** *Dry mouth, unpleasant taste, diarrhea,* constipation, anorexia and weight loss
- **CV:** *Palpitations, tachycardia, hypertension*
- **GU:** Impotence, changes in libido
- **Dermatologic:** Urticaria
- **Endocrine:** Reversible elevations in serum thyroxine with heavy use
- **Other:** Tolerance, psychological dependence, social disability with abuse

Clinically important drug-drug interactions
- Hypertensive crisis and increased CNS effects of dextroamphetamine if given within 14 d of monoamine oxidase inhibitors (MAOIs); DO NOT GIVE DEXTROAMPHETAMINE to patients who are taking or who have recently taken MAOIs • Increased duration of effects of dextroamphetamine if taken with urinary alkalinizers (acetazolamide, sodium bicarbonate), furazolidone • Decreased effects of dextroamphetamine if taken with urinary acidifiers • Decreased efficacy of antihypertensive drugs (guanethidine) given with amphetamines

■ Nursing Considerations

Assessment
- *History:* Hypersensitivity to sympathomimetic amines, tartrazine; advanced arteriosclerosis, symptomatic cardiovascular disease, moderate to severe hypertension, hyperthyroidism, glaucoma, agitated states, history of drug abuse; lactation.
- *Physical:* Body weight; body temperature; skin—color, lesions; orientation, affect, ophthalmic exam (tonometry); P, BP, auscultation; R, adventitious sounds; bowel sounds, normal output; thyroid function tests, blood and urine glucose, baseline ECG

Implementation
- Ensure proper diagnosis before administering to children for behavioral syndromes: drug should not be used until other causes or concomitants of abnormal behavior (learning disability, EEG abnormalities, neurologic deficits) are ruled out.
- Arrange to interrupt drug dosage periodically in children being treated for behavioral disorders to determine if symptoms recur at an intensity that warrants continued drug therapy.
- Monitor growth of children on long-term amphetamine therapy.
- Arrange to discontinue use of amphetamines as anorexiants when tolerance appears to have developed; do not increase dosage.
- Arrange to dispense the least feasible amount of drug at any one time to minimize risk of overdosage.
- Administer drug early in the day to prevent insomnia.
- Monitor blood pressure frequently early in treatment.
- Monitor obese diabetics taking amphetamines closely, and adjust insulin dosage as necessary.

Drug-specific teaching points
- Take this drug exactly as prescribed. If taking this drug as an aid to weight loss, be aware that drug loses efficacy after a short time. Do not increase the dosage without consulting your physician. If the drug appears to be ineffective, consult your nurse or physician.
- Do not crush or chew sustained-release or long-acting tablets.
- Take drug early in the day (especially sustained-release preparations) to avoid night-time sleep disturbance.
- Avoid becoming pregnant while you are taking this drug. This drug has the potential to cause harm to the fetus.
- Know that the following side effects may occur: nervousness, restlessness, dizziness, insomnia, impaired thinking (these effects may become less pronounced after a few days; avoid driving a car or engaging in activities that require alertness if these occur); headache, loss of appetite, dry mouth.
- Report nervousness, insomnia, dizziness, palpitations, anorexia (except in patients

dextromethorphan hydrobromide

(dex troe meth or' fan)

Benylin DM, Congespirin for Children, Delsym, Demo-Cineal (CAN), Hold, Koffex (CAN), Mediquell, Pediacare, Pertussin, Robidex (CAN), St. Joseph Cough, Sedatuss (CAN), Sucrets Cough Control

Pregnancy Category C

Drug classes
Nonnarcotic antitussive

Therapeutic actions
Lacks analgesic and addictive properties; controls cough spasms by depressing the cough center in the medulla; analog of codeine.

Indications
- Control of nonproductive cough

Contraindications/cautions
- Hypersensitivity to any component (check labeling of individual products for flavorings, vehicles); sensitivity to bromides; cough that persists for more than 1 wk, tends to recur, is accompanied by excessive secretions, high fever, rash, nausea, vomiting, or persistent headache (dextromethorphan should not be used; patient should consult a physician); lactation

Dosage
Adult
- **Lozenges, syrup and chewy squares:** 10–30 mg q4–8h PO. Do not exceed 120 mg/24 h.
- **Sustained action liquid:** 60 mg bid PO.

Pediatric
- **Children > 12 y:** As for adults.
- **Children 6–12 y**
  – *Lozenges, syrup, and chewy squares:* 5–10 mg q4h PO or 15 mg q6–8h. Do not exceed 60 mg/24 h.
  – *Sustained-action liquid:* 30 mg bid PO.
- **Children 2–6 y**
  – *Syrup and chewy squares:* 2.5–7.5 mg q4–8h PO. Do not exceed 30 mg/24 h. Do not give lozenges to this age group.
  – *Sustained-action liquid:* 15 mg bid PO.
- **Children < 2 y:** Use only as directed by a physician.

Pharmacokinetics

Route	Onset	Peak	Duration
Oral	15–30 min	2 h	3–6 h

Metabolism: Hepatic; $T_{1/2}$: 2–4 h
Distribution: Crosses placenta; enters breast milk
Excretion: Urine

Adverse effects
- **Respiratory:** Respiratory depression (with overdose)

Nursing Considerations

Assessment
- *History:* Hypersensitivity to any component; sensitivity to bromides; cough that persists for more than 1 wk or is accompanied by excessive secretions, high fever, rash, nausea, vomiting, or persistent headache; lactation
- *Physical:* Body temperature; R, adventitious sounds

Implementation
- Ensure that drug is not taken for longer than recommended or for coughs that may be symptomatic of a serious underlying disorder that should be diagnosed and properly treated; drug may mask symptoms of serious disease.

Drug-specific teaching points
- Take this drug exactly as prescribed. Do not take more than recommended or for longer than recommended.
- Report continued or recurring cough, cough accompanied by fever, rash, persistent headache, nausea, vomiting.

Adverse effects in *Italics* are most common; those in **Bold** are life-threatening.

dextrothyroxine sodium

*(dex troe thye **rox' een**)*
Choloxin

Pregnancy Category C

Drug classes
Antihyperlipidemic agent

Therapeutic actions
Stimulates the liver to increase the breakdown and excretion of cholesterol into the bile and feces; lowers the serum cholesterol and LDLs.

Indications
- Adjunct to diet and other measures for the reduction of elevated serum cholesterol in euthyroid patients with no known cardiovascular disease

Contraindications/cautions
- Contraindicated in the presence of history of organic heart disease, cardiac arrhythmias, rheumatic heart disease, CHF, hypertension, advanced liver or renal disease, pregnancy, lactation, allergy to tartrazine.
- Use caution in the presence of impaired renal or hepatic function; pending surgery (discontinue drug at least 2 wk before surgery).

Dosage
Adult: 1–2 mg/d PO; increase by 1–2 mg at intervals of not less than 1 mo to a maximum of 4–8 mg/d.
- ***Maintenance:*** 4–8 mg/d PO.

Pediatric: 0.05 mg/kg per day PO; increase in up to 0.05 mg/kg per day increments at monthly intervals to a maximum of 0.4 mg/kg per day or 4 mg/d. *Maintenance:* 0.1 mg/kg per day PO.

Pharmacokinetics

Route	Onset
Oral	Gradual

Metabolism: Hepatic; $T_{1/2}$: 18 h

Distribution: Crosses placenta; enters breast milk
Excretion: Urine and feces

Adverse effects
- CNS: Insomnia, nervousness, tremors, headache, tinnitus, dizziness, visual disturbances, exophthalmos, retinopathy, lid lag
- GI: Dyspepsia, nausea, vomiting, constipation, diarrhea, anorexia, weight loss
- CV: Angina, arrhythmias, ischemic myocardial changes, *myocardial infarction*
- Dermatologic: Hair loss, skin rash, itching
- Other: sweating, flushing, hyperthermia, changes in libido, edema

Clinically important drug-drug interactions
- Increased bleeding effects if taken with oral anticoagulants • Increased effects and accumulation of theophyllines if taken with dextrothyroxine • Alteration in serum levels of digitalis glycosides when taken with dextrothyroxine • Increased CNS stimulation when taken with TCAs • Risk of increased drug effects if taken with thyroid hormones

■ Nursing Considerations

Assessment
- *History:* Allergy to tartarzine, history of organic heart disease, cardiac arrhythmias, rheumatic heart disease, CHF, hypertension, liver or renal disease, pregnancy, lactation, scheduled surgery.
- *Physical:* Weight; temperature; skin—color, lesions, hair; reflexes, orientation, eye exam; cardiac evaluation, ECG, liver evaluation; liver and renal function tests, serum cholesterol, LDLs

Implementation
- Arrange for lab tests of serum cholesterol and fractionated lipids before beginning therapy and frequently during therapy.
- Arrange to discontinue drug at least 2 wk before scheduled surgery; notify surgeon of patient's drug therapy in cases of emergency surgery.

Adverse effects in *Italics* are most common; those in **Bold** are life-threatening.

- Discontinue drug and notify physician if any signs of cardiac disease develop.

Drug-specific teaching points
- Take drug as prescribed; monthly blood tests will be needed to monitor your response to the drug and adjust dosage as necessary.
- Know that the following side effects may occur: loss of appetite, nausea, vomiting (small, frequent meals may help); rash, loss of hair (these are effects of the drug; they should pass when the drug is discontinued); dizziness, nervousness, tremors, visual disturbances (use caution if driving or operating dangerous machinery if these effects occur).
- Report chest pain, palpitations, edema, skin rash, diarrhea, headache.

dezocine

(dez' oh seen)
Dalgan

Pregnancy Category C
Pregnancy Category D (labor or delivery)

Drug classes
Narcotic agonist–antagonist analgesic

Therapeutic actions
Acts as an agonist at specific opioid receptors in the CNS to produce analgesia, sedation, but also acts to cause hallucinations; seems to have low abuse potential; not in any schedule of the Federal Controlled Substances Act.

Indications
- Relief of moderate to severe pain in any situation an opiate analgesic is appropriate
- For preoperative or preanesthetic medication to supplement balanced anesthesia and relieve prepartum pain

Contraindications/cautions
- Contraindicated in the presence of hypersensitivity to dezocine, physical dependence on a narcotic analgesic (drug may precipitate withdrawal); pregnancy, lactation.
- Use caution in the presence of bronchial asthma, COPD, respiratory depression, anoxia, increased intracranial pressure, acute MI, ventricular failure, coronary insufficiency, hypertension, biliary tract surgery, renal or hepatic dysfunction.

Dosage
Adult
- ***IM single dose:*** 5–20 mg (usual, 10 mg). Adjust dosage according to patient's weight, age, severity of pain, physical status, and other medications. May be repeated q3–6h as needed. Do not exceed 20 mg/dose. Upper limit is 120 mg/d.
- ***IV:*** 2.5–10 mg repeated q2–4h. Initial dose is usually 5 mg.
- ***SC:*** Not recommended. Repeated injections lead to irritation, inflammation, thrombophlebitis.

Pediatric (< 18 y): Not recommended.

Pharmacokinetics

Route	Onset	Peak
IV	5 min	5–15 min
IM	10–15 min	10–90 min

Metabolism: Hepatic; $T_{1/2}$: 2.4 h
Distribution: Crosses placenta; enters breast milk
Excretion: Urine

IV facts
Preparation: Administer as provided. Store at room temperature; protect from light. Do not use if solution contains precipitate.
Infusion: Infuse slowly.

Adverse effects
- **CNS:** *Sedation, clamminess, sweating, headache, vertigo, floating feeling, dizziness, lethargy, confusion, lightheadedness,* nervousness, unusual dreams, agitation, euphoria, hallucinations
- **GI:** *Nausea, vomiting,* dry mouth
- **CV:** Palpitation, increase or decrease in blood pressure

Adverse effects in *Italics* are most common; those in **Bold** are life-threatening.

- **Respiratory:** Slow, shallow respiration
- **Dermatologic:** Rash, hives, pruritus, flushing, warmth, sensitivity to cold
- **EENT:** Diplopia, blurred vision
- **Local:** *Injection site reactions*

Clinically important drug-drug interactions

- Increased CNS depression if given concurrently with general anesthetics, sedatives, tranquilizers, hypnotics, other opioid analgesics.

■ Nursing Considerations

Assessment

- *History:* Hypersensitivity to dezocine, physical dependence on a narcotic analgesic; bronchial asthma, COPD, respiratory depression, anoxia, increased intracranial pressure, acute MI, ventricular failure, coronary insufficiency, hypertension, biliary tract surgery, renal or hepatic dysfunction; lactation.
- *Physical:* Orientation, reflexes, bilateral grip strength, affect; pupil size, vision; pulse, auscultation, BP; R, adventitious sounds; bowel sounds, normal output; liver, kidney function tests.

Implementation

- Provide narcotic antagonist, facilities for assisted or controlled respiration on standby during parenteral administration.

Drug-specific teaching points

- Incorporate teaching about drug into preoperative teaching when used in the acute setting. For other patients:
- Know that the following side effects may occur: dizziness, sedation, drowsiness, impaired visual acuity (avoid driving a car, performing other tasks that require alertness); nausea, loss of appetite (lying quietly, eating frequent small meals should minimize these effects).
- Report severe nausea, vomiting, palpitations, shortness of breath or difficulty breathing, pain at injection site.

☐ diazepam

(dye az' e pam)
Apo-Diazepam (CAN), Diazemuls (CAN), Valium, Valrelease, Vivol (CAN), Zetran

Pregnancy Category D
C-IV controlled substance

Drug classes
Benzodiazepine
Antianxiety drug
Antiepileptic drug
Centrally acting skeletal muscle relaxant

Therapeutic actions
Exact mechanisms of action not understood; acts mainly at the limbic system and reticular formation; may act in spinal cord and at supraspinal sites to produce skeletal muscle relaxation; potentiates the effects of GABA, an inhibitory neurotransmitter; anxiolytic effects occur at doses well below those necessary to cause sedation, ataxia; has little effect on cortical function.

Indications
- Management of anxiety disorders or for short-term relief of symptoms of anxiety
- Acute alcohol withdrawal; may be useful in symptomatic relief of acute agitation, tremor, delirium tremens, hallucinosis
- Muscle relaxant: adjunct for relief of reflex skeletal muscle spasm due to local pathology (inflammation of muscles or joints) or secondary to trauma; spasticity caused by upper motoneuron disorders (cerebral palsy and paraplegia); athetosis, stiff-man syndrome
- Treatment of tetanus (parenteral)
- **Antiepileptic:** adjunct in status epilepticus and severe recurrent convulsive seizures (parenteral); adjunct in convulsive disorders (oral)
- **Preoperative:** relief of anxiety and tension and to lessen recall in patients prior to surgical procedures, cardioversion, and endoscopic procedures (parenteral)

Adverse effects in *Italics* are most common; those in **Bold** are life-threatening.

- **Unlabeled use**: treatment of panic attacks

Contraindications/cautions
- Contraindicated in the presence of hypersensitivity to benzodiazepines; psychoses, acute narrow-angle glaucoma, shock, coma, acute alcoholic intoxication; pregnancy (cleft lip or palate, inguinal hernia, cardiac defects, microcephaly, pyloric stenosis have been reported when used in first trimester; neonatal withdrawal syndrome reported in babies); lactation.
- Use caution in elderly or debilitated patients; impaired liver or kidney function.

Dosage
Individualize dosage; increase dosage cautiously to avoid adverse effects.

Adult
- **Oral**
  - *Anxiety disorders, skeletal muscle spasm, convulsive disorders:* 2–10 mg bid–qid.
  - *Alcohol withdrawal:* 10 mg tid–qid first 24 h; reduce to 5 mg tid–qid, as needed.
- **Oral sustained release**
  - *Anxiety disorders:* 15–30 mg/d.
  - *Alcohol withdrawal:* 30 mg first 24 h; reduce to 15 mg/d as needed.
- **Parenteral:** Usual dose is 2–20 mg IM or IV. Larger doses may be required for some indications (tetanus). Injection may be repeated in 1 h.
  - *Anxiety:* 2–10 mg IM or IV; repeat in 3–4 h if necessary.
  - *Alcohol withdrawal:* 10 mg IM or IV initially, then 5–10 mg in 3–4 h if necessary.
  - *Endoscopic procedures:* 10 mg or less, up to 20 mg IV just before procedure or 5–10 mg IM 30 min prior to procedure. Reduce or omit dosage of narcotics.
  - *Muscle spasm:* 5–10 mg IM or IV initially, then 5–10 mg in 3–4 h if necessary.
  - *Status epilepticus:* 5–10 mg, preferably by slow IV. May repeat q 5–10 min up to total dose of 30 mg. If necessary, repeat therapy in 2–4 h; other drugs are preferable for long-term control.
  - *Preoperative:* 10 mg IM.
  - *Cardioversion:* 5–15 mg IV 5–10 min before procedure.

Pediatric
- **Oral**
  - *> 6 mo:* 1–2.5 mg PO tid–qid initially. Gradually increase as needed and tolerated. Can be given rectally if needed.
- **Parenteral:** Maximum dose of 0.25 mg/kg IV administered over 3 min; may repeat after 15–30 min if necessary. If no relief of symptoms after three doses, adjunctive therapy is recommended.
  - *Tetanus (> 30 d):* 1–2 mg IM or IV slowly q3–4h as necessary.
  - *Tetanus (5 y or older):* 5–10 mg q 3–4 h.
  - *Status epilepticus (> 30 d but < 5 y):* 0.2–0.5 mg slowly IV q 2–5 min up to a maximum of 5 mg.
  - *Status epilepticus (5 y or older):* 1 mg IV q 2–5 min up to a maximum of 10 mg; repeat in 2–4 h if necessary.

Geriatric patients or those with debilitating disease: 2–2.5 mg PO qd–bid or 2–5 mg parenteral initially. Gradually increase as needed and tolerated.

Pharmacokinetics

Route	Onset	Peak	Duration
Oral	30–60 min	1–2 h	3 h
IM	15–30 min	30–45 min	3 h
IV	1–5 min	30 min	15–60 min

Metabolism: Hepatic; $T_{1/2}$: 20–50 h
Distribution: Crosses placenta; enters breast milk
Excretion: Urine

IV facts
Preparation: Do not mix with other solutions; do not mix in plastic bags or tubing.
Infusion: Inject slowly into large vein; 1 ml/min at most; do not inject intraarterially; if injected into IV tubing, inject as close to vein insertion as possible.
Incompatibilities: Do not mix with other solutions; do not mix with any other drugs.

Adverse effects

- **CNS:** *Transient, mild drowsiness initially; sedation, depression, lethargy, apathy, fatigue, lightheadedness, disorientation, restlessness, confusion,* crying, delirium, headache, slurred speech, dysarthria, stupor, rigidity, tremor, dystonia, vertigo, euphoria, nervousness, difficulty in concentration, vivid dreams, psychomotor retardation, extrapyramidal symptoms; *mild paradoxical excitatory reactions, during first 2 wk of treatment,* visual and auditory disturbances, diplopia, nystagmus, depressed hearing, nasal congestion
- **GI:** *Constipation; diarrhea;* dry mouth; salivation; nausea; anorexia; vomiting; difficulty in swallowing; gastric disorders; elevations of blood enzymes—LDH, alkaline phosphatase, SGOT, SGPT; hepatic dysfunction; jaundice
- **CV:** *Bradycardia, tachycardia,* cardiovascular collapse, hypertension and hypotension, palpitations, edema
- **Hematologic:** Decreased hematocrit, blood dyscrasias
- **GU:** *Incontinence, urinary retention, changes in libido,* menstrual irregularities
- **Dermatologic:** Urticaria, pruritus, skin rash, dermatitis
- **Dependence:** *Drug dependence with withdrawal syndrome* when drug is discontinued (more common with abrupt discontinuation of higher dosage used for longer than 4 mo); IV diazepam: 1.7% incidence of fatalities; oral benzodiazepines ingested alone; no well-documented fatal overdoses
- **Other:** Phlebitis and thrombosis at IV injection sites, hiccups, fever, diaphoresis, paresthesias, muscular disturbances, gynecomastia; pain, burning, and redness after IM injection

Clinically important drug-drug interactions

- Increased CNS depression when taken with alcohol, omeprazole • Increased pharmacologic effects of diazepam when given with cimetidine, disulfiram, oral contraceptives • Decreased effects of diazepam if taken concurrently with theophyllines, ranitidine

■ Nursing Considerations

Assessment

- *History:* Hypersensitivity to benzodiazepines; psychoses, acute narrow-angle glaucoma, shock, coma, acute alcoholic intoxication; elderly or debilitated patients; impaired liver or kidney function; pregnancy, lactation.
- *Physical:* Body weight; skin—color, lesions; orientation, affect, reflexes, sensory nerve function, ophthalmologic exam; P, BP; R, adventitious sounds; bowel sounds, normal output, liver evaluation; normal output; liver and kidney function tests, CBC

Implementation

- Do not administer intra-arterially; may produce arteriospasm, gangrene.
- Arrange to change patients on IV therapy to oral therapy as soon as possible.
- Do not use small veins (dorsum of hand or wrist) for IV injection.
- Arrange to reduce dose of narcotic analgesics in patients receiving IV diazepam; dose should be reduced by at least one-third or eliminated.
- Carefully monitor P, BP, respiration during IV administration.
- Maintain patients receiving parenteral benzodiazepines in bed for 3 h; do not permit ambulatory patients to operate a vehicle following an injection.
- Monitor EEG in patients being treated for status epilepticus; seizures may recur after initial control, presumably because of short duration of drug effect.
- Arrange to monitor liver and kidney function, CBC at intervals during long-term therapy.
- Arrange to taper dosage gradually after long-term therapy, especially in epileptic patients.
- Arrange for epileptic patients to wear medical alert ID indicating that they are epileptics taking this medication.

Adverse effects in *Italics* are most common; those in **Bold** are life-threatening.

Drug-specific teaching points

- Take this drug exactly as prescribed. Do not stop taking this drug (long-term therapy, antiepileptic therapy) without consulting your health care provider.
- Know that the following side effects may occur: drowsiness, dizziness (these may become less pronounced after a few days; avoid driving a car or engaging in other dangerous activities if these occur); GI upset (taking the drug with food may help); dreams, difficulty concentrating, fatigue, nervousness, crying (it may help to know that these are effects of the drug).
- Report severe dizziness, weakness, drowsiness that persists, rash or skin lesions, palpitations, swelling of the ankles, visual or hearing disturbances, difficulty voiding.

❒ diazoxide

(di az ok' sid)
Oral: *Proglycem*
Parenteral: *Hyperstat*
Pregnancy Category C

Drug classes
Glucose-elevating agent (oral)
Antihypertensive
Thiazide (nondiuretic)

Therapeutic actions
Increases blood glucose by decreasing insulin release and decreasing glucose.
Decreases blood pressure by relaxing arteriolar smooth muscle.

Indications
- **Oral diazoxide:** management of hypoglycemia due to hyperinsulinism in infants and children and to inoperable pancreatic islet cell malignancies
- **Parenteral diazoxide:** short-term use in malignant and nonmalignant hypertension, primarily in hospitalized patients

Contraindications/cautions
- Contraindicated in the presence of allergy to thiazides or other sulfonamide derivatives; pregnancy, lactation.
- Use extreme caution in the presence of functional hypoglycemia, decreased cardiac reserve, decreased renal function, gout or hyperurecemia when using oral diazoxide; compensatory hypertension, dissecting aortic aneurysm, pheochromocytoma, decreased cerebral or cardiac circulation, labor and delivery (IV use may stop uterine contractions and cause neonatal hyperbilirubinemia, thrombocytopenia) when using parenteral diazoxide.

Dosage
Oral Diazoxide
- ***Adult:*** 3–8 mg/kg per day PO in two to three doses q8–12h. *Starting dose:* 3 mg/kg per day in three equal doses q8h.
- ***Pediatric:*** 3–8 mg/kg per day PO in two to three doses q8–12h. *Starting dose:* 3 mg/kg per day in three equal doses q8h.
- ***Infants and newborns:*** 8–15 mg/kg per day PO in two to three doses q8–12h. *Starting dose:* 10 mg/kg per day in three equal doses q8h.

Parenteral Diazoxide
- ***Adult:*** 1–3 mg/kg (maximum dose 150 mg) undiluted and rapidly by IV injection in a bolus dose within 30 sec; repeat bolus doses q 5–15 min until desired decrease in BP is achieved. Repeat doses q4–24h until oral antihypertensive medications can be started. Treatment is seldom needed for longer than 4–5 d and should not be continued for more than 10 d.

Pharmacokinetics

Route	Onset	Peak	Duration
Oral	1 h	8 h	
IV	30–60 min	5 min	2–12 h

Metabolism: Hepatic; $T_{1/2}$: 21–45 h
Distribution: Crosses placenta; enters breast milk
Excretion: Urine

IV facts
Preparation: Do not mix or dilute solution. Protect from light.

Infusion: Inject directly as rapid bolus, 30 sec or less; maximum of 150 mg in one injection.

Adverse effects

- CNS: Cerebral ischemia, headache, hearing loss, blurred vision, apprehension, cerebral infarction, coma, convulsions, paralysis, *dizziness, weakness*, altered taste sensation
- GI: **Nausea, vomiting**, hepatotoxicity, anorexia, parotid swelling, constipation, diarrhea, acute pancreatitis
- CV: *Hypotension* (managed by Trendelenburg position or sympathomimetics), occasional hypertension, angina, MI, cardiac arrhythmias, palpitations, *CHF secondary to fluid and sodium retention*
- Respiratory: Dyspnea, choking sensation
- Hematologic: Thrombocytopenia, decreased Hgb, decreased Hct, hyperuricemia
- GU: Renal toxicity
- Dermatologic: Hirsutism, rash
- Metabolic: Hyperglycemia, glycosuria, ketoacidosis, and nonketotic hyperosmolar coma
- Local: Pain at IV injection site

Clinically important drug-drug interactions

- Increased therapeutic and toxic effects of diazoxide if taken concurrently with thiazides • Increased risk of hyperglycemia if taken concurrently with acetohexamide, chlorpropamide, glipizide, glyburide, tolazamide, tolbutamide • Decreased serum levels and effectiveness of hydantoins taken concurrently with diazoxide

Drug-lab test interferences

- Hyperglycemic and hyperuricemic effects of diazoxide prevent testing for disorders of glucose and xanthine metabolism • False-negative insulin response to glucagon

■ Nursing Considerations

Assessment

- *History:* Allergy to thiazides or other sulfonamide derivatives; pregnancy; lactation; functional hypoglycemia, decreased cardiac reserve, decreased renal function, gout or hyperurecemia; compensatory hypertension, dissecting aortic aneurysm, pheochromocytoma; decreased cerebral or cardiac circulation.
- *Physical:* Body weight, skin integrity, swelling or limited motion in joints, earlobes; P, BP, edema, peripheral perfusion; R, pattern, adventitious sounds; intake and output; CBC, blood glucose, serum electrolytes and uric acid, urinalysis, urine glucose and ketones, kidney and liver function tests

Implementation

- Monitor intake and output and weigh patient daily at the same time to check for fluid retention.
- Check urine glucose and ketones daily.
- Have insulin and tolbutamide on standby in case hyperglycemic reaction occurs.
- Have dopamine, norepinephrine on standby in case severe hypotensive reaction occurs.

Oral Diazoxide
- Decrease dose in renal disease.
- Protect oral drug suspensions from light.
- Reassure patient that hirsutism will resolve when drug is discontinued.

Parenteral Diazoxide
- Monitor BP closely during administration until stable and then q$\frac{1}{2}$–1h.
- Protect drug from freezing and light.
- Patient should remain supine for 1 h after last injection.

Drug-specific teaching points

Oral Diazoxide
- Check urine daily for glucose and ketones; report elevated levels as instructed by your nurse.
- Weigh yourself daily at the same time and with the same clothes, and record the results.
- Be aware that you may experience an excessive growth of hair on your forehead, back, or limbs; this will go away shortly after the drug is stopped.

- Report weight gain of more than 5 lb in 2–3 d, increased thirst, nausea, vomiting, confusion, fruity odor on breath, abdominal pain, swelling of extremities, difficulty breathing, bruising, bleeding.

Parenteral Diazoxide
- Report increased thirst, nausea, headache, dizziness, hearing or vision changes, difficulty breathing, pain at injection site.

❏ diclofenac sodium

(dye kloe' fen ak)
Voltaren

diclofenac potassium
Cataflam

Pregnancy Category B

Drug classes
Analgesic (non-narcotic)
Antipyretic
Anti-inflammatory agent
NSAID

Therapeutic actions
Inhibits prostaglandin synthetase to cause antipyretic and anti-inflammatory effects; the exact mechanism of action is not known.

Indications
- Acute or long-term treatment of mild to moderate pain, including dysmenorrhea
- Rheumatoid arthritis
- Osteoarthritis
- Ankylating spondylitis

Contraindications/cautions
- Contraindicated in the presence of significant renal impairment, pregnancy, lactation.
- Use caution in the presence of impaired hearing, allergies, hepatic, cardiovascular, and GI conditions.

Dosage
Adult
- **Pain, including dysmennorhea:** 50 mg tid PO; initial dose of 100 mg may help some patients *(Cataflam)*
- **Osteoarthritis:** 100–150 mg/d PO in divided doses *(Voltaren)*; 50 mg bid–tid PO *(Cataflam)*
- **Rheumatoid arthritis:** 150–200 mg/d PO in divided doses *(Voltaren)*; 50 mg bid–tid PO *(Cataflam)*
- **Ankylosing spondylitis:** 100–125 mg/d PO. Give as 25 mg four times per day, with an extra 25-mg dose at bedtime if necessary *(Voltaren)*; 25 mg qid PO with an additional 25 mg hs if needed *(Cataflam)*

Pediatric: Safety and efficacy not established.

Pharmacokinetics

Route	Onset	Peak	Duration
Oral (sodium)	varies	2–3 h	12–15 h
Oral (potassium)	rapid	20–120 min	12–15 h

Metabolism: Hepatic; $T_{1/2}$: 1.5–2 h
Distribution: Crosses placenta; enters breast milk
Excretion: Urine and feces

Adverse effects
- CNS: *Headache, dizziness,* somnolence, insomnia, fatigue, tiredness, dizziness, tinnitus, ophthamologic effects
- GI: *Nausea, dyspepsia, GI pain, diarrhea,* vomiting, *constipation,* flatulence
- Hematologic: Bleeding, platelet inhibition with higher doses
- GU: Dysuria, renal impairment
- Dermatologic: Rash, pruritus, sweating, dry mucous membranes, stomatitis
- Other: Peripheral edema, anaphylactoid reactions to fatal anaphylactic shock

Clinically important drug-drug interactions
- Increased serum levels and increased risk of lithium toxicity if taken with diclofenac.

■ Nursing Considerations
Assessment
- *History:* Renal impairment; impaired hearing; allergies; hepatic, cardiovascular, and GI conditions; lactation.
- *Physical:* Skin—color and lesions; orientation, reflexes, ophthalmologic and

Adverse effects in *Italics* are most common; those in **Bold** are life-threatening.

audiometric evaluation, peripheral sensation; P, edema; R, adventitious sounds; liver evaluation; CBC, clotting times, renal and liver function tests; serum electrolytes, stool guaiac.

Implementation
- Administer drug with food or after meals if GI upset occurs.
- Arrange for periodic ophthalmologic exam during long term therapy.
- Institute emergency procedures if overdose occurs (gastric lavage, induction of emesis, supportive therapy).

Drug-specific teaching points
- Take drug with food or meals if GI upset occurs.
- Take only the prescribed dosage.
- Know that dizziness, drowsiness can occur (avoid driving or the use of dangerous machinery while on this drug).
- Report sore throat, fever, rash, itching, weight gain, swelling in ankles or fingers, changes in vision; black, tarry stools.

▢ dicloxacillin sodium

*(dye klox a **sill'** in)*
Dynapen, Dycill, Pathocil

Pregnancy Category B

Drug classes
Antibiotic
Penicillinase-resistant pencillin

Therapeutic actions
Bactericidal: inhibits cell wall synthesis of sensitive organisms, causing cell death.

Indications
- Infections due to penicillanase producing staphylococci

Contraindications/cautions
- Contraindicated in the presence of allergies to penicillins, cephalosporins, or other allergens.
- Use caution in the presence of renal disorders, lactation (may cause diarrhea or candidiasis in the infant).

Dosage
Adult: 125 mg q6h PO. Up to 250 mg q6h PO in severe infections.
Pediatric
- ***Less than 40 kg:*** 12.5 mg/kg per day PO in equally divided doses q6h. Up to 25 mg/kg per day PO in equally divided doses q6h in severe infections.

Pharmacokinetics

Route	Onset	Peak	Duration
Oral	Varies	0.5–1 h	4–6 h

Metabolism: Hepatic; $T_{1/2}$: 30–60 min
Distribution: Crosses placenta; enters breast milk
Excretion: Urine

Adverse effects
- **CNS:** Lethargy, hallucinations, seizures, decreased reflexes
- **GI:** *Glossitis, stomatitis, gastritis, sore mouth,* furry tongue, black "hairy" tongue, *nausea, vomiting, diarrhea,* abdominal pain, bloody diarrhea, enterocolitis, pseudomembranous colitis, nonspecific hepatitis
- **Hematologic:** Anemia, thrombocytopenia, leukopenia, neutropenia, prolonged bleeding time, hemorrhagic episodes at high doses
- **GU:** Nephritis: oliguria, proteinuria, hematuria, casts, azotemia, pyuria
- **Hypersensitivity reactions:** *Rash, fever, wheezing,* anaphylaxis
- **Other:** *Superinfections*: oral and rectal moniliasis, vaginitis

Clinically important drug-drug interactions
- Decreased effectiveness if taken with tetracyclines

Clinically important drug-food interactions
- Decreased absorption and decreased serum levels if taken with food

■ Nursing Considerations
Assessment
- *History:* Allergies; renal disorders; lactation

Adverse effects in *Italics* are most common; those in **Bold** are life-threatening.

- *Physical:* Culture infected area; skin—color, lesion; R, adventitious sounds; bowel sounds; CBC, liver and renal function tests, serum electrolytes, hematocrit, urinalysis.

Implementation
- Culture infected area before beginning treatment; reculture area if response is not as expected.
- Administer by oral route only.
- Arrange to continue oral treatment for 10 full d.
- Administer on an empty stomach, 1 h before or 2 h after meals.
- Do not administer with fruit juices or soft drinks; a full glass of water is preferable.

Drug-specific teaching points
- Take drug around the clock as prescribed; take the full course of therapy, usually 10 d.
- Take the drug on an empty stomach, 1 h before or 2 h after meals, with a full glass of water.
- Be aware that this antibiotic is specific for this infection and should not be used to self-treat other infections.
- Know that the following side effects may occur: stomach upset, nausea, diarrhea, mouth sores.
- Report unusual bleeding or bruising, fever, chills, sore throat, hives, rash, severe diarrhea, difficulty breathing.

◻ dicyclomine hydrochloride

(dye sye' kloe meen)

Antispas, Bemote, Bentyl, Bentylol (CAN), Byclomine, Dibent, Formulex (CAN), Neoquess, Spasmoject, Viscerol (CAN)

Pregnancy Category C

Drug classes
Antispasmodic
Anticholinergic
Antimuscarinic
Parasympatholytic

Therapeutic actions
Direct GI smooth muscle relaxant; competitively blocks the effects of acetylcholine at muscarinic cholinergic receptors that mediate the effects of parasympathetic postganglionic impulses, thus relaxing the GI tract.

Indications
- Treatment of functional bowel or irritable bowel syndrome (irritable colon, spastic colon, mucous colitis)

Contraindications/cautions
- Contraindicated in the presence of glaucoma; adhesions between iris and lens, stenosing peptic ulcer, pyloroduodenal obstruction, paralytic ileus, intestinal atony, severe ulcerative colitis, toxic megacolon, symptomatic prostatic hypertrophy, bladder neck obstruction, bronchial asthma, COPD, cardiac arrhythmias, tachycardia, myocardial ischemia; impaired metabolic, liver, or kidney function, myasthenia gravis; lactation.
- Use caution in the presence of Down's syndrome, brain damage, spasticity, hypertension, hyperthyroidism.

Dosage
Adult
- **Oral:** The only effective dose is 160 mg/d PO divided into four equal doses; however, begin with 80 mg/d divided into four equal doses; increase to 160 mg/d unless side effects limit dosage.
- **Parenteral:** 80 mg/d IM in four divided doses; **do not give IV**.

Pediatric: Not recommended for children.

Pharmacokinetics

Route	Onset	Duration
Oral	1–2 h	4 h

Metabolism: Hepatic; $T_{1/2}$: 9–10 h
Distribution: Crosses placenta; enters breast milk
Excretion: Urine

Adverse effects
- CNS: *Blurred vision*, mydriasis, cycloplegia, photophobia, increased intraocular pressure

- GI: *Dry mouth, altered taste perception, nausea, vomiting, dysphagia,* heartburn, constipation, bloated feeling, paralytic ileus, gastroesophageal reflux
- CV: Palpitations, tachycardia
- GU: *Urinary hesitancy and retention;* impotence
- Local: *Irritation at site of IM injection*
- Other: Decreased sweating and predisposition to heat prostration, suppression of lactation

Clinically important drug-drug interactions
- Decreased antipsychotic effectiveness of haloperidol when given with anticholinergic drugs • Decreased effectiveness of phenothiazines given with anticholinergic drugs, but increased incidence of paralytic ileus

■ Nursing Considerations

Assessment
- *History:* Glaucoma; adhesions between iris and lens, stenosing peptic ulcer, pyloroduodenal obstruction, paralytic ileus, intestinal atony, severe ulcerative colitis, toxic megacolon, symptomatic prostatic hypertrophy, bladder neck obstruction, bronchial asthma, COPD, cardiac arrhythmias, myocardial ischemia; impaired metabolic, liver, or kidney function, myasthenia gravis; Down's syndrome, brain damage, spasticity, hypertension, hyperthyroidism; lactation
- *Physical:* Bowel sounds, normal output; normal urinary output, prostate palpation; R, adventitious sounds; pulse, blood pressure; intraocular pressure, vision; bilateral grip strength, reflexes; liver palpation, liver function tests; renal function tests; skin color, lesions, texture.

Implementation
- Ensure adequate hydration; provide environmental control (temperature) to prevent hyperpyrexia.
- Encourage patient to void before each dose of medication if urinary retention becomes a problem.
- Monitor lighting to minimize discomfort of photophobia.

Drug-specific teaching points
- Take drug exactly as prescribed.
- Avoid hot environments while taking this drug (you will be heat intolerant, and dangerous reactions may occur).
- Know that the following side effects may occur: constipation (ensure adequate fluid intake, proper diet); dry mouth (sugarless lozenges, frequent mouth care may help; this effect sometimes lessens with time); blurred vision, sensitivity to light (it may help to know that these are drug effects that will go away when you discontinue the drug; avoid tasks that require acute vision; wear sunglasses when in bright light if these occur); impotence (this is a drug effect that will go away when you discontinue the drug); difficulty in urination (it may help to empty the bladder immediately before taking each dose of drug).
- Report skin rash, flushing, eye pain, difficulty breathing, tremors, loss of coordination, irregular heartbeat, palpitations, headache, abdominal distention, hallucinations, severe or persistent dry mouth, difficulty swallowing, difficulty in urination, severe constipation, sensitivity to light.

🗋 didanosine

*(dye **dan**' oh seen)*

ddl, dideoxyinosine
Videx

Pregnancy Category B

Drug classes
Antiviral

Therapeutic actions
A synthetic nucleoside that inhibits replication of HIV, leading to viral death.

Indications
- Treatment of adult patients with advanced HIV infection who have received prolonged prior zidovudine therapy

Adverse effects in *Italics* are most common; those in **Bold** are life-threatening.

didanosine

- Treatment of adults and children > 6 mo with advanced infection who are intolerant to zidovudine

Contraindications/cautions
- Contraindicated in the presence of allergy to any component of the formulation, lactation.
- Use caution in the presence of impaired hepatic or renal function; history of alcohol abuse.

Dosage
Adult: 125–200 mg PO bid; buffered powder: 167–250 mg PO bid.
Pediatric

Body Surface (m^2)	Tablets (bid)	Pediatric Powder (m^2) Dose (bid)	Vol/ 10 mg/ml (bid)
1.1–1.4	100 mg	125 mg	12.5 ml
0.8–1	75 mg	94 mg	9.5 ml
0.5–0.7	50 mg	62 mg	6 ml
<0.4	25 mg	31 mg	3 ml

Pharmacokinetics

Route	Onset
Onset	Varies

Metabolism: Hepatic; $T_{1/2}$: 1.6 h
Distribution: Crosses placenta; enters breast milk
Excretion: Urine

Adverse effects
- **CNS:** Headache, pain, anxiety, confusion, nervousness, twitching, depression
- **GI:** *Nausea, vomiting, hepatotoxicity, abdominal pain,* **pancreatitis,** stomatitis, oral thrush, melena, dry mouth
- **Hematologic:** *Hemopoietic depression,* elevated bilirubin, elevated uric acid
- **Dermatologic:** Rash, pruritus
- **Other:** Chills, fever, infections, dyspnea, myopathy

Clinically important drug-drug interactions
- Decreased effectiveness of tetracycline, fluoroquinolone antibiotics if taken with didanosine

Clinically important drug-food interactions
- Decreased absorption and effectiveness of didanosine if taken with food

■ Nursing Considerations

Assessment
- *History:* Allergy to any components of formulation, impaired hepatic or renal function, lactation, history of alcohol abuse.
- *Physical:* Weight; temperature; skin—color, lesions; orientation, reflexes, muscle strength, affect; abdominal exam; CBC, pancreatic enzymes, renal and liver function tests

Implementation
- Arrange for lab tests (CBC, SMA 12) before beginning therapy and frequently during therapy.
- Administer drug on an empty stomach, 1 h before or 2 h after meals.
- Instruct patient to chew tablets thoroughly or crush tablets and disperse 2 tablets in at least 1 ounce of water; stir until a uniform dispersion forms. For buffered powder, pour contents of packet into 4 oz of water. Do not mix with fruit juice or acid-containing liquid. Stir until powder completely dissolves; have patient drink entire solution immediately. Pediatric solution should be reconstituted by the pharmacy. Shake admixture thoroughly. Store tightly closed in the refrigerator.
- Avoid generating dust. When cleaning up powdered products, use a wet mop or damp sponge. Clean surface with soap and water. Contain large spills. Avoid inhaling dust.
- Monitor patient for any sign of pancreatitis—abdominal pain, elevated enzymes, nausea, vomiting. Stop drug, and resume only when pancreatitis has been ruled out.
- Monitor patients with hepatic or renal impairment; decreased doses may be needed if toxicity occurs.

Adverse effects in *Italics* are most common; those in **Bold** are life-threatening.

Drug-specific teaching points
- Take drug on an empty stomach, 1 h before or 2 h after meals.
- Chew tablets thoroughly, or crush tablets and disperse 2 tablets in at least 1 ounce of water; stir until a uniform dispersion forms. For buffered powder, pour contents of packet into 4 oz of water. Do not mix with fruit juice or acid-containing liquid. Stir until powder completely dissolves; drink entire solution immediately. Pediatric solution should be reconstituted by the pharmacy. Shake admixture thoroughly. Store tightly closed in the refrigerator.
- Know that the following side effects may occur: loss of appetite, nausea, vomiting (frequent mouth care, small frequent meals may help); rash; chills, fever; headache.
- Arrange to have regular blood tests and physical exams to monitor the drug's effects and progress of disease.
- Report abdominal pain, nausea, vomiting, cough, sore throat, change in color of urine or stools.

☐ dienestrol

(dye en ess' trol)
DV, Ortho Dienestrol
Pregnancy Category X

Drug classes
Estrogen
Hormonal agent

Therapeutic actions
Intravaginal application delivers replacement estrogenic hormone to vulvovaginal area, showing symptomatic epithelial atrophy resulting from the postmenopausal withdrawal of endogenous estrogens; estrogens induce proliferation of vaginal epithelium, deposition of glycogen in vaginal epithelium, cornification of superficial vaginal cells, acidification of vaginal secretions.

Indications
- Treatment of atrophic vaginitis and kraurosis vulvae associated with menopause

Contraindications/cautions
- Contraindicated in the presence of allergy to estrogens or any component of product; pregnancy; lactation.
- Use caution in the presence of endometriosis.

Dosage
Available as topical vaginal cream only. Administer cyclically for short-term use; attempt to discontinue or taper medication at 3- to 6-mo intervals.
Adult: 1–2 applicators intravaginally daily for 1–2 wk; then reduce to half initial dosage or 1 applicator every other day for 1–2 wk. Maintenance dose of 1 applicator one to three times per week after vaginal mucosa is restored.

Pharmacokinetics

Route	Onset
Vaginal	Rapid

Metabolism: Hepatic; $T_{1/2}$: unknown
Distribution: Crosses placenta; enters breast milk

Adverse effects
- **GU:** *Uterine bleeding* (if absorbed through the vaginal mucosa and with sudden discontinuation), serious bleeding in sterilized women with endometriosis, vaginal discharge due to mucus hypersecretion with overdosage
- **Other:** Breast tenderness

■ Nursing Considerations

Assessment
- *History:* Allergy to estrogens or any component of product, endometriosis, pregnancy, lactation.
- *Physical:* Breast exam; pelvic exam; abdominal palpation.

Implementation
- Arrange for complete pelvic exam and Pap smear before beginning therapy and periodically throughout therapy.

Adverse effects in *Italics* are most common; those in **Bold** are life-threatening.

- Administer cyclically and for short terms only; attempt to discontinue or taper medication at 3- to 6-mo intervals.
- Administer high into the vagina with the applicator provided with the product.
- Encourage patient to lie in the recumbent position for 15 min after application.
- Provide patient with pad or protection for clothing after administration.

Drug-specific teaching points
- Apply high into vagina with applicator provided with product; lie down for 15 min after application; you may wish to wear a pad or provide other protection for your clothing after application.
- Do not use this product if you are pregnant; if you think you are pregnant or wish to become pregnant, consult with your physician.
- Report breast tenderness, vaginal bleeding, vaginal discharge.

diethylstilbestrol diphosphate

*(dye eth il stil **bess'trol**)*
DES, , Honvol (CAN), Stilphostrol

Pregnancy Category X

Drug classes
Hormone
Estrogen

Therapeutic actions
Estrogens are endogenous female sex hormones; important in the development of the female reproductive system and secondary sex characteristics; cause capillary dilatation, fluid retention, protein anabolism, and thin cervical mucus; conserve calcium and phosphorus, and encourage bone formation; efficacy as palliation in male patients with androgen-dependent prostatic carcinoma is attributable to their competition with androgens for receptor sites.

Indications
- Palliation in prostatic carcinoma (inoperable and progressing)
- Inoperable and progressing breast cancer

Contraindications/cautions
- Contraindicated in the presence of allergy to estrogens; breast cancer (except in specific, selected patients); estrogen-dependent neoplasm; active thrombophlebitis or thromboembolic disorders or history of such from previous estrogen use; pregnancy.
- Use caution in the presence of metabolic bone disease, renal insufficiency, CHF, lactation.

Dosage
Adult
- **Prostatic cancer**
  - *Oral:* Initially, 50 mg tid PO; increase to > 200 mg tid, depending on patient tolerance. Do not exceed 1 g/d. If relief is not obtained with high oral doses, use IV route. DES (not disphosphate) 3 mg/d PO, average dose 1 mg/d.
  - *Parenteral:* On the first day, give 0.5 g IV dissolved in 250 ml saline or 5% dextrose. On subsequent days, give 1 g dissolved in 250–500 ml of saline or dextrose. Administer slowly (20–30 drops/min) during the first 10–15 min and then adjust flow rate so the entire dose is infused within 1 h. Follow the procedure for > 5 d, depending on the patient response. Then administer 0.25–0.5 g in a similar manner once or twice weekly, or obtain maintenance using oral drug.
- **Inoperable breast cancer (DES, not diphosphate):** 15 mg/d PO.

Pediatric: Not recommended due to effect on the growth of the long bones.

Pharmacokinetics

Route	Onset
Oral	Rapid

Metabolism: Hepatic; $T_{1/2}$: unknowns
Distribution: Crosses placenta; enters breast milk
Excretion: Urine

IV facts
Preparation: Dissolve 0.5 g in 250 ml saline or 5% dextrose; on subsequent days give 1 g dissolved in 250–500 ml saline or dextrose. Store at room temperature, away

from direct light. Stable for 5 d. Do not use if cloudy or precipitates have formed.
Infusion: Administer slowly: 20–30 drops/min during the first 10–15 min and then adjust rate so entire amount is given in 1 h.

Adverse effects

- CNS: *Steepening of the corneal curvature with a resultant change in visual acuity and intolerance to contact lenses, headache,* migraine, dizziness, mental depression, chorea, convulsions
- GI: Hepatic adenoma, *nausea, vomiting, abdominal cramps,* bloating, cholestatic jaundice, colitis, acute pancreatitis
- CV: Increased blood pressure, **thromboembolic and thrombotic disease**, peripheral edema
- Dermatologic: *Photosensitivity,* chloasma, erythema nodosum or multiforme, hemorrhagic eruption, loss of scalp hair, hirsutism, urticaria, dermatitis
- Endocrine: Decreased glucose tolerance, reduced carbohydrate tolerance
- Other: Weight changes, aggravation of porphyria, breast tenderness

Clinically important drug-drug interactions

- Enhanced hepatic metabolism of diethylstilbestrol: barbiturates, phenytoin, rifampin • Increased therapeutic and toxic effects of corticosteroids if taken concurrently.

Drug-lab test interferences

- Increased sulfobromophthalein retention; increased prothrombin and factors VII, VIII, IX, and X; decreased antithrombin III; increased thyroid-binding globulin with increased PBI, T_4, increased uptake of free T_3 resin (free T_4 is unaltered); impaired glucose tolerance; reduced response to metyrapone test; reduced serum folate concentration; increased serum triglycerides and phospholipid concentration.

■ Nursing Considerations

Assessment

- *History:* Allergy to estrogens; breast cancer; estrogen-dependent neoplasm; active thrombophlebitis or thromboembolic disorders; metabolic bone disease, renal insufficiency, CHF, pregnancy, lactation.
- *Physical:* Skin—color, lesions, edema; orientation, affect, reflexes; P, auscultation, BP, peripheral perfusion; R, adventitious sounds; bowel sounds, liver evaluation, abdominal exam; serum calcium, phosphorus; liver and renal function tests; glucose tolerance test.

Implementation

- Caution patient before beginning therapy of the risks involved with estrogen use, including the need for frequent medical followup, need for periodic rests from drug treatment, as appropriate.

Drug-specific teaching points

- Arrange for periodic medical exams because many potentially serious problems have occurred with the use of this drug, including development of cancers, blood clots, liver problems.
- Know that the following side effects may occur: nausea, vomiting, bloating; headache, dizziness, mental depression (use caution if driving or performing tasks that require alertness if this occurs); sensitivity to sunlight (use a sunscreen and wear protective clothing until your tolerance to this effect of the drug is known); skin rash, loss of scalp hair, darkening of the skin on the face.
- Report pain in the groin or calves of the legs, chest pain or sudden shortness of breath, sudden severe headache, dizziness or fainting, changes in vision or speech, weakness or numbness in the arm or leg, severe abdominal pain, yellowing of the skin or eyes, severe mental depression.

☐ diflunisal

*(dye **floo'** ni sal)*
Dolobid

Pregnancy Category C

Drug classes
Analgesic (non-narcotic)
Antipyretic

Adverse effects in *Italics* are most common; those in **Bold** are life-threatening.

diflunisal

Anti-inflammatory agent
NSAID

Therapeutic actions
Exact mechanism of action not known: inhibition of prostaglandin synthetase, the enzyme that breaks down prostaglandins, may account for its antipyretic and anti-inflammatory effects.

Indications
- Acute or long-term treatment of mild to moderate pain
- Rheumatoid arthritis
- Osteoarthritis

Contraindications/cautions
- Contraindicated in the presence of allergy to diflunisalsalicylates or other NSAID, pregnancy, lactation.
- Use caution in the presence of cardiovascular dysfunction, peptic ulceration, GI bleeding, impaired hepatic or renal function.

Dosage
Adult
- ***Mild to moderate pain:*** 1,000 mg PO initially, followed by 500 mg q12h PO.
- ***Osteoarthritis/rheumatoid arthritis:*** 500–1,000 mg/d PO in two divided doses; maintenance dosage should not exceed 1,500 mg/d.

Pediatric: Safety and efficacy has not been established.

Pharmacokinetics

Route	Onset	Peak	Duration
Oral	30–60 min	2–3 h	12 h

Metabolism: Hepatic; $T_{1/2}$: 8–12 h
Distribution: Crosses placenta; enters breast milk
Excretion: Urine

Adverse effects
- **CNS:** *Headache, dizziness, somnolence, insomnia,* fatigue, tiredness, dizziness, tinnitus, ophthamologic effects
- **GI:** *Nausea, dyspepsia, GI pain, diarrhea,* vomiting, constipation, flatulence
- **GU:** Dysuria, renal impairment
- **Hematologic:** Bleeding, platelet inhibition with higher doses
- **Dermatologic:** *Rash,* pruritus, sweating, dry mucous membranes, stomatitis
- **Other:** Peripheral edema, **anaphylactoid reactions to fatal anaphylactic shock**

Clinically important drug-drug interactions
- Decreased absorption of diflunisal if taken with antacids (especially aluminum salts) • Decreased serum diflunisal levels if taken with multiple doses of aspirin

■ Nursing Considerations
Assessment
- *History:* Allergy to diflunisalsalicylates or other NSAID, cardiovascular dysfunction, peptic ulceration, GI bleeding, impaired hepatic or renal function, lactation.
- *Physical:* Skin—color, lesions; temperature; orientation, reflexes, ophthalmologic evaluation; P, BP, edema; R, adventitious sounds; liver evaluation, bowel sounds; CBC, clotting times, urinalysis, renal and liver function tests

Implementation
- Administer drug with food or after meals if GI upset occurs.
- Do not crush, and ensure that patient does not chew tablets.
- Institute emergency procedures if overdose occurs—gastric lavage, induction of emesis, supportive therapy.
- Arrange for ophthalmologic exam if patient offers any eye complaints.

Drug-specific teaching points
- Take the drug only as recommended to avoid overdose.
- Take the drug with food or after meals if GI upset occurs. Swallow the tablet whole; do not chew or crush it.
- Know that the following side effects may occur: nausea, GI upset, dyspepsia (taking the drug with food may help); diarrhea or constipation (ensure ready access to bathroom facilites if diarrhea occurs); dizziness, vertigo, insomnia (use caution

Adverse effects in *Italics* are most common; those in **Bold** are life-threatening.

- if driving or operating dangerous machinery if these occur).
- Report eye changes, unusual bleeding or bruising, swelling of the feet or hands, difficulty breathing, severe GI pain.

☐ digoxin

(di jox' in)

Lanoxicaps, Lanoxin, Novo-Digoxin (CAN)

Pregnancy Category A

Drug classes
Cardiac glycoside
Cardiotonic drug

Therapeutic actions
Increases intracellular calcium and allows more calcium to enter the myocardial cell during depolarization via a sodium–potassium pump mechanism; this increases force of contraction (positive inotropic effect), increases renal perfusion (seen as diuretic effect in patients with CHF), decreases heart rate (negative chronotropic effect), and decreases AV node conduction velocity.

Indications
- CHF
- Atrial fibrillation
- Atrial flutter
- Paroxysmal atrial tachycardia

Contraindications/cautions
- Contraindicated in allergy to digitalis preparations, ventricular tachycardia, ventricular fibrillation, heart block, sick sinus syndrome, IHSS, acute MI, renal insufficiency and electrolyte abnormalities (decreased K^+, decreased Mg^{++}, increased Ca^{++}).
- Use caution in the presence of pregnancy and lactation.

Dosage
Patient response to digoxin has been found to be quite variable. Careful patient assessment and evaluation are needed to determine the appropriate dose for each individual patient.

Adult
- **Loading dose:** 0.75–1.25 mg PO or 0.125–0.25 mg IV.
- **Maintenance dose:** 0.125–0.25 mg/d PO.

Pediatric
- **Maintenance dose:** 25%–35% of loading dose in divided daily doses.

	Loading Dose	
	Oral	IV
Premature	20–30 mcg/kg	15–25 mcg/kg
Neonate	25–35 mcg/kg	20–30 mcg/kg
1–24 mo	35–60 mcg/kg	30–50 mcg/kg
2–5 y	30–40 mcg/kg	25–35 mcg/kg
5–10 y	20–35 mcg/kg	15–30 mcg/kg
>10 y	10–15 mcg/kg	8–12 mcg/kg

Geriatric patients with impaired renal function

Creatinine Clearance	Dose
10–25 ml/min	0.125 mg/d
26–49 ml/min	0.1875 mg/d
50–79 ml/min	0.25 mg/d

Note: Lanoxicaps have a greater bioavailability than standard oral preparations. The 0.2-mg Lanoxicap is equivalent to the 0.25 mg tablets; the 0.1-mg Lanoxicap is equivalent to the 0.125-mg tablets, and so forth. Adjust dosage accordingly.

Pharmacokinetics

Route	Onset	Peak	Duration
Oral	30–120 min	2–6 h	6–8 d
IV	5–30 min	1–5 h	4–5 d

Metabolism: Some Hepatic; $T_{1/2}$: 30–40 h
Distribution: May cross placenta; enters breast milk
Excretion: Largely unchanged in the urine

IV facts
Preparation: Give undiluted or diluted in fourfold or greater volume of Sterile Water for Injection, 0.9% Sodium Chloride Injection, 5% Dextrose Injection or Lactated

Ringer's Injection. Use diluted product promptly. Do not use if solution contains precipitates.
Infusion: Inject slowly over 5 min or longer.

Adverse effects
- CNS: *Headache, weakness*, drowsiness, visual disturbances
- GI: *GI upset*, anorexia
- CV: *Arrhythmias*

Clinically important drug-drug interactions
- Increased therapeutic and toxic effects of digoxin if taken concurrently with thioamines, verapamil, amiodarone, quinidine, quinine, erythromycin, cyclosporine (a decrease in digoxin dosage may be necessary to prevent toxicity; when the interacting drug is discontinued, an increase in the digoxin dosage may be necessary) • Increased incidence of cardiac arrhythmias if taken with potassium-losing (loop and thiazide) diuretics • Increased absorption or increased bioavailability of oral digoxin, leading to increased effects if taken with tetracyclines, erythromycin • Decreased therapeutic effects of digoxin if taken with thyroid hormones, metoclopramide, penicillamine • Decreased absorption of oral digoxin if taken with cholestyramine, charcoal, colestipol, antineoplastic agents (eg, bleomycin, cyclophosphamide, methotrexate) • Increased or decreased effects of oral digoxin (it may be necessary to adjust the dose of digoxin during concomitant therapy) if taken with oral aminoglycosides.

■ Nursing Considerations

Assessment
- *History:* Allergy to digitalis preparations, ventricular tachycardia, ventricular fibrillation, heart block, sick sinus syndrome, IHSS, acute MI, renal insufficiency, decreased K^+, decreased Mg^{++}, increased Ca^{++}
- *Physical:* Body weight; orientation, affect, reflexes, vision; P, BP, baseline ECG, cardiac auscultation, peripheral pulses, peripheral perfusion, edema; R, adventitious sounds; abdominal percussion, bowel sounds, liver evaluation; urinary output; electrolyte levels, liver and renal function tests

Implementation
- Monitor apical pulse or ECG before administering.
- Check dosage and preparation carefully.
- Avoid IM injections, which may be very painful.
- Follow diluting instructions carefully, and use diluted solution promptly.
- Avoid giving with meals; this will delay absorption.
- Have emergency equipment readily available; have potassium salts, lidocaine, phenytoin, atropine, cardiac monitor on standby in case toxicity develops.

Drug-specific teaching points
- Do not stop taking this drug without notifying your health care provider.
- Take your pulse at the same time each day, and record it on a calendar (normal pulse for you is —).
- Weigh yourself every other day with the same clothing and at the same time during the day. Record this on the calendar.
- Wear or carry a medical alert tag stating that you are on this drug.
- Have regular medical checkups, which may include blood tests, to evaluate the effects and dosage of this drug.
- Report unusually slow pulse, irregular pulse, rapid weight gain, loss of appetite, nausea, vomiting, blurred or "yellow" vision, unusual tiredness and weakness, swelling of the ankles, legs or fingers, difficulty breathing.

❑ digoxin immune fab (ovine)

*(di **jox**' in)*
digoxin-specific antibody fragments

Digibind

Pregnancy Category C

Adverse effects in *Italics* are most common; those in **Bold** are life-threatening.

digoxin immune fab (ovine)

Drug classes
Antidote

Therapeutic actions
Antigen-binding fragments (fab) derived from specific antidigoxin antibodies; binds molecules of digoxin, making them unavailable at the site of action; fab-fragment complex accumulates in the blood and is excreted by the kidneys.

Indications
- Treatment of life-threatening digoxin intoxication (serum digoxin levels > 10 ng/ml, serum K^+ > 5 mEq/L in setting of digitalis intoxication)
- Treatment of life-threatening digitoxin overdose

Contraindications/cautions
- Contraindicated in the presence of allergy to sheep products.
- Use caution during pregnancy or lactation.

Dosage
Adult: Dosage is determined by serum digoxin level or estimate of the amount of digoxin ingested. If no estimate of the amount of digoxin ingested is available and serum digoxin levels cannot be obtained, use 800 mg (20 vials), which should treat most life-threatening ingestions in adults and children.

Estimated fab fragment dose based on amount of digoxin ingested:

Est. # of 0.25 mg caps ingested	Dose in mg	# of vials
25	340	8.5
50	680	17
75	1000	25
100	1360	34
150	2000	50
200	2680	67

Estimated fab fragments dose based on serum digoxin concentration:

	Serum digoxin concentration (ng/ml)					
wt (kg)	1	2	4	8	12	16
Infants/Children			Dose as mg			
1	0.5	1	1.5	3	5	6
3	1	2	5	9	13	18
5	2	4	8	15	22	30
10	4	8	15	30	40	60
20	8	15	30	60	80	120
Adults			Dose as vials			
40	0.5	1	2	3	5	6
60	0.5	1	2	5	7	9
70	1	2	3	5	8	11

Equations also are available for calculating exact dosage from serum digoxin or digitoxin concentration.

Pharmacokinetics

Route	Onset	Duration
IV	15–30 min	4–6 h

Metabolism: $T_{1/2}$: 15–20 h
Distribution: Crosses placenta; enters breast milk
Excretion: Urine

IV facts
Preparation: Dissolve the contents in each vial with 4 ml of Sterile Water for Injection. Mix gently to give an approximate isosmotic solution with a protein concentration of 10 mg/ml. Use reconstituted solution promptly. Store in refrigerator for up to 4 h. Discard after that time. Reconstituted solution may be further diluted with Sterile Isotonic Saline.
Infusion: Administer IV over 30 min through a 0.22-μm filter; administer as a bolus injection if cardiac arrest is imminent.

Adverse effects
- **CV:** *Low cardiac output states*, CHF, rapid ventricular response in patients with atrial fibrillation
- **Hematologic:** Hypokalemia due to reactivation of Na, K ATPase

Adverse effects in *Italics* are most common; those in **Bold** are life-threatening.

- **Hypersensitivity:** Allergic reactions: drug fever to **anaphylaxis**

■ Nursing Considerations
Assessment
- *History:* Allergy to sheep products, digoxin drug history, lactation
- *Physical:* P, BP, auscultation, baseline ECG, serum digoxin levels, serum electrolytes

Implementation
- Arrange for serum digoxin concentration determinations before administration.
- Monitor continuously patient's cardiac response to digoxin overdose and therapy—cardiac rhythm, serum electrolytes, body temperature, BP.
- Maintain life-support equipment and emergency drugs (IV inotropes) on standby for severe overdose.
- Do not redigitalize patient until digoxin immune-fab has been cleared from the body; several days to a week or longer in cases of renal insufficiency. Serum digoxin levels will be very high and will be unreliable for up to 3 days after administration.

Drug-specific teaching points
- Report muscle cramps, dizziness, palpitations.

▢ dihydroergotamine mesylate

(dye hye droe er got' a meen)

DHE 45, Dihydroergotamine-Sandoz (CAN)

Pregnancy Category X

Drug classes
Ergot derivative
Antimigraine drug

Therapeutic actions
Mechanism of action not understood; constricts cranial blood vessels; decreases pulsation in cranial arteries and decreases hyperperfusion of basilar artery vascular bed.

Indications
- Rapid control of vascular headaches
- Prevention or abortion of vascular headaches when other routes of administration are not feasible (parenteral)

Contraindications/cautions
- Contraindicated in the presence of allergy to ergot preparations, peripheral vascular disease, severe hypertension, coronary artery disease, impaired liver or renal function, sepsis, pruritus, malnutrition, pregnancy.
- Use extreme caution if lactating.

Dosage
Adult: 1 mg IM at first sign of headache; repeat at 1-h intervals to a total of 3 mg. Use the minimum effective dose based on patient's experience. For IV use, administer up to a maximum of 2 mg; do not exceed 6 mg/wk.
Pediatric: Safety and efficacy not established.

Pharmacokinetics

Route	Onset	Peak	Duration
IM	15–30 min	2 h	3–4 h
IV	Immediate	1–2 h	3–4 h

Metabolism: Hepatic; $T_{1/2}$: 21–32 h
Distribution: Crosses placenta; enters breast milk
Excretion: Bile

IV facts
Preparation: No preparation necessary.
Infusion: Administer by direct IV injection, or inject into running IV. Administer a maximum of 2 mg.

Adverse effects
- **CNS:** *Numbness, tingling of fingers and toes*
- **GI:** *Nausea, vomiting*
- **CV:** Pulselessness, weakness in the legs; precordial distress and pain; transient tachycardia, bradycardia; localized

edema and itching; increased arterial pressure, arterial insufficiency, coronary vasoconstriction, bradycardia; hypoperfusion, chest pain, blood pressure changes, confusion
- **Other:** Muscle pain in the extremities; ergotism (nausea, vomiting, diarrhea, severe thirst); drug dependency and abuse with extended use

Clinically important drug-drug interactions
- Increased bioavailability of ergotamine if taken concurrently with nitroglycerin, nitrates • Increased risk of peripheral ischemia if taken concurrently with beta-blockers

■ Nursing Considerations
Assessment
- *History:* Allergy to ergot preparations, peripheral vascular disease, severe hypertension, coronary artery disease, impaired liver or renal function, sepsis, pruritus, malnutrition, pregnancy, lactation.
- *Physical:* Skin—color, edema, lesions; peripheral sensation; P, BP, peripheral pulses, peripheral perfusion; liver evaluation, bowel sounds; CBC, liver and renal function tests

Implementation
- Avoid prolonged administration or excessive dosage.
- Arrange for use of atropine or phenothiazine antiemetics if nausea and vomiting are severe.
- Assess extremities carefully to ensure there is no gangrene or decubitus ulcer formation.

Drug-specific teaching points
- Take this drug as soon as possible after the first symptoms of an attack.
- Know that the following side effects may occur: nausea, vomiting (if this becomes severe, medication may be ordered to help); numbness, tingling, loss of sensation in the extremities (use caution to avoid injury, and examine extremities daily to ensure that no injury has occurred).
- This drug cannot be taken during pregnancy; if you become pregnant or desire to become pregnant, consult with your physician.
- Report irregular heartbeat, pain or weakness of extremities, severe nausea or vomiting, numbness or tingling of fingers or toes.

☐ dihydroxyaluminum sodium carbonate

*(dye hi drox ee a **loo'** mi num)*
Rolaids Antacid

Pregnancy Category C

Drug classes
Antacid

Therapeutic actions
Neutralizes or reduces gastric acidity, resulting in an increase in the pH of the stomach and duodenal bulb and inhibiting the proteolytic activity of pepsin, protecting the lining of the stomach and duodenum.

Indications
- Symptomatic relief of upset stomach associated with hyperacidity
- Hyperacidity associated with peptic ulcer, gastritis, peptic esophagitis, gastric hyperacidity, and hiatal hernia

Contraindications/cautions
- Allergy to aluminum products.
- Use caution in the presence of gastric outlet obstruction (aluminum may inhibit gastric emptying); hypertension, CHF (sodium content is fairly high, especially extra strength suspension of aluminum carbonate); hypophosphatemia (aluminum decreases phosphate absorption); lactation.

Dosage
Adult: Chew 1–2 tablets as needed to relieve stomach upset.
Pediatric: Not recommended.

Adverse effects in *Italics* are most common; those in **Bold** are life-threatening.

Pharmacokinetics

Route	Onset
Oral	Varies

Metabolism: Hepatic metabolism
Distribution: With chronic use, small amounts may be absorbed systemically, cross the placenta, and enter breast milk
Excretion: GI bound in the feces

Adverse effects

- **GI:** *Constipation,* intestinal obstruction, decreased absorption of fluoride, accumulation of aluminum in serum, bone and CNS
- **MS:** Osteomalacia and chronic phosphate deficiency with bone pain, malaise, muscular weakness

Clinically important drug-drug interactions

• Do not administer other oral drugs within 1–2 h of antacid administration; change in gastric pH may interfere with absorption of oral drugs • Decreased pharmacologic effect of corticosteroids, difluinisal, digoxin, iron, isoniazid, penicillamine, phenothiazines, ranitidine, tetracyclines if given concomitantly • Increased pharmacologic effect of benzodiazepines if given concomitantly

■ Nursing Considerations

Assessment

- *History:* Allergy to aluminum products; gastric outlet obstruction; hypertension, CHF; hypophosphatemia; lactation
- *Physical:* Bone strength, muscle strength; P, auscultation, BP, peripheral edema; abdominal exam, bowel sounds; serum phosphorous, serum fluoride; bone x-ray is appropriate

Implementation

- Do not administer oral drugs within 1–2 h of antacid administration.
- Administer drug between meals and at bedtime.
- Monitor bowel function, and take appropriate action to establish bowel program if constipation occurs.

Drug-specific teaching points

- Take this drug between meals and at bedtime.
- Do not take this drug with any other oral medications; absorption of those medications can be inhibited; take other oral medications at least 1–2 h after aluminum salt.
- Know that constipation may occur as a result of drug therapy.
- Report constipation; bone pain, muscle weakness; coffee ground vomitus, black tarry stools; no relief from symptoms being treated.

▢ diltiazem hydrochloride

(dil tye' a zem)
Apo-Diltiaz (CAN), Cardizem, Cardizem CD, Cardizem SR, Dilacor XR, Novo-Diltazem (CAN), Nu-Diltiaz (CAN), Syn-Diltiazem (CAN)

Pregnancy Category C

Drug classes
Calcium channel-blocker
Antianginal drug
Antihypertensive

Therapeutic actions
Inhibits the movement of calcium ions across the membranes of cardiac and arterial muscle cells, which results in the depression of impulse formation in specialized cardiac pacemaker cells, slowing of the velocity of conduction of the cardiac impulse, depression of myocardial contractility, and dilation of coronary arteries and arterioles and peripheral arterioles; these effects lead to decreased cardiac work, decreased cardiac energy consumption, and in patients with vasospastic (Prinzmetal's) angina, increased delivery of oxygen to myocardial cells.

Indications
- Angina pectoris due to coronary artery spasm (Prinzmetal's variant angina)

Adverse effects in *Italics* are most common; those in **Bold** are life-threatening.

diltiazem hydrochloride

- Effort-associated angina; chronic stable angina in patients not controlled by beta-adrenergic blockers, nitrates
- Essential hypertension (sustained release)
- Paroxysmal supraventricular tachycardia (parenteral)

Contraindications/cautions

- Allergy to diltiazem, impaired hepatic or renal function, sick sinus syndrome, heart block (second or third degree), lactation.

Dosage

Careful patient assessment and evaluation are needed to determine the appropriate dose of this drug.
Adult: Initially 30 mg PO qid before meals and at bedtime; gradually increase dosage at 1- to 2-d intervals to 180–360 mg PO in three to four divided doses.

- ***Sustained release:*** *Cardizem SR:* Initially 60–120 mg PO bid; adjust dosage when maximum antihypertensive effect is achieved (around 14 d); optimum range is 240–360 mg/d. *Cardizem CD:* 180–240 mg qid PO for hypertension; 120–180 mg qd PO for angina. *Dilacor XR:* 180–240 mg qd PO as needed; up to 480 mg has been used.
- ***IV:*** Direct IV bolus—0.25 mg/kg (20 mg for the average patient); second bolus of 0.35 mg/kg. *Continuous IV infusion*: 5–10 mg/h with increases up to 15 mg/h; may be continued for up to 24 h.

Pediatric: Safety and efficacy not established.

Pharmacokinetics

Route	Onset	Peak
Oral	30–60 min	2–3 h
SR	30–60 min	6–11 h
IV	Immediate	2–3 min

Metabolism: Hepatic; $T_{1/2}$: 3½–6 h; 5–7 h (SR)
Distribution: Crosses placenta; enters breast milk
Excretion: Urine

IV facts

Preparation: For continuous infusion, transfer appropriate quantity to desired volume of Normal Saline, D5W, D5W/0.45% NaCl (see below). Mix thoroughly. Use within 24 h. Keep refrigerated until use.

Diluent Volume (ml)	Quantity of Injection	Final Conc (mg/ml)	Dose (mg/h)	Infusion Rate (ml/h)
100	125 mg (25 ml)	1	10	10
			15	15
250	250 mg (50 ml)	0.83	10	12
			15	18
500	250 mg (50 ml)	0.45	10	22
			15	33

Infusion: Administer bolus dose over 2 min. For continuous infusion, rate of 10 ml/h is the recommended rate. Do not use continuous infusion longer than 24 h.
Incompatibilities: Do not mix in the same solution with furosemide solution.

Adverse effects

- **CNS:** *Dizziness, lightheadedness, headache, asthenia,* fatigue
- **GI:** *Nausea,* hepatic injury
- **CV:** *Peripheral edema,* hypotension, arrhythmias, **bradycardia, AV block,** asystole
- **Dermatologic:** *Flushing,* rash

Clinically important drug-drug interactions

- Increased serum levels and toxicity of cyclosporine if taken concurrently with diltiazem

■ Nursing Considerations

Assessment

- *History:* Allergy to diltiazem, impaired hepatic or renal function, sick sinus syndrome, heart block, lactation
- *Physical:* Skin—lesions, color, edema; P, BP, baseline ECG, peripheral perfusion, auscultation; R, adventitious sounds; liver evaluation, normal output; liver and renal function tests, urinalysis

Implementation

- Monitor patient carefully (BP, cardiac rhythm, and output) while drug is being

Adverse effects in *Italics* are most common; those in **Bold** are life-threatening.

titrated to therapeutic dose; dosage may be increased more rapidly in hospitalized patients under close supervision.
- Monitor BP carefully if patient is on concurrent doses of nitrates.
- Monitor cardiac rhythm regularly during stabilization of dosage and periodically during long-term therapy.

Drug-specific teaching points
- Know that the following side effects may occur: nausea, vomiting (small, frequent meals may help); headache (monitor the lighting, noise, and temperature; medication may be ordered if this becomes severe).
- Report irregular heart beat, shortness of breath, swelling of the hands or feet, pronounced dizziness, constipation.

▢ dimenhydrate

(dye men hye' dri nate)

Oral preparations: Calm-X, Dimentabs, Dramamine, Gravol (CAN), Nauseatol (CAN), Travel Aid (CAN), Travel Eze (CAN), Travel Tabs (CAN)

Parenteral preparations: Dinate, Dramamine, Dramanate, Dramocen, Dramoject, Dymenate, Hydrate

Pregnancy Category B

Drug classes
Antimotionsickness drug (antihistamine, anticholinergic)

Therapeutic actions
Antihistamine with antiemetic and anticholinergic activity; depresses hyperstimulated labyrinthine function; probably acts at least partly by blocking synapses in the vomiting center; peripheral anticholinergic effects may contribute to antimotion sickness efficacy.

Indications
- Prevention and treatment of nausea, vomiting, or vertigo of motion sickness

Contraindications/cautions
- Contraindicated in the presence of allergy to dimenhydrinate or its components, lactation.
- Use caution in the presence of narrow-angle glaucoma, stenosing peptic ulcer, symptomatic prostatic hypertrophy, bronchial asthma, bladder neck obstruction, pyloroduodenal obstruction, cardiac arrhythmias.

Dosage
Adult
- **Oral:** 50–100 mg q4–6h PO; for prophylaxis, first dose should be taken $\frac{1}{2}$ h before exposure to motion. Do not exceed 400 mg in 24 h.
- **Parenteral:** 50 mg IM as needed; 50 mg in 10 ml Sodium Chloride Injection given IV over 10 min.

Pediatric
- *6–12 y:* 25–50 mg PO q6–8h, not to exceed 150 mg/24 h.
- *2–6 y:* Up to 25 mg PO q6–8h, not to exceed 75 mg/24 h.
- *< 2 y:* Only on advice of physician; 1.25 mg/kg IM qid, not to exceed 300 mg/24 h.
- *Neonates:* Not recommended.

Geriatric: More likely to cause dizziness, sedation, syncope, toxic confusional states and hypotension in elderly patients; use with caution.

Pharmacokinetics

Route	Onset	Peak	Duration
Oral	15–30 min	2 h	3–6 h
IM	20–30 min	1–2 h	3–6 h
IV	Immediate	1–2 h	3–6 h

Metabolism: Hepatic; $T_{1/2}$: unknown
Distribution: Crosses placenta; enters breast milk
Excretion: Urine

IV facts
Preparation: Dilute 50 mg in 10 ml Sodium Chloride Injection.
Infusion: Administer by direct IV injection over 2 min.

Adverse effects
- CNS: *Drowsiness, confusion, nervousness, restlessness, headache, dizziness, vertigo, lassitude, tingling, heaviness and weakness of hands; insomnia* and excitement (especially in children), hallucinations, convulsions, **death**, blurring of vision, diplopia
- GI: Epigastric distress, anorexia, nausea, vomiting, diarrhea or constipation; dryness of mouth, nose, and throat
- CV: Hypotension, palpitations, tachycardia
- Respiratory: Nasal stuffiness, chest tightness, thickening of bronchial secretions
- Dermatologic: Urticaria, drug rash, photosensitivity

Clinically important drug-drug interactions
- Increased depressant effects if taken concurrently with alcohol, other CNS depressants

■ Nursing Considerations

Assessment
- *History:* Allergy to dimenhydrinate or its components, lactation, narrow-angle glaucoma, stenosing peptic ulcer, symptomatic prostatic hypertrophy, bronchial asthma, bladder neck obstruction, pyloroduodenal obstruction, cardiac arrhythmias
- *Physical:* Skin—color, lesions, texture; orientation, reflexes, affect; vision exam; P, BP; R, adventitious sounds; bowel sounds; prostate palpation; CBC

Implementation
- Maintain epinephrine 1:1,000 readily available when using parenteral preparations; hypersensitivity reactions, including anaphylaxis, have occurred.

Drug-specific teaching points
- Take drug as prescribed; avoid excessive dosage.
- Use drug before motion sickness occurs; antimotion sickness drugs work best if used prophylactically.
- Know that the following side effects may occur: dizziness, sedation, drowsiness (use caution if driving or performing tasks that require alertness if these occur); epigastric distress, diarrhea or constipation (taking the drug with food may help); dry mouth (frequent mouth care, sucking sugarless lozenges may help); thickening of bronchial secretions, dryness of nasal mucosa (another type of motion sickness remedy may be preferable).
- Avoid alcohol while taking this drug; serious sedation could occur.
- Report difficulty breathing, hallucinations, tremors, loss of coordination, unusual bleeding or bruising, visual disturbances, irregular heartbeat.

dimercaprol

*(dye mer **kap'** role)*
BAL in Oil, British Anti-Lewisite

Pregnancy Category D

Drug classes
Antidote
Chelating agent

Therapeutic actions
Forms complexes with arsenic, gold, mercury, which increase the urinary and fecal elimination of these metals.

Indications
- Treatment of arsenic, gold, and mercury poisoning
- Acute lead poisoning when used with calcium edetate disodium
- Acute mercury poisoning if therapy is begun within 1–2 h

Contraindications/cautions
- Contraindicated in the presence of hepatic insufficiency; iron, cadmium, or selenium poisoning.

Dosage
Adult
- ***Mild arsenic or gold poisoning:*** 2.5 mg/kg qid IM for 2 d, then two times

on the third day; once daily thereafter for 10 d.
- **Severe arsenic or gold poisoning:** 3 mg/kg q4h IM for 2 d, then four times on the third day, then bid for 10 d.
- **Mercury poisoning:** 5 mg/kg IM followed by 2.5 mg/kg one to two times per day for 10 d.
- **Acute lead encephalopathy:** 3–4 mg/kg IM and then at 4-h intervals in combination with calcium edetate disodium. Maintain treatment for 2–7 d.

Pediatric: Same dosage as adults, but use caution—fever and decreased white cells may occur.

Pharmacokinetics

Route	Onset	Peak	Duration
IM	Rapid	30–60 min	3–4 h

Metabolism: Hepatic; $T_{1/2}$: short
Distribution: Crosses placenta; may enter breast milk
Excretion: Feces and urine

Adverse effects
- GI: *Nausea, vomiting,* burning of lips and throat, salivation, abdominal pain, anxiety, weakness, unrest
- CNS: *Headache,* conjunctivitis, lacrimation, tingling of hands
- CV: *Rise in BP, tachycardia*
- Other: Burning sensation in penis, sweating of forehead and hands, feeling of constriction in chest, throat, *pain at site of injection,* **renal damage**

Clinically important drug-drug interactions
- Increased risk of toxicity if taken with iron

■ Nursing Considerations

Assessment
- *History:* Hepatic insufficiency; iron, cadmium or selenium poisoning
- *Physical:* Skin—color, edema, lesions; peripheral sensation; P, BP, abdominal exam; CBC, liver function tests, serum levels of heavy metals

Implementation
- Administer by deep IM injection only.
- Begin therapy as soon as possible after poisoning.
- Monitor BP and P when treatment has begun, increased BP and P can occur.
- Alkalinize urine to increase excretion of chelated complex.
- Monitor intake and output to detect any alteration in renal function.

Drug-specific teaching points
- Know that treatment will need to be continued for 2–10 d, as appropriate. Drug can be given only IM.
- Know that the following side effects may occur: nausea, vomiting (if this becomes severe, medication may be ordered to help); numbness, tingling, loss of sensation in the extremities (use caution to avoid injury, and examine extremities daily to ensure that no injury has occurred); headache; pain at site of injection.
- Report irregular heartbeat, pain or weakness of extremities, severe nausea or vomiting, severe pain at injection site; changes in voiding patterns.

☐ dinoprostone

*(dye noe **prost**' one)*
prostaglandin E_2
Prepidil Gel (CAN), Prostin E2

Pregnancy Category C

Drug classes
Prostaglandin
Abortifacient

Therapeutic actions
Stimulates the myometrium of the pregnant uterus to contract, similar to the contractions of the uterus during labor, thus evacuating the contents of the uterus.

Indications
- Termination of pregnancy 12–20 wk from the first day of the last menstrual period

Adverse effects in *Italics* are most common; those in **Bold** are life-threatening.

dinoprostone

- Evacuation of the uterus in the management of missed abortion or intrauterine fetal death up to 28 wk gestational age
- Management of nonmetastatic gestational trophoblastic disease (benign hydatidiform mole)
- **Unlabeled use:** induction of labor, initiation of cervical ripening (low dose, 3-mg vaginal suppositories)

Contraindications/cautions
- Contraindicated in the presence of allergy to prostaglandin preparations, acute pelvic inflammatory disease, active cardiac, hepatic, pulmonary, renal disease.
- Use caution in the presence of history of asthma; hypotension; hypertension; cardiovascular, adrenal, renal, or hepatic disease; anemia; jaundice; diabetes; epilepsy; scarred uterus; cervicitis, infected endocervical lesions, acute vaginitis.

Dosage
Available as vaginal suppository only.
Adult: Insert one suppository (20 mg) high into the vagina; patient should remain supine for 10 min following insertion. Additional suppositories may be administered at 3- to 5-h intervals based on uterine response and patient tolerance. Do not administer longer than 2 d.

Pharmacokinetics

Route	Onset	Peak	Duration
Intravaginal	10 min	15 min	2–3 h

Metabolism: Tissue; $T_{1/2}$: 5–10 h
Distribution: Crosses placenta; enters breast milk
Excretion: Urine

Adverse effects
- **CNS:** *Headache,* paresthesias, anxiety, weakness, syncope, dizziness
- **GI:** *Vomiting, diarrhea, nausea*
- **CV:** *Hypotension,* arrhythmias, chest pain
- **Respiratory:** Coughing, dyspnea
- **GU:** Endometritis, perforated uterus, uterine rupture, uterine or vaginal pain, incomplete abortion
- **Other:** Chills, diaphoresis, backache, breast tenderness, eye pain, skin rash, pyrexia

■ Nursing Considerations

Assessment
- *History:* Allergy to prostaglandin preparations; acute PID; active cardiac, hepatic, pulmonary, renal disease; history of asthma; hypotension; hypertension; anemia; jaundice; diabetes; epilepsy; scarred uterus; cervicitis, infected endocervical lesions, acute vaginitis
- *Physical:* Body temperature; BP, P, auscultation; R, adventitious sounds; bowel sounds, liver evaluation; vaginal discharge, pelvic exam, uterine tone; liver and renal function tests, WBC, urinalysis, CBC

Implementation
- Administer as vaginal suppository only.
- Store vaginal suppositories in freezer; bring to room temperature before insertion.
- Arrange for pretreatment or concurrent treatment with antiemetic and antidiarrheal drugs to decrease the incidence of GI side effects.
- Ensure that abortion is complete or that other measures are used to complete the abortion if drug effects are not sufficient.
- Monitor body temperature, using care to differentiate prostaglandin-induced pyrexia from postabortion endometritis pyrexia.
- Monitor uterine tone and vaginal discharge throughout procedure and several days after the procedure to assess drug effects and recovery.
- Ensure adequate hydration throughout procedure.

Drug-specific teaching points
Teaching about dinoprostone should be incorporated into the total teaching plan for the patient undergoing the abortion; specific information that should be included follows:
- If the patient has never had a vaginal suppository, explain the administration

Adverse effects in *Italics* are most common; those in **Bold** are life-threatening.

procedure and tell her she will need to lie down for 10 min after insertion.
- Know that the following side effects may occur: nausea, vomiting, diarrhea, uterine or vaginal pain, fever, headache, weakness, dizziness.
- Report severe pain, difficulty breathing, palpitations, eye pain, rash.

▫ diphenhydramine hydrochloride

(dye fen hye' dra meen)

Oral: Beldin, Benadryl, Benylin Cough, Bydramine, Compoz, Diphen Cough, Dormarex 2, Nervine, Nytol, Sleep-Eze 3, Sominex 2

Oral prescription preparations: Benadryl

Parenteral preparations: Benadryl, Benahist, Benoject, Diphenacen

Pregnancy Category B

Drug classes
Antihistamine (ethanolamine type)
Antimotionsickness drug
Sedative
Antiparkinsonism drug
Cough suppressant

Therapeutic actions
Competitively blocks the effects of histamine at H_1 receptor sites, has atropine-like, antipruritic, and sedative effects.

Indications
- Symptomatic relief of symptoms associated with perennial and seasonal allergic rhinitis; vasomotor rhinitis; allergic conjunctivitis; mild, uncomplicated urticaria and angioedema; amelioraton of allergic reactions to blood or plasma; dermatographism; adjunctive therapy in anaphylactic reactions
- Active and prophylactic treatment of motion sickness
- Nighttime sleep aid
- Parkinsonism (including drug-induced parkinsonism and extrapyramidal reactions) in the elderly intolerant of more potent agents, for milder forms of the disorder in other age groups, and in combination with centrally acting anticholinergic antiparkinsonism drugs
- Suppression of cough due to colds or allergy (syrup formulation)

Contraindications/cautions
- Contraindicated in the presence of allergy to any antihistamines, third trimester of pregnancy, lactation.
- Use caution in the presence of narrow-angle glaucoma, stenosing peptic ulcer, symptomatic prostatic hypertrophy, asthmatic attack, bladder neck obstruction, pyloroduodenal obstruction, pregnancy.

Dosage
Adult
- **Oral:** 25–50 mg q4–6h PO.
  – *Motion sickness:* Give full dose prophylactically ½ h before exposure to motion, and repeat before meals and at bedtime.
  – *Nighttime sleep aid:* 50 mg PO at bedtime.
  – *Cough suppression:* 25 mg q4h PO, not to exceed 150 mg in 24 h.
- **Parenteral:** 10–50 mg IV or deep IM or up to 100 mg if required. Maximum daily dose is 400 mg.

Pediatric (> 10 kg, 20 lb)
- **Oral:** 12.5–25 mg tid–qid PO or 5 mg/kg per day PO or 150 mg/m² per day PO. Maximum daily dose 300 mg.
  – *Motion sickness:* Give full dose prophylactically ½ h before exposure to motion and repeat before meals and at bedtime.
  – *Cough suppression (6–12 y):* 12.5 mg q4h PO, not to exceed 75 mg in 24 h. *2–6 y:* 6.25 mg q4h, not to exceed 25 mg in 24 h.
- **Parenteral:** 5 mg/kg per day or 150 mg/m² per day IV or by deep IM injection. Maximum daily dose is 300 mg divided into four doses.

Geriatric: More likely to cause dizziness, sedation, syncope, toxic confusional states, and hypotension in elderly patients; use with caution.

Pharmacokinetics

Route	Onset	Peak	Duration
Oral	15–30 min	1–4 h	4–7 h
IM	20–30 min	1–4 h	4–8 h
IV	Rapid	30–60 min	4–8 h

Metabolism: Hepatic; $T_{1/2}$: 2.5–7 h
Distribution: Crosses placenta; enters breast milk
Excretion: Urine

IV facts
Preparation: No additional preparation required.
Infusion: Administer slowly by direct injection or into tubing of running IV.

Adverse effects
- **CNS:** *Drowsiness, sedation, dizziness, disturbed coordination*, fatigue, confusion, restlessness, excitation, nervousness, tremor, headache, blurred vision, diplopia
- **GI:** *Epigastric distress*, anorexia, increased appetite and weight gain, nausea, vomiting, diarrhea or constipation
- **CV:** Hypotension, palpitations, bradycardia, tachycardia, extra systoles
- **Respiratory:** *Thickening of bronchial secretions*, chest tightness, wheezing, nasal stuffiness, dry mouth, dry nose, dry throat, sore throat
- **Hematologic:** Hemolytic anemia, hypoplastic anemia, thrombocytopenia, leukopenia, agranulocytosis, pancytopenia
- **GU:** Urinary frequency, dysuria, urinary retention, early menses, decreased libido, impotence
- **Other:** Urticaria, rash, **anaphylactic shock**, photosensitivity, excessive perspiration

Clinically important drug-drug interactions
- Possible increased and prolonged anticholinergic effects if taken with MAO inhibitors

■ Nursing Considerations
Assessment
- *History:* Allergy to any antihistamines, narrow-angle glaucoma, stenosing peptic ulcer, symptomatic prostatic hypertrophy, asthmatic attack, bladder neck obstruction, pyloroduodenal obstruction, third trimester of pregnancy, lactation
- *Physical:* Skin—color, lesions, texture; orientation, reflexes, affect; vision exam; P, BP; R, adventitious sounds; bowel sounds; prostate palpation; CBC with differential

Implementation
- Administer with food if GI upset occurs.
- Administer syrup form if patient is unable to take tablets.
- Monitor patient response, and arrange for adjustment of dosage to lowest possible effective dose.

Drug-specific teaching points
- Take as prescribed; avoid excessive dosage.
- Take with food if GI upset occurs.
- Know that the following side effects may occur: dizziness, sedation, drowsiness (use caution if driving or performing tasks that require alertness if these occur); epigastric distress, diarrhea or constipation (taking the drug with meals may help); dry mouth (frequent mouth care, sucking sugarless lozenges may help); thickening of bronchial secretions, dryness of nasal mucosa (use of a humidifier may help if this becomes a problem).
- Avoid alcohol while on this drug; serious sedation could occur.
- Report difficulty breathing, hallucinations, tremors, loss of coordination, unusual bleeding or bruising, visual disturbances, irregular heartbeat.

❒ diphenidol

*(di **phen'** i dol)*
Vontrol

Pregnancy Category C

Drug classes
Antiemetic
Antivertigo

Adverse effects in *Italics* are most common; those in **Bold** are life-threatening.

Therapeutic actions
Acts specifically on the vestibular apparatus to control vertigo; works on the CTZ to control nausea and vomiting.

Indications
- Labryinthine vertigo and associated nausea and vomiting; Meniere's disease; middle and inner ear surgery
- Control of nausea and vomiting in postoperative states, malignant neoplasms, and labyrinthine disorders

Contraindications/cautions
- Contraindicated in the presence of allergy to diphenidol, tartrazine sensitivity, anuria, nausea and vomiting of pregnancy.
- Use caution in the presence of glaucoma, obstructive lesion of the GI or GU tract, organic cardiospasm.

Dosage
Adult: 25 mg qid PO; up to 50 mg qid may be used.
Pediatric: 0.4 mg/lb (0.88 mg/kg); usual dose is 25 mg PO. Do not give more than q4h. Do not exceed 2.5 mg/lb per 24 h.

Pharmacokinetics

Route	Onset	Peak
Oral	Slow	1½–3 h

Metabolism: Hepatic; $T_{1/2}$: 4 h
Distribution: May cross placenta; enters breast milk
Excretion: Urine

Adverse effects
- **CNS:** Auditory and visual hallucinations; disorientation; confusion; drowsiness; overstimulation; depression; sleep disturbance; blurred vision, dizziness, malaise
- **GI:** *Dry mouth,* nausea, indigestion, heartburn
- **CV:** Slight, transient lowering of blood pressure
- **Dermatologic:** Skin rash

■ Nursing Considerations
Assessment
- *History:* Allergy to diphenidol, tartrazine sensitivity, anuria, nausea and vomiting of pregnancy, glaucoma, obstructive lesion of the GI or GU tract, organic cardiospasm
- *Physical:* Skin—lesions, color; orientation, affect, reflexes, vision; P, BP, renal function tests

Implementation
- Monitor patient closely during administration; hallucinations or confusion are common. Should be used only in patients who are hospitalized or constantly monitored.
- Administer drug with meals if GI upset occurs.

Drug-specific teaching points
- Take the drug with food if GI upset occurs.
- Know that the following side effects may occur: nausea, dry mouth (taking the drug with meals may help); hallucinations, disorientation, confusion, drowsiness (do not drive or try to participate in any activities that could be dangerous; someone should be with you at all times).
- Report hallucinations, visual changes, rash.

▢ dipyridamole

(dye peer id' a mole)
Persantine, Persantine IV

Pregnancy Category B

Drug classes
Antianginal drug
Antiplatelet drug

Therapeutic actions
Decreases coronary vascular resistance and increases coronary blood flow without increasing myocardial oxygen consumption; inhibits platelet aggregation.

Indications
- "Possibly effective" for long-term therapy of angina pectoris; use withdrawn by the FDA; further hearings are pending

dipyridamole

- With warfarin to prevent thromboembolism in patients with prosthetic heart valves
- Unlabeled use: prevention of myocardial reinfarction or reduction of mortality post-MI
- Unlabeled use: with aspirin to prevent coronary bypass graft occlusion
- IV use: diagnostic aid in evaluation of CAD in patients who cannot exercise, as an alternative to exercise in thallium myocardial perfusion imaging studies

Contraindications/cautions
- Contraindicated in the presence of allergy to dipyridamole, pregnancy, lactation.
- Use caution in the presence of hypotension (drug can cause peripheral vasodilation that could exacerbate hypotension).

Dosage
Adult
- ***Angina:*** 50 mg tid PO at least 1 h before meals. Clinical response may not be evident before second or third month of therapy.
- ***Prophylaxis in thromboembolism following cardiac valve surgery:*** 75–100 mg qid PO as an adjunct to warfarin therapy.
- ***Diagnostic agent in thallium myocardial perfusion imaging:*** 0.142 mg/kg per minute (0.57 mg total) infused over 4 min. Inject thallium-201 within 5 min following the 4-min infusion of dipyridamole.

Pharmacokinetics

Route	Onset	Peak	Duration
Oral	Varies	75 min	3–4 h
IV	Rapid	6.5 min	30 min

Metabolism: Hepatic; $T_{1/2}$: 40 min, then 10 h
Distribution: Crosses placenta; enters breast milk
Excretion: Bile

IV facts
Preparation: Dilute dose based on weight in at least a 1:2 ration with 0.5N Sodium Chloride Injection, 1N Sodium Chloride Injection, or 5% Dextrose Injection for a total volume of about 20–50 ml. Protect from direct light.
Infusion: Infuse slowly over 4 min. Do not infuse undiluted drug; local irritation can occur.

Adverse effects
- CNS: *Headache, dizziness,* weakness, syncope, flushing
- GI: Nausea, *GI distress,* constipation, diarrhea
- CV: **Fatal and nonfatal MI, ventricular fibrillation** (IV)
- Respiratory: **Bronchospasm** (IV)
- GU: Possible decreased fertility and loss of eggs in women
- Dermatologic: *Skin rash,* pruritus
- Local: Pain and burning at injection site

Clinically important drug-drug interactions
- Decreased coronary vasodilation effects if IV use with theophylline

■ Nursing Considerations

Assessment
- *History:* Allergy to dipyridamole, hypotension, lactation
- *Physical:* Skin—color, temperature, lesions; orientation, reflexes, affect; P, BP, orthostatic BP, baseline ECG, peripheral perfusion; R, adventitious sounds

Implementation
- Provide continual monitoring of ECG, BP, and orientation during administration of IV dipyridamole.
- Administer at least 1 h before meals with a full glass of fluid.

Drug-specific teaching points
- Take dipyridamole at least 1 h before meals with a full glass of fluid.
- Know that the following side effects may occur: dizziness, lightheadedness (this may pass as you adjust to the drug; use care to change positions slowly; lie down or sit down when you take your dose to decrease the risk of falling); headache

---

Adverse effects in *Italics* are most common; those in **Bold** are life-threatening.

(lying down in a cool environment and resting may help; OTC preparations may help); flushing of the neck or face (this usually passes as the drug's effects pass); nausea, gastric distress (small, frequent meals may help).
- Report skin rash, chest pain, fainting, severe headache; pain at injection site (IV).

disopyramide phosphate

*(dye soe **peer**' a mide)*
Norpace, Norpace CR, Rythmodan (CAN)

Pregnancy Category C

Drug classes
Antiarrhythmic

Therapeutic actions
Type 1a antiarrhythmic: decreases rate of diastolic depolarization, decreases automaticity, decreases the rate of rise of the action potential, prolongs the refractory period of cardiac muscle cells.

Indications
- Treatment of documented ventricular arrhythmias considered to be life threatening
- **Unlabeled use**: treatment of paroxysmal supraventricular tachycardia

Contraindications/cautions
- Allergy to disopyramide, congestive heart failure, hypotension, cardiac conduction abnormalities (eg, Wolff-Parkinson-White syndrome, sick sinus syndrome, heart block), cardiac myopathies, urinary retention, glaucoma, myasthenia gravis, renal or hepatic disease, potassium imbalance, pregnancy, lactation.

Dosage
Careful patient assessment and evaluation with close monitoring of cardiac response are necessary for determining the correct dosage for each patient.

Adult: 400–800 mg/d PO given in divided doses q6h or q12h if using the controlled-release products.
Pediatric: Give in equal, divided doses q6h PO, titrating the dose to the patient's need.

Age	Daily Dosage
<1 y	10–30 mg/kg
1–4 y	10–20 mg/kg
4–12 y	10–15 mg/kg
12–18 y	6–15 mg/kg

Geriatric: Loading dose of 150 mg PO may be given, followed by 100 mg at the intervals shown.

Creatinine Clearance	Interval
40–30 ml/min	q8h
30–15 ml/min	q12h
<15 ml/min	q24h

Pharmacokinetics

Route	Onset	Peak	Duration
Oral	30–60 min	2 h	1.5–8.5 h

Metabolism: Hepatic; $T_{1/2}$: 4–10 h
Distribution: Crosses placenta; enters breast milk
Excretion: Urine

Adverse effects
- **CNS**: Dizziness, fatigue, headache, *blurred vision*
- **CV**: Congestive heart failure, hypotension, cardiac conduction disturbances
- **GI**: *Dry mouth, constipation,* nausea, abdominal pain, gas
- **GU**: *Urinary hesitancy and retention, impotence*
- **Other**: *Dry mose, eyes, and throat;* rash; itching; *muscle weakness; malaise; aches and pains*

Clinically important drug-drug interactions
- Decreased disopyramide plasma levels if used with phenytoins, rifampin

■ Nursing Considerations
Assessment
- *History:* Allergy to disopyramide, CHF, hypotension, Wolff-Parkinson-White syn-

---
Adverse effects in *Italics* are most common; those in **Bold** are life-threatening.

drome, sick sinus syndrome, heart block, cardiac myopathies, urinary retention, glaucoma, myasthenia gravis, renal or hepatic disease, potassium imbalance, labor or delivery, lactation
- **Physical:** Weight; orientation, reflexes; P, BP, auscultation, ECG, edema; R, adventitious sounds; bowel sounds, liver evaluation; urinalysis, renal and liver function tests, blood glucose, serum K^+

Implementation

- Check that patients with supraventricular tachyarrhythmias have been digitalized before starting disopyramide.
- Reduce dosage in patients less than 110 lb.
- Reduce dosage in patients with hepatic or renal failure.
- Monitor continuously patients with severe refractory tachycardia who may be given up to 1,600 mg/d.
- Make a pediatric suspension form (1–10 mg/ml) by adding the contents of the immediate release capsule to cherry syrup, NF if desired. Store in dark bottle, and refrigerate. Shake well before using. Stable for 1 mo.
- Take care to differentiate the controlled release form from the immediate-release preparation.
- Monitor blood pressure, orthostatic pressure.
- Evaluate for safe and effective serum levels (2–8 μg/ml).

Drug-specific teaching points

- Know that you will require frequent monitoring of cardiac rhythm, blood pressure.
- Know that the following side effects may occur: dry mouth (frequent mouth care, sucking sugarless lozenges may help); constipation (laxatives may be ordered); difficulty voiding (emptying the bladder before taking the drug may help); muscle weakness or aches and pains.
- Do not stop taking this drug for any reason without checking with your health care provider.
- Return for regular follow-up visits to check your heart rhythm and blood pressure.
- Report swelling of fingers or ankles, difficulty breathing, dizziness, urinary retention, severe headache or visual changes.

▢ disulfiram

(dye sul' fi ram)
Antabuse
Pregnancy Category C

Drug classes
Antialcoholic
Enzyme inhibitor

Therapeutic actions
Inhibits the enzyme aldehyde dehydrogenase, blocking oxidation of alcohol and allowing acetaldehyde to accumulate to concentrations in the blood 5–10 times higher than normally achieved during alcohol metabolism; accumulation of acetaldehyde produces the highly unpleasant reaction described below that deters consumption of alcohol.

Indications

- Aids in the management of selected chronic alcoholics who want to remain in a state of enforced sobriety

Contraindications/cautions

- Contraindicated in the presence of allergy to disulfiram or other thiuram derivatives used in pesticides and rubber vulcanization, severe myocardial disease or coronary occlusion; psychoses, current or recent treatment with metrondiazole, paraldehyde, alcohol, alcohol-containing preparations (eg, cough syrups, tonics).
- Use caution in the presence of diabetes mellitus, hypothyroidism, epilepsy, cerebral damage, chronic and acute nephritis, hepatic cirrhosis or dysfunction.

Dosage
Never administer to an intoxicated patient or without the patient's knowledge. Do not administer until patient has abstained from alcohol for at least 12 h.

Adult
- **Initial dosage:** Administer maximum of 500 mg/d PO in a single dose

for 1–2 wk. If a sedative effect occurs, administer at bedtime or decrease dosage.
- ***Maintenance regimen:*** 125–500 mg/d PO. Do not exceed 500 mg/d. Continue use until patient is fully recovered socially and a basis for permanent self-control is established.
- ***Trial with alcohol (do not administer to anyone > 50 y):*** After 1–2 wk of therapy with 500 mg/d PO, a drink of 15 ml of 100 proof whiskey or its equivalent is taken slowly. Dose may be repeated once, if patient is hospitalized and supportive facilities are available.

Pharmacokinetics

Route	Onset	Peak	Duration
Oral	Slow	12 h	1–2 wk

Metabolism: Hepatic; $T_{1/2}$: unclear
Distribution: Crosses placenta; enters breast milk
Excretion: Feces, lungs

Adverse effects
- Disulfiram-alcohol reaction: Flushing, throbbing in head and neck, throbbing headaches, respiratory difficulty, nausea, copious vomiting, sweating, thirst, chest pain, palpitations, dyspnea, hyperventilation, tachycardia, hypotension, syncope, weakness, vertigo, blurred vision, confusion; severe reactions may include arrhythmias, cardiovascular collapse, acute congestive heart failure, unconsciousness, convulsions, myocardial infarction, **death**

Adverse Effects of Disulfiram Alone
- **CNS:** *Drowsiness, fatigability, headache,* restlessness, peripheral neuropathy, optic or retrobulbar neuritis
- **GI:** *Metallic or garliclike aftertaste,* hepatotoxicity
- **Dermatologic:** *Skin eruptions,* anceiform eruptions, allergic dermatitis

Clinically important drug-drug interactions
- Increased serum levels and risk of toxicity of phenytoin and its congeners, diazepam, chlordiazepoxide • Increased therapeutic and toxic effects of theophyllines if taken concurrently with disulfiram • Increased prothrombin time caused by disulfiram may lead to a need to adjust dosage of oral anticoagulants • Severe alcohol-intolerance reactions if taken with any alcohol-containing liquid medications (eg, elixirs, tinctures) • Acute toxic psychosis if taken concurrently with metronidazole

■ Nursing Considerations
Assessment
- *History:* Allergy to disulfiram or other thiuram derivatives; severe myocardial disease or coronary occlusion; psychoses; current or recent treatment with metronidazole, paraldehyde, alcohol, alcohol-containing preparations (eg, cough syrups, tonics); diabetes mellitus, hypothyroidism, epilepsy, cerebral damage, chronic and acute nephritis, hepatic cirrhosis or dysfunction
- *Physical:* Skin—color, lesions; thyroid palpation; orientation, affect, reflexes; P, auscultation, BP ; R, adventitious sounds; liver evaluation; renal and liver function tests, CBC, SMA-12

Implementation
- Do not administer until patient has abstained from alcohol for at least 12 h.
- Administer orally; tablets may be crushed and mixed with liquid beverages.
- Arrange to monitor liver function tests before beginning therapy, in 10–14 d, and every 6 mo during therapy to evaluate for hepatic dysfunction.
- Arrange to monitor CBC, SMA-12 before beginning therapy and every 6 mo during therapy.
- Inform patient of the seriousness of disulfiram-alcohol reaction and the potential consequences of alcohol use: disulfiram should not be taken for at least 12 h after alcohol ingestion, and a reaction may occur up to 2 wk after disulfiram therapy is stopped; all forms of alcohol must be avoided.
- Arrange for treatment with antihistamines if skin reaction occurs.

Adverse effects in *Italics* are most common; those in **Bold** are life-threatening.

Drug-specific teaching points
- Take drug daily; if drug makes you dizzy or tired, take it at bedtime. Tablets may be crushed and mixed with liquid.
- Abstain from forms of alcohol (eg, beer, wine, liquor, vinegars, cough mixtures, sauces, aftershave lotions, liniments, colognes). Taking alcohol while on this drug can cause severe, unpleasant reactions—flushing, copious vomiting, throbbing headache, difficulty breathing, even death.
- Wear or carry a medical identification alert while you are on this drug to notify any medical personnel who may care for you in an emergency that you are on this drug.
- Arrange to have periodic blood tests while on this drug to evaluate its effects on the liver.
- Know that the following side effects may occur: drowsiness, headache, fatigue, restlessness, blurred vision (use caution if driving or performing tasks that require alertness if this occurs); metallic aftertaste (this usually passes after the first few weeks of therapy).
- Report unusual bleeding or bruising, yellowing of skin or eyes, chest pain, difficulty breathing, ingestion of any alcohol.

❒ dobutamine hydrochloride

(doe' byoo ta meen)
Dobutrex

Pregnancy Category C

Drug classes
Sympathomimetic drug
Beta-1 adrenergic agonist

Therapeutic actions
Positive inotropic effects are mediated by beta-1 adrenergic receptors in the heart; increases the force of myocardial contraction with relatively minor effects on heart rate, arrhythmogenesis; has minor effects on blood vessels.

Indications
- For inotropic support in the short-term treatment of adults with cardiac decompensation due to depressed contractility, resulting from either organic heart disease or from cardiac surgical procedures
- Investigational use in children with congenital heart disease undergoing diagnostic cardiac catheterization, to augment cardiovascular function

Contraindications/cautions
- Contraindicated in the presence of IHSS; hypovolemia (dobutamine is not a substitute for blood, plasma, fluids, electrolytes, which should be restored promptly when loss has occurred and in any case before treatment with dobutamine); acute myocardial infarction (may increase the size of an infarct by intensifying ischemia); general anesthesia with halogenated hydrocarbons or cyclopropane, which sensitize the myocardium to catecholamines.
- Use caution in the presence of diabetes, lactation.

Dosage
Administer only by IV infusion. Rate of administration is titrated on the basis of the patient's hemodynamic/renal response. Close monitoring is necessary.
Adult: 2.5–10 μg/kg/min IV is usual rate of administration to increase cardiac output; rarely, rates up to 40 μg/kg per minute are needed.
Pediatric: Safety and efficacy not established. When used investigationally in children undergoing cardiac catheterization (see above), doses of 2.0 and 7.75 μg/kg per minute were infused for 10 min.

Pharmacokinetics

Route	Onset	Peak	Duration
IV	1–2 min	10 min	Length of infusion

Metabolism: Hepatic; $T_{1/2}$: 2 min
Distribution: Crosses placenta; enters breast milk
Excretion: Urine

dopamine hydrochloride ■ 405

IV facts

Preparation: Reconstitute by adding 10 ml Sterile Water for Injection or 5% Dextrose Injection to 250-mg vial. If material is not completely dissolved, add 10 ml of diluent. Further dilute to at least 50 ml with 5% Dextrose Injection, 0.9% Sodium Chloride Injection, or Sodium Lactate Injection before administering. Store reconstituted solution under refrigeration for 48 h or at room temperature for 6 h. Store final diluted solution for infusion in glass or Viaflex container at room temperature. Stable for 24 h. Do not freeze. (Note: drug solutions may exhibit a color that increases with time; this indicates oxidation of the drug, not a loss of potency.)

Infusion: May be administered through common IV tubing with dopamine, lidocaine, tobramycin, nitroprusside, potassium chloride, or protamine sulfate.

Incompatibilities: Do *not* mix drug with alkaline solutions, such as 5% Sodium Bicarbonate Injection; do *not* mix with hydrocortisone sodium succinate, cefazolin, cefamandole, neutral cephalothin, penicillin, sodium ethacrynate; sodium heparin.

Adverse effects

- CNS: *Headache*
- GI: *Nausea*
- CV: *Increase in heart rate, increase in systolic blood pressure, increase in ventricular ectopic beats (PVCs)*, anginal pain, palpitations, shortness of breath

Clinically important drug-drug interactions

• Increased effects when given with TCAs (eg, imipramine), furazolidone, methyldopa • Risk of severe hypertension if taken concurrently with rauwolfia alkaloids, beta-blockers (alseroxylon, deserpidine, rescinnamine, reserpine) • Decreased effects of guanethidine if taken with dobutamine

■ Nursing Considerations

Assessment

- *History:* IHSS, hypovolemia, acute MI, general anesthesia with halogenated hydrocarbons or cyclopropane, diabetes, lactation
- *Physical:* Body weight, skin—color, temperature; P, BP, pulse pressure, auscultation; R, adventitious sounds; urine output; serum electrolytes, Hct, ECG

Implementation

- Arrange to digitalize patients who have atrial fibrillation with a rapid ventricular rate before giving dobutamine—dobutamine facilitates AV conduction.
- Monitor urine flow, cardiac output, pulmonary wedge pressure, ECG, and blood pressure closely during infusion.

Drug-specific teaching points

- Because this drug is used only in acute emergency care situations, teaching will depend on patient's awareness and will relate primarily to the indication for the drug rather than to the drug itself.

❒ dopamine hydrochloride

(doe' pa meen)
Intropin, Revimine (CAN)

Pregnancy Category C

Drug classes

Sympathomimetic drug
Alpha-adrenergic agonist
Beta-1 adrenergic agonist
Dopaminergic agonist

Therapeutic actions

Drug acts directly and by the release of norepinephrine from sympathetic nerve terminals; dopaminergic receptors mediate dilation of vessels in the renal and splanchnic beds, which maintains renal perfusion and function; alpha receptors, which are activated by higher doses of dopamine, mediate vasoconstriction, which can override the vasodilating effects; beta-1 receptors mediate a positive inotropic effect on the heart.

Adverse effects in *Italics* are most common; those in **Bold** are life-threatening.

dopamine hydrochloride

Indications
- Correction of hemodynamic imbalances present in the shock syndrome due to MI, trauma, endotoxic septicemia, open heart surgery, renal failure, and chronic cardiac decompensation in congestive failure

Contraindications/cautions
- Contraindicated in the presence of pheochromocytoma, tachyarrhythmias, ventricular fibrillation, hypovolemia (dopamine is not a substitute for blood, plasma, fluids, electrolytes, which should be restored promptly when loss has occurred), general anesthesia with halogenated hydrocarbons or cyclopropane, which sensitize the myocardium to catecholamines.
- Use caution in the presence of atherosclerosis, arterial embolism, Reynaud's disease, cold injury, frostbite, diabetic endarteritis, Buerger's disease (closely monitor skin color and temperature of the extremities).

Dosage
Dilute before using; administer only by IV infusion, using a metering device to control the rate of flow. Rate of administration is titrated on the basis of the patient's hemodynamic/renal response. Close monitoring is necessary. In titrating to the desired systolic blood pressure response, the optimum administration rate for renal response may be exceeded, thus necessitating a reduction in rate after hemodynamic stabilization.

Adult
- ***Patients likely to respond to modest increments of cardiac contractility and renal perfusion:*** Initially, 2–5 µg/kg per min IV.
- ***Patients who are more seriously ill:*** Initially, 5 µg/kg per min IV. Increase in increments of 5–10 µg/kg per minute up to a rate of 20–50 µg/kg per minute. Check urine output frequently if doses > 16 µg/kg per minute are needed.

Pediatric: Safety and efficacy not established.

Pharmacokinetics

Route	Onset	Peak	Duration
IV	1–2 min	10 min	Length of infusion

Metabolism: Hepatic; $T_{1/2}$: 2 min
Distribution: Crosses placenta; enters breast milk
Excretion: Urine

IV facts
Preparation: Prepare solution for IV infusion as follows: Add 200–400 mg dopamine to 250–500 ml of one of the following IV solutions: Sodium Chloride Injection; 5% Dextrose Injection; 5% Dextrose and 0.45% or 0.9% Sodium Chloride Solution; 5% Dextrose in Lactated Ringer's Solution; Sodium Lactate (⅙ Molar) Injection; Lactated Ringer's Injection. Commonly used concentrations are 800 µg/ml (200 mg in 250 ml) and 1,600 µg/ml (400 mg in 250 ml). The 160 mg/ml concentrate may be preferred in patients with fluid retention. Protect drug solutions from light; drug solutions should be clear and colorless.
Infusion: Determine infusion rate based on patient response.
Incompatibilities: Do *not* mix with other drugs; do *not* add to 5% Sodium Bicarbonate or other alkaline IV solutions, oxidizing agents, or iron salts because drug is inactivated in alkaline solution (solutions become pink to violet).

Adverse effects
- GI: *Nausea, vomiting*
- CV: *Ectopic beats, tachycardia, anginal pain, palpitations, hypotension, vasoconstriction, dyspnea,* bradycardia, hypertension, widened QRS
- Other: Headache, piloerection, azotemia, gangrene with prolonged use

Clinically important drug-drug interactions
- Increased effects when given with MAO inhibitors, TCAs (eg, imipramine) • In-

Adverse effects in *Italics* are most common; those in **Bold** are life-threatening.

creased risk of hypertension if given with alseroxylon, deserpidine, rauwolfia, rescinnamine, reserpine, furazolidone, methyldopa • Seizures, hypotension, bradycardia when infused with phenytoin • Decreased cardiostimulating effects when given with guanethidine

■ Nursing Considerations

Assessment
- *History:* Pheochromocytoma, tachyarrhythmias, ventricular fibrillation, hypovolemia, general anesthesia with halogenated hydrocarbons or cyclopropane, occlusive vascular disease, labor and delivery
- *Physical:* Body weight; skin—color, temperature; P, BP, pulse pressure; R, adventitious sounds; urine output; serum electrolytes, Hct, ECG

Implementation
- Exercise extreme caution in calculating and preparing doses; dopamine is a very potent drug; small errors in dosage can cause serious adverse effects. Drug should always be diluted before use if not prediluted.
- Arrange to reduce initial dosage by $\frac{1}{10}$ in patients who have been on MAO inhibitors.
- Administer into large veins of the antecubital fossa in preference to veins in hand or ankle.
- Provide phentolamine on standby in case extravasation occurs (infiltration with 10–15 ml saline containing 5–10 mg phentolamine is effective).
- Monitor urine flow, cardiac output, and blood pressure closely during infusion.

Drug-specific teaching points
- Because dopamine is used only in acute emergency situations, patient teaching will depend on patient's awareness and will relate mainly to patient's status, monitors, rather than specifically to therapy with dopamine. Instruct patient to report any pain at injection site.

▢ dornase alfa

(door' nace)
recombinant human deoxyribonuclease, DNase
Pulmozyme

Pregnancy Category B

Drug classes
Cystic fibrosis agent

Therapeutic actions
Breaks down DNA molecules in sputum, resulting in a break up of thick, sticky mucus that clogs airways.

Indications
- Management of respiratory symptoms associated with cystic fibrosis

Contraindications/cautions
- Contraindicated in presence of dornase, Chinese Hamster Ovary products
- Use caution in lactation.

Dosage
2.5 mg qid inhaled through nebulizer for adults and children > 5 y with cystic fibrosis; may increase to 2.5 mg bid.

Pharmacokinetics

Route	Onset	Peak	Duration
Inhal.	Slow	3–4 h	Up to 1 wk

Metabolism: Tissue; $T_{1/2}$: unknown

Adverse effects
- **Respiratory:** Increased cough, dyspnea, hemoptysis, *pharyngitis*, rhinitis, sputum increase, wheezes, voice changes
- **Other:** Conjunctivitis, chest pain

■ Nursing Considerations

Assessment
- *History:* Diagnosis of cystic fibrosis, allergy to dornase, Chinese hamster ovary cell products; lactation
- *Physical:* R, auscultation

Implementation
- Store drug in refrigerator and protect from.

Adverse effects in *Italics* are most common; those in **Bold** are life-threatening.

- Monitor patient closely during administration.
- Ensure proper use of inhalation device.

Drug-specific teaching points
- Be aware that this drug does not cure the disease but will help improve the respiratory symptoms of disease.
- Review the use of nebulizer with health care provider; store in refrigerator and protect from light.
- Report worsening of disease, difficulty breathing, increased productive cough.

doxapram hydrochloride

(docks' a pram)
Dopram

Pregnancy Category B

Drug classes
Analeptic

Therapeutic actions
Stimulates the peripheral carotid chemoreceptors to cause an increase in tidal volume and slight increase in respiratory rate; this stimulation also has a pressor effect.

Indications
- To stimulate respiration in patients with drug-induced postanesthesia respiratory depression or apnea; also used to "stir up" patients in combination with oxygen postoperatively.
- To stimulate respiration, hasten arousal in patients experiencing drug-induced CNS depression.
- As a temporary measure in hospitalized patients with acute respiratory insufficiency superimposed on COPD
- **Unlabeled use**: treatment of apnea of prematurity when methylxanthines have failed

Contraindications/cautions
- Contraindicated in the presence newborns (contains benzyl alcohol), epilepsy, incompetence of the ventilatory mechanism, flail chest, hypersensitivity to doxapram, head injury, pneumothorax, acute bronchial asthma, pulmonary fibrosis, severe hypertension, CVA.
- Use caution in the presence of pregnancy, lactation.

Dosage
Adult
- ***Postanesthetic use:*** Single injection of 0.5–1 mg/kg IV; do not exceed 1.5 mg/kg as a total single injection or 2 mg/kg when given as mutiple injections at 5-min intervals. *Infusion:* 250 mg in 250 ml of dextrose or saline solution; initiate at 5 mg/min until response is seen; maintain at 1–3 mg/min; recommended total dose is 300 mg.
- ***Management of drug-induced CNS depression***
  – *Intermittent injection:* Priming dose of 2 mg/kg IV; repeat in 5 min. Repeat every 1–2 h until patient awakens; if relapse occurs, repeat at 1–2 h intervals.
  – *Intermittent IV infusion:* Priming dose of 2 mg/kg IV; if no response, infuse 250 mg in 250 ml of dextrose or saline solution at a rate of 1–3 mg/min, discontinue at end of 2 h if patient awakens; repeat in ½–2 h if relapse occurs; do not exceed 3 g/d.
- ***Chronic obstructive pulmonary disease associated with acute hypercapnia:*** Mix 400 mg in 180 ml of IV infusion; start infusion at 1–2 mg/min (0.5–1 ml/min); check blood gases, and adjust rate accordingly. Do not use for longer than 2 h.

Pediatric: Do not give to children younger than 12 y.

Pharmacokinetics

Route	Onset	Peak	Duration
IV	20–40 sec	1–2 min	5–12 min

Metabolism: Hepatic; $T_{1/2}$: 2.4–4.1 h
Distribution: May cross placenta; may enter breast milk
Excretion: Urine

IV facts

Preparation: Add 250 mg doxapram to 250 ml of 5% or 10% Dextrose in Water of normal saline.

Infusion: Initiate infusion at 5 mg/min; once response is seen, 1–3 mg/min is satisfactory.

Incompatibilities: Do not mix in alkaline solutions—precipitate or gas may form.

Adverse effects

- CNS: Headache, dizziness, apprehension, disorientation, pupillary dilation, *increased reflexes*, hyperactivity, **convulsions**, muscle spasticity, clonus, pyrexia, flushing, sweating
- GI: Nausea, vomiting, diarrhea
- CV: Arrhythmias, chest pain, tightness in the chest, *increased blood pressure*
- Respiratory: Cough, dyspnea, tachypnea, laryngospasm, **bronchospasm**, hiccups, rebound hyperventilation
- Hematologic: Decreased hemoglobin, hematocrit
- GU: Urinary retention, spontaneous voiding, proteinuria

Clinically important drug-drug interactions

- Increased pressor effect if given with sympathomimetics, MAO inhibitors • Increased effects if given to patients receiving halothane, cyclopropane, enflurane (delay treatment for at least 10 min after discontinuance of anesthesia)

■ Nursing Considerations

Assessment

- *History:* Epilepsy, incompetence of the ventilatory mechanism, flail chest, hypersensitivity to doxapram, head injury, pneumothorax, acute bronchial asthma, pulmonary fibrosis, severe hypertension, CVA, lactation
- *Physical:* Temperature; skin—color; weight; R, adventitious sounds; P, BP, ECG; reflexes; urinary output; arterial blood gases, CBC

Implementation

- Administer IV only.
- Monitor injection site for extravasation. Discontinue infusion immediately, and restart in another vein; apply cold compresses to the area.
- Monitor patient carefully during infusion and until patient is fully awake—P, PB, ECG, reflexes and respiratory status. Patients with COPD should have arterial blood gases monitored during drug use.
- Do not use longer than 2 h.
- Discontinue drug and notify physician if deterioration, sudden hypotension, dyspnea occur.

Drug-specific teaching points

- As doxapram is used in emergency situations, patient teaching should be incorporated into the general teaching plan associated with the condition being treated or procedure being done.

☐ doxazosin mesylate

(dox ay' zoe sin)
Cardura

Pregnancy Category B

Drug classes
Alpha adrenergic-blocking agent
Antihypertensive

Therapeutic actions
Reduces total peripheral resistance through alpha$_1$-blockade; does not affect cardiac output or heart rate; increases HDL and the HDL to cholesterol ratio, while lowering total cholesterol and LDL, making it desirable for patients with atherosclerosis or hyperlipidemia.

Indications
- Treatment of mild to moderate hypertension

Contraindications/cautions
- Contraindicated when lactating.
- Use caution in the presence of allergy to doxazosin, CHF, renal failure, hepatic impairment.

Adverse effects in *Italics* are most common; those in **Bold** are life-threatening.

410 ■ doxepin hydrochloride

Dosage
Adult: Initially 1–16 mg qd PO, given once daily. *Maintenance:* 2–4 mg qid PO, given once a day.
Pediatric: Safety and efficacy not established.

Pharmacokinetics

Route	Onset	Peak
Oral	Varies	2–3 h

Metabolism: Hepatic; $T_{1/2}$: 22 h
Distribution: Crosses placenta; enters breast milk
Excretion: Bile/feces, urine

Adverse effects
- CNS: *Headache, fatigue, dizziness, postural dizziness, lethargy, vertigo,* rhinitis, asthemia, anxiety, parasthesia, increased sweating, muscle cramps, insomnia, eye pain, conjunctivitis
- GI: *Nausea, dyspepsia, diarrhea,* abdominal pain, flatulence, constipation
- CV: *Tachycardia, palpitations, edema, orthostatic hypotension,* chest pain
- GU: *Sexual dysfunction,* increased urinary frequency
- Other: Dyspnea, increased sweating, rash

Clinically important drug-drug interactions
- Increased hypotensive effects if taken with alcohol, nitrates, other antihypertensives

■ Nursing Considerations
Assessment
- *History:* Allergy to doxazosin, CHF, renal failure, hepatic impairment, lactation
- *Physical:* Body weight; skin—color, lesions; orientation, affect, reflexes; ophthalmologic exam; P, BP, orthostatic BP, supine BP, perfusion, edema, auscultation; R, adventitious sounds, status of nasal mucous membranes; bowel sounds, normal output; voiding pattern, normal output; kidney function tests, urinalysis

Implementation
- Monitor edema, body weight in patients with incipient cardiac decompensation, and arrange to add a thiazide diuretic to the drug regimen if sodium and fluid retention, signs of impending CHF occur.
- Monitor patient carefully with first dose; chance of orthostatic hypotension, dizziness and syncope are great with the first dose. Establish safety precautions as appropriate.

Drug-specific teaching points
- Take this drug exactly as prescribed, once a day. Use care when beginning therapy; the chance of dizziness, syncope, are greatest at the beginning of therapy. Change position slowly to avoid increased dizziness.
- Know that the following side effects may occur: dizziness, weakness (these are more likely to occur when you change position, in the early morning, after exercise, in hot weather, and when you have consumed alcohol; some tolerance may occur after you have taken the drug for a while; avoid driving a car or engaging in tasks that require alertness while you are experiencing these symptoms; remember to change position slowly, use caution in climbing stairs, lie down for a while if dizziness persists); GI upset (frequent, small meals may help); impotence; stuffy nose; most of these effects gradually disappear with continued therapy.
- Report frequent dizziness or fainting.

❐ doxepin hydrochloride

(dox' e pin)

Novo-Doxepin (CAN),
Sinequan, Triadapin (CAN)

Pregnancy Category C

Drug classes
TCA (tertiary amine)
Antianxiety drug

Therapeutic actions
Mechanism of action unknown; TCAs inhibit the reuptake of the neurotransmit-

Adverse effects in *Italics* are most common; those in **Bold** are life-threatening.

doxepin hydrochloride ■ 411

ters norepinephrine and serotonin, leading to an increase in their effects; anticholinergic at CNS and peripheral receptors; sedative.

Indications
- Relief of symptoms of depression (endogenous depression most responsive); sedative effects of tertiary amine TCAs may be helpful in patients whose depression is associated with anxiety and sleep disturbance
- Treatment of depression in patients with manic-depressive illness
- Antianxiety agent

Contraindications/cautions
- Contraindicated in the presence of hypersensitivity to any tricyclic drug; concomitant therapy with an MAO inhibitor; recent MI; myelography within previous 24 h or scheduled within 48 h; lactation.
- Use caution in the presence of electroshock therapy; preexisting cardiovascular disorders (severe coronary heart disease, progressive heart failure, angina pectoris, paroxysmal tachycardia); angle-closure glaucoma, increased intraocular pressure, urinary retention, ureteral or urethral spasm; seizure disorders; hyperthyroidism; impaired hepatic, renal function; psychiatric patients (schizophrenic or paranoid patients may exhibit a worsening of psychosis with TCA therapy); manic-depressive patients; elective surgery (TCAs should be discontinued as long as possible before surgery).

Dosage
Adult
- ***Mild to moderate anxiety or depression:*** Initially 25 mg tid PO; individualize dosage. Usual optimum dosage is 75–150 mg/d; alternatively, total daily dosage, up to 150 mg, may be given at bedtime.
- ***More severe anxiety or depression:*** Initially 50 mg tid PO; if needed, may gradually increase to 300 mg/d.
- ***Mild symptomatology or emotional symptoms accompanying organic disease:*** 25–50 mg PO is often effective.

Pediatric: Not recommended in children < 12 y.

Pharmacokinetics

Route	Onset	Peak
Oral	Varies	2–8 h

Metabolism: Hepatic; $T_{1/2}$: 8–25 h
Distribution: Crosses placenta; enters breast milk
Excretion: Urine

Adverse effects
- **CNS:** *Sedation and anticholinergic (atropine-like) effects; confusion* (especially in elderly), *disturbed concentration*, hallucinations, disorientation, decreased memory, feelings of unreality, delusions, anxiety, nervousness, restlessness, agitation, panic, insomnia, nightmares, hypomania, mania, exacerbation of psychosis, drowsiness, weakness, fatigue, headache, numbness, tingling, paresthesias of extremities, incoordination, motor hyperactivity, akathisia, ataxia, tremors, peripheral neuropathy, extrapyramidal symptoms, seizures, speech blockage, dysarthria, tinnitus, altered EEG
- **GI:** *Dry mouth, constipation,* paralytic ileus, *nausea,* vomiting, anorexia, epigastric distress, diarrhea, flatulence, dysphagia, peculiar taste, increased salivation, stomatitis, glossitis, parotid swelling, abdominal cramps, black tongue, hepatitis, jaundice (rare); elevated transaminase, altered alkaline phosphatase
- **CV:** *Orthostatic hypotension,* hypertension, syncope, tachycardia, palpitations, MI, arrhythmias, heart block, precipitation of CHF, stroke
- **Hematologic:** Bone marrow depression, including agranulocytosis; eosinophila, purpura, thrombocytopenia, leukopenia
- **GU:** Urinary retention, delayed micturition, dilation of the urinary tract, gynecomastia, testicular swelling in men; breast enlargement, menstrual irregularity and

Adverse effects in *Italics* are most common; those in **Bold** are life-threatening.

doxepin hydrochloride

galactorrhea in women; increased or decreased libido; impotence
- **Endocrine:** Elevated or depressed blood sugar; elevated prolactin levels; inappropriate ADH secretion
- **Hypersensitivity:** Skin rash, pruritus, vasculitis, petechiae, photosensitization, edema (generalized or of face and tongue), drug fever
- **Withdrawal:** Symptoms on abrupt discontinuation of prolonged therapy: nausea, headache, vertigo, nightmares, malaise
- **Other:** Nasal congestion, excessive appetite, weight gain or loss; sweating (paradoxical effect in a drug with prominent anticholinergic effects), alopecia, lacrimation, hyperthermia, flushing, chills

Clinically important drug-drug interactions

- Increased TCA levels and pharmacologic (especially anticholinergic) effects when given with cimetidine, fluoxetine • Increased TCA levels (due to decreased metabolism) when given with methylphenidate, phenothiazines, oral contraceptives, disulfiram • Hyperpyretic crises, severe convulsions, hypertensive episodes and deaths when MAO inhibitors, furazolidone are given with TCAs • Increased antidepressant response and cardiac arrhythmias when given with thyroid medication • Increased or decreased effects of TCAs given with estrogens • Delirium when TCAs are given with disulfiram • Sympathetic hyperactivity, sinus tachycardia, hypertension, agitation when TCAs are given with levodopa • Increased biotransformation of TCAs in patients who smoke cigarettes • Increased sympathomimetic (especially α-adrenergic) effects of direct-acting sympathomimetic drugs (norepinephrine, epinephrine) when given with TCAs (due to inhibition of uptake into adrenergic nerves) • Increased anticholinergic effects of anticholinergic drugs (including anticholinergic antiparkinsonism drugs) when given with TCAs • Increased response (especially CNS depression) to barbiturates • Increased effects of dicumarol (oral anticoagulant) when given with TCAs • Decreased antihypertensive effect of guanethidine, clonidine, other antihypertensives when given with TCAs (because the uptake of the antihypertensive drug into adrenergic neurons is inhibited) • Decreased effects of indirect-acting sympathomimetic drugs (ephedrine) when given with TCAs (because of inhibition of uptake into adrenergic nerves)

■ Nursing Considerations

Assessment
- *History:* Hypersensitivity to any tricyclic drug; concomitant therapy with an MAO inhibitor; recent MI; myelography within previous 24 h or scheduled within 48 h; lactation; electroshock therapy; preexisting cardiovascular disorders; angle-closure glaucoma, increased intraocular pressure, urinary retention, ureteral or urethral spasm; seizure disorders; hyperthyroidism; impaired hepatic, renal function; psychiatric patients; manic-depressive patients; elective surgery
- *Physical:* Body weight; temperature; skin—color, lesions; orientation, affect, reflexes, vision and hearing; P, BP, orthostatic BP, perfusion; bowel sounds, normal output, liver evaluation; urine flow, normal output; usual sexual function, frequency of menses, breast and scrotal exam; liver function tests, urinalysis, CBC, ECG

Implementation
- Ensure that depressed and potentially suicidal patients have access to only limited quantities of drug.
- Administer major portion of dose at bedtime if drowsiness, severe anticholinergic effects occur.
- Dilute oral concentrate with approximately 120 ml of water, milk, or fruit juice just prior to administration; do not prepare or store bulk dilutions.
- Expect clinical antianxiety response to be rapidly evident, although antidepressant response may require 2–3 wk.

Adverse effects in *Italics* are most common; those in **Bold** are life-threatening.

- Arrange to reduce dosage if minor side effects develop; arrange to discontinue the drug if serious side effects occur.
- Arrange for CBC if patient develops fever, sore throat, or other sign of infection during therapy.

Drug-specific teaching points
- Take drug exactly as prescribed; do not stop taking this drug abruptly or without consulting the physician or nurse.
- Avoid alcohol, other sleep-inducing drugs, OTC drugs while on this drug.
- Avoid prolonged exposure to sunlight or sunlamps; use a sunscreen or protective garments if long exposure to sunlight is unavoidable.
- Know that the following side effects may occur: headache, dizziness, drowsiness, weakness, blurred vision (these effects are reversible; safety measures may need to be taken if these become severe, and you should avoid driving an automobile or performing tasks that require alertness while these persist); nausea, vomiting, loss of appetite, dry mouth (small frequent meals, frequent mouth care, and sucking sugarless candies may help); nightmares, inability to concentrate, confusion; changes in sexual function.
- Report dry mouth, difficulty in urination, excessive sedation.

☐ doxorubicin hydrochloride

*(dox oh **roo'** bi sin)*
ADR
Adriamycin

Pregnancy Category D

Drug classes
Antibiotic
Antineoplastic agent

Therapeutic actions
Cytotoxic: binds to DNA and inhibits DNA synthesis in susceptible cells, causing cell death.

Indications
- To produce regression in the following neoplasms: acute lymphoblastic leukemia, acute myeloblastic leukemia, Wilm's tumor, neuroblastoma, soft tissue and bone sarcoma, breast carcinoma, ovarian carcinoma, transitional cell bladder carcinoma, thyroid carcinoma, Hodgkin's and non-Hodgkin's lymphomas, bronchogenic carcinoma

Contraindications/cautions
- Contraindicated in the presence of allergy to doxorubicin hydrochloride, malignant melanoma, kidney carcinoma, large bowel carcinoma, brain tumors, CNS metastases, myelosuppression, cardiac disease (may predispose to cardiac toxicity) pregnancy, lactation.
- Use caution in the presence of impaired hepatic function, previous courses of doxorubicin or daunorubicin therapy (may predispose to cardiac toxicity), prior mediastinal irradiation, concurrent cyclophosphamide therapy (predispose to cardiac toxicity).

Dosage
Adult: 60–75 mg/m^2 as a single IV injection administered at 21-d intervals. Alternate schedule: 30 mg/m^2 IV on each of 3 successive days, repeated every 4 wk.
- ***Patients with elevated bilirubin:*** *Serum bilirubin 1.2–3.0 mg/100 ml:* 50% of normal dose. *Serum bilirubin > 3 mg/100 ml:* 25% of normal dose

Pharmacokinetics

Route	Onset	Peak	Duration
IV	Rapid	2 h	24–36 h

Metabolism: Hepatic; $T_{1/2}$: 12 min then 3.3 h then 29.6 h
Distribution: Crosses placenta; enters breast milk
Excretion: Bile/feces and urine

IV facts
Preparation: Reconstitute the 10-mg vial with 5 ml, the 50-mg vial with 25 ml of 0.9% Sodium Chloride or Sterile Water for Injection to give a concentration of 2

mg/ml doxorubicin. Reconstituted solution is stable for 24 h at room temperature or 48 h if refrigerated. Protect from sunlight.
Infusion: Administer slowly into tubing of a freely running IV infusion of Sodium Chloride Injection or 5% Dextrose Injection; attach the tubing to a butterfly needle inserted into a large vein; avoid veins over joints or in extremities with poor perfusion. Rate of administration will depend on the vein and dosage; do not give in less than 3–5 min; red streaking over the vein and facial flushing are often signs of too rapid administration.

Incompatibilities: Heparin, cephalothin, dexamethasone sodium phosphatase (a precipitate forms and the IV solution must not be used), aminophylline, and 5–fluorouracil (doxorubicin decomposes) denoted by a color change from red to blue-purple.

Adverse effects

- GI: *Nausea, vomiting, mucositis,* anorexia, diarrhea
- CV: Cardiac toxicity, CHF, phlebosclerosis
- Hematologic: *Myelosuppression*, hyperuricemia due to cell lysis
- GU: *Red urine*
- Dermatologic: *Complete but reversible alopecia*; hyperpigmentation of nailbeds and dermal creases, facial flushing
- Local: **Severe local cellulitis**, vesication and tissue necrosis if extravasation occurs
- Hypersensitivity: Fever, chills, urticaria, anaphylaxis
- Other: Carcinogenesis (documented in experimental models)

Clinically important drug-drug interactions

- Decreased serum levels and actions of digoxin if taken concurrently with doxorubicin

■ Nursing Considerations

Assessment

- *History:* Allergy to doxorubicin hydrochloride, malignant melanoma, kidney carcinoma, large bowel carcinoma, brain tumors, CNS metastases, myelosuppression, cardiac disease, impaired hepatic function, previous courses of doxorubicin or daunorubicin therapy, prior mediastinal irradiation, concurrent cyclophosphamide therapy, lactation.
- *Physical:* Temperature; skin—color, lesions; weight; hair; nailbeds; local injection site; auscultation, peripheral perfusion, pulses, ECG; R, adventitious sounds; liver evaluation, mucus membranes; CBC, liver function tests, uric acid levels.

Implementation

- Do not administer IM or SC because severe local reaction and tissue necrosis occur.
- Monitor injection site for extravasation: reports of burning or stinging. Discontinue infusion immediately, and restart in another vein. Local SC extravasation: local infiltration with corticosteroid may be ordered; flood area with normal saline; apply cold compress to area. If ulceration begins, arrange consultation with plastic surgeon.
- Monitor patient's response to therapy frequently at beginning of therapy: serum uric acid level, cardiac output (listen for S_3); CBC changes may require a decrease in the dose; consult with physician.
- Record doses received to monitor total dosage; toxic effects are often dose related, as total dose approaches 550 mg/m^2.
- Ensure adequate hydration during the course of therapy to prevent hyperuricemia.

Drug-specific teaching points

- Prepare a calendar of days to return for drug therapy.
- Know that the following side effects may occur: rash, skin lesions, loss of hair, changes in nails (you may want to invest in a wig before hair loss occurs; skin care may help somewhat); loss of appetite, nausea, mouth sores (frequent mouth care, small frequent meals may help; try to maintain good nutrition if at all

possible; a dietician may be able to help; an antiemetic also may be ordered); red urine (this is a result of drug therapy and will pass after a few days).
- Arrange for regular medical followup, which will include blood tests to monitor the drug's effects.
- Report difficulty breathing, sudden weight gain, swelling, burning or pain at injection site, unusual bleeding or bruising.

☐ doxycycline

(dox i sye' kleen)
Apo-Doxy (CAN), Doryx, Doxy-Caps, Doxycin (CAN), Doxychel Hyclate, Vibra-Tabs, Vibramycin

Pregnancy Category D

Drug classes
Antibiotic
Tetracycline

Therapeutic actions
Bacteriostatic: inhibits protein synthesis of susceptible bacteria, causing cell death.

Indications
- Infections caused by rickettsiae; *M. pneumoniae;* agents of psittacosis, ornithosis, lymphogranuloma venereum and granuloma inguinale; *B. recurrhoeas; H. ducreyi; P. pestis; P. tularensis; B. bacilliformis; Bacteroides; V. comma; V. fetus; Brucella; E. coli; E. aerogenes; Shigella; A. calcoaceticus; H. influenzae; Klebsiella; D. pneumoniae; S. aureus*
- When penicillin is contraindicated, infections caused by *N. gonorrhoeae, T. pallidum, T. pertenue, L. monocytogenes, Clostridium, B. anthracis,* As an adjunct to amebicides in acute intestinal amebiasis
- Oral tetracyclines are indicated for treatment of acne, uncomplicated urethral, endocervical or rectal infections in adults caused by *C. trachomatis*
- Unlabeled use: prevention of "traveler's diarrhea" commonly caused by enterotoxigenic *E. coli*

Contraindications/cautions
- Allergy to tetracyclines, renal or hepatic dysfunction, pregnancy, lactation.

Dosage
Adult: 200 mg IV in one or two infusions (each over 1–4 h) on the first treatment day, followed by 100–200 mg/d IV, depending on the severity of the infection.
- ***Primary or secondary syphilis:*** 300 mg/d IV for 10 d; or 100 mg q12h PO on the first day of treatment, followed by 100 mg/d as one dose or 50 mg q12h PO.
- ***Acute gonococcal infection:*** 200 mg PO, then 100 mg at bedtime, followed by 100 mg bid for 3 d; or 300 mg PO followed by 300 mg in 1 h.
- ***Primary and secondary syphilis:*** 300 mg/d PO in divided doses for at least 10 d.
- ***Traveler's diarrhea:*** 100 mg/d PO as prophylaxis.
- ***CDC recommendations for sexually transmitted diseases:*** 100 mg bid PO for 7–10 d.

Pediatric
- ***> 8 y and less than 100 lb:*** 4.4 mg/kg, IV in one or two infusions, followed by 2.2—4.4 mg/kg per day IV in one or two infusions; or 4.4 mg/kg, PO in two divided doses the first day of treatment, followed by 2.2–4.4 mg/kg per day on subsequent days.
- ***More than 100 lbs:*** Give adult dose. Not recommended for children < 8 y.

Geriatric or renal failure patients: IV doses of doxycycline are not as toxic as other tetracyclines in these patients.

Pharmacokinetics

Route	Onset	Peak
Oral	Varies	1.5–4 h
IV	Rapid	End of infusion

Metabolism: $T_{1/2}$: 15–25 h
Distribution: Crosses placenta; enters breast milk
Excretion: Urine and feces

IV facts
Preparation: Prepare solution of 10 mg/ml reconstitute with 10 (100-mg vial):

20 ml (200 mg vial) of Sterile Water for Injection; dilute further with 100–1,000 ml (100-mg vial) or 200–2,000 ml (200-mg vial) of Sodium Chloride Injection, 5% Dextrose Injection, Ringer's Injection, 10% Invert Sugar in Water, Lactated Ringer's Injection, 5% Dextrose in Lactated Ringer's, Normosol-M in D5-W, Normosol-R in D5-W, or Plasma-Lyte 56 or 148 in 5% Dextrose. If mixed in Lactated Ringer's or 5% Dextrose in Lactated Ringer's, infusion must be completed within 6 h after reconstitution; otherwise, may be stored up to 72 h if refrigerated and protected from light, but infusion should then be completed within 12 h; discard solution after that time.

Infusion: Infuse slowly over 1–4 h.

Adverse effects
- **GI:** Fatty liver, **liver failure**, *anorexia, nausea, vomiting, diarrhea, glossitis,* dysphagia, enterocolitis, esophageal ulcer
- **Hematologic:** Hemolytic anemia, thrombocytopenia, neutropenia, eosinophilia, leukocytosis, leukopenia
- **Dermatologic:** *Phototoxic reactions, rash,* exfoliative dermatitis (more frequent and more severe with this tetracycline than with any others)
- **Dental:** *Discoloring and inadequate calcification of primary teeth of fetus if used by pregnant women, discoloring and inadequate calcification of permanent teeth if used during period of dental development*
- **Local:** Local irritation at injection site
- **Other:** Superinfections, nephrogenic diabetes insipidus syndrome

Clinically important drug-drug interactions
- Decreased absorption of doxycycline if taken with antacids, iron, alkali • Decreased therapeutic effects of doxycycline if taken with barbiturates, carbamazepine, phenytoins • Increased digoxin toxicity if taken with doxycycline • Increased nephrotoxicity if taken with methoxyflurane • Decreased activity of penicillins if taken with doxycycline.

Clinically important drug-food interactions
- Decreased effectiveness of doxycycline if taken with food, dairy products

Drug-lab test interferences
- Interference with culture studies for several days following therapy

■ Nursing Considerations
Assessment
- *History:* Allergy to tetracyclines, renal or hepatic dysfunction, pregnancy, lactation.
- *Physical:* Skin status, R and sounds, GI function and liver evaluation, urinary output and concentration, urinalysis and BUN, liver and renal function tests; culture infected area before beginning therapy.

Implementation
- Administer the oral medication without regard to food or meals; if GI upset occurs, give with meals.
- Protect patient from light and sun exposure.

Drug-specific teaching points
- Take drug throughout the day for best results; if GI upset occurs, take drug with food.
- Know that the following side effects may occur: sensitivity to sunlight (wear protective clothing, and use a sunscreen), diarrhea.
- Report rash, itching; difficulty breathing; dark urine or light-colored stools; pain at injection site.

❒ dronabinol

(droe **nab'** i nol)
delta-9-tetrahydrocannabinol, delta-9-THC

Marinol

Pregnancy Category B
C-II controlled substance

Adverse effects in *Italics* are most common; those in **Bold** are life-threatening.

dronabinol

Drug classes
Antiemetic

Therapeutic actions
Principal psychoactive substance in marijuana; has complex CNS effects; mechanism of action as antiemetic is not understood.

Indications
- Treatment of nausea and vomiting associated with cancer chemotherapy in patients who have failed to respond adequately to conventional antiemetic treatment (should be used only under close supervision by a responsible individual because of potential to alter the mental state)
- Treatment of anorexia associated with weight loss in patients with AIDS

Contraindications/cautions
- Contraindicated in the presence of allergy to dronabinol or sesame oil vehicle in capsules, nausea and vomiting arising from any cause other than cancer chemotherapy, lactation.
- Use caution in the presence of hypertension; heart disease; manic, depressive, schizophrenic patients (dronabinol may unmask symptoms of these disease states).

Dosage
Adult
- ***Antiemetic:*** Initially, 5 mg/m^2 PO 1–3 h prior to the administration of chemotherapy. Repeat dose q2–4h after chemotherapy is given, for a total of four to six doses per day. If the 5 mg/m^2 dose is ineffective and there are no significant side effects, increase dose by 2.5 mg/m^2 increments to a maximum of 15 mg/m^2 per dose.
- ***Appetite stimulation:*** Initially give 2.5 mg PO bid before lunch and supper. May reduce dose to 2.5 mg/d as a single bedtime dose; up to 10 mg PO bid has been tolerated.

Pharmacokinetics

Route	Onset	Peak	Duration
Oral	30–60 min	2–4 h	4–6 h

Metabolism: Hepatic; T$_{1/2}$: 25–36 h
Distribution: Crosses placenta; enters breast milk
Excretion: Bile/feces and urine

Adverse effects
- **CNS:** *Drowsiness; easy laughing, elation, heightened awareness, often termed a "high;" dizziness; anxiety; muddled thinking; perceptual difficulties; impaired coordination; irritability, weird feeling, depression; weakness, sluggishness, headache;* hallucinations, memory lapse; unsteadiness, ataxia; paresthesia, visual distortions; paranoia, depersonalization; disorientation, confusion; tinnitus, nightmares, speech difficulty
- **GI:** *Dry mouth*
- **CV:** Tachycardia, postural hypotension; syncope
- **GU:** Decrease in pregnancy rate, spermatogenesis when doses higher than those used clinically were given in preclinical studies
- **Dermatologic:** Facial flushing, perspiring
- **Dependence:** Psychological and physical dependence; tolerance to CVS and subjective effects after 30 d of use; withdrawal syndrome (irritability, insomnia, restlessness, hot flashes, sweating, rhinorrhea, loose stools, hiccups, anorexia) beginning 12 h and ending 96 h after discontinuation of high doses of the drug

Clinically important drug-drug interactions
- Do not give with alcohol, sedatives, hypnotics, other psychotomimetic substances

■ Nursing Considerations

Assessment
- *History:* Allergy to dronabinol or sesame oil vehicle in capsules, nausea and vomiting arising from any cause other than cancer chemotherapy, hypertension, heart disease, manic, depressive, schizophrenic patients, lactation.
- *Physical:* Skin—color, texture; orientation, reflexes, bilateral grip strength, af-

Adverse effects in *Italics* are most common; those in **Bold** are life-threatening.

fect; P, BP, orthostatic BP; status of mucous membranes.

Implementation
- Store capsules in refrigerator.
- Arrange to limit prescriptions for dronabinol to the minimum necessary for a single cycle of chemotherapy because of abuse potential.
- Warn patient about drug's profound effects on mental status, abuse potential before administering drug; patient should be fully informed to participate in the decision regarding the use of this drug.
- Warn patient about drug's potential effects on mood and behavior to prevent panic in case these occur.
- Arrange for patient to remain under supervision of responsible adult while taking this drug; determine duration of patient supervision required by very close monitoring, preferably in an inpatient setting, during the first cycle of chemotherapy in which dronabinol is used.
- Arrange to discontinue drug at least temporarily in any patient who has a psychotic reaction; observe patient closely, and do not reinstitute therapy until patient has been evaluated and counseled; patient should participate in decision about further use of drug, perhaps at lower dosage.

Drug-specific teaching points
- Take drug exactly as prescribed; a responsible adult should be with you at all times while you are taking this drug.
- Avoid alcohol, sedatives, OTC drugs, including nose drops, cold remedies, while you are taking this drug.
- Know that the following side effects may occur: mood changes (euphoria, laughing, feeling "high," anxiety, depression, weird feeling, hallucinations, memory lapse, impaired thinking; it may help to know that these are drug effects that will go away when you stop taking the drug); weakness, faintness when you get up out of bed or out of a chair (change postion slowly to avoid injury); dizziness, drowsiness (do not drive a car or perform tasks that require alertness if you experience these effects).
- Report bizarre thoughts, uncontrollable behavior or thought processes, fainting, dizziness, irregular heart beat.

☐ dyphylline

(dye' fi lin)
dihydroxypropyl theophyllin
Dilor, Dyflex, Dy-Phyl-Lin, Lufyllin, Neothylline, Protophylline (CAN)

Pregnancy Category C

Drug classes
Bronchodilator
Xanthine

Therapeutic actions
A theophylline derivative that is not metabolized to theophylline; relaxes bronchial smooth muscle, causing bronchodilation and increasing vital capacity, which has been impaired by bronchospasm and air trapping; at high doses it also inhibits the release of slow reacting substance of anaphylaxis and histamine.

Indications
- Symptomatic relief or prevention of bronchial asthma and reversible bronchospasm associated with chronic bronchitis and emphysema

Contraindications/cautions
- Contraindicated in the presence of hypersensitivity to any xanthine or to ethylenediamine, peptic ulcer, active gastritis.
- Use caution in the presence of cardiac arrhythmias, acute myocardial injury, CHF, cor pulmonale, severe hypertension, severe hypoxemia, renal or hepatic disease, hyperthyroidism, alcoholism, labor, lactation.

Dosage
Individualize dosage, basing adjustments on clinical responses with monitoring of serum dyphylline levels; serum theophylline levels do *not* measure dyphylline; the

amount of dyphylline equivalent to a given amount of theophylline is not known.

Adult: Up to 15 mg/kg, PO qid or 250–500 mg injected slowly IM (not for IV use); do not exceed 15 mg/kg per 6 h.

Pediatric: Use in children < 6 mo not recommended; children are very sensitive to CNS stimulant action of xanthines. Use caution in younger children who cannot complain of minor side effects. 2–3 mg/lb (4.4–6.6 mg/kg) daily in divided doses.

Geriatric or impaired adult: Use caution, especially in elderly men and in patients with cor pulmonale, CHF, kidney disease.

Pharmacokinetics

Route	Peak	Duration
Oral	1 h	6 h
IM	30–45 min	6 h

Metabolism: Hepatic; $T_{1/2}$: 2 h
Distribution: Crosses placenta; enters breast milk
Excretion: Urine

Adverse effects

- CNS: *Headache, insomnia,* irritability; restlessness, dizziness, muscle twitching, convulsions, severe depression, stammering speech; abnormal behavior characterized by withdrawal, mutism, and unresponsiveness alternating with hyperactive periods, brain damage, **death**
- GI: *Nausea, vomiting, diarrhea,* loss of appetite, hematemesis, epigastric pain, gastroesophageal reflux during sleep, increased SGOT
- CV: Palpitations, sinus tachycardia, ventricular tachycardia, **life-threatening ventricular arrhythmias**, circulatory failure, hypotension
- **Respiratory:** Tachypnea, respiratory arrest
- GU: Proteinuria, increased excretion of renal tubular cells and RBCs; diuresis (dehydration), urinary retention in men with prostate enlargement
- Other: Fever, flushing, hyperglycemia, SIADH, rash

Clinically important drug-drug interactions

- Increased effects of dyphylline when given with probenecid, mexiletine • Increased cardiac toxicity when given with halothane • Decreased effects of benzodiazepines, nondepolarizing neuromuscular blockers given with dyphylline • Mutually antagonistic effects of beta-blockers and dyphylline

■ Nursing Considerations

Assessment

- *History:* Hypersensitivity to any xanthine or to ethylenediamine, peptic ulcer, active gastritis, cardiac arrhythmias, acute myocardial injury, CHF, cor pulmonale, severe hypertension, severe hypoxemia, renal or hepatic disease, hyperthyroidism, alcoholism, labor, lactation.
- *Physical:* Bowel sounds, normal output; P, auscultation, BP, perfusion, ECG; R, adventitious sounds; frequency, voiding, normal output pattern, urinalysis, renal function tests; liver palpation, liver function tests; thyroid function tests; skin color, texture, lesions; reflexes, bilateral grip strength, affect, EEG.

Implementation

- Give oral dosage forms with food if GI effects occur.
- Monitor patient carefully for clinical signs of adverse effects.
- Maintain diazepam on standby to treat seizures.

Drug-specific teaching points

- Take this drug exactly as prescribed; it may be necessary to take this drug around the clock for adequate control of asthma attacks.
- Avoid excessive intake of coffee, tea, cocoa, cola beverages, chocolate.
- Keep all appointments for monitoring of response to this drug.
- Know that the following side effects may occur: nausea, loss of appetite (taking this drug with food may help); difficulty sleeping, depression, emotional lability

Adverse effects in *Italics* are most common; those in **Bold** are life-threatening.

edetate calcium disodium

(it may be reassuring to know that these are drug effects).
- Report nausea, vomiting, severe GI pain, restlessness, convulsions, irregular heartbeat.

edetate calcium disodium

(ed' e tate)
calcium EDTA
Calcium Disodium Versenate

edetate disodium
Disotate, Endrate
Pregnancy Category C

Drug classes
Antidote

Therapeutic actions
Calcium in this compound is easily displaced by heavy metals, such as lead, to form stable complexes that are excreted in the urine; edetate disodium has strong affinity to calcium, lowering calcium levels and pulling calcium out of extracirculatory stores during slow infusion.

Indications
- Acute and chronic lead poisoning and lead encephalopathy (edetate calcium disodium)
- Emergency treatment of hypercalcemia (edetate disodium)
- Control of ventricular arrhythmias associated with digitalis toxicity (edetate disodium)

Contraindications/cautions
- Contraindicated in the presence of sensitivity to EDTA preparations, anuria, increased intracranial pressure (rapid IV infusion).
- Use caution in the presence of cardiac disease, CHF, lactation.

Dosage
Effective by IM, SC, IV routes. IM route is safest in children and patients with lead encephalopathy.

Adult
- **Lead poisoning:** Edetate calcium disodium.
- *IV:* Asymptomatic patients: 5 ml diluted IV bid for up to 5 d. Interrupt therapy for 2 d; follow with another 5 d of treatment if indicated. Do not exceed 50 mg/kg per day. Symptomatic adults: Keep fluids to basal levels; administer above dilution over 2 h. Give second daily infusion 6 h or more after the first.
- *IM:* Do not exceed 35 mg/kg bid, total of approximately 75 mg/kg per day.
- **Hypercalcemia, treatment of ventricular arrhythmias due to digitalis toxicity:** Edetate disodium: Administer 50 mg/kg per day IV to a maximum dose of 3 g in 24 h. A suggested regimen includes five consecutive daily doses followed by 2 d without medication. Repeat courses as necessary to a total of 15 doses.

Pediatric
- **Lead poisoning:** Edetate calcium disodium.
- *IM:* Do not exceed 35 mg/kg bid, total of approximately 75 mg/kg per day. In mild cases do not exceed 50 mg/kg per day. For younger children, give total daily dose in divided doses q8–12h for 3–5 d. Give a second course after a rest period of 4 d or more.
- **Lead encephalopathy:** Use above IM dosage. If used in combination with dimercaprol, give at separate deep IM sites.
- **Hypercalcemia, treatment of ventricular arrhythmias due to digitalis toxicity:** Edetate disodium. Administer 40 mg/kg per day IV to a maximum dose of 70 mg/kg per day, or give 15–50 mg/kg per day to a maximum of 3 g/d, allowing 5 d between courses of therapy.

Pharmacokinetics

Route	Onset	Peak
IM/IV	1 h	24–48 h

Metabolism: $T_{1/2}$: 20–60 min (IV), 90 min (IM)
Excretion: Urine

IV facts

Preparation: Lead poisoning: Dilute the 5-ml ampul with 250–500 ml of Normal Saline or 5% Dextrose Solution. Hypercalcemia: Dissolve dose in 500 ml of 5% Dextrose Injection or 0.9% Sodium Chloride Injection. Pediatric: Dissolve dose in a sufficient volume of 5% Dextrose Injection or 0.9% Sodium Chloride Injection to bring the final concentration to not more than 3%.

Infusion: Lead poisoning: Administer prepared solution over at least 1 h. Hypercalcemia: Infuse over 3 h or more, and do not exceed the patient's cardiac reserve. Pediatric: Infuse over 3 h or more. Do not exceed patient's cardiac reserve.

Adverse effects

- **CNS:** Headache, transient circumoral paresthesia, numbness
- **GI:** *Nausea, vomiting, diarrhea* (edetate disodium)
- **CV:** CHF, blood pressure changes, thrombophlebitis
- **Hematologic:** *Electrolyte imbalance* (hypocalcemia, hypokalemia, hypomagnesemia, altered blood sugar)
- **GU:** Renal tubular necrosis

■ Nursing Considerations

Assessment
- *History*: Sensitivity to EDTA preparations; anuria; increased intracranial pressure; cardiac disease, CHF, lactation
- *Physical:* Pupillary reflexes, orientation; P, BP; urinalysis, BUN, serum electrolytes

Implementation
- Administer edetate calcium disodium IM for safest and most convenient route.
- Avoid rapid IV infusion, which can cause fatal increases in intracranial pressure or fatal hypocalcemia with edetate disodium.
- Avoid excess fluids in patients with lead encephalopathy and increased intracranial pressure; for these patients, mix edetate calcium disodium 20% solution with procaine to give a final concentration of 0.5% procaine, and administer IM.
- Monitor patient response and electrolytes carefully during slow IV infusion of edetate disodium.
- Establish urine flow by IV infusion before administering the first dose to patients who are dehydrated from vomiting. Once urine flow is established, restrict further IV fluid to basal water and electrolyte requirements. Stop EDTA when urine flow ceases.
- Arrange for periodic BUN and serum electrolyte determinations before and during each course of therapy. Arrange to stop drug if signs of increasing renal damage occur.
- Do not administer in larger than recommended doses.
- Arrange for cardiac monitoring if edetate disodium is being used to treat digitalis-induced ventricular arrhythmias. Patient should be carefully monitored for signs of CHF and other adverse effects as digitalis is withdrawn.
- Arrange for patient to remain supine for a short period because of the possibility of postural hypotension.
- Do not administer edetate disodium as a chelating agent for treatment of atherosclerosis; such therapy is not approved and is suspect.

Drug-specific teaching points
- Prepare a schedule of rest and drug days.
- Arrange for periodic blood tests during the course of therapy.
- Be aware that constant monitoring of heart rhythm may be needed during drug administration.
- Report pain at injection site, difficulty voiding.

▢ edrophonium chloride

*(ed roe **foe'** nee um)*
Enlon, Tensilon

Pregnancy Category C

Drug classes
Cholinesterase inhibitor (anticholinesterase)

Adverse effects in *Italics* are most common; those in **Bold** are life-threatening.

edrophonium chloride

Diagnostic agent
Antidote

Therapeutic actions
Increases the concentration of acetylcholine at the sites of cholinergic transmission; prolongs and exaggerates the effects of acetylcholine by reversibly inhibiting the enzyme acetylcholinesterase, facilitating transmission at the skeletal neuromuscular junction.

Indications
- Differential diagnosis and adjunct in evaluating treatment of myasthenia gravis
- Antidote for nondepolarizing neuromuscular junction blockers (curare, tubocurarine, gallamine) after surgery

Contraindications/cautions
- Contraindicated in the presence of hypersensitivity to anticholinesterases, intestinal or urogenital tract obstruction, peritonitis, lactation.
- Use caution in the presence of asthma, peptic ulcer, bradycardia, cardiac arrhythmias, recent coronary occlusion, vagotonia, hyperthyroidism, epilepsy, pregnancy near term.

Dosage
Adult
- ***Differential diagnosis of myasthenia gravis***
  - *IV:* Prepare tuberculin syringe containing 10 mg edrophonium with IV needle. Inject 2 mg IV in 15–30 sec; leave needle in vein. If no reaction occurs after 45 sec, inject the remaining 8 mg. If a cholinergic reaction (parasympathomimetic effects, muscle fasciculations, or increased muscle weakness) occurs after 2 mg, discontinue the test, and administer atropine sulfate 0.4–0.5 mg IV. May repeat test after ½ h.
  - *IM:* If veins are inaccessible, inject 10 mg IM. Patients who demonstrate cholinergic reaction (see above) should be retested with 2 mg IM after ½ h to rule out false-negative results.
- ***Evaluation of treatment requirements in myasthenia gravis:*** 1–2 mg IV 1 h after oral intake of the treatment drug. Responses are summarized below:

Response to Edrophonium Test	Myasthenic (Under-treated)	Cholinergic (Over-treated)
Muscle strength ptosis, diplopia, respiration, limb strength	Increased	Decreased
Fasciculations orbicularis oculi, facial and limb muscles	Absent	Present or absent
Side reactions lacrimation, sweating, salivating, nausea, vomiting, diarrhea, abdominal cramps	Absent	Severe

- ***Edrophonium test in crisis:*** Secure controlled respiration immediately if patient is apneic, then administer test. If patient is in cholinergic crisis, administration of edrophonium will increase oropharyngeal secretions and further weaken respiratory muscles. If crisis is myasthenic, administration of edrophonium will improve respiration, and patient can be treated with longer-acting IV anticholinesterase medication.
- To administer the test, draw up no more than 2 mg edrophonium into the syringe. Give 1 mg IV initially. Carefully observe cardiac response. If after 1 min this dose does not further impair the patient, inject the remaining 1 mg. If after a 2-mg dose no clear improvement in respiration occurs, discontinue all anticholinesterase drug therapy, and control ventilation by tracheostomy and assisted respiration.
- ***Antidote for curare:*** 10 mg given slowly IV over 30–45 sec so that onset of cholinergic reaction can be detected; repeat when necessary. Maximal dose for any patient is 40 mg.

Pediatric
- ***Differential diagnosis of myasthenia gravis***

edrophonium chloride ■ 423

– *IV: Children up to 75 lb (34 kg)*: 1 mg. Children over 75 lb: 2 mg. *Infants*: 0.5 mg. If children do not respond in 45 sec, dose may be titrated up to 5 mg in children under 75 lb, up to 10 mg in children over 75 lb, given in increments of 1 mg q 30–45 sec.
– *IM:* Up to 75 lb (34 kg): 2 mg. Over 75 lb: 5 mg. A delay of 2–10 min occurs until reaction.

Pharmacokinetics

Route	Onset	Duration
IM	2–10 min	5–30 min
IV	30–60 sec	5–10 min

Metabolism: $T_{1/2}$: 5–10 min
Distribution: Crosses placenta; enters breast milk
Excretion: Unknown

IV facts

Preparation: Drug is used directly; no preparation is required.
Infusion: Rate of infusion varies with reason for administration; see above.

Adverse effects
Parasympathomimetic Effects

- GI: *Salivation, dysphagia, nausea, vomiting, increased peristalsis, abdominal cramps,* flatulence, diarrhea
- CV: *Bradycardia, cardiac arrhythmias, AV block and nodal rhythm, cardiac arrest;* decreased cardiac output, leading to hypotension, syncope
- Respiratory: *Increased pharyngeal and tracheobronchial secretions,* laryngospasm, bronchospasm, bronchiolar constriction, dyspnea
- GU: *Urinary frequency and incontinence,* urinary urgency
- EENT: *Lacrimation, miosis,* spasm of accommodation, diplopia, conjunctival hyperemia
- Dermatologic: Diaphoresis, flushing

Skeletal Muscle Effects

- CNS: Convulsions, dysarthria, dysphonia, drowsiness, dizziness, headache, loss of consciousness
- **Respiratory**: **Respiratory muscle paralysis, central respiratory paralysis**
- Peripheral: Skeletal muscle weakness, fasciculations, muscle cramps, arthralgia

Other

- Dermatologic: Skin rash, urticaria, anaphylaxis
- Local: Thrombophlebitis after IV use

Clinically important drug-drug interactions

- Risk of profound muscular depression refractory to anticholinesterases if given concurrently with corticosteroids, succinylcholine.

■ Nursing Considerations

Assessment

Note: The administration of edrophonium for diagnostic purposes would generally be supervised by a neurologist or other physician skilled and experienced in dealing with myasthenic patients; the administration of edrophonium to reverse neuromuscular blocking agents would generally be supervised by an anesthesiologist. The following are points that any nurse participating in the care of a patient receiving anticholinesterases should keep in mind.

- *History:* Hypersensitivity to anticholinesterases; intestinal or urogenital tract obstruction, peritonitis, lactation, asthma, peptic ulcer, cardiac arrhythmias, recent coronary occlusion, vagotonia, hyperthyroidism, epilepsy, pregnancy near term
- *Physical:* Bowel sounds, normal output; frequency, voiding pattern, normal output; R, adventitious sounds; P, auscultation, blood pressure; reflexes, bilateral grip strength, EEG; thyroid function tests; skin color, texture, lesions

Implementation

- Administer IV slowly with constant monitoring of patient's response.
- Be aware that overdosage with anticholinesterase drugs can cause muscle weakness (cholinergic crisis) that is difficult to differentiate from myasthenic weakness; edrophonium is used to help make this

Adverse effects in *Italics* are most common; those in **Bold** are life-threatening.

diagnostic distinction. The administration of atropine may mask the parasympathetic effects of anticholinesterases and confound the diagnosis.
- Maintain atropine sulfate on standby as an antidote and antagonist to edrophonium.

Drug-specific teaching points
- The patient should know what to expect during diagnostic test with edrophonium (patients receiving drug to reverse neuromuscular blockers will not be aware of drug effects and do not require specific teaching about the drug).

☐ enalapril maleate

*(e **nal'** a pril)*
Vasotec

enalaprilat
Vasotec I.V.

Pregnancy Category C

Drug classes
Antihypertensive
Angiotensin-converting enzyme inhibitor

Therapeutic actions
Renin, synthesized by the kidneys, is released into the circulation where it acts on a plasma precursor to produce angiotensin I, which is converted by angiotensin-converting enzyme to angiotensin II, a potent vasoconstrictor that also causes release of aldosterone from the adrenals; both of these actions increase blood pressure. Enalapril blocks the conversion of angiotensin I to angiotensin II, decreasing blood pressure, decreasing aldosterone secretion, slightly increasing serum potassium levels, and causing sodium and fluid loss; increased prostaglandin synthesis also may be involved in the antihypertensive action.

Indications
- Treatment of hypertension alone or in combination with thiazide-type diuretics
- Treatment of acute and chronic CHF

Contraindications/cautions
- Contraindicated in the presence of allergy to enalapril.
- Use caution in the presence of impaired renal function; salt/volume depletion—hypotension may occur; lactation.

Dosage
Adult
- **Hypertension**
– *Oral:* Patients not taking diuretics: Initial dose—5 mg/d PO. Adjust dosage based on patient response. Usual range is 10–40 mg/d as a single dose or in two divided doses. *Patient taking diuretics:* Discontinue diuretic for 2–3 d if possible. If it is not possible to discontinue diuretic, give initial dose of 2.5 mg, and monitor for excessive hypotension. *Converting to oral therapy from IV therapy:* 5 mg qd with subsequent doses based on patient response.
– *Parenteral:* Give IV only. 1.25 mg q6h given IV over 5 min. A response is usually seen within 15 min, but peak effects may not occur for 4h. *Converting to IV therapy from oral therapy:* 1.25 mg q6h; monitor patient response. *Patients taking diuretics:* 0.625 mg IV over 5 min. If adequate response is not seen after 1 h, repeat the 0.625-mg dose. Give additional doses of 1.25 mg q6h.

- **Heart failure**
– *Oral:* 2.5 mg qd or bid in conjunction with diuretics and digitalis. Maintenance dose is 5–20 mg/d given in two divided doses. Maximum daily dose is 40 mg.

Pediatric: Safety and efficacy not established.

Geriatric and renal impaired: Excretion is reduced in renal failure; use smaller initial dose, and titrate upward to a maximum of 40 mg/d PO.

Creatinine Clearance (ml/min)	Serum Creatinine	Initial Dose
>80		5 mg/d
≤80 to >30	<3 mg/dl	5 mg/d
≤30	>3 mg/dl	2.5 mg/d
Dialysis		2.5 mg on dialysis days

enalapril maleate ■ 425

– *IV:* Give 0.625 mg, which may be repeated. Additional doses of 1.25 mg q6h may be given with careful patient monitoring.

Pharmacokinetics

Route	Onset	Peak	Duration
Oral	60 minutes	4–6 h	24 h
IV	15 min	3–4 h	6 h

Metabolism: $T_{1/2}$: 11 h
Distribution: Crosses placenta; enters breast milk
Excretion: Urine

IV facts
Preparation: Enalaprilat can be given as supplied or mixed with up to 50 ml of 5% Dextrose Injection, 0.9% Sodium Chloride Injection, 0.9% Sodium Chloride Injection in 5% Dextrose, 5% Dextrose in Lactated Ringer's, Isolyte E. Stable at room temperature for 24 h.
Infusion: Give by slow IV infusion over at least 5 min.

Adverse effects
- CNS: *Headache, dizziness, fatigue,* insomnia, paresthesias
- GI: Gastric irritation, *nausea,* vomiting, *diarrhea,* abdominal pain, dyspepsia, elevated liver enzymes
- CV: Syncope, chest pain, palpitations, hypotension in salt/volume depleted patients
- Hematologic: *Decreased hematocrit and hemoglobin*
- GU: Proteinuria, renal insufficiency, renal failure, polyuria, oliguria, urinary frequency, impotence
- Other: *Cough,* muscle cramps, hyperhidrosis

Clinically important drug-drug interactions
- Decreased hypotensive effect if taken concurrently with indomethacin

■ Nursing Considerations
Assessment
- *History:* Allergy to enalapril, impaired renal function, salt/volume depletion, lactation

- *Physical:* Skin—color, lesions, turgor; body temperature; orientation, reflexes, affect, peripheral sensation; P, BP, peripheral perfusion; mucous membranes, bowel sounds, liver evaluation; urinalysis, renal and liver function tests, CBC, and differential

Implementation
- Alert surgeon, and mark patient's chart with notice that enalapril is being taken; the angiotensin II formation subsequent to compensatory renin release during surgery will be blocked; hypotension may be reversed with volume expansion.
- Monitor patients on diuretic therapy for excessive hypotension following the first few doses of enalapril.
- Monitor patient closely in any situation that may lead to a fall in blood pressure secondary to reduced fluid volume (excessive perspiration and dehydration, vomiting, diarrhea) because excessive hypotension may occur.
- Arrange for reduced dosage in patients with impaired renal function.
- Monitor patient receiving enalaprilat carefully because peak effect may not be seen for 4 h. Do not administer second dose until checking blood pressure.

Drug-specific teaching points
- Do not stop taking the medication without consulting your physician.
- Know that the following side effects may occur: GI upset, loss of appetite, change in taste perception (these may be limited effects that will pass with time; mouth sores (frequent mouth care may help); skin rash; fast heart rate; dizziness, lightheadedness (this usually passes after the first few days of therapy; if it occurs, change position slowly, and limit your activities to those that do not require alertness and precision).
- Be careful in any situation that may lead to a drop in blood pressure (diarrhea, sweating, vomiting, dehydration).
- Avoid OTC medications while you are on this drug, especially cough, cold, allergy

Adverse effects in *Italics* are most common; those in **Bold** are life-threatening.

medications that may contain ingredients that will interact with this drug.
- Report mouth sores; sore throat, fever, chills; swelling of the hands, feet; irregular heartbeat, chest pains; swelling of the face, eyes, lips, tongue, difficulty breathing.

◻ enoxacin

(en ox' a sin)
Penetrex

Pregnancy Category C

Drug classes
Antibacterial drug

Therapeutic actions
Bactericidal: interferes with DNA replication in susceptible gram-negative bacteria, preventing cell reproduction.

Indications
- For the treatment of infections in adults caused by susceptible organisms: sexually transmitted diseases caused by *Neisseria gonorrhoeae*; urinary tract infections due to *Escherichia coli, Staphylococcus epidermidis, Klebsiella pneumoniae, Proteus mirabilis, Pseudomonas aeruginosa, Enterobacter cloacae*

Contraindications/cautions
- Contraindicated in the presence of allergy to enoxacin, norfloxacin; syphilis; pregnancy; lactation.
- Use caution in the presence of renal dysfunction, seizures.

Dosage
Adult
- ***Uncomplicated urinary tract infections:*** 200 mg q12h PO for 7 d.
- ***Complicated urinary tract infections:*** 400 mg q12h PO for 14 d.
- ***Sexually transmitted diseases:*** 400 mg qd PO once.

Pediatric: Not recommended for children younger than 18 y; produced lesions of joint cartilage in immature experimental animals.

Impaired renal function: Creatinine clearance < 30 ml/min/1.73 m^2; after a normal dose, use a 12-h interval and half the recommended dose.

Pharmacokinetics

Route	Onset	Peak	Duration
Oral	Varies	1–1½ h	4–5 h

Metabolism: Hepatic, T$_{1/2}$: 4–6 h
Distribution: Crosses placenta; enters breast milk
Excretion: Urine and bile

Adverse effects
- **CNS:** *Headache, dizziness,* insomnia, fatigue, somnolence, depression, blurred vision
- **GI:** *Nausea, vomiting,* dry mouth, diarrhea, abdominal pain
- **Hematologic:** Elevated BUN, SGOT, SGPT, serum creatinine and alkaline phosphatase; decreased WBC, neutrophil count, hematocrit
- **Other:** Fever, rash, photosensitivity

Clinically important drug-drug interactions
- Decreased therapetic effect of enoxacin if taken concurrently with iron salts • Decreased absorption of enoxacin if taken with antacids • Increased serum levels and toxic effects of theophyllines if taken concurrently with enoxacin

■ Nursing Considerations

Assessment
- *History:* Allergy to enoxacin, ciprofloxacin, norfloxacin; renal dysfunction; seizures; lactation
- *Physical:* Skin—color, lesions; body temperature; orientation, reflexes, affect; mucous membranes, bowel sounds; renal and liver function tests

Implementation
- Arrange for culture and sensitivity tests before beginning therapy.
- Continue therapy for 2 d after the signs and symptoms of infection have disappeared.

Adverse effects in *Italics* are most common; those in **Bold** are life-threatening.

- Administer oral drug 1 h before or 2 h after meals with a glass of water.
- Ensure that patient is well hydrated during course of drug therapy.
- Administer antacids, if needed, at least 2 h after dosing.
- Monitor clinical response; if no improvement is seen or a relapse occurs, repeat culture and sensitivity.
- Encourage patient to complete full course of therapy.

Drug-specific teaching points
- Take oral drug on an empty stomach, 1 h before or 2 h after meals. If an antacid is needed, do not take it within 2 h of enoxacin dose.
- Drink plenty of fluids while you are on this drug.
- Know that the following side effects may occur: nausea, vomiting, abdominal pain (small, frequent meals may help); drowsiness, blurring of vision, dizziness (use caution if driving or using dangerous equipment).
- Report rash, visual changes, severe GI problems, weakness, tremors.

▢ enoxaparin

*(en **ocks**' a pear in)*

Lovenox

Pregnancy Category B

Drug classes
Anticoagulant

Therapeutic actions
Low molecular weight heparin that inhibits thrombus and clot formation by blocking factor Xa, factor IIa, preventing the formation of clots.

Indications
- Prevention of deep vein thrombosis, which may lead to pulmonary embolism following hip replacement
- Unlabeled use: prevention of deep vein thrombosis following knee surgery

Contraindications/cautions
- Contraindicated in the presence of hypersensitivity to enoxaparin, heparin, pork products; severe thrombocytopenia; uncontrolled bleeding.
- Use caution in the presence of pregnancy or lactation, history of GI bleed.

Dosage
Adult: 30 mg SC bid with the initial dose given as soon as possible after surgery, not more than 24 h. Continue treatment throughout the postoperative period. Up to 14 d may be needed.
Pediatric: Safety and efficacy not established.

Pharmacokinetics

Route	Onset	Peak	Duration
SC	20–60 min	3–5 h	12 h

Metabolism: $T_{1/2}$: 4½ h
Distribution: May cross placenta; may enter breast milk
Excretion: Urine

Adverse effects
- **Hematologic:** Hemorrhage; *bruising;* thrombocytopenia; elevated SGOT, SGPT levels; hyperkalemia
- **Hypersensitivity:** Chills, fever, urticaria, asthma
- **Other:** Fever; pain; local irritation, hematoma, erythema at site of injection

Clinically important drug-drug interactions
- Increased bleeding tendencies with oral anticoagulants, salicylates, penicillins, cephalosporins

Drug-lab test interferences
- Increased AST, ALT levels

■ Nursing Considerations

Assessment
- *History:* Recent surgery or injury; sensitivity to heparin, pork products, enoxaparin; lactation; history of GI bleed
- *Physical:* Peripheral perfusion, R, stool guaiac test, PTT or other tests of blood

coagulation, platelet count, kidney function tests

Implementation
- Arrange to give drug as soon as possible after hip surgery.
- Give deep subcutaneous injections; *do not* give enoxaparin by IM injection.
- Administer by deep SC injection; patient should be lying down. Alternate administration between the left and right anterolateral and left and right posterolateral abdominal wall. Introduce the whole length of the needle into a skin fold held between the thumb and forefinger; hold the skin fold throughout the injection.
- Apply pressure to all injection sites after needle is withdrawn; inspect injection sites for signs of hematoma; do not massage injection sites.
- Do not mix with other injections or infusions.
- Store at room temperature; fluid should be clear, colorless to pale yellow.
- Provide for safety measures (electric razor, soft toothbrush) to prevent injury to patient who is at risk for bleeding.
- Check patient for signs of bleeding; monitor blood tests.
- Alert all health care providers that patient is on enoxaparin.
- Discontinue and initiate appropriate therapy if thromboembolic episode occurs despite enoxaparin therapy.
- Have protamine sulfate (enoxaparin antidote) on standby in case of overdose.
- Treat overdose as follows: Protamine sulfate (1% solution). Each mg of protamine neutralizes 1 mg enoxaparin. Give very slowly IV over 10 min.

Drug-specific teaching points
- Arrange for periodic blood tests that will be needed to monitor your response to this drug.
- Avoid injury while you are on this drug: Use an electric razor; avoid activities that might lead to injury.
- Report nose bleed, bleeding of the gums, unusual bruising, black or tarry stools, cloudy or dark urine, abdominal or lower back pain, severe headache.

▢ ephedrine sulfate (parenteral)

(e fed' rin)

Nasal decongestant:
Kondon's Nasal, Pretz-D, Vicks Va-Tro-Nol Nose Drops

Pregnancy Category C

Drug classes
Sympathomimetic drug
Vasopressor
Bronchodilator
Antiasthmatic drug
Nasal decongestant

Therapeutic actions
Peripheral effects are mediated by receptors in target organs and are due in part to the release of norepinephrine from nerve terminals. Effects mediated by these receptors include vasoconstriction (increased blood pressure, decreased nasal congestion alpha receptors); cardiac stimulation (beta-1), and bronchodilation (beta-2). Longer acting but less potent than epinephrine; also has CNS stimulant properties.

Indications
- Treatment of hypotensive states, especially those associated with spinal anesthesia; Stokes-Adams syndrome with complete heart block; CNS stimulant in narcolepsy and depressive states; acute bronchospasm (parenteral)
- Pressor agent in hypotensive states following sympathectomy, overdosage with ganglionic-blocking agents, antiadrenergic agents, or other drugs used for lowering blood pressure (parenteral)
- Relief of acute bronchospasm (parenteral; epinephrine is the preferred drug)
- Treatment of allergic disorders, such as bronchial asthma, and local treatment of nasal congestion in acute coryza, vasomotor rhinitis, acute sinusitis, hay fever (oral)
- Symptomatic relief of nasal and nasopharyngeal mucosal congestion due to the common cold, hay fever, or other respiratory allergies (topical)

- Adjunctive therapy of middle ear infections by decreasing congestion around the eustachian ostia (topical)

Contraindications/cautions
- Contraindicated in the presence of allergy to ephedrine, angle-closure glaucoma, anesthesia with cyclopropane or halothane, thyrotoxicosis, diabetes, hypertension, cardiovascular disorders, women in labor whose BP < 130/80.
- Use caution in the presence of angina, arrhythmias, prostatic hypertrophy, unstable vasomotor syndrome, lactation.

Dosage
Parenteral preparations may be given IM, SC, or slow IV.
Adult
- ***Hypotensive episodes, allergic disorders, asthma:*** 25–50 mg IM (fast absorption), SC (slower absorption), or IV (emergency administration).
- ***Labor:*** Titrate parenteral doses to maintain blood pressure at or below 130/80 mm Hg.
- ***Acute asthma:*** Administer the smallest effective dose (0.25–0.5 ml or 12.5–25 mg).
- ***Maintenance dosage—allergic disorders, asthma:*** 25–50 mg PO q3–4h as necessary.
- ***Topical nasal decongestant:*** Instill solution or apply a small amount of jelly in each nostril q4h. Do not use longer than 3–4 consecutive days.

Pediatric: 25–100 mg/m^2 IM or SC divided into four to six doses; 3 mg/kg per day or 100 mg/m^2 per day divided into four to six doses, PO, SC, or IV for bronchodilation.
- ***Topical nasal decongestant (older than 6 y):*** Instill solution or apply a small amount of jelly in each nostril q4h. Do not use for longer than 3–4 consecutive d. Do not use in children younger than 6 y unless directed by physician.

Geriatric: These patients are more likely to experience adverse reactions; use with caution.

Pharmacokinetics

Route	Onset	Duration
Oral	15–60 min	3–5 h
SC	30–40 min	1 h
IM	10–20 min	1 h
IV	Instant	1 h
Nasal	Rapid	4–6 h

Metabolism: Hepatic, T$_{1/2}$: 3–6 h
Distribution: Crosses placenta; enters breast milk
Excretion: Urine

IV facts
Preparation: Administer as provided; no preparation required.
Infusion: Administer directly into vein or tubing or running IV; administer slowly.

Adverse effects
Systemic effects are less likely with topical administration than with systemic administration, but because systemic absorption can take place, the systemic effects should be considered.
- **CNS:** *Fear, anxiety, tenseness, restlessness, headache, lightheadedness, dizziness,* drowsiness, tremor, insomnia, hallucinations, psychological disturbances, convulsions, CNS depression, weakness, blurred vision, ocular irritation, tearing, photophobia, symptoms of paranoid schizophrenia
- **GI:** *Nausea,* vomiting, anorexia
- **CV:** Arrhythmias, hypertension resulting in intracranial hemorrhage, cardiovascular collapse with hypotension, palpitations, tachycardia, precordial pain in patients with ischemic heart disease
- **GU:** Constriction of renal blood vessels and *decreased urine formation* (initial parenteral administration), *dysuria, vesical sphincter spasm* resulting in difficult and painful urination, urinary retention in males with prostatism
- **Local:** *Rebound congestion* with topical nasal application
- **Other:** *Pallor,* respiratory difficulty, orofacial dystonia, sweating

Adverse effects in *Italics* are most common; those in **Bold** are life-threatening.

Clinically important drug-drug interactions
- Severe hypertension when taken with MAO-inhibitors, tricyclic antidepressants, furazolidone • Additive effects and increased risk of toxicity if taken with urinary alkalinizers • Decreased vasopressor response if taken with reserpine, methyldopa, urinary acidifiers • Decreased hypotensive action of guanethidine if taken with ephedrine

■ Nursing Considerations

Assessment
- *History:* Allergy to ephedrine; angle-closure glaucoma; anesthesia with cyclopropane or halothane; thyrotoxicosis, diabetes, hypertension, cardiovascular disorders; prostatic hypertrophy, unstable vasomotor syndrome; lactation.
- *Physical:* Skin—color, temperature; orientation, reflexes, peripheral sensation, vision; P, BP, auscultation, peripheral perfusion; R, adventitious sounds; urinary output pattern, bladder percussion, prostate palpation

Implementation
- Protect parenteral solution from light; do not administer unless solution is clear; discard any unused portion.
- Monitor urine output with parenteral administration; initially renal blood vessels may be constricted and urine formation decreased.
- Do not use nasal decongestant for longer than 3–5 d.
- Avoid prolonged use of systemic ephedrine (a syndrome resembling an anxiety effect may occur); temporary cessation of the drug usually reverses this syndrome.
- Monitor cardiovascular effects carefully; patients with hypertension who take this drug may experience changes in blood pressure because of the additional vasoconstriction. If a nasal decongestant is needed, pseudoephedrine is the drug of choice.

Drug-specific teaching points
- Do not exceed recommended dose. Demonstrate proper administration technique for topical nasal application. Avoid prolonged use because underlying medical problems can be disguised. Use nasal decongestant no longer than 3–5 d.
- Avoid OTC medications while you are on this drug. Many of them contain the same or similar drugs and serious overdosage can occur.
- Know that the following side effects may occur: dizziness, weakness, restlessness, lightheadedness, tremor (avoid driving or operating dangerous equipment when these effects occur); urinary retention (emptying the bladder before taking the drug may help).
- Report nervousness, palpitations, sleeplessness, sweating.

□ epinephrine

*(ep i **nef** rin)*
adrenaline

Injection: Sus-Phrine

epinephrine bitartrate
Aerosols: AsthmaHaler, Bronitin, Bronkaid Mist, Medihaler-Epi, Primatene Mist

epinephrine borate
Ophthalmic solution: Epinal, Eppy

epinephrine hydrochloride
Injection, OTC nasal solution: Adrenalin Chloride

Ophthalmic solution: Epifrin, Glaucon

Insect sting emergencies: EpiPen Auto-Injector (delivers 0.3 mg IM adult dose), EpiPen Jr. Auto-Injector (delivers 0.15 mg IM for children).

OTC solutions for nebulization: AsthmaNefrin, microNefrin, Nephron, S-2, Vaponefrin

Pregnancy Category C

Drug classes
Sympathomimetic drug
Alpha-adrenergic agonist

epinephrine ■ 431

Beta-1 and beta-2 adrenergic agonist
Cardiac stimulant
Vasopressor
Bronchodilator
Antiasthmatic drug
Nasal decongestant
Mydriatic
Antiglaucoma drug

Therapeutic actions
Naturally occurring neurotransmitter, the effects of which are mediated by alpha or beta receptors in target organs. Effects on alpha receptors include vasoconstriction, contraction of dilator muscles of iris. Effects on beta receptors include positive chronotropic and inotropic effects on the heart (beta-1 receptors); bronchodilation, vasodilation, and uterine relaxation (beta-2 receptors); decreased production of aqueous humor.

Indications
- *Epinephrine, intravenous*: In ventricular standstill after other measures have failed to restore circulation, given by trained personnel by intracardiac puncture and intramyocardial injection; treatment and prophylaxis of cardiac arrest and attacks of transitory AV heart block with syncopal seizures (Stokes-Adams syndrome); syncope due to carotid sinus syndrome; acute hypersensitivity (anaphylactoid) reactions, serum sickness, urticaria, angioneurotic edema; treatment of acute asthmatic attacks to relieve bronchospasm not controlled by inhalation or SC injection of the drug; relaxation of uterine musculature; additive to local anesthetic solutions for injection to prolong their duration of action and limit systemic absorption (other sympathomimetics may be preferred for some of these indications)
- *Injection:* Relief from respiratory distress of bronchial asthma, chronic bronchitis, emphysema, other COPD
- *Aerosols and solutions for nebulization:* Temporary relief from acute attacks of bronchial asthma
- *Topical nasal solution:* Temporary relief from nasal and nasopharyngeal mucosal congestion due to a cold, sinusitis, hay fever, or other upper respiratory allergies; adjunctive therapy in middle ear infections by decreasing congestion around eustachian ostia
- *0.25%–2% ophthalmic solutions:* Management of open-angle (chronic simple) glaucoma, often in combination with miotics or other drugs
- *0.1% ophthalmic solution:* Conjunctivitis, during eye surgery to control bleeding, to produce mydriasis

Contraindications/cautions
- Contraindicated in the presence of allergy or hypersensitivity to epinephrine or components of drug preparation (many of the inhalant and ophthalmic products contain sulfites: sodium bisulfite, sodium or potassium metabisulfite; check label before using any of these products in a sulfite-sensitive patient); narrow-angle glaucoma; shock other than anaphylactic shock; hypovolemia; general anesthesia with halogenated hydrocarbons or cyclopropane; organic brain damage, cerebral arteriosclerosis; cardiac dilation and coronary insufficiency; tachyarrhythmias; ischemic heart disease; hypertension; renal dysfunction (drug may initially decrease renal blood flow); COPD patients who have developed degenerative heart disease; diabetes mellitus; hyperthyroidism; lactation.
- Use caution in the presence of prostatic hypertrophy (may cause bladder sphincter spasm, difficult and painful urination), history of seizure disorders, psychoneurotic individuals, labor and delivery (may delay second stage of labor; can accelerate fetal heart beat; may cause fetal and maternal hypoglycemia), children (syncope has occurred when epinephrine has been given to asthmatic children).
- Route-specific contraindications for ophthalmic preparations: wearing contact lenses (drug may discolor the contact lens), aphakic patients (maculopathy with decreased visual acuity may occur)

Dosage
Adult
- ***Epinephrine injection***
  – ***Cardiac arrest:*** 0.5–1.0 mg (5–10 ml

of 1:10,000 solution) IV or by intracardiac injection into left ventricular chamber; during resuscitation, 0.5 mg q5 min.
- *Intraspinal:* 0.2–0.4 ml of a 1:1,000 solution added to anesthetic spinal fluid mixture.
- *Other use with local anesthetic:* Concentrations of 1:100,000–1:20,000 are usually used.
- *1:1,000 solution*
  – *Respiratory distress:* 0.3–0.5 ml of 1:1,000 solution (0.3–0.5 mg), SC or IM, q20 min for 4 h.
- *1:200 suspension (for SC administration only)*
  – *Respiratory distress:* 0.1–0.3 ml (0.5–1.5 mg) SC.
- *Inhalation (aerosol):* Begin treatment at first symptoms of bronchospasm. Individualize dosage. Wait 1–5 min between inhalations to avoid overdose.
- *Inhalation (nebulization):* Place 8–15 drops into the nebulizer reservoir. Place nebulizer nozzle into partially opened mouth. Patient inhales deeply while bulb is squeezed one to three times. If no relief in 5 min, give 2–3 additional inhalations. Use four to six times per day usually maintains comfort.
- *Topical nasal solution:* Apply locally as drops or spray or with a sterile swab, as required.
- *Ophthalmic solution for glaucoma:* Instill 1–2 drops into affected eye(s) qd–bid. May be given as infrequently as every 3 d; determine frequency by tonometry. When used in conjunction with miotics, instill miotic first.
- *Ophthalmic solution for vasoconstriction, mydriasis:* Instill 1–2 drops into the eye(s); repeat once if necessary.

Pediatric
- *Epinephrine injection:* 1:1,000 solution, children and infants except premature infants and full-term newborns: 0.01 mg/kg or 0.3 ml/m^2 (0.01 mg/kg or 0.3 mg/m^2) SC q20 min (or more often if needed) for 4 h. Do not exceed 0.5 ml (0.5 mg) in a single dose. 1:200 suspension, infants and children (1 mo–1 y): 0.005 ml/kg (0.025 mg/kg) SC. Children 30 kg or less: Maximum single dose is 0.15 ml (0.75 mg). Administer subsequent doses only when necessary and not more often than q6h.
- *Topical nasal solution (children older than 6 y):* Apply locally as drops or spray or with a sterile swab, as required.
- *Ophthalmic solutions:* Safety and efficacy for use in children not established.

Geriatric or renal failure patients: Use with caution; patients older than 60 y are more likely to develop adverse effects.

Pharmacokinetics

Route	Onset	Peak	Duration
SC	5–10 min	20 min	20–30 min
IM	5–10 min	20 min	20–30 min
IV	instant	20 min	20–30 min
Inhal.	3–5 min	20 min	1–3 h
Eye	< 1 h	4–8 h	24 h

Metabolism: Neural
Distribution: Crosses placenta; passes into breast milk

IV facts
Preparation: 0.5 ml dose may be diluted to 10 ml with Sodium Chloride Injection for direct injection; prepare infusion by mixing 1 mg in 250 ml 5% Dextrose in Water (4 µg/ml)
Infusion: Administer by direct IV injection or into the tubing of a running IV, or run infusion at 1–4 µg/min (15–60 ml/h)

Adverse effects
Systemic Administration
- CNS: *Fear, anxiety, tenseness, restlessness, headache, lightheadedness, dizziness,* drowsiness, tremor, insomnia, hallucinations, psychological disturbances, convulsions, **CNS depression,** weakness, blurred vision, ocular irritation, tearing, photophobia, symptoms of paranoid schizophrenia
- GI: *Nausea,* vomiting, anorexia

- **CV:** Arrhythmias, hypertension resulting in intracranial hemorrhage, cardiovascular collapse with hypotension, palpitations, tachycardia, precordial pain in patients with ischemic heart disease
- **GU:** Constriction of renal blood vessels and *decreased urine formation* (initial parenteral administration), *dysuria, vesical sphincter spasm* resulting in difficult and painful urination, urinary retention in males with prostatism
- **Other:** *Pallor*, respiratory difficulty, orofacial dystonia, sweating

Local Injection
- **Local:** Necrosis at sites of repeat injections (due to intense vasoconstriction)

Nasal Solution
- **Local:** Rebound congestion, local burning and stinging

Ophthalmic Solutions
- **CNS:** *Headache, browache, blurred vision,* photophobia, difficulty with night vision, pigmentary (adrenochrome) deposits in the cornea, conjunctiva, or lids with prolonged use
- **Local:** *Transitory stinging on initial instillation,* eye pain or ache, conjunctival hyperemia

Clinically important drug-drug interactions

- Increased sympathomimetic effects when given with other tricyclic antidepressants (eg, imipramine), rauwolfia alkaloids
- Excessive hypertension when epinephrine is given with propranolol, beta-blocker, furazolidone • Decreased cardiostimulating and bronchodilating effects when given with beta-adrenergic blockers (eg, propranolol)
- Decreased vasopressor effects when given with chlorpromazine, phenothiazines
- Decreased antihypertensive effect of guanethidine, methyldopa, when given with epinephrine

■ Nursing Considerations

Assessment
- *History:* Allergy or hypersensitivity to epinephrine or components of drug preparation; narrow-angle glaucoma; shock other than anaphylactic shock; hypovolemia; general anesthesia with halogenated hydrocarbons or cyclopropane; oganic brain damage, cerebral arteriosclerosis; cardiac dilation and coronary insufficiency; tachyarrhythmias; ischemic heart disease; hypertension; renal dysfunction; COPD; diabetes mellitus; hyperthyroidism; prostatic hypertrophy; history of seizure disorders; psychoneuroses; labor and delivery; lactation; contact lens use, aphakic patients (ophthalmic prep)
- *Physical:* Body weight; skin—color, temperature, turgor; orientation, reflexes, intraocular pressure; P, BP; R, adventitious sounds; prostate palpation, normal urine output; urinalysis, kidney function tests, blood and urine glucose, serum electrolytes, thyroid function tests, ECG

Implementation
- Use extreme caution when calculating and preparing doses; epinephrine is a very potent drug; small errors in dosage can cause serious adverse effects. Double-checking of pediatric dosage is recommended.
- Use minimal doses for minimal periods of time; "epinephrine-fastness" (a form of drug tolerance) can occur with prolonged use.
- Protect drug solutions from light, extreme heat, and freezing; do not use pink or brown solutions. Drug solutions should be clear and colorless (does not apply to suspension for injection).
- Shake the suspension for injection well before withdrawing the dose.
- Rotate SC injection sites to prevent necrosis; monitor injection sites frequently.
- Maintain a rapidly acting alpha-adrenergic blocker (phentolamine) or a vasodilator (such as a nitrite) on standby in case of excessive hypertensive reaction.
- Maintain an alpha-adrenergic blocker or facilities for intermittent positive pressure breathing on standby in case pulmonary edema occurs.
- Maintain a beta-adrenergic blocker (propranolol; a cardioselective beta-blocker,

Adverse effects in *Italics* are most common; those in **Bold** are life-threatening.

such as atenolol, should be used in patients with respiratory distress) on standby in case cardiac arrhythmias occur.
- Do not exceed recommended dosage of inhalation products; administer pressurized inhalation drug forms during second half of inspiration, because the airways are open wider and the aerosol distribution is more extensive. If a second inhalation is needed, administer at peak effect of previous dose, 3–5 min.
- Use topical nasal solutions only for acute states; do not use for longer than 3–5 d, and do not exceed recommended dosage. Rebound nasal congestion can occur after vasoconstriction subsides.

Drug-specific teaching points
- Do not exceed recommended dosage; adverse effects or loss of effectiveness may result. Read the instructions that come with the product (respiratory inhalant products), and consult your health care provider or pharmacist if you have any questions.
- Administer eye drops as follows: Lie down or tilt head backward, and look at ceiling. Hold dropper above eye; drop medicine inside lower lid while looking up. Do not touch dropper to eye, fingers, or any surface. Release lower lid; keep eye open, and do not blink for at least 30 sec. Apply gentle pressure with fingers to inside corner of the eye for about 1 min; wait at least 5 min before using other eye drops.
- Know that the following side effects may occur: dizziness, drowsiness, fatigue, apprehension (use caution if driving or performing tasks that require alertness if these effects occur); anxiety, emotional changes; nausea, vomiting, change in taste (small, frequent meals may help; fast heart rate,. *Nasal solution:* burning or stinging when first used (these effects are transient and usually cease to be a problem after several treatments). *Ophthalmic solution:* slight stinging when first used (this is usually transient and usually ceases to be a problem after several uses); headache or browache (this usually occurs only during the first few days of therapy).
- Report chest pain, dizziness, insomnia, weakness, tremor or irregular heart beat (respiratory inhalant products, nasal solution), difficulty breathing, productive cough, failure to respond to usual dosage (respiratory inhalant products), decrease in visual acuity (ophthalmic preparations).

⬜ epoetin alfa

(e poe e' tin)
EPO
Epogen, Procrit

Pregnancy Category C

Drug classes
Recombinant human erythropoietin

Therapeutic actions
A natural glycoprotein produced in the kidneys, which stimulates red blood cell production in the bone marrow.

Indications
- Treatment of anemia associated with chronic renal failure, including patients on dialysis
- Treatment of anemia related to therapy with AZT in HIV-infected patients
- Treatment of anemia related to chemotherapy in cancer patients (*Procrit* only)
- Unlabeled use: increasing the procurement of autologous blood in patients about to undergo elective surgery

Contraindications/cautions
- Uncontrolled hypertension; hypersensitivity to mammalian cell-derived products or to albumin human; lactation.

Dosage
Adult: Starting dose: 50–100 U/kg three times weekly, IV for dialysis patients and IV or SC for nondialysis patients. Reduce dose if Hct increases > 4 points in any 2-wk period. Increase dose if Hct does not increase by 5–6 points after 8 wk of therapy. Maintenance dose: individualize based on

Hct, generally 25 U/kg three times weekly. Target Hct range 30%–33%.
- **HIV-infected patients on AZT therapy:** Patients receiving < 4,200 mg/wk with serum erythropoietin levels < 500 mU/ml: 100 U/kg IV or SC three times weekly for 8 wk; when desired response is achieved, titrate dose to maintain hematocrit with lowest possible dose.
- **Cancer patients on chemotherapy (Procrit only):** 150 U/kg SC three times per week; after 8 wk, can be increased to 300 U/kg.

Pediatric: Safety and efficacy not established.

Pharmacokinetics

Route	Onset	Peak	Duration
SC	7–14 d	5–24 h	24 h

Metabolism: Serum, $T_{1/2}$: 4–13 h
Distribution: Crosses placenta; enters breast milk
Excretion: Urine

IV facts
Preparation: Administer as provided; no additional preparation needed. Enter vial only once; discard any unused solution. Refrigerate.
Infusion: Administer by direct IV injection or into tubing of running IV.
Incompatibilities: Do not mix with any other drug solution.

Adverse effects
- **CNS:** *Headache, arthralgias, fatigue, asthenia, dizziness,* seizure, **CVA/TIA**
- **GI:** *Nausea, vomiting, diarrhea*
- **CV:** *Hypertension, edema, chest pain*
- **Other:** Clotting of access line

■ Nursing Considerations
Assessment
- *History:* Uncontrolled hypertension, hypersensitivity to mammalian cell-derived products or to albumin human, lactation
- *Physical:* Reflexes; affect; BP, P; urinary output, renal function; tests, CBC, Hct, iron levels, electrolytes

Implementation
- Ensure chronic, renal nature of anemia. Epoetin is not intended as a treatment of severe anemia and is not a substitute for emergency transfusion.
- Prepare solution with gentle mixing. Do not shake; shaking may denature the glycoprotein. Use only one dose per vial; do not reenter the vial. Discard unused portions.
- Do not administer in conjunction with any other drug solution.
- Administer dose three times weekly. If administered independent of dialysis, administer into venous access line. If patient is not on dialysis, administer IV or SC.
- Monitor access lines for signs of clotting.
- Arrange for Hct reading before administration of each dose to determine appropriate dosage. If patient fails to respond within 8 wk of therapy, evaluate patient for other etiologies of the problem.
- Evaluate iron stores prior to and periodically during therpy. Supplemental iron may need to be ordered.
- Maintain seizure precautions on standby during administration.

Drug-specific teaching points
- Know that the drug will need to be given three times a week and can only be given IV or SC or into a dialysis access line. Prepare a schedule of administration dates.
- Keep appointments for blood tests; frequent blood tests are necessary to determine the effects of the drug on your blood count and to determine the appropriate dosage needed.
- Know that the following side effects may occur: dizziness, headache, seizures (avoid driving a car or performing hazardous tasks); fatigue, joint pain (medications may be available to help); nausea, vomiting, diarrhea (proper nutrition is important; ensure ready access to bathroom facilities).

Adverse effects in *Italics* are most common; those in **Bold** are life-threatening.

- Report difficulty breathing, numbness or tingling, chest pain, seizures, severe headache.
- Maintain all of the usual activities and restrictions that apply to your chronic renal failure. If this becomes difficult, consult with your nurse or physician.

☐ ergonovine maleate

(er goe noe' veen)

Ergotrate Maleate

Pregnancy Category Unknown

Drug classes
Oxytocic

Therapeutic actions
Increases the strength, duration, and frequency of uterine contractions, and decreases postpartum uterine bleeding by direct effects at neuroreceptor sites.

Indications
- Prevention and treatment of postpartum and postabortal hemorrhage due to uterine atony
- Migraine headache, especially if use of ergotamine, which is generally more effective, has been accompanied by paresthesias
- Unlabeled use: diagnostic test for Printzmetal's angina; doses of 0.05–0.2 mg IV during coronary arteriography provoke coronary artery spasm (reversible with nitroglycerin; arrhythmias, ventricular tachycardia, MI have occurred)

Contraindications/cautions
- Contraindicated in the presence of allergy to ergonovine, induction of labor, threatened spontaneous abortion.
- Use caution in the presence of hypertension, heart disease, venoatrial shunts, mitral-valve stenosis, obliterative vascular disease, sepsis, hepatic or renal impairment, lactation.

Dosage
Adult
- ***Parenteral:*** 0.2 mg IM (IV in emergency situations). Severe bleeding may require repeat doses q2–4h.
- ***Oral:*** 1–2 tablets q6–12h until the danger of uterine atony has passed, usually 48 h. May be given sublingually.
- ***Diagnostic:*** 0.1–0.4 mg IV.

Pharmacokinetics

Route	Onset	Duration
Oral	5–15 min	3 h
IM	2–5 min	3 h
IV	Immediate	45 min

Metabolism: Hepatic, $T_{1/2}$: 0.5–2 h
Distribution: Crosses placenta; enters breast milk
Excretion: Feces, urine

IV facts
Preparation: No preparation required.
Infusion: Administer by direct IV injection or into tubing of running IV; reserve IV use for emergency situation or diagnostic test.

Adverse effects
- CNS: *Dizziness, headache*, ringing in the ears
- GI: *Nausea, vomiting*, diarrhea
- CV: Elevation of blood pressure—more common with ergonovine than other oxytocics
- Hypersensitivity: Allergic response, including shock
- Other: Ergotism—nausea, blood pressure changes, weak pulse, dyspnea, chest pain, numbness and coldness of the extremities, confusion, excitement, delirium, hallucinations, convulsions, coma

■ Nursing Considerations

Assessment
- *History:* Allergy to ergonovine, induction of labor, threatened spontaneous abortion, hypertension, heart disease, venoatrial shunts, obliterative vascular disease,

Adverse effects in *Italics* are most common; those in **Bold** are life-threatening.

sepsis, hepatic or renal impairment, lactation
- *Physical:* Uterine tone; orientation, reflexes, affect; P, BP, edema; R, adventitious sounds; CBC, renal and liver function tests

Implementation

- Administer parenteral preparation by IM injection unless emergency requires IV use; complications are more frequent with IV use.
- Administer oral ergonovine to minimize postpartum bleeding; abdominal cramping is evidence of effectiveness but may require a reduction of dosage.
- Monitor postpartum women for BP changes and amount and character of vaginal bleeding.
- Arrange for discontinuation of drug if signs of ergotism occur.
- Avoid prolonged use of the drug.

Drug-specific teaching points

- The patient receiving a parenteral oxytocic is usually receiving it as part of an immediate medical situation, and the drug teaching should be incorporated into the teaching about the complication of delivery or abortion that is involved. The patient needs to know the name of the drug and what she can expect once it is administered.
- Take 1–2 tablets q6–12h until the danger of uterine bleeding has passed, usually only 48 h.
- Know that the following side effects may occur: nausea, vomiting, dizziness, headache, ringing in the ears (the drug is only given for a short time, so these may be tolerable.
- Report difficulty breathing, headache, numb or cold extremities, severe abdominal cramping.

☐ ergotamine tartrate

(er got' a meen)
Sublingual preparations:
Ergostat, Gynergen (CAN)
Pregnancy Category X

Drug classes
Ergot derivative
Antimigraine drug

Therapeutic actions
Mechanism of action not understood; constricts cranial blood vessels; decreases pulsation in cranial arteries, and decreases hyperperfusion of basilar artery vascular bed.

Indications
- Prevention or abortion of vascular headaches, such as migraine, migraine variant, cluster headache

Contraindications/cautions
- Allergy to ergot preparations; peripheral vascular disease, severe hypertension, coronary artery disease, impaired liver or renal function, sepsis, pruritus, malnutrition; pregnancy; lactation (can cause ergotism—vomiting, diarrhea, seizures—in infant).

Dosage
Adult
- *Sublingual:* 1 tablet under the tongue as soon as possible after the first symptoms of an attack; take subsequent doses at $\frac{1}{2}$-h intervals if necessary. Do not exceed 3 tablets/d; do not exceed 10 mg/wk.

Pediatric: Safety and efficacy not established.

Pharmacokinetics

Route	Onset	Peak
Sublingual	Rapid	$\frac{1}{2}$–3 h

Metabolism: Hepatic, $T_{1/2}$: 2.7 h, then 21 h
Distribution: Crosses placenta; enters breast milk
Excretion: Feces

Adverse effects
- CNS: *Numbness, tingling of fingers and toes, muscle pain in the extremities*
- GI: *Nausea, vomiting* (drug stimulates CTZ)
- CV: *Pulselessness, weakness in the legs; precordial distress and pain, transient tachycardia, bradycardia, localized*

edema and itching; increased arterial pressure, arterial insufficiency, coronary vasoconstriction, bradycardia
- **Other:** Ergotism—nausea, vomiting, diarrhea, severe thirst, hypoperfusion, chest pain, blood pressure changes, confusion—with prolonged use; drug dependency and abuse—with extended use, patients may require progressively increasing doses for relief of headaches and for prevention of dysphoric effects that occur with drug withdrawal

Clinically important drug-drug interactions
- Peripheral ischemia manifested by cold extremities; possible peripheral gangrene if taken concurrently with beta-blockers

■ Nursing Considerations
Assessment
- *History:* Allergy to ergot preparations, peripheral vascular disease, severe hypertension, coronary artery disease, impaired liver or renal function, sepsis, pruritus, malnutrition, pregnancy, lactation
- *Physical:* Skin—color, edema, lesions; body temperature; peripheral sensation; P, BP, peripheral pulses, peripheral perfusion; liver evaluation, bowel sounds; CBC, liver and renal function tests

Implementation
- Avoid prolonged administration or excessive dosage.
- Arrange for use of atropine or phenothiazine antiemetics if nausea and vomiting are severe.
- Assess extremities carefully to ensure there is no gangrene or decubitus ulcer formation.
- Provide supportive measures if acute overdose occurs.

Drug-specific teaching points
- Take the drug as soon as possible after the first symptoms of an attack. Do not exceed the recommended dosage; if relief is not obtained, contact your physician.
- Know that the following side effects may occur: nausea, vomiting (if this becomes severe, medication may be ordered to help); numbness, tingling, loss of sensation in the extremities (use caution to avoid injury and examine extremities daily to ensure that no injury has occurred).
- Do not take this drug during pregnancy. If you become pregnant or desire to become pregnant, consult with your physician.
- Report irregular heartbeat, pain or weakness of extremities, severe nausea or vomiting, numbness or tingling of fingers or toes.

❒ erythrityl tetranitrate

(e ri' thri till)
Cardilate

Pregnancy Category C

Drug classes
Antianginal drug
Nitrate

Therapeutic actions
Relaxes vascular smooth muscle, decreasing venous return and decreasing arterial blood pressure, which reduces left ventricular work load and decreases myocardial oxygen consumption.

Indications
- Prophylaxis and long-term treatment of anginal pain and reduced exercise tolerance associated with angina pectoris

Contraindications/cautions
- Allergy to nitrates; severe anemia; head trauma, cerebral hemorrhage (drug increases intracranial pressure); hypertrophic cardiomyopathy; lactation.

Dosage
Adult
- ***Sublingual:*** 5–10 mg prior to anticipated physical or emotional stress that may cause anginal attack.
- ***Chewable or oral:*** 10 mg before meals, midmorning and midafternoon. Additional dose may be given at bedtime

if nocturnal angina occurs. Up to 100 mg/d is usually well tolerated.
Pediatric: Safety and efficacy not established.

Pharmacokinetics

Route	Onset	Peak	Duration
Oral	15–30 min	1 h	6 h
Sublingual	5 min	15 min	3 h

Metabolism: Hepatic
Distribution: Crosses placenta; enters breast milk
Excretion: Urine

Adverse effects

- **CNS:** *Headache, apprehension, restlessness, weakness,* vertigo, dizziness, faintness
- **GI:** *Nausea, vomiting,* incontinence, abdominal pain
- **CV:** *Tachycardia,* retrosternal discomfort, palpitations, hypotension, syncope, collapse, postural hypotension, angina
- **Dermatologic:** Rash, exfoliative dermatitis, cutaneous vasodilation with flushing
- **Other:** Muscle twitching, pallor, perspiration, cold sweat

Clinically important drug-drug interactions

- Increased blood pressure and lack of antianginal effects if taken concurrently with ergot alkaloids

Drug-lab test interferences

- False report of decreased serum cholesterol if done by the Zlatkis-Zak color reaction

■ Nursing Considerations

Assessment

- *History:* Allergy to nitrates, severe anemia, head trauma, cerebral hemorrhage, hypertrophic cardiomyopathy, lactation
- *Physical:* Skin—color, temperature, lesions; orientation, reflexes, affect; P, BP, orthostatic BP, baseline ECG, peripheral perfusion; R, adventitious sounds; liver evaluation, normal GI output; CBC, hemoglobin

Implementation

- Administer sublingual preparations under the tongue or in the buccal pouch; encourage the patient not to swallow.
- Administer oral preparations with meals.
- Monitor patient for nocturnal angina; have additional dosage available at bedtime for these patients.
- Maintain life support equipment on standby if overdose occurs or cardiac condition worsens.
- Arrange for gradual reduction in dose if anginal treatment is being terminated; rapid discontinuation can lead to problems of withdrawal.

Drug-specific teaching points

- Place sublingual tablets under your tongue or in your cheek. Do not chew or swallow these tablets. Take the drug before chest pain begins, when you anticipate that your activities or situation may precipitate an attack. Take before meals and at other prescribed times.
- Be aware that if pain is not relieved within 5 min by one sublingual tablet, you should dissolve a second tablet. Repeat in 5 min if needed. If pain is not relieved by 3 tablets or if it intensifies, notify physician immediately, or go to nearest hospital emergency room.
- Know that the following side effects may occur: dizziness, lightheadedness (this may pass as you adjust to the drug; use care to change positions slowly); headache (lying down in a cool environment and resting may help, OTC preparations also may help); flushing of the neck or face (this usually passes as the drug's effects pass).
- Report blurred vision, persistent or severe headache, skin rash, more frequent or more severe angina attacks, fainting.

❒ erythromycin base

*(er ith roe **mye' **sin)*

Oral, ophthalmic ointment, topical dermatologic solution for acne, topical dermatologic ointment:

Adverse effects in *Italics* are most common; those in **Bold** are life-threatening.

erythromycin base

AK-Mycin, Akne-mycin, A/T/S, E-Mycin, Eryc, Eryderm, Erymax, Ery-Tab, Ilotycin, Ilotycin Ophthalmic, Novorythro (CAN), Robimycin, Staticin, T-Stat

erythromycin estolate
Oral: Ilosone, Novorythro (CAN)

erythromycin ethylsuccinate
Oral: E.E.S., E-Mycin, EryPed

erythromycin gluceptate
Parenteral, IV: Ilotycin Gluceptate

erythromycin lactobionate, erythromycin stearate
Oral: Eramycin

Pregnancy Category B

Drug classes
Macrolide antibiotic

Therapeutic actions
Bacteriostatic or bactericidal in susceptible bacteria; binds to cell membrane, causing change in protein function, leading to cell death.

Indications
Systemic Administration
- Acute infections caused by sensitive strains of *Streptococcus pneumoniae, Mycoplasma pneumoniae, Listeria monocytogenes, Legionella pneumophila*
- URIs, LRIs, skin and soft-tissue infections caused by group A beta-hemolytic streptococci when oral treatment is preferred to injectable benzathine penicillin
- PID caused by *N. gonorrhoeae* in patients allergic to penicillin
- In conjunction with sulfonamides in URIs caused by *Haemophilus influenzae*
- As an adjunct to antitoxin in infections caused by *Corynebacterium diphtheriae* and *Corynebacterium minutissimum*
- Prophylaxis against alpha-hemolytic streptococcal endocarditis before dental or other procedures in patients allergic to penicillin who have valvular heart disease

Oral Erythromycin
- Treatment of intestinal amebiasis caused by *Entamoeba histolytica*; infections in the newborn and in pregnancy that are caused by *Chlamydia trachomatis* and in adult chlamydial infections when tetracycline cannot be used; primary syphilis (*Treponema pallidum*) in penicillin-allergic patients; eliminating *Bordetella pertussis* organisms from the nasopharynx of infected individuals and as prophylaxis in exposed and susceptible individuals.
- Unlabeled uses: erythromycin base is used with neomycin before colorectal surgery to reduce wound infection; treatment of severe diarrhea associated with *Campylobacter* enteritis or enterococolitis; treatment of genital, inguinal, or anorectal lymphogranuloma venereum infection; treatment of *Haemophilus ducreyi* (chancroid)

Ophthalmic Ointment
- Treatment of superficial ocular infections caused by susceptible strains of microorganisms; prophylaxos of ophthalmia neonatorum caused by *N. gonorrhoeae* or *C. trachomatis*

Topical Dermatologic Solutions for Acne
- Treatment of acne vulgaris

Topical Dermatologic Ointment
- Prophylaxis against infection in minor skin abrasions
- Treatment of skin infections caused by sensitive microorganisms

Contraindications/cautions
Systemic Administration
- Contraindicated in the presence of allergy to erythromycin.
- Use caution in the presence of hepatic dysfunction, lactation (secreted and may be concentrated in breast milk; may modify bowel flora of nursing infant and interfere with fever workups).

erythromycin base

Ophthalmic Ointment
- Contraindicated in the presence of allergy to erythromycin; viral, fungal, mycobacterial infections of the eye.

Dosage

Systemic administration: Oral preparations of the different erythromycin salts differ in pharmacokinetics: 400 mg erythromycin ethylsuccinate produces the same free erythromycin serum levels as 250 mg of erythromycin base, sterate, or estolate.

- ***Adult:*** 15–20 mg/kg per day in continuous IV infusion or up to 4 g/d in divided doses q6h; 250 mg (400 mg of ethylsuccinate) q6h PO or 500 mg q12h PO or 333 mg q8h PO, up to 4 g/d, depending on the severity of the infection.
  - *Streptococcal infections:* 20–50 mg/kg per day PO in divided doses (for group A beta-hemolytic streptococcal infections, continue therapy for at least 10 d).
  - *Legionnaire's disease:* 1–4 g/d PO or IV in divided doses (ethylsuccinate 1.6 g/d; optimal doses not established).
  - *Dysenteric amebiasis:* 250 mg (400 mg of ethylsuccinate) PO qid or 333 mg q8h for 10–14 d.
  - *Acute pelvic inflammatory disease (N. gonorrhoeae):* 500 mg of lactobionate or gluceptate IV q6h for 3 d and then 250 mg stearate or base PO q6h or 333 mg q8h for 7 d.
  - *Pertussis:* 40–50 mg/kg per day PO in divided doses for 5–14 d (optimal dosage not established).
  - *Prophylaxis against bacterial endocarditis before dental or upper respiratory procedures:* 1 g (1.6 g of ethylsuccinate) 6 h later.
  - *Chlamydial infections:* Urogenital infections during pregnancy: 500 mg PO qid or 666 mg q8h for at least 7 d; 250 mg qid or 333 mg q8h for at least 14 d if intolerant to first regimen. Urethritis in males: 800 mg of ethylsuccinate PO tid for 7 d.
  - *Primary syphilis:* 30–40 g (48–64 g of ethylsuccinate) in divided doses over 10–15 d.
  - *CDC recommendations for sexually transmitted diseases:* 500 mg PO qid for 7–30 d, depending on the infection involved.
- ***Pediatric:*** 30–50 mg/kg per day PO in divided doses. Specific dosage should be determined by severity of infection, age and body weight of child.
  - *Dysenteric amebiasis:* 30–50 mg/kg per day in divided doses for 10–14 d.
  - *Prophylaxis against bacterial endocarditis:* 20 mg/kg before procedure and then 10 mg/kg 6 h later.
  - *Chlamydial infections:* 50 mg/kg per day PO in divided doses, for at least 2 (conjunctivitis of newborn) or 3 (pneumonia of infancy) wk.

Ophthalmic ointment: ½-in ribbon instilled into conjunctival sac of affected eye two to six times per day, depending on severity of infection.

Topical dermatologic solution of acne: Apply to affected areas morning and evening.

Topical dermatologic ointment: Apply to affected area one to five times per day.

Pharmacokinetics

Route	Onset	Peak
Oral	1–2 h	1–4 h
IV	Rapid	1 h

Metabolism: Hepatic, $T_{1/2}$: 3–5 h
Distribution: Crosses placenta; enters breast milk
Excretion: Bile and urine

IV facts

Preparation: Reconstitute powder for IV infusion only with Sterile Water for Injection without preservatives—10 ml for 250- and 500-mg vials, 20 ml for 1-g vials. Prepare intermittent infusion as follows: Dilute 250–500 mg in 100–250 ml of 0.9% Sodium Chloride Injection or 5% Dextrose in Water. Prepare for continuous infusion by adding reconstituted drug to 0.9% Sodium Chloride Injection, Lactated Ringer's injection, or 5% Dextrose in Water that will make a solution of 1 g/L.

Infusion: Intermittent infusion: administer over 20–60 min qid; infuse slowly to avoid vein irritation. Administer continuous infusion within 4 h, or buffer the solution to neutrality if the period of administration is prolonged.

Adverse effects
Systemic Administrations
- CNS: Reversible hearing loss, confusion, uncontrollable emotions, abnormal thinking
- GI: *Abdominal cramping, anorexia, diarrhea, vomiting*, pseudomembranous colitis, hepatotoxicity
- Hypersensitivity: Allergic reactions ranging from rash to anaphylaxis
- Other: *Superinfections*

Ophthalmic Ointment
- Dermatologic: Edema, utricaria, dermatitis, angioneurotic edema
- Local: *Irritation, burning, itching* at site of application

Topical Dermatologic Preparations
- Local: *Superinfections*, particularly with long-term use

Clinically important drug-drug interactions
Systemic Administration
- Increased serum levels of digoxin if taken with erythromycin • Increased effects of oral anticoagulants, theophyllines, carbamazepine • Increased therapeutic and toxic effects of corticosteroids • Increased levels of cyclosporine and risk of renal toxicity when taken concurrently with erythromycin • Potentially fatal cardiac arrhythmias if taken with astemizde, terfenadine

Topical Dermatologic Solution for Acne
- Increased irritant effects with peeling, desquamating, or abrasive agents

Drug-lab test interferences
Systemic Administration
- Interferes with fluorometric determination of urinary catecholamines • Decreased urinary estriol levels due to inhibition of hydrolysis of steroids in the gut

■ Nursing Considerations
Assessment
- *History:* Allergy to erythromycin, hepatic dysfunction, lactation; viral, fungal, mycobacterial infections of the eye (ophthalmologic)
- *Physical:* Site of infection; skin—color, lesions; orientation, affect, hearing tests; R, adventitious sounds; GI output, bowel sounds, liver evaluation; culture and sensitivity tests of infection, urinalysis, liver function tests

Implementation
Systemic Administration
- Culture site of infection before beginning therapy.
- Administer oral erythromycin base or stearate on an empty stomach, 1 h before or 2–3 h after meals, with a full glass of water (oral erythromycin estolate, ethylsuccinate, and certain enteric-coated tablets [see manufacturer's instructions] may be given without regard to meals).
- Administer drug around the clock to maximize therapeutic effect; scheduling may have to be adjusted to minimize sleep disruption.
- Monitor liver function in patients on prolonged therapy.
- Give some preparations (see above) with meals, or it may be possible to substitute one of these preparations, if GI upset occurs with oral therapy.

Topical Dermatologic Solution for Acne
- Wash affected area, rinse well, and dry before application.

Ophthalmic and Topical Dermatologic Preparation
- Use topical erythromycin products only when clearly needed. Sensitization produced by the topical use of an antibiotic may preclude its later systemic use in serious infections. Topical preparations that contain antibiotics not normally used systemically are therefore preferable.

Adverse effects in *Italics* are most common; those in **Bold** are life-threatening.

- Culture site of infection before beginning therapy.
- Cover the affected area with a sterile bandage if needed (topical dermatologic preparations).

Drug-specific teaching points
Systemic Administration
- Take oral drug on an empty stomach, 1 h before or 2–3 h after meals, with a full glass of water, or drug may be taken without regard to meals, as appropriate. The drug should be taken around the clock; schedule to minimize sleep disruption. It is important that you finish the *full course* of the drug therapy.
- Know that the following side effects may occur: stomach cramping, discomfort (taking the drug with meals, if appropriate, may alleviate this problem); uncontrollable emotions, crying, laughing, abnormal thinking (these will go away when the drug is stopped).
- Report severe or watery diarrhea, severe nausea or vomiting, dark urine, yellowing of the skin or eyes, loss of hearing, skin rash or itching.

Ophthalmic Ointment
- Pull the lower eyelid down gently and squeeze a ½-in ribbon of the ointment into the sac that is formed, using care to avoid touching the eye or lid. A mirror may be helpful. Gently close the eye, and roll the eyeball in all directions.
- Know that drug may cause temporary blurring of vision, stinging, or itching.
- Report stinging or itching that becomes pronounced.

Topical Dermatologic Solution for Acne
- Wash and rinse area, and pat it dry before applying solution.
- Use fingertips or an applicator to apply; wash hands thoroughly after application.

☐ esmolol hydrochloride

(ess' moe lol)
Brevibloc
Pregnancy Category C

Drug classes
Beta-adrenergic blocking agent (β_1 selective)

Therapeutic actions
Blocks beta-adrenergic receptors in the heart and juxtaglomerular apparatus, reducing the influence of the sympathetic nervous system on these tissues; decreasing the excitability of the heart, cardiac output, and release of renin; and lowering blood pressure. At low doses, esmolol acts relatively selectively at the β_1-adrenergic receptors of the heart; has very rapid onset and short duration.

Indications
- Supraventricular tachycardia, when rapid but short-term control of ventricular rate is desirable (eg, patients with atrial fibrillation, flutter, in perioperative or postoperative situations)
- Noncompensatory tachycardia when heart rate requires specific intervention

Contraindications/cautions
- Because this drug is reserved for emergency situations, there are no contraindications to its use.

Dosage
Adult: Individualize dosage by titration, in which each step consists of a loading dose followed by a maintenance dose: initial loading dose of 500 μg/kg per minute IV for 1 min followed by a maintenance dose of 50 μg/kg per minute for 4 min. If adequate response is not observed within 5 min, repeat loading dose and follow with maintenance infusion of 100 μg/kg per minute. Repeat titration as necessary, increasing rate of maintenance dose in increments of 50 μg/kg per minute. As desired heart rate or safe end point is approached, omit loading infusion and decrease incremental dose in maintenance infusion to 25 μg/kg per minute (or less), or increase interval between titration steps from 5 to 10 min. Infusions for up to 24 h have been used; infusions up to 48 h may be well tolerated.
Pediatric: Safety and efficacy not established.

Pharmacokinetics

Route	Onset	Peak	Duration
IV	< 5 min	10–20 min	10–30 min

Metabolism: RBC esterases, $T_{1/2}$: 9 min
Distribution: Crosses placenta; enters breast milk
Excretion: Urine

IV facts

Preparation: Dilute drug before infusing as follows: Add the contents of 2 ampuls of esmolol (2.5 g) to 20 ml of a compatible diluent: 5% Dextrose Injection, 5% Dextrose in Ringer's Injection; 5% Dextrose and 0.9% or 0.45% Sodium Chloride Injection; Lactated Ringer's Injection; 0.9% or 0.45% Sodium Chloride Injection to make a drug solution with a concentration of 10 mg/ml. Diluted solution is stable for 24 h at room temperature. May be further diluted with same solution for continuous infusion.

Infusion: Rate of infusion is determined by patient response.

Adverse effects

- CNS: *Light-headedness, speech disorder, midscapular pain, weakness, rigors,* somnolence, confusion
- GI: *Taste perversion*
- CV: *Hypotension,* pallor
- GU: *Urinary retention*
- Local: *Inflammation,* induration, edema, erythema, burning at the site of infusion
- Other: Fever, rhonchi, flushing

Clinically important drug-drug interactions

- Increased therapeutic and toxic effects of esmolol if taken with verapamil • Impaired antihypertensive effects if taken with ibuprofen, indomethacin, piroxicam

■ Nursing Considerations

Assessment

- *History:* Cardiac disease, cerebrovascular disease
- *Physical:* P, BP, ECG; orientation, reflexes; R, adventitious sounds; urinary output

Implementation

- Ensure that drug is not used in chronic settings when transfer to another agent is anticipated.
- Do not give undiluted drug.
- Do not mix esmolol with sodium bicarbonate; do not mix undiluted esmolol with other drug solutions.
- Monitor BP closely.

Drug-specific teaching points

- This drug is reserved for emergency use; it is best to incorporate any information about this drug into an overall teaching program.

❒ estazolam

*(es **taz**' e lam)*
ProSom

Pregnancy Category X
C-IV controlled substance

Drug classes

Benzodiazepine
Sedative/hypnotic

Therapeutic actions

Exact mechanisms of action not understood; acts mainly at subcortical levels of the CNS, leaving the cortex relatively unaffected; potentiates the effects of GABA, an inhibitory neurotransmitter.

Indications

- Insomnia characterized by difficulty in falling asleep, frequent nocturnal awakenings, or early morning awakening
- Recurring insomnia or poor sleeping habits
- Acute or chronic medical situations requiring restful sleep

Contraindications/cautions

- Contraindicated in the presence of hypersensitivity to benzodiazepines, psychoses, acute narrow-angle glaucoma, shock, coma, acute alcoholic intoxication with depression of vital signs, pregnancy (increased risk of congenital malformations, neonatal withdrawal syndrome), labor

Adverse effects in *Italics* are most common; those in **Bold** are life-threatening.

estazolam ■ 445

and delivery ("floppy infant" syndrome reported when mothers were given benzodiazepines during labor), lactation (secreted in breast milk; chronic administration of diazepam, another benzodiazepine, to nursing mothers has caused infants to become lethargic and lose weight).
- Use caution in the presence of impaired liver or kidney function, debilitation, depression, suicidal tendencies.

Dosage
Individualize dosage.
Adult: 1 mg PO before bedtime; up to 2 mg may be needed in some patients.
Pediatric: Not for use in children younger than 15 y.
Geriatric patients or those with debilitating disease: 1 mg PO if healthy; starting dose of 0.5 mg in debilitated patients.

Pharmacokinetics

Route	Onset	Peak
Oral	45–60 min	2 h

Metabolism: Hepatic, $T_{1/2}$: 10–24 h
Distribution: Crosses placenta; enters breast milk
Excretion: Urine

Adverse effects
- CNS: *Transient, mild drowsiness initially; sedation, depression, lethargy, apathy, fatigue, lightheadedness, disorientation, restlessness, asthenia,* crying, delirium, headache, slurred speech, dysarthria, stupor, rigidity, tremor, dystonia, vertigo, euphoria, nervousness, difficulty in concentration, vivid dreams, psychomotor retardation, extrapyramidal symptoms, *mild paradoxical excitatory reactions, during first 2 wk of treatment* (especially in psychiatric patients, aggressive children, and with high dosage), visual and auditory disturbances, diplopia, nystagmus, depressed hearing, nasal congestion
- GI: *Constipation, diarrhea, dyspepsia,* dry mouth, salivation, nausea, anorexia, vomiting, difficulty in swallowing, gastric disorders, elevations of blood enzymes: LDH, alkaline phosphatase, SGOT, SGPT, hepatic dysfunction, jaundice
- CV: *Bradycardia, tachycardia,* cardiovascular collapse, hypertension and hypotension, palpitations, edema
- Hematologic: Decreased hematocrit, blood dyscrasias
- GU: *Incontinence, urinary retention, changes in libido,* menstrual irregularities
- Dermatologic: Urticaria, pruritus, skin rash, dermatitis
- Dependence: *Drug dependence with withdrawal syndrome* when drug is discontinued (more common with abrupt discontinuation of higher dosage used for longer than 4 mo)
- Other: Hiccups, fever, diaphoresis, paresthesias, muscular disturbances, gynecomastia

Clinically important drug-drug interactions
- Increased CNS depression when taken with alcohol, omeprazole • Increased pharmacologic effects of estazolam when given with cimetidine • Decreased sedative effects of estazolam if taken concurrently with theophylline, aminophylline, dyphylline, oxitriphylline

■ Nursing Considerations
Assessment
- *History:* Hypersensitivity to benzodiazepines; psychoses; acute narrow-angle glaucoma; shock; coma; acute alcoholic intoxication; pregnancy; labor; lactation; impaired liver or kidney function, debilitation, depression, suicidal tendencies.
- *Physical:* Skin—color, lesions; body temperature; orientation, reflexes, affect, ophthalmologic exam; P, BP; R, adventitious sounds; liver evaluation, abdominal exam, bowel sounds, normal output; CBC, liver and renal function tests.

Implementation
- Arrange to monitor liver and kidney function, CBC at intervals during long-term therapy.

Adverse effects in *Italics* are most common; those in **Bold** are life-threatening.

- Arrange to taper dosage gradually after long-term therapy, especially in epileptic patients.

Drug-specific teaching points
- Take drug exactly as prescribed; do not stop taking this drug (long-term therapy) without consulting the health care provider.
- Avoid alcohol, sleep-inducing, or OTC drugs while on this drug.
- Know that the following side effects may occur: drowsiness, dizziness (these may become less pronounced after a few days; avoid driving a car or engaging in other dangerous activities if these occur); GI upset (taking the drug with water may help); depression, dreams, emotional upset, crying; nocturnal sleep may be disturbed for several nights after discontinuing the drug.
- Report severe dizziness, weakness, drowsiness that persists, rash or skin lesions, palpitations, swelling of the extremities, visual changes, difficulty voiding.

☐ estradiol oral

*(ess tra **dye**' ole)*
Estrace

estradiol transdermal system: *Estraderm*

estradiol topical vaginal cream: *Estrace*

estradiol cypionate in oil
Depo-Estradiol Cypionate, dep Gynogen, Depogen, Dura-Estrin, Estra-D, Estro-Cyp, Estroject-L.A., Estronol-LA,

estradiol valerate in oil
Deladiol, Delestrogen, Dioval, Duragen, Estra-L 40, Gynogen L.A. 20, Valergen

Pregnancy Category X

Drug classes
Hormone
Estrogen

Therapeutic actions
Estradiol is the most potent endogenous female sex hormone. Estrogens are important in the development of the female reproductive system and secondary sex characteristics; affect the release of pituitary gonadotropins; cause capillary dilatation, fluid retention, protein anabolism and thin cervical mucus; conserve calcium and phosphorus and encourage bone formation; inhibit ovulation and prevent postpartum breast discomfort. They are responsible for the proliferation of the endometrium; absence or decline of estrogen produces signs and symptoms of menopause on the uterus, vagina, breasts, cervix; efficacy as palliation in male patients with androgen-dependent prostatic carcinoma; is attributable to their competition with androgens for receptor sites, thus decreasing the influence of androgens.

Indications
- Palliation of moderate to severe vasomotor symptoms, atrophic vaginitis or kraurosis vulvae associated with menopause (estradiol oral, transdermal, cream, estradiol valerate)
- Treatment of female hypogonadism, female castration, primary ovarian failure (estradiol oral, transdermal, estradioll cypionate, valerate)
- Palliation of inoperable prostatic cancer (estradiol oral, estradiol valerate)
- Palliation of inoperable, progressing breast cancer (estradiol oral)
- Prevention of postpartum breast engorgement (estradiol valerate)

Contraindications/cautions
- Contraindicated in the presence of allergy to estrogens, allergy to tartrazine (in 2-mg oral tablets), breast cancer (except in specific, selected patients), estrogen-dependent neoplasm, undiagnosed abnormal genital bleeding, active thrombophlebitis or thromboembolic disorders or history of such from previous estrogen use, pregnancy (associated with serious fetal defects; women of childbearing age

should be advised of the potential risks and birth control measures suggested).
- Use caution in the presence of metabolic bone disease, renal insufficiency, CHF, lactation.

Dosage
Adult
- ***Moderate to severe vasomotor symptoms, atrophic vaginitis, kraurosis vulvae associated with menopause:*** 1–2 mg/d PO. Adjust dose to control symptoms. Cyclic therapy (3 wk on and 1 wk off drug therapy) is recommended, especially in women who have not had a hysterectomy. 1–5 mg estradiol cypionate in oil IM every 3–4 wk. 10–20 mg estradiol valerate in oil IM, every 4 wk. 0.05-mg system applied to the skin twice weekly. If women have been on oral estrogens, start transdermal system 1 wk after withdrawal of oral form. Therapy is usually given on a cyclic schedule, 3 wk of therapy followed by 1 wk of rest. Attempt to taper or discontinue medication every 3–6 mo.
- *Vaginal cream:* 2–4 g intravaginally daily for 1–2 wk, then reduce to ½ dosage for similar period followed by maintenance doses of 1 g one to three times a week thereafter. Discontinue or taper at 3- to 6-mo intervals.
- ***Female hypogonadism, female castration, primary ovarian failure:*** 1–2 mg/d PO. Adjust dose to control symptoms. Cyclic therapy (3 wk on and 1 wk off drug therapy) is recommended. 1.5–2 mg estradiol cypionate in oil IM at monthly intervals. 10–20 mg estradiol valerate in oil IM every 4 wk. 0.05 mg system applied to skin twice weekly as above.
- ***Prostatic cancer (inoperable):*** 1–2 mg PO tid. Administer chronically. 30 mg or more estradiol valerate in oil IM every 1–2 wk.
- ***Breast cancer (inoperable, progressing):*** 10 mg tid PO for at least 3 mo.
- ***Prevention of postpartum breast engorgement:*** 10–25 mg estradiol valerate in oil IM as a single injection at the end of the first stage of labor.

Pediatric: Not recommended due to effect on the growth of the long bones.

Pharmacokinetics

Route	Onset	Peak
Oral	Slow	Days

Metabolism: Hepatic, $T_{1/2}$: not known
Distribution: Crosses placenta; enters breast milk
Excretion: Urine

Adverse effects
- **CNS:** Steepening of the corneal curvature with a resultant change in visual acuity and intolerance to contact lenses, *headache*, migraine, dizziness, mental depression, chorea, convulsions
- **GI:** Gallbladder disease (in postmenopausal women), **hepatic adenoma,** *nausea, vomiting, abdominal cramps, bloating,* cholestatic jaundice, colitis, acute pancreatitis
- **CV:** Increased blood pressure, thromboembolic and thrombotic disease
- **Hematologic:** Hypercalcemia, decreased glucose tolerance
- **GU:** Increased risk of endometrial cancer in postmenopausal women, *breakthrough bleeding, change in menstrual flow, dysmenorrhea, premenstrual-like syndrome,* amenorrhea, vaginal candidiasis, cystitis-like syndrome, endometrial cystic hyperplasia
- **Dermatologic:** *Photosensitivity, peripheral edema, chloasma,* erythema nodosum or multiforme, hemorrhagic eruption, loss of scalp hair, hirsutism, urticaria, dermatitis
- **Local:** *Pain at injection site,* sterile abscess, postinjection flare
- **Other:** Weight changes, reduced carbohydrate tolerance, aggravation of por-

Adverse effects in *Italics* are most common; those in **Bold** are life-threatening.

phyria, edema, changes in libido, breast tenderness

Topical Vaginal Cream
Systemic absorption may cause uterine bleeding in menopausal women and may cause serious bleeding of remaining endometrial foci in sterilized women with endometriosis.

Clinically important drug-drug interactions
- Increased therapeutic and toxic effects of corticosteroids if taken concurrently with estradiol • Decreased serum levels of estradiol if taken with drugs that enhance hepatic metabolism of the drug: barbiturates, phenytoin, rifampin

Drug-lab test interferences
- Increased sulfobromophthalein retention; prothrombin and factors VII, VIII, IX, and X; thyroid-binding globulin with increased PBI, T_4, increased uptake of free T_3 resin (free T_4 is unaltered), serum triglycerides and phospholipid concentration • Decreased antithrombin III, pregnanediol excretion, response to metyrapone test, serum folate concentration • Impaired glucose tolerance

■ Nursing Considerations

Assessment
- *History:* Allergy to estrogens, tartrazine; breast cancer, estrogen-dependent neoplasm; undiagnosed abnormal genital bleeding; active or previous thrombophlebitis or thromboembolic disorders; pregnancy; lactation; metabolic bone disease; renal insufficiency; CHF
- *Physical:* Skin—color, lesions, edema; breast exam; injection site; orientation, affect, reflexes; P, auscultation, BP, peripheral perfusion; R, adventitious sounds; bowel sounds, liver evaluation, abdominal exam; pelvic exam; serum calcium, phosphorus; liver and renal function tests; Pap smear; glucose tolerance test

Implementation
- Arrange for pretreatment and periodic (at least annual) history and physical, which should include BP, breasts, abdomen, pelvic organs, and a Pap smear.
- Caution patient, before beginning therapy, of the risks involved with estrogen use, the need to prevent pregnancy during treatment, the need for frequent medical follow-up, the need for periodic rests from drug treatment (as appropriate).
- Administer cyclically for short-term only when treating postmenopausal conditions because of the risk of endometrial neoplasm; taper to the lowest effective dose, and provide a drug-free week each month if at all possible.
- Apply transdermal system to a clean, dry area of skin on the trunk of the body, preferably the abdomen; do not apply to breasts; rotate the site with an interval of at least 1 wk between applications to the same site; avoid the waistline because tight or constrictive clothing may rub the system off; apply immediately after opening and compress for about 10 sec to ensure that it is attached.
- Arrange for the concomitant use of progestin therapy during chronic estrogen therapy in women; this will mimic normal physiologic cycling and allow for a cyclic uterine bleeding, which may decrease the risk of endometrial cancer.
- Administer parenteral preparations by deep IM injection only. Monitor injection sites for the development of abscesses; rotate injection sites with each injection to decrease development of abscesses.

Drug-specific teaching points
- Use this drug in cycles or short term; prepare a calendar of drug days, rest days, and drug-free periods.
- Learn the proper application of transdermal system, proper use of vaginal cream.
- Know that many potentially serious problems have occurred with the use of this drug, including development of cancers, blood clots, liver problems; it is very important that you have periodic medical exams throughout therapy.

Adverse effects in *Italics* are most common; those in **Bold** are life-threatening.

- Know that this drug cannot be given to pregnant women because of serious toxic effects to the baby.
- Know that the following side effects may occur: nausea, vomiting, bloating; headache, dizziness, mental depression (use caution if driving or performing tasks that require alertness if this occurs); sensitivity to sunlight (use a sunscreen and wear protective clothing until your tolerance to this effect of the drug is known); skin rash, loss of scalp hair, darkening of the skin on the face; changes in menstrual patterns.
- Report pain in the groin or calves of the legs, chest pain or sudden shortness of breath, abnormal vaginal bleeding, lumps in the breast, sudden severe headache, dizziness or fainting, changes in vision or speech, weakness or numbness in the arm or leg, severe abdominal pain, yellowing of the skin or eyes, severe mental depression, pain at injection site.

▢ estramustine phosphate sodium

*(ess tra **muss' ** teen)*
Emcyt

Pregnancy Category X

Drug classes
Hormonal agent
Estrogen
Antineoplastic agent

Therapeutic actions
Estradiol and an alkylating agent are linked in each molecule of drug; the drug binds somewhat preferentially to cells with estrogen (steroid) receptors, where alkylating effect is enhanced and cell death occurs.

Indications
- Palliative treatment of metastatic or progressive carcinoma of the prostate

Contraindications/cautions
- Contraindicated in the presence of allergy to estradiol or nitrogen mustard; active thrombophlebitis or thromboembolic disorders (except when the tumor mass is the cause of the thromboembolic phenomenon, and the benefits outweigh the risks).
- Use caution in the presence of cerebral vascular and coronary artery disorders; epilepsy, migraine, renal dysfunction, CHF; impaired hepatic function; metabolic bone diseases with hypercalcemia; diabetes mellitus.

Dosage
Adult: 10–16 mg/kg per day PO in three to four divided doses. Treat for 30–90 d before assessing the possible benefits. Continue therapy as long as response is favorable.

Pharmacokinetics

Route	Onset	Peak
Oral	Varies	2–3 h

Metabolism: Hepatic, $T_{1/2}$: 20 h
Excretion: Feces

Adverse effects
- CNS: *Lethargy, emotional lability, insomnia, headache, anxiety*, chest pain, tearing of the eyes
- GI: *Nausea, vomiting, diarrhea, anorexia*, flatulence, GI bleeding, burning throat, thirst
- CV: Cerebrovascular accident, myocardial infarction, thrombophlebitis, pulmonary emboli, *CHF, edema, dyspnea, leg cramps, elevated blood pressure*
- **Respiratory:** Upper respiratory discharge, hoarseness
- **Hematologic:** Leukopenia, thrombopenia, abnormalities in bilirubin, LDH, SGOT; decreased glucose tolerance
- **Dermatologic:** *Rash, pruritus, dry skin, peeling skin or fingertips*, easy bruising, flushing, thinning hair
- **Other:** *Breast tenderness, mild to moderate breast enlargement*, carcinoma of the liver, breast

Adverse effects in *Italics* are most common; those in **Bold** are life-threatening.

Nursing Considerations

Assessment
- *History:* Allergy to estradiol or nitrogen mustard; active thrombophlebitis or thromboembolic disorder; cerebrovascular and coronary artery disorders; epilepsy, migraine, renal dysfunction, CHF; impaired hepatic function; metabolic bone diseases with hypercalcemia; diabetes mellitus
- *Physical:* Skin—lesions, color, turgor; hair; breast exam; body weight; orientation, affect, reflexes; P, BP, auscultation, peripheral pulses, edema; R, adventitious sounds; liver evaluation, bowel sounds; stool guaiac, renal and liver function tests, blood glucose

Implementation
- Administer the drug for 30–90 d before assessing the possible benefits of continued therapy; therapy can be continued as long as response is favorable.
- Refrigerate capsules; capsules may be left out of the refrigerator for up to 48 h without loss of potency.
- Monitor diabetic patients carefully, because glucose tolerance may change, changing the need for insulin.
- Arrange to monitor hepatic function periodically during therapy.
- Monitor BP regularly as therapy begins and periodically throughout therapy.
- Caution patient to use some contraceptive method while on this drug, because mutagenesis has been reported.

Drug-specific teaching points
- Know that the effects may not be seen for several weeks. Capsules should be stored in the refrigerator; they will be stable for up to 48 h out of the refrigerator if necessary.
- Know that the following side effects may occur: nausea, vomiting, diarrhea, flatulence; dry, peeling skin and rash (skin care may be necessary); headache, emotional lability, lethargy (it may help just to know that these are drug effects).
- Use contraceptive measures; there is a risk of producing deformed babies while on this drug.
- Report pain or swelling in the legs, chest pain, difficulty breathing, edema, leg cramps.

☐ estrogens, conjugated

(ess' troe jenz)
Oral, topical vaginal cream:
C.E.S. (CAN), C.S.D. (CAN), Premarin
Parenteral: Premarin Intravenous

Pregnancy Category X

Drug classes
Hormone
Estrogen

Therapeutic actions
Estrogens are endogenous female sex hormones important in the development of the female reproductive system and secondary sex characteristics. They affect the release of pituitary gonadotropins; cause capillary dilatation, fluid retention, protein anabolism, and thin cervical mucus; conserve calcium and phosphorus; encourage bone formation; inhibit ovulation and prevent postpartum breast discomfort. They are responsible for the proliferation of the endometrium; absence or decline of estrogen produces signs and symptoms of menopause on the uterus, vagina, breasts, cervix. Their efficacy as palliation in male patients with androgen-dependent prostatic carcinoma is attributable to their competition with androgens for receptor sites, thus decreasing the influence of androgens.

Indications
- *Oral:* palliation of moderate to severe vasomotor symptoms, atrophic vaginitis, or kraurosis vulvae associated with menopause
- Treatment of female hypogonadism; female castration; primary ovarian failure
- Osteoporosis: to retard progression
- Palliation of inoperable prostatic cancer

estrogens, conjugated ■ 451

- Palliation of mammary cancer
- Prevention of postpartum breast engorgement
- Unlabeled use: postcoital contraceptive
- *Parenteral:* treatment of uterine bleeding due to hormonal imbalance in the absence of organic pathology
- *Vaginal cream:* treatment of atrophic vaginitis and kraurosis vulvae associated with menopause

Contraindications/cautions

- Contraindicated in the presence of allergy to estrogens, breast cancer (except in specific, selected patients), estrogen-dependent neoplasm, undiagnosed abnormal genital bleeding, active thrombophlebitis or thromboembolic disorders or history of such from previous estrogen use, pregnancy (associated with serious fetal defects; women of childbearing age should be advised of the potential risks and birth control measures suggested).
- Use caution in the presence of metabolic bone disease, renal insufficiency, CHF, lactation.

Dosage

Oral drug should be given cyclically (3 wk of daily estrogen, 1 wk off) except in selected cases of carcinoma and prevention of postpartum breast engorgement.

Adult

- ***Moderate to severe vasomotor symptoms associated with menopause and to retard progression of osteoporosis:*** 1.25 mg/d PO. If patient has not menstruated in 2 mo, start at any time. If patient is menstruating, start therapy on day 5 of bleeding.
- ***Atrophic vaginitis, kraurosis vulvae associated with menopause:*** 0.3–1.25 mg/day PO or more if needed. 2–4 g vaginal cream daily intravaginally or topically, depending on severity of condition. Taper or discontinue at 3- to 6-mo intervals.
- ***Female hypogonadism:*** 2.5–7.5 mg/d PO in divided doses for 20 d followed by 10 d of rest. If bleeding does not appear at the end of this time, repeat course. If bleeding does occur before the end of the 10-d rest, begin a 20-d 2.5–7.5 mg estrogen with oral progestin given during the last 5 d of therapy. If bleeding occurs before this cycle is finished, restart course of day 5 of bleeding.
- ***Female castration, primary ovarian failure:*** 1.25 mg/d PO. Adjust dosage by patient response to lowest effective dose.
- ***Prostatic cancer (inoperable):*** 1.25–2.5 mg tid PO. Judge effectiveness by phosphatase determinations and by symptomatic improvement.
- ***Breast cancer (inoperable, progressing):*** 10 mg tid PO for at least 3 mo.
- ***Prevention of postpartum breast engorgement:*** 3.75 mg q4h PO for 5 doses, or 1.25 mg q4h for 5 d.
- ***Abnormal uterine bleeding due to hormonal imbalance:*** 25 mg IV or IM. Repeat in 6–12 h as needed. IV route provides a more rapid response.
- ***Postcoital contraceptive:*** 30 mg/d PO in divided doses for 5 consecutive days beginning within 72 h after intercourse.

Pediatric: Not recommended due to effect on the growth of the long bones.

Pharmacokinetics

Route	Onset	Peak
Oral	Slow	Days
IV	Gradual	Hours

Metabolism: Hepatic, $T_{1/2}$: not known
Distribution: Crosses placenta; enters breast milk
Excretion: Urine

IV facts

Preparation: Reconstitute with provided diluent; add to Normal Saline, dextrose, and invert sugar solutions. Refrigerate unreconstituted parenteral solution; use reconstituted solution within a few hours. Refrigerated reconstituted solution is stable for 60 d; do not use solution if darkened or precipitates have formed.
Infusion: Infuse slowly.

Incompatibilities: Do *not* mix with protein hydrolysate, ascorbic acid or any solution with an acid pH.

Adverse effects
- CNS: Steepening of the corneal curvature with a resultant change in visual acuity and intolerance to contact lenses, *headache*, migraine, dizziness, mental depression, chorea, convulsions
- GI: Gallbladder disease (in postmenopausal women), **hepatic adenoma,** *nausea, vomiting, abdominal cramps, bloating,* cholestatic jaundice, colitis, acute pancreatitis
- CV: Increased blood pressure, thromboembolic and thrombotic disease
- Hematologic: Hypercalcemia, decreased glucose tolerance
- GU: Increased risk of endometrial cancer in postmenopausal women, *breakthrough bleeding, change in menstrual flow, dysmenorrhea, premenstrual-like syndrome,* amenorrhea, vaginal candidiasis, cystitis-like syndrome, endometrial cystic hyperplasia
- Dermatologic: *Photosensitivity, peripheral edema, chloasma,* erythema nodosum or multiforme, hemorrhagic eruption, loss of scalp hair, hirsutism, urticaria, dermatitis
- Local: *Pain at injection site,* sterile abscess, postinjection flare
- Other: Weight changes, reduced carbohydrate tolerance, aggravation of porphyria, edema, changes in libido, breast tenderness

Topical Vaginal Cream
Systemic absorption may cause uterine bleeding in menopausal women and may cause serious bleeding of remaining endometrial foci in sterilized women with endometriosis.

Clinically important drug-drug interactions
- Increased therapeutic and toxic effects of corticosteroids if taken concurrently with estrogen • Decreased serum levels of estrogen if taken with drugs that enhance hepatic metabolism of the drug: barbiturates, phenytoin, rifampin

Drug-lab test interferences
- Increased sulfobromophthalein retention; prothrombin and factors VII, VIII, IX, and X; thyroid-binding globulin with increased PBI, T_4, increased uptake of free T_3 resin (free T_4 is unaltered), serum triglycerides and phospholipid concentration
- Decreased antithrombin III, pregnanediol excretion, response to metyrapone test, serum folate concentration • Impaired glucose tolerance

■ Nursing Considerations
Assessment
- *History:* Allergy to estrogens; breast cancer, estrogen-dependent neoplasm; undiagnosed abnormal genital bleeding; active or previous thrombophlebitis or thromboembolic disorders; pregnancy; lactation; metabolic bone disease; renal insufficiency; CHF
- *Physical:* Skin—color, lesions, edema; breast exam; injection site; orientation, affect, reflexes; P, auscultation, BP, peripheral perfusion; R, adventitious sounds; bowel sounds, liver evaluation, abdominal exam; pelvic exam; serum calcium, phosphorus; liver and renal function tests; Pap smear; glucose tolerance test

Implementation
- Arrange for pretreatment and periodic (at least annual) history and physical, which should include BP, breasts, abdomen, pelvic organs, and a Pap smear.
- Caution patient, before beginning therapy, of the risks involved with estrogen use, the need to prevent pregnancy during treatment, the need for frequent medical follow-up; the need for periodic rests from drug treatment (as appropriate).
- Administer cyclically for short term only when treating postmenopausal conditions because of the risk of endometrial neoplasm; taper to the lowest effective dose, and provide a drug-free week each month if at all possible.

- Refrigerate unreconstituted parenteral solution; use reconstituted solution within a few hours.
- Refrigerated reconstituted solution is stable for 60 d; do not use solution if darkened or precipitates have formed.
- Arrange for the concomitant use of progestin therapy during chronic estrogen therapy in women; this will mimic normal physiologic cycling and allow for cyclic uterine bleeding, which may decrease the risk of endometrial cancer.

Drug-specific teaching points

- Use this drug cyclically or short term; prepare a calendar of drug days, rest days, and drug-free periods.
- Learn the proper application of transdermal system, proper use of vaginal cream.
- Know that many potentially serious problems have occurred with the use of this drug, including development of cancers, blood clots, liver problems; it is very important that you have periodic medical exams throughout therapy.
- Know that this drug cannot be given to pregnant women because of serious toxic effects to the baby.
- Know that the following side effects may occur: nausea, vomiting, bloating; headache, dizziness, mental depression (use caution if driving or performing tasks that require alertness if this occurs); sensitivity to sunlight (use a sunscreen and wear protective clothing until your tolerance to this effect of the drug is known); skin rash, loss of scalp hair, darkening of the skin on the face; changes in menstrual patterns.
- Report pain in the groin or calves of the legs, chest pain or sudden shortness of breath, abnormal vaginal bleeding, lumps in the breast, sudden severe headache, dizziness or fainting, changes in vision or speech, weakness or numbness in the arm or leg, severe abdominal pain, yellowing of the skin or eyes, severe mental depression, pain at injection site.

☐ estrogens, esterified

(*ess' troe jenz*)
Climestrone (CAN), Estratab, Estromed (CAN), Menest

Pregnancy Category X

Drug classes
Hormone
Estrogen

Therapeutic actions
Estrogens are endogenous female sex hormones important in the development of the female reproductive system and secondary sex characteristics. They cause capillary dilatation, fluid retention, protein anabolism, and thin cervical mucus; conserve calcium and phosphorus and encourage bone formation; inhibit ovulation and prevent postpartum breast discomfort. They are responsible for the proliferation of the endometrium; absence or decline of estrogen produces signs and symptoms of menopause on the uterus, vagina, breasts, cervix. Their efficacy as palliation in male patients with androgen-dependent prostatic carcinoma is attributable to their competition for androgen receptor sites, decreasing the influence of androgens.

Indications
- Palliation of moderate to severe vasomotor symptoms, atrophic vaginitis, or kraurosis vulvae associated with menopause
- Treatment of female hypogonadism; female castration; primary ovarian failure
- Palliation of inoperable prostatic cancer
- Palliation of inoperable, progressing breast cancer in men, postmenopausal women

Contraindications/cautions
- Contraindicated in the presence of allergy to estrogens, breast cancer (except in specific, selected patients), estrogen-dependent neoplasm, undiagnosed abnormal genital bleeding, active thrombophlebitis or thromboembolic disorders or history of such from previous estrogen use, pregnancy (associated with serious

454 ■ estrogens, esterified

fetal defects; women of childbearing age should be advised of the potential risks and birth control measures suggested).
- Use caution in the presence of metabolic bone disease, renal insufficiency, CHF, lactation.

Dosage

Administer PO only.

Adult

- ***Moderate to severe vasomotor symptoms, atrophic vaginitis, kraurosis vulvae associated with menopause:*** 0.3–1.25 mg/d PO. Adjust to lowest effective dose. Cyclic therapy (3 wk of daily estrogen followed by 1 wk of rest from drug therapy) is recommended.
- ***Female hypogonadism:*** 2.5–7.5 mg/d PO in divided doses for 20 d followed by 10 d of rest. If bleeding does not occur by the end of that period, repeat the same dosage schedule. If bleeding does occur before the end of the 10-d rest, begin a 20-d estrogen-progestin cyclic regimen with progestin given orally during the last 5 d of estrogen therapy. If bleeding occurs before end of 10-d rest period, begin a 20-d estrogen-progestin cyclic regimen.
- ***Female castration, primary ovarian failure:*** Begin a 20-d estrogen-progestin regimen of 2.5–7.5 mg/d PO estrogen in divided doses for 20 d with oral progestin given during the last 5 d of estrogen therapy. If bleeding occurs before the regimen is completed, discontinue therapy and resume on the fifth day of bleeding.
- ***Prostatic cancer (inoperable):*** 1.25–2.5 mg tid PO. Chronic therapy: judge effectiveness by symptomatic response and serum phosphatase determinations.
- ***Breast cancer (inoperable, progressing):*** 10 mg tid PO for at least 3 mo in selected men and postmenopausal women.

Pediatric: Not recommended due to effect on the growth of the long bones.

Pharmacokinetics

Route	Onset	Peak
Oral	Slow	Days

Metabolism: Hepatic, $T_{1/2}$: not known
Distribution: Crosses placenta; enters breast milk
Excretion: Urine

Adverse effects

- **CNS:** Steepening of the corneal curvature with a resultant change in visual acuity and intolerance to contact lenses, *headache*, migraine, dizziness, mental depression, chorea, convulsions
- **GI:** Gallbladder disease (in postmenopausal women), hepatic adenoma (rarely occurs, but may rupture and cause death), *nausea, vomiting, abdominal cramps, bloating,* cholestatic jaundice, colitis, acute pancreatitis
- **CV:** Increased blood pressure, thromboembolic and thrombotic disease (with high doses in certain groups of susceptible women and in men receiving estrogens for prostatic cancer)
- **Hematologic:** Hypercalcemia (in breast cancer patients with bone metastases), decreased glucose tolerance
- **GU:** Increased risk of endometrial cancer in postmenopausal women, *breakthrough bleeding, change in menstrual flow, dysmenorrhea, premenstrual-like syndrome,* amenorrhea, vaginal candidiasis, cystitis-like syndrome, endometrial cystic hyperplasia
- **Dermatologic:** *Photosensitivity, peripheral edema, chloasma,* erythema nodosum or multiforme, hemorrhagic eruption, loss of scalp hair, hirsutism, urticaria, dermatitis
- **Other:** Weight changes, reduced carbohydrate tolerance, aggravation of porphyria, edema, changes in libido, breast tenderness

Adverse effects in *Italics* are most common; those in **Bold** are life-threatening.

Clinically important drug-drug interactions
- Increased therapeutic and toxic effects of corticosteroids if taken concurrently with estrogen
- Decreased serum levels of estrogen if taken with drugs that enhance hepatic metabolism of the drug: barbiturates, phenytoin, rifampin

Drug-lab test interferences
- Increased sulfobromophthalein retention; prothrombin and factors VII, VIII, IX, and X; thyroid-binding globulin with increased PBI, T_4, increased uptake of free T_3 resin (free T_4 is unaltered), serum triglycerides and phospholipid concentration
- Decreased antithrombin III, pregnanediol excretion, response to metyrapone test, serum folate concentration
- Impaired glucose tolerance

■ Nursing Considerations

Assessment
- *History:* Allergy to estrogens; breast cancer, estrogen-dependent neoplasm; undiagnosed abnormal genital bleeding; thrombophlebitis or thromboembolic disorders; pregnancy; lactation; metabolic bone disease; renal insufficiency; CHF
- *Physical:* Skin—color, lesions, edema; breast exam; injection site; orientation, affect, reflexes; P, auscultation, BP, peripheral perfusion; R, adventitious sounds; bowel sounds, liver evaluation, abdominal exam; pelvic exam; serum calcium, phosphorus; liver and renal function tests; Pap smear; glucose tolerance test

Implementation
- Arrange for pretreatment and periodic (at least annual) history and physical, which should include BP, breasts, abdomen, pelvic organs, and a Pap smear.
- Caution patient, before beginning therapy, of the risks involved with estrogen use; the need to prevent pregnancy during treatment; the need for frequent medical follow-up; the need for periodic rests from drug treatment (as appropriate).
- Administer cyclically for short term only when treating postmenopausal conditions because of the risk of endometrial neoplasm; taper to the lowest effective dose, and provide a drug-free week each month if at all possible.
- Arrange for the concomitant use of progestin therapy during chronic estrogen therapy in women; this will mimic normal physiologic cycling and allow for cyclic uterine bleeding, which may decrease the risk of endometrial cancer.

Drug-specific teaching points
- Use this drug in cycles or short term; prepare a calendar of drug days, rest days, and drug-free periods.
- Know that many potentially serious problems have occurred with the use of this drug, including development of cancers, blood clots, liver problems; it is very important that you have periodic medical exams throughout therapy.
- Know that this drug cannot be given to pregnant women because of serious toxic effects to the baby.
- Know that the following side effects may occur: nausea, vomiting, bloating; headache, dizziness, mental depression (use caution if driving or performing tasks that require alertness if this occurs); sensitivity to sunlight (use a sunscreen and wear protective clothing until your tolerance to this effect of the drug is known); skin rash, loss of scalp hair, darkening of the skin on the face; changes in menstrual patterns.
- Report pain in the groin or calves of the legs, chest pain or sudden shortness of breath, abnormal vaginal bleeding, lumps in the breast, sudden severe headache, dizziness or fainting, changes in vision or speech, weakness or numbness in the arm or leg, severe abdominal pain, yellowing of the skin or eyes, severe mental depression.

❒ estrone

(ess' trone)

Femogen (CAN), Kestrone 5, Theelin Aqueous (aqueous suspension)

estrogenic substance (mainly estrone)

Wehgen (aqueous suspension)

Pregnancy Category X

Drug classes
Hormone
Estrogen

Therapeutic actions
Estrogens are endogenous female sex hormones important in the development of the female reproductive system and secondary sex characteristics. They cause capillary dilatation, fluid retention, protein anabolism, and thin cervical mucus; conserve calcium and phosphorus and encourage bone formation; inhibit ovulation and prevent postpartum breast discomfort. They are responsible for the proliferation of the endometrium; absence or decline of estrogen produces signs and symptoms of menopause on the uterus, vagina, breasts, cervix. Their efficacy as palliation in male patients with androgen-dependent prostatic carcinoma is attributable to their competition with androgens for receptor sites, decreasing the influence of androgens.

Indications
- Palliation of moderate to severe vasomotor symptoms, atrophic vaginitis or kraurosis vulvae associated with menopause
- Treatment of female hypogonadism, female castration, primary ovarian failure
- Palliation of inoperable prostatic cancer

Contraindications/cautions
- Contraindicated in the presence of allergy to estrogens, breast cancer (except in specific, selected patients), estrogen-dependent neoplasm, undiagnosed abnormal genital bleeding, active or previous thrombophlebitis or thromboembolic disorders from estrogen use, pregnancy (associated with serious fetal defects; women of childbearing age should be advised of the potential risks and birth control measures suggested).
- Use caution in the presence of metabolic bone disease, renal insufficiency, CHF, lactation.

Dosage
Administer IM only.
Adult
- ***Moderate to severe vasomotor symptoms, atrophic vaginitis, kraurosis vulvae associated with menopause:*** 0.1–0.5 mg two to three times per wk IM.
- ***Female hypogonadism, female castration, primary ovarian failure:*** Initially, 0.1–1 mg/wk in single or divided doses IM. 0.5–2 mg/wk has been used in some cases.
- ***Prostatic cancer (inoperable):*** 2–4 mg, two to three times per wk IM. Response should occur within 3 mo. If a response does occur, continue drug until disease is again progressive.

Pediatric: Not recommended due to effect on the growth of the long bones.

Pharmacokinetics

Route	Onset	Peak
IM	Slow	Days

Metabolism: Hepatic, $T_{1/2}$: not known
Distribution: Crosses placenta; enters breast milk
Excretion: Urine

Adverse effects
- **CNS:** Steepening of the corneal curvature with a resultant change in visual acuity and intolerance to contact lenses, *headache,* migraine, dizziness, mental depression, chorea, convulsions
- **GI:** Gallbladder disease (in postmenopausal women), **hepatic adenoma,** *nausea, vomiting, abdominal cramps, bloating,* cholestatic jaundice, colitis, acute pancreatitis
- **CV:** Increased blood pressure, thromboembolic and thrombotic disease
- **Hematologic:** Hypercalcemia, decreased glucose tolerance

Adverse effects in *Italics* are most common; those in **Bold** are life-threatening.

- **GU:** Increased risk of endometrial cancer in postmenopausal women, *breakthrough bleeding, change in menstrual flow, dysmenorrhea, premenstrual-like syndrome*, amenorrhea, vaginal candidiasis, cystitis-like syndrome, endometrial cystic hyperplasia
- **Dermatologic:** *Photosensitivity, peripheral edema, chloasma*, erythema nodosum or multiforme, hemorrhagic eruption, loss of scalp hair, hirsutism, urticaria, dermatitis
- **Local:** *Pain at injection site*, sterile abscess, postinjection flare
- **Other:** weight changes, reduced carbohydrate tolerance, aggravation of porphyria, edema, changes in libido, breast tenderness

Clinically important drug-drug interactions
- Increased therapeutic and toxic effects of corticosteroids if taken concurrently with estrogens • Decreased serum levels of estrogens if taken with drugs that enhance hepatic metabolism of the drug: barbiturates, phenytoin, rifampin

Drug-lab test interferences
- Increased sulfobromophthalein retention; prothrombin and factors VII, VIII, IX, and X; thyroid-binding globulin with increased PBI, T_4, increased uptake of free T_3 resin (free T_4 is unaltered), serum triglycerides and phospholipid concentration • Decreased antithrombin III, pregnanediol excretion, response to metyrapone test, serum folate concentration • Impaired glucose tolerance

■ Nursing Considerations

Assessment
- *History:* Allergy to estrogens; breast cancer, estrogen-dependent neoplasm; undiagnosed abnormal genital bleeding; thrombophlebitis or thromboembolic disorders; pregnancy; lactation; metabolic bone disease; renal insufficiency; CHF
- *Physical:* Skin—color, lesions, edema; breast exam; injection site; orientation, affect, reflexes; P, auscultation, BP, peripheral perfusion; R, adventitious sounds; bowel sounds, liver evaluation, abdominal exam; pelvic exam; serum calcium, phosphorus; liver and renal function tests; Pap smear; glucose tolerance test

Implementation
- Arrange for pretreatment and periodic (at least annual) history and physical, which should include BP, breasts, abdomen, pelvic organs, and a Pap smear.
- Caution patient, before beginning therapy, of the risks involved with estrogen use, the need to prevent pregnancy during treatment, the need for frequent medical follow-up, the need for periodic rests from drug treatment, as appropriate.
- Administer cyclically for short term only when treating postmenopausal conditions because of the risk of endometrial neoplasm. Taper to the lowest effective dose, and provide a drug-free week each month if at all possible.
- Arrange for the concomitant use of progestin therapy during chronic estrogen therapy in women; this will mimic normal physiologic cycling and allow for a cyclic uterine bleeding, which may decrease the risk of endometrial cancer.
- Administer by deep IM injection only; monitor injection sites for the development of abscesses. Rotate injection sites with each injection to decrease development of abscesses.

Drug-specific teaching points
- Be aware that this drug can only be given IM. Prepare a calendar of drug days, rest days, and drug-free periods for the patient (as appropriate).
- Know that many potentially serious problems have occurred with the use of this drug, including development of cancers, blood clots, liver problems; it is very important that you have periodic medical exams throughout therapy.
- Know that this drug cannot be given to pregnant women because of serious toxic effects to the baby.

Adverse effects in *Italics* are most common; those in **Bold** are life-threatening.

- Know that the following side effects may occur: nausea, vomiting, bloating; headache, dizziness, mental depression (use caution if driving or performing tasks that require alertness if this occurs); sensitivity to sunlight (use a sunscreen and wear protective clothing until your tolerance to this effect of the drug is known); skin rash, loss of scalp hair, darkening of the skin on the face; changes in menstrual patterns.
- Report pain in the groin or calves of the legs, chest pain or sudden shortness of breath, abnormal vaginal bleeding, lumps in the breast, sudden severe headache, dizziness or fainting, changes in vision or speech, weakness or numbness in the arm or leg, severe abdominal pain, yellowing of the skin or eyes, severe mental depression, pain at injection site.

☐ estropipate

(ess' troe pi' pate)

piperazine estrone sulfate
Ogen, Ortho-Est

Pregnancy Category X

Drug classes
Hormone
Estrogen

Therapeutic actions
Estrogens are endogenous female sex hormones important in the development of the female reproductive system and secondary sex characteristics. They cause capillary dilatation, fluid retention, protein anabolism, and thin cervical mucus; conserve calcium and phosphorus and encourage bone formation; inhibit ovulation and prevent postpartum breast discomfort. They are responsible for the proliferation of the endometrium; absence or decline of estrogen produces signs and symptoms of menopause on the uterus, vagina, breasts, cervix. Their efficacy as palliation in male patients with androgen-dependent prostatic carcinoma is attributable to their competition with androgens for receptor sites, decreasing the influence of androgens.

Indications
- Palliation of moderate to severe vasomotor symptoms, atrophic vaginitis, or kraurosis vulvae associated with menopause
- Treatment of female hypogonadism, female castration, primary ovarian failure
- Prevention of osteoporosis

Contraindications/cautions
- Contraindicated in the presence of allergy to estrogens, breast cancer (except in specific, selected patients), estrogen-dependent neoplasm, undiagnosed abnormal genital bleeding, active thrombophlebitis or thromboembolic disorders or history of such from previous estrogen use, pregnancy (associated with serious fetal defects; women of childbearing age should be advised of the potential risks and birth control measures suggested).
- Use caution in the presence of metabolic bone disease, renal insufficiency, CHF, lactation.

Dosage
Adult
- ***Moderate to severe vasomotor symptoms, atrophic vaginitis, kraurosis vulvae associated with menopause:*** 0.625–5 mg/d PO given cyclically.
- ***Female hypogonadism, female castration, primary ovarian failure:*** 1.25–7.5 mg/d PO for the first 3 wk, followed by a rest period of 8–10 d. Repeat if bleeding does not occur at end of rest period.
- ***Prevention of osteoporosis:*** 0.625 mg qd PO for 25 d of a 31-d cycle per month

Pediatric: Not recommended due to effect on the growth of the long bones.

Pharmacokinetics

Route	Onset	Peak
PO	Slow	Days

Metabolism: Hepatic, $T_{1/2}$: not known
Distribution: Crosses placenta; enters breast milk
Excretion: Urine

Adverse effects
- CNS: Steepening of the corneal curvature with a resultant change in visual acuity and intolerance to contact lenses, *headache*, migraine, dizziness, mental depression, chorea, convulsions
- GI: Gallbladder disease (in postmenopausal women), **hepatic adenoma**, *nausea, vomiting, abdominal cramps, bloating*, cholestatic jaundice, colitis, acute pancreatitis
- CV: Increased blood pressure, thromboembolic and thrombotic disease
- Hematologic: Hypercalcemia, decreased glucose tolerance
- GU: Increased risk of endometrial cancer in postmenopausal women, *breakthrough bleeding, change in menstrual flow, dysmenorrhea, premenstrual-like syndrome*, amenorrhea, vaginal candidiasis, cystitis-like syndrome, endometrial cystic hyperplasia
- Dermatologic: *Photosensitivity, peripheral edema, chloasma*, erythema nodosum or multiforme, hemorrhagic eruption, loss of scalp hair, hirsutism, urticaria, dermatitis
- Other: Weight changes, reduced carbohydrate tolerance, aggravation of porphyria, edema, changes in libido, breast tenderness

Clinically important drug-drug interactions
- Increased therapeutic and toxic effects of corticosteroids if taken concurrently with estrogens • Decreased serum levels of estrogens if taken with drugs that enhance hepatic metabolism of the drug: barbiturates, phenytoin, rifampin

Drug-lab test interferences
- Increased sulfobromophthalein retention; prothrombin and factors VII, VIII, IX, and X; thyroid-binding globulin with increased PBI, T_4, increased uptake of free T_3 resin (free T_4 is unaltered), serum triglycerides and phospholipid concentration •-
Decreased antithrombin III, pregnanediol excretion, response to metyrapone test, serum folate concentration • Impaired glucose tolerance

■ Nursing Considerations
Assessment
- *History:* Allergy to estrogens; breast cancer, estrogen-dependent neoplasm; undiagnosed abnormal genital bleeding; thrombophlebitis or thromboembolic disorders; pregnancy; lactation; metabolic bone disease; renal insufficiency; CHF
- *Physical:* Skin—color, lesions, edema; breast exam; injection site; orientation, affect, reflexes; P, auscultation, BP, peripheral perfusion; R, adventitious sounds; bowel sounds, liver evaluation, abdominal exam; pelvic exam; serum calcium, phosphorus; liver and renal function tests; Pap smear; glucose tolerance test

Implementation
- Arrange for pretreatment and periodic (at least annual) history and physical, which should include BP, breasts, abdomen, pelvic organs, and a Pap smear.
- Caution patient, before beginning therapy, of the risks involved with estrogen use, the need to prevent pregnancy during treatment, the need for frequent medical follow-up, the need for periodic rests from drug treatment (as appropriate).
- Administer cyclically for short term only when treating postmenopausal conditions because of the risk of endometrial neoplasm. Taper to the lowest effective dose and provide a drug-free week each month if at all possible.
- Arrange for the concomitant use of progestin therapy during chronic estrogen therapy in women; this will mimic normal physiologic cycling and allow for a cyclic uterine bleeding, which may decrease the risk of endometrial cancer.

Drug-specific teaching points
- Prepare a calendar of drug days, rest days, and drug-free periods (as appropriate).
- Know that many potentially serious problems have occurred with the use of this

Adverse effects in *Italics* are most common; those in **Bold** are life-threatening.

460 ▪ ethacrynic acid

drug, including development of cancers, blood clots, liver problems; it is very important that you have periodic medical exams throughout therapy.
- Know that this drug cannot be given to pregnant women because of serious toxic effects to the baby.
- Know that the following side effects may occur: nausea, vomiting, bloating; headache, dizziness, mental depression (use caution if driving or performing tasks that require alertness if this occurs); sensitivity to sunlight (use a sunscreen and wear protective clothing until your tolerance to this effect of the drug is known); skin rash, loss of scalp hair, darkening of the skin on the face; changes in menstrual patterns.
- Report pain in the groin or calves of the legs, chest pain or sudden shortness of breath, abnormal vaginal bleeding, lumps in the breast, sudden severe headache, dizziness or fainting, changes in vision or speech, weakness or numbness in the arm or leg, severe abdominal pain, yellowing of the skin or eyes, severe mental depression.

▢ ethacrynic acid

(eth a **krin' ik**)
Edecrin

ethacrynate sodium
Sodium Edecrin

Pregnancy Category B

Drug classes
Loop (high ceiling) diuretic

Therapeutic actions
Inhibits the reabsorption of sodium and chloride from the proximal and distal renal tubules and the loop of Henle, leading to a sodium-rich diuresis.

Indications
- Edema associated with CHF, cirrhosis, renal disease
- Acute pulmonary edema (IV)
- Ascites due to malignancy, idiopathic edema, lymphedema
- Short-term management of pediatric patients with congenital heart disease

Contraindications/cautions
- Contraindicated in the presence of allergy to ethacrynic acid, electrolyte depletion, anuria, severe renal failure, hepatic coma, SLE, gout, diabetes mellitus, lactation.
- Use caution in the presence of hypoproteinemia (reduces response to drug).

Dosage
Adult
- **Edema:** Initial dose: 50–100 mg/d PO. Adjust dose in 25- to 50-mg intervals. Higher doses, up to 200 mg/d, may be required in refractory patients. Intermittent dosage schedule is preferred for maintenance. When used with other diuretics, give initial dose of 25 mg/d and adjust dosage in 25-mg increments.
- **Parenteral therapy:** Do not give IM or SC—causes pain and irritation. Usual adult dose is 50 mg or 0.5–1 mg/kg run slowly through IV tubing or by direct injection over several minutes. *Not recommended for pediatric patients.*

Pediatric: Initial dose of 25 mg PO with careful adjustment of dose by 25-mg increment. Maintain at lowest effective dose. Avoid use in infants.

Pharmacokinetics

Route	Onset	Peak	Duration
Oral	30 min	2 h	6–8 h
IV	5 min	15–30 min	2 h

Metabolism: Hepatic, $T_{1/2}$: 30–70 min
Distribution: Crosses placenta; enters breast milk
Excretion: Urine and bile

IV facts
Preparation: Add 50 ml of 5% Dextrose Injection or Sodium Chloride Injection to the vial of parenteral solution; do not use solution diluted with dextrose if it appears hazy or opalescent. Dextrose solutions may have a low pH. Discard unused solution after 24 h.

ethacrynic acid 461

Infusion: Give slowly over several minutes by direct IV injection or into the tubing of actively running IV.
Incompatibilities: Do not mix IV solution with whole blood or its derivatives.

Adverse effects

- **CNS:** *Dizziness, vertigo, paresthesias, confusion,* apprehension, fatigue, nystagmus, weakness, headache, drowsiness, blurred vision, tinnitus, irreversible hearing loss
- **GI:** *Nausea, anorexia, vomiting, GI bleeding, dysphagia; sudden, profuse watery diarrhea,* acute pancreatitis, jaundice
- **CV:** *Orthostatic hypotension,* volume depletion, cardiac arrhythmias, thrombophlebitis
- **Hematologic:** Leukopenia, anemia, thrombocytopenia, fluid and electrolyte imbalances (hyperuricemia, metabolic alkalosis, hypokalemia, hyponatremia, hypochloremia, hypocalcemia, hyperuricemia, hyperglycemia, increased serum creatinine)
- **GU:** *Polyuria, nocturia, glycosuria,* hematuria
- **Dermatologic:** *Photosensitivity, rash,* pruritus, urticaria, purpura
- **Other:** Muscle cramps and muscle spasms

Clinically important drug-drug interactions

- Increased risk of cardiac glycoside (digitalis) toxicity (secondary to hypokalemia)
- Increased risk of ototoxicity if taken with aminoglycoside antibiotics, cisplatin
- Decreased diuretic effect if taken concurrently with NSAIDs

■ Nursing Considerations

Assessment

- *History:* Allergy to ethacrynic acid; electrolyte depletion; anuria, severe renal failure; hepatic coma; SLE; gout; diabetes mellitus; hypoproteinemia; lactation
- *Physical:* Skin—color, lesions, edema; orientation, reflexes, hearing; P, baseline ECG, BP, orthostatic BP, perfusion; R, pattern, adventitious sounds; liver evaluation, bowel sounds; output patterns; CBC, serum electrolytes (including calcium), blood sugar, liver and renal function tests, uric acid, urinalysis

Implementation

- Administer oral doses with food or milk to prevent GI upset.
- Mark calendars or other reminders of drug days for outpatients if every other day or 3–5 d/wk therapy is the most effective for treating edema.
- Administer early in the day so that increased urination does not disturb sleep.
- Avoid IV use if oral use is at all possible.
- Change injection sites to prevent thrombophlebitis if more than one IV injection is needed.
- Measure and record regular body weights to monitor fluid changes.
- Arrange to monitor serum electrolytes, hydration, liver function during long-term therapy.
- Provide potassium-rich diet or supplemental potassium.

Drug-specific teaching points

- Record alternate day therapy on calendar or dated envelopes prepared for the patient. Take the drug early in the day, as increased urination will occur. The drug should be taken with food or meals to prevent GI upset.
- Weigh yourself on a regular basis at the same time of the day and in the same clothing, and record the weight on your calendar.
- Know that the following side effects may occur: increased volume and frequency of urination (have ready access to a bathroom when drug effect is greatest); dizziness, feeling faint on arising, drowsiness (if these changes occur, avoid rapid position changes; hazardous activities, like driving a car; and consumption of alcohol, which can intensify these problems); sensitivity to sunlight (use sunglasses, wear protective clothing, or use a sunscreen when outdoors); increased

Adverse effects in *Italics* are most common; those in **Bold** are life-threatening.

thirst (sucking on sugarless lozenges may help to alleviate the thirst; frequent mouth care also may help); loss of body potassium (a potassium-rich diet or even a potassium supplement will be necessary).
- Report loss or gain of more than 3 lb in one day, swelling in your ankles or fingers, unusual bleeding or bruising, dizziness, trembling, numbness, fatigue, muscle weakness or cramps.

☐ ethambutol hydrochloride

(e tham' byoo tole)
Etibi (CAN), Myambutol

Pregnancy Category B

Drug classes
Antituberculous drug ("second line")

Therapeutic actions
Inhibits the synthesis of metabolites in growing mycobacterium cells, impairing cell metabolism, arresting cell multiplication, and causing cell death.

Indications
- Treatment of pulmonary tuberculosis in conjunction with at least one other antituberculous drug

Contraindications/cautions
- Contraindicated in the presence of allergy to ethambutol; optic neuritis; pregnancy (the safest antituberculous regimen for use in pregnancy is considered to be ethambutol, isoniazid, and rifampin).
- Use caution in the presence of impaired renal function.

Dosage
Ethambutol is not administered alone; use in conjunction with four other antituberculosis agents.
Adult: Initial treatment: 15 mg/kg per day PO as a single daily oral dose. Continue therapy until bacteriologic conversion has become permanent and maximal clinical improvement has occurred. *Retreatment:* 25 mg/kg per day as a single daily oral dose. After 60 d, reduce dose to 15 mg/kg per day as a single daily dose.
Pediatric: Not recommended for children younger than 13 y.

Pharmacokinetics

Route	Onset	Peak	Duration
Oral	Rapid	2–4 h	20–24 h

Metabolism: Hepatic, $T_{1/2}$: 3.3 h
Distribution: Crosses placenta; enters breast milk
Excretion: Urine, feces

Adverse effects
- **CNS:** *Optic neuritis* (loss of visual acuity, changes in color perception), *fever, malaise, headache,* dizziness, mental confusion, disorientation, hallucinations, peripheral neuritis
- **GI:** *Anorexia, nausea, vomiting,* GI upset, abdominal pain, transient liver impairment
- **Hypersensitivity:** Allergic reactions—dermatitis, pruritus, anaphylactoid reaction
- **Other:** Toxic epidermal necrolysis, thrombocytopenia, joint pain, acute gout

Clinically important drug-drug interactions
- Decreased absorption of ethambutol in the presence of aluminum salts

■ Nursing Considerations

Assessment
- *History:* Allergy to ethambutol, optic neuritis, impaired renal function
- *Physical:* Skin—color, lesions; temperature; orientation, reflexes, ophthalmologic examination; liver evaluation, bowel sounds; CBC, liver and renal function tests

Implementation
- Administer with food if GI upset occurs.
- Administer in a single daily dose; must be used in combination with other antituberculous agents.

Adverse effects in *Italics* are most common; those in **Bold** are life-threatening.

- Arrange for follow-up of liver and renal function tests, CBC, ophthalmologic examinations.

Drug-specific teaching points
- Take drug in a single daily dose; it may be taken with meals if GI upset occurs.
- Take this drug regularly; avoid missing doses. *Do not* discontinue this drug without first consulting your physician.
- Know that the following side effects may occur: nausea, vomiting, epigastric distress; skin rashes or lesions; disorientation, confusion, drowsiness, dizziness (use caution if driving a car or operating dangerous machinery; use precautions to avoid injury).
- Arrange to have periodic medical checkups, which will include an eye examination and blood tests to evaluate the drug effects.
- Report changes in vision (blurring, altered color perception), skin rash.

▢ ethchlorvynol

(eth klor vi' nole)
Placidyl

Pregnancy Category C
C-IV controlled substance

Drug classes
Sedative-hypnotic (nonbarbiturate)

Therapeutic actions
Has sedative-hypnotic, anticonvulsant and muscle relaxant properties; produces EEG patterns similar to those produced by the barbiturates.

Indications
- Short-term hypnotic therapy for periods up to 1 wk in the management of insomnia; retreat only after drug free interval of 1 or more wk and only after further evaluation of the patient
- Unlabeled use: sedative: dosage of 100–200 mg bid–tid PO

Contraindications/cautions
- Contraindicated in the presence of hypersensitivity to ethchlorvynol, allergy to tartrazine (in 750-mg capsules), acute intermittent porphyria, insomnia in the presence of pain, lactation.
- Use caution in the presence of patients who exhibit unpredictable behavior or paradoxical restlessness or excitement in response to barbiturates or alcohol, impaired hepatic or renal function, addiction-prone patients, emotionally depressed patients with or without suicidal tendencies.

Dosage
Adult: Individualize dosage. Usual hypnotic dosage is 500 mg PO at bedtime. 750–1,000 mg may be needed for severe insomnia. May supplement with 200 mg PO to reinstitute sleep in patients who awaken during early morning hours after the original bedtime dose of 500 or 750 mg. Do not prescribe for longer than 1 wk.
Pediatric: Safety and efficacy not established; not recommended.
Geriatric or debilitated: Give the smallest effective dose.

Pharmacokinetics

Route	Onset	Peak	Duration
Oral	15–60 min	2 h	5 h

Metabolism: Hepatic, $T_{1/2}$: 10–20 h
Distribution: Crosses placenta; enters breast milk
Excretion: Urine

Adverse effects
- CNS: *Dizziness, facial numbness, transient giddiness and ataxia*, mild hangover, blurred vision
- GI: *Vomiting, gastric upset, nausea*, aftertaste, cholestatic jaundice
- **Hematologic:** Thrombocytopenia
- **Dermatologic:** Urticaria, rash
- **Other:** Idiosyncratic reactions: syncope without marked hypotension; mild stimulation; marked excitement, hysteria; prolonged hypnosis; profound muscular weakness; physical, psychological dependence; tolerance; withdrawal reaction

Adverse effects in *Italics* are most common; those in **Bold** are life-threatening.

Clinically important drug-drug interactions

- Decreased prothrombin time response to coumarin anticoagulants; dosage adjustment may be necessary when ethchlorvynol therapy is inititated or discontinued
- Exaggerated depressant effects if taken with alcohol, barbiturates, narcotics

■ Nursing Considerations

Assessment

- *History:* Hypersensitivity to ethchlorvynol, tartrazine, acute intermittent porphyria, insomnia in the presence of pain, unpredictable behavior or paradoxical restlessness or excitement in response to barbiturates or alcohol, impaired hepatic or renal function, addiction-prone patients, emotionally depressed patients with or without suicidal tendencies, lactation
- *Physical:* Skin—color, lesions; orientation, affect, reflexes, vision exam; P, BP; bowel sounds, normal output, liver evaluation; CBC with differential, hepatic and renal function tests

Implementation

- Supervise carefully dose and amount of drug prescribed in patients who are addiction prone or likely to increase dosage on their own initiative.
- Dispense least amount of drug feasible to patients who are depressed or suicidal.
- Withdraw drug gradually if patient has used drug long term or if patient has developed tolerance; supportive therapy similar to that for withdrawal from barbiturates may be necessary to prevent dangerous withdrawal symptoms.

Drug-specific teaching points

- Take this drug exactly as prescribed. Take drug with food to reduce GI upset, giddiness, ataxia. Do not exceed prescribed dosage.
- Avoid alcohol, sleep-inducing, or OTC drugs while you are on this drug; these could cause dangerous effects.
- Know that the following side effects may occur: drowsiness, dizziness, blurred vision (avoid driving a car or performing other tasks requiring alertness or visual acuity if these occur), GI upset (frequent small meals may help).
- Report skin rash, yellowing of the skin or eyes, bruising.

❒ ethionamide

*(e thye on **am'** ide)*
Trecator S.C.

Pregnancy Category D

Drug classes
Antituberculous drug ("third line")

Therapeutic actions
Bacteriostatic against *Mycobacterium tuberculosis*; mechanism of action is not known.

Indications
- Tuberculosis— any form that is not responsive to first-line antituberculous agents—in conjunction with other antituberculous agents

Contraindications/cautions
- Contraindicated in the presence of allergy to ethionamide, pregnancy.
- Use caution in the presence of hepatic impairment, diabetes mellitus.

Dosage
Adult: Always use with at least one other antituberculous agent: 0.5–1.0 g/d in divided doses PO. Concomitant administration with pyridoxine is recommended
Pediatric: 15–20 mg/kg per day PO; maximum dose of 1 g/d.

Pharmacokinetics

Route	Peak	Duration
Oral	3 h	9 h

Metabolism: Hepatic, $T_{1/2}$: h
Distribution: Crosses placenta; enters breast milk
Excretion: Urine

Adverse effects
- CNS: *Depression, drowsiness, asthenia*, convulsions, peripheral neuritis, neurop-

Adverse effects in *Italics* are most common; those in **Bold** are life-threatening.

athy, olfactory disturbances, blurred vision, diplopia, optic neuritis, dizziness, headache, restlessness, tremors, psychosis
- **GI:** *Anorexia, nausea, vomiting, diarrhea, metallic taste,* stomatitis, hepatitis
- **CV:** Postural hypotension
- **Dermatologic:** Skin rash, acne, alopecia, thrombocytopenia, pellagra-like syndrome
- **Other:** Gynecomastia, impotence, menorrhagia, difficulty managing diabetes mellitus

■ Nursing Considerations

Assessment
- *History:* Allergy to ethionamide; hepatic impairment, diabetes mellitus; pregnancy
- *Physical:* Skin—color, lesions; orientation, reflexes, ophthalmologic exam, affect; BP, orthostatic BP; liver evaluation; liver function tests, blood and urine glucose

Implementation
- Arrange for culture and sensitivity tests before use.
- Administer only in conjunction with other antituberculous agent.
- Arrange for follow-up of liver function tests prior to and every 2–4 wk during therapy.

Drug-specific teaching points
- Take drug three to four times each day; take with food if GI upset occurs.
- Take this drug regularly; avoid missing doses. *Do not* discontinue this drug without first consulting your physician.
- Know that the following side effects may occur: loss of appetite, nausea, vomiting, metallic taste in mouth, increased salivation (taking the drug with food, frequent mouth care, small frequent meals may help) diarrhea (ensure ready access to bathroom facilities); drowsiness, depression, dizziness, blurred vision (use caution if operating a car or dangerous machinery; change position slowly; take special precautions to avoid injury); impotence, menstrual difficulties.
- Arrange to have regular, periodic medical checkups, which will include blood tests to evaluate the drug effects.
- Report unusual bleeding or bruising, severe GI upset, severe changes in vision.

❒ ethosuximide

*(eth oh **sux**' i mide)*
Zarontin

Pregnancy Category C

Drug classes
Antiepileptic
Succinimide

Therapeutic actions
Suppresses the EEG pattern associated with lapses of consciousness in absence (petit mal) seizures; reduces frequency of attacks; mechanism of action not understood, but may act in inhibitory neuronal systems.

Indications
- Control of absence (petit mal) seizures

Contraindications/cautions
- Contraindicated in the presence of hypersensitivity to succinimides, lactation.
- Use caution in the presence of hepatic, renal abnormalities; pregnancy.

Dosage
Adult: Initial dosage is 500 mg/d PO. Increase by small increments to maintenance dosage. One method is to increase the daily dose by 250 mg every 4–7 d until control is achieved with minimal side effects. Administer dosages > 1.5 g/d in divided doses only under strict supervision (compatible with other antiepileptics when other forms of epilepsy coexist with absence seizures).
Pediatric: 3–6 y: Initial dose is 250 mg/d PO. Increase as described for adults above. > 6 y: Adult dosage.

Adverse effects in *Italics* are most common; those in **Bold** are life-threatening.

466 ■ ethosuximide

Pharmacokinetics

Route	Peak
Oral	3–7 h

Metabolism: Hepatic, $T_{1/2}$: 30 h in children, 60 h in adults

Distribution: Crosses placenta; enters breast milk

Excretion: Urine, bile

Adverse effects
Succinimides
- CNS: *Drowsiness, ataxia, dizziness, irritability, nervousness, headache, blurred vision,* myopia, photophobia, hiccups, euphoria, dreamlike state, lethargy, hyperactivity, fatigue, insomnia, increased frequency of grand mal seizures may occur when used alone in some patients with mixed types of epilepsy, confusion, instability, mental slowness, depression, hypochondriacal behavior, sleep disturbances, night terrors, aggressiveness, inability to concentrate
- GI: *Nausea, vomiting, vague gastric upset, epigastric and abdominal pain, cramps, anorexia, diarrhea, constipation, weight loss,* swelling of tongue, gum hypertrophy
- Hematologic: Eosinophilia, granulocytopenia, leukopenia, agranulocytosis, aplastic anemia, monocytosis, **pancytopenia**
- Dermatologic: *Pruritus, urticaria,* Stevens-Johnson syndrome, pruritic erythematous rashes, skin eruptions, erythema multiforme, systemic lupus erythematosus, alopecia, hirsutism
- Other: Vaginal bleeding, periorbital edema, hyperemia, muscle weakness, abnormal liver and kidney function tests

Clinically important drug-drug interactions
- Decreased serum levels of primidone if administered with ethosuximide

■ Nursing Considerations
Assessment
- *History:* Hypersensitivity to succinimides; hepatic, renal abnormalities; lactation
- *Physical:* Skin—color, lesions; orientation, affect, reflexes, bilateral grip strength, vision exam; bowel sounds, normal output, liver evaluation; liver and kidney function tests, urinalysis, CBC with differential, EEG

Implementation
- Arrange to reduce dosage, discontinue ethosuximide, or substitute other antiepileptic medication gradually; abrupt discontinuation may precipitate absence (petit mal) status.
- Monitor CBC and differential before therapy is instituted, and frequently during therapy.
- Arrange to discontinue drug if skin rash, depression of blood count, or unusual depression, aggressiveness, or behavioral alterations occur.
- Arrange for appropriate counseling for women of childbearing age who need chronic maintenance therapy with antiepileptic drugs and who wish to become pregnant.
- Evaluate for therapeutic serum levels (40–100 µg/ml).

Drug-specific teaching points
- Take this drug exactly as prescribed.
- Do not discontinue this drug abruptly or change dosage, except on the advice of your physician.
- Avoid alcohol, sleep-inducing, or OTC drugs while you are on this drug; these could cause dangerous effects.
- Arrange for frequent checkups to monitor your response to this drug; it is important that you keep all appointments for checkups.
- Know that the following side effects may occur: drowsiness, dizziness, confusion, blurred vision (avoid driving a car or performing other tasks requiring alertness or visual acuity if these occur); GI upset (taking the drug with food or milk and eating frequent small meals may help).
- Wear a medical alert tag at all times so that any emergency medical personnel taking care of you will know that you

Adverse effects in *Italics* are most common; those in **Bold** are life-threatening.

are an epileptic taking antiepileptic medication.
- Report skin rash, joint pain, unexplained fever, sore throat, unusual bleeding or bruising, drowsiness, dizziness, blurred vision, pregnancy.

▢ ethotoin

(eth' i toe in)
Peganone
Pregnancy Category D

Drug classes
Antiepileptic
Hydantoin

Therapeutic actions
Has antiepileptic activity without causing general CNS depression; stabilizes neuronal membranes and prevents hyperexcitability caused by excessive stimulation; limits the spread of seizure activity from an active focus.

Indications
- Control of grand mal (tonic-clonic) and psychomotor seizures

Contraindications/cautions
- Contraindicated in the presence of hypersensitivity to hydantoins, pregnancy, lactation, hepatic abnormalities, hematologic disorders.
- Use caution in the presence of acute intermittent porphyria; hypotension, severe myocardial insufficiency; diabetes mellitus, hyperglycemia.

Dosage
Administer in four to six divided doses daily. Take after eating; space as evenly as possible.
Adult: Initial dose should be < 1 g/d PO. Increase gradually over several days; maintenance from 2–3 g/d PO; < 2 g/d is ineffective in most adults. If replacing another drug, reduce the dose of the other drug gradually as ethotoin dose is increased.
Pediatric: Initial dose should not exceed 750 mg/d PO; maintenance doses range from 500 mg/d to 1 g/d PO.

Pharmacokinetics

Route	Onset	Peak
Oral	Rapid	1–3 h

Metabolism: Hepatic, $T_{1/2}$: 3–9 h
Distribution: Crosses placenta; enters breast milk
Excretion: Urine

Adverse effects
- **CNS:** *Nystagmus, ataxia, dysarthria, slurred speech, mental confusion, dizziness, drowsiness, insomnia, transient nervousness, motor twitchings, fatigue, irritability, depression, numbness, tremor, headache,* photophobia, diplopia, conjunctivitis
- **GI:** *Nausea,* vomiting, diarrhea, constipation, *gingival hyperplasia,* toxic hepatitis, liver damage, sometimes fatal; hypersensitivity reactions with hepatic involvement, including hepatocellular degeneration and fatal hepatocellular necrosis
- **Respiratory: Pulmonary fibrosis**, acute pneumonitis
- **Hematologic:** Hematopoietic complications, sometimes fatal: thrombocytopenia, leukopenia, granulocytopenia, agranulocytosis, pancytopenia; macrocytosis and megaloblastic anemia that usually respond to folic acid therapy; eosinophilia, monocytosis, leukocytosis, simple anemia, hemolytic anemia, aplastic anemia, hyperglycemia
- **GU:** Nephrosis
- **Dermatologic:** Scarlatiniform, morbilliform, maculopapular, urticarial and nonspecific rashes; also serious and sometimes fatal dermatologic reactions: bullous, exfoliative, or purpuric dermatitis, lupus erythematosus, and Stevens-Johnson syndrome; toxic epidermal necrolysis, hirsutism, alopecia, coarsening of the facial features, enlargement of the lips, Peyronie's disease
- **Other:** Lymph node hyperplasia, sometimes progressing to frank malignant lymphoma, monoclonal gammopathy and multiple myeloma (prolonged ther-

Adverse effects in *Italics* are most common; those in **Bold** are life-threatening.

apy), polyarthropathy, osteomalacia, weight gain, chest pain, periarteritis nodosa

Clinically important drug-drug interactions

- Increased pharmacologic effects of hydantoins when given with chloramphenicol, cimetidine, disulfiram, isoniazid, phenacemide, phenylbutazone, sulfonamides, trimethoprim • Complex interactions and effects when hydantoins and valproic acid are given together: toxicity with apparently normal serum ethotoin levels; decreased plasma levels of valproic acid given with hydantoins; breakthrough seizures when the two drugs are given together • Decreased pharmacologic effects of hydantoins when given with antineoplastics, diazoxide, folic acid, rifampin, theophyllines • Increased pharmacologic effects and toxicity when primidone, oxyphenbutazone, fluconazole, amiodarone are given concurrently with hydantoins • Increased hepatotoxicity if given concurrently with acetaminophen • Decreased pharmacologic effects of the following drugs when given with hydantoins: corticosteroids, cyclosporine, dicumarol, disopyramide, doxycycline, estrogens, levodopa, methadone, metyrapone, mexiletine, oral contraceptives, quinestrol, carbamazepine

Drug-lab test interferences

- Interference with the metyrapone and the 1-mg dexamethasone tests; avoid the use of hydantoins for at least 7 d prior to metyrapone testing

■ Nursing Considerations

Assessment

- *History:* Hypersensitivity to hydantoins; hepatic abnormalities; hematologic disorders; acute intermittent porphyria; hypotension, severe myocardial insufficiency; diabetes mellitus, hyperglycemia; pregnancy; lactation
- *Physical:* Body temperature; skin—color, lesions; lymph node palpation; orientation, affect, reflexes, vision exam; P, BP; R, adventitious sounds; bowel sounds, normal output, liver evaluation; periodontal exam; liver function tests, urinalysis, CBC and differential, blood proteins, blood and urine glucose, EEG and ECG

Implementation

- Give after food to enhance absorption and reduce GI upset.
- Administer with other anticonvulsants to regulate seizures; not compatible with phenacemide.
- Arrange to reduce dosage, discontinue ethotoin, or substitute other antiepileptic medication gradually; abrupt discontinuation may precipitate status epilepticus.
- Arrange to discontinue drug if skin rash, depression of blood count, enlarged lymph nodes, hypersensitivity reaction, signs of liver damage, or Peyronie's disease (induration of the corpora cavernosa of the penis) occurs. Arrange to institute another antiepileptic drug promptly.
- Monitor hepatic function periodically during chronic therapy; monitor blood counts, urinalysis monthly.
- Monitor urine sugar of patients with diabetes mellitus regularly. Adjustment of dosage of hypoglycemic drug may be necessary because antiepileptic drug may inhibit insulin release and induce hyperglycemia.
- Arrange to have lymph node enlargement occurring during therapy evaluated carefully. Lymphadenopathy, which simulates Hodgkin's disease, has occurred. Lymph node hyperplasia may progress to lymphoma.
- Monitor blood proteins, as appropriate, to detect early malfunction of the immune system (eg, multiple myeloma).
- Arrange dental consultation to instruct patients on long-term hydantoin therapy in proper oral hygiene technique to prevent development of gum hyperplasia.
- Arrange for appropriate counseling for women of childbearing age who need chronic maintenance therapy with antiepileptic drugs and who wish to become pregnant.

Drug-specific teaching points

- Take this drug exactly as prescribed, after food to enhance absorption and reduce GI upset. Be especially careful

not to miss a dose if you are on once-a-day therapy.
- Do not discontinue this drug abruptly or change dosage, except on the advice of your physician.
- Maintain good oral hygiene—regular brushing and flossing—to prevent gum disease while you are taking this drug.
- Arrange frequent dental checkups to prevent serious gum disease.
- Arrange for frequent checkups to monitor your response to this drug; it is important that you keep all appointments for checkups.
- Monitor your urine sugar regularly, and report any abnormality to your nurse or physician if you are a diabetic.
- Use some form of contraception, other than birth control pills, while you are on this drug. This drug is not recommended for use during pregnancy. If you wish to become pregnant, consult with your physician.
- Know that the following side effects may occur: drowsiness, dizziness, confusion, blurred vision (avoid driving a car or performing other tasks requiring alertness or visual acuity if these occur); GI upset (taking the drug with food and eating frequent small meals may help).
- Wear a medical alert tag at all times so that any emergency medical personnel taking care of you will know that you are an epileptic taking antiepileptic medication.
- Report skin rash, severe nausea or vomiting, drowsiness, slurred speech, impaired coordination (ataxia), swollen glands, bleeding, swollen or tender gums, yellowish discoloration of the skin or eyes, joint pain, unexplained fever, sore throat, unusual bleeding or bruising, persistent headache, malaise, any indication of an infection or bleeding tendency, abnormal erection, pregnancy.

⬜ etodolac

*(ee toe **doe'** lak)*

Lodine

Pregnancy Category C

Drug classes
Analgesic (non-narcotic)
Antipyretic
NSAID

Therapeutic actions
Inhibits prostaglandin synthetase to cause antipyretic and anti-inflammatory effects; the exact mechnanism of action is not known.

Indications
- Acute or long-term use in the management of signs and symptoms of osteoarthritis
- Management of pain
- Unlabeled uses: ankylosing spondylitis, rheumatoid arthritis, tendinitis, bursitis, gout

Contraindications/cautions
- Contraindicated in the presence of significant renal impairment, pregnancy, lactation.
- Use caution in the presence of impaired hearing, allergies, hepatic, cardiovascular, and GI conditions.

Dosage
Adult
- ***Osteoarthritis:*** Initially 800–1,200 mg/d PO in divided doses; maintenance ranges 600–1,200 mg/d in divided doses. Do not exceed 1,200 mg/d. Patients < 60 kg: Do not exceed 20 mg per kg.
- ***Analgesia, acute pain:*** 200–400 mg q6–8h PO. Do not exceed 1,200 mg/d. Patients < 60 kg: Do not exceed 20 mg per kg.

Pediatric: Safety and efficacy not established.

Pharmacokinetics

Route	Onset	Peak
Oral	Varies	1–2 h

Metabolism: Hepatic, $T_{1/2}$: 7.3 h
Distribution: Crosses placenta; enters breast milk
Excretion: Urine and feces

etoposide

(e toe **poe'** side)

VP-16-213

Vepesid

Pregnancy Category D

Drug classes
Mitotic inhibitor
Antineoplastic agent

Therapeutic actions
G_2 specific cell toxic: lyses cells entering mitosis; inhibits cells from entering prophase; inhibits DNA synthesis, leading to cell death.

Indications
- Refractory testicular tumors as part of combination therapy
- Treatment of small cell lung carcinoma as part of combination therapy

Contraindications/cautions
- Allergy to etoposide, bone marrow suppression, pregnancy, lactation.

Dosage
Modify dosage based on myelosuppression.
Adult
- ***Testicular cancer:*** 50–100 mg/m^2 per day IV on days 1 to 5 or 100 mg per m^2 per day IV on days 1, 3, and 5, every 3–4 wk in combination with other agents.
- ***Small-cell lung cancer:*** 35 mg/m^2 per day IV for 4 d to 50 mg/m^2 for day for 5 d; repeat every 3–4 wk after recovery from toxicity.
- *Oral:* Two times the IV dose rounded to the nearest 50 mg.

Pediatric: Safety and efficacy not established.

Pharmacokinetics

Route	Onset	Peak	Duration
Oral	30–60 min	1–1½ h	20–30 h
IV	30 min	60 min	20–30 h

Metabolism: Hepatic, $T_{1/2}$: 4–11 h

Adverse effects
- CNS: *Dizziness*, somnolence, insomnia, fatigue, tiredness, dizziness, tinnitus, ophthalmologic effects
- GI: *Nausea, dyspepsia, GI pain, diarrhea*, vomiting, *constipation*, flatulence
- Hematologic: Bleeding, platelet inhibition with higher doses
- GU: Dysuria, renal impairment
- Dermatologic: Rash, pruritus, sweating, dry mucous membranes, stomatitis
- Other: Peripheral edema, **anaphylactoid reactions** to fatal anaphylactic shock

Nursing Considerations

Assessment
- *History:* Renal impairment, impaired hearing, allergies, hepatic, cardiovascular, and GI conditions, lactation
- *Physical:* Skin color and lesions; orientation, reflexes, ophthalmologic and audiometric evaluation, peripheral sensation; P, edema; R, adventitious sounds; liver evaluation; CBC, clotting times, renal and liver function tests; serum electrolytes, stool guaiac

Implementation
- Administer drug with food or after meals if GI upset occurs.
- Arrange for periodic ophthalmologic examination during long-term therapy.
- Institute emergency procedures if overdose occurs (gastric lavage, induction of emesis, supportive therapy).

Drug-specific teaching points
- Take drug with food or meals if GI upset occurs.
- Take only the prescribed dosage.
- Know that dizziness, drowsiness can occur (avoid driving or the use of dangerous machinery while on this drug).
- Report sore throat, fever, rash, itching, weight gain, swelling in ankles or fingers; changes in vision; black, tarry stools.

Adverse effects in *Italics* are most common; those in **Bold** are life-threatening.

Distribution: Crosses placenta; enters breast milk
Excretion: Urine and bile

IV facts
Preparation: Dilute with 5% Dextrose Injection or 0.9% Sodium Chloride Injection to give a concentration of 0.2 or 0.4 mg/ml. Unopened vials are stable at room temperature for 2 y; diluted solutions are stable at room temperature for 2 (0.4 mg/ml) or 4 (0.2 mg/ml) d.

Infusion: Administer slowly over 30–60 min. *Do not give by rapid IV push.*

Adverse effects
- CNS: *Somnolence, fatigue,* peripheral neuropathy
- GI: *Nausea, vomiting, anorexia, diarrhea,* stomatitis, aftertaste, liver toxicity
- CV: Hypotension (after rapid IV administration)
- Hematologic: *Myelotoxicity*
- Dermatologic: *Alopecia*
- Hypersensitivity: Chills, fever, tachycardia, bronchospasm, dyspnea, anaphylactic-like reaction
- Other: Potentially, carcinogenesis

■ Nursing Considerations
Assessment
- *History:* Allergy to etoposide; bone marrow suppression; pregnancy; lactation
- *Physical:* Temperature; weight; hair; orientation, reflexes; BP, P; mucous membranes, abdominal exam; CBC

Implementation
- Do not administer IM or SC because severe local reaction and tissue necrosis occur.
- Avoid skin contact with this drug. The use of rubber gloves is suggested while using this drug; if contact occurs, immediately wash with soap and water.
- Monitor blood pressure during administration; if hypotension occurs, discontinue dose and consult with physician. Fluids and other supportive therapy may be needed.
- Monitor patient's response to therapy before starting therapy and prior to each dose: platelet count, hemoglobin, WBC count, differential. If severe response occurs, discontinue therapy and consult with physician.
- Arrange for an antiemetic for severe nausea and vomiting.
- Arrange for wig or other suitable head covering before alopecia occurs. Teach patient the importance of covering the head at extremes of temperature.

Drug-specific teaching points
- Prepare a calendar for specific treatment days and additional courses of drug therapy.
- Know that the following side effects may occur: loss of appetite, nausea, vomiting, mouth sores (frequent mouth care, small frequent meals may help; you will need to try to maintain good nutrition if at all possible; a dietician may be able to help, and an antiemetic may be ordered); loss of hair (you might like to arrange for a wig or other suitable head covering before the hair loss occurs; it is important to keep the head covered at extremes of temperature).
- Arrange to have regular blood tests to monitor the drug's effects.
- Report severe GI upset, diarrhea, vomiting, unusual bleeding or bruising, fever, chills, sore throat, difficulty breathing.

❐ etretinate

(e tret' i nate)

Tegison

Pregnancy Category X

Drug classes
Antipsoriatic (systemic)

Therapeutic actions
Related to retinoic acid vitamin A; mechanism of action is not known, but improvement seems to be related to a decrease in scale, erythema, and thickness

Adverse effects in *Italics* are most common; those in **Bold** are life-threatening.

of lesions; normalization of epidermal differentiation; and decreased inflammation in the epidermis and dermis.

Indications
- Treatment of severe recalcitrant psoriasis in patients who are unresponsive to standard treatment

Contraindications/cautions
- Contraindicated in the presence of allergy to etretinate, retinoids, pregnancy, lactation.
- Use caution in the presence of cardiovascular disease (drug increases triglycerides); diabetes mellitus, obesity, increased alcohol intake, familial history of these conditions (these patients have a tendency to develop hypertriglyceridemia and may be at greater risk of developing this condition in association with etretinate therapy); pregnancy (caused severe fetal malformations and spontaneous abortions); lactation.

Dosage
Adult: Individualize dosage based on side effects and disease response. *Initial dose:* 0.75–1 mg/kg per day PO in divided doses. Maximum daily dose: 1.5 mg/kg. Erythrodermic psoriasis may respond to lower initial doses of 0.25 mg/kg per day, PO increased by 0.25 mg/kg per day each wk until optimal initial response is attained. Maintenance doses of 0.5–0.75 mg/kg per day PO may be initiated after initial response, generally after 8–16 wk of therapy. Therapy is usually terminated in patients whose lesions have sufficiently resolved; relapses may be treated as for initial therapy.
Pediatric: Use only if all other treatments have proven unsuccessful; may cause premature closure of the epiphyses.

Pharmacokinetics

Route	Onset	Peak	Duration
Oral	Slow	2–6 h	Weeks–months

Metabolism: Hepatic, $T_{1/2}$: 120 d
Distribution: Crosses placenta; may enter breast milk
Excretion: Bile and urine

Adverse effects
- **CNS:** *Lethargy, insomnia, fatigue, headache, fever, dizziness, amnesia,* abnormal thinking, pseudotumor cerebri
- **GI:** *Cheilitis, chapped lips; dry mouth, thirst; sore mouth and tongue, gingival bleeding and inflammation, nausea,* vomiting, abdominal pain, anorexia, inflammatory bowel disease, **hepatitis** (including fatalities)
- **CV:** *Cardiovascular, thrombotic or obstructive events,* edema, *dyspnea*
- **Hematologic:** Elevated mean corpuscular hemoglobin concentration, mean corpuscular hemoglobin, reticulocytes, partial thromboplastin time, erythrocyte sedimentation rate; decreased Hgb/Hct, RBC and mean corpuscular volume, increased platelets, *increased or decreased WBC or prothrombin time,* elevated triglycerides, AST, ALT, alkaline phosphatase, GGTP, globulin, cholesterol, bilirubin abnormal liver function tests, increased fasting serum glucose, increased BUN and creatinine, increased or decreased potassium
- **GU:** *White cells in the urine, proteinuria, red blood cells in the urine, hematuria,* glycosuria, aceetonuria
- **MS:** *Skeletal hyperostosis, arthralgia, muscle cramps,* bone and joint pain and stiffness
- **EENT:** Epistaxis, *dry nose, eye irritation, conjunctivitis, corneal opacities, eyeball pain; abnormalities of eyelid, cornea, lens, and retina; decreased visual acuity, double vision;* abnormalities of lacrimation, vision, extraocular musculature, ocular tension, pupil and vitreous, earache, otitis externa
- **Dermatologic:** *Skin fragility, dry skin, pruritus, rash, thinning of hair, peeling of palms and soles,* skin infections, nail brittleness, petechiae, sunburn, changes in perspiration

Clinically important drug-food interactions
- Increased absorption of etretinate if taken concurrently with milk

Nursing Considerations

Assessment
- *History:* Allergy to etretinate, retinoids; cardiovascular disease; diabetes mellitus, obesity, increased alcohol intake; pregnancy, lactation
- *Physical:* Body weight; skin—color, lesions, turgor, texture; joints—range of motion; orientation, reflexes, affect, ophthalmologic exam; mucous membranes, bowel sounds; hepatic function tests (AST, ALT, LDH), serum triglycerides, cholesterol, HDL, sedimentation rate, CBC and differential, urinalysis, serum electrolytes, pregnancy test

Implementation
- Ensure that patient is not pregnant before administering; arrange for a pregnancy test 2 wk before beginning therapy. Advise patient to use contraceptive measures during treatment and for an indefinite period after treatment is discontinued (the exact length of time after treatment when pregnancy should be avoided is not known; etretinate has been detected in the blood of some patients 2–3 y after therapy was discontinued).
- Arrange for patient to have hepatic function tests prior to therapy and at 1- to 2-wk intervals for the first 1–2 mo of therapy and at intervals of 1–3 mo thereafter.
- Arrange for patient to have blood lipid determinations before therapy and at intervals of 1 or 2 wk until the lipid response is established (usually within 4–8 wk). If elevations occur, institute other measures to lower serum triglycerides: weight reduction, reduction in dietary fat, exercise, increased intake of insoluble fiber, decreased alcohol consumption.
- Administer drug with meals; do not crush capsules.
- Discontinue drug if signs of papilledema occur, and arrange for patient to consult a neurologist for further care.
- Discontinue drug if visual disturbances occur, and arrange for an ophthalmologic exam.
- Discontinue drug if abdominal pain, rectal bleeding, or severe diarrhea occurs, and consult with physician.
- Do not allow blood donation from patients taking etretinate due to the teratogenic effects of the drug.

Drug-specific teaching points
- Take drug with meals. Do not crush capsules.
- Be aware that this drug has been associated with severe birth defects and miscarriages, it is contraindicated in pregnant women. It is important to use contraceptive measures during treatment and for 1 mo after treatment is discontinued. If you think that you have become pregnant, consult with your physician immediately.
- Do not take vitamin A supplements while you are taking this drug.
- Do not donate blood while on this drug because of its possible effects on the fetus of a blood recipient.
- Know that the following side effects may occur: exacerbation of psoriasis during initial therapy; dizziness, lethargy, headache, visual changes (avoid driving or performing tasks that require alertness if these occur); sensitivity to the sun (avoid sunlamps, exposure to the sun; use sunscreens, protective clothing if it cannot be avoided); diarrhea, abdominal pain, loss of appetite (taking the drug with meals may help); dry mouth (sucking sugarless lozenges is often helpful); eye irritation and redness, inability to wear contact lenses; dry skin, itching, redness.
- Report headache with nausea and vomiting, yellowing of the skin, eyes; pale stools, visual difficulties.

factor IX complex

(fac' tor nin)

Konyne-HT, Profilnine Heat-Treated, Proplex T
Pregnancy Category C

Drug classes
Antihemophilic agent

factor IX complex

Therapeutic actions
Human factor IX complex consists of plasma fractions involved in the intrinsic pathway of blood coagulation; causes an increase in blood levels of clotting factors II, VII, IX, and X.

Indications
- Factor IX deficiency (hemophilia B, Christmas disease) to prevent or control bleeding
- Bleeding episodes in patients with inhibitors to factor VIII
- Reversal of coumarin anticoagulant-induced hemorrhage; if prompt reversal is required, use fresh, frozen plasma
- Prevention or control of bleeding episodes in patients with factor VII deficiency (*Proplex T* only)

Contraindications/cautions
- Factor VII deficiencies (except as listed above for *Proplex T*); liver disease with signs of intravascular coagulation or fibrinolysis

Dosage
Dosage depends on severity of deficiency and severity of bleeding; follow treatment carefully with factor IX level assays. To calculate dosage, use the following formula: Dose = 1 U/kg × body weight (kg) × desired increase (% of normal). Administer qd–bid (once every 2–3 d may suffice to maintain lower effective levels) IV.

Surgery: Maintain levels > 25% for at least 1 wk. Calculate dose to raise level to 40%–60% of normal.

Hemarthroses: In hemophiliacs with inhibitors to factor VIII, dosage levels approximate 75 U/kg IV. Give a second dose after 12 h if needed.

Maintainence dose: Dose is usually 10–20 U/kg per day IV. Individualize dose based on patient response.

Inhibitor patients (hemophilia A patients with inhibitors to factor VIII): 75 U/kg IV; give a second dose after 12 h if needed.

Reversal of coumadin effect: 15 U/kg IV is suggested.

Prophylaxis: 10–20 U/kg IV once or twice a week may prevent spontaneous bleeding in hemophilia B patients. Inidividualize dose. Increase dose if patient is exposed to trauma or surgery.

Pharmacokinetics

Route	Onset	Duration
IV	Immediate	1–2 d

Metabolism: Plasma, $T_{1/2}$: 24–32 h
Distribution: Crosses placenta; enters breast milk

IV facts
Preparation: Prepare using diluents and needles supplied with product. Refrigerate.
Infusion: Infuse slowly. 100 U/min and 2–3 ml/min have been suggested. Do not exceed 3 ml/min, and stop or slow the infusion at any sign of headache, pulse, or BP changes.

Adverse effects
- CNS: *Headache,* flushing, chills, tingling, somnolence, lethargy
- GI: *Nausea,* vomiting, hepatitis—risk associated with use of blood products
- Hematologic: *Thrombosis,* disseminated intravascular coagulation, AIDS—risk associated with use of blood products
- Other: Chills, fever; blood pressure changes, urticaria

■ Nursing Considerations

Assessment
- *History:* Factor VII deficiencies; liver disease with signs of intravascular coagulation or fibrinolysis
- *Physical:* Skin—color, lesions; body temperature; orientation, reflexes, affect; P, BP, peripheral perfusion; clotting factors levels, liver function tests

Implementation
- Administer by IV route only.
- Decrease rate of infusion if headache, flushing, fever, chills, tingling, urticaria

occur; in some individuals, the drug will need to be discontinued.
- Monitor patient's clinical response and factors IX, II, VII, X levels regularly, and regulate dosage based on response.
- Monitor patient for any sign of thrombosis; use comfort and preventive measures when possible (exercise, support stockings, ambulation, positioning).

Drug-specific teaching points
- Know that dosage varies at different times and in different situations. All known safety precautions are taken to ensure that this blood product is pure and the risk of AIDS and hepatitis is as minimal as possible.
- Wear or carry a medical alert tag to alert medical personnel who may be taking care of you in an emergency that you require this treatment.
- Report headache, rash, chills, calf pain, swelling, unusual bleeding, or bruising.

❏ famciclovir sodium

(fam sye' kloe vir)
Famvir

Pregnancy Category C

Drug classes
Antiviral drug

Therapeutic actions
Antiviral activity; inhibits viral DNA replication in acute herpes zoster.

Indications
- Management of acute herpes zoster (shingles)

Contraindications/cautions
- Contraindicated in the presence of hypersensitivity to famciclovir or acyclovir, lactation.
- Use caution in the presence of cytopenia, history of cytopenic reactions, impaired renal function.

Dosage
Adult: 500 mg q8h PO for 7 d.
Pediatric: Safety and efficacy not established.

Pharmacokinetics

Route	Onset	Peak
Oral	Varies	0.5–1 h

Metabolism: $T_{1/2}$: 2 h
Distribution: Crosses placenta; may enter breast milk
Excretion: Urine

Adverse effects
- **CNS:** Dreams, ataxia, coma, confusion, dizziness, *headache*
- **GI:** Abnormal liver function tests, nausea, vomiting, anorexia, *diarrhea*, abdominal pain
- **CV:** Arrhythmia, hypertension, hypotension
- **Hematologic:** Granulocytopenia, thrombocytopenia, anemia
- **Dermatologic:** *Rash,* alopecia, pruritus, urticaria
- **Other:** *Fever*, chills, **cancer, sterility**

Clinically important drug-drug interactions
- Use with extreme caution with cytotoxic drugs because the accumulation effect could cause severe bone marrow depression and other GI and dermatologic problems

■ Nursing Considerations

Assessment
- *History:* Hypersensitivity to famciclovir or acyclovir; cytopenia; impaired renal function; lactation
- *Physical:* Skin—color, lesions; orientation; BP, P, auscultation, perfusion, edema; R, adventitious sounds; urinary output; CBC, Hct, BUN, creatinine clearance, liver function tests

Implementation
- Arrange for decreased dosage in patients with impaired renal function.
- Arrange for CBC before beginning therapy and every 2 d during daily dosing and at least weekly thereafter. Consult with

Adverse effects in Italics are most common; those in Bold are life-threatening.

476 ■ famotidine

physician, and arrange for reduced dosage if WBCs or platelets fall.

Drug-specific teaching points
- Take this drug for 7 full days as prescribed.
- Know that the following side effects may occur: decreased blood count leading to susceptibility to infection (blood tests may be needed; avoid crowds and exposure to disease as much as possible), headache (analgesics may be ordered), diarrhea (maintain ready access to bathroom facililites).
- Report bruising, bleeding, worsening of condition, fever, infection.

☐ famotidine

(fa moe' ti deen)
Pepcid

Pregnancy Category B

Drug classes
Histamine₂ (H₂) antagonist

Therapeutic actions
Competitively blocks the action of histamine at the histamine (H₂) receptors of the parietal cells of the stomach; inhibits basal gastric acid secretion and chemically induced gastric acid secretion.

Indications
- Short-term treatment and maintenance of duodenal ulcer
- Short-term treatment of benign gastric ulcer
- Treatment of pathologic hypersecretory conditions
- Short-term treatment of gastroesophageal reflux disease (GERD), esophagitis due to GERD

Contraindications/cautions
- Allergy to famotidine; renal failure; pregnancy; lactation.

Dosage
Adult
- ***Active duodenal ulcer:*** 40 mg PO or IV at bedtime *or* 20 mg bid PO or IV. Therapy at full dosage should generally be discontinued after 6–8 wk.
- ***Maintenance therapy, duodenal ulcer:*** 20 mg PO at bedtime.
- ***Benign gastric ulcer:*** 40 mg PO qd at bedtime.
- ***Hypersecretory syndrome:*** 20 mg q6h PO initially. Doses up to 160 mg q6h have been administered.
- ***GERD:*** 20 mg bid PO for up to 6 wk.
- ***Esophagitis:*** 20–40 mg bid PO for up to 12 wk.

Pediatric: Safety and efficacy not established.

Geriatric or renal insufficiency: Reduce dosage to 20 mg PO at bedtime *or* 40 mg PO q36–48h.

Pharmacokinetics

Route	Onset	Peak	Duration
Oral	Slow	1–3 h	6–12 h
IV	< 1 h	½–3 h	8–15 h

Metabolism: Hepatic, $T_{1/2}$: 2 1/22–3 1/2 h
Distribution: Crosses placenta; enters breast milk
Excretion: Urine

IV facts
Preparation: For direct injection, dilute 2 ml (solution contains 10 mg/ml) with 0.9% Sodium Chloride Injection, Water for Injection, 5% or 10% Dextrose Injection, Lactated Ringer's Injection, or 5% Sodium Bicarbonate Injection to a total volume of 5–10 ml. For infusion, 2 ml diluted with 100 ml 5% Dextrose Solution or other IVs. Stable for 48 h at room temperature, 14 d if refrigerated.

Infusion: Inject directly slowly, over not less than 2 min. Infuse over 15–30 min; continuous infusion: 40 mg/24 hr.

Adverse effects
- CNS: *Headache,* malaise, *dizziness,* somnolence, insomnia
- GI: *Diarrhea, constipation,* anorexia, abdominal pain
- Dermatologic: Skin rash

Adverse effects in *Italics* are most common; those in **Bold** are life-threatening.

- **Other:** Muscle cramp, increase in total bilirubin, sexual impotence

■ Nursing Considerations

Assessment
- *History:* Allergy to famotidine; renal failure; lactation
- *Physical:* Skin—lesions; liver evaluation, abdominal exam, normal output; renal function tests, serum bilirubin

Implementation
- Administer drug at bedtime.
- Arrange for decreased doses in patients with renal failure.
- Arrange for administration of concurrent antacid therapy to relieve pain.

Drug-specific teaching points
- Take this drug at bedtime (or in the morning and at bedtime). Therapy may continue for 4–6 wk or longer.
- Be aware that if you are also on an antacid, you should take it exactly as it has been prescribed, being careful of the times of administration.
- Arrange to have regular medical follow-up while you are on this drug to evaluate your response.
- Know that the following side effects may occur: constipation or diarrhea; loss of libido or impotence (these are reversible and will pass when the drug therapy has been discontinued); headache (monitoring lights, temperature, noise levels may help).
- Report sore throat, fever, unusual bruising or bleeding, severe headache, muscle or joint pain.

☐ fat emulsion, intravenous

*(fat ee **mul'** shun)*
Intralipid 10%, 20%, Liposyn II 10%, 20%, Liposyn III 10%, 20%

Pregnancy Category C

Drug classes
Caloric agent

Therapeutic actions
A preparation from soybean or safflower oil that provides neutral triglycerides, mostly unsaturated fatty acids; these are used as a source of energy, causing an increase in heat production, decrease in respiratory quotient, and increase in oxygen consumption.

Indications
- Source of calories and essential fatty acids for patients requiring parental nutrition for extended periods
- Source of essential fatty acids when a deficiency occurs

Contraindications/cautions
- Contraindicated in the presence of disturbance of normal fat metabolism (hyperlipemia, lipoid nephrosis, acute pancreatitis), allergy to eggs.
- Use caution in the presence of severe liver damage, pulmonary disease, anemia, blood coagulation disorders, pregnancy, jaundiced or premature infants.

Dosage
Parenteral nutrition: Should not comprise more than 60% of total calorie intake. *10%:* infuse IV at 1 ml/min for the first 15–30 min; may be increased to 2 ml/min. Infuse only 500 ml the first day, and increase the following day. Do not exceed 2.5 g/kg per day. *20%:* infuse at 0.5 ml/min for the first 15–30 min; infuse only 250 ml *Liposyn II* or 500 ml Intralipid the first day, and increase the following day. Do not exceed 3 g/kg per day.
Fatty acid deficiency: Supply 8%–10% of the caloric intake by IV fat emulsion.
Pediatric parenteral nutrition: Should not comprise more than 60% of total calorie intake. *10%:* initial IV infusion rate is 0.1 ml/min for the first 10–15 min. *20%:* initial infusion rate is 0.05 ml/min for the first 10–15 min. If no untoward reactions occur, increase rate to 1 g/kg in 4 h. Do not exceed 3 g/kg per day.

Adverse effects in *Italics* are most common; those in **Bold** are life-threatening.

Pharmacokinetics

Route	Onset
IV	Rapid

Metabolism: Hepatic and tissue, T$_{1/2}$: varies
Distribution: Crosses placenta; may enter breast milk

IV facts

Preparation: Supplied in single-dose containers; do not store partially used bottles; do not resterilize for later use; do not use with filters; do not use any bottle in which there appears to be separation from the emulsion.

Infusion: Infusion rate is 1 ml/min for 10% solution, monitor for 15–30 min; if no adverse reaction occurs, may be increased to 2 ml/min; 0.5 ml/min for 20% solution, may be increased if no adverse reactions. May be infused simultaneously with Amino Acid-Dextrose mixtures by means of Y-connector located near the infusion site using separate flow rate; keep the Lipid Solution higher than the Amino Acid-Dextrose line.

Incompatibilities: Do not mix with amikacin, tetracycline. Monitor electrolyte and acid content; fat emulsion seperates in acid solution.

Adverse effects

- CNS: *Headache,* flushing, fever, sweating, sleepiness, pressure over the eyes, dizziness
- GI: *Nausea,* vomiting
- Hematologic: *Thrombophlebitis,* **sepsis**, hyperlipemia, hypercoagulability, thrombocytopenia, leukopenia, elevated liver enzymes
- Other: Irritation at infusion site, brown pigmentation in RES (IV fat pigment), cyanosis

■ Nursing Considerations

Assessment

- *History:* Disturbance of normal fat metabolism, allergy to eggs, severe liver damage, pulmonary disease, anemia, blood coagulation disorders, pregnancy, jaundiced or premature infants
- *Physical:* Skin—color, lesions; body temperature; orientation; P, BP, peripheral perfusion; CBC, plasma lipid profile, clotting factors levels, liver function tests

Implementation

- Administer by IV route only.
- Inspect admixture for TPN for any sign of "breaking or oiling out" of the emulsion—a separation of the emulsion seen as a yellow streaking or accumulation of yellow droplets in the admixture—or for the formation of any particulates; discard any admixture if these occur.
- Monitor patient carefully for any sign of fluid or fat overloading during infusion: diluted serum electrolytes, overhydration, pulmonary edema, elevated JVP, metabolic acidosis, impaired pulmonary diffusion capacity. Discontinue the infusion; reevaluate patient before restarting infusion at a lower rate.
- Monitor patient's clinical response, serum lipid profile, weight gain, improved nitrogen balance.
- Monitor patient for any sign of thrombosis or sepsis; use comfort and preventive measures when possible (exercise, support stockings, ambulation, positioning).

Drug-specific teaching points

- Report pain at infusion site, difficulty breathing, chest pain, calf pain, excessive sweating.

❒ felodipine

(fell ob' di peen)
Plendil

Pregnancy Category C

Drug classes
Calcium channel-blocker
Antihypertensive

Therapeutic actions
Inhibits the movement of calcium ions across the membranes of cardiac and arterial muscle cells; inhibition of transmembrane calcium flow results in the

Adverse effects in *Italics* are most common; those in **Bold** are life-threatening.

depression of impulse formation in specialized cardiac pacemaker cells, slowing of the velocity of conduction of the cardiac impulse, the depression of myocardial contractility, and the dilation of coronary arteries and arterioles and peripheral arterioles; these effects lead to decreased cardiac work, decreased cardiac energy consumption, and decreased blood pressure.

Indications
- Essential hypertension, alone or in combination with other antihypertensives

Contraindications/cautions
- Allergy to felodipine or other calcium channel-blockers, impaired hepatic or renal function, sick sinus syndrome, heart block (second or third degree), lactation.

Dosage
Adult: Initially 5 mg PO qd; dosage may be gradually increased over 10–14 d to an average 10–15 mg PO qd. Maximum effective dose is 20 mg qd.
Pediatric: Safety and efficacy not established.
Geriatric or hepatic impairment: Carefully monitor; do not exceed 10 mg qd PO.

Pharmacokinetics

Route	Onset	Peak
Oral	120–130 min	2½–5 h

Metabolism: Hepatic metabolism, $T_{1/2}$: 11–16 h
Distribution: Crosses placenta; may pass into breast milk
Excretion: Urine

Adverse effects
- CNS: *Dizziness, lightheadedness, headache,* asthenia, *fatigue, lethargy*
- GI: *Nausea,* abdominal discomfort
- CV: *Peripheral edema,* arrhythmias
- Dermatologic: *Flushing,* rash

Clinically important drug-drug interactions
- Decreased serum levels of felodipine if taken with barbiturates, hydantoins • Increased serum levels and toxicity of felodipine if taken with erythromycin, cimetidine, ranitidine

■ Nursing Considerations
Assessment
- *History:* Allergy to felodipine, impaired hepatic or renal function, sick sinus syndrome, heart block, lactation
- *Physical:* Skin—lesions, color, edema; P, BP, baseline ECG, peripheral perfusion, auscultation, R, adventitious sounds; liver evaluation, GI normal output; liver function tests, renal function tests, urinalysis

Implementation
- Have patient swallow tablet whole; do not chew or crush.
- Monitor patient carefully (BP, cardiac rhythm and output) while drug is being titrated to therapeutic dose.
- Monitor cardiac rhythm regularly during stabilization of dosage and periodically during long-term therapy.
- Administer drug without regard to meals.

Drug-specific teaching points
- Take this drug with meals if upset stomach occurs.
- Know that the following may occur as a result of drug therapy: nausea, vomiting (small, frequent meals may help); headache (monitor the lighting, noise, and temperature; medication may be ordered if this becomes severe).
- Report irregular heart beat, shortness of breath, swelling of the hands or feet, pronounced dizziness, constipation.

❒ fenofibrate

(feen noh fye' brate)
Lipidil

Pregnancy Category C

Drug classes
Antihyperlipidemic agent

Therapeutic actions
Stimulates the liver to increase breakdown of VLDL to LDL; decreases liver synthesis

Adverse effects in Italics *are most common; those in* **Bold** *are life-threatening.*

of VLDL; inhibits cholesterol formation, lowering serum lipid levels; has antiplatelet effect.

Indications
- Adjunctive therapy to diet for treatment of adult patients with very high elevations of serum triglyceride levels (types IV and I hyperlipidemia) who are at risk of pancreatitis and who do not respond adequately to a determined dietary effort.

Contraindications/cautions
- Allergy to fenofibrate, hepatic or renal dysfunction, primary biliary cirrhosis, peptic ulcer, pregnancy, lactation.

Dosage
Adult: 100 mg/d PO in divided doses as a recommended starting dose.
Pediatric: Safety and efficacy not established.

Pharmacokinetics

Route	Onset	Peak	Duration
Oral	Varies	3–6 h	Weeks

Metabolism: Hepatic, $T_{1/2}$: 15 h
Distribution: Crosses placenta; enters breast milk
Excretion: Urine

Adverse effects
- GI: *Nausea*, vomiting, diarrhea, dyspepsia, flatulence, bloating, stomatitis, gastritis, gallstones, peptic ulcer, GI hemorrhage
- CV: Angina, arrhythmias, swelling, phlebitis, thrombophlebitis, pulmonary emboli
- GU: *Impotence, decreased libido*, dysuria, hematuria, proteinuria, decreased urine output
- Hematologic: Leukopenia, anemia, eosinophilia, increased SGOT and SGPT, increased thymol turbidity, increased CPK, BSP retention
- Dermatologic: *Skin rash*, alopecia, dry skin, dry and brittle hair, pruritus, urticaria
- Other: *Myalgia, "flu-like" syndromes,* arthralgia, weight gain, polyphagia, increased perspiration, systemic lupus erythematosus, blurred vision, gynecomastia

Clinically important drug-drug interactions
- Increased bleeding tendencies if oral anticoagulants are given with fenofibrate—reduce dosage of anticoagulant, usually by 50% • Increased pharmacologic effects of sulfonylureas, insulin with resultant increased risk of hypoglycemia if given concurrently with fenofibrate

■ Nursing Considerations

Assessment
- *History:* Allergy to fenofibrate, hepatic or renal dysfunction, primary biliary cirrhosis, peptic ulcer, lactation
- *Physical:* Skin—lesions, color, temperature; P, BP, auscultation, baseline ECG, peripheral perfusion, edema; bowel sounds, normal output, liver evaluation; normal output; lipid studies, CBC, clotting profile, liver and renal function tests, urinalysis

Implementation
- Administer drug with meals or milk if GI upset occurs.
- Arrange for regular follow-up, including blood tests for lipids, liver function, CBC during long-term therapy.

Drug-specific teaching points
- Take the drug with meals or with milk if GI upset occurs.
- Know that the following side effects may occur: diarrhea, loss of appetite (ensure ready access to the bathroom if this occurs; small frequent meals may help); dry skin, dry and brittle hair, excessive sweating (frequent skin care, use of nonabrasive lotion may help); loss of libido, impotence.
- Arrange to have regular follow-up visits to your doctor for blood tests.
- Report chest pain, shortness of breath, palpitations, severe stomach pain with nausea and vomiting, fever and chills or sore throat, blood in the urine, little urine output, swelling of the ankles or legs, unusual weight gain.

Adverse effects in *Italics* are most common; those in **Bold** are life-threatening.

☐ fenoprofen

*(fen oh **proe'** fen)*
Nalfon

Pregnancy Category B

Drug classes
NSAID
Analgesic (non-narcotic)
Propionic acid derivative

Therapeutic actions
Analgesic, anti-inflammatory, and antipyretic activities largely related to inhibition of prostaglandin synthesis; exact mechanisms of action are not known.

Indications
- Acute and long-term treatment of signs and symptoms of rheumatoid arthritis and osteoarthritis
- Mild to moderate pain

Contraindications/cautions
- Contraindicated in the presence of significant renal impairment, pregnancy, lactation.
- Use caution in the presence of impaired hearing, allergies, hepatic, cardiovascular, and GI conditions.

Dosage
Do not exceed 3,200 mg/d.
Adult
- ***Rheumatoid arthritis/osteoarthritis:*** 300–600 mg PO tid or qid. 2–3 wk may be required to see improvement.
- ***Mild to moderate pain:*** 200 mg q4–6h PO, as needed.

Pediatric: Safety and efficacy have not been established.

Pharmacokinetics

Route	Onset	Peak
Oral	30–60 min	1–2 h

Metabolism: Hepatic, $T_{1/2}$: 2–3 h

Distribution: Crosses placenta; enters breast milk
Excretion: Urine

Adverse effects
NSAIDs
- CNS: *Headache, dizziness, somnolence, insomnia,* fatigue, tiredness, dizziness, tinnitus, ophthalmologic effects
- GI: *Nausea, dyspepsia, GI pain,* diarrhea, vomiting, *constipation,* flatulence
- **Respiratory:** Dyspnea, hemoptysis, pharyngitis, bronchospasm, rhinitis
- **Hematologic:** Bleeding, platelet inhibition with higher doses, neutropenia, eosinophilia, leukopenia, pancytopenia, thrombocytopenia, agranulocytosis, granulocytopenia, aplastic anemia, decreased hemoglobin or hematocrit, bone marrow depression, menorrhagia
- GU: Dysuria, **renal impairment** (fenoprofen is one of the most nephrotoxic NSAIDs)
- Dermatologic: *Rash,* pruritus, sweating, dry mucous membranes, stomatitis
- Other: Peripheral edema, **anaphylactoid reactions to fatal anaphylactic shock**

■ Nursing Considerations

Assessment
- *History:* Renal impairment, impaired hearing, allergies, hepatic, cardiovascular, and GI conditions, lactation
- *Physical:* Skin—color and lesions; orientation, reflexes, ophthalmologic and audiometric evaluation, peripheral sensation; P, edema; R, adventitious sounds; liver evaluation; CBC, clotting times, renal and liver function tests; serum electrolytes, stool guaiac

Implementation
- Administer drug with food or after meals if GI upset occurs.
- Arrange for periodic ophthalmologic examination during long-term therapy.
- Institute emergency procedures if overdose occurs—gastric lavage, induction of emesis, supportive therapy.

Adverse effects in *Italics* are most common; those in **Bold** are life-threatening.

Drug-specific teaching points
- Take drug with food or meals if GI upset occurs.
- Take only the prescribed dosage.
- Know that dizziness, drowsiness can occur (avoid driving or the use of dangerous machinery while on this drug).
- Report sore throat, fever, rash, itching, weight gain, swelling in ankles or fingers; changes in vision, black, tarry stools.

☐ fentanyl

(fen' ta nil)
Duragesic, Fentanyl Oralet, Sublimaze

Pregnancy Category B
C-II Controlled Substance

Drug classes
Narcotic agonist analgesic

Therapeutic actions
Acts at specific opioid receptors, causing analgesia, respiratory depression, physical depression, euphoria.

Indications
- Analgesic action of short duration during anesthesia and in the immediate postoperative period
- Analgesic supplement in general or regional anesthesia
- Administration with a neuroleptic as an anesthetic premedication, for induction of anesthesia, and as an adjunct in maintenance of general and regional anesthesia
- For use as an anesthetic agent with oxygen in selected high-risk patients
- Transdermal system: management of chronic pain in patients requiring opioid analgesia

Contraindications/cautions
- Contraindicated in the presence of hypersensitivity to narcotics, diarrhea caused by poisoning, acute bronchial asthma, upper airway obstruction, pregnancy.
- Use caution in the presence of bradycardia, history of seizures, lactation.

Dosage
Individualize dosage; monitor vital signs routinely.
Adult
- ***Premedication:*** 0.05–0.1 mg IM 30–60 min prior to surgery.
- ***Adjunct to general anesthesia:*** Total dosage is 0.002 mg/kg. Maintenance dose: 0.025–0.1 mg IV or IM when changes in vital signs indicate surgical stress or lightening of analgesia.
- ***With oxygen for anesthesia:*** Total high dose is 0.05–0.1 mg/kg IV; up to 0.12 mg/kg may be necessary.
- ***Adjunct to regional anesthesia:*** 0.05–0.1 mg IM or slowly IV over 1–2 min.
- ***Postoperatively:*** 0.05–0.1 mg IM for the control of pain, tachypnea or emergence delirium; repeat in 1–2 h if needed.
- ***Transdermal:*** Apply to nonirritated and nonirradiated skin on a flat surface of the upper torso; may require replacement in 72 h if pain has not subsided.
- ***Lozenges:*** Place in mouth and suck, 20–40 min before desired efect.

Pediatric (2–12 y): 2–3 μg/kg IV as vital signs indicate.

Pharmacokinetics

Route	Onset	Duration
IM	7–8 min	1–2 h
Transdermal	Gradual	72 h

Metabolism: Plasma, $T_{1/2}$: $1\frac{1}{2}$–6 h
Distribution: Crosses placenta; enters breast milk

IV facts
Preparation: Protect vials from light.
Infusion: Administer slowly by direct injection or into running IV tubing.

Adverse effects
- CNS: *Sedation, clamminess, sweating, headache, vertigo, floating feeling, dizziness, lethargy, confusion, lightheadedness,* nervousness, unusual dreams, agitation, euphoria, hallucinations, de-

Adverse effects in *Italics* are most common; those in **Bold** are life-threatening.

lirium, insomnia, anxiety, fear, disorientation, impaired mental and physical performance, coma, mood changes, weakness, headache, tremor, convulsions
- **GI:** *Nausea, vomiting,* dry mouth, anorexia, constipation, biliary tract spasm
- **CV:** Palpitation, increase or decrease in blood pressure, circulatory depression, **cardiac arrest**, **shock**, tachycardia, bradycardia, arrhythmia, palpitations
- **Respiratory:** Slow, shallow respiration, apnea, suppression of cough reflex, laryngospasm, bronchospasm
- **GU:** Ureteral spasm, spasm of vesical sphincters, urinary retention or hesitancy, oliguria, antidiuretic effect, reduced libido or potency
- **EENT:** Diplopia, blurred vision
- **Dermatologic:** Rash, hives, pruritus, flushing, warmth, sensitivity to cold
- **Local:** Phlebitis following IV injection, pain at injection site; tissue irritation and induration (SC injection)
- **Other:** Physical tolerance and dependence, psychological dependence; local skin irritation with transdermal system

Clinically important drug-drug interactions
- Potentiation of effects of fentanyl when given with barbiturate anesthetics; decrease dose of fentanyl when coadministering

Drug-lab test interferences
- Elevated biliary tract pressure may cause increases in plasma amylase, lipase; determinations of these levels may be unreliable for 24 h after administration of narcotics

■ Nursing Considerations

Assessment
- *History:* Hypersensitivity to fentanyl or narcotics, physical dependence on a narcotic analgesic, pregnancy, labor, lactation, COPD, respiratory depression, anoxia, increased intracranial pressure, acute MI, ventricular failure, coronary insufficiency, hypertension, biliary tract surgery, renal or hepatic dysfunction
- *Physical:* Orientation, reflexes, bilateral grip strength, affect; pupil size, vision; P,

auscultation, BP; R, adventitious sounds; bowel sounds, normal output; liver and kidney function tests

Implementation
- Administer to women who are nursing a baby 4–6 h before the next scheduled feeding to minimize the amount in milk.
- Provide narcotic antagonist, facilities for assisted or controlled respiration on standby during parenteral administration.
- Prepare site by clipping (not shaving) hair at site; do not use soap, oils, lotions, alcohol; allow skin to dry completely before application. Apply immediately after removal from the sealed package; firmly press the transdermal system in place with the palm of the hand for 10–20 sec, making sure the contact is complete. Must be worn continually for 72 h.

Drug-specific teaching points
- Know that the following side effects may occur: dizziness, sedation, drowsiness, impaired visual acuity (ask for assistance if you need to move); nausea, loss of appetite (lying quietly, eating frequent small meals should minimize these effects); constipation (notify your nurse or physician if this is severe; a laxative may help).
- Report severe nausea, vomiting, palpitations, shortness of breath or difficulty breathing.

❒ ferrous fumarate

(fair' us)

Feostat, Fersamal (CAN), Fumerin, Fumasorb, Hemocyte, Ircon, Novofumar (CAN), Palafer (CAN)

ferrous gluconate

Fergon, Ferralet, Fertinic (CAN), Novoferrogluc (CAN), Simron

ferrous sulfate

Feosol, Fer-In-Sol, Fer-Iron, Fero-Gradumet Filmtabs, Ferospace, Fesofor (CAN),

Adverse effects in *Italics* are most common; those in **Bold** are life-threatening.

ferrous fumarate

Mol-Iron, Novoferrosulfa (CAN)

ferrous sulfate exsiccated
Feosol, Fer-In-Sol, Ferralyn Lanacaps, Slow FE

Pregnancy Category A

Drug classes
Iron preparation

Therapeutic actions
Elevates the serum iron concentration and is then converted to hemoglobin or trapped in the reticuloendothelial cells for storage and eventual conversion to a usable form of iron.

Indications
- Prevention and treatment of iron deficiency anemias
- Unlabeled use: supplemental use during epoetin therapy to ensure proper hematologic response to epoetin

Contraindications/cautions
- Allergy to any ingredient; tartrazine allergy (tartrazine is contained in timed-release capsules marketed as *Mol-Iron*); sulfite allergy; hemochromatosis, hemosiderosis, hemolytic anemias; normal iron balance; peptic ulcer, regional enteritis, ulcerative colitis

Dosage
Adult
- ***Daily requirements:*** Males, 10 mg/d PO; females, 18 mg/d PO; pregnancy and lactation, 30–60 mg/d PO.
- ***Replacement in deficiency states:*** 90–300 mg/d (6 mg/kg per day) PO for approximately 6–10 mo may be required.

Pediatric: Daily requirement: 10–15 mg/d PO.

Pharmacokinetics

Route	Onset	Peak	Duration
Oral	4 d	7–10 d	2–4 mo

Metabolism: Recycled for use, $T_{1/2}$: not known
Distribution: Crosses placenta; enters breast milk

Adverse effects
- CNS: CNS toxicity, acidosis, **coma and death—overdose**
- GI: *GI upset, anorexia, nausea, vomiting, constipation*, diarrhea, dark stools, temporary staining of the teeth (liquid preparations)

Clinically important drug-drug interactions
- Decreased anti-infective response to ciprofloxacin, enoxacin, norfloxacin, ofloxacin if taken with iron • Decreased absorption of iron if taken with antacids, cimetidine • Decreased effects of levodopa if taken with iron • Increased serum iron levels if taken with chloramphenicol

Clinically important drug-food interactions
- Decreased absorption of iron if taken with antacids, eggs or milk, coffee and tea; space administration to avoid concurrent administration of any of these.

■ Nursing Considerations

Assessment
- *History*: Allergy to any ingredient, sulfite; hemochromatosis, hemosiderosis, hemolytic anemias; normal iron balance; peptic ulcer, regional enteritis, ulcerative colitis
- *Physical*: Skin—lesions, color; gums, teeth (color); bowel sounds; CBC, hemoglobin, Hct, serum ferritin assays

Implementation
- Ensure that patient does have iron deficiency anemia before treatment.
- Administer drug with meals (avoiding milk, eggs, coffee, and tea) if GI discomfort is severe, and slowly increase to the recommended dose to help build up tolerance to the effects.
- Administer liquid preparations in water or juice to mask the taste and prevent

Adverse effects in *Italics* are most common; those in **Bold** are life-threatening.

staining of teeth; have the patient drink solution with a straw.
- Caution patient that stool may be dark or green.
- Arrange for periodic monitoring of hematocrit and hemoglobin levels.

Drug-specific teaching points
- Take drug on an empty stomach with water. Take after meals if GI upset is severe (avoid milk, eggs, coffee, and tea at the meals involved).
- Take liquid preparations diluted in water or juice and sipped through a straw to prevent staining of the teeth.
- Be aware that treatment may no longer be necessary if cause of anemia can be corrected. Treatment may be needed for several months to reverse the anemia.
- Arrange periodic blood tests during therapy to follow your response to the drug and determine the appropriate dosage for you.
- Do not take this preparation with antacids or tetracyclines. If these drugs are needed, they will be prescribed at intervals that will be less likely to cause problems.
- Know that the following side effects may occur: GI upset, nausea, vomiting (taking the drug with meals may help); diarrhea or constipation; dark or green stools.
- Report severe GI upset, lethargy, rapid respirations, constipation.

☐ fibrinolysin and desoxyribonuclease

(fye brin oh lye' sin and dez ox ee rye boe nuke' lee ase)
Elase

Drug classes
Enzyme

Therapeutic actions
Fibrinolysin attacks fibrin of blood clots and exudates; desoxyribonuclease attacks DNA found in purulent exudates.

Indications
- Débriding agent in general surgical wounds; ulcerative lesions; second- and third-degree burns; circumcision; episiotomy
- Cervicitis and vaginitis
- Irrigation agent for infected wounds, superficial hematomas, otorhinolaryngologic wounds

Contraindications/cautions
- Allergy to any component of the preparation, bovine products.

Dosage
Apply a thin layer of ointment, and cover with petrolatum gauze or other nonadhering agent two to three times per day, *or* mix solution and saturate strips of gauze. Pack ulcerated area with gauze; allow to dry, 6–8 h. Remove dry gauze; repeat three to four times per day.
Intravaginal: Apply 5 g of ointment deep into vagina at bedtime for five applications. In severe cases, insert 10 ml of solution intravaginally, wait 1–2 min, then insert cotton tampon. Remove tampon the next day.
Abscesses: Irrigate with solution; drain and replace solution every 6–10 h.

Pharmacokinetics

Route	Onset	Duration
Topical	Slow	24 h
Negligible systemic absorption.		

Adverse effects
- *Local:* Hyperemia with high concentrations

■ Nursing Considerations
Assessment
- *History*: Allergy to bovine products, drug or components of preparation
- *Physical*: Affected site—lesions, color, edema

Implementation
- Clean wound with water, peroxide, or normal saline, and dry area gently. Surgically remove dense, dry eschar before applying ointment. Apply a thin layer

Adverse effects in *Italics* are most common; those in **Bold** are life-threatening.

of ointment, and cover with petrolatum gauze or other nonadhering dressing. Change dressing at least once a day, preferably two to three times. Flush away the necrotic debris and fibrinous exudates with saline, peroxide, or warm water.
- Prepare solution by reconstituting contents of each vial with 10 ml isotonic sodium chloride solution. Higher or lower concentrations can be made by varying diluent. Solutions should be prepared fresh before each use; refrigerate for up to 24 h; discard after that time.
- Prepare wet to dry dressing by mixing 1 vial of powder with 10–50 ml saline, and saturate strips of fine-mesh gauze or unfolded sterile gauze sponge with solution. Pack area with gauze, and allow to dry. Remove dried gauze; this débrides the area. Repeat three to four times per day. After 2–4 d, the area will be clean and will begin to fill in with granulation tissue.
- Apply vaginally very high in the vagina, preferably at bedtime when patient will be supine for a long period of time.
- Irrigate abscesses as above. Traces of blood in discharge with irrigation usually indicates active filling of the cavity.
- Maintain epinephrine 1:1,000 on standby in case of severe allergic reaction.

Drug-specific teaching points
- Incorporate teaching about this drug into the explanation of wound care while changing dressing, irrigating, and so forth.
- Insert high into vagina just before bedtime. You may wish to wear a sanitary pad to protect clothing while using this drug.
- Be aware that some discomfort may occur at site of infection.
- Report difficulty breathing, fast heart rate, pain at site of infection.

☐ filgrastim

(fill grass' stim)
granulocyte colony-stimulating factor, G-CS
Neupogen

Pregnancy Category C

Drug classes
Colony-stimulating factor

Therapeutic actions
Human granulocyte colony-stimulating factor produced by recombinant DNA technology; increases the production of neutrophils within the bone marrow with little effect on the production of other hematopoietic cells.

Indications
- To decrease the incidence of infection in patients with nonmyeloid malignancies receiving myelosuppressive anticancer drugs associated with a significant incidence of severe neutropenia with fever
- Orphan drug uses: treatment of muelodysplastic syndrome, severe chronic neutropenia, neutropenia associated with bone marrow transplants, AIDS patients with CMV retinitis being treated with ganciclovir

Contraindications/cautions
- Contraindicated in the presence of hypersensitivity to *Escherichia coli* products, pregnancy.
- Use caution in the presence of lactation.

Dosage
Adult: Starting dose is 5 μg/kg per day SC or IV as a single daily injection. May be increased in increments of 5 μg/kg for each chemotherapy cycle. 4–8 μg/kg per day is usually effective.
Pediatric: Safety and efficacy not established.

Pharmacokinetics

Route	Peak	Duration
SC	8 h	4 d
IV	2 h	4 d

Metabolism: Unknown; $T_{1/2}$: 210–231 min
Distribution: Crosses placenta; may enter breast milk

IV facts
Preparation: No special preparation required. Refrigerate; avoid shaking. Prior to injection, allow to warm to room temperature. Discard vial after one use, and do not

reenter vial; discard any vial that has been at room temperature > 6 h.
Infusion: Inject directly IV slowly, or inject slowly into tubing of running IV.

Adverse effects
- CNS: Headache, fever, generalized weakness, fatigue
- GI: *Nausea, vomiting*, stomatitis, anorexia, *diarrhea*, constipation
- Dermatologic: *Alopecia*, rash, mucositis
- Other: *Bone pain*, generalized pain, sore throat, cough

■ Nursing Considerations

Assessment
- *History:* Hypersensitivity to *E. coli* products, pregnancy, lactation.
- *Physical:* Skin—color, lesions, hair; body temperature; abdominal exam, status of mucous membranes; CBC, platelets

Implementation
- Obtain CBC and platelet count prior to and twice weekly during therapy; doses may be increased after chemotherapy cycles according to the duration and severity of bone marrow suppression.
- Administer no earlier than 24 h after cytotoxic chemotherapy and not in the period of 24 h before the administration of chemotherapy.
- Give daily for up to 2 wk until the neutrophil count is 10,000/mm^3; discontinue therapy if this number is exceeded.
- Store in refrigerator; allow to warm to room temperature before use; if vial is at room temperature for > 6 h, discard the vial. Use each vial for one dose; do not reenter the vial. Discard any unused drug.
- Do not shake vial before use. If SC dose exceeds 1 ml, consider using two sites.

Drug-specific teaching points
- Store drug in refrigerator; do not shake vial. Each vial can be used only once; do not reuse syringes or needles (proper container for disposal will be provided). Another person should be instructed in the proper administration technique. Use sterile technique.
- Avoid exposure to infection while you are receiving this drug (eg, crowds).
- Know that the following side effects may occur: bone pain (analgesia may be ordered), nausea and vomiting (small, frequent meals may help), loss of hair (you may want to arrange for appropriate head covering; it is very important to cover head in very cold or very hot temperatures).
- Arrange to keep appointments for frequent blood tests that will be needed to evaluate the effects of this drug on your blood count.
- Report fever, chills, severe bone pain, sore throat, weakness, pain or swelling at injection site.

▢ finasteride

*(fin **as'** teh ride)*
Proscar

Pregnancy Category X

Drug classes
Androgen hormone inhibitor

Therapeutic actions
Inhibits the intracellular enzyme that coverts testosterone into a potent androgen (DHT); does not affect androgen receptors in the body; the prostate gland depends on DHT for its development and maintenance.

Indications
- Treatment of symptomatic benign prostatic hyperplasia (BPH); most effective with long-term use
- Unlabeled uses: adjuvant monotherapy following radical prostatectomy; prevention of the progression of first-stage prostate cancer; treatment of male pattern baldness, acne, hirsutism

Contraindications/cautions
- Contraindicated in the presence of allergy to finasteride or any component of the product, pregnancy, lactation.

Adverse effects in *Italics* are most common; those in **Bold** are life-threatening.

- Use caution in the presence of hepatic impairment.

Dosage
Adult: 5 mg qd PO with or without meals; 6–12 mo may be needed to see the actual response.
Pediatric: Safety and efficacy not established.
Geriatric or renal insufficiency: No dosage adjustment is needed.

Pharmacokinetics

Route	Onset	Peak	Duration
Oral	Rapid	8 h	24 h

Metabolism: Hepatic, $T_{1/2}$: 6 h
Distribution: Crosses placenta; may enter breast milk (but not indicated for use in women)
Excretion: Feces and urine

Adverse effects
- **GI**: Abdominal upset
- **GU**: Impotence, decreased libido, decreased volume of ejaculation

Clinically important drug-drug interactions
- Possible decreased levels of theophylline if taken with finasteride

Drug-lab test interferences
- Decreased PSA levels when measured while taking finasteride; false decrease in PSA does not mean that patient is free of risk of prostate cancer

■ Nursing Considerations

Assessment
- *History*: Allergy to finasteride or any component of the product, hepatic impairment
- *Physical*: Liver evaluation, abdominal exam; renal function tests, normal urine output, prostate exam

Implementation
- Assess patient to ensure that problem is BPH, and other disorders (eg, prostate cancer, infection, strictures, hypotonic bladder) have been ruled out.
- Administer without regard to meals.
- Arrange for regular follow-up, including prostate exam, PSA levels, and evaluation of urine flow.
- Monitor urine flow and output; increase in urine flow may not occur in all patients.
- Do not allow pregnant women to handle finasteride tablets or crushed tablets, because of risk of inadvertent absorption, which would adversely affect the fetus.
- Caution male patients that if their sexual partner is or may become pregnant, she should be protected from exposure to his semen, which will contain finasteride, which could adversely affect the fetus. The patient should use a condom or discontinue finasteride therapy.
- Alert patient that libido may be decreased as well as the volume of ejaculate; these are usually reversible when the drug is stopped.

Drug-specific teaching points
- Take this drug once a day without regard to meals.
- Arrange to have regular medical follow-up while you are on this drug to evaluate your response.
- Know that the following side effects may occur: loss of libido, impotence, decreased amount of ejaculate (these effects are usually reversible when the drug is stopped).
- Be aware that this drug has serious adverse effects on unborn babies. Do not allow a pregnant woman to handle the drug; if your sexual partner is or may become pregnant, protect her from exposure to semen by using a condom. You may need to discontinue the drug if this is not acceptable.
- Report inability to void, groin pain, sore throat, fever, weakness

❒ flavoxate hydrochloride

(fla vox' ate)
Urispas

Pregnancy Category C

Adverse effects in *Italics* are most common; those in **Bold** are life-threatening.

flecainide acetate ■ 489

Drug classes
Urinary antispasmodic
Parasympathetic blocking agent

Therapeutic actions
Counteracts smooth muscle spasm of the urinary tract by relaxing the detrusor and other smooth muscles through action at the parasympathetic receptors; also has local anesthetic and analgesic properties.

Indications
- Symptomatic relief of dysuria, urgency, nocturia, suprapubic pain, frequency and incontinence due to cystitis, prostatitis, urethritis, urethrocystitis/urethrotrigonitis

Contraindications/cautions
- Contraindicated in the presence of allergy to flavoxate, pyloric or duodenal obstruction, obstructive intestinal lesions or ileus, achalasia, GI hemorrhage, obstructive uropathies of the lower urinary tract.
- Use caution in the presence of glaucoma.

Dosage
Adult and pediatric older than 12 y: 100–200 mg PO tid or qid. Reduce dose when symptoms improve. Use of up to 1,200 mg/d has been reported in severe urinary urgency following pelvic radiotherapy.
Pediatric (younger than 12 y): Safety and efficacy not established.

Pharmacokinetics

Route	Onset	Duration
Oral	Slow	6 h

Metabolism: $T_{1/2}$: 2–3 h
Distribution: May cross placenta
Excretion: Urine

Adverse effects
- GI: *Nausea, vomiting, dry mouth*
- CNS: *Nervousness, vertigo, headache, drowsiness,* mental confusion, hyperpyrexia, *blurred vision,* increased ocular tension, disturbance in accommodation
- Dermatologic: Urticaria, dermatoses
- GU: Dysuria
- CV: Tachycardia, palpitations
- Hematologic: Eosinophilia, leukopenia

■ Nursing Considerations
Assessment
- *History*: Allergy to flavoxate, pyloric or duodenal obstruction, obstructive intestinal lesions or ileus, achalasia, GI hemorrhage, obstructive uropathies of the lower urinary tract, glaucoma
- *Physical*: Skin—color, lesions; body temperature; orientation, affect, reflexes, ophthalmic exam, ocular pressure measurement; P; bowel sounds, oral mucous membranes; CBC, stool guaiac

Implementation
- Arrange for definitive treatment of urinary tract infections causing the symptoms being managed by flavoxate.
- Arrange for ophthalmic exam before beginning therapy and periodically during therapy.

Drug-specific teaching points
- Take drug three to four times a day.
- Be aware that this drug is meant to relieve the symptoms you are experiencing; other medications will be used to treat the cause of the symptoms.
- Know that the following side effects may occur: dry mouth, GI upset (sucking on sugarless lozenges and frequent mouth care may help); drowsiness, blurred vision (avoid driving or performing tasks that require alertness while on this drug).
- Report blurred vision, fever, skin rash, nausea, vomiting.

❒ flecainide acetate

*(fle **kay**' nide)*
Tambocor

Pregnancy Category C

Drug classes
Antiarrhythmic

Therapeutic actions
Type 1c antiarrhythmic: acts selectively to depress fast sodium channels, decreasing

Adverse effects in *Italics* are most common; those in **Bold** are life-threatening.

flecainide acetate

the height and rate of rise of cardiac action potentials and slowing conduction in all parts of the heart.

Indications
- Treatment of documented life-threatening ventricular arrhythmias, such as sustained ventricular tachycardia (not recommended for patients with less severe ventricular arrhythmias)
- Prevention of paroxysmal atrial fibrillation/flutter (PAF) associated with symptoms and paroxysmal supraventricular tachycardias (PSVT), including atrioventricular nodal reentrant tachycardia, atrioventricular reentrant tachycardia, and other supraventricular tachycardias of unspecified mechanism associated with disabling symptoms in patients without structural heart disease

Contraindications/cautions
- Contraindicated in the presence of allergy to flecainide; CHF; cardiogenic shock; cardiac conduction abnormalities (heart blocks of any kind, unless an artificial pacemaker is present to maintain heart beat); sick sinus syndrome; lactation.
- Use caution in the presence of endocardial pacemaker (permanent or temporary—stimulus parameters may need to be increased); hepatic or renal disease; potassium imbalance.

Dosage
Careful patient assessment and evaluation with close monitoring of cardiac response are necessary for determining the correct dosage for each patient.

Adult
- **PSVT and PAF:** Starting dose of 50 mg q12h PO; may be increased in increments of 50 mg bid q4d until efficacy is achieved; maximum dose is 300 mg/d.
- ***Sustained ventricular tachycardia:*** 100 mg q12h PO. Increase in 50-mg increments twice a day every fourth day until efficacy is achieved. Maximum dose is 400 mg/d.
- **Recent MI or CHF:** Initial dose of no more than 100 mg q12h PO. May increase in 50-mg increments twice daily every fourth day to a maximum of 200 mg/d; higher doses are associated with increased CHF.

Pediatric: Safety and efficacy in children younger than 18 y has not been established.
Geriatric and renal impaired: Initial dose: 100 mg qd PO or 50 mg q12h. Wait about 4 d to reach a steady state and then increase dose cautiously. Creatinine clearance < 20 ml/min: decrease dose by 25%–50%.

Transfer to flecainide: Allow at least 2–4 plasma half-lives to elapse for the drug being discontinued before starting flecainide at the usual dosage. Consider hospitalization of patients in whom withdrawal of a previous antiarrhythmic is likely to produce life-threatening arrhythmias.

Pharmacokinetics

Route	Onset	Peak	Duration
Oral	30–60 min	3 h	24 h

Metabolism: Hepatic, $T_{1/2}$: 20 h
Distribution: Crosses placenta; may enter breast milk
Excretion: Urine and feces

Adverse effects
- **CNS:** *Dizziness, fatigue, drowsiness, visual changes, headache*, tinnitus, paresthesias
- **GI:** *Nausea, vomiting, abdominal pain, constipation*, diarrhea
- **CV:** *Cardiac arrhythmias*, congestive heart failure, slowed cardiac conduction, *palpitations, chest pain*
- **GU:** Polyuria, urinary retention, decreased libido
- **Other:** *Dyspnea*, sweating, hot flashes, night sweats, leukopenia

■ Nursing Considerations

Assessment
- *History:* Allergy to flecainide, CHF, cardiogenic shock, cardiac conduction abnormalities, sick sinus syndrome, endocardial pacemaker, hepatic or renal disease, potassium imbalance, lactation

Adverse effects in *Italics* are most common; those in **Bold** are life-threatening.

- *Physical:* Weight; orientation, reflexes, vision; P, BP, auscultation, ECG, edema, R, adventitious sounds; bowel sounds, liver evaluation; urinalysis, CBC, serum electrolytes, liver and renal function tests

Implementation
- Monitor patient response carefully, especially when beginning therapy.
- Reduce dosage in patients with renal disease, hepatic failure, CHF, or recent MI.
- Check serum K^+ levels before administration.
- Monitor cardiac rhythm carefully.
- Evaluate for therapeutic serum levels of 0.2–1 μg/ml.
- Provide life support equipment, including pacemaker, on standby in case serious CVS, CNS effects occur—also dopamine, dobutamine, isoproterenol, or other positive inotropic agents.

Drug-specific teaching points
- Be aware that you will need frequent monitoring of cardiac rhythm.
- Know that the following side effects may occur: drowsiness, dizziness, numbness, visual disturbances (avoid driving or working with dangerous machinery until you know your response to the drug); nausea, vomiting (small, frequent meals may help); diarrhea, polyuria (have bathroom facilities available after taking the drug); sweating, night sweats, hot flashes, loss of libido (these resolve within a few weeks of stopping the drug).
- Do not stop taking this drug for any reason without checking with your health care provider. Because the drug is taken at 12-h intervals, work out a schedule that will allow you to take the drug as prescribed without waking up at night.
- Return for regular follow-up visits to check your heart rhythm. You also may have a blood test to check your blood levels of this drug.
- Report swelling of ankles or fingers, palpitations, fainting, chest pain.

floxuridine

(flox yoor' i deen)
FUDR
Pregnancy Category D

Drug classes
Antimetabolite
Antineoplastic drug

Therapeutic actions
Converted in the body to fluorouracil, another antineoplastic drug; inhibits the enzyme thymidylate synthetase, leading to inhibition of DNA synthesis.

Indications
- Palliative management of GI adenocarcinoma metastatic to the liver in patients considered to be incurable by surgery or other means (given only by regional intra-arterial perfusion)

Contraindications/cautions
- Allergy to floxuridine; poor nutritional status; serious infections; hematopoietic depression secondary to radiation or chemotherapy; impaired liver function; pregnancy; lactation.

Dosage
Adult: Given by intra-arterial infusion only: continuous arterial infusion of 0.1–0.6 mg/kg per day (larger doses of 0.4–0.6 mg/kg per day are used for infusion into the hepatic artery as the liver metabolizes the drug). Continue until adverse reactions occur; resume therapy when side effects subside. Maintain use as long as patient is responding to therapy.

Pharmacokinetics

Route	Onset	Peak	Duration
Intra-arterial	Immediate	1–2 h	3 h

Metabolism: Hepatic, $T_{1/2}$: 20 h
Distribution: Crosses placenta; enter breast milk
Excretion: Urine

Adverse effects
- CNS: *Lethargy, malaise, weakness,* euphoria, acute cerebellar syndrome, pho-

Adverse effects in *Italics* are most common; those in **Bold** are life-threatening.

tophobia, lacrimation, decreased vision, nystagmus, diplopia, fever, epistaxis
- **GI:** *Diarrhea, anorexia, nausea, vomiting*, cramps, enteritis, duodenal ulcer, duodenitis, gastritis, glossitis, stomatitis, pharyngitis, esophagopharyngitis
- **CV:** Myocardial ischemia, angina
- **Hematologic:** *Leukopenia, thrombocytopenia*, elevations of alkaline phosphatase, serum transaminase, serum bilirubin, lactic dehydrogenase
- **Dermatologic:** *Alopecia, dermatitis*, maculopapular rash, photosensitivity, nail changes, including nail loss, dry skin, fissures
- **Regional arterial infusion:** Arterial aneurysm, arterial ischemia, arterial thrombosis, bleeding at catheter site, embolism, fibromyositis, abscesses, infection at catheter site, thrombophlebitis

Drug-lab test interferences
- 5-hydroxyindoleacetic acid (5-HIAA) urinary excretion may increase • Plasma albumin may decrease due to protein malabsorption

■ Nursing Considerations

Assessment
- *History:* Allergy to floxuridine, poor nutritional status, serious infections, hematopoietic depression secondary to radiation or chemotherapy, impaired liver function, pregnancy, lactation
- *Physical:* Weight; temperature; skin—lesions, color; hair; vision, speech, orientation, reflexes, sensation; R, adventitious sounds; mucous membranes, liver evaluation, abdominal exam; CBC, differential; renal and liver function tests; urinalysis, chest x-ray

Implementation
- Arrange for tests to evaluate hematologic status before beginning therapy and before each dose.
- Arrange for discontinuation of drug therapy if any sign of toxicity occurs (stomatitis, esophagopharyngitis, rapidly falling WBC count, intractable vomiting, diarrhea, GI ulceration and bleeding, thrombocytopenia, hemorrhage); consult with physician. Reconstitute powder with 5 ml sterile water. Refrigerate reconstituted vials for no more than 2 wk.
- Administer by intra-arterial line only; use an infusion pump to ensure continual delivery and overcome pressure of arteries.

Drug-specific teaching points
- Prepare a calendar of treatment days.
- Know that the following side effects may occur: nausea, vomiting, loss of appetite (medication may be ordered to help; small, frequent meals also may help; it is very important to maintain your nutrition while you are on this drug); decreased vision, tearing, double vision, malaise, weakness, lethargy (these are all effects of the drug; it is advisable to avoid driving or operating dangerous machinery if these occur); mouth sores (frequent mouth care will be needed); diarrhea (ensure ready access to bathroom facilities if these occur); loss of hair (you may wish to obtain a wig or other suitable head covering; it is important to keep the head covered in extremes of temperature); skin rash, sensitivity of skin and eyes to sunlight and ultraviolet light (avoid exposure to the sun; use a sunscreen and protective clothing if exposed to sun).
- Use birth control while on this drug; this drug may cause birth defects or miscarriages.
- Arrange to have frequent, regular medical follow-up, including frequent blood tests to follow the effects of the drug on your body.
- Report black, tarry stools; fever; chills; sore throat; unusual bleeding or bruising; chest pain; mouth sores.

❒ fluconazole

*(floo **kon**' a zole)*
Diflucan
Pregnancy Category C

Drug classes
Antifungal agent

Therapeutic actions
Binds to sterols in the fungal cell membrane, changing membrane permeability; fungicidal or fungistatic depending on concentration and organism.

Indications
- Treatment of oropharyngeal and esophageal candidiasis
- Treatment of cryptococcal meningitis
- Treatment of systemic fungal infections

Contraindications/cautions
- Contraindicated in the presence of hypersensitivity to fluconazole, lactation.
- Use caution in the presence of renal impairment.

Dosage
Individualize dosage. Dosage is the same for oral or IV routes because of rapid and almost complete absorption.

Adult
- ***Oropharyngeal candidiasis:*** 200 mg PO or IV on the first day, followed by 100 mg qd. Continue treatment for at least 2 wk to decrease likelihood of relapse.
- ***Esophageal candidiasis:*** 200 mg PO or IV on the first day, followed by 100 mg qd. Dosage up to 400 mg/d may be used in severe cases. Treat for at least 3 wk or 2 wk following resolution of symptoms.
- ***Systemic candidiasis:*** 400 mg PO or IV on the first day, followed by 200 mg qd. Treat for a minimum of 4 wk for at least 2 wk after resolution of symptoms.
- ***Vaginal candidiasis:*** 150 mg PO as a single dose.
- ***Cryptococcal meningitis:*** 400 mg PO or IV on the first day, followed by 200 mg qd. 400 mg qd may be needed. Continue treatment for 10–12 wk.
- ***Suppression of cryptococcal meningitis in AIDS patients:*** 200 mg qd PO or IV.

Pediatric: Safety and efficacy not established.

Geriatric or renal impaired: Initial dose of 50–400 mg PO or IV. If creatinine clearance > 50 ml/min, use 100% recommended dose; creatinine clearance 21–50 ml/min, use 50% of the recommended dose; creatinine clearance 11–20, use 25% of recommended dose; patients on hemodialysis, use one dose after each dialysis.

Pharmacokinetics

Route	Onset	Peak	Duration
Oral	Slow	1–2 h	2–4 d
IV	Rapid	1 h	2–4 d

Metabolism: Hepatic, $T_{1/2}$: 30 h
Distribution: Crosses placenta; may enter breast milk
Excretion: Urine

IV facts
Preparation: Do not remove overwrap until ready for use. Inner bag maintains sterility of product. Do not use plastic containers in series connections. Tear overwrap down side at slit, and remove solution container. Some opacity of plastic may occur; check for minute leaks, squeezing bag firmly. Discard solution if any leaks are found.
Infusion: Infuse at a maximum rate of 200 mg/h given as a continuous infusion.
Incompatibilities: Do not add any supplementary medications.

Adverse effects
- CNS: *Headache*
- GI: *Nausea, vomiting, diarrhea, abdominal pain*
- Other: Skin rash

Clinically important drug-drug interactions
- Increased serum levels and therefore therapeutic and toxic effects of cyclosporine, phenytoin, oral hypoglycemics, warfarin anticoagulants if taken concurrently with fluconazole • Decreased serum levels of

Adverse effects in *Italics* are most common; those in **Bold** are life-threatening.

fluconazole if taken concurrently with rifampin

■ Nursing Considerations
Assessment
- *History:* Hypersensitivity to fluconazole, renal impairment, lactation
- *Physical:* Skin—color, lesions; body temperature; injection site; orientation, reflexes, affect; bowel sounds; renal function tests; CBC and differential; culture of area involved

Implementation
- Arrange for appropriate culture of infection before beginning therapy; treatment should begin, however, before laboratory results are returned.
- Arrange for decreased dosage in cases of renal failure.
- Infuse IV only; not intended for IM or SC use.
- Do not add any supplementary medication to the fluconazole.
- Administer through sterile equipment at a maximum rate of 200 mg/h given as a continuous infusion.
- Monitor renal function tests weekly, discontinue or decrease dosage of drug at any sign of increased renal toxicity.

Drug-specific teaching points
- Be aware that the drug may be given orally or IV as needed, depending on your condition. The drug will need to be taken for the full course that has been prescribed. Therapy may need to be long term.
- Use hygiene measures to prevent reinfection or spread of infection.
- Arrange for frequent follow-up while you are on this drug. Be sure to keep all appointments, which may include blood tests.
- Know that the following side effects may occur: nausea, vomiting, diarrhea (small frequent meals may help); headache (analgesics may be ordered).
- Report rash, changes in stool or urine color, difficulty breathing, increased tears or salivation.

☐ flucytosine

(floo sye' toe seen)
5-FC, 5-fluorocytosine

Ancobon, Ancotil (CAN)
Pregnancy Category C

Drug classes
Antifungal

Therapeutic actions
Affects cell membranes of susceptible fungi to cause fungus death; exact mechanism of action is not understood.

Indications
- Treatment of serious infections caused by susceptible strains of *Candida, Cryptococcus*
- Unlabeled use: treatment of chromomycosis

Contraindications/cautions
- Contraindicated in the presence of allergy to flucytosine, pregnancy, lactation.
- Use caution in the presence of renal impairment (drug accumulation and toxicity may occur), bone marrow depression.

Dosage
Adult: 50–150 mg/kg per day PO at 6-h intervals.
Geriatric or renal impaired: Initial dose should be at the lower level.

Pharmacokinetics

Route	Onset	Peak	Duration
Oral	Varies	2 h	10–12 h

Metabolism: $T_{1/2}$: 2–5 h
Distribution: Crosses placenta; may enter breast milk
Excretion: Urine and feces

Adverse effects
- CNS: Confusion, hallucinations, headache, sedation, vertigo
- GI: *Nausea, vomiting, diarrhea*

Adverse effects in *Italics* are most common; those in **Bold** are life-threatening.

- Hematologic: *Anemia, leukopenia, thrombopenia*, elevation of liver enzymes, BUN and creatinine
- Dermatologic: *Rash*

Nursing Considerations

Assessment
- *History*: Allergy to flucytosine, renal impairment, bone marrow depression, lactation
- *Physical*: Skin—color, lesions; orientation, reflexes, affect; bowel sounds, liver evaluation; renal and liver function tests; CBC and differential

Implementation
- Administer capsules a few at a time over a 15-min period to decrease the GI upset and diarrhea.
- Arrange to monitor hepatic and renal function tests and hematologic function periodically throughout treatment.

Drug-specific teaching points
- Take the capsules a few at a time over a 15-min period to decrease GI upset.
- Know that the following side effects may occur: nausea, vomiting, diarrhea (taking the capsules a few at a time over a 15-min period will help); sedation, dizziness, confusion (avoid driving or performing tasks that require alertness if these occur).
- Report skin rash, severe nausea, vomiting, diarrhea, fever, sore throat, unusual bleeding or bruising.

fludarabine

*(floo **dar**' a been)*
Fludara

Pregnancy Category D

Drug classes
Antimetabolite
Antineoplastic drug

Therapeutic actions
Inhibits DNA polymerase alpha, ribonucleotid reductase and DNA primase, which inhibits DNA synthesis and prevents cell replication.

Indications
- Chronic lymphocytic leukemia (CLL); treatment of patients with B-cell CLL who have not responded to or have progressed during treatment with at least one standard regimen that contains an alkylating agent
- Unlabeled uses: non-Hodgkin's lymphoma, macroglobulinemic lymph-oma, prolymphocytic leukemia or prolymphocytoid variant of CLL, mycosis fungoides, hairy-cell leukemia, Hodgkin's disease.

Contraindications/cautions
- Contraindicated in the presence of allergy to fludarabine or any component, lactation, pregnancy, severe bone marrow depression.
- Use caution in the presence of renal impairment.

Dosage
Adult: 25 mg/m^2 IV over a 30-min period for 5 consecutive d. Commence each 5-d course every 28 d. It is recommended that three additional cycles be given following the achievement of a maximal response, then discontinue drug.

Pharmacokinetics

Route	Onset	Peak
IV	Rapid	1–2 h

Metabolism: Hepatic, T$_{1/2}$: 10 h
Distribution: Crosses placenta; enters breast milk
Excretion: Urine

IV facts
Preparation: Reconstitute with 2 ml of Sterile Water for Injection; the solid cake should dissolve in < 15 sec; each ml of resulting solution will contain 25 mg fludarabine, 25 mg mannitol and sodium hydroxide; may be further diluted in 100 or 125 ml of 5% Dextrose Injection or 0.9% Sodium Chloride; use within 8 h of reconstitution; discard after that time. Store unreconstituted drug in refrigerator.

Adverse effects in *Italics* are most common; those in **Bold** are life-threatening.

Infusion: Infuse slowly over no less than 30 min.

Adverse effects

- CNS: *Weakness, paresthesia, headache, visual disturbance*, hearing loss, sleep disorder, depression, **CNS toxicity**
- GI: *Diarrhea, anorexia, nausea, vomiting, stomatitis*, esophagopharyngitis, GI bleeding, mucositis
- CV: *Edema*, angina
- Respiratory: *Cough, pneumonia, dyspnea, sinusitis*, upper respiratory infection, epistaxis, bronchitis, hypoxia
- Hematologic: *Bone marrow toxicity*
- GU: Dysuria, urinary infection, hematuria, **renal failure**
- Dermatologic: *Rash, pruritus*, seborrhea
- General: *Fever, chills, fatigue, infection, pain, malaise*, diaphoresis, hemorrhage, myalgia, arthralgia, osteoporosis, **tumor lysis syndrome**

■ Nursing Considerations

Assessment

- *History:* Allergy to fludarabine or any component, lactation, pregnancy, severe bone marrow depression, renal impairment
- *Physical:* Weight; temperature; skin—lesions, color, edema; hair; vision, speech, orientation, reflexes, sensation; R, adventitious sounds; mucous membranes, liver evaluation, abdominal exam; CBC, differential; renal and liver function tests; urinalysis, chest x-ray

Implementation

- Arrange for tests to evaluate hematologic status before beginning therapy and before each dose.
- Arrange for discontinuation of drug therapy if any sign of toxicity occurs (CNS complaints, stomatitis, esophagopharyngitis, rapidly falling WBC count, intractable vomiting, diarrhea, GI ulceration and bleeding, thrombocytopenia, hemorrhage); consult with physician.
- Caution patient to avoid pregnancy while on this drug.

Drug-specific teaching points

- Prepare a calendar of treatment days.
- Know that the following side effects may occur: nausea, vomiting, loss of appetite (medication may be ordered to help; small, frequent meals may also help; it is very important to maintain your nutrition while you are on this drug); headache, fatigue, malaise, weakness, lethargy (these are all effects of the drug; it is advisable to avoid driving or operating dangerous machinery if these occur); mouth sores (frequent mouth care will be needed); diarrhea (ensure ready access to bathroom facilities if these occur); increased susceptibility to infection (avoid crowded areas, exposure to anyone with an infection; consult with your nurse or physician at any sign of infection, eg, fever, fatigue)
- Use birth control while on this drug; this drug may cause birth defects or miscarriages.
- Arrange to have frequent, regular medical follow-up, including frequent blood tests to follow the effects of the drug on your body.
- Report black, tarry stools; fever; chills; sore throat; unusual bleeding or bruising; chest pain; mouth sores; changes in vision; dizziness.

☐ fludrocortisone acetate

*(floo droe **kor**' ti sone)*
Florinef Acetate

Pregnancy Category C

Drug classes

Corticosteroid
Mineralocorticoid
Hormonal agent

Therapeutic actions

Increases sodium reabsorption in renal tubules and increases potassium and hydrogen excretion, leading to sodium and water retention.

Adverse effects in *Italics* are most common; those in **Bold** are life-threatening.

fludrocortisone acetate

Indications
- Partial replacement therapy in primary and secondary cortical insufficiency and for the treatment of salt-losing adrenogenital syndrome (therapy must be accompanied by adequate doses of glucocorticoids).
- Unlabeled use: management of servere orthostatic hypotension

Contraindications/cautions
- Contraindicated in the presence of CHF, hypertension, cardiac disease.
- Use caution in the presence of infections, high sodium intake, lactation.

Dosage
Adult
- ***Addison's disease:*** 0.1 mg/d (range 0.1 mg three times per week to 0.2 mg/d) PO. Reduce dose to 0.05 mg/d if transient hypertension develops. Administration with hydrocortisone (10–30 mg/d) or cortisone (10.0–37.5 mg/d) is preferable.
- ***Salt-losing adrenogenital syndrome:*** 0.1–0.2 mg/d PO.

Pediatric: Safety and efficacy not established. If infants or children are maintained on prolonged therapy, their growth and development must be carefully observed.

Pharmacokinetics

Route	Onset	Peak	Duration
Oral	Gradual	1.7 h	18–36 h

Metabolism: Hepatic, $T_{1/2}$: $3\frac{1}{2}$ h
Distribution: Crosses placenta; enters breast milk

Adverse effects
- CNS: *Frontal and occipital headaches, arthralgia,* tendon contractures, weakness of extremities with ascending paralysis
- CV: *Increased blood volume, edema, hypertension,* CHF, cardiac arrhythmias, enlargement of the heart
- Hypersensitivity: Rash to **anaphylaxis**

Clinically important drug-drug interactions
- Decreased effects of fludrocortisone if taken with barbiturates, hydantoins, rifampin • Decreased effects of anticholinesterases with resultant muscular depression in myasthenia gravis • Decreased serum levels and effectiveness of salicylates if taken with fludrocortisone

■ Nursing Considerations

Assessment
- *History:* CHF, hypertension, cardiac disease, infections, high sodium intake, lactation
- *Physical:* P, BP, chest sounds, body weight and temperature, tissue turgor, reflexes and bilateral grip strength, serum electrolytes

Implementation
- Use only in conjunction with glucocorticoid therapy and control of electrolytes and infection.
- Arrange for increased dosage during times of stress to prevent drug-induced adrenal insufficiency.
- Monitor BP and serum electrolytes regularly to prevent overdosage.
- Arrange to have drug discontinued if signs of overdosage (hypertension, edema, excessive weight gain, increased heart size) appear.
- Arrange for treatment of muscle weakness due to excessive potassium loss with potassium supplements.
- Restrict sodium intake if edema develops.

Drug-specific teaching points
- Learn range-of-motion exercises, positioning to help you deal with musculoskeletal effects of the drug.
- Take drug exactly as prescribed, and do not to stop taking this drug without notifying health care provider; if a dose is missed, take it as soon as possible unless it is almost time for the next dose—do not double the next dose.
- Arrange to keep appointments for frequent follow-up visits so that drug re-

---

Adverse effects in *Italics* are most common; those in **Bold** are life-threatening.

sponse may be determined and the dosage adjusted if necessary.
- Wear a medical alert ID so that any emergency medical personnel will know about this drug therapy.
- Report unusual weight gain, swelling of the lower extremities, muscle weakness, dizziness, and severe or continuing headache.

flumazenil

(floo maz' eh nill)
Romazicon

Pregnancy Category C

Drug classes
Antidote
Benzodiazepine receptor antagonist

Therapeutic actions
Antagonizes the actions of benzodiazepines on the CNS and inhibits activity at GABA/benzodiazepine receptor sites.

Indications
- Complete or partial reversal of the sedative effects of benzodiazepines when general anesthesia has been induced or maintained with benzodiazepines, when sedation has been produced with benzodiazepines for diagnostic and therapeutic procedures, and for the management of benzodiazepine overdose.

Contraindications/cautions
- Contraindicated in the presence of hypersensitivity to flumazenil or benzodiazepines; patients who have been given benzodiazepines to control potentially life threatening conditions; patients showing signs of serious cyclic antidepressant overdose.
- Use caution in the presence of history of seizures, hepatic impairment, panic disorders, head injury, history of drug or alcohol dependence.

Dosage
Use the smallest dose possible to achieve the desired effect.

Adults
- ***Reversal of conscious sedation or in general anesthesia:*** Initial dose of 0.2 mg (2 ml) IV; wait 45 sec; if desired effect does not occur, repeat dose at 60-sec intervals. Maximum dose of 1 mg (10 ml).
- ***Management of suspected benzodiazepine overdose:*** Initial dose of 0.2 mg IV; repeat with 0.3 mg IV q30 sec, up to a maximum dose of 3 mg.

Pediatric: Safety and efficacy not established.
Geriatric: No reduction of dosage is required.

Pharmacokinetics

Route	Onset	Peak	Duration
IV	20–30 sec	6–10 min	72 h

Metabolism: Hepatic, $T_{1/2}$: 7–15 min, then 41–79 min
Distribution: Crosses placenta; may enter breast milk

IV facts
Preparation: Can be drawn into syringe with 5% Dextrose in Water, Lactated Ringer's, and normal saline solutions. Discard within 24 h if mixed in solution. Do not remove from vial until ready for use.
Infusion: Infuse slowly over 15 sec for general anesthesia, over 30 sec for overdose. To reduce pain of injection, administer through a freely running IV infusion in a large vein.

Adverse effects
- CNS: *Dizziness, vertigo,* agitation, nervousness, dry mouth, tremor, palpitations, emotional lability, confusion, crying, vision changes
- GI: *Nausea, vomiting,* hiccups
- CV: Vasodilation, flushing, arrhythmias, chest pain
- Other: *Headache, pain at injection site, increased sweating,* fatigue

Adverse effects in *Italics* are most common; those in **Bold** are life-threatening.

Clinically important drug-food interactions

- Ingestion of food during IV infusion decreases flumazenil serum levels and effectiveness

■ Nursing Considerations

Assessment

- *History:* Hypersensitivity to flumazenil or benzodiazepines; use of benzodiazepines for control of potentially life threatening conditions; signs of serious cyclic antidepressant overdose, history of seizures, hepatic impairment, panic disorders, head injury, history of drug or alcohol dependence
- *Physical:* Skin—color, lesions; body temperature; orientation, reflexes, affect; P, BP, peripheral perfusion; serum drug levels

Implementation

- Administer by IV route only.
- Ensure emergency equipment, secure airway during administration.
- Monitor clinical response carefully to determine effects of drug and need for repeated doses.
- Inject into actively running IV in a large vein to decrease pain of injection.
- Provide patient with written information after use; amnesia may be long-term, and teaching may not be remembered, including safety measures.

Drug-specific teaching points

- Know that drug may cause changes in vision, dizziness, changes in alertness (avoid driving a car or operating machinery that may be dangerous for at least 18–24 h after drug use).
- Do not use any alcohol or OTC drugs for 18–24 h after use of this drug.
- Report difficulty breathing, pain at IV site, changes in vision, severe headache.

☐ flunisolide

*(floo **niss'** oh lide)*
AeroBid, Nasalide

Pregnancy Category C

Drug classes
Corticosteroid
Glucocorticoid
Hormonal Agent

Therapeutic actions
Anti-inflammatory effect; local administration into lower respiratory tract or nasal passages maximizes beneficial effects on these tissues while decreasing the likelihood of adverse effects from systemic absorption.

Indications
- Respiratory inhalant: control of bronchial asthma that requires corticosteroids in conjunction with other therapy
- Intranasal: relief of symptoms of seasonal or perennial rhinitis that respond poorly to other treatments

Contraindications/cautions
- Presence of systemic fungal infections, untreated local nasal infections, epistaxis, nasal trauma, septal ulcers, recent nasal surgery, lactation.

Dosage
Respiratory inhalant: Each actuation delivers 250 µg.
- *Adult:* Two inhalants (500 µg) bid morning and evening (total dose 1 mg), not to exceed 4 inhalations bid (2 mg).
- *Pediatric (6–12 y):* Two inhalants bid morning and evening. Do not use in children younger than 6 y.

Intranasal: Each actuation of the inhaler delivers 25 µg.
- *Adult:* Initial dosage 2 sprays (50 µg) in each nostril bid (total dose 200 µg/d); may be increased to 2 sprays in each nostril tid (total dose 300 µg/d). Maximum daily dose, 8 sprays in each nostril (400 µg/d).
- *Pediatric (6–14 y):* Initial dosage 1 spray in each nostril tid or 2 sprays in each nostril bid (total dose 150–200 µg/d). Maximum daily dose 4 sprays in each nostril (200 µg/d). Not recommended for children younger than 6 y.

Maintenance dosage: Reduce dosage to smallest amount needed to control symptoms. Discontinue therapy after 3 wk in the absence of significant symptomatic improvement.

Pharmacokinetics

Route	Onset	Peak	Duration
Intranasal	Slow	10–30 min	4–6 h

Metabolism: Hepatic, $T_{1/2}$: 1–2 h
Distribution: Crosses placenta; enters breast milk
Excretion: Urine and feces

Adverse effects
Respiratory Inhalant
- Endocrine: Suppression of hypothalamic-pituitary-adrenal (HPA) function due to systemic absorption
- Local: *Oral, laryngeal, pharyngeal irritation*; fungal infections

Intranasal
- CNS: *Headache*
- GI: Nausea
- Respiratory: *Epistaxis, rebound congestion*, perforation of the nasal septum, anosmia
- Dermatologic: Urticaria
- Endocrine: HPA suppression, Cushing's syndrome with overdosage
- Local: *Nasal irritation, fungal infection*

■ Nursing Considerations
Assessment
- *History:* Systemic fungal infections, untreated local nasal infections, epistaxis, nasal trauma, septal ulcers, recent nasal surgery, lactation
- *Physical:* Body weight, temperature; BP, P, auscultation, R, adventitious sounds, examination of nares

Implementation
- Do not use the respiratory inhalant product during an acute asthmatic attack or to manage status asthmaticus.
- Arrange to taper systemic steroids carefully during transfer to inhalational steroids; deaths from adrenal insufficiency have occurred.
- Arrange for use of decongestant nose drops to facilitate penetration if edema, excessive secretions are present.

Drug-specific teaching points
- Do not use this drug more often than prescribed.
- Do not stop using this drug without consulting your health care provider.
- Be aware that if using the oral inhalant, you should administer the inhalational bronchodilator drug first if receiving concomitant bronchodilator therapy. Allow at least 1 min between puffs.
- Rinse your mouth after using the inhalant.
- Be aware that if using the intranasal preparation, you should administer decongestant nose drops first if nasal passages are blocked.
- Know that the following side effects may occur: local irritation (make sure you are using your device correctly), headache (if this becomes severe, consult with your nurse or physician).
- Report sore mouth, sore throat.

☐ fluorouracil

(flure oh yoor' a sill)

5-fluorouracil, 5-FU
Adrucil, Efudex, Fluoroplex

Pregnancy Category D

Drug classes
Antimetabolite
Antineoplastic drug

Therapeutic actions
Inhibits thymidylate synthetase, leading to inhibition of DNA synthesis and cell death.

Indications
- Palliative management of carcinoma of the colon, rectum, breast, stomach, pancreas in selected patients considered incurable by surgery or other means (parenteral)
- Topical treatment of multiple actinic or solar keratoses
- Topical treatment of superficial basal cell carcinoma

Adverse effects in *Italics* are most common; those in **Bold** are life-threatening.

fluorouracil

- Unlabeled use: topical treatment of condylomata acuminata
- Orphan drug uses: in combination with interferon alpha 2-a recombinant for esophageal and advanced colorectal carcinoma; with leucovorin for colon/rectum metastatic adenocarcinoma

Contraindications/cautions
- Allergy to fluorouracil; poor nutritional status; serious infections; hematopoietic depression secondary to radiation or chemotherapy; impaired liver function; pregnancy; lactation.

Dosage
Adult: Initial dosage: 12 mg/kg IV once daily for 4 successive d; do not exceed 800 mg/d. If no toxicity occurs, give 6 mg/kg on the sixth, eighth, 10th, and 12th day with no drug therapy on days 5, 7, 9, and 11. Discontinue therapy at end of 12th day, even if no toxicity is apparent.
- ***Poor-risk patients, undernourished:*** 6 mg/kg per day IV for 3 d. If no toxicity develops, give 3 mg/kg on the fifth, seventh, and ninth days. No drug is given on days 4, 6, and 8. Do not exceed 400 mg/d.
- ***Maintenance therapy:*** Continue therapy on one of the following schedules: 1. If toxicity is not a problem, repeat dosage of first course every 30 d after the last day of the previous course of treatment. 2. If toxicity develops from first course, give 10–15 mg/kg per week as a single dose after signs of toxicity subside. Do not exceed 1 g/wk. Consider patient response, and adjust dosage accordingly; therapy may be prolonged (12–60 mo).
- ***Hepatic failure:*** If serum bilirubin > 5, do not administer fluorouracil.
- ***Topical use:*** *Actinic or solar keratoses:* Apply bid to cover lesions. Continue until inflammatory response reaches erosion, necrosis, and ulceraton stage, then discontinue use. Usual course of therapy is 2–6 wk. Complete healing may not be evident for 1–2 mo after cessation of therapy. *Superficial basal cell carcinoma:* Apply 5% strength bid in an amount sufficient to cover the lesions. Continue treatment for at least 3–6 wk. Treatment may be required for 10–12 wk.

Pharmacokinetics

Route	Onset	Peak	Duration
IV	Immediate	1–2 h	6 h
Topical	Minimal absorption		

Metabolism: Hepatic, $T_{1/2}$: 18–20 min
Distribution: Crosses placenta; enters breast milk
Excretion: Urine and lungs

IV facts
Preparation: Store vials at room temperature; solution may discolor during storage with no adverse effects. Protect ampule from light. Precipitate may form during storage, heat to 60°C, and shake vigorously to dissolve. Cool to body temperature before administration. No dilution is required.
Infusion: Infuse slowly; inject into tubing of running IV to avoid pain on injection.
Incompatibilities: Do not mix with IV additives or other chemotherapeutic agents.

Adverse effects
Parenteral
- CNS: *Lethargy, malaise, weakness,* euphoria, acute cerebellar syndrome, photophobia, lacrimation, decreased vision, nystagmus, diplopia
- GI: *Diarrhea, anorexia, nausea, vomiting, cramps, enteritis, duodenal ulcer, duodenitis, gastritis, glossitis, stomatitis,* pharyngitis, esophagopharyngitis
- CV: Myocardial ischemia, angina
- Hematologic: *Leukopenia, thrombocytopenia,* elevations in alkaline phosphatase, serum transaminase, serum bilirubin, lactic dehydrogenase
- Dermatologic: *Alopecia, dermatitis, maculopapular rash, photosensitivity,* nail changes including nail loss, dry skin, fissures
- Other: Fever, epistaxis

Adverse effects in *Italics* are most common; those in **Bold** are life-threatening.

Topical
- Hematologic: Leukocytosis, thrombocytopenia, toxic granulation, eosinophilia
- Local: *Local pain, pruritus, hyperpigmentation, irritation, inflammation and burning at the site of application,* allergic contact dermatitis, scarring, soreness, tenderness, suppuration, scaling and swelling

Drug-lab test interferences
- 5-hydroxyindoleacetic acid (5-HIAA) urinary excretion may increase • Plasma albumin may decrease due to protein malabsorption

■ Nursing Considerations
Assessment
- *History:* Allergy to fluorouracil, poor nutritional status, serious infections, hematopoietic depression, impaired liver function, pregnancy, lactation
- *Physical:* Weight; temperature; skin—lesions, color; hair; vision; speech, orientation, reflexes, sensation; R, adventitious sounds; mucous membranes, liver evaluation, abdominal exam; CBC, differential; renal and liver function tests; urinalysis, chest x-ray

Implementation
- Arrange for tests to evaluate hematologic status before beginning therapy and before each dose.
- Arrange for discontinuation of drug therapy if any sign of toxicity occurs (stomatitis, esophagopharyngitis, rapidly falling WBC count, intractable vomiting, diarrhea, GI ulceration and bleeding, thrombocytopenia, hemorrhage); consult with physician.
- Arrange for biopsies of skin lesions to rule out frank neoplasm before beginning topical therapy and in all patients who do not respond to topical therapy.
- Wash hands thoroughly immediately after application of topical preparations. Use caution if applying to areas near the nose, eyes, and mouth.
- Avoid the use of occlusive dressings with topical application; the incidence of inflammatory reactions in adjacent skin areas is increased with these dressings. Use porous gauze dressings for cosmetic reasons if desired.

Drug-specific teaching points
- Prepare a calendar of treatment days to follow. If using the topical application, wash hands thoroughly after application. Do not use occlusive dressings, a porous gauze dressing may be used for cosmetic reasons if desired.
- Know that the following side effects may occur: nausea, vomiting, loss of appetite (medication may be ordered to help; small, frequent meals also may help; it is very important to maintain your nutrition while you are on this drug); decreased vision, tearing, double vision, malaise, weakness, lethargy (these are all effects of the drug; it is advisable to avoid driving or operating dangerous machinery if these occur); mouth sores (frequent mouth care will be needed); diarrhea (ensure ready access to bathroom facilities if these occur); loss of hair (you may wish to obtain a wig or other suitable head covering; it is important to keep the head covered in extremes of temperature); skin rash, sensitivity of skin and eyes to sunlight and ultraviolet light (avoid exposure to the sun; use a sunscreen and protective clothing if exposed to sun; this is especially important with the topical application; ultraviolet light will increase the severity of the local reaction); birth defects or miscarriages (it is advisable to use birth control while on this drug); unsightly local reaction to topical application (this may continue for several weeks following cessation of therapy; a porous gauze dressing may be used to cover these areas; do not use occlusive dressings); pain, burning, stinging, swelling at local application.
- Arrange to have frequent, regular medical follow-up, including frequent blood tests to follow the effects of the drug on your body.

Adverse effects in *Italics* are most common; those in **Bold** are life-threatening.

fluoxetine hydrochloride ■ 503

- Report black, tarry stools; fever; chills; sore throat; unusual bleeding or bruising; chest pain; mouth sores; severe pain; tenderness; scaling at sight of local application.

☐ fluoxetine hydrochloride

(floo ox' e teen)
Prozac

Pregnancy Category B

Drug classes
Antidepressant
SSRI

Therapeutic actions
Acts as an antidepressant by inhibiting CNS neuronal uptake of serotonin; blocks uptake of serotonin with little effect on norepinephrine; also thought to antagonize muscarinic, histaminergic and α_1-adrenergic receptors.

Indications
- Treatment of depression; most effective in patients with major depressive disorder
- Unlabeled uses: treatment of obesity, treatment of bulimia and obsessive-compulsive disorders

Contraindications/cautions
- Contraindicated in the presence of hypersensitivity to fluoxetine; pregnancy.
- Use caution in the presence of impaired hepatic or renal function, diabetes mellitus, lactation.

Dosage
Adult: The full antidepressant effect may not be seen for up to 4 wk. Initial: 20 mg/d PO in the morning. If no clinical improvement is seen, increase dose after several weeks. Administer doses > 20 mg/d on a bid schedule. Do not exceed 80 mg/d.
Pediatric: Safety and efficacy not established.
Geriatric or renal impaired: Administer a lower or less frequent dose in these patients. Monitor response as a guide for dosage.

Pharmacokinetics

Route	Onset	Peak
Oral	Slow	6–8 h

Metabolism: Hepatic, $T_{1/2}$: 2–3 d
Distribution: Crosses placenta; enters breast milk
Excretion: Urine and feces

Adverse effects
- **CNS:** *Headache, nervousness, insomnia, drowsiness, anxiety, tremor, dizziness, lightheadedness,* agitation, sedation, abnormal gait, **convulsions**
- **GI:** *Nausea, vomiting, diarrhea, dry mouth, anorexia, dyspepsia, constipation, taste changes,* flatulence, gastroenteritis, dysphagia, gingivitis
- **CV:** Hot flashes, palpitations
- **Respiratory:** *Upper respiratory infections, pharyngitis,* cough, dyspnea, bronchitis, rhinitis
- **GU:** *Painful menstruation, sexual dysfunction, frequency,* cystitis, impotence, urgency, vaginitis
- **Dermatologic:** *Sweating, rash, pruritus,* acne, alopecia, contact dermatitis
- **Other:** *Weight loss, asthenia, fever*

Clinically important drug-drug interactions
- Increased therapeutic and toxic effects of tricyclic antidepressants if taken concurrently with fluoxetine • Decreased therapeutic effects if taken with cyproheptadine

■ Nursing Considerations
Assessment
- *History:* Hypersensitivity to fluoxetine, impaired hepatic or renal function, diabetes mellitus, lactation, pregnancy
- *Physical:* Weight, temperature; skin—rash, lesions; reflexes, affect; bowel sounds, liver evaluation; P, peripheral perfusion; urinary output, renal function; renal and liver function tests, CBC

Implementation
- Arrange for lower dose or less frequent administration in elderly patients and patients with hepatic or renal impairment.

Adverse effects in *Italics* are most common; those in **Bold** are life-threatening.

- Establish suicide precautions for severely depressed patients. Dispense only a small number of capsules at a time to these patients.
- Administer drug in the morning. If dose of > 20 mg/d is needed, administer in divided doses.
- Monitor patient response for up to 4 wk before increasing dose because of lack of therapeutic effect.

Drug-specific teaching points

- Be aware that it may take up to 4 wk to get a full antidepressant effect from this drug. The drug should be taken in the morning (or in divided doses if necessary).
- Know that the following side effects may occur: dizziness, drowsiness, nervousness, insomnia (avoid driving a car or performing hazardous tasks); nausea, vomiting, weight loss (small, frequent meals may help; monitor your weight loss); sexual dysfunction (it may help to know that this is a drug effect); flulike symptoms.
- Do not take this drug during pregnancy. If you think that you are pregnant or wish to become pregnant, consult with your physician.
- Report rash, mania, seizures, severe weight loss.
- Keep this drug, and all medications, out of the reach of children.

☐ fluoxymesterone

(floo ox i mes' te rone)
Android-F, Halotestin

Pregnancy Category X
C-III Controlled substance

Drug classes
Androgen
Hormonal agent

Therapeutic actions
Analog of testosterone, the primary natural androgen; endogenous androgens are responsible for growth and development of male sex organs and the maintenance of secondary sex characteristics; administration of androgen analogs increases the retention of nitrogen, sodium, potassium, phosphorus, and decreases urinary excretion of calcium; increases protein anabolism and decreases protein catabolism; stimulates the production of red blood cells.

Indications
- Male: replacement therapy in hypogonadism—primary hypogonadism, hypogonadotropic hypogonadism, delayed puberty
- Female: metastatic cancer—breast cancer in women who are 1–5 years postmenopausal, postpartum breast pain/engorgement

Contraindications/cautions
- Contraindicated in the presence of known sensitivity to androgens, allergy to tartrazine or aspirin (in products marketed under the brand name *Halotestin*), prostate or breast cancer in males, pregnancy, lactation.
- Use caution in the presence of MI, liver disease.

Dosage
Hypogonadism: 5–20 mg/d PO.
Delayed puberty: 2.5–20 mg/d PO, although generally 2.5–10 mg/d PO for 4–6 mo is sufficient.
Postpartum breast pain/engorgement: 2.5 mg PO shortly after delivery, then 5–10 mg/d PO in divided doses for 4–5 d.
Carcinoma of the breast: 10–40 mg/d PO in divided doses. Continue for 1 mo for a subjective response and 2–3 mo for an objective response.

Pharmacokinetics

Route	Onset	Peak
Oral	Rapid	2 h

Metabolism: Hepatic, $T_{1/2}$: 9.5 h
Distribution: Crosses placenta; enters breast milk
Excretion: Urine and feces

fluoxymesterone ■ 505

Adverse effects
- CNS: *Dizziness, headache, sleep disorders, fatigue,* tremor, sleeplessness, generalized paresthesia, sleep apnea syndrome, CNS hemorrhage
- GI: *Nausea, hepatic dysfunction;* hepatocellular carcinoma, **potentially life threatening peliosis hepatitis**
- Hematologic: *Polycythemia, leukopenia,* hypercalcemia, altered serum cholesterol levels; retention of sodium, chloride, water, potassium, phosphates, and calcium
- GU: Fluid retention, decreased urinary output
- Dermatologic: *Rash,* dermatitis, anaplylactoid reactions
- Endocrine: *Androgenic effects* (acne, edema, mild hirsutism, decrease in breast size, deepening of the voice, oily skin or hair, weight gain, clitoral hypertrophy or testicular atrophy), *hypoestrogenic effects* (flushing, sweating, vaginitis, nervousness, emotional lability)
- Other: Chills, premature closure of the epiphyses

Clinically important drug-drug interactions
- Potentiation of oral anticoagulants if taken with androgens; anticoagulant dosage may need to be decreased

Drug-lab test interferences
- Altered glucose tolerance tests • Decrease in thyroid function tests, which may persist for 2–3 wk after stopping therapy • Suppression of clotting factors II, V, VII, and X • Increased creatinine, creatinine clearance, which may last for 2 wk after therapy

■ Nursing Considerations

Assessment
- *History:* Sensitivity to androgens, allergy to tartrazine or aspirin, prostate or breast cancer in males, MI, liver disease, pregnancy, lactation
- *Physical:* Skin—color, lesions, texture; hair distribution pattern; affect, orientation, peripheral sensation; abdominal exam, liver evaluation; serum electrolytes, serum cholesterol levels, liver function tests, glucose tolerance tests, thyroid function tests, long bone x-ray (in children)

Implementation
- Administer drug with meals or snacks to decrease GI upset.
- Monitor effect on children with long bone x-rays every 3–6 mo during therapy. Discontinue drug well before the bone age reaches the norm for the patient's chronologic age.
- Monitor patient for occurrence of edema; arrange for appropriate diuretic therapy as needed.
- Arrange to monitor liver function, serum electrolytes periodically during therapy, and consult with physician for appropriate corrective measures as needed.
- Arrange to measure cholesterol levels periodically in patients who are at high risk for coronary artery disease.
- Monitor diabetic patients closely as glucose tolerance may change. Adjustments may be needed in insulin, oral hypoglycemic dosage, and diet.
- Arrange for periodic monitoring of urine and serum calcium during treatment of disseminated breast carcinoma, and arrange for appropriate treatment or discontinuation of the drug.
- Monitor geriatric males for prostatic hypertrophy and carcinoma.
- Discontinue drug and arrange for appropriate consultation if abnormal vaginal bleeding occurs.

Drug-specific teaching points
- Take drug with meals or snacks to decrease the GI upset.
- Know that the following side effects may occur: body hair growth, baldness, deepening of the voice, loss of libido, impotence (most of these effects will be reversible when the drug is stopped); excitation, confusion, insomnia (avoid driving, performing tasks that require alertness if these effects occur); swelling of the

Adverse effects in *Italics* are most common; those in **Bold** are life-threatening.

ankles, fingers (medication may be ordered to help).
- Be aware that diabetic patients need to monitor urine sugar closely as glucose tolerance may change. Report any abnormalities to physician, so corrective action can be taken.
- Report ankle swelling, nausea, vomiting, yellowing of skin or eyes, unusual bleeding or bruising, penile swelling or pain, hoarseness, body hair growth, deepening of the voice, acne, menstrual irregularities (women).

☐ fluphenazine decanoate

*(floo **fen'** a zeen)*
Injection: Modecate Deconoate (CAN), Prolixin Decanoate

fluphenazine enanthate
Injection: Moditen Enanthate (CAN), Prolixin Enanthate

fluphenazine hydrochloride
Oral tablets, concentrate, elixir, injection: Apo-Fluphenazine (CAN), Moditen Hydrochloride (CAN), Permitil, Prolixin

Pregnancy Category C

Drug classes
Phenothiazine (piperazine)
Dopaminergic blocking drug
Antipsychotic drug

Therapeutic actions
Mechanism of action not fully understood: antipsychotic drugs block postsynaptic dopamine receptors in the brain, depress the reticular activating system, including the parts of the brain involved with wakefulness and emesis; anticholinergic, antihistaminic (H_1), and alpha-adrenergic blocking activity also may contribute to some of its therapeutic (and adverse) actions.

Indications
- Management of manifestations of psychotic disorders; the longer acting parenteral dosage forms, fluphenazine enanthate and fluphenazine decanoate, indicated for management of patients (eg, chronic schizophrenics) who require prolonged parenteral therapy

Contraindications/cautions
- Contraindicated in the presence of coma or severe CNS depression, bone marrow depression, blood dyscrasia, circulatory collapse, subcortical brain damage, Parkinson's disease, liver damage, cerebral arteriosclerosis, coronary disease, severe hypotension or hypertension.
- Use caution in the presence of respiratory disorders ("silent pneumonia" may develop); glaucoma, prostatic hypertrophy (anticholinergic effects may exacerbate glaucoma and urinary retention); epilepsy or history of epilepsy (drug lowers seizure threshold); breast cancer (elevations in prolactin may stimulate a prolactin-dependent tumor); thyrotoxicosis; peptic ulcer, decreased renal function; myelography within previous 24 h or myelography scheduled within 48 h; exposure to heat or phosphorous insecticides; pregnancy; lactation; children younger than 12 y, especially those with chickenpox, CNS infections (children are especially susceptible to dystonias that may confound the diagnosis of Reye's syndrome).

Dosage
Full clinical effects may require 6 wk–6 mo of therapy.
Fluphenazine hydrochloride
Patients who have never taken phenothiazines, "poor-risk" patients (those disorders that predispose to undue reactions) should be treated initially with this shorter acting dosage form and then switched to the longer acting parenteral forms, fluphenazine enanthate or decanoate, if this is deemed desirable.
- ***Adult:*** Individualize dosage, beginning with low dosage and gradually increasing.

- **Oral:** 0.5–10.0 mg/d in divided doses q6–8h; usual daily dose is less than 3 mg. Give daily doses greater than 20 mg with caution. When symptoms are controlled, gradually reduce dosage.
- **IM:** Average starting dose is 1.25 mg (range 2.5–10.0 mg), divided and given q6–8h; parenteral dose is one-third to one-half the oral dose. Give daily doses greater than 10 mg with caution.
- **Pediatric:** Generally not recommended for children younger than 12 y.
- **Geriatric:** Initial oral dose is 1.0–2.5 mg/d.

Fluphenazine enanthate, fluphenazine decanoate

The duration of action of the estrified forms of fluphenazine is *markedly* longer than those of fluphenazine hydrochloride; the duration of action of fluphenazine enanthate is estimated to be 1–3 wk; the duration of action of fluphenazine decanoate is estimated to be 4 wk. No precise formula is available for the conversion of fluphenazine hydrochloride dosage to fluphenazine dicanoate dosage, but one study suggests that 20 mg of fluphenazine hydrochloride daily was equivalent to 25 mg decanoate every 3 wk.

- **Adult:** Initial dose 12.5–25.0 mg IM or SC; determine subsequent doses and dosage interval in accordance with patient response. Dose should not exceed 100 mg.

Pharmacokinetics

Route	Onset	Peak	Duration
Oral	60 min	2 h	6–8 h
IM (HCl)	60 min	1–2 h	6–8 h
IM (enanthate)	24–72 h		2 wk
IM (decanoate)	24–72 h		1–6 wk

Metabolism: Hepatic, $T_{1/2}$: 4.5–15.3 h (fluphenazine), 3.7 d (fluphenazine enanthate), 6.8–9.6 d (fluphenazine decanoate)

Distribution: Crosses placenta; enters breast milk
Excretion: Unchanged in the urine

Adverse effects

- CNS: *Drowsiness*, insomnia, vertigo, headache, weakness, tremor, ataxia, slurring, cerebral edema, seizures, exacerbation of psychotic symptoms, extrapyramidal syndromes *(pseudoparkinsonism); dystonias; akathisia*, tardive dyskinesias, potentially irreversible, neuroleptic malignant syndrome (extrapyramidal symptoms), hyperthermias, **autonomic disturbances** (rare, but 20% fatal)
- CV: Hypotension, orthostatic hypotension, hypertension, tachycardia, bradycardia, cardiac arrest, CHF, cardiomegaly, **refractory arrhythmias** (some fatal), pulmonary edema
- Respiratory: Bronchospasm, laryngospasm, dyspnea; suppression of cough reflex and potential for aspiration **(sudden death related to asphyxia or cardiac arrest has been reported)**
- Hematologic: Eosinophilia, leukopenia, leukocytosis, anemia; aplastic anemia; hemolytic anemia; thrombocytopenic or nonthrombocytopenic purpura; pancytopenia
- Hypersensitivity: Jaundice, urticaria, angioneurotic edema, laryngeal edema, photosensitivity, eczema, asthma, anaphylactoid reactions, exfoliative dermatitis
- Endocrine: Lactation, breast engorgement in females, galactorrhea; syndrome of inappropriate ADH secretion; amenorrhea, menstrual irregularities; gynecomastia in males; changes in libido; hyperglycemia or hypoglycemia; glycosuria; hyponatremia; pituitary tumor with hyperprolactinemia; inhibition of ovulation, infertility, pseudopregnancy; reduced urinary levels of gonadotropins, estrogens, progestins
- Autonomic: Dry mouth, salivation, nasal congestion, nausea, vomiting, anorexia, fever, pallor, flushed facies, sweating, constipation, paralytic ileus, urinary re-

Adverse effects in *Italics* are most common; those in **Bold** are life-threatening.

tention, incontinence, polyuria, enuresis, priapism, ejaculation inhibition, male impotence

Clinically important drug-drug interactions
- Additive CNS depression with alcohol
- Additive anticholinergic effects and possibly decreased antipsychotic efficacy with anticholinergic drugs
- Increased likelihood of seizures with metrizamide (contrast agent used in myelography)
- Decreased antihypertensive effect of guanethidine when taken with antipsychotic drugs

Drug-lab test interferences
- False-positive pregnancy tests (less likely if serum test is used)
- Increase in protein-bound iodine, not attributable to an increase in thyroxine

■ Nursing Considerations

Assessment
- *History:* Coma or severe CNS depression; bone marrow depression; blood dyscrasia; circulatory collapse; subcortical brain damage; Parkinson's disease; liver damage; cerebral arteriosclerosis; coronary disease; severe hypotension or hypertension; respiratory disorders; glaucoma, prostatic hypertrophy; epilepsy; breast cancer; thyrotoxicosis; peptic ulcer, decreased renal function; myelography within previous 24 h or myelography scheduled within 48 h; exposure to heat or phosphorous insecticides; children younger than 12 y, chickenpox, CNS infections
- *Physical:* Body weight, temperature; reflexes, orientation, intraocular pressure; P, BP, orthostatic BP; R, adventitious sounds; bowel sounds and normal output, liver evaluation; urinary output, prostate size; CBC, urinalysis, thyroid, liver and kidney function tests

Implementation
- Arrange to use the oral elixir or the oral concentrate for patients who cannot or will not swallow tablets.
- Dilute the oral concentrate *only* in one of the following: water, saline, Seven-Up, homogenized milk, carbonated orange beverage, and pineapple, apricot, prune, orange, V-8, tomato, and grapefruit juices.
- Do *not* mix the oral concentrate with beverages containing caffeine (coffee, cola), tannics (tea), or pectinates (apple juice), because drug may be physically incompatible with these liquids.
- Avoid skin contact with oral solution; contact dermatitis has occurred.
- Arrange for discontinuation of drug if serum creatinine, BUN become abnormal or if WBC count is depressed.
- Monitor elderly patients for dehydration, and institute remedial measures promptly. Sedation and decreased sensation of thirst related to CNS effects of drug can lead to severe dehydration.
- Consult physician regarding appropriate warning of patient or patient's guardian about tardive dyskinesias.
- Consult physician about dosage reduction, use of anticholinergic antiparkinsonian drugs (controversial) if extrapyramidal effects occur.

Drug-specific teaching points
- Take drug exactly as prescribed.
- Avoid driving a car or engaging in other dangerous activities if CNS, vision changes occur.
- Avoid prolonged exposure to sun, or use a sunscreen or covering garments if exposure is unavoidable.
- Maintain fluid intake, and use precautions against heatstroke in hot weather.
- Report sore throat, fever, unusual bleeding or bruising, rash, weakness, tremors, impaired vision, dark urine (pink or reddish brown urine is to be expected), pale stools, yellowing of the skin or eyes.

☐ flurazepam hydrochloride

(flur az' e pam)
Dalmane, Somnal (CAN)

Pregnancy Category X
C-IV controlled substance

flurazepam hydrochloride

Drug classes
Benzodiazepine
Sedative/hypnotic

Therapeutic actions
Exact mechanisms of action not understood; acts mainly at subcortical levels of the CNS, leaving the cortex relatively unaffected; potentiates the effects of gamma-aminobutyrate, an inhibitory neurotransmitter.

Indications
- Insomnia characterized by difficulty in falling asleep, frequent nocturnal awakenings, or early morning awakening
- Recurring insomnia or poor sleeping habits
- Acute or chronic medical situations requiring restful sleep

Contraindications/cautions
- Contraindicated in the presence of hypersensitivity to benzodiazepines, psychoses, acute narrow-angle glaucoma, shock, coma, acute alcoholic intoxication with depression of vital signs, pregnancy (increased risk of congenital malformations, neonatal withdrawal syndrome), labor and delivery ("floppy infant" syndrome reported when mothers were given benzodiazepines during labor), lactation (secreted in breast milk; chronic administration of diazepam, another benzodiazepine, to nursing mothers has caused infants to become lethargic and lose weight).
- Use caution in the presence of impaired liver or kidney function, debilitation, depression, suicidal tendencies.

Dosage
Individualize dosage.
Adult: 30 mg PO before bedtime; 15 mg may suffice.
Pediatric: Not for use in children younger than 15 y.
Geriatric patients or those with debilitating disease: Initially, 15 mg; adjust as needed and tolerated.

Pharmacokinetics

Route	Onset	Peak
Oral	Varies	30–60 min

Metabolism: Hepatic, $T_{1/2}$: 47–100 h
Distribution: Crosses placenta; enters breast milk
Excretion: Urine

Adverse effects
- **CNS:** *Transient, mild drowsiness initially; sedation, depression, lethargy, apathy, fatigue, lightheadedness, disorientation, restlessness, asthenia,* crying, delirium, headache, slurred speech, dysarthria, stupor, rigidity, tremor, dystonia, vertigo, euphoria, nervousness, difficulty in concentration, vivid dreams, psychomotor retardation, extrapyramidal symptoms; *mild paradoxical excitatory reactions during first 2 wk of treatment* (especially in psychiatric patients, aggressive children, and with high dosage), visual and auditory disturbances, diplopia, nystagmus, depressed hearing, nasal congestion
- **GI:** *Constipation, diarrhea, dyspepsia,* dry mouth, salivation, nausea, anorexia, vomiting, difficulty in swallowing, gastric disorders, elevations of blood enzymes: LDH, alkaline phosphatase, SGOT, SGPT, hepatic dysfunction, jaundice
- **CV:** *Bradycardia, tachycardia,* cardiovascular collapse, hypertension and hypotension, palpitations, edema
- **Hematologic:** Decreased hematocrit, blood dyscrasias
- **GU:** *Incontinence, urinary retention, changes in libido,* menstrual irregularities
- **Dermatologic:** Urticaria, pruritus, skin rash, dermatitis
- **Dependence:** *Drug dependence with withdrawal syndrome* when drug is discontinued (more common with abrupt discontinuation of higher dosage used for longer than 4 mo)
- **Other:** Hiccups, fever, diaphoresis, paresthesias, muscular disturbances, gynecomastia

Adverse effects in *Italics* are most common; those in **Bold** are life-threatening.

Clinically important drug-drug interactions

- Increased CNS depression when taken with alcohol, omeprazole • Increased pharmacologic effects of chlordiazepoxide when given with cimetidine, disulfiram, oral contraceptives • Decreased sedative effects of chlordiazepoxide if taken concurrently with theophylline, aminophylline, dyphylline, oxitriphylline

■ Nursing Considerations

Assessment
- *History:* Hypersensitivity to benzodiazepines; psychoses; acute narrow-angle glaucoma; shock; coma; acute alcoholic intoxication; pregnancy; labor; lactation; impaired liver or kidney function, debilitation, depression, suicidal tendencies
- *Physical:* Skin—color, lesions; body temperature; orientation, reflexes, affect, ophthalmologic exam; P, BP;R, adventitious sounds; liver evaluation, abdominal exam, bowel sounds, normal output; CBC, liver and renal function tests

Implementation
- Arrange to monitor liver and kidney function, CBC at intervals during long-term therapy.
- Arrange to taper dosage gradually after long-term therapy, especially in epileptic patients.

Drug-specific teaching points
- Take drug exactly as prescribed.
- Do not stop taking this drug (long-term therapy) without consulting the health care provider.
- Know that the following side effects may occur: drowsiness, dizziness (these may become less pronounced after a few days; avoid driving a car or engaging in other dangerous activities if these occur); GI upset (taking the drug with water may help); depression, dreams, emotional upset, crying; nocturnal sleep may be disturbed for several nights after discontinuing the drug.
- Report severe dizziness, weakness, drowsiness that persists, rash or skin lesions, palpitations, swelling of the extremities, visual changes, difficulty voiding.

❑ flurbiprofen

(flure bi' proe fen)
Ophthalmic solution: Ocufen
Oral: Ansaid
Pregnancy Category B

Drug classes
NSAID
Analgesic (non-narcotic)
Anti-inflammatory agent

Therapeutic actions
Analgesic, anti-inflammatory, and antipyretic activities largely related to inhibition of prostaglandin synthesis; exact mechanisms of action are not known.

Indications
- Acute or long-term treatment of the signs and symptoms of rheumatoid arthritis and osteoarthritis (oral)
- Inhibition of intraoperative miosis (ophthalmic solution)
- Unlabeled uses of ophthalmic solution: topical treatment of cystoid macular edema, inflammation after cataract surgery and uveitis syndromes

Contraindications/cautions
- Contraindicated in the presence of significant renal impairment, pregnancy, lactation.
- Use caution in the presence of impaired hearing, allergies, hepatic, cardiovascular, and GI conditions.

Dosage
Adult
- **Oral:** Initial recommended daily dose of 200—300 mg PO, administered in divided doses two, three, or four times per day. Largest recommended single dose is 100 mg. Doses above 300 mg/d PO are not recommended. Taper to lowest possible dose.
- **Ophthalmic solutions:** Instill 1 drop approximately every ½ h, beginning 2 h before surgery (total of 4 drops).

Pediatric: Safety and efficacy not established.

Pharmacokinetics

Route	Onset	Peak
Oral	30–60 min	1½ h
Ophthalmologic	Minimal systemic absorption	

Metabolism: Hepatic, $T_{1/2}$: 5.7 h
Distribution: Crosses placenta; enters breast milk
Excretion: Urine

Adverse effects
NSAIDs
- **CNS:** *Headache, dizziness, somnolence, insomnia,* fatigue, tiredness, dizziness, tinnitus, ophthamological effects
- **GI:** *Nausea, dyspepsia, GI pain,* diarrhea, vomiting, *constipation,* flatulence
- **Respiratory:** Dyspnea, hemoptysis, pharyngitis, bronchospasm, rhinitis
- **Hematologic:** Bleeding, platelet inhibition with higher doses, neutropenia, eosinophilia, leukopenia, pancytopenia, thrombocytopenia, agranulocytosis, granulocytopenia, aplastic anemia, decreased hemoglobin or hematocrit, bone marrow depression, menorrhagia
- **GU:** Dysuria, **renal impairment**
- **Dermatologic:** *Rash,* pruritus, sweating, dry mucous membranes, stomatitis
- **Other:** Peripheral edema, **anaphylactoid reactions to fatal anaphylactic shock**

Ophthalmic Solution
- **Local:** *Transient stinging and burning on instillation, ocular irritation*

■ Nursing Considerations

Assessment
- *History:* Renal impairment; impaired hearing; allergies; hepatic, cardiovascular, and GI conditions; lactation
- *Physical:* Skin—color and lesions; orientation, reflexes, ophthalmologic and audiometric evaluation, peripheral sensation; P, edema; R, adventitious sounds; liver evaluation; CBC, clotting times, renal and liver function tests; serum electrolytes, stool guaiac

Implementation
- Administer drug with food or after meals if GI upset occurs.
- Assess patient receiving ophthalmic solutions for systemic effects, because absorption does occur.
- Arrange for periodic ophthalmologic examination during long-term therapy.
- Institute emergency procedures if overdose occurs: gastric lavage, induction of emesis, supportive therapy.

Drug-specific teaching points
- Take drug with food or meals if GI upset occurs; take only the prescribed dosage.
- Know that dizziness, drowsiness can occur (avoid driving or the use of dangerous machinery while on this drug).
- Report sore throat, fever, rash, itching, weight gain, swelling in ankles or fingers, changes in vision, black, tarry stools.

☐ flutamide

(floo' ta mide)
Eulexin

Pregnancy Category D

Drug classes
Antiandrogen

Therapeutic actions
A nonsteroidal agent, it exerts potent antiandrogenic activity by inhibiting androgen uptake or by inhibiting nuclear binding of androgen in target tissues.

Indications
- Treatment of metastatic prostatic carcinoma in combination with LHRH agonistic analogs (leuprolide acetate)

Contraindications/cautions
- Hypersensitivity to flutamide or any component of the preparation, pregnancy, lactation.

Dosage
Adult: Two capsules three times per day PO at 8-h intervals; total daily dosage of 750 mg.
Pediatric: Safety and efficacy not established.

Adverse effects in *Italics* are most common; those in **Bold** are life-threatening.

Pharmacokinetics

Route	Onset	Peak	Duration
Oral	Varies	2 h	72 h

Metabolism: Hepatic, $T_{1/2}$: 6 h
Distribution: Crosses placenta; enters breast milk
Excretion: Urine

Adverse effects

- **CNS:** Drowsiness, confusion, depression, anxiety, nervousness
- **GI:** *Nausea, vomiting, diarrhea, GI disturbances*, jaundice, hepatitis, hepatic necrosis
- **Hematologic:** *Anemia, leukopenia,* thrombocytopenia, elevated AST, ALT
- **GU:** *Impotence, loss of libido*
- **Dermatologic:** *Rash,* photosensitivity
- **Endocrine:** *Gynecomastia, hot flashes*
- **Other:** Carcinogenesis, mutagenesis

■ Nursing Considerations

Assessment

- *History*: Hypersensitivity to flutamide or any component of the preparation, pregnancy, lactation
- *Physical:* Skin—color, lesions; reflexes; affect; urinary output; bowel sounds, liver evaluation; CBC, Hct, electrolytes, liver function tests

Implementation

- Administer flutamide concomitantly with other drugs used for medical castration.
- Arrange for periodic monitoring of liver function tests during long-term therapy.

Drug-specific teaching points

- Take this drug concomitantly with other drugs to treat your problem. Do not interrupt dosing or stop taking these medications without consulting your health care provider.
- Know that periodic blood tests will be necessary to monitor the drug effects. It is important that you keep appointments for these tests.
- Know that the following side effects may occur: dizziness, drowsiness (avoid driving a car or performing hazardous tasks); nausea, vomiting, diarrhea (proper nutrition is important; consult with your dietician to maintain nutrition); impotence, loss of libido (it may help to know that these are drug effects).
- Report change in stool or urine color, yellow skin, difficulty breathing, malaise.

☐ fluvastatin

*(flue va **sta'** tin)*
Lescol

Pregnancy Category X

Drug classes
Antihyperlipidemic agent

Therapeutic actions
A fungal metabolite that inhibits the enzyme HMG-CoA that catalyzes the first step in the cholesterol synthesis pathway, resulting in a decrease in serum cholesterol, serum LDLs (associated with increased risk of coronary artery disease), and either an increase or no change in serum HDLs (associated with decreased risk of coronary artery disease).

Indications

- As an adjunct to diet in the treatment of elevated total cholestrol and LDL cholesterol in patients with primary hypercholesterolemia (types IIa and IIb) whose response to dietary restriction of satruated fat and cholesterol and other nonpharmacologic measures has not been adequate.

Contraindications/cautions

- Contraindicated in the presence of allergy to lovastatin, fungal byproducts, pregnancy, lactation.
- Use caution in the presence of impaired hepatic function, cataracts.

Dosage
Adult: Initial dosage: 20 mg/d PO administered in the evening. Maintenance doses: 20–40 mg/d PO as a single evening dose.

Adverse effects in *Italics* are most common; those in **Bold** are life-threatening.

Pediatric: Safety and efficacy not established.

Pharmacokinetics

Route	Onset	Peak
Oral	Slow	4–6 wk

Metabolism: Hepatic, $T_{1/2}$: unknown
Distribution: Crosses placenta; enters breast milk
Excretion: Bile and feces

Adverse effects

- **CNS:** *Headache, blurred vision,* dizziness, insomnia, fatigue, muscle cramps, cataracts
- **GI:** *Flatulence, abdominal pain, cramps, constipation, nausea,* dyspepsia, heartburn
- **Hematologic:** Elevations of CPK, alkaline phosphatase and transaminiases

Clinically important drug-drug interactions

- Possible severe myopathy or rhabdomyolysis if taken with cyclosporine, erythromycin, gemfibrozil, niacin

■ Nursing Considerations

Assessment

- *History:* Allergy to fluvastatin, fungal byproducts; impaired hepatic function; cataracts (use caution); pregnancy; lactation
- *Physical:* Orientation, affect, ophthalmologic exam; liver evaluation; lipid studies, liver function tests

Implementation

- Administer drug in the evening; highest rates of cholesterol synthesis are between midnight and 5 AM.
- Arrange for regular follow-up during long-term therapy.
- Arrange for periodic ophthalmologic exam to check for cataract development.

Drug-specific teaching points

- Take drug in the evening.
- Institute appropriate diet changes that need to be made.

- Know that the following side effects may occur: nausea (small, frequent meals may help); headache, muscle and joint aches and pains (these may lessen with time).
- Arrange to have periodic ophthalmic exams while you are on this drug.
- Report severe GI upset, changes in vision, unusual bleeding or bruising, dark urine or light-colored stools.

☐ fluvoxamine maleate

*(floo **vox'** a meen)*

Luvox

Pregnancy Category C

Drug classes

SSRI (Selective serotonin reuptake inhibitor)

Therapeutic actions

Selectively inhibits CNS neuronal uptake of serotonin; blocks uptake of serotonin with little effect on norepinephrine; also thought to antagonize muscarinic, histaminergic and a_1-adrenergic receptors.

Indications

- Treatment of obsessive-compulsive disorder

Contraindications/cautions

- Contraindicated in the presence of hypersensitivity to fluvoxamine, lactation.
- Use caution in the presence of impaired hepatic or renal function, suicidal tendencies, seizures, mania, ECT therapy, cardiovascular disease, labor and delivery, pregnancy.

Dosage

Adult: Initially 50 mg PO at bedtime. Increase in 50 mg increments at 4–7 d intervals. Usual range 100–300 mg/d. Divide doses over 100 mg and give larger dose at bedtime.
Pediatric: Safety and efficacy not established for < 18 y.
Geriatric or hepatic impaired: Administer a reduced dose, and titrate more slowly.

Adverse effects in *Italics* are most common; those in **Bold** are life-threatening.

514 ■ folic acid

Pharmacokinetics

Route	Onset	Peak
Oral	Rapid	2–8 h

Metabolism: Hepatic metabolism; $T_{1/2}$: 15 h
Distribution: Crosses placenta; passes into breast milk
Excretion: Urine

Adverse effects

- **CNS:** *Headache, nervousness, insomnia, drowsiness, anxiety, tremor, dizziness, lightheadedness,* agitation, sedation, abnormal gait, convulsions
- **GI:** *Nausea, vomiting, diarrhea, dry mouth, anorexia, dyspepsia, constipation, taste changes,* flatulence, gastroenteritis, dysphagia, gingivitis
- **Dermatologic:** *Sweating, rash, pruritus,* acne, alopecia, contact dermatitis
- **Respiratory:** *Upper respiratory infections, pharyngitis,* cough, dyspnea, bronchitis, rhinitis
- **GU:** *sexual dysfunction, frequency,* cystitis, impotence, urgency, vaginitis

Clinically important drug-drug interactions

- Do not administer to any patient concurrently taking terfenadine, astemizole, MAO inhibitors (during or within 14 d). • Increased effects of triazolam, alprazolam, warfarin, carbamazepine, methadone, beta blockers, diltiazem. Reduced dosages of these drugs will be needed. • Decreased effects of fluvoxamine due to increased metabolism in cigarette smokers.

■ Nursing Considerations

Assessment

- *History:* Hypersensitivity to fluvoxamine; lactation; impaired hepatic or renal function; suicidal tendencies; seizures; mania; ECT therapy; cardiovascular disease; labor and delivery; pregnancy
- *Physical:* Weight; temperature; skin—rash, lesions; **reflexes; affect; bowel sounds; liver evaluation; P, peripheral perfusion; urinary output; renal function; renal and liver function tests; CBC**

Implementation

- Arrange for lower dose or less frequent administration in elderly patients, and patients with hepatic or renal impairment.
- Establish suicide precautions for severly depressed patients. Dispense only a small number of capsules at a time to these patients.
- Administer drug at bedtime, if dose exceeds 100 mg, divide dose and administer the largest dose at bedtime.
- Monitor patient response for up to 4–7 d before increasing dose because of lack of therapeutic effect.

Drug-specific teaching points

- Take this drug at bedtime; if a large dose is needed, the dose may be divided, but take the largest dose at bedtime.
- Know that the following side effects may occur: dizziness, drowsiness, nervousness, insomnia (avoid driving a car or performing hazardous tasks), nausea, vomiting, weight loss (small frequent meals may help), sexual dysfunction (it may help to know that this is a drug effect.)
- Report rash, mania, seizures, severe weight loss.

❑ folic acid

(foe' lik)
folacin, pteroylglutamic acid, folate

Folvite, Novofolacid (CAN)

Pregnancy Category A

Drug classes
Folic acid

Therapeutic actions
Active reduced form of folic acid; required for nucleoprotein synthesis and maintenence of normal erythropoiesis.

Indications
- Treatment of megoblastic anemias due to sprue, nutritional deficiency, pregnancy, infancy, and childhood

Adverse effects in *Italics* are most common; those in **Bold** are life-threatening.

Contraindications/cautions
- Contraindicated in the presence of allergy to folic acid preparations; pernicious, aplastic, normocytic anemias.
- Use caution during lactation.

Dosage
Administer orally unless severe intestinal malabsorption is present.

Adult
- ***Therapeutic dose:*** Up to 1 mg/d PO, IM, IV, or SC. Larger doses may be needed in severe cases.
- ***Maintainence dose:*** 0.4 mg/d.
- ***Pregnancy and lactation:*** 0.8 mg/d.

Pediatric
- ***Maintenance:*** *Infants:* 0.1 mg/d; younger than 4 y: up to 0.3 mg/d; older than 4 y: 0.4 mg/d.

Pharmacokinetics

Route	Onset	Peak
Oral, IM, SC, IV	Varies	30–60 min

Metabolism: Hepatic, $T_{1/2}$: unknown
Distribution: Crosses placenta; enters breast milk
Excretion: Urine

IV facts
Preparation: Solution is yellow to yellow-orange; may be added to hyperalimentation solution or dextrose solutions.
Infusion: Infuse at rate of 5 mg/min by direct IV injection; may be diluted in hyperalimentation for continuous infusion.

Adverse effects
- **Hypersensitivity:** Allergic reactions
- **Local:** *Pain and discomfort at injection site*

Clinically important drug-drug interactions
- Decrease in serum phenytoin and subsequent increase in seizure activity when taken concurrently with folic acid preparations • Decreased absorption of folic acid if taken concurrently with sulfasalazine, aminosalicyclic acid

■ Nursing Considerations

Assessment
- *History:* Allergy to folic acid preparations; pernicious, aplastic, normocytic anemias; lactation
- *Physical:* Skin—lesions, color; R, adventitious sounds; CBC, hemoglobin, hematocrit, serum folate levels, serum vitamin B_{12} levels, Schilling test

Implementation
- Administer orally if at all possible. If severe GI malabsorption exists or disease is very severe, may be given IM, SC, or IV.
- Ensure that patient does not have pernicious anemia by using Schilling test and serum vitamin B_{12} levels before beginning treatment. Therapy may mask the signs of pernicious anemia while the neurologic deterioration continues.
- Use caution when administering the parenteral preparations to premature infants. These preparations contain benzyl alcohol, which has been associated with a fatal gasping syndrome in premature infants.
- Monitor patient for hypersensitivity reactions, especially if patient has received the drug before. Maintain supportive equipment and emergency drugs on standby in case of serious allergic response.

Drug-specific teaching points
- Know that when the reason for the megaloblastic anemia has been treated or passes (eg, infancy, pregnancy), the need for this drug also may pass as folic acid is normally found in sufficient quantities in the diet.
- Report rash, difficulty breathing, pain or discomfort at injection site.

☐ foscarnet sodium

*(foss **kar**' net)*
Foscavir
Pregnancy Category C

Adverse effects in *Italics* are most common; those in **Bold** are life-threatening.

foscarnet sodium

Drug classes
Antiviral

Therapeutic actions
Inhibits replication of all known herpesviruses by selectively inhibiting specific DNA and RNA enzymes.

Indications
- Treatment of CMV retinitis in patients with AIDS

Contraindications/cautions
- Contraindicated in the presence of allergy to foscarnet.
- Use caution during lactation.

Dosage
Induction: 60 mg/kg q8h IV for 2–3 wk.
Maintenance: 90–120 mg/kg IV.
Geriatric or renal impaired: Monitor patient carefully; if Ccr falls below 0.4 ml/min/kg, discontinue therapy.

Pharmacokinetics

Route	Onset
IV	Immediate

Metabolism: $T_{1/2}$: 1.4–3 h
Distribution: Crosses placenta; enters breast milk
Excretion: Urine

IV facts
Preparation: Administer with Normal Saline, 5% Dextrose Solution.
Infusion: Infuse slowly. Induction dose over a minimum of 1 h using an infusion pump. Maintenance dose: infuse over 2 h using an infusion pump to control rate.
Incompatibilities: Do not mix in the same catheter with anything but Normal Saline or 5% Dextrose Solution. Incompatible with 30% Dextrose, amphotericin B, solutions containing calcium; acyclovir sodium, ganciclovir, trimetrexate, pentamidine, vancomycin, trimethoprim/sulfamethoxazole, diazepam, disazolam, digoxin, phenytoin, leucovorin, prochlorperazine.

Adverse effects
- CNS: *Headache, seizures,* paresthesia, tremor, ataxia, abnormal coordination, **coma, death**, depression, confusion, anxiety, insomnia, nervousness, emotional lability, vision changes, taste abnormalities
- GI: *Nausea, vomiting, diarrhea,* abdominal pain, dry mouth, melena, pancreatitis
- Respiratory: Cough, dyspnea, pneumonia, sinusitis, pharyngitis
- Hematologic: **Bone marrow suppression**, *anemia,* mineral and electrolyte imbalance
- Renal: **Acute renal failure,** *abnormal renal funtions,* dysuria, polyuria, urinary retention, urinary tract infections
- Other: *Fever;* fatigue, rash, pain, edema, pain at site of injection

Clinically important drug-drug interactions
- Increased risk of renal problems if taken with other renal toxic drugs • Risk of hypocalcemia if given with pentamidine

■ Nursing Considerations

Assessment
- *History:* Presence of allergy to foscarnet, lactation
- *Physical:* Skin—color, lesions; body temperature; orientation, reflexes, affect; urinary output; R, adventitious sounds; CBC, serum electrolytes, renal function tests

Implementation
- Administer by IV route only; do administer by bolus or rapid injection.
- Monitor serum creatinine and renal function carefully during treatment; dosage adjustment may be necessary.
- Stop infusion immediately at any report of tingling, paresthesias, numbness. Monitor electrolytes as appropriate.
- Ensure adequate hydration during treatment; push fluids to ensure diuresis and decrease the risk of renal impairment.
- Arrange for periodic ophthalmic exams for retinitis; foscarnet is not a cure.

Adverse effects in *Italics* are most common; those in **Bold** are life-threatening.

Drug-specific teaching points
- Be aware that this drug must be given IV using a special pump.
- Know that foscarnet is not a cure for retinitis; symptoms may continue while on therapy. It is important to arrange for periodic ophthalmic exams.
- Drink a lot of fluids, and know that a lot of IV fluids may be given to you during therapy.
- Arrange for periodic medical exams, including blood tests, while on this drug.
- Know that the following side effects may occur: fever, headache (appropriate medication may be arranged); dizziness, fatigue, vision changes (do not drive or operate dangerous machinery while these effects occur); nausea, vomiting, diarrhea (ensure ready access to bathroom facilities).
- Report tingling around the mouth, numbness, "heavy" extremities, difficulty breathing, leg cramps, tremors, pain at injection site.

☐ fosinopril sodium

(foh sin' oh pril)
Monopril
Pregnancy Category D

Drug classes
Antihypertensive
Angiotensin-converting enzyme inhibitor

Therapeutic actions
Renin, synthesized by the kidneys, is released into the circulation where it acts on a plasma precursor to produce angiotensin I, which is converted by angiotensin-converting enzyme to angiotensin II, a potent vasoconstrictor that also causes release of aldosterone from the adrenals; benazepril blocks the conversion of angiotensin I to angiotensin II, leading to decreased blood pressure, decreased aldosterone secretion, a small increase in serum potassium levels, and sodium and fluid loss; increased prostaglandin synthesis also may be involved in the antihypertensive action.

Indications
- Treatment of hypertension, alone or in combination with thiazide-type diuretics

Contraindications/cautions
- Contraindicated in the presence of allergy to fosinopril or other ACE inhibitors.
- Use caution with impaired renal function, CHF, salt/volume depletion, lactation.

Dosage
Adult: Initial dose: 10 mg PO qd. Maintenance dose: 20–40 mg/d PO as a single dose or two divided doses. Patients on diuretics should discontinue the diuretic 2–3 d before beginning fosinopril therapy. If blood pressure is not controlled, add diuretic slowly. If diuretic cannot be discontinued, begin fosinopril therapy with 10 mg.
Pediatric: Safety and efficacy not established.

Pharmacokinetics

Route	Onset	Peak	Duration
Oral	1 h	3 h	24 h

Metabolism: Hepatic, $T_{1/2}$: 12 h
Distribution: Crosses placenta; enters breast milk
Excretion: Urine and feces

Adverse effects
- **GI:** *Nausea,* abdominal pain, vomiting, diarrhea
- **CV:** Angina pectoris, orthostatic hypotension in salt/volume depleted patients, palpitations
- **Respiratory:** *Cough,* asthma, bronchitis, dyspnea, sinusitis
- **Dermatologic:** Rash, pruritus, diaphoresis, flushing
- **Other:** Angioedema, asthenia, myalgia, arthralgia

■ Nursing Considerations
Assessment
- *History:* Allergy to fosinopril and other ACE inhibitors, impaired renal function, CHF, salt/volume depletion, lactation

Adverse effects in *Italics* are most common; those in **Bold** are life-threatening.

- *Physical:* Skin—color, lesions, turgor; body temperature; P, BP, peripheral perfusion; mucous membranes, bowel sounds, liver evaluation; urinalysis, renal and liver function tests, CBC, and differential

Implementation
- Alert surgeon and mark patient's chart with notice that fosinopril is being taken; the angiotensin II formation subsequent to compensatory renin release during surgery will be blocked; hypotension may be reversed with volume expansion.
- Monitor patient closely in any situation that may lead to a fall in blood pressure secondary to reduction in fluid volume (excessive perspiration and dehydration, vomiting, diarrhea) because excessive hypotension may occur.

Drug-specific teaching points
- Do not stop taking the medication without consulting your prescriber.
- Know that the following side effects may occur: GI upset, loss of appetite (these may be limited effects that will pass with time); lightheadedness (this usually passes after the first few days of therapy; if it occurs, change position slowly and limit your activities to those that do not require alertness and precision); dry cough (this is irritating but not harmful).
- Be careful in any situation that may lead to a drop in blood pressure (diarrhea, sweating, vomiting, dehydration); if lightheadedness or dizziness occurs, consult your care provider.
- Report mouth sores; sore throat, fever, chills; swelling of the hands, feet; irregular heartbeat, chest pains; swelling of the face, eyes, lips, tongue, difficulty in breathing, persistent cough.

☐ furosemide

(fur ob' se mide)
Lasix, Novosemide (CAN), Uritol (CAN)

Pregnancy Category C

Drug classes
Loop (high-ceiling) diuretic

Therapeutic actions
Inhibits the reabsorption of sodium and chloride from the proximal and distal renal tubules and the loop of Henle, leading to a sodium-rich diuresis.

Indications
- Edema associated with CHF, cirrhosis, renal disease (oral, IV)
- Acute pulmonary edema (IV)
- Hypertension (oral)

Contraindications/cautions
- Contraindicated in the presence of allergy to furosemide, sulfonamides; allergy to tartrazine (in oral solution); electrolyte depletion; anuria, severe renal failure; hepatic coma; pregnancy; lactation.
- Use caution in the presence of SLE, gout, diabetes mellitus.

Dosage
Adult
- ***Edema:*** Initially, 20–80 mg/d PO as a single dose. If needed, a second dose may be given in 6–8 h. If response is unsatisfactory, dose may be increased in 20- to 40-mg increments at 6- to 8-h intervals. Up to 600 mg/d may be given. Intermittent dosage schedule (2–4 consecutive d/wk) is preferred for maintenance, *or* 20–40 mg IM or IV (slow IV injection over 1–2 min). May increase dose in increments of 20 mg in 2 h. High-dose therapy should be given as infusion at rate not exceeding 4 mg/min.
- ***Acute pulmonary edema:*** 40 mg IV over 1–2 min. May be increased to 80 mg IV given over 1–2 min if response is unsatisfactory after 1 h.
- ***Hypertension:*** 40 mg bid PO. If needed, additional antihypertensive agents may be added at 50% usual dosage.

Pediatric: Avoid use in premature infants: stimulates PGE_2 synthesis and may increase incidence of patent ductus arteriosus and complicate respiratory distress syndrome.
- ***Hypertension:*** Initially, 2 mg/kg per day PO. If needed, increase by 1–2

furosemide ■ 519

mg/kg in 6–8 h. *Do not exceed* 6 mg/kg. Adjust maintenance dose to lowest effective level.
- ***Edema:*** 1 mg/kg IV or IM. May increase by 1 mg/kg in 2 h until the desired effect is seen. *Do not exceed* 6 mg/kg.

Geriatric or renal impaired: Up to 2–2.5 g/d has been tolerated. IV bolus injection should not exceed 1 g/d given over 30 min.

Pharmacokinetics

Route	Onset	Peak	Duration
Oral	60 min	60–120 min	6–8 h
IV/IM	5 min	30 min	2 h

Metabolism: Hepatic, $T_{1/2}$: 120 min
Distribution: Crosses placenta; enters breast milk
Excretion: Urine

IV facts

Preparation: Store at room temperature; exposure to light may slightly discolor solution.
Infusion: Inject directly or into tubing of actively running IV; inject slowly over 1–2 min.
Incompatibilites: Do not mix with acidic solutions, isotonic saline, Lactated Ringer's Injection, and 5% Dextrose Injection may be used after pH has been adjusted (if necessary); precipitates form with gentamicin, netilimicin, milrinone in 5% Dextrose, 0.9% Sodium Chloride.

Adverse effects

- CNS: *Dizziness, vertigo, paresthesias, xanthopsia, weakness,* headache, drowsiness, fatigue, blurred vision, tinnitus, **irreversible hearing loss**
- GI: *Nausea, anorexia, vomiting, oral and gastric irritation, constipation;* diarrhea, acute pancreatitis, jaundice
- CV: *Orthostatic hypotension,* volume depletion, cardiac arrhythmias, *thrombophlebitis*
- Hematologic: *Leukopenia, anemia, thrombocytopenia,* fluid and electrolyte imbalances
- GU: Polyuria, nocturia, *glycosuria, urinary bladder spasm*
- Dermatologic: *Photosensitivity, rash, pruritus, urticaria,* purpura, exfoliative dermatitis, erythema multiforme
- Other: *Muscle cramps and muscle spasms*

Clinically important drug-drug interactions

• Increased risk of cardiac arrhythmias if taken concurrently with digitalis glycosides (due to electrolyte imbalance) • Increased risk of ototoxicity if taken with aminoglycoside antibiotics, cisplatin • Decreased absorption of furosemide if taken with phenytoin • Decreased natriuretic and antihypertensive effects of furosemide if taken with indomethacin, ibuprofen, other NSAIDs • Decreased GI absorption of furosemide if taken with charcoal

■ Nursing Considerations

Assessment

- *History*: Allergy to furosemide, sulfonamides, tartrazine; electrolyte depletion anuria, severe renal failure; hepatic coma; SLE; gout; diabetes mellitus; lactation
- *Physical*: Skin—color, lesions, edema; orientation, reflexes, hearing; pulses, baseline ECG, BP, orthostatic BP, perfusion; R, pattern, adventitious sounds; liver evaluation, bowel sounds; urinary output patterns; CBC, serum electrolytes (including calcium), blood sugar, liver and renal function tests, uric acid, urinalysis

Implementation

- Administer with food or milk to prevent GI upset.
- Reduce dosage if given concurrently with other antihypertensives; readjust dosages gradually as blood pressure responds.
- Administer early in the day if possible so that increased urination will not disturb sleep.
- Avoid IV use if oral use is at all possible.
- Do not mix parenteral solution with highly acidic solutions with pH below 3.5.

Adverse effects in *Italics* are most common; those in **Bold** are life-threatening.

- Do not expose to light, which may discolor tablets or solution; do not use discolored drug or drug solutions.
- Discard diluted solution after 24 h.
- Refrigerate oral solution.
- Measure and record regular body weights to monitor fluid changes.
- Arrange to monitor serum electrolytes, hydration, liver function during long-term therapy.
- Arrange for potassium-rich diet or supplemental potassium as needed.

Drug-specific teaching points

- Record intermittent therapy on a calendar or dated envelopes. When possible, take the drug early in the day so increased urination will not disturb sleep. The drug should be taken with food or meals to prevent GI upset.
- Weigh yourself on a regular basis, at the same time of the day and in the same clothing, and record the weight on your calendar.
- Know that the following side effects may occur: increased volume and frequency of urination (ensure access to a bathroom when drug effect is greatest); dizziness, feeling faint on arising, drowsiness (if these changes occur, avoid rapid position changes; hazardous activities, like driving a car; and consumption of alcohol, which can intensify these problems); sensitivity to sunlight (use sunglasses, wear protective clothing, or use a sunscreen when outdoors); increased thirst (sucking on sugarless lozenges may help to alleviate the thirst; frequent mouth care also may help); loss of body potassium (a potassium-rich diet, or even a potassium supplement, will be necessary).
- Report loss or gain of more than 3 lb in one day, swelling in your ankles or fingers, unusual bleeding or bruising, dizziness, trembling, numbness, fatigue, muscle weakness or cramps.

▢ gabapentin

*(gab ah **pen**' tin)*
Neurontin

Pregnancy Category C

Drug classes
Antiepileptic

Therapeutic actions
Mechanism of action not understood; antiepileptic activity may be related to its ability to inhibit polysynaptic responses and block post-tetanic potentiation.

Indications
- Adjunctive therapy in the treatment of partial seizures with and without secondary generalization in adults with epilepsy

Contraindications/cautions
- Hypersensitivity to gabapentin, lactation.

Dosage
Adult: 900–1,800 mg/d PO in divided doses three times per day PO; maximum time between doses should not exceed 12 h. Up to 2,400–3,600 mg/d has been used. Initial dose of 300 mg/d PO; 300 mg bid PO on day 2; 300 tid PO on day 3.
Pediatric: Safety and efficacy not established.
Geriatric or renal impaired: Creatinine clearance > 60 ml/min: 400 mg tid PO; 30–60 ml/min: 300 mg bid PO; 15–30 ml/min: 300 mg qd PO; < 15 ml/min: 300 mg qod PO; dialysis: 200–300 mg PO following each 4 h of dialysis.

Pharmacokinetics

Route	Onset	Duration
Oral	Varies	6–8 h

Metabolism: $T_{1/2}$: 5–7 h
Distribution: Crosses placenta; enters breast milk
Excretion: Urine

Adverse effects
- **CNS:** *Dizziness, insomnia,* nervousness, fatigue, *somnolence, ataxia,* diplopia
- **GI:** Dyspepsia, vomiting, nausea, constipation
- **Respiratory:** Rhinitis, pharyngitis
- **Dermatologic:** Pruritus, abrasion
- **Other:** Weight gain, facial edema, cancer, impotence

Clinically important drug-drug interactions
- Decreased serum levels of gabapentin if given with antacids

■ Nursing Considerations
Assessment
- *History:* Hypersensitivity to gabapentin; lactation
- *Physical:* Body weight; body temperature; skin—color, lesions; orientation, affect, reflexes; P; R, adventitious sounds; bowel sounds, normal output

Implementation
- Give drug with food to prevent GI upset.
- Arrange for consultation with support groups for epileptics as needed.

Drug-specific teaching points
- Take this drug exactly as prescribed; do not discontinue this drug abruptly or change dosage, except on the advice of your physician.
- Know that the following side effects may occur: dizziness, blurred vision (avoid driving a car or performing other tasks requiring alertness or visual acuity if this occurs); GI upset (taking the drug with food or milk and eating frequent small meals may help); headache, nervousness, insomnia, fatigue (periodic rest periods may be helpful).
- Wear a medical alert tag at all times so that any emergency medical personnel taking care of you will know that you are an epileptic taking antiepileptic medication.
- Report severe headache, sleepwalking, skin rash, severe vomiting, chills, fever, difficulty breathing.

❒ gallium nitrate

(gal' ee um)
Ganite

Pregnancy Category C

Drug classes
Antihypercalcemic drug

Therapeutic actions
Inhibits calcium resorption from bone, reduces bone turnover, resulting in lower serum calcium levels.

Indications
- Treatment of cancer-related hypercalcemia (clearly symptomatic) unresponsive to adequate hydration

Contraindications/cautions
- Contraindicated in the presence of severe renal impairment, lactation.
- Use caution in the presence of asymptomatic or mild to moderate hypocalcemia, visual and auditory disturbances, pregnancy.

Dosage
Adult: 200 mg/m^2 IV per day for 5 consecutive d; 100 mg/m^2 IV per day may be effective in mild hypercalcemia.
Pediatric: Safety and efficacy not established.

Pharmacokinetics

Route	Onset	Peak	Duration
IV	Slow	2 d	3–4 d

Metabolism: T$_{1/2}$: unknown
Distribution: May cross placenta; may enter breast milk
Excretion: Urine

IV facts
Preparation: Dilute daily dose in in 1 L 0.9% Sodium Chloride Injection or 5% Dextrose Injection. Stable for 48 h at room temperature and 7 d refrigerated; discard any unused portion after that time.
Infusion: Infuse slowly over 24 h.
Incompatibilities: Do not mix with IV anesthetics; precipitates may form.

Adverse effects
- CNS: Acute optic neuritis, visual impairment, decreased hearing
- GI: Nausea, vomiting, diarrhea, constipation

Adverse effects in *Italics* are most common; those in **Bold** are life-threatening.

- **GU:** *Rising BUN, creatinine;* **acute renal failure**
- **CV:** Tachycardia, edema, decreased blood pressure
- **Respiratory:** Dyspnea, rales and rhonchi, pleural effusion, pulmonary infiltrates
- **Metabolic:** *Hypocalcemia; decreased serum bicarbonate*

Clinically important drug-drug interactions

- Increased risk of nephrotoxicity if taken with other nephrotoxic drugs: aminoglycosides, amphotericin B

■ Nursing Considerations

Assessment

- *History:* Severe renal impairment, lactation, hypocalcemia, visual and auditory disturbances, pregnancy
- *Physical:* Body weight, skin condition, hydration, reflexes, P, BP, R and adventitious sounds, kidney function tests, serum electrolytes, especially calcium, phosphorus

Implementation

- Monitor serum calcium, phosphorus, renal function daily during therapy and twice weekly thereafter.
- Arrange to discontinue gallium if serum creatinine exceeds 2.5 mg/dl.
- Arrange to discontinue gallium therapy if serum calcium levels return to normal before the 5-d course is finished.
- Maintain adequate hydration during therapy; use caution to avoid overhydraton if patient is cardiac compromised.

Drug-specific teaching points

- Know that the drug can be given only IV and must be given for 5 consecutive d; frequent blood tests will be needed to evaluate the effects of the drug on your body.
- Report difficulty breathing, very slow breathing, changes in vision or hearing, numbness or tingling.

⬜ ganciclovir sodium

(gan sye' kloe vir)

DHPG

Cytovene

Pregnancy Category C

Drug classes
Antiviral drug

Therapeutic actions
Antiviral activity; inhibits viral DNA replication in cytomegalovirus (CMV).

Indications

- Treatment of CMV retinitis in immunocompromised patients, including patients with AIDS (safety and efficacy for treatment of other CMV infections and congenital or neonatal CMV disease has not been established)

Contraindications/cautions

- Contraindicated in the presence of hypersensitivity to ganciclovir or acyclovir, lactation.
- Use caution in the presence of cytopenia, history of cytopenic reactions, impaired renal function.

Dosage

Adult

- ***Initial dose:*** 5 mg/kg given IV at a constant rate over 1 h, q12h for 14–21 d.
- ***Maintenance:*** 5 mg/kg given by IV infusion over 1 h once/d, 7 d/wk *or* 6 mg/kg once/d, 5 d/wk.

Pediatric: Safety and efficacy not established. Use only if benefit outweighs potential carcinogenesis and reproductive toxicity.

Geriatric or renal impaired: Reduce initial dose by up to 50%, monitoring patient response. *Maintenance dose:*

Creatinine Clearance	Dose (mg/kg)	Dosing Intervals (h)
≥80	5	12
50–79	2.5	12
25–49	2.5	24
<25	1.25	24

Adverse effects in *Italics* are most common; those in **Bold** are life-threatening.

ganciclovir sodium ■ 523

Pharmacokinetics

Route	Onset	Peak
IV	Slow	1 h

Metabolism: $T_{1/2}$: 2–4 h
Distribution: Crosses placenta; may enter breast milk
Excretion: Urine

IV facts
Preparation: Reconstitute vial by injecting 10 ml of Sterile Water for Injection into vial; *do not* use Bacteriostatic Water for Injection; shake vial to dissolve the drug. Discard vial if any particulate matter or discoloration is seen. Reconstituted solution in the vial is stable at room temperature for 12 h. *Do not refrigerate* reconstituted solution.
Infusion: Infuse slowly over 1 h.
Compatibilities: Compatible with 0.9% Sodium Chloride, 5% Dextrose, Ringer's Injection, and Lactated Ringer's Injection.

Adverse effects
- CNS: Dreams, ataxia, coma, confusion, dizziness, headache
- GI: *Abnormal liver function tests*, nausea, vomiting, anorexia, diarrhea, abdominal pain
- CV: Arrhythmia, hypertension, hypotension
- Hematologic: *Granulocytopenia, thrombocytopenia, anemia*
- Dermatologic: *Rash,* alopecia, pruritus, urticaria
- Local: *Pain, inflammation at injection site*, phlebitis
- Other: *Fever*, chills, **cancer, sterility**

Clinically important drug-drug interactions
• Increased ganciclovir effects if taken with probenecid • Use with extreme caution with cytotoxic drugs because the accumulation effect could cause severe bone marrow depression and other GI and dermatologic problems • Increased risk of seizures if taken concurrently with imipenem-cilastatin • Extreme drowsiness and risk of bone marrow depression if taken with zidovudine

■ Nursing Considerations

Assessment
- *History:* Hypersensitivity to ganciclovir or acyclovir; cytopenia; impaired renal function; lactation
- *Physical:* Skin color, lesions; orientation; BP, P, auscultation, perfusion, edema; R, adventitious sounds; urinary output; CBC, Hct, BUN, creatinine clearance, liver function tests

Implementation
- Administer by IV infusion only. Do not give IM or SC because the drug can be very irritating to the tissues.
- Do not exceed the recommended dosage, frequency, or infusion rates.
- Monitor infusion carefully; infuse at concentrations no greater than 10 mg/ml.
- Arrange for decreased dosage in patients with impaired renal function.
- Arrange for CBC before beginning therapy and every 2 d during daily dosing and at least weekly thereafter. Consult with physician and arrange for reduced dosage if WBCs or platelets fall.
- Consult with pharmacy for proper disposal of unused solution. Precautions are required for disposal of nucleoside analogues.
- Provide patient with a calendar of drug days, and help to arrange convenient times for the IV infusion in outpatients.
- Arrange for periodic ophthalmic examinations during therapy. Drug is not a cure for the disease, and deterioration may occur.
- Advise patients that ganciclovir can decrease sperm production in men and cause birth defects in the fetuses of pregnant women. Advise the patient to use some form of contraception during ganciclovir therapy. Men receiving ganciclovir therapy should use some form of barrier contraception during and for at least 90 d after ganciclovir therapy.

Adverse effects in *Italics* are most common; those in **Bold** are life-threatening.

524 ■ gemfibrozil

- Advise patient that ganciclovir has caused cancer in animals and that risk is possible in humans.

Drug-specific teaching points

- Know that this drug will need to be given daily and can be given only through an IV line. Appointments will be made for outpatients. Long-term therapy is frequently needed.
- Know that frequent blood tests will be necessary to determine the effects of the drug on your blood count and to determine the appropriate dosage needed. It is important that you keep appointments for these tests.
- Arrange for periodic ophthalmic examinations during therapy to evaluate progress of the disease. This drug is not a cure for your retinitis.
- Be aware that if you also are receiving zidovudine, the two drugs cannot be given concomitantly; severe adverse effects may occur.
- Know that the following side effects may occur: rash, fever, pain at injection site; decreased blood count leading to susceptibility to infection (frequent blood tests will be needed; avoid crowds and exposure to disease as much as possible); birth defects and decreased sperm production (the drug cannot be taken during pregnancy; if you think you are pregnant or wish to become pregnant, consult with your physician; use some form of contraception during drug therapy; male patients should use a form of barrier contraception during drug therapy and for at least 90 d after therapy).
- Report bruising, bleeding, pain at injection site, fever, infection.

▢ gemfibrozil

(jem fi' broe zil)
Lopid

Pregnancy Category B

Drug classes
Antihyperlipidemic agent

Therapeutic actions
Inhibits peripheral lipolysis and decreases the hepatic excretion of free fatty acids; this reduces hepatic triglyceride production; inhibits synthesis of VLDL carrier apolipoprotein; decreases VLDL production; increases HDL concentration.

Indications
- Hypertriglyceridemia in adult patients with triglyceride levels > 750 mg/dl (type IV and V hyperlipidemia) at risk of abdominal pain and pancreatitis who do not respond to diet therapy
- Reduction of coronary heart disease risk, possibly effective

Contraindications/cautions
- Allergy to gemfibrozil, hepatic or renal dysfunction, primary biliary cirrhosis, gallbladder disease, pregnancy, lactation.

Dosage
Adult: 1,200 mg/d PO in two divided doses, 30 min before morning and evening meals. Adjust dosage to patient response; dosages may range from 900–1,500 mg/d. *Caution:* Use this drug only if strongly indicated and lipid studies show a definite response; hepatic tumorigenicity occurs in laboratory animals.
Pediatric: Safety and efficacy not established.

Pharmacokinetics

Route	Onset	Peak
Oral	Varies	1–2 h

Metabolism: Hepatic, $T_{1/2}$: 1½ h
Distribution: Crosses placenta; enters breast milk
Excretion: Urine and feces

Adverse effects
- **CNS:** *Headache, dizziness, blurred vision*, vertigo, insomnia, paresthesia, tinnitus, *fatigue*, malaise, syncope
- **GI:** *Abdominal pain, epigastric pain, diarrhea, nausea, vomiting*, flatulence, dry mouth, constipation, anorexia, *dyspepsia*, cholelithiasis

Adverse effects in *Italics* are most common; those in **Bold** are life-threatening.

- **Hematologic:** Anemia, eosinophilia, leukopenia, hypokalemia, liver function changes, hyperglycemia
- **GU:** Impairment of fertility
- **Dermatologic:** *Eczema, rash*, dermatitis, pruritus, urticaria
- **Other:** Painful extremities, back pain, arthralgia, muscle cramps, myalgia, swollen joints

■ Nursing Considerations

Assessment
- *History:* Allergy to gemfibrozil, hepatic or renal dysfunction, primary biliary cirrhosis, gallbladder disease, pregnancy, lactation
- *Physical:* Skin—lesions, color, temperature; gait, range of motion; orientation, affect, reflexes; bowel sounds, normal output, liver evaluation; lipid studies, CBC, liver and renal function tests, blood glucose

Implementation
- Administer drug with meals or milk if GI upset occurs.
- Arrange for regular follow-up, including blood tests for lipids, liver function, CBC, blood glucose during long-term therapy.

Drug-specific teaching points
- Take the drug with meals or with milk if GI upset occurs; diet changes will need to be made.
- Know that the following side effects may occur: diarrhea, loss of appetite, flatulence (ensure ready access to the bathroom if diarrhea occurs; small, frequent meals may help); muscular aches and pains, bone and joint discomfort; dizziness, faintness, blurred vision (use caution if driving or operating dangerous equipment).
- Arrange for regular follow-up visits to your doctor for blood tests to evaluate the effectiveness of this drug.
- Report severe stomach pain with nausea and vomiting, fever and chills or sore throat, severe headache, vision changes.

▢ gentamicin sulfate

(jen ta mye' sin)

Parenteral, intrathecal:
Alcomicin (CAN), Cidomycin (CAN), Garamycin, Jenamicin

Topical dermatologic cream, ointment: Garamycin

Ophthalmic: Garamycin, Gentak, Gentacidin, Genoptic

Gentamicin impregnated PMMA beads: Septopal, Gentamicin liposome injection

Pregnancy Category C

Drug classes
Aminoglycoside antibiotic

Therapeutic actions
Bactericidal: inhibits protein synthesis in susceptible strains of gram-negative bacteria; appears to disrupt functional integrity of bacterial cell membrane, causing cell death.

Indications
Parenteral
- Serious infections caused by susceptible strains of *Pseudomonas aeruginosa, Proteus, Escherichia coli, Klebsiella- Enterobacter-Serratia* species, *Citrobacter*, staphylococci
- In serious infections when causative organisms are not known (often in conjunction with a penicillin or cephalosporin)
- Unlabeled use: with clindamycin as alternative regimen in pelvic inflammatory disease (PID)

Intrathecal
- For serious CNS infections caused by susceptible *Pseudomonas* species

Ophthalmic Preparations
- Treatment of superficial ocular infections due to strain of microorganisms susceptible to gentamicin

Topical Dermatologic Preparation
- Infection prophylaxis in minor skin abrasions and treatment of superficial infec-

Adverse effects in *Italics* are most common; those in **Bold** are life-threatening.

tions of the skin due to susceptible organisms amenable to local treatment

Gentamicin-Impregnated PMAA Beads on Surgical Wire

- Orphan drug use: treatment of chronic osteomyelitis of post-traumatic, postoperative, or hematogenous origin

Gentamicin Liposome Injection

- Orphan drug use: treatment of disseminated *Myobacterium avium-intracellulare* infection

Contraindications/cautions

- Contraindicated in the presence of allergy to any aminoglycosides; renal or hepatic disease; preexisting hearing loss; active infection with herpes, vaccinia, varicella, fungal infections, myobacterial infections (ophthalmic preparations); myasthenia gravis; parkinsonism; infant botulism; lactation.
- Use caution during pregnancy.

Dosage

Adult: 3 mg/kg per day in three equal doses q8h IM or IV. Up to 5 mg/kg per day in three to four equal doses in severe infections. For IV use, a loading dose of 1–2 mg/kg may be infused over 30–60 min, followed by a maintenance dose.

- ***PID:*** 2 mg/kg IV followed by 1.5 mg/kg tid plus clindamycin 600 mg IV qid. Continue for at least 4 d and at least 48 h after patient improves, then continue clindamycin 450 mg orally qid for 10–14 d total therapy.
- ***Surgical prophylaxis regimens:*** Several complex, multidrug prophylaxis regimens are available for preoperative use; consult manufacturer's instructions.

Pediatric: 2–2.5 mg/kg q8h IM or IV. Infants and neonates: 2.5 mg/kg q8h. Premature or full-term neonates: 2.5 mg/kg q12h.

Geriatric or renal failure patients: Reduce dosage or extend time dosage intervals, and carefully monitor serum drug levels and renal function tests throughout treatment.

- *Ophthalmic solution:* 1–2 drops into affected eye(s) q4h; up to 2 drops hourly in severe infections.
- *Ophthalmic ointment:* Apply small amount to affected eye bid–tid.
- *Dermatologic preparations:* Apply one to five times per day. Cover with sterile bandage if needed.

Pharmacokinetics

Route	Onset	Peak
IM/IV	Rapid	30–90 min

Metabolism: $T_{1/2}$: 2–3 h
Distribution: Crosses placenta; enters breast milk
Excretion: Urine

IV facts

Preparation: Dilute single dose in 50–200 ml of sterile isotonic saline or 5% Dextrose in Water. Do not mix in solution with any other drugs.

Infusion: Infuse over $1/2$–2 h.

Incompatibilities: Do not mix in solution with any other drugs.

Adverse effects

- CNS: Ototoxicity—*tinnitus, dizziness, ringing in the ears,* vertigo, **deafness** (partially reversible to irreversible), vestibular paralysis, confusion, disorientation, depression, lethargy, nystagmus, visual disturbances, headache, *numbness, tingling,* tremor, paresthesias, muscle twitching, convulsions, muscular weakness, neuromuscular blockade
- GI: Hepatic toxicity, *nausea, vomiting, anorexia,* weight loss, stomatitis, increased salivation
- CV: Palpitations, hypotension, hypertension
- Hematologic: *Leukemoid reaction,* agranulocytosis, granulocytosis, leukopenia, leukocytosis, thrombocytopenia, eosinophilia, pancytopenia, anemia, hemolytic anemia, increased or decreased reticulocyte count, electrolyte disturbances
- GU: *Nephrotoxicity*

Adverse effects in *Italics* are most common; those in **Bold** are life-threatening.

- Hypersensitivity: *Purpura, rash,* urticaria, exfoliative dermatitis, itching
- Local: *Pain, irritation, arachnoiditis at IM injection sites*
- Other: Fever, apnea, splenomegaly, joint pain, *superinfections*

Ophthalmic Preparations
- Local: *Transient irritation, burning, stinging, itching,* angioneurotic edema, urticaria, vesicular and maculopapular dermatitis

Topical Dermatologic Preparations
- Local: *photosensitization,* superinfections

Clinically important drug-drug interactions
- Increased ototoxic, nephrotoxic, neurotoxic effects if taken with other aminoglycosides, cephalothin, potent diuretics • Increased neuromuscular blockade and muscular paralysis when given with anesthetics, nondepolarizing neuromuscular blocking drugs, succinylcholine, citrate-anticoagulated blood • Potential inactivation of both drugs if mixed with beta-lactam-type antibiotics (space doses when patient is receiving concomitant therapy) • Increased bactericidal effect if combined with penicillins, cephalopsorins (when used to treat some gram-negative organisms and enterococci) carbenicillin, ticarcillin (when used to treat *Pseudomonas* infections)

■ Nursing Considerations

Assessment
- *History:* Allergy to any aminoglycosides; renal or hepatic disease; preexisting hearing loss; active infection with herpes, vaccinia, varicella, fungal infections, myobacterial infections (ophthalmic preparations); myasthenia gravis; parkinsonism; infant botulism; lactation
- *Physical:* Site of infection; skin—color, lesions; orientation, reflexes, eighth cranial nerve function; P, BP ; R, adventitious sounds; bowel sounds, liver evaluation; urinalysis, BUN, serum creatinine, serum electrolytes, liver function tests, CBC

Implementation
- Administer by IM route if at all possible; give by deep IM injection.
- Culture infected area before beginning therapy.
- Use 2 mg/ml intrathecal preparation without preservatives, for intrathetal use.
- Cleanse area before application of dermatologic preparations.
- Ensure adequate hydration of patient before and during therapy.
- Arrange for monitoring of renal function tests, complete blood counts, serum drug levels during long-term therapy. Consult with prescriber to adjust dosage accordingly.

Drug-specific teaching points
- Apply ophthalmic preparations by tilting head back; place medications into conjunctival sac and close eye; apply light pressure on lacrimal sac for 1 min. Cleanse area before applying dermatologic preparations; cover if necessary.
- Know that the following side effects may occur: ringing in the ears, headache, dizziness (these effects are reversible; safety measures may need to be taken if these become severe); nausea, vomiting, loss of appetite (small frequent meals, frequent mouth care may help); burning, blurring of vision with ophthalmic preparations (avoid driving or performing dangerous activities if visual effects occur); photosensitization with dermatologic preparations (wear a sunscreen, and wear protective clothing to protect the skin).
- Report pain at injection site, severe headache, dizziness, loss of hearing, changes in urine pattern, difficulty breathing, rash or skin lesions; itching or irritation (ophthalmic preparations); worsening of the condition, rash, irritation (dermatologic preparation).

❑ glipizide

(glip' i zide)
Glucotrol

Pregnancy Category C

Adverse effects in *Italics* are most common; those in **Bold** are life-threatening.

Drug classes
Antidiabetic agent
Sulfonylurea, second generation

Therapeutic actions
Stimulates insulin release from functioning beta cells in the pancreas; may improve binding between insulin and insulin receptors or increase the number of insulin receptors; more potent in effect than first-generation sulfonylureas.

Indications
- Adjunct to diet to lower blood glucose in patients with non–insulin-dependent diabetes mellitus (Type II)
- Adjunct to insulin therapy in the stabilization of certain cases of insulin-dependent maturity-onset diabetes, reducing the insulin requirement and decreasing the chance of hypoglycemic reactions

Contraindications/cautions
- Allergy to sulfonylureas; diabetes complicated by fever, severe infections, severe trauma, major surgery, ketosis, acidosis, coma (insulin is indicated in these conditions); Type I or juvenile diabetes, serious hepatic impairment, serious renal impairment, uremia, thyroid or endocrine impairment, glycosuria, hyperglycemia associated with primary renal disease; labor and delivery (if glipizide is used during pregnancy, discontinue drug at least 1 mo before delivery); lactation.

Dosage
Give approximately 30 min before meal to achieve greatest reduction in postprandial hyperglycemia.
Adult
- *Initial therapy:* 5 mg PO before breakfast. Adjust dosage in increments of 2.5–5 mg as determined by blood glucose response. At least several days should elapse between titration steps. Maximum once-daily dose should not exceed 15 mg; above 15 mg, divide dose, and administer before meals. Do not exceed 40 mg/d.
- *Maintenance therapy:* Total daily doses above 15 mg PO should be divided; total daily doses above 30 mg are given in divided doses bid.

Pediatric: Safety and efficacy not established.

Geriatric and hepatic impaired: Geriatric patients tend to be more sensitive to the drug. Start with initial dose of 2.5 mg/d PO. Monitor for 24 h and gradually increase dose after several days as needed.

Pharmacokinetics

Route	Onset	Peak	Duration
Oral	1–1.5 h	1–3 h	10–16 h

Metabolism: Hepatic, $T_{1/2}$: 2–4 h
Distribution: Crosses placenta; enters breast milk
Excretion: Bile and urine

Adverse effects
- **GI**: *Anorexia, nausea*, vomiting, *epigastric discomfort, heartburn, diarrhea*
- **CV:** Increased risk of cardiovascular mortality
- **Hematologic:** Leukopenia, thrombocytopenia, anemia
- **Hypersensitivity:** *Allergic skin reactions*, eczema, pruritus, erythema, urticaria, photosensitivity, fever, eosinophilia, jaundice
- **Endocrine:** *Hypoglycemia*

Clinically important drug-drug interactions
- Increased risk of hypoglycemia if glipizide is taken concurrently with sulfonamides, chloramphenicol, fenfluramine, oxyphenbutazone, phenylbutazone, salicylates, clofibrate • Decreased effectiveness of glipizide and diazoxide if taken concurrently • Increased risk of hyperglycemia if glipizide is taken with rifampin, thiazides
- Risk of hypoglycemia and hyperglycemia if glipizide is taken with ethanol; "disulfiram reaction" also has been reported

■ Nursing Considerations

Assessment
- *History:* Allergy to sulfonylureas; diabetes with complications; Type I or juvenile diabetes, serious hepatic or renal impair-

Adverse effects in *Italics* are most common; those in **Bold** are life-threatening.

ment, uremia, thyroid or endocrine impairment, glycosuria, hyperglycemia associated with primary renal disease
- *Physical:* Skin—color, lesions; body temperature; orientation, reflexes, peripheral sensation; R, adventitious sounds; liver evaluation, bowel sounds; urinalysis, BUN, serum creatinine, liver function tests, blood glucose, CBC

Implementation
- Administer drug in the morning before breakfast; if severe GI upset occurs or more than 15 mg/d is required, dose may be divided and given before meals.
- Monitor urine and serum glucose levels frequently to determine effectiveness of drug and dosage being used.
- Arrange for transfer to insulin therapy during periods of high stress (eg, infections, surgery, trauma).
- Arrange for use of IV glucose if severe hypoglycemia occurs as a result of overdose.

Drug-specific teaching points
- Do not discontinue this medication without consulting physician.
- Monitor urine or blood for glucose and ketones as prescribed.
- Do not use this drug during pregnancy.
- Avoid alcohol while on this drug.
- Report fever, sore throat, unusual bleeding or bruising, skin rash, dark urine, light-colored stools, hypoglycemic or hyperglycemic reactions.

▢ glucagon

(gloo' ka gon)
Pregnancy Category B

Drug classes
Glucose elevating agent
Hormone
Diagnostic agent

Therapeutic actions
Accelerates the breakdown of glycogen to glucose (glycogenolysis) in the liver, causing an increase in blood glucose level; relaxes smooth muscle of the GI tract.

Indications
- Hypoglycemia: counteracts severe hypoglycemic reactions in diabetic patients or during insulin shock therapy in psychiatric patients
- Diagnostic aid in the radiologic examination of the stomach, duodenum, small bowel, or colon when a hypotonic state is advantageous

Contraindications/cautions
- Insulinoma (drug releases insulin), pheochromocytoma (drug releases cathecholamines), pregnancy, lactation.

Dosage
Adult
- ***Hypoglycemia:*** 0.5–1.0 mg SC, IV, or IM. Response is usually seen in 5–20 min. If response is delayed, dose may be repeated one to two times.
- ***Insulin shock therapy:*** 0.5–1.0 mg SC, IV, or IM after 1 h of coma. Dose may be repeated if no response.
- ***Diagnostic aid:*** Suggested dose, route, and timing of dose vary with the segment of GI tract to be examined and duration of effect needed. Carefully check manufacturer's literature before use.

Pharmacokinetics

Route	Onset	Peak	Duration
IV	1 min	15 min	9–20 min
IM	8–10 min	20–30 min	19–32 min

Metabolism: Hepatic, $T_{1/2}$: 3–10 min
Distribution: Crosses placenta; enters breast milk
Excretion: Bile and urine

IV facts
Preparation: Reconstitute with vial provided. Use immediately; refrigerated solution stable for 48 h. If doses higher than 2 mg, reconstitute with Sterile Water for Injection and use immediately.
Infusion: Inject directly into the IV tubing of an IV drip infusion.
Incompatibilities: Compatible with dextrose solutions, but precipitates may form in solutions of sodium chloride, potassium chloride, or calcium chloride.

Adverse effects
- GI: *Nausea, vomiting*
- Hematologic: Hypokalemia in overdose
- Hypersensitivity: Urticaria, respiratory distress, hypotension

Clinically important drug-drug interactions
- Increased anticoagulant effect and risk of bleeding if taken concurrently with oral anticoagulants

■ Nursing Considerations

Assessment
- *History:* Insulinoma, pheochromocytoma, lactation
- *Physical:* Skin—color, lesions, temperature; orientation, reflexes; P, BP, peripheral perfusion; R; liver evaluation, bowel sounds; blood and urine glucose, serum potassium

Implementation
- Arouse hypoglycemic patient as soon as possible after drug injection, and provide supplemental carbohydrates to restore liver glycogen and prevent secondary hypoglycemia.
- Arouse patient from insulin shock therapy as soon as possible, and provide oral carbohydrates and reinstitute regular dietary regimen.
- Arrange for evaluation of insulin dosage in cases of hypoglycemia as a result of insulin overdosage; insulin dosage may need to be adjusted.

Drug-specific teaching points
- Family members of some diabetic patients learn to administer the drug SC in case of hypoglycemia. These patients and their families will need to learn drug administration and appropriate use and notification of physician.

☐ glutethimide

*(gloo **teth**' i mide)*

Pregnancy Category C
C-II controlled substance

Drug classes
Sedative/hypnotic (nonbarbiturate)

Therapeutic actions
Mechanism by which CNS is affected is not known; causes CNS depression similar to barbiturates; anticholinergic.

Indications
- Short-term relief of insomnia (3–7 d); not indicated for chronic administration; allow a drug-free interval of 1 wk or more before retreatment

Contraindications/cautions
- Hypersensitivity to glutethimide, porphyria, lactation.

Dosage
Adult: Usual dosage: 250–500 mg PO at bedtime.
Pediatric: Not recommended.
Geriatric or debilitated: Initial daily dosage should not exceed 500 mg PO at bedtime to avoid oversedation.

Pharmacokinetics

Route	Onset	Peak
Oral	Erratic	1–6 h

Metabolism: Hepatic, $T_{1/2}$: 10–12 h
Distribution: Crosses placenta; enters breast milk
Excretion: Urine

Adverse effects
- CNS: *Drowsiness, hangover,* suppression of REM sleep; REM rebound when drug is discontinued, mydriasis
- GI: *Nausea,* dry mouth, decreased intestinal motility
- Hematologic: Porphyria, blood dyscrasias
- Dermatologic: *Skin rash*
- Other: Physical, psychological dependence; tolerance; withdrawal reaction

Clinically important drug-drug interactions
- Additive CNS depression when given with alcohol • Increased metabolism and decreased effectiveness of oral (coumarin) anticoagulants given with glutethimide • Re-

532 ■ glycerin

Geriatric: Geriatric patients tend to be more sensitive to the drug; start with initial dose of 1.25 mg/d PO. Monitor for 24 h, and gradually increase dose after at least 1 wk as needed.

Pharmacokinetics

Route	Onset	Duration
Oral	1 h	24 h

Metabolism: Hepatic, $T_{1/2}$: 4 h
Distribution: Crosses placenta; enters breast milk
Excretion: Bile and urine

Adverse effects

- GI: *Anorexia, nausea,* vomiting, *epigastric discomfort, heartburn, diarrhea*
- CV: Increased risk of cardiovascular mortality
- Hematologic: Leukopenia, thrombocytopenia, anemia
- Hypersensitivity: *Allergic skin reactions,* eczema, pruritus, erythema, urticaria, photosensitivity, fever, eosinophilia, jaundice
- Endocrine: *Hypoglycemia*

Clinically important drug-drug interactions

- Increased risk of hypoglycemia if glyburide is taken concurrently with sulfonamides, chloramphenicol, fenfluramine, oxyphenbutazone, phenylbutazone, salicylates, clofibrate • Decreased effectiveness of glyburide and diazoxide if taken concurrently • Increased risk of hyperglycemia if glyburide is taken with rifampin, thiazides • Risk of hypoglycemia and hyperglycemia if glyburide is taken with ethanol; "disulfiram reaction" has been reported

■ Nursing Considerations

Assessment

- *History:* Allergy to sulfonylureas; diabetes with complications; Type I or juvenile diabetes, serious hepatic or renal impairment, uremia, thyroid or endocrine impairment, glycosuria, hyperglycemia associated with primary renal disease
- *Physical:* Skin—color, lesions; body temperature; orientation, reflexes, peripheral sensation; R, adventitious sounds; liver evaluation, bowel sounds; urinalysis, BUN, serum creatinine, liver function tests, blood glucose, CBC

Implementation

- Administer drug in the morning before breakfast. If severe GI upset occurs, dose may be divided and given before meals.
- Monitor urine and serum glucose levels frequently to determine effectiveness of drug and dosage being used.
- Arrange for transfer to insulin therapy during periods of high stress (eg, infections, surgery, trauma).
- Arrange for use of IV glucose if severe hypoglycemia occurs as a result of overdose.

Drug-specific teaching points

- Do not discontinue this medication without consulting physician.
- Monitor urine or blood for glucose and ketones as prescribed.
- Do not use this drug during pregnancy.
- Avoid alcohol while on this drug.
- Report fever, sore throat, unusual bleeding or bruising, skin rash, dark urine, light-colored stools, hypoglycemic or hyperglycemic reactions.

☐ glycerin

(gli' ser in)

glycerol

Fleet Babylax, Osmoglyn, Sani-Supp

Pregnancy Category C

Drug classes
Osmotic diuretic
Hyperosmolar laxative

Therapeutic actions
Elevates the osmolarity of the glomerular filtrate, thereby hindering the reabsorption of water and leading to a loss of

Adverse effects in *Italics* are most common; those in **Bold** are life-threatening.

duced absorption and decreased circulating levels of glutethimide if taken concurrently with charcoal interactants

■ Nursing Considerations

Assessment
- *History:* Hypersensitivity to glutethimide, porphyria, lactation
- *Physical:* Skin—color, lesions; orientation, affect, reflexes; bowel sounds

Implementation
- Supervise dose and amount of drug prescribed carefully in patients who are addiction prone or alcoholic; normally a week's supply of drug is sufficient; patient should then be reevaluated.
- Dispense least amount of drug feasible to patients who are depressed or suicidal.
- Withdraw drug gradually if patient has used drug long term or if patient has developed tolerance; supportive therapy similar to that for withdrawal from barbiturates may be necessary to prevent dangerous withdrawal symptoms (nausea, abdominal discomfort, tremors, convulsions, delirium).
- Arrange for reevaluation of patients with prolonged insomnia. Therapy of the underlying cause of insomnia (eg, pain, depression) is preferable to prolonged therapy with sedative/hypnotic drugs.

Drug-specific teaching points
- Take this drug exactly as prescribed. Do not exceed prescribed dosage; this drug should be used for no longer than 1 wk.
- Do not discontinue the drug abruptly; consult your nurse or physician if you wish to discontinue the drug before you are instructed to do so.
- Avoid alcohol, sleep-inducing, or OTC drugs while you are on this drug; these could cause dangerous effects.
- Know that the following side effects may occur: drowsiness, dizziness, blurred vision (avoid driving a car or performing other tasks requiring alertness or visual acuity if these occur), GI upset (frequent small meals may help).
- Report skin rash.

▢ glyburide

(glye' byoor ide)
Diabeta, Micronase

Pregnancy Category B

Drug classes
Antidiabetic agent

Therapeutic actions
Stimulates insulin release from functioning beta cells in the pancreas; may improve binding between insulin and insulin receptors or increase the number of insulin receptors; more potent in effect than first-generation sulfonylureas.

Indications
- Adjunct to diet to lower blood glucose in patients with non–insulin-dependent diabetes mellitus (type II)
- Adjunct to insulin therapy in the stabilization of certain cases of insulin-dependent, maturity-onset diabetes, reducing the insulin requirement, and decreasing the chance of hypoglycemic reactions

Contraindications/cautions
- Allergy to sulfonylureas; diabetes complicated by fever, severe infections, severe trauma, major surgery, ketosis, acidosis, coma (insulin is indicated in these conditions); type I or juvenile diabetes, serious hepatic or renal impairment, uremia, thyroid or endocrine impairment, glycosuria, hyperglycemia associated with primary renal disease; labor and delivery (if glyburide is used during pregnancy, discontinue drug at least 1 mo before delivery); lactation.

Dosage
Adult
- *Initial therapy:* 2.5–5 mg PO with breakfast.
- *Maintenance therapy:* 1.25–20 mg/d PO given as a single dose or in divided doses. Increase in increments of no more than 2.5 mg at weekly intervals based on patient's blood glucose response.

Pediatric: Safety and efficacy not established.

glycerin ■ 533

water, sodium, and chloride; creates an osmotic gradient in the eye between plasma and ocular fluids, thereby reducing intraocular pressure; causes the local absorption of sodium and water in the stool, leading to a more liquid stool and local intestinal movement.

Indications
- Glaucoma: to interrupt acute attacks, or when a temporary drop in intraocular pressure is required (*Osmoglyn*)
- Prior to ocular surgery performed under local anesthetic when a reduction in intraocular pressure is indicated (*Osmoglyn*)
- Temporary relief of constipation
- Unlabeled use: IV (with proper preparation) to lower intracranial or intraocular pressure

Contraindications/cautions
- Contraindicated in the presence of hypersensitivity to glycerin.
- Use caution in the presence of hypervolemia, CHF, confused mental states, severe dehydration, elderly, senility, diabetes, lactation.

Dosage
Adult: *Osmoglyn: Given PO only:* 1–1.5 g/kg, 1–1½ h prior to surgery.
- ***Laxative:*** Insert one suppository high in rectum and retain 15 min; rectal liquid: insert stem with tip pointing toward navel; squeeze unit until nearly all liquid is expelled, then remove.

Pediatric: Safety and efficacy not established.

Pharmacokinetics

Route	Onset	Peak	Duration
Oral *(Osmoglyn)*	Varies	1 h	5 h

Metabolism: T$_{1/2}$: 2–3 h
Distribution: Crosses placenta; may enter breast milk
Excretion: Urine

Adverse effects
- **CNS:** *Confusion, headache, syncope,* disorientation
- **GI:** *Nausea, vomiting*
- **CV:** Cardiac arrhythmias
- **Endocrine:** Hyperosmolar nonketotic coma
- **Other:** Severe dehydration, weight gain with continued use

■ Nursing Considerations

Assessment
- *History:* Hypersensitivity to glycerin, hypervolemia, CHF, confused mental states, severe dehydration, elderly, senility, diabetes, lactation
- *Physical:* Skin—color, edema; orientation, reflexes, muscle strength, pupillary reflexes; P, BP, perfusion; R, pattern, adventitious sounds; urinary output patterns; serum electrolytes, urinalysis

Implementation
- Administer Osmoglyn orally only; not for injection.
- Administer laxative as follows: Insert one suppository high in rectum, and have patient retain 15 min; rectal liquid—insert stem with tip pointint toward navel; squeeze unit until nearly all liquid is expelled, then remove.
- Monitor urinary output carefully.
- Monitor BP regularly.

Drug-specific teaching points
- Administer laxative as follows: Insert one suppository high in rectum and retain 15 min; rectal liquid—insert stem with tip pointing toward navel; squeeze unit until nearly all liquid is expelled, then remove.
- Know that the following side effects may occur: increased urination (bathroom facilities will be made readily available), GI upset (small frequent meals may help), dry mouth (sugarless lozenges to suck may help this problem), headache, blurred vision (use caution when moving around; ask for assistance).
- Report severe headache, chest pain, confusion, rapid respirations, violent diarrhea.

Adverse effects in *Italics* are most common; those in **Bold** are life-threatening.

glycopyrrolate

*(glye koe **pye'** roe late)*
Robinul

Pregnancy Category C (parenteral)
Pregnancy Category B

Drug classes
Anticholinergic (quaternary)
Antimuscarinic
Parasympatholytic
Antispasmodic

Therapeutic actions
Competitively blocks the effects of acetylcholine at receptors that mediate the effects of parasympathetic postganglionic impulses; depresses salivary and bronchial secretions; dilates the bronchi; inhibits vagal influences on the heart; relaxes the GI and GU tracts; inhibits gastric acid secretion.

Indications
- Adjunctive therapy in the treatment of peptic ulcer (oral)
- Reduction of salivary, tracheobronchial, and pharyngeal secretions preoperatively; reduction of the volume and free acidity of gastric secretions; and blocking of cardiac vagal inhibitory reflexes during induction of anesthesia and intubation; may be used intraoperatively to counteract drug-induced or vagal traction reflexes with the associated arrhythmias (parenteral)
- Protection against the peripheral muscarinic effects (eg, bradycardia, excessive secretions) of cholinergic agents, such as neostigmine, pyridostigmine, that are used to reverse the neuromuscular blockade produced by nondepolarizing neuromuscular junction blockers (parenteral)

Contraindications/cautions
- Contraindicated in the presence of glaucoma; adhesions between iris and lens; stenosing peptic ulcer; pyloroduodenal obstruction; paralytic ileus; intestinal atony; severe ulcerative colitis; toxic megacolon; symptomatic prostatic hypertrophy; bladder neck obstruction; bronchial asthma; COPD; cardiac arrhythmias; tachycardia; myocardial ischemia; lactation; impaired metabolic, liver, or kidney function; myasthenia gravis.
- Use caution in the presence of Down's syndrome, brain damage, spasticity, hypertension, hyperthyroidism.

Dosage
Adult
- **Oral:** 1 mg tid or 2 mg bid–tid; maintenance: 1 mg bid.
- **Parenteral**
- *Peptic ulcer:* 0.1–0.2 mg IM or IV tid–qid.
- *Preanesthetic medication:* 0.004 mg/kg (0.002 mg/lb) IM 30 min to 1 h prior to anesthesia.
- *Intraoperative:* 0.1 mg IV; repeat as needed at 2- to 3-min intervals. With neostigmine, pyridostigmine: 0.2 mg for each 1 mg neostigmine or 5 mg pyridostigmine; administer IV simultaneously.

Pediatric: Not recommended for children younger than 12 y for peptic ulcer.
- **Parenteral**
- *Preanesthetic medication (younger than 2 y):* 0.004 mg/lb IM 30 min to 1 h prior to anesthesia. Younger than 12 y: 0.002–0.004 mg/lb IM.
- *Intraoperative:* 0.004 mg/kg (0.002 mg/lb) IV, not to exceed 0.1 mg in a single dose. May be repeated at 2- to 3-min intervals.
- *With neostigmine, pyridostigmine:* 0.2 mg for each 1 mg neostigmine or 5 mg pyridostigmine. Administer IV simultaneously.

Pharmacokinetics

Route	Onset	Peak	Duration
Oral	60 min	60 min	8–12 h
IM/SC	15–30 min	30–45 min	2–7 h
IV	1 min		

Metabolism: Hepatic, $T_{1/2}$: 2.5 h
Crosses placenta; enters breast milk
Excretion: Urine

IV facts
Preparation: No additional preparation required.

gold sodium thiomalate (gold) ■ 535

Infusion: Administer slowly into tubing of a running IV.

Adverse effects
- CNS: *Blurred vision*, mydriasis, cycloplegia, photophobia, increased intraocular pressure
- GI: *Dry mouth, altered taste perception, nausea, vomiting, dysphagia*, heartburn, constipation, bloated feeling, paralytic ileus, gastroesophageal reflux
- CV: Palpitations, tachycardia
- GU: *Urinary hesitancy and retention*, impotence
- Local: *Irritation at site of IM injection*
- Other: Decreased sweating and predisposition to heat prostration, suppression of lactation, nasal congestion

Clinically important drug-drug interactions
- Decreased antipsychotic effectiveness of haloperidol when given with anticholinergic drugs

■ Nursing Considerations

Assessment
- *History:* Glaucoma; adhesions between iris and lens, stenosing peptic ulcer, pyloroduodenal obstruction, paralytic ileus, intestinal atony, severe ulcerative colitis, toxic megacolon, symptomatic prostatic hypertrophy, bladder neck obstruction, COPD, cardiac arrhythmias, myocardial ischemia, impaired metabolic, liver or kidney function, myasthenia gravis; lactation; Down syndrome, brain damage, spasticity, hypertension, hyperthyroidism
- *Physical:* Bowel sounds, normal output; normal urinary output, prostate palpation; R, adventitious sounds; pulse, blood pressure; intraocular pressure, vision; bilateral grip strength, reflexes; hepatic palpation, liver and renal function tests; skin color, lesions, texture

Implementation
- Ensure adequate hydration; provide environmental control (temperature) to prevent hyperpyrexia.
- Encourage patient to void before each dose of medication if urinary retention becomes a problem.

Drug-specific teaching points
- Take this drug exactly as prescribed.
- Avoid hot environments while taking this drug (you will be heat-intolerant, and dangerous reactions may occur).
- Know that the following side effects may occur: constipation (ensure adequate fluid intake, proper diet); dry mouth (sugarless lozenges, frequent mouth care may help; this effect sometimes lessens with time); blurred vision, sensitivity to light (it may help to know that these are drug effects that will go away when you discontinue the drug; avoid tasks that require acute vision; wear sunglasses when in bright light if these occur); impotence (this is a drug effect that will go away when you discontinue the drug); difficulty in urination (it may help to empty the bladder immediately before taking each dose of drug).
- Report skin rash, flushing, eye pain, difficulty breathing, tremors, loss of coordination, irregular heartbeat, palpitations, headache, abdominal distention, hallucinations, severe or persistent dry mouth, difficulty swallowing, difficulty urinating, severe constipation, sensitivity to light.

❐ gold sodium thiomalate (gold)

Myochrysine

Pregnancy Category C

Drug classes
Antirheumatic agent
Gold compound

Therapeutic actions
Suppresses and prevents arthritis and synovitis: taken up by macrophages, this results in inhibition of phagocytosis and inhibition of activities of lysosomal enzymes; decreases concentrations of rheumatoid factor and immunoglobulins.

Adverse effects in *Italics* are most common; those in **Bold** are life-threatening.

gold sodium thiomalate (gold)

Indications
- Treatment of selected cases of adult and juvenile rheumatoid arthritis; most effective early in disease; late in the disease when damage has occurred, gold can only prevent further damage.

Contraindications/cautions
- Allergy to gold preparations, uncontrolled diabetes mellitus, severe debilitation, renal disease, hepatic dysfunction, history of infectious hepatitis, marked hypertension, uncontrolled CHF, SLE, agranulocytosis, hemorrhagic diathesis, blood dyscrasias, recent radiation treatment, previous toxic response to gold or heavy metals (urticaria, eczema, colitis), pregnancy, lactation.

Dosage
Contains approximately 50% gold. Administer by IM injection only, preferably intragluteally.

Adult
- **Weekly injections:** First injection, 10 mg, IM; Second injection, 25 mg, IM; Third and subsequent injections, 25–50 mg IM until major clinical improvement is seen, toxicity occurs, or cumulative dose reaches 1 g.
- **Maintenance:** 25–50 mg IM every other week for 2–20 wk. If clinical course remains stable, give 25–50 mg every third and then every fourth week indefinitely. Some patients require maintenance intervals of 1–3 wk. If arthritis is exacerbated, resume weekly injections. In severe cases, dosage can be increased by 10-mg increments; do not exceed 100 mg in a single injection.

Pediatric: Initial test dose of 10 mg IM, then give 1 mg/kg, not to exceed 50 mg as a single injection. Adult guidelines for dosage apply.

Geriatric: Monitor patients carefully; tolerance to gold decreases with age.

Pharmacokinetics

Route	Onset	Peak
IM	Slow	3–6 h

Metabolism: $T_{1/2}$: 14–40 d, then 168 d
Distribution: Crosses placenta; enters breast milk
Excretion: Urine and feces

Adverse effects
- **GI:** *Stomatitis, glossitis, gingivitis*, metallic taste, pharyngitis, gastritis, colitis, tracheitis, nausea, vomiting, anorexia, abdominal cramps, *diarrhea*, hepatitis with jaundice
- **Respiratory:** Gold bronchitis, interstitial pneumonitis and fibrosis, cough, shortness of breath
- **Hematologic:** Granulocytopenia, thrombocytopenia, leukopenia, eosinophilia, anemias
- **GU:** Vaginitis, nephrotic syndrome or glomerulitis with proteinuria and hematuria, acute tubular necrosis and renal failure
- **Dermatologic:** *Dermatitis; pruritus, erythema, exfoliative dermatitis*, chrysiasis (gray-blue color to the skin due to gold deposition), rash
- **Hypersensitivity:** Nitritoid or allergic reactions: flushing, fainting, dizziness, sweating, nausea, vomiting, malaise, weakness
- **Immediate postinjection effects: Anaphylactic shock**, syncope, bradycardia, thickening of the tongue, dysphagia, dyspnea, angioneurotic edema
- **Other:** Fever, nonvasomotor postinjection reaction: arthralgia for 1–2 d after the injection, usually subsides after the first few injections; carcinogenesis, mutagenesis, impairment of fertility (reported in preclinical studies)

■ Nursing Considerations

Assessment
- *History:* Allergy to gold preparations, uncontrolled diabetes mellitus, severe debilitation, renal or hepatic dysfunction, history of infectious hepatitis, marked hypertension, uncontrolled CHF, SLE, hemorrhagic diathesis, blood dyscrasias, recent radiation treatment, previous toxic response to gold or heavy metals, lactation

Adverse effects in *Italics* are most common; those in **Bold** are life-threatening.

- *Physical:* Skin—color, lesions; body temperature; edema; P, BP; R, adventitious sounds; mucous membranes, bowel sounds; liver evaluation; CBC, renal and liver function tests, chest x-ray

Implementation
- Do not administer drug to patients with history of idiosyncratic or severe reactions to gold therapy.
- Monitor hematologic status, liver and kidney function, respiratory status regularly during the course of drug therapy.
- Do not use if material has darkened; color should be a pale yellow.
- Administer by intragluteal IM injection; have patient remain recumbent for 10 min after injection.
- Arrange for discontinuation of drug at first sign of toxic reaction.
- Arrange for use of systemic corticosteroids for treatment of severe stomatitis, dermatitis, renal, hematologic, pulmonary, enterocolitic complications.
- Protect patient from exposure to sunlight or ultraviolet light to decrease risk of chrysiasis.

Drug-specific teaching points
- Prepare a calendar of projected injection dates. This drug's effects are not seen immediately; several months of therapy are needed to see results. You will be asked to stay in the recumbent position for about 10 min after each injection.
- Be aware that this drug does not cure the disease, but only stops its effects.
- Know that the following side effects may occur: increased joint pain for 1–2 d after injection (this usually subsides after the first few injections); diarrhea (ensure ready access to bathroom facilities); mouth sores, metallic taste (frequent mouth care will help); rash, gray-blue color to the skin (avoid exposure to the sun or ultraviolet light to help to decrease this effect); nausea, loss of appetite (small, frequent meals may help).
- Do not become pregnant while on this drug; if you decide to become pregnant, consult with physician about discontinuing drug.
- Report unusual bleeding or bruising, sore throat, fever, severe diarrhea, skin rash, mouth sores.

☐ gonadorelin acetate

(goe nad oh rell' in)
GnRH
Lutrepulse

gonadorelin hydrochloride
Factrel

Pregnancy Category B

Drug classes
Gonadotropin releasing hormone
Hormone
Diagnostic agent

Therapeutic actions
A synthetic polypeptide that is identical to gonadotropic releasing hormone (GnRH) which is released from the hypothalamus in a pulsatile fashion to stimulate LH (leutinizing hormone) and FSH (follicle stimulating hormone) release from the pituitary; these hormones in turn are responsible for regulating reproductive status.

Indications
- Treatment of primary hypothalamic amenorrhea (gonadorelin acetate)
- Evaluation of functional capacity and response of the gonadotropes of the anterior pituitary; testing suspected gonadotropin deficiency; evaluating residual gonadotropic function of the pituitary following removal of a pituitary tumor by surgery or irradiation (gonadorelin hydrochloride)
- Unlabeled uses of gonadorelin hydrochloride: induction of ovulation (by IV, SC, and intranasal routes); ovulation inhibition; treatment of precocious puberty

Contraindications/cautions
- Hypersensitivity to gonadorelin or any of the components; ovarian cyst, causes of anovulation other than those of hypothalamic origin; hormone-dependent tumors; lactation.

Dosage
Adult (gonadorelin acetate)
- **Primary hypothalamic amenorrhea:** 5 μg q90 min (range 1–20 μg). This is delivered by the *Lutrepulse* pump using the 0.8-mg solution at 50 μl per pulse; 68% of the 5 μg q90 min regimens induced ovulation. For individualization of dose, see manufacturer's instructions.

Pediatric (gonadorelin acetate): Safety and efficacy not established.

Adult (gonadorelin hydrochloride): 100 μg SC or IV. In females, perform the test in the early follicular phase (days 1–7) of the menstrual cycle.

Pharmacokinetics

Route	Onset	Duration
IV, SC	Slow	3–5 h

Metabolism: Plasma, $T_{1/2}$: 10–40 min
Distribution: Crosses placenta; enters breast milk
Excretion: Urine

IV facts
Preparation: Reconstitute gonadorelin acetate using aseptic technique with 8 ml of diluent immediately prior to use, and transfer to plastic reservoir. Shake for a few seconds to produce a clear, colorless solution with no particulate matter. Prepare gonadorelin hydrochloride by reconstituting 100-μg vial with 1 ml and the 500-μg vial with 2 ml of the accompanying diluent. Prepare immediately before use. Store at room temperature; use within 1 d. Discard any unused solution and diluent.

Infusion: Administer gonadorelin acetate IV using the Lutrepulse pump set at pulse period of 1 min at a frequency of 90 min. The 8-ml solution will supply 90-min pulsatile doses for approximately 7 consecutive d. Inject gonadorelin HCl directly into vein or into tubing of running IV.

Adverse effects
- **CNS:** Headache, lightheadedness
- **GI:** Nausea, abdominal discomfort
- **GU:** *Ovarian hyperstimulation, multiple pregnancies* (gonadorelin acetate)
- **Local:** *Inflammation, infection, mild phlebitis, hematoma at injection site*

■ Nursing Considerations
Assessment
- *History:* Hypersensitivity to gonadorelin or any of the components, ovarian cyst, hormone-dependent tumors, lactation
- *Physical:* Reflexes, affect; Pap smear, pelvic exam; pregnancy test

Implementation
- Ensure cause of amenorrhea before treatment begins.
- Monitor for response to gonadorelin acetate within 2–3 wk after therapy started. Continue infusion pump for another 2 wk to maintain the corpus luteum.
- Monitor injection sites; pump access line for signs of local irritation and inflammation.
- Monitor patients on infusion pumps for any sign of infection; change the cannula and IV sites q48h.

Drug-specific teaching points
Gonadorelin HCl
- Patients receiving gonadorelin hydrochloride for diagnostic testing should have information about the drug included as part of their teaching about their condition and testing.
- Report difficulty breathing, rash, pain, or inflammation at the injection site.

Gonadorelin acetate
- Know that gonadorelin acetate needs to be delivered in a pulsating fashion using the Lutrepulse pump. Care of the pump and injection site will be covered in the information kit provided by the manufacturer.
- Be aware that ovulation may occur within 2–3 wk of the beginning of therapy. You will need to be followed closely to determine these effects. If pregnancy does occur, the therapy will be continued for 2 wk to help maintain the pregnancy.
- Know that the following side effects may occur: headache, abdominal discomfort;

Adverse effects in *Italics* are most common; those in **Bold** are life-threatening.

goserelin acetate

(*goe' se rel in*)
Zoladex

Pregnancy Category X

Drug classes
Antineoplastic agent
Hormonal agent

Therapeutic actions
An analog of lutenizing hormone-releasing hormone (LHRH or GnRH); potent inhibitor of pituitary gonadotropin secretion; initial administration causes increase in FSH and LH and resultant increase in testosterone levels; with chronic administration, these hormone levels fall to levels normally seen with surgical castration within 2–4 wk, as pituitary is inhibited.

Indications
- Palliative treatment of advanced prostatic cancer when orchiectomy or estrogen administration is not indicated or is unacceptable to the patient
- Management of endometriosis, including pain relief and reduction of endometriotic lesions

Contraindications/cautions
- Pregnancy, lactation, hypersensitivity to LHRH or any component.

Dosage
Adult: 3.6 mg SC every 28 d into the upper abdominal wall.
- ***Prostatic carcinoma:*** long-term use
- ***Endometriosis:*** Continue therapy for 6 mo.

Pediatric: Safety and efficacy not established.

Pharmacokinetics

Route	Onset	Peak
SC	Slow	12–15 d

Metabolism: Hepatic, $T_{1/2}$: 4.2 h
Distribution: Crosses placenta; may enter breast milk
Excretion: Urine

Adverse effects
- **CNS:** Insomnia, dizziness, lethargy, anxiety, depression
- **GI:** Nausea, anorexia
- **CV:** CHF, edema, hypertension, arrhythmia, chest pain
- **GU:** *Hot flashes, sexual dysfunction, decreased erections, lower urinary tract symptoms*
- **Other:** Rash, sweating, cancer

■ Nursing Considerations

Assessment
- *History:* Pregnancy, lactation
- *Physical:* Skin—temperature, lesions; reflexes, affect; BP, P; urinary output; pregnancy test if appropriate

Implementation
- Use syringe provided. Discard if package is damaged. Remove sterile syringe immediately before use.
- Arrange for use of a local anesthetic prior to injection to decrease pain and discomfort.
- Administer using aseptic technique under the supervision of a physician familiar with the implant technique.
- Bandage area after implant has been injected.
- Ensure repeat injection in 28 d; it is important to keep as close to this schedule as possible.

Drug-specific teaching points
- Be aware that this drug will need to be implanted into your upper abdomen every 28 d. It is important to stick to this schedule as closely as possible. Mark a calendar of injection dates.
- Know that the following side effects may occur: hot flashes (a cool temperature

may help you to cope with this); sexual dysfunction—regression of sex organs, impaired fertility, decreased erections (it may help to know that these are drug effects); pain at injection site (a local anesthetic will be used at the time of implantation, which will help to alleviate the pain; if the discomfort becomes severe, analgesics may be ordered).
- Do not take this drug if pregnant; if you are pregnant or wish to become pregnant, consult with your physician (female patients only).
- Report chest pain, increased signs and symptoms of your cancer, difficulty breathing, dizziness, severe pain at injection site.

☐ granisetron hydrochloride

(gran iz' e tron)
Kytril

Pregnancy Category B

Drug classes
Antiemetic

Therapeutic actions
Selectively binds to serotonin receptors in the CTZ, blocking the nausea and vomiting caused by the release of serotonin by mucosal cells during chemotherapy, which stimulates the CTZ and causes nausea and vomiting.

Indications
- Prevention and treatment of nausea and vomiting associated with emetogenic chemotherapy

Contraindications/cautions
- Contraindicated in pregnancy, lactation.

Dosage
Adult and pediatric older than 2 y: 10 μg/kg IV over 5 min starting within 30 min of beginning of chemotherapy; only on days of chemotherapy.

Pediatric: Younger than 2 y: not recommended.

Pharmacokinetics

Route	Onset	Peak
IV	Rapid	30–45 min

Metabolism: Hepatic, $T_{1/2}$: unknown
Distribution: Crosses placenta; enters breast milk
Excretion: Urine

IV facts
Preparation: No additional preparation necessary.
Infusion: Inject slowly over 5 min.

Adverse effects
- CNS: *Headache,* asthenia, somnolence
- GI: Diarrhea or constipation
- CV: Hypertension
- Other: Fever

■ Nursing Considerations

Assessment
- *History:* Allergy to granisetron, pregnancy, lactation, liver or renal impairment
- *Physical:* Orientation, reflexes, affect; BP; bowel sounds; body temperature

Implementation
- Provide mouth care, sugarless lozenges to suck to help alleviate nausea.

Drug-specific teaching points
- Be aware that this drug must be given IV when you are receiving your chemotherapy; it will help decrease nausea and vomiting.
- Know that the following side effects may occur: lack of sleep, drowsiness (use caution if driving or performing tasks that require alertness if these occur); diarrhea or constipation; headache (appropriate medication will be arranged to alleviate this problem).
- Report severe headache, fever, numbness or tingling, severe diarrhea or constipation.

Adverse effects in *Italics* are most common; those in **Bold** are life-threatening.

guaifenesin

(gwye fen' e sin)

Anti-tuss, Breonesin, Genatuss, GG-Cen, Glyate, Guaituss, Halotussin, Hytuss 2X, Humibid Sprinkle, Malotuss, Mytussin, Naldecon-EX, Robitussin, Scot-tussin Expertorant, Uni-tussin

Pregnancy Category C

Drug classes
Expectorant

Therapeutic actions
Enhances the output of respiratory tract fluid by reducing adhesiveness and surface tension, facilitating the removal of viscous mucus.

Indications
- Symptomatic relief of respiratory conditions characterized by dry, nonproductive cough and in the presence of mucus in the respiratory tract.

Contraindications/cautions
- Allergy to guaifenesin.

Dosage
Adult and pediatric older than 12 y: 100–400 mg PO q4h. Do not exceed 2.4 g/d.
Pediatric: 6–12 y: 100–200 mg PO q4h. Do not exceed 1.2 g/d. *2–6 y:* 50–100 PO q4h. Do not exceed 600 mg/d.

Pharmacokinetics

Route	Onset	Duration
Oral	30 min	4–6 h

Metabolism: Not known, $T_{1/2}$: not known
Distribution and Excretion: Unknown

Adverse effects
- **CNS:** Headache, dizziness
- **GI:** *Nausea, vomiting*
- **Dermatologic:** Rash

Drug-lab test interferences
- Color interference and false results of 5-HIAA and VMA urinary determinations

■ Nursing Considerations
Assessment
- *History:* Allergy to guaifenesin; persistent cough due to smoking, asthma, or emphysema; very productive cough
- *Physical:* Skin—lesions, color; body temperature; orientation, affects; R, adventitious sounds

Implementation
- Monitor reaction to drug; persistent cough for more than 1 wk, fever, rash, or persistent headache may indicate a more serious condition.

Drug-specific teaching points
- Do not take for longer than 1 wk; if fever, rash, headache occur, consult physician.
- Know that the following side effects may occur: nausea, vomiting (small, frequent meals may help); dizziness, headache (if these occur, avoid driving a car or operating dangerous machinery while taking this drug).
- Report fever, rash, severe vomiting, persistent cough.

guanabenz acetate

(gwahn' a benz)

Wytensin

Pregnancy Category C

Drug classes
Antihypertensive drug
Centrally acting sympatholytic drug

Therapeutic actions
Stimulates central (CNS) alpha$_2$-adrenergic receptors, reduces sympathetic nerve impulses from the vasomotor center to the heart and blood vessels, decreases peripheral vascular resistance, and lowers systemic blood pressure.

Indications
- Management of hypertension, alone or in combination with a thiazide diuretic

Adverse effects in *Italics* are most common; those in **Bold** are life-threatening.

- Unlabeled use: opiate detoxification, relief of chronic pain

Contraindications/cautions
- Contraindicated in the presence of hypersensitivity to guanabenz, lactation.
- Use caution in the presence of severe coronary insufficiency, recent MI, cerebrovascular disease, severe renal or hepatic failure, pregnancy.

Dosage
Adult: Individualize dosage. Initial dose of 4 mg PO bid, whether used alone or with a thiazide diuretic; increase in increments of 4–8 mg/d every 1–2 wk. Maximum dose studied has been 32 mg bid, but doses this high are rarely needed.
Pediatric: Safety and efficacy not established for children younger than 12 y; therefore, not recommended for use in this age group.

Pharmacokinetics

Route	Onset	Peak	Duration
Oral	45–60 min	2–5 h	6–12 h

Metabolism: Unknown, $T_{1/2}$: 6 h
Distribution: Crosses placenta; enters breast milk
Excretion: Urine and feces

Adverse effects
- **CNS:** *Sedation, weakness, dizziness, headache*
- **GI:** *Dry mouth*
- **CV:** Chest pain, edema, **arrhythmias**

■ Nursing Considerations

Assessment
- *History:* Hypersensitivity to guanabenz; severe coronary insufficiency, cerebrovascular disease, severe renal or hepatic failure; lactation
- *Physical:* Orientation, affect, reflexes; P, BP, orthostatic BP, perfusion, auscultation; liver and kidney function tests, ECG

Implementation
- Store tightly sealed, protected from light.
- Do not discontinue drug abruptly; discontinue therapy by reducing the dosage gradually over 2–4 d to avoid rebound hypertension, increased blood and urinary catecholamines, anxiety, nervousness, and other subjective effects.
- Assess compliance with drug regimen in a nonthreatening, supportive manner.

Drug-specific teaching points
- Take this drug exactly as prescribed; it is important that you not miss doses. Do not discontinue the drug unless instructed to do so. Do not discontinue abruptly. Store tightly sealed, protected from light.
- Know that the following side effects may occur: drowsiness, dizziness, lightheadedness, headache, weakness (these are often transient symptoms that go away after 4–6 wk of treatment; observe caution while driving or performing other tasks that require alertness or physical dexterity while you are experiencing these symptoms).
- Report persistent or severe drowsiness, dry mouth.

▢ guanadrel sulfate

(gwahn' a drel)
Hylorel

Pregnancy Category B

Drug classes
Antihypertensive drug
Adrenergic neuron blocking drug

Therapeutic actions
Antihypertensive effects depend on inhibition of norepinephrine release and depletion of norepinephrine from postganglionic sympathetic adrenergic nerve terminals.

Indications
- Treatment of hypertension in patients not responding adequately to a thiazide-type diuretic

Contraindications/cautions
- Contraindicated in the presence of hypersensitivity to guanadrel; known or sus-

pected pheochromocytoma, frank CHF not due to hypertension; lactation.
- Use caution in the presence of coronary artery disease with insufficiency or recent MI, cerebrovascular disease (these patients are at special risk if orthostatic hypotension occurs); history of bronchial asthma; active peptic ulcer, ulcerative colitis (these conditions may be aggravated by a relative increase in parasympathetic tone); renal dysfunction (drug-induced hypotension may further compromise renal function).

Dosage

Individualize dosage.

Adult: Usual starting dose is 10 mg/d PO. Most patients will require a daily dosage of 20–75 mg, usually in twice daily doses. For larger doses, three to four times daily dosing may be needed. Administer in divided doses; adjust the dosage weekly or monthly until blood pressure is controlled. With long-term therapy, some tolerance may occur, and dosage may need to be increased.

Pediatric: Safety and efficacy not established.

Geriatric or renal impaired: Reduce initial dosage to 5 mg q24h PO for Ccr of 30–60 ml/min; Ccr < 30 ml/min: give 5 mg q48h PO. Cautiously adjust dosage at intervals of 7–14 d.

Pharmacokinetics

Route	Onset	Peak	Duration
Oral	1½–2 h	4–6 h	4–14 h

Metabolism: $T_{1/2}$: 10 h
Distribution: May cross placenta; may enter breast milk
Excretion: Urine

Adverse effects

Incidence is higher during the first 8 wk of therapy.
- **CNS:** *Fatigue, headache, faintness, drowsiness, visual disturbances, paresthesias, confusion,* psychological problems
- **GI:** *Increased bowel movements, gas pain/indigestion, constipation, anorexia,* glossitis
- **CV/Respiratory:** *Shortness of breath on exertion,* **palpitations,** *chest pain, coughing,* shortness of breath at rest
- **GU:** *Nocturia, urinary urgency or frequency, peripheral edema, ejaculation disturbances,* impotence
- **Other:** *Excessive weight loss, excessive weight gain, aching limbs,* leg cramps

■ Nursing Considerations

Assessment
- *History:* Hypersensitivity to guanadrel; known or suspected pheochromocytoma; frank CHF; coronary artery disease, cerebrovascular disease; history of bronchial asthma; active peptic ulcer, ulcerative colitis; renal dysfunction; lactation
- *Physical:* Body weight; skin—color, lesions; orientation, affect, reflexes; P, BP, orthostatic BP, supine BP, perfusion, edema, auscultation; R, adventitious sounds, status of nasal mucous membranes; bowel sounds, normal output, palpation of salivary glands; voiding pattern, normal output; kidney function tests, urinalysis

Implementation
- Arrange to discontinue drug if diarrhea is severe.
- Arrange to discontinue guanadrel therapy 48–72 h prior to surgery to reduce the possibility of vascular collapse and cardiac arrest during anesthesia.
- Note prominently on patient's chart that patient is receiving guanadrel if emergency surgery is needed; a reduced dosage of preanesthetic medication and anesthetics will be needed.
- Monitor patient for orthostatic hypotension, which is most marked in the morning, and is accentuated by hot weather, alcohol, exercise.
- Monitor edema, body weight in patients with incipient cardiac decompensation, and arrange to add a thiazide diuretic to the drug regimen if sodium and fluid retention, signs of impending CHF, occur.

Adverse effects in *Italics* are most common; those in **Bold** are life-threatening.

Drug-specific teaching points
- Take this drug exactly as prescribed.
- Do not get out of bed without help while dosage is being adjusted.
- Know that the following side effects may occur: dizziness, weakness (these are more likely to occur when you change position, in the early morning, after exercise, in hot weather, and when you have consumed alcohol; some tolerance may occur after you have taken the drug for a while; avoid driving a car or engaging in tasks that require alertness while you are experiencing these symptoms; remember to change position slowly; use caution when climbing stairs); diarrhea; GI upset (frequent small meals may help); impotence, failure of ejaculation; emotional depression (it may help to know that this may be a drug effect); stuffy nose.
- Report severe diarrhea, frequent dizziness or fainting.

❒ guanethidine monosulfate

(gwahn eth' i deen)

Ismelin

Pregnancy Category C

Drug classes
Antihypertensive drug
Adrenergic neuron blocking drug

Therapeutic actions
Antihypertensive effects depend on inhibition of norepinephrine release and depletion of norepinephrine from postganglionic sympathetic adrenergic nerve terminals.

Indications
- Moderate to severe hypertension either alone or as an adjunct
- Renal hypertension, including that secondary to pyelonephritis, renal amyloidosis, and renal artery stenosis
- Orphan drug use: treatment of moderate to severe reflex sympathetic dystrophy and causalgia

Contraindications/cautions
- Contraindicated in the presence of hypersensitivity to guanethidine; known or suspected pheochromocytoma; frank CHF; lactation.
- Use caution in the presence of coronary artery disease with insufficiency or recent MI; cerebrovascular disease, especially with encephalopathy; history of bronchial asthma (these patients are likely to be hypersensitive to catecholamine depletion); active peptic ulcer, ulcerative colitis (these conditions may be aggravated by a relative increase in parasympathetic tone); renal dysfunction (drug-induced hypotension may further compromise renal function).

Dosage
Initial doses should be small, and dosage should be increased slowly. It may take 2 wk to adequately evaluate the response to daily administration.

Adult
- ***Ambulatory patients:*** 10 mg/d PO initially. Do not increase dosage more often than every 5–7 d. Take blood pressure in supine position, after standing for 10 min, and immediately after exercise if feasible. Increase dosage only if there has been no decrease in standing BP from the previous levels. Average dose is 25–50 mg qd. Reduce dosage in any of the following: normal supine pressure, excessive orthostatic fall in pressure, severe diarrhea.
- ***Hospitalized patients:*** Initial dose of 25–50 mg PO. Increase by 25 or 50 mg daily or every other day as indicated.
- ***Combination therapy:*** Diuretics enhance guanethidine effectiveness, may reduce incidence of edema, and may allow reduction of guanethidine dosage. Withdraw MAO inhibitors at least 1 wk before starting guanethidine. It may be advisable to withdraw ganglionic blockers gradually to prevent spiking BP response during the transfer.

Pediatric: Initial dose of 0.2 mg/kg per hour (6 mg/m^2 per 24 h) as a single oral dose. Increase by 0.2 mg/kg per 24 h PO

every 7–10 d. Maximum dosage: 3 mg/kg per 24 h PO.
Geriatric or impaired renal function: Use reduced dosage.

Pharmacokinetics

Route	Onset	Peak	Duration
Oral	Slow	1–3 wk	up to 2 wk

Metabolism: Hepatic, $T_{1/2}$: 4–8 d
Distribution: Crosses placenta; enters breast milk
Excretion: Urine

Adverse effects

- CNS: *Dizziness, weakness, lassitude, syncope resulting from either postural or exertional hypotension,* fatigue, myalgia, muscle tremor, emotional depression, ptosis of the lids and blurring of vision
- GI: *Increase in bowel movements and diarrhea,* nausea, vomiting, dry mouth, parotid tenderness
- CV: *Bradycardia,* angina, chest paresthesias, *fluid retention and edema with occasional development of* **CHF**
- **Respiratory**: Dyspnea, nasal congestion, asthma,
- GU: *Inhibition of ejaculation,* nocturia, urinary incontinence
- **Dermatologic**: Dermatitis, alopecia

Clinically important drug-drug interactions

• Decreased antihypertensive effect of guanethidine when given with anorexiants (eg, amphetamines), tricyclic antidepressants (imipramine, etc), phenothiazines (chlorpromazine), indirect-acting sympathomimetics (ephedrine, phenylpropanolamine, pseudoephedrine) • Increased pressor response and arrhythmogenic potential of direct-acting sympathomimetics (epinephrine, norepinephrine, phenylephrine), metaraminol, methoxamine

■ Nursing Considerations

Assessment

- *History:* Hypersensitivity to guanethidine; known or suspected pheochromocytoma; frank CHF; coronary artery disease; cerebrovascular disease; history of bronchial asthma; active peptic ulcer, ulcerative colitis; renal dysfunction; lactation
- *Physical:* Body weight; skin—color, lesions; orientation, affect, reflexes; P, BP, orthostatic BP, supine BP, perfusion, edema, auscultation; R, adventitious sounds, status of nasal mucous membranes; bowel sounds, normal output, palpation of salivary glands; voiding pattern, normal output; kidney function tests, urinalysis

Implementation

- Arrange to discontinue drug if diarrhea is severe.
- Arrange to discontinue guanethidine therapy at least 2 wk prior to surgery to reduce the possibility of vascular collapse and cardiac arrest during anesthesia.
- Note prominently on patient's chart that patient is receiving guanethidine if emergency surgery is needed; a reduced dosage of preanesthetic medication and anesthetics will be needed.
- Arrange to decrease dosage in the presence of fever, which decreases drug requirements.
- Monitor patient for orthostatic hypotension, which is most marked in the morning and is accentuated by hot weather, alcohol, exercise.
- Monitor edema, body weight in patients with incipient cardiac decompensation, and arrange to add a thiazide diuretic to the drug regimen if sodium and fluid retention, signs of impending CHF, occur.

Drug-specific teaching points

- Take this drug exactly as prescribed.
- Do not get out of bed without help while dosage is being adjusted.
- Know that the following side effects may occur: dizziness, weakness (these are more likely to occur when you change position, in the early morning, after exercise, in hot weather, and when you have consumed alcohol; some tolerance may occur after you have taken the drug for a while, but avoid driving a car or engag-

Adverse effects in *Italics* are most common; those in **Bold** are life-threatening.

ing in tasks that require alertness while you are experiencing these symptoms; remember to change positions slowly; use caution in climbing stairs); diarrhea; GI upset (frequent small meals may help); impotence, failure of ejaculation; emotional depression (it may help to know that this may be a drug effect); stuffy nose.
- Report severe diarrhea, frequent dizziness or fainting.

☐ guanfacine hydrochloride

(gwahn' fa seen)
Tenex

Pregnancy Category B

Drug classes
Antihypertensive drug
Centrally acting sympatholytic drug

Therapeutic actions
Stimulates central (CNS) alpha$_2$-adrenergic receptors, reduces sympathetic nerve impulses from the vasomotor center to the heart and blood vessels, decreases peripheral vascular resistance, and lowers systemic blood pressure.

Indications
- Management of hypertension; as monotherapy or in the presence of a thiazide diuretic
- Unlabeled use: amelioration of withdrawal symptoms in heroin withdrawal

Contraindications/cautions
- Contraindicated in the presence of hypersensitivity to guanfacine, labor and delivery, lactation.
- Use caution in the presence of severe coronary insufficiency, recent MI, cerebrovascular disease, chronic renal or hepatic failure, pregnancy.

Dosage
Adult: Recommended dose is 1 mg/d PO given at bedtime to minimize somnolence. If 1 mg/d does not give a satisfactory result after 3–4 wk of therapy, doses of 2 mg and then 3 mg may be given, although most of the drug's effect is seen at 1 mg. If blood pressure rises toward the end of the dosing interval, divided dosage should be used. Higher daily doses (rarely up to 40 mg/d in divided doses) have been used, but adverse reactions increase with doses > 3 mg/d, and there is no evidence of increased efficacy.
Pediatric: Safety and efficacy not established for children younger than 12 y; therefore, not recommended for use in this age group.

Pharmacokinetics

Route	Onset	Peak	Duration
Oral	2 h	1–4 h	24 h

Metabolism: Hepatic, T$_{1/2}$: 10–30 h
Distribution: Crosses placenta; enters breast milk
Excretion: Urine

Adverse effects
- **CNS:** *Sedation, weakness, dizziness,* headache, insomnia, amnesia, confusion, depression, conjunctivitis, iritis, vision disturbance, malaise, paresthesia, paresis, taste perversion, tinnitus, hypokinesia
- **GI:** *Dry mouth, constipation,* abdominal pain, diarrhea, dyspepsia, dysphagia, nausea
- **CV:** Bradycardia, palpitations, substernal pain
- **GU:** *Impotence,* libido decrease, testicular disorder, urinary incontinence
- **Dermatologic:** Dermatitis, pruritus, purpura, sweating
- **Other:** Rhinitis, leg cramps

■ Nursing Considerations
Assessment
- *History:* Hypersensitivity to guanfacine; severe coronary insufficiency, cerebrovascular disease; chronic renal or hepatic failure; pregnancy; lactation
- *Physical:* Skin—color, lesions; orientation, affect, reflexes; ophthalmologic exam; P, BP, orthostatic BP, perfusion, auscultation; R, adventitious sounds;

bowel sounds, normal output; normal urinary output, voiding pattern; liver and kidney function tests, ECG

Implementation

- Do not discontinue drug abruptly; discontinue therapy by reducing the dosage gradually over 2–4 d to avoid rebound hypertension (much less likely than with clonidine; BP usually returns to pretreatment levels in 2–4 d without ill effects).
- Assess compliance with drug regimen in a nonthreatening, supportive manner.

Drug-specific teaching points

- Take this drug exactly as prescribed; it is important that you do not miss doses. Do not discontinue the drug unless instructed to do so. Do not discontinue abruptly.
- Know that the following side effects may occur: drowsiness, dizziness, lightheadedness, headache, weakness (these are often transient symptoms that go away after 4–6 wk of treatment; observe caution while driving or performing other tasks that require alertness or physical dexterity while you are experiencing these symptoms); dry mouth (sucking on sugarless lozenges or ice chips may help); GI upset (frequent small meals may help); dizziness, lightheadedness when you change position (get up slowly; use caution when climbing stairs); impotence, other sexual dysfunction, decreased libido; palpitations.
- Report urinary incontinence, changes in vision, skin rash.

❒ halazepam

(hal az' e pam)
Paxipam

Pregnancy Category D
C-IV controlled substance

Drug classes
Benzodiazepine
Antianxiety drug

Therapeutic actions
Exact mechanisms of action not understood; acts mainly at subcortical levels of the CNS, leaving the cortex relatively unaffected; main sites of action may be the limbic system and reticular formation; benzodiazepines potentiate the effects of GABA, an inhibitory neurotransmitter; anxiolytic effects occur at doses well below those necessary to cause sedation, ataxia.

Indications
- Management of anxiety disorders or for short-term relief of symptoms of anxiety

Contraindications/cautions
- Contraindicated in the presence of hypersensitivity to benzodiazepines; psychoses; acute narrow-angle glaucoma; shock; coma; acute alcoholic intoxication; pregnancy (increased risk of congenital malformations, neonatal withdrawal syndrome); labor and delivery ("floppy infant" syndrome reported when mothers were given benzodiazepines during labor); lactation.
- Use caution in the presence of impaired liver or kidney function, debilitation.

Dosage
Increase dosage gradually to avoid adverse effects.
Adult: Usual dose is 20–40 mg PO tid–qid. Optimal dosage usually ranges from 80–160 mg daily.
Geriatric patients (70 y or older) or those with debilitating disease: Initially, 20 mg PO qd–bid. Adjust as needed and tolerated.

Pharmacokinetics

Route	Onset	Peak
Oral	Slow	1–3 h

Metabolism: Hepatic, $T_{1/2}$: 14 h
Distribution: Crosses placenta; enters breast milk
Excretion: Urine

Adverse effects
- **CNS:** *Transient, mild drowsiness initially; sedation, depression, lethargy,*

Adverse effects in *Italics* are most common; those in **Bold** are life-threatening.

548 ■ haloperidol

- *apathy, fatigue, lightheadedness, disorientation, anger, hostility,* episodes of mania and hypomania, *restlessness, confusion, crying,* delirium, *headache,* slurred speech, dysarthria, stupor, rigidity, tremor, dystonia, vertigo, euphoria, nervousness, difficulty in concentration, vivid dreams, psychomotor retardation, extrapyramidal symptoms; *mild paradoxical excitatory reactions, during first 2 wk of treatment*
- GI: *Constipation, diarrhea, dry mouth,* salivation, *nausea,* anorexia, vomiting, difficulty in swallowing, gastric disorders, hepatic dysfunction
- CV: Bradycardia, tachycardia, cardiovascular collapse, hyper- and hypotension, palpitations, edema
- Hematologic: elevations of blood enzymes: LDH, alkaline phosphatase, SGOT, SGPT; blood dyscrasias: agranulocytosis, leukopenia
- GU: Incontinence, urinary retention, changes in libido, menstrual irregularities
- EENT: Visual and auditory disturbances, diplopia, nystagmus, depressed hearing, nasal congestion
- Dermatologic: Urticaria, pruritus, skin rash, dermatitis
- Other: Hiccups, fever, diaphoresis, paresthesias, muscular disturbances, gynecomastia. *Drug dependence with withdrawal syndrome when drug is discontinued; more common with abrupt discontinuation of higher dosage used for longer than 4 mo.*

Clinically important drug-drug interactions

- Increased CNS depression when taken with alcohol, omeprazole • Increased pharmacologic effects of halazepam when given with cimetidine, disulfiram, oral contraceptives • Decreased effects of halazepam if taken concurrently with theophyllines

■ Nursing Considerations
Assessment

- *History:* Hypersensitivity to benzodiazepines; psychoses, acute narrow-angle glaucoma, shock, coma, acute alcoholic intoxication; elderly or debilitated patients; impaired liver or kidney function; pregnancy, lactation
- *Physical:* Body weight; skin—color, lesions; orientation, affect, reflexes, sensory nerve function, ophthalmologic exam; P, BP; R, adventitious sounds; bowel sounds, normal output, liver evaluation; normal output; liver and kidney function tests, CBC

Implementation

- Arrange to taper dosage gradually after long-term therapy, especially in epileptic patients.

Drug-specific teaching points

- Take this drug exactly as prescribed. Do not stop taking this drug (long-term therapy) without consulting your health care provider.
- Know that the following side effects may occur: drowsiness, dizziness (these may become less pronounced after a few days; avoid driving a car or engaging in other dangerous activities if these occur); GI upset (taking the drug with food may help); dreams, difficulty concentrating, fatigue, nervousness, crying (it may help to know that these are effects of the drug).
- Report severe dizziness, weakness, drowsiness that persists, rash or skin lesions, palpitations, swelling of the ankles, visual or hearing disturbances, difficulty voiding.

❒ haloperidol

*(ha loe **per**' i dole)*

haloperidol decanoate, haloperidol lactate

Apo-Haloperidol (CAN), Haldol, Haldol Decanoate, Haldol LA (CAN), Novoperidol (CAN), Peridol (CAN)

Pregnancy Category C

Drug classes
Dopaminergic blocking drug
Antipsychotic drug
Butyrophenone (not a phenothiazine)

Adverse effects in *Italics* are most common; those in **Bold** are life-threatening.

Therapeutic actions

Mechanism of action not fully understood: antipsychotic drugs block postsynaptic dopamine receptors in the brain, depress the reticular activating system, including those parts of the brain involved with wakefulness and emesis; chemically resembles the phenothiazines.

Indications

- Management of manifestations of psychotic disorders
- Control of tics and vocalizations in Gilles de la Tourette's syndrome in adults and children
- Short-term treatment of hyperactive children who also show impulsivity, difficulty sustaining attention, aggressivity, mood lability, or poor frustration tolerance
- Prolonged parenteral therapy of chronic schizophrenia (haloperidol decanoate)
- Unlabeled uses: control of nausea and vomiting, control of acute psychiatric situations (IV use)

Contraindications/cautions

- Contraindicated in the presence of coma or severe CNS depression, bone marrow depression, blood dyscrasia, circulatory collapse, subcortical brain damage, Parkinson's disease, liver damage, cerebral arteriosclerosis, coronary disease, severe hypotension or hypertension.
- Use caution in the presence of respiratory disorders ("silent pneumonia" may develop); glaucoma, prostatic hypertrophy (anticholinergic effects may exacerbate glaucoma and urinary retention); epilepsy or history of epilepsy (drug lowers seizure threshold); breast cancer (elevations in prolactin may stimulate a prolactin-dependent tumor); thyrotoxicosis; peptic ulcer, decreased renal function; myelography within previous 24 h or scheduled within 48 h; exposure to heat or phosphorous insecticides; lactation; children younger than 12 y, especially those with chickenpox, CNS infections (children are especially susceptible to dystonias that may confound the diagnosis of Reye's syndrome); allergy to aspirin if giving the 1-, 2-, 5-, and 10-mg tablets (these tablets contain tartrazine).

Dosage

Full clinical effects may require 6 wk–6 mo of therapy. Children, debilitated and geriatric patients, and patients with a history of adverse reactions to neuroleptic drugs may require lower dosage.

Adult

- ***Initial oral dosage range:*** 0.5–2.0 mg bid–tid PO for patients with moderate symptoms; 3–5 mg bid–tid PO for more resistant patients. Daily dosages up to 100 mg/d (or more) have been used, but safety of prolonged use of such doses has not been demonstrated. For maintenance, reduce dosage to lowest effective level.
- ***IM, haloperidol lactate injection:*** 2–5 mg (up to 10–30 mg) q30–60 min or q4–8h IM as necessary for prompt control of acutely agitated patients with severe symptoms. Switch to oral dosage as soon as feasible, using total IM dosage in previous 24 h as a guide to total daily oral dosage.
- ***IV, haloperidol lactate injection, unlabeled use for acute situations:*** 2–25 mg q30 IV or more min at a rate of 5 mg/min.
- ***Haloperidol decanoate injection (IM):*** Initial dose: 10–15 times the daily oral dose; repeat at 4-wk intervals.

Pediatric: Children 3–12 y or 15–40 kg weight: Initial dose of 0.5 mg/d PO; may increase in increments of 0.5 mg q5–7 d as needed. Total daily dose may be divided and given bid–tid.

- ***Psychiatric disorders:*** 0.05–0.15 mg/kg per day. Severely disturbed psychotic children may require higher dosage. There is little evidence that behavior is further improved by doses greater than 6 mg/d.
- ***Nonpsychotic and Gilles de la Tourette's syndromes:*** 0.05–0.075 mg/kg per day.

Geriatric: Use lower doses (0.5–2.0 mg bid–tid), and increase dosage more gradually than in younger patients.

Pharmacokinetics

Metabolism: Hepatic, $T_{1/2}$: 21–24 h, 3 wk for decanoate

550 ■ haloperidol

Distribution: Crosses placenta; enters breast milk
Excretion: Urine and bile

Route	Onset	Peak
Oral	Varies	3–5 h
IM	Rapid	20 min
IM, decanoate	Slow	4–11 d

Adverse effects

Not all effects have been reported with haloperidol; however, because haloperidol has certain pharmacologic similarities to the phenothiazine class of antipsychotic drugs, all adverse effects associated with phenothiazine therapy should be kept in mind when haloperidol is used.

- CNS: *Drowsiness*, insomnia, vertigo, headache, weakness, tremor, ataxia, slurring, cerebral edema, seizures, exacerbation of psychotic symptoms, extrapyramidal syndromes—*pseudoparkinsonism; dystonias; akathisia,* tardive dyskinesias, potentially irreversible (no known treatment), **neuroleptic malignant syndrome**—extrapyramidal symptoms, hyperthermia, autonomic disturbances
- CV: Hypotension, orthostatic hypotension, hypertension, tachycardia, bradycardia, cardiac arrest, CHF, cardiomegaly, **refractory arrhythmias** (some fatal), pulmonary edema
- Respiratory: Bronchospasm, laryngospasm, dyspnea; **suppression of cough reflex and potential for aspiration**
- Hematologic: Eosinophilia, leukopenia, leukocytosis, anemia; aplastic anemia; hemolytic anemia; thrombocytopenic or nonthrombocytopenic purpura; pancytopenia
- Hypersensitivity: Jaundice, urticaria, angioneurotic edema, laryngeal edema, photosensitivity, eczema, asthma, **anaphylactoid reactions**, exfoliative dermatitis
- Endocrine: Lactation, breast engorgement in females, galactorrhea; SIADH; amenorrhea, menstrual irregularities; gynecomastia in males; changes in libido; hyperglycemia or hypoglycemia; glycosuria; hyponatremia; pituitary tumor with hyperprolactinemia; inhibition of ovulation, infertility, pseudopregnancy
- Autonomic: Dry mouth, salivation, nasal congestion, nausea, vomiting, anorexia, fever, pallor, flushed facies, sweating, constipation, paralytic ileus, urinary retention, incontinence, polyuria, enuresis, priapism, ejaculation inhibition

Clinically important drug-drug interactions

- Additive anticholinergic effects and possibly decreased antipsychotic efficacy with anticholinergic drugs • Increased risk of toxic side effects if taken concurrently with lithium • Decreased effectiveness of haloperidol if taken concurrently with carbamazepine

Drug-lab test interferences

- False-positive pregnancy tests (less likely if serum test is used) • Increase in protein-bound iodine, not attributable to an increase in thyroxine

■ Nursing Considerations

Assessment

- *History:* Severe CNS depression; bone marrow depression; blood dyscrasia; circulatory collapse; subcortical brain damage; Parkinson's disease; liver damage; cerebral arteriosclerosis; coronary disease; severe hypotension or hypertension; respiratory disorders; glaucoma, prostatic hypertrophy; epilepsy or history of epilepsy; breast cancer; thyrotoxicosis; peptic ulcer, decreased renal function; myelography within previous 24 h or scheduled within 48 h; exposure to heat or phosphorus insecticides; children younger than 12 y, especially those with chickenpox, CNS infections; allergy to aspirin
- *Physical:* Body weight, temperature; reflexes, orientation, intraocular pressure; P, BP, orthostatic BP; R, adventitious sounds; bowel sounds and normal output, liver evaluation; urinary output, prostate size, CBC, urinalysis, thyroid, liver and kidney function tests

Adverse effects in *Italics* are most common; those in **Bold** are life-threatening.

Implementation
- Do not give children IM injections.
- Do not use haloperidol decanoate for IV injections.
- Arrange for gradual drug withdrawal when patient has been on maintenance therapy to avoid withdrawal-emergent dyskinesias.
- Arrange for discontinuation of drug if serum creatinine, BUN become abnormal or if WBC count is depressed.
- Monitor elderly patients for dehydration, and institute remedial measures promptly; sedation and decreased sensation of thirst related to CNS effects of drug can lead to severe dehydration.
- Consult physician regarding appropriate warning of patient or patient's guardian about tardive dyskinesias.
- Consult physician about dosage reduction, use of anticholinergic antiparkinsonian drugs (controversial) if extrapyramidal effects occur.

Drug-specific teaching points
- Take this drug exactly as prescribed.
- Avoid driving a car or engaging in other dangerous activities if CNS, vision changes occur.
- Avoid prolonged exposure to sun, or use a sunscreen or covering garments if exposure is unavoidable.
- Maintain fluid intake, and use precautions against heatstroke in hot weather.
- Report sore throat, fever, unusual bleeding or bruising, rash, weakness, tremors, impaired vision, dark-colored urine (pink or reddish brown urine is to be expected), pale stools, yellowing of the skin or eyes.

❏ heparin calcium injection

(hep' ah rin)
Calcilean (CAN), Calciparine

heparin sodium injection
Hepalean (CAN), Lipo-Hepin, Liquaemin Sodium

heparin sodium and 0.9% sodium chloride, heparin sodium lock flush solution
Heparin Lock Flush, Hep-Lock

Pregnancy Category C

Drug classes
Anticoagulant

Therapeutic actions
Inhibits thrombus and clot formation by blocking the conversion of prothrombin to thrombin and fibrinogen to fibrin, the final steps in the clotting process.

Indications
- Prevention and treatment of venous thrombosis and pulmonary embolism
- Treatment of atrial fibrillation with embolization
- Diagnosis and treatment of disseminated intravascular coagulation
- Prevention of clotting in blood samples and heparin lock sets and during dialysis procedures
- Unlabeled uses: adjunct in therapy of coronary occlusion with acute MI, prevention of left ventricular thrombi and CVA post-MI, prevention of cerebral thrombosis in the evolving stroke

Contraindications/cautions
- Hypersensitivity to heparin; severe thrombocytopenia; uncontrolled bleeding; any patient who cannot be monitored regularly with blood coagulation tests; labor and immediate postpartum period; women older than 60 y are at high risk for hemorrhaging; dysbetalipoproteinemia; recent surgery or injury.

Dosage
Adjust dosage according to results of coagulation tests. Dosage is adequate when WBCT = 2.5—three times control—or APTT = 1.5—two times control value. The following are to be used as guidelines to dosage:
Adult
- ***For general anticoagulation***
- *SC (deep SC injection):* IV loading dose of 5,000 U and then 10,000–20,000

heparin calcium injection

U SC followed by 8,000–10,000 U q8h or 15,000–20,000 U q12h.
- *Intermittent IV:* Initial dose of 10,000 U and then 5,000–10,000 U q4–6h.
- *Continuous IV infusion:* Loading dose of 5,000 U and then 20,000–40,000 U/d.
- **Prophylaxis of postoperative thromboembolism:** 5,000 U by deep SC injection 2 h before surgery and q8–12h thereafter for 7 d or until patient is fully ambulatory.
- **Surgery of heart and blood vessels for patients undergoing total body perfusion:** Not less than 150 U/kg; guideline often used is 300 U/kg for procedures less than 60 min, 400 U/kg for longer procedures.
- **Clot prevention in blood samples:** 70–150 U/10–20 ml of whole blood.
- **Heparin lock and extracorporal dialysis:** See manufacturer's instructions.

Pediatric: Initial IV bolus of 50 U/kg and then 100 U/kg IV q4h, or 20,000 U/m^2 per 24 h by continuous IV infusion.

Pharmacokinetics

Route	Onset	Peak	Duration
IV	Immediate	Minutes	2–6 h
SC	20–60 min	2–4 h	8–12 h

Metabolism: T$_{1/2}$: 30–180 min
Distribution: Does not cross placenta, does not enter breast milk; broken down in liver
Excretion: Urine

IV facts

Continuous infusion: can be mixed in Normal Saline, D5W, Ringer's; mix well; invert bottle numerous times to ensure adequate mixing. Monitor patient closely; infusion pump is recommended. Single dose: direct, undiluted IV injection of up to 5,000 U (adult) or 50 U/kg (pediatric), given over 60 seconds.

Monitoring: blood should be drawn for coagulation testing 30 min before each intermittent IV dose or q4h if patient is on continuous infusion pump.

Incompatibilities: Heparin should *not* be mixed in solution with any other drug unless specifically ordered; direct incompatibilities in solution seen with amikacin, codeine, chlorpromazine, cytarabine, diazepam, dobutamine, doxorubicin, droperidol, ergotamine, erythromycin, gentamicin, haloperidol, nyaluronidase, hydrocortisone, kanamycin, levorphanol, meperidine, methadone, methicillin, methotrimeprazine, morphine, netilimicin, pentazocine, phenytoin, polymyxin B, promethazine, streptomycin, tetracycline, tobramycin, triflupromazine, vancomycin

Adverse effects
- Hematologic: *Hemorrhage; bruising;* thrombocytopenia; elevated SGOT, SGPT levels, hyperkalemia
- Dermatologic: Loss of hair
- Hypersensitivity: Chills, fever, urticaria, asthma
- Other: Osteoporosis, suppression of renal function (long-term, high-dose therapy)
- Treatment of overdose: Protamine sulfate (1% solution). Each mg of protamine neutralizes 100 USP heparin U. Give very slowly IV over 10 min, not to exceed 50 mg. Establish dose based on blood coagulation studies.

Clinically important drug-drug interactions
- Increased bleeding tendencies with oral anticoagulants, salicylates, penicillins, cephalosporins • Decreased anticoagulation effects if taken concurrently with nitroglycerin

Drug-lab test interferences
- Increased AST, ALT levels • Increased thyroid function tests • Altered blood gas analyses, especially levels of carbon dioxide, bicarbonate concentration, and base excess

■ Nursing Considerations
Assessment
- *History:* Recent surgery or injury; sensitivity to heparin; hyerlipidemia

Adverse effects in *Italics* are most common; those in **Bold** are life-threatening.

- *Physical:* Peripheral perfusion, R, stool guaiac test, PTT or other tests of blood coagulation, platelet count, kidney function tests

Implementation
- Adjust dose according to results of coagulation test results determined just before injection (30 min before each intermittent dose or q4h if continuous IV dose). Therapeutic range is 1.5–2.5 times control.
- Use heparin lock needle to avoid repeated injections.
- Give deep subcutaneous injections; *do not* give heparin by IM injection.
- Do not give IM injections to patients on heparin therapy (heparin predisposes to hematoma formation).
- Apply pressure to all injection sites after needle is withdrawn; inspect injection sites for signs of hematoma; do not massage injection sites.
- Mix well when adding heparin to IV infusion.
- Do not add heparin to infusion lines of other drugs, and do not piggyback other drugs into heparin line. If this must be done, ensure drug compatibility.
- Provide for safety measures (electric razor, soft toothbrush) to prevent injury to patient who is at risk for bleeding.
- Check patient for signs of bleeding; monitor blood tests.
- Alert all health care providers that patient is on heparin.
- Have protamine sulfate (heparin antidote) on standby in case of overdose.

Drug-specific teaching points
- Know that this drug must be given by a parenteral route (cannot be taken orally).
- Know that frequent blood tests are necessary to determine that your blood clotting time is within the correct range.
- Be careful to avoid injury while you are on this drug; use an electric razor, avoid contact sports, avoid activities that might lead to injury.
- Know that side effects may include the loss of hair.
- Report nose bleed, bleeding of the gums, unusual bruising, black or tarry stools, cloudy or dark urine, abdominal or lower back pain, severe headache.

❒ hetastarch

(bet' a starch)

hydroxyethyl starch, HES
Hespan

Pregnancy Category C

Drug classes
Plasma expander

Therapeutic actions
Complex mixture of various molecules with colloidal properties that raise human plasma volume when administered IV; increases the erythrocyte sedimentation rate and improves the efficiency of granulocyte collection by centrifugal means.

Indications
- Adjunctive therapy for plasma volume expansion in shock due to hemorrhage, burns, surgery, sepsis, trauma
- Adjunctive therapy in leukapheresis to improve harvesting and increase the yield of granulocytes

Contraindications/cautions
- Contraindicated in the presence of allergy to hetastarch, severe bleeding disorders, severe cardiac congestion, renal failure or anuria.
- Use caution in the presence of liver dysfunction, pregnancy.

Dosage
Adult
- ***Plasma volume expansion:*** 500–1,000 ml IV. Do not usually exceed 1,500 ml/d. In acute hemorrhagic shock, rates approaching 20 ml/kg per hour are often needed.
- ***Leukapheresis:*** 250–700 ml hetastarch infused at a constant fixed ratio of 1:8 to venous whole blood. Safety of up to 2 procedures per week and a total of 7–10 procedures using hetastarch have been established.

554 ■ histrelin acetate

Pediatric: Safety and efficacy have not been established.

Pharmacokinetics

Route	Onset	Peak	Duration
IV	Immediate	24 h	24–36 h

Metabolism: Hepatic, $T_{1/2}$: 17 d, then 48 d
Distribution: Crosses placenta; enters breast milk
Excretion: Urine

IV facts
Preparation: Use as prepared by manufacturer; store at room temperature; do not use if turbid deep brown or if crystalline precipitate forms.
Infusion: Rate of infusion should be determined by patient response.

Adverse effects
- CNS: *Headache*, muscle pain
- GI: *Vomiting, submaxillary and parotid glandular enlargement*
- Hematologic: Prolongation of prothrombin time, partial thromboplastin time; **bleeding and increased clotting times**
- Hypersensitivity: Periorbital edema, urticaria, wheezing
- Other: *Mild temperature elevations, chills, itching, mild influenza-like symptoms*, peripheral edema of the lower extremities

■ Nursing Considerations

Assessment
- *History:* Allergy to hetastarch, severe bleeding disorders, severe cardiac congestion, renal failure or anuria; liver dysfunction
- *Physical:* Body temperature; submaxillary and parotid gland evaluation; P, BP, adventitious sounds, peripheral and periorbital edema; R, adventitious sounds; liver evaluation; urinalysis, renal and liver function tests, clotting times, PT, PTT, hemoglobin, hematocrit

Implementation
- Administer by IV infusion only; monitor rates based on patient response.
- Maintain life support equipment on standby in cases of shock.

Drug-specific teaching points
- Know that this drug can only be given IV.
- Report difficulty breathing, headache, muscle pain, skin rash, unusual bleeding or bruising.

❒ histrelin acetate

(his trell' in)
Supprelin

Pregnancy Category X

Drug classes
Gonadotropin-releasing hormone (GnRH) agonist

Therapeutic actions
GnRH or LHRH agonist; inhibits gonadotropin secretion in chronic administration, resulting in decreased sex steroid levels and regression of secondary sexual characteristics.

Indications
- Control of the biochemical and clinical manifestations of central precocious puberty

Contraindications/cautions
- Hypersensitivity to histrelin or any of the components; pregnancy; congenital adrenal hyperplasia; steroid-secreting tumors.

Dosage
Pediatric: 10 μg/kg SC as a single daily injection. If response is not as anticipated within 3 mo, reevaluate therapy

Pharmacokinetics

Route	Onset	Duration
SC	Slow	3 mo

Metabolism: Plasma, $T_{1/2}$: unknown

Adverse effects in *Italics* are most common; those in **Bold** are life-threatening.

Distribution: Crosses placenta; may enter breast milk
Excretion: Unknown

Adverse effects
- CNS: *Headache*, lightheadedness, mood changes, libido changes, depression, ear pain
- GI: Nausea, vomiting, abdominal pain, flatulence, dyspepsia, anorexia
- CV: *Vasodilitation*, edema, palpitations
- GU: *Vaginal dryness, irritation, odor*; leukorrhea; metrorrhagia; *vaginal bleeding* (within first 1–3 wk)
- Endocrine: Breast pain/discharge, goiter, tenderness of female genitalia
- Respiratory: URI, cough, asthma
- Other: *Chills, pyrexia, malaise*, weight gain, viral infections, joint stiffness, muscle pain
- Local: *Inflammation, infection at injection site*

■ Nursing Considerations

Assessment
- *History:* Hypersensitivity to histrelin or any of the components, pregnancy, congenital adrenal hyperplasia, steroid-secreting tumors, lactation
- *Physical:* Height and weight; temperature; skin—color, lesions; P; R, adventitious sounds; reflexes; affect; abdominal exam; injection site; wrist and hand x-rays; steroid levels; GnRH stimulation test; tomography of the head; pelvic/adrenal/testicular ultrasounds; beta-human chorionic gonadotropin levels; GnRH levels

Implementation
- Ensure patient has only central precocious puberty before treatment: wrist and hand x-rays; steroid levels; GnRH stimulation test; tomography of the head; pelvic/adrenal/testicular ultrasounds; beta-human chorionic gonadotropin levels to rule out other problems.
- Monitor for response to drug, including GnRH levels. If appropriate response is not seen within 3 mo, consider alternate therapy.
- Rotate injection sites daily. Monitor sites for inflammation, pain, infection. Arrange for appropriate treatment if needed (eg, hot soaks, steroids).
- Instruct patient and significant others in the proper techniques for SC injection.
- Refrigerate vials; use each vial only once and discard. Allow vial to warm to room temperature before injection.
- Arrange to discontinue therapy at any sign of hypersensitivity: difficulty breathing, swallowing; rash, fever, chills; tachycardia.

Drug-specific teaching points
- Know that histrelin must be given by single, daily SC injections. Learn the proper technique for administering this drug. Refrigerate vials. Warm vial to room temperature before injection. Use each vial only once and then discard.
- Administer drug each day. Failure to inject daily may result in failure of therapy and return to pubertal state.
- Rotate injection sites daily. Monitor sites for any sign of infection—swelling, pain, redness.
- Arrange for regular medical follow-up while on this drug; this will include blood tests, x-rays of bones, and monitoring of sexual development.
- Know that the following side effects may occur: headache, abdominal discomfort (medications may be available to help); vaginal bleeding (during the first 1–3 wk of therapy); vaginal pain, irrititation, odor; nausea, loss of appetite, vomiting (small, frequent meals may help); flushing, red face (cool environment, avoiding exposure to heat will help).
- Report difficulty breathing, rash, swelling, rapid heartbeat, difficulty swallowing, irritation or redness of injection sites that does not go away.

❏ hyaluronidase

*(bye al yoor **on'** i dase)*
Wydase

Pregnancy Category C

Adverse effects in *Italics* are most common; those in **Bold** are life-threatening.

hyaluronidase

Drug classes
Enzyme

Therapeutic actions
Spreading factor that promotes diffusion and absorption of fluid injected in the subcutaneous tissues by breaking down the viscous substance, hyaluronic acid, that is in the interstices of tissues.

Indications
- Adjuvant to increase absorption and dispersion of injected drugs
- Hypodermoclysis
- Adjunct in SC urography to improve resorption of radiopaques

Contraindications/cautions
- Contraindicated in the presence of allergy to bovine products; acutely inflamed or cancerous areas (avoid injection into these areas).
- Use caution if lactating.

Dosage
Adult
- ***Absorption and dispersion of injected drugs:*** Add 150 U hyaluronidase to the vehicle containing the other medication.
- ***Hypodermoclysis:*** Inject hyaluronidase solution into rubber tubing close to needle inserted between skin and muscle, *or* inject hyaluronidase SC before clysis; 150 U will facilitate absorption of 1,000 ml or more of solution. Individualize dose, rate of injection, and type of solution (saline, glucose, Ringer's).

Pediatric
- ***Hypodermoclysis:*** *For children younger than 3 y:* limit the volume of a single clysis to 200 ml; in premature infants or neonates, the daily dosage should not exceed 25 ml/kg; rate should not be greater than 2 ml/min.
- ***Subcutaneous urography:*** With the patient prone, inject 75 U hyaluronidase SC over each scapula. Inject the contrast medium at the same sites.

Geriatric: Do not exceed the rate and volume of administration used for IV infusion.

Pharmacokinetics

Route	Onset	Duration
SC	Rapid	36–40 h

Metabolism: Tissue, $T_{1/2}$: unknown
Distribution: May cross placenta or enter breast milk

Adverse effects
- **Hematologic:** *Hypovolemia* (if solutions devoid of inorganic electrolytes are given by hypodermoclysis)
- **Hypersensitivity:** Occurs infrequently (drug is a protein and potential antigen)

■ Nursing Considerations

Assessment
- *History:* Allergy to bovine products, acutely inflamed or cancerous areas
- *Physical:* Skin—injection sites; turgor; P, BP, JVP to monitor hypovolemia

Implementation
- Perform a preliminary skin test in patients prone to sensitivity reactions: intradermal injection of 0.02 ml solution. Positive reaction consists of a wheal with pseudopods appearing within 5 min and persisting for 20–30 min with itching.
- Prepare lyphilized powder for injection by adding 1 ml of 0.9% sodium chloride to a vial containing 150 U hyaluronidase and 10 ml 0.9% sodium chloride to 1,500 U hyaluronidase; resulting solution contains 150 U/ml. Refrigerate prepared solution.
- Monitor patients given hyaluronidase with epinephrine for the systemic effects of epinephrine.
- Monitor for hypovolemia throughout therapy; can be corrected through change in solution.

Drug-specific teaching points
- Know that there may be some discomfort at the injection site.
- Report itching, pain at injection site, shortness of breath, dizziness.

Adverse effects in *Italics* are most common; those in **Bold** are life-threatening.

☐ hydralazine hydrochloride

*(hye **dral**' a zeen)*
Apresoline

Pregnancy Category C

Drug classes
Antihypertensive drug
Vasodilator

Therapeutic actions
Acts directly on vascular smooth muscle to cause vasodilation, primarily arteriolar; maintains or increases renal and cerebral blood flow.

Indications
- Oral: essential hypertension alone or in combination with other agents
- Parenteral: severe essential hypertension when the drug cannot be given orally or when the need to lower blood pressure is urgent
- Unlabeled uses: reducing afterload in the treatment of CHF, severe aortic insufficiency, and after valve replacement (doses up to 800 mg tid)

Contraindications/cautions
- Contraindicated in the presence of hypersensitivity to hydralazine, tartrazine (in 100-mg tablets marketed as *Apresoline*); coronary artery disease, mitral valvular rheumatic heart disease (drug has been implicated in MI).
- Use caution in the presence of cerebrovascular accidents; increased intracranial pressure (drug-induced BP fall may increase cerebral ischemia); severe hypertension with uremia; advanced renal damage; slow acetylators (higher plasma levels may be achieved; lower dosage may be adequate); lactation.

Dosage
Adult
- ***Oral:*** Inititate therapy with gradually increasing dosages. Start with 10 mg qid PO for the first 2–4 d; increase to 25 mg qid PO for the balance of the first week. Second and subsequent weeks: 50 mg qid. Maintenance: Adjust to lowest effective dosage; twice daily dosage may be adequate. Some patients may require up to 300 mg/d. Incidence of toxic reactions, particularly the LE syndrome, is high in patients receiving large doses.
- ***Parenteral:*** Patient should be hospitalized. Give IV or IM. Use parenteral therapy only when drug cannot be given orally. Usual dose is 20–40 mg, repeated as necessary. Monitor BP frequently; average maximal decrease occurs in 10–80 min.

Pediatric: Although safety and efficacy have not been established by controlled clinical trials, there is experience with the use of hydralazine in children.
- ***Oral:*** 0.75–3 mg/kg per 24 h PO, given in divided doses q6–12h. Dosage may be gradually increased over the next 3–4 wk to a maximum of 7.5 mg/kg per 24 h PO or 200 mg/24 h PO.
- ***Parenteral:*** 1.7–3.5 mg/kg per 24 h IV or IM, divided into four to six doses.

Pharmacokinetics

Route	Onset	Peak	Duration
Oral	Varies	1–2 h	6–12 h
IM/IV	Rapid	10–20 min	2–4 h

Metabolism: Hepatic, $T_{1/2}$: 3–7 h
Distribution: Crosses placenta; may enter breast milk
Excretion: Urine

IV facts
Preparation: No further preparation required, use as provided.
Infusion: Inject slowly, directly into vein or into tubing of running IV; monitor BP response continually.

Adverse effects
- CNS: *Headache,* lacrimation, conjunctivitis, peripheral neuritis, dizziness, tremors; psychotic reactions characterized by depression, disorientation, or anxiety
- GI: *Anorexia, nausea, vomting, diarrhea,* constipation, paralytic ileus

Adverse effects in *Italics* are most common; those in **Bold** are life-threatening.

558 ■ hydralazine hydrochloride

- **CV:** *Palpitations, tachycardia, angina pectoris,* hypotension, paradoxical pressor response
- **GU:** Difficult micturition, impotence
- **Hypersensitivity:** Rash, urticaria, pruritus; fever, chills, arthralgia, eosinophilia; rarely, hepatitis and obstructive jaundice
- **Hematologic:** Blood dyscrasias
- **Other:** Nasal congestion, flushing, edema, muscle cramps, lymphadenopathy, splenomegaly, dyspnea, lupus-like (LE) syndrome, possible carcinogenesis

Clinically important drug-drug interactions
- Increased bioavailability of oral hydralazine given with food • Increased pharmacologic effects of beta-adrenergic blockers and hydralazine when given concomitantly; dosage of beta-blocker may need adjusting

■ Nursing Considerations

Assessment
- *History:* Hypersensitivity to hydralazine, tartrazine; heart disease; cerebrovascular accidents; increased intracranial pressure; severe hypertension; advanced renal damage; slow acetylators; lactation
- *Physical:* Body weight; body temperature; skin—color, lesions; lymph node palpation; orientation, affect, reflexes; exam of conjunctiva; P, BP, orthostatic BP, supine BP, perfusion, edema, auscultation; R, adventitious sounds, status of nasal mucous membranes; bowel sounds, normal output; voiding pattern, normal output; CBC with differential, LE cell preparations, antinuclear antibody (ANA) determinations, kidney function tests, urinalysis

Implementation
- Administer oral drug with food to increase bioavailability (drug should be given in a consistent relationship to ingestion of food for consistent response to therapy).
- Use parenteral hydralazine immediately after opening ampul. Use as quickly as possible after drawing through a needle into a syringe. Hydralazine changes color after contact with metal, and discolored solutions should be discarded.
- Arrange to withdraw drug gradually, especially from patients who have experienced marked blood pressure reduction. Rapid withdrawal may cause a possible sudden increase in BP.
- Arrange for CBC, LE cell preparations, ANA titers before and periodically during prolonged therapy, even in the asymptomatic patient. Arrange to discontinue drug if blood dyscrasias occur. Arrange to reevaluate therapy if ANA or LE tests are positive.
- Arrange to discontinue or reevaluate drug therapy if patient develops arthralgia, fever, chest pain, continued malaise.
- Arrange for pyridoxine therapy if patient develops symptoms of peripheral neuritis.
- Monitor patient for orthostatic hypotension, which is most marked in the morning and is accentuated by hot weather, alcohol, exercise.

Drug-specific teaching points
- Take this drug exactly as prescribed. Take with food. Do not discontinue this drug or reduce the dosage without consulting your nurse or physician.
- Know that the following side effects may occur: dizziness, weakness (these are more likely to occur when you change position, in the early morning, after exercise, in hot weather, and when you have consumed alcohol; some tolerance may occur after you have taken the drug for a while; avoid driving a car or engaging in tasks that require alertness while you are experiencing these symptoms; remember to change position slowly; use caution in climbing stairs; lie down for a while if dizziness persists); GI upset (frequent, small meals may help); constipation; impotence; numbness, tingling (a vitamin supplement may be prescribed to ameliorate these symptoms); stuffy nose.
- Report persistent or severe constipation; unexplained fever or malaise, muscle or

Adverse effects in *Italics* are most common; those in **Bold** are life-threatening.

Pharmacokinetics

Route	Onset	Peak
Oral	10–20 min	30–60 min

Metabolism: Hepatic, $T_{1/2}$: 3.8 h
Distribution: Crosses placenta; enters breast milk
Excretion: Urine

Adverse effects

- **CNS:** *Sedation, clamminess, sweating, headache, vertigo, floating feeling, dizziness, lethargy, confusion, lightheadedness*
- **GI:** Dry mouth, anorexia, *constipation, nausea*, biliary tract spasm
- **Dermatologic:** Rash, hives, pruritus, flushing, warmth, sensitivity to cold

Clinically important drug-drug interactions

- Potentiation of effects of codeine when given with barbiturate anesthetics; decrease dose of hydrocodone when coadministering.

Drug-lab test interferences

- Elevated biliary tract pressure may cause increases in plasma amylase, lipase; determinations of these levels may be unreliable for 24 h after administration of narcotics.

■ Nursing Considerations

Assessment

- *History:* Hypersensitivity to codeine, hydrocodone, physical dependence on a narcotic analgesic, pregnancy, labor, lactation, COPD, respiratory depression, anoxia, increased intracranial pressure, recent surgery
- *Physical:* Orientation, reflexes, bilateral grip strength, affect; pupil size, vision; P, auscultation, BP; R, adventitious sounds; bowel sounds, normal output; liver and kidney function tests

Implementation

- Administer to women who are nursing a baby 4–6 h before the next scheduled feeding to minimize the amount in milk.
- Provide narcotic antagonist, facilities for assisted or controlled respiration on standby during parenteral administration.
- Instruct postoperative patients in pulmonary toilet; drug suppresses cough reflex.

Drug-specific teaching points

- Take drug exactly as prescribed.
- Know that the following side effects may occur: dizziness, sedation, drowsiness, impaired visual acuity (avoid driving a car, performing other tasks that require alertness); nausea, loss of appetite (lying quietly, eating frequent small meals should minimize these effects); constipation (a laxative may help).
- Report severe nausea, vomiting, palpitations, shortness of breath or difficulty breathing.

☐ hydrocortisone butyrate

Dermatologic ointment and cream: Locoid

hydrocortisone cypoinate

Oral suspension: Cortef, Hycort (CAN)

hydrocortisone sodium phosphate

IV, IM, or SC injection: Hydrocortisone phosphate

hydrocortisone sodium succinate

IV, IM injection: A-hydroCort, Solu-Cortef

hydrocortisone valerate

Dermatologic cream, ointment, lotion: Westcort

Pregnancy Category C

Drug classes

Corticosteroid, short acting
Glucocorticoid
Mineralocorticoid
Adrenal cortical hormone (hydrocortisone)
Hormonal agent

Adverse effects in *Italics* are most common; those in **Bold** are life-threatening.

Therapeutic actions

Enters target cells and binds to cytoplasmic receptors; initiates many complex reactions that are responsible for its anti-inflammatory, immunosuppressive (glucocorticoid), and salt-retaining (mineralocorticoid) actions. Some of these actions are considered undesirable, depending on the indication for which the drug is being used.

Indications

- Replacement therapy in adrenal cortical insufficiency
- Hypercalcemia associated with cancer
- Short-term management of various inflammatory and allergic disorders, such as rheumatoid arthritis, collagen diseases (eg, SLE), dermatologic diseases (eg, pemphigus), status asthmaticus, and autoimmune disorders
- Hematologic disorders—thrombocytopenic purpura, erythroblastopenia
- Trichinosis with neurologic or myocardial involvement
- Ulcerative colitis, acute exacerbations of multiple sclerosis, and palliation in some leukemias and lymphomas
- Intra-articular or soft-tissue administration: Arthritis, psoriatic plaques, and so forth.
- Retention enema: For ulcerative colitis/proctitis
- Dermatologic preparations: To relieve inflammatory and pruritic manifestations of dermatoses that are steroid responsive
- Anorectal cream, suppositories: To relieve discomfort of hemorrhoids and perianal itching or irritation
- Note that synthetic analogues with weaker mineralocorticoid activity may be preferable to hydrocortisone, except for replacement therapy. Local administration to the affected site (eg, by the use of ophthalmic corticosteroid preparations for eye disorders) may be preferable to systemic use.

Contraindications/cautions

- Systemic administration: infections, especially tuberculosis, fungal infections, amebiasis, hepatitis B, vaccinia, or varicella, and antibiotic-resistant infections; kidney disease (predisposes to edema); liver disease, cirrhosis, hypothyroidism; ulcerative colitis with impending perforation; diverticulitis; recent GI surgery; active or latent peptic ulcer; inflammatory bowel disease (drug may cause exacerbations or bowel perforation); hypertension, CHF; thromboembolitic tendencies, thrombophlebitis, osteoporosis, convulsive disorders, metastatic carcinoma, diabetes mellitus; lactation.
- Retention enemas, intrarectal foam: systemic fungal infections, recent intestinal surgery, extensive fistulas.
- Topical dermatologic administration: fungal, tubercular, herpes simplex skin infections; vaccinia, varicella; ear application when eardrum is perforated; lactation.

Dosage

Adult: Individualize dosage, depending on the severity of the condition and the patient's response. Administer daily dose before 9 AM to minimize adrenal suppression. If long-term therapy is needed, alternate-day therapy should be considered. After long-term therapy, withdraw drug slowly to avoid adrenal insufficiency. For maintenance therapy, reduce initial dose in small increments at intervals until the lowest dose that maintains satisfactory clinical response is reached.

- ***IM, IV (hydrocortisone sodium succinate):*** 100–500 mg initially and q2–6h, depending on patient's condition and response.
- *Acute adrenal insufficiency (hydrocortisone sodium phosphate):* 100 mg IV followed by 100 mg q8h in IV fluids.

Pediatric: Individualize dosage on the basis of the severity of the condition and the patient's response rather than by strict adherence to formulae that correct adult doses for age or body weight. Carefully observe growth and development in infants and children on prolonged therapy.

- ***Oral (hydrocortisone and cypionate):*** 20–240 mg/d in single or divided doses.

- **IM or SC (hydrocortisone and sodium phosphate):** 20–240 mg/d usually in divided doses q12h.
- **IM, IV (hydrocortisone sodium succinate):** Reduce dose, depending on condition and response, but give no less than 25 mg/d.
- *Acute adrenal insufficiency (hydrocortisone sodium phosphate):* Older children: 1–2 mg/kg IV bolus; then 150–250 mg/kg per day in divided doses. Infants: 1–2 mg/kg IV bolus; then 25–150 mg/kg per day in divided doses.
- **Retention enema (hydrocortisone):** 100 mg nightly for 21 d.
- **Intrarectal foam (hydrocortisone acetate):** 1 applicator qd or bid for 2 wk and every second day thereafter.
- **Intra-articular, intralesional (hydrocortisone acetate):** 5–25 mg, depending on joint or soft-tissue injection site.
- **Topical dermatologic preparations:** Apply sparingly to affected area bid–qid.

Pharmacokinetics

Route	Onset	Peak	Duration
Oral	1–2 h	1–2 h	1–1½ d
IM	Rapid	4–8 h	1–1½ d
IV	Immediate		1–1½ d
PR	Slow	3–5 d	4–6 d

Metabolism: Hepatic, $T_{1/2}$: 80–120 min
Distribution: Crosses placenta; enters breast milk
Excretion: Urine

IV facts

Preparation: Give directly or dilute in Normal Saline or D5W. Administer within 24 h of diluting.

Infusion: Inject slowly, directly or dilute, and infuse at a rate of 25 mg/min.

Incompatibilities: Do not mix with amobarbital, ampicillin, bleomycin, colistimethate, dimenhydrinate, doxapram, doxorubicin, ephedrine, ergotamine, heparin, hydralazine, metaraminol, methicillin, nafcillin, pentobarbital, phenobarbital, phenytoin, prochloperazine, promethazine, secobarbital, tetracyclines.

Adverse effects

Systemic
- CNS: *Vertigo, headache,* paresthesias, insomnia, convulsions, psychosis
- GI: *Peptic or esophageal ulcer, pancreatitis,* abdominal distention, nausea, vomiting, increased appetite and weight gain (long-term therapy)
- CV: *Hypotension, shock,* hypertension and CHF secondary to fluid retention, thromboembolism, thrombophlebitis, fat embolism, cardiac arrhythmias secondary to electrolyte disturbances
- Hematologic: *Na^+ and fluid retention, hypokalemia,* hypocalcemia, increased blood sugar, increased serum cholesterol, decreased serum T_3 and T_4 levels
- MS: *Muscle weakness,* steroid myopathy and loss of muscle mass, osteoporosis, spontaneous fractures (long-term therapy)
- EENT: Cataracts, glaucoma (long-term therapy), increased intraocular pressure
- Dermatologic: *Thin, fragile skin; petechiae; ecchymoses;* purpura; striae; subcutaneous fat atrophy
- Hypersensitivity: Anaphylactoid or hypersensitivity reactions
- Endocrine: *Amenorrhea, irregular menses,* growth retardation, decreased carbohydrate tolerance and diabetes mellitus, cushingoid state (long-term therapy), hypothalamic-pituitary-adrenal (HPA) suppression systemic with therapy longer than 5 d
- Other: *Immunosuppression, aggravation or masking of infections, impaired wound healing*

Adverse Effects Related to Specific Routes of Administration
- IM repository injections: Atrophy at injection site
- Retention enema: Local pain, burning; rectal bleeding; systemic absorption and adverse effects (above)

Adverse effects in *Italics* are most common; those in **Bold** are life-threatening.

- **Intra-articular:** Osteonecrosis, tendon rupture, infection
- **Intraspinal:** Meningitis, adhesive arachnoiditis, conus medullaris syndrome
- **Intralesional therapy, head and neck:** Blindness (rare)
- **Intrathecal administration:** Arachnoiditis
- **Topical dermatologic ointments, creams, sprays:** Local burning, irritation, acneiform lesions, striae, skin atrophy

Systemic absorption can lead to HPA suppression (see above), growth retardation in children, and other systemic adverse effects. Children may be at special risk of systemic absorption because of their larger skin surface area to body weight ratio.

Clinically important drug-drug interactions

- Increased steroid blood levels if taken concurrently with oral contraceptives, troleandomycin • Decreased steroid blood levels if taken concurrently with phenytoin, phenobarbital, rifampin, cholestyramine • Decreased serum level of salicylates if taken concurrently with hydrocortisone • Decreased effectiveness of anticholinesterases (ambenonium, edrophonium, neostigmine, pyridostigmine) if taken concurrently with hydrocortisone

Drug-lab test interferences

- False-negative nitroblue-tetrazolium test for bacterial infection (with systemic absorption) • Suppression of skin test reactions

■ Nursing Considerations

Assessment

- *History:* Infections; kidney disease; liver disease, hypothyroidism; ulcerative colitis with impending perforation; diverticulitis; recent GI surgery; active or latent peptic ulcer; inflammatory bowel disease; hypertension; CHF; thromboembolitic tendencies, thrombophlebitis, osteoporosis, convulsive disorders, metastatic carcinoma, diabetes mellitus; lactation. *Retention enemas, intrarectal foam:* Systemic fungal infections; recent intestinal surgery, extensive fistulas. *Topical dermatologic administration:* Fungal, tubercular, herpes simplex skin infections; vaccinia, varicella; ear application when eardrum is perforated
- *Physical: Systemic administration:* body weight, temperature; reflexes, affect, bilateral grip strength, ophthalmologic exam; BP, P, auscultation, peripheral perfusion, discoloration, pain or prominence of superficial vessels; R, adventitious sounds, chest x-ray; upper GI x-ray (history or symptoms of peptic ulcer), liver palpation; CBC, serum electrolytes, 2-h postprandial blood glucose, urinalysis, thyroid function tests, serum cholesterol. *Topical, dermatologic preparations:* Affected area, integrity of skin

Implementation

Systemic Administration

- Administer once-a-day before 9 AM to mimic normal peak diurnal corticosteroid levels and minimize HPA suppression.
- Space multiple doses evenly throughout the day.
- Do not give IM injections if patient has thrombocytopenic purpura.
- Rotate sites of IM repository injections to avoid local atrophy.
- Use minimal doses for minimal duration of time to minimize adverse effects.
- Arrange to taper doses when discontinuing high-dose or long-term therapy.
- Arrange for increased dosage when patient is subject to unusual stress.
- Use alternate-day maintenance therapy with short-acting corticosteroids whenever possible.
- Do not give live virus vaccines with immunosuppressive doses of hydrocortisone.
- Provide antacids between meals to help avoid peptic ulcer.

Topical Dermatologic Administration

- Use caution with occlusive dressings, tight or plastic diapers over affected area; these can increase systemic absorption.

Adverse effects in *Italics* are most common; those in **Bold** are life-threatening.

- Avoid prolonged use, especially near eyes, in genital and rectal areas, on face, and in skin creases.

Drug-specific teaching points

Systemic Administration
- Take this drug exactly as prescribed. Do not stop taking this drug without notifying your health care provider; drug dosage must be slowly tapered to avoid problems.
- Take with meals or snacks if GI upset occurs.
- Take single daily or alternate-day doses before 9 AM; mark calendar or use other measures as reminder of treatment days.
- Do not overuse joint after intra-articular injections, even though pain may be gone.
- Arrange for frequent follow-up visits to your health care provider so that your response to the drug may be determined and the dosage adjusted if necessary.
- Know that the following side effects may occur: increase in appetite, weight gain (some of the weight gain may be from fluid retention; watching calories may be helpful); heartburn, indigestion (small, frequent meals, use of antacids between meals may help); increased susceptibility to infection (avoid crowded areas during peak cold or flu seasons, and avoid contact with anyone with a known infection); poor wound healing (if you have an injury or wound, consult your health care provider); muscle weakness, fatigue (frequent rest periods may help).
- Wear a medical alert ID (applies to patients on chronic therapy) so that any emergency medical personnel will know that you are taking this drug.
- Report unusual weight gain, swelling of lower extremities, muscle weakness, black or tarry stools, vomiting of blood, epigastric burning, puffing of face, menstrual irregularities, fever, prolonged sore throat, cold or other infection, worsening of symptoms.
- Know that with dosage reductions you may experience signs of adrenal insufficiency. Report any of the following: fatigue, muscle and joint pains, anorexia, nausea, vomiting, diarrhea, weight loss, weakness, dizziness, low blood sugar (if you monitor blood sugar).

Intra-articular, Intra-lesional Administration
- Do not overuse the injected joint even if the pain is gone. Follow directions you have been given for proper rest and exercise.

Topical Dermatologic Administration
- Apply sparingly, and rub in lightly
- Avoid eye contact.
- Report burning, irritation, or infection of the site, worsening of the condition.
- Avoid prolonged use.

Anorectal Preparations
- Maintain normal bowel function with proper diet, adequate fluid intake, and regular exercise.
- Use stool softeners or bulk laxatives if needed.
- Notify your health care provider if symptoms do not improve in 7 d or if bleeding, protrusion, or seepage occurs.

hydroflumethiazide

(bye droe floo me thye' a zide)
Diucardin, Saluron

Pregnancy Category C

Drug classes
Thiazide diuretic

Therapeutic actions
Inhibits reabsorption of sodium and chloride in distal renal tubule, increasing the excretion of sodium, chloride, and water by the kidney.

Indications
- Adjunctive therapy in edema associated with CHF, cirrhosis, corticosteroid, and estrogen therapy; renal dysfunction
- Hypertension, as sole therapy or in combination with other antihypertensives
- Unlabeled uses: calcium nephrolithiasis alone or with amiloride or allopurinal to prevent recurrences in hypercalciuric or normal calciuric patients, diabetes in-

sipidus, especially nephrogenic diabetes insipidus, osteoporosis

Contraindications/cautions

- Contraindicated in the presence of allergy to thiazides, sulfonamides; fluid or electrolyte imbalance; renal disease (risk of azotemia); liver disease (may precipitate hepatic coma); gout (risk of precipitation of attack); SLE; glucose tolerance abnormalities, diabetes mellitus; hyperparathyroidism; manic-depressive disorder (aggravated by hypercalcemia); pregnancy; lactation.

Dosage

Adult

- **Edema:** 50 mg qd–bid PO. Maintenance: 25–200 mg qd PO; divide doses if dose exceeds 100 mg/d
- **Hypertension:** 50 mg PO bid. Maintenance: 50–100 mg/d PO. Do not exceed 200 mg/d.

Pharmacokinetics

Route	Onset	Peak	Duration
Oral	2 h	4 h	6–12 h

Metabolism: Hepatic, $T_{1/2}$: 17 h
Distribution: Crosses placenta; enters breast milk
Excretion: Urine

Adverse effects

- **CNS:** *Dizziness, vertigo,* paresthesias, weakness, headache, drowsiness, fatigue, leukopenia, thrombocytopenia, agranulocytosis, aplastic anemia, neutropenia
- **GI:** *Nausea, anorexia, vomiting, dry mouth,* diarrhea, constipation, jaundice, hepatitis, pancreatitis
- **CV:** Orthostatic hypotension, venous thrombosis, volume depletion, cardiac arrhythmias, chest pain
- **GU:** *Polyuria, nocturia,* impotence, loss of libido
- **Dermatologic:** Photosensitivity, rash, purpura, exfoliative dermatitis, hives
- **Other:** Muscle cramps and muscle spasms, fever, gouty attacks, flushing, weight loss, rhinorrhea

Clinically important drug-drug interactions

- Increased thiazide effects if taken with diazoxide • Decreased absorption with cholestyramine, colestipol • Increased risk of cardiac glycoside toxicity if hypokalemia occurs • Increased risk of lithium toxicity • Decreased effectiveness of antidiabetic agents when taken concurrently with hydrochlorothiazide

Drug-lab test interferences

- Decreased PBI levels without clinical signs of thyroid disturbance

■ Nursing Considerations

Assessment

- *History:* Allergy to thiazides, sulfonamides; fluid or electrolyte imbalance; renal or liver disease; gout; SLE; glucose tolerance abnormalities; hyperparathyroidism; manic-depressive disorders; lactation
- *Physical:* Skin—color, lesions, edema; orientation, reflexes, muscle strength; pulses, baseline ECG, BP, orthostatic BP, perfusion; R, pattern, adventitious sounds; liver evaluation, bowel sounds, urinary output patterns; CBC, serum electrolytes, blood glucose, liver and renal function tests, serum uric acid, urinalysis

Implementation

- Administer with food or milk if GI upset occurs.
- Mark calendars or other reminders of drug days for outpatients if every other day or 3–5 d/wk therapy is the most advantageous for treating edema.
- Reduce dosage of other antihypertensive drugs by at least 50% if given concurrently with thiazides; readjust dosages gradually as blood pressure responds.
- Administer early in the day so increased urination will not disturb sleep.
- Measure and record regular body weights to monitor fluid changes.

Drug-specific teaching points

- Record intermittent therapy on a calendar, or use prepared, dated envelopes. Take the drug early in the day so in-

Adverse effects in *Italics* are most common; those in **Bold** are life-threatening.

creased urination will not disturb sleep. The drug may be taken with food or meals if GI upset occurs.
- Weigh yourself on a regular basis, at the same time of the day and in the same clothing, and record the weight on your calendar.
- Know that the following side effects may occur: increased volume and frequency of urination (have ready access to a bathroom when drug effect is greatest); dizziness, feeling faint on arising, drowsiness (if these changes occur, avoid rapid position changes; hazardous activities, like driving a car; and alcohol, which can intensify these problems); sensitivity to sunlight (use sunglasses, wear protective clothing, or use a sunscreen when outdoors); decrease in sexual function; increased thirst (sucking on sugarless lozenges may help to alleviate the thirst; frequent mouth care also may help).
- Report loss or gain of more than 3 lb in one day, swelling in your ankles or fingers, unusual bleeding or bruising, dizziness, trembling, numbness, fatigue, muscle weakness or cramps.

hydromorphone hydrochloride

(bye droe mor' fone)
Dilaudid

Pregnancy Category C
Pregnancy Category D
(labor & delivery)
C-II controlled substance

Drug classes
Narcotic agonist analgesic

Therapeutic actions
Acts as agonist at specific opioid receptors in the CNS to produce analgesia, euphoria, sedation; the receptors mediating these effects are thought to be the same as those mediating the effects of endogenous opioids (enkephalins, endorphins).

Indications
- Relief of moderate to severe pain

Contraindications/cautions
- Contraindicated in the presence of hypersensitivity to narcotics, tartrazine (in the 1-, 2-, and 4-mg tablets marketed as *Dilaudid*); physical dependence on a narcotic analgesic (drug may precipitate withdrawal); lactation.
- Use caution in the presence of pregnancy (readily crosses placenta; neonatal withdrawal may occur in infants born to mothers who used this drug during pregnancy); labor or delivery (safety to mother and fetus has not been established); bronchial asthma, COPD, respiratory depression, anoxia, increased intracranial pressure, acute MI, ventricular failure, coronary insufficiency, hypertension, biliary tract surgery, renal or hepatic dysfunction.

Dosage
Adult
- **Oral:** 2–4 mg q4–6h.
- **Parenteral:** 2–4 mg IM, SC q4–6h as needed. May be given by slow IV injection if no other route is tolerated.
- **Rectal:** 3 mg q6–8h.

Pediatric: Safety and efficacy not established. Contraindicated in premature infants.

Geriatric or impaired adult: Use caution; respiratory depression may occur in elderly, the very ill, those with respiratory problems. Reduced dosage may be necessary.

Pharmacokinetics

Route	Onset	Peak	Duration
Oral	Varies	30–60 min	4–5 h
IM	15–30 min	30–60 min	4–5 h

Metabolism: Hepatic, $T_{1/2}$: 2–3 h
Distribution: Crosses placenta; enters breast milk
Excretion: Urine

IV facts
Preparations: Administer undiluted or diluted in Normal Saline or D5W.
Infusion: Inject slowly, directly into vein or into tubing of running IV.

Adverse effects

- **CNS:** *Lightheadedness, dizziness, sedation,* euphoria, dysphoria, delirium, insomnia, agitation, anxiety, fear, hallucinations, disorientation, drowsiness, lethargy, impaired mental and physical performance, coma, mood changes, weakness, headache, tremor, convulsions, miosis, visual disturbances, suppression of cough reflex
- **GI:** *Nausea, vomiting,* dry mouth, anorexia, constipation, biliary tract spasm; increased colonic motility in patients with chronic ulcerative colitis
- **CV:** Facial flushing, peripheral circulatory collapse, tachycardia, bradycardia, arrhythmia, palpitations, chest wall rigidity, hypertension, hypotension, orthostatic hypotension, syncope
- **GU:** Ureteral spasm, spasm of vesical sphincters, urinary retention or hesitancy, oliguria, antidiuretic effect, reduced libido or potency
- **Dermatologic:** Pruritus, urticaria, laryngospasm, bronchospasm, edema
- **Hypersensitivity:** Anaphylactoid reactions (IV administration)
- **Local:** Phlebitis following IV injection pain at injection site; tissue irritation and induration (SC injection)
- **Major hazards: Respiratory depression, apnea, circulatory depression, respiratory arrest, shock, cardiac arrest**
- **Other:** *Sweating,* physical tolerance and dependence, psychological dependence

Clinically important drug-drug interactions

- Potentiation of effects of hydromorphone when given with barbiturate anesthetics; decrease dose of hydromorphone when coadministering.

Drug-lab test interferences

- Elevated biliary tract pressure (an effect of narcotics) may cause increases in plasma amylase, lipase; determinations of these levels may be unreliable for 24 h after administration of narcotics.

■ Nursing Considerations

Assessment

- *History:* Hypersensitivity to narcotics, tartrazine, physical dependence on a narcotic analgesic; pregnancy; lactation; COPD, respiratory depression, anoxia, increased intracranial pressure, acute MI, ventricular failure, coronary insufficiency, hypertension, biliary tract surgery, renal or hepatic dysfunction
- *Physical:* Orientation, reflexes, bilateral grip strength, affect; pupil size, vision; P, auscultation, BP; R, adventitious sounds; bowel sounds, normal output; thyroid, liver, kidney function tests

Implementation

- Administer to women who are nursing a baby 4–6 h before the next scheduled feeding to minimize the amount in milk.
- Provide narcotic antagonist, facilities for assisted or controlled respiration on standby during parenteral administration.
- Use caution when injecting SC into chilled body areas or in patients with hypotension or in shock; impaired perfusion may delay absorption. With repeated doses, an excessive amount may be absorbed when circulation is restored.
- Refrigerate rectal suppositories.

Drug-specific teaching points

- Learn how to administer rectal suppositories; refrigerate suppositories.
- Take drug exactly as prescribed.
- Avoid alcohol, antihistamines, sedatives, tranquilizers, OTC drugs while taking this drug.
- Know that the following side effects may occur: nausea, loss of appetite (taking the drug with food and lying quietly, eating frequent small meals should minimize these effects); constipation (a laxative may help); dizziness, sedation, drowsiness, impaired visual acuity (avoid driving a car, performing other tasks that require alertness, visual acuity).

Adverse effects in *Italics* are most common; those in **Bold** are life-threatening.

hydroxocobalamin crystalline

- Do not take any leftover medication for other disorders, and do not let anyone else take the prescription.
- Report severe nausea, vomiting, constipation, shortness of breath or difficulty breathing.

hydroxocobalamin crystalline

*(hye drox oh koe **bal'** a min)*

Vitamin B$_{12a}$

Hydrobexan, Hydro-Crysti 12, LA-12

Pregnancy Category C

Drug classes
Vitamin

Therapeutic actions
Essential to growth, cell reproduction, hematopoiesis, and nucleoprotein and myelin synthesis; physiologic function is associated with nucleic acid and protein synthesis; acts the same way as cyanocobalamin.

Indications
- Vitamin B$_{12}$ deficiency due to malabsorption; GI pathology, dysfunction, or surgery; fish tapeworm; gluten enteropathy, sprue; small bowel bacterial overgrowth; folic acid deficiency
- Increased vitamin B$_{12}$ requirements—pregnancy, thyrotoxicosis, hemolytic anemia, hemorrhage, malignancy, hepatic and renal disease
- Unlabeled use: prevention and treatment of cyanide toxicity associated with sodium nitroprusside (forms cyanocobalamin with the cyanide, thus lowering plasma and RBC cyanide concentrations)

Contraindications/cautions
- Contraindicated in the presence of allergy to cobalt, vitamin B$_{12}$, or any component of these medications; Leber's disease.
- Use caution in the presence of pregnancy (safety not established, but is an essential vitamin required during pregnancy—4 µg/d); lactation—secreted in breast milk (required nutrient during lactation—4 µg/d).

Dosage
For IM use only; folic acid therapy should be given concurrently if needed.
Adult: 30 µg/d for 5–10 d IM, followed by 100–200 µg/mo.
Pediatric: 1–5 mg over 2 or more wk in doses of 100 µg IM, then 30–50 µg every 4 wk for maintainence.

Pharmacokinetics

Route	Onset	Peak
IM	Intermediate	60 min

Metabolism: Hepatic, T$_{1/2}$: 24–36 h
Distribution: Crosses placenta; enters breast milk
Excretion: Urine

Adverse effects
- **CNS:** Severe and swift optic nerve atrophy (patients with early Leber's disease)
- **GI:** *Mild, transient diarrhea*
- **CV:** Pulmonary edema, congestive heart failure, peripheral vascular thrombosis
- **Hematologic:** Polycythemia vera
- **Dermatologic:** *Itching, transitory exanthema*, urticaria
- **Hypersensitivity: Anaphylactic shock and death**
- **Local:** *Pain at injection site*
- **Other:** Feeling of total body swelling; hypokalemia

Drug-lab test interferences
- Invalid folic acid and vitamin B$_{12}$ diagnostic blood assays if patient is taking methotrexate, pyrimethamine, most antibiotics

■ Nursing Considerations

Assessment
- *History:* Allergy to cobalt, vitamin B$_{12}$, or any component of these medications; Leber's disease
- *Physical:* Skin—color, lesions; ophthalmic exam; P, BP, peripheral perfusion; R, adventitious sounds; CBC, hematocrit,

Adverse effects in *Italics* are most common; those in **Bold** are life-threatening.

hemoglobin, vitamin B_{12}, and folic acid levels

Implementation
- Administer in parenteral form for pernicious anemia.
- Administer with folic acid if needed; check serum levels.
- Monitor serum potassium levels, especially during the first few days of treatment; arrange for appropriate treatment of hypokalemia.
- Maintain emergency drugs and life support equipment on standby in case of severe anaphylactic reaction.
- Arrange for periodic checks for stomach cancer in patients with pernicious anemia; risk is three times greater in these patients.

Drug-specific teaching points
- Know that the IM route is the only one available. Monthly injections will be needed for life in patients with pernicious anemia. Without it, anemia will return and irreversible neurologic damage will develop.
- Know that the following side effects may occur: mild diarrhea (this usually passes after a few doses); rash, itching; pain at injection site.
- Report swelling of the ankles, leg cramps, fatigue, difficulty breathing, pain at injection site.

❐ hydroxychloroquine sulfate

*(bye drox ee **klor'** oh kwin)*
Plaquenil Sulfate

Pregnancy Category C

Drug classes
Antimalarial
Antirheumatic agent
4-aminoquinoline

Therapeutic actions
Inhibits protozoal reproduction and protein synthesis, preventing the replication of DNA, the transcription of RNA, and the synthesis of protein. Anti-inflammatory action in rheumatoid arthritis, lupus: mechanism of action is not known but is thought to involve the suppression of the formation of antigens, which cause hypersensitivity reactions and symptoms.

Indications
- Suppression and treatment of acute attacks of malaria caused by susceptible strains of plasmodia
- Treatment of acute or chronic rheumatoid arthritis
- Treatment of chronic discoid and systemic lupus erythematosus
- *Note:* Radical cure of vivax malaria requires concomitant primaquine therapy; some strains of *Plasmodium falciparum* are resistant to chloroquine and related drugs.

Contraindications/cautions
- Contraindicated in the presence of allergy to 4-aminoquinolines, porphyria, psoriasis, retinal disease (irreversible retinal damage may occur); pregnancy.
- Use caution in the presence of hepatic disease, alcoholism, G-6-PD deficiency.

Dosage
200 mg hydroxychloroquine sulfate is equivalent to 155 mg hydroxychloroquine base.

Adult
- ***Suppression of malaria:*** 310 mg base/wk PO on the same day each week, beginning 2 wk prior to exposure and continuing for 6–8 wk after leaving the endemic area. If suppressive therapy is not begun prior to exposure, double the initial loading dose (620 mg base), and give in two doses, 6 h apart.
- ***Acute attack of malaria***

Dose	Time	Dosage (mg Base)
Initial	Day 1	620 mg
2nd dose	6 h later	310 mg
3rd dose	Day 2	310 mg
4th dose	Day 3	310 mg

- ***Rheumatoid arthritis:*** Initial dosage 400–600 mg/d PO taken with meals or a glass of milk. From 5–10 d later, gradually increase dosage to optimum effectiveness.

hydroxychloroquine sulfate ■ 571

– **Maintenance dosage:** When good response is obtained (usually 4–12 wk), reduce dosage to 200–400 mg/d PO.
- **Lupus erythematosus:** 400 mg qd–bid PO continued for several weeks or months; for prolonged use, 200–400 mg/d may be sufficient.

Pediatric
- **Suppression of malaria:** 5 mg base/kg weekly PO as described above for adults.
- **Acute attack of malaria**

Dose	Time	Dosage (mg Base)
Initial	Day 1	10 mg/kg
2nd dose	6 h later	5 mg/kg
3rd dose	Day 2	5 mg/kg
4th dose	Day 3	5 mg/kg

Pharmacokinetics

Route	Onset	Peak
Oral	Varies	1–6 h

Metabolism: Hepatic, $T_{1/2}$: 70–120 h
Distribution: Crosses placenta; enters breast milk
Excretion: Urine

Adverse effects

- **CNS:** Ringing in the ears, loss of hearing (ototoxicity), exacerbation of porphyria, muscle weakness, absent or hypoactive deep tendon reflexes, irritability, nervousness, emotional changes, nightmares, psychosis, headache, dizziness, vertigo, nystagmus, convulsions, ataxia
- **GI:** *Nausea, vomiting, diarrhea*, abdominal cramps, loss of appetite
- **Hematologic:** **Blood dyscrasias**, immunoblastic lymphadenopathy, hemolysis in patients with G-6-PD deficiency
- **EENT:** *Retinal changes, corneal changes*—edema, opacities, decreased sensitivity; ciliary body changes—disturbance of accommodation, blurred vision
- **Dermatologic:** *Pruritus, bleaching of hair,* alopecia, skin and mucosal pigmentation, skin eruptions, psoriasis, exfoliative dermatitis

■ Nursing Considerations

Assessment
- *History:* Allergy to 4-aminoquinolines, porphyria, psoriasis, retinal disease, hepatic disease, alcoholism, G-6-PD deficiency
- *Physical:* Skin—color, lesions; hair; reflexes, muscle strength, auditory and ophthalmological screening, affect, reflexes; liver palpation, abdominal exam, mucous membranes; CBC, G-6-PD in deficient patients, liver function tests

Implementation
- Administer with meals or milk.
- Titrate long-term therapy to smallest effective dose; incidence of retinopathy increases with larger doses.
- Schedule malaria suppressive doses for weekly same-day therapy on a calendar.
- Double check pediatric doses; children are very susceptible to overdosage.
- Arrange for administration of ammonium chloride (8 g/d in divided doses for adults) 3–4 d/wk for several months after therapy has been stopped if serious toxic symptoms occur.
- Arrange for ophthalmologic examinations during long-term therapy.

Drug-specific teaching points
- Take full course of drug therapy as prescribed.
- Take drug with meals or milk.
- Mark your calendar with the drugs days for malarial prophylaxis.
- Know that the following side effects may occur: stomach pain, loss of appetite, nausea, vomiting or diarrhea; irritability, emotional changes, nightmares, headache (it may help to know that these are drug effects).
- Arrange for regular ophthalmologic exams if long-term use is indicated.
- Report blurring of vision, loss of hearing, ringing in the ears, muscle weakness, skin rash or itching, unusual bleeding

Adverse effects in *Italics* are most common; those in **Bold** are life-threatening.

or bruising, yellow color of eyes or skin, mood swings or mental changes.

☐ hydroxyprogesterone caproate in oil

(bye drox' ee proe jess' te rone)
Duralutin, Gesterol L.A. Hylutin, Hyprogest

Pregnancy Category X

Drug classes
Hormonal agent
Progestin

Therapeutic actions
Progesterone derivative. Endogenous progesterone transforms proliferative endometrium into secretory endometrium; inhibits the secretion of pituitary gonadotropins, which prevents follicular maturation and ovulation; and inhibits spontaneous uterine contraction. Progestins have varying profiles of estrogenic, antiestrogenic, anabolic, and androgenic activity.

Indications
- Treatment of amenorrhea (primary or secondary); abnormal uterine bleeding due to hormonal imbalance
- Production of secretory endometrium and desquamation

Contraindications/cautions
- Contraindicated in the presence of allergy to progestins; thrombophlebitis, thromboembolic disorders, cerebral hemorrhage, or history of these conditions; hepatic disease, carcinoma of the breast or genital organs, undiagnosed vaginal bleeding, missed abortion; pregnancy (fetal abnormalities, including masculinization of the female fetus have been reported); lactation.
- Use caution in the presence of epilepsy, migraine, asthma, cardiac or renal dysfunction.

Dosage
Administer IM only.
Adult
- ***Amenorrhea; abnormal uterine bleeding:*** 375 mg IM at any time. After 4 d of desquamation or if no bleeding occurs in 21 d after hydroxyprogesterone alone, start cyclic therapy (administer 20 mg estradiol valerate on day 1 of each cycle; 2 wk after day 1, administer 250 mg hydroxyprogesterone caproate and 5 mg estradiol valerate; 4 wk after day 1 is day 1 of the next cycle). Repeat every 4 wk, and stop after four cycles. Observe patient for onset of normal cycling for two to three cycles after cessation of therapy.
- ***Production of secretory endometrium and desquamation:*** Start cyclic therapy any time (see above); repeat every 4 wk until no longer required. Give 125–250 mg IM given on 10th day of cycle; repeat q7 d until suppression is no longer necessary.

Pharmacokinetics

Route	Onset	Duration
IM	Slow	9–17 d

Metabolism: Hepatic, $T_{1/2}$: unknown
Distribution: Crosses placenta; enters breast milk
Excretion: Urine

Adverse effects
- **CNS:** Sudden, partial or complete loss of vision, proptosis, diplopia, migraine, precipitation of acute intermittent porphyria, mental depression, pyrexia, insomnia, somnolence
- **GI:** Cholestatic jaundice, nausea
- **CV:** Thrombophlebitis, cerebrovascular disorders, retinal thrombosis, pulmonary embolism, thromboembolic and thrombotic disease, increased blood pressure
- **GU:** *Breakthrough bleeding, spotting, change in menstrual flow, amenorrhea,* changes in cervical erosion and cervical secretions, breast tenderness and secretion

Adverse effects in *Italics* are most common; those in **Bold** are life-threatening.

- **Dermatologic:** *Rash with or without pruritus, acne,* melasma or chloasma, alopecia, hirsutism, photosensitivity
- **General:** *Fluid retention, edema, increase or decrease in weight*
- **Other:** Decreased glucose tolerance

Drug-lab test interferences
- Inaccurate tests of hepatic and endocrine function

■ Nursing Considerations
Assessment
- *History:* Allergy to progestins; thromboembolic disorders, cerebral hemorrhage; hepatic disease, carcinoma of the breast or genital organs, undiagnosed vaginal bleeding, missed abortion; epilepsy, migraine, asthma, cardiac or renal dysfunction
- *Physical:* Skin—color, lesions, turgor; hair; breasts; pelvic exam; orientation, affect; ophthalmologic exam; P, auscultation, peripheral perfusion, edema; R, adventitious sounds; liver evaluation; liver and renal function tests, glucose tolerance, Pap smear

Implementation
- Arrange for pretreatment and periodic (at least annual) history and physical, which should include BP, breasts, abdomen, pelvic organs, and a Pap smear.
- Caution patient before beginning therapy of the need to prevent pregnancy during treatment, the need for frequent medical follow-up.
- Administer IM only.
- Arrange to discontinue medication and consult physician if sudden partial or complete loss of vision occurs; if papilledema or retinal vascular lesions are present on exam, the drug should be discontinued.
- Arrange to discontinue medication and consult physician at the first sign of thromboembolic disease (leg pain, swelling, peripheral perfusion changes, shortness of breath).

Drug-specific teaching points
- Prepare a calendar of drug days to remind you about doses.
- Know that this drug can be given only by IM injection.
- Know that the following side effects may occur: sensitivity to light (avoid exposure to the sun; use sunscreen and protective clothing if exposure is necessary); dizziness, sleeplessness, depression (use caution if driving or performing tasks that require alertness if these occur); skin rash, color changes, loss of hair; fever; nausea.
- Do not take this drug during pregnancy; serious fetal abnormalities have been reported.
- Report pain or swelling and warmth in the calves, acute chest pain or shortness of breath, sudden severe headache or vomiting, dizziness or fainting, visual disturbances, numbness or tingling in the arm or leg.

◻ hydroxyurea

(bye drox ee yoor ee′ a)

Hydrea

Pregnancy Category D

Drug classes
Antineoplastic agent

Therapeutic actions
Cytotoxic: inhibits an enzyme that is crucial for DNA synthesis, but exact mechanism of action is not fully understood.

Indications
- Melanoma
- Resistant chronic myelocytic leukemia
- Recurrent, metastatic, or inoperable ovarian cancer
- Concomitant therapy with irradiation for primary squamous cell carcinoma of the head and neck, excluding the lip
- Treatment of sickle cell anemia

Contraindications/cautions
- Allergy to hydroxyurea, irradiation, leukopenia, impaired hepatic and renal function, pregnancy, lactation.

Dosage
Adult: Base dosage on ideal or actual body weight, whichever is less. Interrupt therapy if WBC falls below 2,500/mm³ or

platelet count below 100,000/mm^3. Recheck in 3 d and resume therapy when counts approach normal.
- **Solid tumors:** Intermittent therapy: 80 mg/kg PO as a single dose every third day. Continuous therapy: 20–30 mg/kg PO as a single daily dose.
- **Concomitant therapy with irradiation:** 80 mg/kg as a single daily dose every third day. Begin hydroxyurea 7 d before irradiation, and continue during and for a prolonged period after radiotherapy.
- **Resistant chronic myelocytic leukemia:** 20–30 mg/kg as a single daily dose.

Pediatric: Dosage regimen not established.

Pharmacokinetics

Route	Onset	Peak	Duration
Oral	Varies	2 h	18–20 h

Metabolism: Hepatic, T$_{1/2}$: 3–4 h
Distribution: Crosses placenta; enters breast milk
Excretion: Urine

Adverse effects
- CNS: *Headache, dizziness,* disorientation, hallucinations
- GI: *Stomatitis, anorexia, nausea, vomiting,* diarrhea, constipation, elevated hepatic enzymes
- Hematologic: **Bone marrow depression**
- GU: Impaired renal tubular function
- Dermatologic: Maculopapular rash, facial erythema
- Local: Mucositis at the site, especially in combination with irradiation
- Other: Fever, chills, malaise

Drug-lab test interferences
- Serum uric acid, BUN, and creatinine levels may increase with hydroxyurea therapy • Drug causes self-limiting abnormalities in erythrocytes that resemble those of pernicious anemia but are not related to vitamin B$_{12}$ or folate deficiency

■ Nursing Considerations

Assessment
- *History:* Allergy to hydroxyurea, irradiation, leukopenia, impaired hepatic and renal function, lactation
- *Physical:* Weight; temperature; skin—color, lesions; reflexes, orientation, affect; mucous membranes, abdominal exam; CBC, renal and liver function tests

Implementation
- Administer in oral form only. If patient is unable to swallow capsules, empty capsules into a glass of water, and administer immediately (inert products may not dissolve).
- Encourage patient to drink 10–12 glasses of fluid each day.
- Arrange for and check CBC before administration of each dose of drug.

Drug-specific teaching points
- Prepare a calendar for dates to return for diagnostic testing on treatment days. If you are unable to swallow the capsule, empty the capsule into a glass of water, and take immediately (some of the material may not dissolve).
- Know that the following side effects may occur: loss of appetite, nausea, vomiting, mouth sores (frequent mouth care, small frequent meals may help; you will need to try to maintain good nutrition if at all possible; an antiemetic also may be ordered); constipation or diarrhea (a bowel program may be established to help out with this problem; ensure ready access to bathroom facilties if diarrhea occurs); disorientation, dizziness, headache (take special precautions to avoid injury if these occur); red face, rash (these are effects of the drug; they should pass when the drug is discontinued).
- Arrange for regular blood tests to monitor the drug's effects.
- Drink at least 10–12 glasses of fluid each day while on this drug.
- Report fever, chills, sore throat, unusual bleeding or bruising, severe nausea, vomiting, loss of appetite, sores in the mouth

hydroxyzine hydrochloride

(bye drox' i zeen)

Oral preparations: Anxanil, Atarax, Vistaril

Parenteral preparations: E-Vista, Hydroxacen, Hyzine, Multipax (CAN), Quiess, Vistacon, Vistaject, Vistaquel, Vistaril

hydroxyzine pamoate

Oral preparations: Vistaril

Pregnancy Category C

Drug classes
Antianxiety drug
Antihistamine
Antiemetic

Therapeutic actions
Mechanisms of action not understood; actions may be due to suppression of subcortical areas of the CNS; has clinically demonstrated antihistaminic, analgesic, antispasmodic, antiemetic, mild antisecretory, and bronchodilator activity.

Indications
- Symptomatic relief of anxiety and tension associated with psychoneurosis; adjunct in organic disease states in which anxiety is manifested; alcoholism and asthma
- Management of pruritus due to allergic conditions, such as chronic urticaria, atopic and contact dermatosis, and in histamine-mediated pruritus
- Sedation when used as premedication and following general anesthesia
- Management of the acutely disturbed or hysterical patient; the acute or chronic alcoholic with anxiety withdrawal symptoms or delirium tremens; as preoperative and postoperative and prepartum and postpartum adjunctive medication to permit reduction in narcotic dosage, allay anxiety, and control emesis (IM administration)

Contraindications/cautions
- Allergy to hydroxyzine; uncomplicated vomiting in children (may contribute to development of Reye's syndrome or unfavorably influence its outcome; extrapyramidal effects of drugs may obscure diagnosis of Reye's syndrome); pregnancy; lactation.

Dosage
Start patients on IM therapy; use oral therapy for maintenance. Adjust dosage to patient's response.

Adult
- **Oral**
  - *Symptomatic relief of anxiety:* 50–100 mg qid.
  - *Management of pruritus:* 25 mg tid–qid.
  - *Sedative (preoperative and postoperative):* 50–100 mg.
- **IM**
  - *Psychiatric and emotional emergencies, including alcoholism:* 50–100 mg immediately and q4–6h as needed.
  - *Nausea and vomiting:* 25–100 mg.
  - *Preoperative and postoperative, prepartum and postpartum:* 25–100 mg.

Pediatric
- **Oral**
  - *Anxiety, pruritus:* Older than 6 y: 50–100 mg/d in divided doses. *Younger than 6 y:* 50 mg/d in divided doses.
  - *Sedative:* 0.6 mg/kg.
- **IM**
  - *Nausea, preoperative and postoperative:* 1.1 mg/kg (0.5 mg/lb).

Pharmacokinetics

Route	Onset	Peak	Duration
Oral/IM	15–30 min	3 h	4–6 h

Metabolism: Hepatic, $T_{1/2}$: 3 h
Distribution: Crosses placenta; may enter breast milk
Excretion: Urine

Adverse effects
- **CNS:** *Drowsiness*, involuntary motor activity, including tremor and convulsions

---
Adverse effects in *Italics* are most common; those in **Bold** are life-threatening.

576 ■ ibuprofen

- GI: *Dry mouth*
- Hypersensitivity: Wheezing, dyspnea, chest tightness

■ Nursing Considerations
Assessment
- *History:* Allergy to hydroxyzine, uncomplicated vomiting in children, lactation
- *Physical:* Skin—color, lesions, texture; orientation, reflexes, affect; R, adventitious sounds

Implementation
- Attempt to determine and arrange treatment for underlying cause of vomiting. Drug may mask signs and symptoms of serious conditions, such as brain tumor, intestinal obstruction, appendicitis.
- Do not administer parenteral solution SC, IV or intra-arterially; tissue necrosis has occurred with SC and intra-arterial injection, hemolysis with IV injection.
- Administer IM injections deep into a large muscle: adults—upper outer quadrant of buttocks or midlateral thigh; children—midlateral thigh muscles; use deltoid area only if well developed.

Drug-specific teaching points
- Take this drug as prescribed. Avoid excessive dosage.
- Know that the following side effects may occur: dizziness, sedation, drowsiness (use caution if driving or performing tasks that require alertness if these occur); avoid alcohol, sedatives, sleep aids while you are taking this drug (serious overdosage could result); dry mouth (frequent mouth care, sucking sugarless lozenges may help).
- Report difficulty breathing, tremors, loss of coordination, sore muscles, or muscle spasms.

❒ ibuprofen

(eye byoo' proe fen)

Aches-N-Pain, Advil, Amersol (CAN), Excedrin IB, Genpril, Haltran, Ibuprin, Ibuprohm, Ibu-Tab, Medipren, Midol, Motrin, Nuprin, Pamprin-IB, Pediaprofen, Rufen, Saleto-200, Trendar

Pregnancy Category B

Drug classes
NSAID
Non-narcotic analgesic
Propionic acid derivative

Therapeutic actions
Anti-inflammatory, analgesic, and antipyretic activities largely related to inhibition of prostaglandin synthesis; exact mechanisms of action are not known.

Indications
- Relief of signs and symptoms of rheumatoid arthritis and osteoarthritis
- Relief of mild to moderate pain
- Treatment of primary dysmenorrhea
- Fever reduction
- Unlabeled use: treatment of juvenile rheumatoid arthritis

Contraindications/cautions
- Contraindicated in the presence of allergy to ibuprofen, salicylates, or other NSAIDs (more common in patients with rhinitis, asthma, chronic urticaria, nasal polyps); cardiovascular dysfunction, hypertension; peptic ulceration, GI bleeding; pregnancy; lactation.
- Use caution in the presence of impaired hepatic or renal function.

Dosage
Do not exceed 3200 mg/d.
Adult
- ***Mild to moderate pain:*** 400 mg q4–6h PO.
- ***Osteoarthritis/rheumatoid arthritis:*** 1,200–3,200 mg/d PO (300 mg qid or 400, 600, 800 mg tid or qid; individualize dosage. Therapeutic response may occur in a few days, but often takes 2 wk).
- ***Primary dysmenorrhea:*** 400 mg q4h PO.

Adverse effects in *Italics* are most common; those in **Bold** are life-threatening.

ibuprofen ■ 577

- **OTC use:** 200–400 mg q4–6h PO while symptoms persist; do not exceed 1,200 mg/d. Do not take for more than 10 d for pain or 3 d for fever, unless so directed by health care provider.

Pediatric
- **Juvenile arthritis:** 30–40 mg/kg per day PO in three to four divided doses; 20 mg/kg per day for milder disease.
- **Fever:** 5–10 mg/kg PO q6–8h; do not exceed 40 mg/kg per day.

Pharmacokinetics

Route	Onset	Peak	Duration
Oral	30 min	1–2 h	4–6 h

Metabolism: Hepatic; $T_{1/2}$: 1.8–2½ h
Distribution: Crosses placenta; may enter breast milk
Excretion: Urine

Adverse effects
NSAIDs
- CNS: *Headache, dizziness, somnolence, insomnia,* fatigue, tiredness, dizziness, tinnitus, ophthalmologic effects
- GI: *Nausea, dyspepsia, GI pain,* diarrhea, vomiting, *constipation,* flatulence
- Respiratory: Dyspnea, hemoptysis, pharyngitis, bronchospasm, rhinitis
- Hematologic: Bleeding, platelet inhibition with higher doses, neutropenia, eosinophilia, leukopenia, pancytopenia, thrombocytopenia, agranulocytosis, granulocytopenia, aplastic anemia, decreased hemoglobin or hematocrit, bone marrow depression, menorrhagia
- GU: Dysuria, renal impairment
- Dermatologic: *Rash,* pruritus, sweating, dry mucous membranes, stomatitis
- Other: Peripheral edema, anaphylactoid reactions to fatal anaphylactic shock

Clinically important drug-drug interactions
- Increased toxic effects of lithium if taken with ibuprofen • Decreased diuretic effect if taken concurrently with loop diuretics: bumetanide, furosemide, ethacrynic acid
- Potential decrease in antihypertensive effect of beta-adrenergic blocking agents

■ Nursing Considerations
Assessment
- *History:* Allergy to ibuprofen, salicylates or other NSAIDs; cardiovascular dysfunction, hypertension; peptic ulceration, GI bleeding; impaired hepatic or renal function; pregnancy; lactation
- *Physical:* Skin—color, lesions; temperature; orientation, reflexes, ophthalmologic evaluation, audiometric evaluation, peripheral sensation; P, BP, edema; R, adventitious sounds; liver evaluation, bowel sounds; CBC, clotting times, urinalysis, renal and liver function tests, serum electrolytes, stool guaiac

Implementation
- Administer drug with food or after meals if GI upset occurs.
- Arrange for periodic ophthalmologic examination during long-term therapy.
- Arrange for discontinuation of drug if eye changes, symptoms of liver dysfunction, renal impairment occur.
- Institute emergency procedures if overdose occurs: gastric lavage, induction of emesis, supportive therapy.

Drug-specific teaching points
- Use the drug only as suggested; avoid overdose. Take the drug with food or after meals if GI upset occurs. Do not exceed the prescribed dosage.
- Know that the following side effects may occur: nausea, GI upset, dyspepsia (taking the drug with food may help); diarrhea or constipation; drowsiness, dizziness, vertigo, insomnia (use caution when driving or operating dangerous machinery if these occur).
- Avoid OTC drugs while you are taking this drug. Many of these drugs contain similar medications, and serious overdosage can occur.
- Report sore throat, fever, rash, itching, weight gain, swelling in ankles or fingers, changes in vision, black or tarry stools.

Adverse effects in *Italics* are most common; those in **Bold** are life-threatening.

idarubicin hydrochloride

(eye da roo' bi sin)

Idamycin

Pregnancy Category D

Drug classes
Antibiotic (anthracycline)
Antineoplastic agent

Therapeutic actions
Cytotoxic: binds to DNA and inhibits DNA synthesis in susceptible cells.

Indications
- In combination with other approved antileukemic drugs for the treatment of acute myeloid leukemia (AML) in adults
- Orphan drug uses: acute nonlymphocytic leukemia, acute lymphoblastic leukemia in pediatric patients

Contraindications/cautions
- Contraindicated in the presence of allergy to idarubicin, other anthracycline antibiotics; myelosuppression; cardiac disease; pregnancy; lactation.
- Use caution in the presence of impaired hepatic or renal function.

Dosage
Adult
- ***Induction therapy in adults with AML:*** 12 mg/m^2 daily for 3 d by slow IV injections in combination with *Ara-C;* 100 mg/m^2 daily given by continuous infusion for 7 d or as a 25-mg/m^2 IV bolus followed by 200 mg/m^2 daily for 5 d by continuous infusion. A second course may be administered when toxicity has subsided, if needed.

Pediatric: Safety and efficacy not established.

Geriatric, renal or hepatic impairment: Reduce dosage by 25%. Do not administer if bilirubin level is > 5 mg/dl.

Pharmacokinetics

Route	Onset	Peak
IV	Rapid	Minutes

Metabolism: Hepatic; T$_{1/2}$: 22 h
Distribution: Crosses placenta; enters breast milk
Excretion: Bile and urine

IV facts
Preparation: Reconstitute the 5- and 10-mg vials with 5 and 10 ml, respectively of 0.9% Sodium Chloride Injection to give a final concentration of 1 mg/ml. Do not use bacteriostatic diluents. Use extreme caution when preparing drug. Use of goggles and gloves is recommended as drug can cause severe skin reactions. If skin is accidently exposed to idarubicin, wash with soap and water; use standard irrigation techniques if eyes are contaminated. Vials are under pressure; use care when inserting needle to minimize inhalation of any aerosol that is released. Reconstituted solution is stable for 7 d if refrigerated and 72 h at room temperature.

Infusion: Administer slowly (over 10–15 min) into tubing of a freely running IV infusion of Sodium Chloride Injection or 5% Dextrose Injection. Attach the tubing to a butterfly needle inserted into a large vein; avoid veins over joints or in extremities with poor perfusion.

Incompatibilities: Do not mix idarubicin with other drugs, especially heparin (a precipitate forms, and the IV solution must not be used) and any alkaline solution.

Adverse effects
- **GI:** *Nausea, vomiting, mucositis,* anorexia, diarrhea
- **CV:** Cardiac toxicity, CHF, phlebosclerosis
- **Hematologic:** *Myelosuppression,* hyperuricemia due to cell lysis
- **Dermatologic:** *Complete but reversible alopecia,* hyperpigmentation of nailbeds and dermal creases, facial flushing
- **Hypersensitivity:** Fever, chills, urticaria, anaphylaxis
- **Local:** Severe local cellulitis, vesication and tissue necrosis if extravasation occurs
- **Other:** Carcinogenesis, infertility

Adverse effects in *Italics* are most common; those in **Bold** are life-threatening.

Nursing Considerations

Assessment
- *History:* Allergy to idarubicin, other anthracycline antibiotics; myelosuppression; cardiac disease; impaired hepatic or renal function; pregnancy; lactation
- *Physical:* Temperature; skin—color, lesions; weight; hair; nailbeds; local injection site; cardiac auscultation, peripheral perfusion, pulses, ECG; R, adventitious sounds; liver evaluation, mucous membranes; CBC, liver and renal function tests, uric acid levels

Implementation
- Do not administer IM or SC because severe local reaction and tissue necrosis occur. Give IV only.
- Monitor injection site for extravasation: reports of burning or stinging. Discontinue infusion immediately, and restart in another vein. For local SC extravasation, local infiltration with corticosteroid may be ordered; flood area with normal saline, and apply cold compress to area. If ulceration begins, arrange consultation with plastic surgeon.
- Monitor patient's response to therapy frequently at beginning of therapy: serum uric acid level, cardiac output (listen for S_3). CBC changes may require a decrease in the dose; consult with physician.
- Ensure adequate hydration during the course of therapy to prevent hyperuricemia.

Drug-specific teaching points
- Prepare a calendar for days to return for drug therapy. Drug can only be given IV.
- Know that the following side effects may occur: rash, skin lesions, loss of hair, changes in nails (you may want to invest in a wig before hair loss occurs; skin care may help somewhat); loss of appetite, nausea, mouth sores (frequent mouth care, small frequent meals may help; you will need to try to maintain good nutrition if at all possible; a dietician may be able to help; an antiemetic may be ordered); red urine (this is a result of drug therapy and will pass after a few days).
- Arrange for regular medical follow-up, which will include blood tests to monitor the drug's effects.
- Report difficulty breathing, sudden weight gain, swelling, burning or pain at injection site, unusual bleeding or bruising.

❏ ifosfamide

(eye foss' fa mide)
Ifex

Pregnancy Category D

Drug classes
Alkylating agent
Nitrogen mustard
Antineoplastic drug

Therapeutic actions
Cytotoxic: Exact mechanism of action is not known, though metabolite of ifosfamide alkylates DNA, interferes with the replication of susceptible cells; immunosuppressive: lymphocytes are especially sensitive to drug effects.

Indications
- In combination with other approved neoplastic agents for third-line chemotherapy of germ cell testicular cancer; should be used with an agent for hemorrhagic cystitis
- Unlabeled uses: possible effectiveness in the treatment of lung, breast, ovarian, pancreatic and gastric cancer, sarcomas, acute leukemias, malignant lymphomas
- Orphan drug uses: third-line chemotherapy in the treatment of germ cell testicular cancer, bone sarcomas, soft-tissue sarcomas

Contraindications/cautions
- Allergy to ifosfamide, hematopoietic depression, impaired hepatic or renal function, pregnancy, lactation.

Dosage
Adult: Administer IV at a dose of 1.2 mg/m^2 per day for 5 consecutive d. Treatment is repeated every 3 wk or after recovery from hematologic toxicity.

Pediatric: Safety and efficacy not established.
Geriatric or renal or hepatic impaired: Data not available on appropriate dosage. Reduced dosage is advisable.

Pharmacokinetics

Route	Onset
IV	Rapid

Metabolism: Hepatic; $T_{1/2}$: 15 h
Distribution: Crosses placenta; enters breast milk
Excretion: Urine

IV facts

Preparation: Add Sterile Water for Injection or Bacteriostatic Water for Injection to the vial, and shake gently. Use 20 ml diluent with 1-g vial, giving a final concentration of 50 mg/ml, or use 60-ml diluent with 3-g vial, giving a final concentration of 50 mg/ml. Solutions may be further diluted to achieve concentrations of 0.6–20 mg/ml in 5% Dextrose Injection, 0.9% Sodium Chloride Injection, Lactated Ringer's Injection, and Sterile Water for Injection. Solution is stable for at least 1 wk at room temperature or 6 wk if refrigerated. Dilutions not prepared with Bacteriostatic Water for Injection should be refrigerated and used within 6 h.

Infusion: Administer as a slow IV infusion lasting a minimum of 30 min.

Adverse effects

- **CNS:** *Somnolence, confusion, hallucinations,* coma, depressive psychosis, dizziness, seizures
- **GI:** *Anorexia, nausea, vomiting,* diarrhea, stomatitis
- **Hematologic:** *Leukopenia,* thrombocytopenia, anemia (rare), increased serum uric acid levels
- **GU:** *Hemorrhagic cystitis,* bladder fibrosis, *hematuria* to potentially fatal hemorrhagic cystitis, increased urine uric acid levels, gonadal suppression
- **Dermatologic:** *Alopecia,* darkening of skin and fingernails
- **Other:** Immunosuppression, secondary neoplasia

■ Nursing Considerations

Assessment
- *History:* Allergy to ifosfamide, hematopoietic depression, impaired hepatic or renal function, pregnancy, lactation
- *Physical:* Reflexes, affect; skin—lesions, hair; urinary output, renal function; renal and hepatic function tests, CBC, Hct

Implementation
- Arrange for blood tests to evaluate hematopoietic function before beginning therapy and weekly during therapy.
- Arrange for extensive hydration consisting of at least 2 L of oral or IV fluid per day to prevent bladder toxicity.
- Arrange to administer a protector, such as mesna, to prevent hemorrhagic cystitis.
- Counsel male patients not to father a child during or immediately after therapy; infant cardiac and limb abnormalities have occurred. Counsel female patients not to become pregnant while on this drug; severe birth defects have occurred.

Drug-specific teaching points
- Know that this drug can only be given IV.
- Arrange for frequent blood tests to monitor your response to this drug. All appointments for follow-up should be kept.
- Know that the following side effects may occur: nausea, vomiting, loss of appetite (taking the drug with food, small frequent meals may help); try to maintain your fluid intake and nutrition while on this drug (drink at least 10–12 glassses of fluid each day); darkening of the skin and fingernails, loss of hair (you may wish to obtain a wig or arrange for some other head covering before the loss of hair occurs; keep the head covered in extremes of temperature).
- Use birth control methods while on this drug and for a time afterwards (male and female patients); this drug can cause severe birth defects.

Adverse effects in *Italics* are most common; those in **Bold** are life-threatening.

- Report unusual bleeding or bruising, fever, chills, sore throat, cough, shortness of breath, blood in the urine, painful urination, unusual lumps or masses, flank, stomach or joint pain, sores in mouth or on lips, yellow discoloration of skin or eyes.

☐ imipramine hydrochloride

(im ip' ra meen)

Apo-Imipramine (CAN), Impril (CAN), Janimine, Novopramine (CAN), Tipramine, Tofranil

imipramine pamoate

Tofranil-PM

Pregnancy Category B

Drug classes
Tricyclic antidepressant (TCA; tertiary amine)

Therapeutic actions
Mechanism of action unknown; the TCAs are structurally related to the phenothiazine antipsychotic drugs (eg, chlorpromazine), but unlike the phenothiazines, TCAs inhibit the presynaptic reuptake of the neurotransmitters norepinephrine and serotonin; anticholinergic at CNS and peripheral receptors; sedative; the relation of these effects to clinical efficacy is unknown.

Indications
- Relief of symptoms of depression (endogenous depression most responsive); sedative effects of tertiary amine TCAs may be helpful in patients whose depression is associated with anxiety and sleep disturbance
- Enuresis in children 6 y or older
- Unlabeled use: control of chronic pain (eg, intractable pain of cancer, peripheral neuropathies, postherpetic neuralgia, tic douloureux, central pain syndromes)

Contraindications/cautions
- Contraindicated in the presence of hypersensitivity to any tricyclic drug or to tartrazine (in preparations marketed as *Janimine, Tofranil, Tofranil PM*; patients with aspirin allergy are often allergic to tartrazine); concomitant therapy with an MAO inhibitor; electroshock therapy with coadministration of TCAs; recent MI; myelography within previous 24 h or scheduled within 48 h; pregnancy; lactation.
- Use caution in the presence of preexisting cardiovascular disorders; seizure disorders (TCAs lower the seizure threshold); hyperthyroidism; angle-closure glaucoma, increased intraocular pressure, urinary retention, ureteral or urethral spasm; impaired hepatic, renal function; psychiatric patients (schizophrenic or paranoid patients may exhibit a worsening of psychosis with TCA therapy; manic-depressive patients may shift to hypomanic or manic phase); elective surgery.

Dosage
Adult
- **Depression:** *Hospitalized patients:* Initially, 100–150 mg/d PO in divided doses. Gradually increase to 200 mg/d as required. If no response after 2 wk, increase to 250–300 mg/d. Total daily dosage may be administered at bedtime. *May be given IM initially only in patients unable or unwilling to take drug PO:* up to 100 mg/d in divided doses. Replace with oral medication as soon as possible. Outpatients: Initially, 75 mg/d PO, increasing to 150 mg/d. Dosages > 200 mg/d not recommended. Total daily dosage may be administered at bedtime. Maintenance dose is 50–150 mg/d.
- **Chronic pain:** 50–200 mg/d PO.

Pediatric adolescent patients: 30–40 mg/d PO; doses > 100mg/d generally are not needed.
- **Childhood enuresis (6 y or older):** Initially, 25 mg/d 1 h before bedtime. If response is not satisfactory after 1 wk, increase to 50 mg nightly in children younger than 12 y, 75 mg nightly in children older than 12 y. Doses > 75 mg/d do not have greater efficacy but are more likely to increase side effects. Do not exceed 2.5 mg/kg per day. Early night bedwetters may be more effec-

tively treated with earlier and divided dosage (25 mg midafternoon, repeated at bedtime). Institute drug-free period after successful therapy, gradually tapering dosage.
Geriatric: 30–40 mg/day PO; doses > 100 mg/d generally are not needed.

Pharmacokinetics

Route	Onset	Peak
Oral	Varies	2–4 h

Metabolism: Hepatic; $T_{1/2}$: 8–16 h
Distribution: Crosses placenta; enters breast milk
Excretion: Urine

Adverse effects
Adult Use
- CNS: *Sedation and anticholinergic effects*—dry mouth, blurred vision, disturbance of accommodation for near vision, mydriasis, increased intraocular pressure; *confusion, disturbed concentration,* hallucinations, disorientation, decreased memory, feelings of unreality, delusions, anxiety, nervousness, restlessness, agitation, panic, insomnia, nightmares, hypomania, mania, exacerbation of psychosis, drowsiness, weakness, fatigue, headache, numbness, tingling, paresthesias of extremities, incoordination, motor hyperactivity, akathisia, ataxia, tremors, peripheral neuropathy, extrapyramidal symptoms, *seizures,* speech blockage, dysarthria, tinnitus, altered EEG
- GI: *Dry mouth, constipation,* paralytic ileus, *nausea,* vomiting, anorexia, epigastric distress, diarrhea, flatulence, dysphagia, peculiar taste, increased salivation, stomatitis, glossitis, parotid swelling, abdominal cramps, black tongue, hepatitis
- CV: *Orthostatic hypotension,* hypertension, syncope, tachycardia, palpitations, MI, arrhythmias, heart block, precipitation of CHF, stroke
- Hematologic: Bone marrow depression, including agranulocytosis; eosinophila, purpura, thrombocytopenia, leukopenia
- GU: Urinary retention, delayed micturition, dilation of the urinary tract, gynecomastia, testicular swelling in men; breast enlargement, menstrual irregularity and galactorrhea in women; increased or decreased libido; impotence
- Hypersensitivity: Skin rash, pruritus, vasculitis, petechiae, photosensitization, edema (generalized or of face and tongue), drug fever
- Endocrine: Elevated or depressed blood sugar, elevated prolactin levels, inappropriate ADH secretion
- Withdrawal: Symptoms with abrupt discontinuation of prolonged therapy: nausea, headache, vertigo, nightmares, malaise
- Other: Nasal congestion, excessive appetite, weight gain or loss; sweating (paradoxical effect in a drug with prominent anticholinergic effects), alopecia, lacrimation, hyperthermia, flushing, chills

Pediatric Use for Enuresis
- CNS: *Nervousness, sleep disorders, tiredness,* convulsions, anxiety, emotional instability, syncope, collapse
- GI: Constipation, *mild GI disturbances*
- CV: ECG changes of unknown significance when given in doses of 5 mg/kg per day
- Other: Adverse reactions reported with adult use

Clinically important drug-drug interactions
- Increased TCA levels and pharmacologic (especially anticholinergic) effects when given with cimetidine, fluoxetine, ranitidine • Increased serum levels and risk of bleeding if taken concurrently with oral anticoagulants • Altered response, including dysrhythmias and hypertension if taken with sympathomimetics • Risk of severe hypertension when taken concurrently with clonidine • Hyperpyretic crises, severe convulsions, hypertensive episodes, and deaths when MAO inhibitors are given with TCAs • Decreased hypotensive activity of guanethidine if taken concurrently with imipramine • *Note:* MAOIs and tricyclic antide-

pressants have been used successfully in some patients resistant to therapy with single agents; however, case reports indicate that the combination can cause serious and potentially fatal adverse effects.

■ Nursing Considerations

Assessment
- *History:* Hypersensitivity to any tricyclic drug or to tartrazine; concomitant therapy with an MAO inhibitor; electroshock therapy with coadministration of TCAs; recent MI; myelography within previous 24 h or scheduled within 48 h; preexisting cardiovascular disorders; seizure disorders; hyperthyroidism; angle-closure glaucoma, increased intraocular pressure, urinary retention, ureteral or urethral spasm; impaired hepatic, renal function; psychiatric patients; elective surgery; pregnancy; lactation
- *Physical:* Body weight; temperature; skin—color, lesions; orientation, affect, reflexes, vision and hearing; P, BP, auscultation, orthostatic BP, perfusion; bowel sounds, normal output, liver evaluation; urine flow, normal output; usual sexual function, frequency of menses, breast and scrotal examination; liver function tests, urinalysis, CBC, ECG

Implementation
- Ensure that depressed and potentially suicidal patients have access to only limited quantities of the drug.
- Administer IM only when oral therapy is impossible. Do not administer IV.
- Administer major portion of dose at bedtime if drowsiness, severe anticholinergic effects occur (note that the elderly may not tolerate single daily dose therapy).
- Arrange to reduce dosage if minor side effects develop; arrange to discontinue the drug if serious side effects occur.
- Arrange for CBC if patient develops fever, sore throat, or other sign of infection during therapy.

Drug-specific teaching points
- Take drug exactly as prescribed. Do not stop taking this drug abruptly or without consulting your physician or nurse.
- Avoid prolonged exposure to sunlight or sunlamps; use a sunscreen or protective garments if you must be in sunlight for long periods of time.
- Know that the following side effects may occur: headache, dizziness, drowsiness, weakness, blurred vision (these effects are reversible; safety measures may need to be taken if these become severe; avoid driving an automobile or performing tasks that require alertness while these persist); nausea, vomiting, loss of appetite (small frequent meals, frequent mouth care may help); dry mouth (sucking sugarless candies may help); disorientation, difficulty concentrating, emotional changes (it may help to know that these are drug effects); changes in sexual function, impotence, changes in libido.
- Report dry mouth, difficulty in urination, excessive sedation, fever, chills, sore throat, palpitations.

▢ indapamide

*(in **dap**' a mide)*
Lozol

Pregnancy Category B

Drug classes
Thiazide-like diuretic (actually an indoline)

Therapeutic actions
Inhibits reabsorption of sodium and chloride in distal renal tubule, increasing excretion of sodium, chloride, and water by the kidney.

Indications
- Edema associated with CHF
- Hypertension, as sole therapy or in combination with other antihypertensives
- Unlabeled use: diabetes insipidus, especially nephrogenic diabetes insipidus

Contraindications/cautions
- Contraindicated in the presence of allergy to thiazides, sulfonamides; fluid or electrolyte imbalance; renal disease (risk of azotemia); liver disease (may precipitate hepatic coma); gout (risk of precipitation

indapamide

of attack); SLE; glucose tolerance abnormalities, diabetes mellitus; hyperparathyroidism; manic-depressive disorder (aggravated by hypercalcemia); pregnancy; lactation.

Dosage
Adult
- **Edema:** 2.5 mg/d PO as single dose in the morning. May be increased up to 5 mg/d if patient's response is not satisfactory after 1 wk.
- **Hypertension:** 2.5 mg/d PO. May be increased up to 5 mg/d if response is not satisfactory after 4 wk. If combination antihypertensive therapy is needed, reduce the dosage of other agents by 50%, then adjust according to patient's response.

Pharmacokinetics

Route	Onset	Peak	Duration
Oral	1–2 h	2 h	36 h

Metabolism: Hepatic; $T_{1/2}$: 14 h
Distribution: Crosses placenta; enters breast milk
Excretion: Urine

Adverse effects
- **CNS:** *Dizziness, vertigo,* paresthesias, weakness, headache, drowsiness, fatigue, leukopenia, thrombocytopenia, agranulocytosis, aplastic anemia, neutropenia
- **GI:** *Nausea, anorexia, vomiting, dry mouth,* diarrhea, constipation, jaundice, hepatitis, pancreatitis
- **CV:** Orthostatic hypotension, venous thrombosis, volume depletion, cardiac arrhythmias, chest pain
- **GU:** *Polyuria, nocturia,* impotence, loss of libido
- **Dermatologic:** Photosensitivity, rash, purpura, exfoliative dermatitis, hives
- **Other:** Muscle cramps and muscle spasms, fever, gouty attacks, flushing, weight loss, rhinorrhea

Clinically important drug-drug interactions
- Increased thiazide effects if taken with diazoxide • Decreased absorption with cholestyramine, colestipol • Increased risk of cardiac glycoside toxicity if hypokalemia occurs • Increased risk of lithium toxicity • Decreased effectiveness of antidiabetic agents when taken concurrently with indapamide

Drug-lab test interferences
- Decreased PBI levels without clinical signs of thyroid disturbance

■ Nursing Considerations
Assessment
- *History:* Allergy to thiazides, sulfonamides; fluid or electrolyte imbalance; renal or liver disease; gout; SLE; glucose tolerance abnormalities, diabetes mellitus; hyperparathyroidism; manic-depressive disorders; lactation
- *Physical:* Skin color, lesions, edema; orientation, reflexes, muscle strength; pulses, baseline ECG, BP, orthostatic BP, perfusion; R, pattern, adventitious sounds; liver evaluation, bowel sounds, urinary output patterns; CBC, serum electrolytes, blood glucose, liver and renal function tests, serum uric acid, urinalysis

Implementation
- Administer with food or milk if GI upset occurs.
- Mark calendars or provide other reminders of drug days for outpatients on every other day or 3–5 d/wk therapy.
- Administer early in the day so increased urination will not disturb sleep.
- Measure and record regular body weights to monitor fluid changes.

Drug-specific teaching points
- Record intermittent therapy on a calendar, or use prepared, dated envelopes. Take the drug early in the day so increased urination will not disturb sleep. The drug may be taken with food or meals if GI upset occurs.
- Weigh yourself on a regular basis, at the same time of the day and in the same clothing, and record the weight on your calendar.
- Know that the following side effects may occur: increased volume and frequency

Adverse effects in Italics *are most common; those in* **Bold** *are life-threatening.*

of urination; dizziness, feeling faint on arising, drowsiness (if these changes occur, avoid rapid position changes; hazardous activities, like driving a car, and alcohol; which can intensify these problems); sensitivity to sunlight (use sunglasses, wear protective clothing, or use a sunscreen when outdoors); decrease in sexual function; increased thirst (sucking on sugarless lozenges may help to alleviate the thirst; frequent mouth care also may help).
- Report loss or gain of more than 3 lb in one day, swelling in your ankles or fingers, unusual bleeding or bruising, dizziness, trembling, numbness, fatigue, muscle weakness or cramps.

indomethacin

(in doe meth' a sin)

Apo-Indomethacin (CAN), Indometh, Indocin, Indo-Lemmon, Indocin-SR, Inocid (CAN), Novomethacin (CAN)

indomethacin sodium trihydrate

Apo-Indomethacin (CAN), Indocin I.V., Novomethacin (CAN)

Pregnancy Category B
Category D in third trimester

Drug classes
NSAID

Therapeutic actions
Anti-inflammatory, analgesic, and antipyretic activities largely related to inhibition of prostaglandin synthesis; exact mechanisms of action are not known.

Indications
Oral, Topical, Suppositories
- Relief of signs and symptoms of moderate to severe rheumatoid arthritis and moderate to severe osteoarthritis, moderate to severe ankylosing spondylitis, acute painful shoulder (bursitis, tendinitis), acute gouty arthritis (*not* sustained-release form)

- Unlabeled uses for oral form: pharmacologic closure of persistent patent ductus arteriosus in premature infants; suppression of uterine activity to prevent premature labor; juvenile rheumatoid arthritis
- Unlabeled use of topical eye drops: cystoid macular edema

IV Preparation
- Closure of hemodynamically significant patent ductus arteriosus in premature infants weighing between 500–1,750 g, if 48 h of usual medical management is not effective

Contraindications/cautions
- Oral and rectal preparations: allergy to indomethacin, salicylates or other NSAIDs; cardiovascular dysfunction, hypertension; peptic ulceration, GI bleeding; history of proctitis or rectal bleeding; impaired hepatic or renal function; pregnancy; labor and delivery; lactation. IV preparations: proven or suspected infection; bleeding, thrombocytopenia, coagulation defects; necrotizing enterocolitis; renal impairment; local irritation if extravasation occurs.

Dosage
Adult
- *Osteoarthritis/rheumatoid arthritis, ankylosing spondylitis:* 25 mg PO bid or tid. If tolerated, increase dose by 25- or 50-mg increments if needed up to total daily dose of 150–200 mg/d PO.
- *Acute painful shoulder:* 75–150 mg/d PO, in three to four divided doses. Discontinue drug after inflammation is controlled, usually 7–14 d.
- *Acute gouty arthritis:* 50 mg PO, tid until pain is tolerable, then rapidly decrease dose until no longer needed, usually within 3–5 d.

Pediatric: Safety and efficacy have not been established. When special circumstances warrant use in children older than 2 y, initial dose is 2 mg/kg per day in divided doses PO. Do not exceed 4 mg/kg per day or 150–200 mg/d, whichever is less.

— *IV:* Three IV doses given at 12- to 24-h intervals is a course of therapy.

indomethacin

Age	1st dose	2nd dose	3rd dose
<48 h	0.2 mg/kg	0.1 mg/kg	0.1 mg/kg
2–7 d	0.2 mg/kg	0.2 mg/kg	0.2 mg/kg
>7 d	0.2 mg/kg	0.25 mg/kg	0.25 mg/kg

If marked anuria or oliguria occurs, do not give additional doses. If ductus reopens, course of therapy may be repeated at 12- to 24-h intervals.

Pharmacokinetics

Route	Onset	Peak	Duration
Oral	30 min	1–2 h	4–6 h
IV	Immediate		15–30 min

Metabolism: Hepatic; $T_{1/2}$: 4½–6 h
Distribution: Crosses placenta; enters breast milk
Excretion: Urine

IV facts

Preparation: Reconstitute solution with 1–2 ml of 0.9% Sodium Chloride Injection or Water for Injection; diluents should be preservative free. If 1 ml of diluent is used, concentration is 0.1 mg/0.1 ml. If 2 ml of diluent is used, concentration is 0.05 mg/0.1 ml. Discard any unused portion of the solution; prepare fresh solution before each dose.

Infusion: Inject reconstituted solution IV over 5–10 sec; further dilution is not recommended.

Adverse effects
NSAIDs: Oral, Suppositories

- CNS: *Headache, dizziness, somnolence, insomnia,* fatigue, tiredness, dizziness, tinnitus, ophthalmologic effects
- GI: *Nausea, dyspepsia, GI pain,* diarrhea, vomiting, *constipation,* flatulence
- Respiratory: Dyspnea, hemoptysis, pharyngitis, bronchospasm, rhinitis
- Hematologic: Bleeding, platelet inhibition with higher doses, neutropenia, eosinophilia, leukopenia, pancytopenia, thrombocytopenia, agranulocytosis, granulocytopenia, aplastic anemia, decreased hemoglobin or hematocrit, bone marrow depression, mennorhagia
- GU: Dysuria, renal impairment
- Dermatologic: *Rash,* pruritus, sweating, dry mucous membranes, stomatitis
- Other: Peripheral edema, **anaphylactoid reactions to fatal anaphylactic shock**

Intravenous Preparation

- GI: *GI bleeding, vomiting,* abdominal distention, transient ileus
- Respiratory: *Apnea, exacerbation of pulmonary infection,* pulmonary hemorrhage
- Hematologic: *Increased bleeding problems,* including intracranial bleed, disseminated intravascular coagulopathy, hyponatremia, hyperkalemia, hypoglycemia, fluid retention
- GU: Renal dysfunction
- Other: Retrolental fibroplasia

Clinically important drug-drug interactions

- Increased toxic effects of lithium if taken with indomethacin • Decreased diuretic effect if taken concurrently with loop diuretics: bumetanide, furosemide, ethacrynic acid • Potential decrease in antihypertensive effect of beta-adrenergic blocking agents, captopril, lisinopril, enalapril

■ Nursing Considerations

Assessment

- *History:* Oral and rectal preparations: allergy to indomethacin, salicylates or other NSAIDs; cardiovascular dysfunction, hypertension; peptic ulceration, GI bleeding; history of proctitis or rectal bleeding; impaired hepatic or renal function; pregnancy; labor & delivery. IV preparations: proven or suspected infection; bleeding, thrombocytopenia, coagulation defects; necrotizing enterocolitis; renal impairment; local irritation if extravasation occurs
- *Physical:* Skin—color, lesions; temperature; orientation, reflexes, ophthalmological evaluation, audiometric evaluation, peripheral sensation; P, BP, edema; R, adventitious sounds; liver evaluation, bowel sounds; CBC, clotting times, uri-

Adverse effects in *Italics* are most common; those in **Bold** are life-threatening.

nalysis, renal and liver function tests, serum electrolytes, stool guaiac

Implementation

Oral and Rectal Preparations
- Administer drug with food or after meals if GI upset occurs.
- Do not administer sustained-release tablets for gouty arthritis.
- Arrange for periodic ophthalmologic examination during long-term therapy.
- Arrange for discontinuation of drug if eye changes, symptoms of liver or renal dysfunction occur.
- Institute emergency procedures if overdose occurs: gastric lavage, induction of emesis, support.
- Arrange for renal function tests between doses of indomethacin. If severe renal impairment is noted, do not give the next dose.

Drug-specific teaching points
- Use the drug only as suggested; avoid overdose. Take the drug with food or after meals if GI upset occurs. Do not exceed the prescribed dosage
- Know that the following side effects may occur: nausea, GI upset, dyspepsia (taking the drug with food may help); diarrhea or constipation (ensure ready access to bathroom facilites if these problems occur); drowsiness, dizziness, vertigo, insomnia (use caution if driving or operating dangerous machinery if these occur).
- Report sore throat, fever, rash, itching, weight gain, swelling in ankles or fingers, changes in vision, black, tarry stools.
- Parents of infants receiving IV therapy of indomethacin for PDA will need support and encouragement and an explanation of the drug's action; this is best incorporated into the teaching about the disease.

▢ insulin

(in' su lin)

Insulin injection: Humulin R, Novolin R, Regular Iletin I, Velosulin

Insulin zinc suspension, prompt (Semilente): Semilente Iletin I, Semilente Insulin

Isophane insulin suspension (NPH): Humulin N, Insulatard NPH, Novolin N, NPH Insulin

Isophane insulin suspension and insulin injection: Mixtard

Insulin zinc suspension (Lente): Lente Insulin, Novolin L

Protamine zinc suspension (PZI): Iletin PZI (CAN)

Insulin zinc suspension, extended (Ultralente): Ultralente Insulin

Insulin injection concentrated: Regular Iletin II U-500 (Rx preparation)

Pregnancy Category B

Drug classes
Antidiabetic agent
Hormonal agent

Therapeutic actions
Insulin is a hormone that, by receptor-mediated effects, promotes the storage of the body's fuels, facilitating the transport of metabolites and ions (potassium) through cell membranes and stimulating the synthesis of glycogen from glucose, of fats from lipids, and proteins from amino acids.

Indications
- Treatment of diabetes mellitus type I
- Treatment of diabetes mellitus type II that cannot be controlled by diet
- Treatment of severe ketoacidosis or diabetic coma (regular insulin injection)
- Treatment of hyperkalemia with infusion of glucose to produce a shift of potassium into the cells
- Highly purified and human insulins promoted for short courses of therapy (surgery, intercurrent disease), newly diagnosed patients, patients with poor metabolic control, and patients with gestational diabetes
- Insulin injection concentrated indicated for treatment of diabetic patients with marked insulin resistance (requirements of > 200 U/d)

Contraindications/cautions
- Allergy to beef, pork products (varies with preparations; use of human insulin removes this caution); pregnancy (keep patients under close supervision; rigid control is desired; following delivery, requirements may drop for 24–72 h, rising to normal levels during next 6 wk); lactation (monitor mother carefully; insulin requirements may decrease during lactation).

Dosage
Adult and Pediatric: The number and size of daily doses, times of administration, and type of insulin preparation are all determined under close medical supervision in conjunction with considerations of the patient's blood and urine glucose, diet, exercise, and intercurrent infections and other stresses. Usually given SC. Regular insulin may be given IV or IM in diabetic coma or ketoacidosis. Insulin injection concentrated may be given SC or IM, but do not administer IV.

Pharmacokinetics

Type	Onset	Peak	Duration
Regular	30–60 min		6–8 h
Semilente	1–1.5 h	5–10 h	12–16 h
NPH	1–1.5 h	4–12 h	24 h
Lente	1–2.5 h	7–15 h	24 h
PZ	4–8 h	14–24 h	36 h
Ultralente	4–8 h	10–30 h	>36 h

Metabolism: Cellular; $T_{1/2}$: varies with preparation
Distribution: Crosses placenta; does not enter breast milk

IV facts
Preparation: May be mixed with standard IV solutions; use of plastic tubing or bag will change the amount of insulin delivered.
Infusion: Use of a monitored delivery system is suggested. Rate should be determined by patient response and glucose levels.

Adverse effects
- **Hypersensitivity:** Rash, **anaphylaxis** or **angioedema**, may be life threatening
- **Metabolic:** Hypoglycemia; ketoacidosis
- **Local:** Allergy—local reactions at injection site—redness, swelling, itching; usually resolves in a few days to a few weeks; a change in type or species source of insulin may be tried

Clinically important drug-drug interactions
- Increased hypoglycemic effects of insulin if taken with monoamine oxidase inhibitors, beta blockers, salicylates, alcohol • Altered insulin requirements in diabetics secondary to use of fenfluramine, requiring cautious administration of insulin and regular monitoring of glucose levels
- Delayed recovery from hypoglycemic episodes and masked signs and symptoms of hypoglycemia if taken with beta-adrenergic blocking agents

■ Nursing Considerations

Assessment
- *History:* Allergy to beef, pork products; pregnancy; lactation
- *Physical:* Skin—color, lesions; eyeball turgor; orientation, reflexes, peripheral sensation; P, BP, adventitious sounds; R, adventitious sounds; urinalysis, blood glucose

Implementation
- Ensure uniform dispersion of insulin suspensions by rolling the vial gently between hands; avoid vigorous shaking.
- Administer maintenance doses SC, rotating injection sites regularly to decrease the incidence of lipodystrophy; give regular insulin IV or IM in severe ketoacidosis or diabetic coma.
- Monitor patients receiving insulin IV carefully; plastic IV infusion sets have been reported to remove 20%–80% of the insulin; dosage delivered to the patient will vary.
- Do not administer insulin injection concentrated IV; severe anaphylactic reactions can occur.
- Use caution when mixing two types of insulin; always draw the regular insulin into the syringe first; use mixtures of

regular and NPH or regular and lente insulins within 5–15 min of combining them.
- Be advised to double-check, or even to have a colleague check, the dosage drawn up for pediatric patients, for patients receiving concentrated insulin injection, or patients receiving very small doses; even small errors in dosage can cause serious problems in these patients.
- Monitor patients being switched from one type of insulin to another carefully; dosage adjustments are often needed. Human insulins often require smaller doses than beef or pork insulin; use careful monitoring and caution if patients are switched.
- Store insulin in a cool place away from direct sunlight. Refrigeration is preferred. Do not freeze insulin. Insulin prefilled in glass or plastic syringes is stable for 1 wk refrigerated; this is often a safe way of ensuring adequate dosage for patients with limited vision or who have problems with the mechanics of drawing up insulin.
- Monitor urine and serum glucose levels frequently to determine effectiveness of drug and dosage being used. Patients can learn to adjust insulin dosage on the "sliding scale" based on results of these tests.
- Monitor insulin needs during times of trauma or severe stress; dosage adjustments may be needed.
- Maintain life support equipment, glucose on standby to deal with ketoacidosis or hypoglycemic reactions.

Drug-specific teaching points
- Use the same type and brand of syringe; use the same type and brand of insulin to avoid dosage errors.
- Do not change the order of mixing insulins. Rotate injection sites regularly (it is a good idea to keep a chart) to prevent breakdown at injection sites. Dosage may vary with activities, stress, diet. Monitor blood or urine glucose levels, and consult physician if problems arise. Store drug in the refrigerator or in a cool place out of direct sunlight; do not freeze insulin.
- Monitor your urine or blood for glucose and ketones as prescribed.
- Wear a medical alert tag stating that you are diabetic and taking insulin so that medical personnel will be prepared to take proper care of you in an emergency.
- Avoid alcohol while on this drug; serious reactions can occur.
- Report fever, sore throat, vomiting, hypoglycemic or hyperglycemic reactions, skin rash.

interferon alfa-2a

(in ter feer' on)
IFLrA, rIFN-A
Roferon-A

Pregnancy Category C

Drug classes
Antineoplastic agent
Interferon

Therapeutic actions
Inhibits growth of tumor cells: mechanism of action is not clearly understood; prevents tumor cells from multiplying and modulates host immune response. Interferons are produced by human leukocytes in response to viral infections and other stimuli. Interferon alfa-2a is produced by recombinant DNA technology using *Escherichia coli*.

Indications
- Hairy cell leukemia in selected patients 18 y and older
- AIDS-related Kaposi's sarcoma in selected patients 18 y and older
- Unlabeled uses: treatment of several malignant and viral conditions, phase I AIDS, ARC
- Orphan drug uses: treatment of chronic myelogenous leukemia, advanced colorectal cancer, esophageal carcinoma, metastatic malignant melanoma, renal cell carcinoma

Contraindications/cautions
- Contraindicated in the presence of allergy to interferon-α or any components of the product, pregnancy, lactation.

interferon alfa-2a

- Use caution in the presence of pancreatitis, hepatic or renal disease, seizure disorders, compromised CNS function, cardiac disease or history of cardiac disease, bone marrow depression.

Dosage
Adult
- **Hairy cell leukemia:** Induction dose: 3 million IU/d SC or IM for 16–24 wk. Maintenance dose: 3 million IU/d three times per week. Treat patient for approximately 6 mo then decide on basis of response whether to continue therapy. Treatment for up to 20 mo has been reported. Dosage may need to be adjusted downward based on adverse reactions.
- **AIDS-related Kaposi's sarcoma:** 36 million IU daily for 10–12 wk IM or SC. Maintenance: 36 million IU three times per week. Dose reductions by one-half or withholding of individual doses may be required when severe adverse reactions occur. Treatment should continue until no evidence of tumor or until discontinuation is required.

Pediatric (younger than 18 y): Safety and efficacy not established.

Pharmacokinetics

Route	Onset	Peak
IM	Rapid	3.8 h
SC	Slow	7.3 h

Metabolism: Hepatic and renal; $T_{1/2}$: 3.7–8.5 h

Distribution: Crosses placenta; may enter breast milk

Excretion: Urine

Adverse effects
- **CNS:** *Dizziness, confusion,* paresthesias, numbness, lethargy, decreased mental status, depression, visual disturbances, sleep disturbances, nervousness
- **CV:** Hypotension, edema, hypertension, chest pain, arrhythmias, palpitations
- **GI:** *Anorexia, nausea,* diarrhea, vomiting, change in taste
- **Hematologic:** Leukopenia, neutropenia, thrombocytopenia, anemia, decreased hemoglobin; increased levels of SGOT, LDH, alkaline phosphatase, bilirubin, uric acid, serum creatinine, BUN, blood sugar, serum phosphorus, neutralizing antibodies; hypocalcemia
- **GU:** Impairment of fertility in women, transient impotence in men
- **Dermatologic:** Rash, dryness or inflammation of the oropharnyx, dry skin, pruritus, partial alopecia
- **General:** *Flulike syndrome,* weight loss, diaphoresis, arthralgia

■ Nursing Considerations

Assessment
- *History:* Allergy to interferon-α or any components of the product, pancreatitis, hepatic or renal disease, seizure disorders, compromised CNS function, cardiac disease or history of cardiac disease, bone marrow depression, pregnancy, lactation
- *Physical:* Weight; temperature; skin—color, lesions; orientation, reflexes; P, BP, edema, ECG; liver evaluation; CBC, blood glucose, liver and renal function tests, urinalysis

Implementation
- Arrange for laboratory tests (CBC, differential, granulocytes and hairy cells, bone marrow hairy cells, and liver function tests) before beginning therapy and monthly during therapy.
- Monitor for severe reactions of any kind; notify physician immediately; dosage reduction or discontinuation of drug may be necessary.
- Refrigerate solution; do not shake. Use reconstituted powder within 30 d.
- Ensure that patient is well hydrated, especially during initiation of treatment.
- Provide small, frequent meals if GI problems occur.
- Counsel female patients to use some form of birth control while on this drug. Drug is contraindicated in pregnancy.
- Assure patient that all steps possible are taken to ensure that there is little risk of hepatitis, AIDS from use of human blood products.

Adverse effects in *Italics* are most common; those in **Bold** are life-threatening.

Drug-specific teaching points
- Prepare a calendar to check off as drug is given. You and a significant other should learn the proper technique for SC or IM injection for outpatient use. Do not change brands of interferon without consulting with physician.
- Refrigerate solution; do not shake. Use reconstituted powder within 30 d.
- Know that the following side effects may occur: loss of appetite, nausea, vomiting (frequent mouth care, small frequent meals may help; try to maintain good nutrition if at all possible; a dietician may be able to help; an antiemetic also may be ordered); fatigue, confusion, dizziness, numbness, visual disturbances, depression (it may help to know that these are drug effects; use special precautions to avoid injury if these occur; avoid driving a car or using dangerous machinery if these effects occur); impotence (usually transient and will pass when the drug is discontinued); fetal deformities or death (use some form of birth control while you are on this drug).
- Arrange for regular blood tests to monitor the drug's effects.
- Report fever, chills, sore throat, unusual bleeding or bruising, chest pain, palpitations, dizziness, changes in mental status.

❒ interferon alfa-2b

(in ter feer' on)
IFN-alpha 2, rIFN-a2, a-2-interferon

Intron-A

Pregnancy Category C

Drug classes
Antineoplastic agent
Interferon

Therapeutic actions
Inhibits growth of tumor cells; mechanism of action is not clearly understood; prevents the replication of tumor cells and enhances host immune response. Interferons are produced by human leukocytes in response to viral infections and other stimuli. Interferon alfa-2b is produced by recombinant DNA technology using *E. coli*.

Indications
- Hairy cell leukemia
- Intralesional treatment of condylomata acuminata
- AIDS-related Kaposi's sarcoma
- Treatment of chronic hepatitis, non-A, non B/C
- Treatment of chronic hepatitis B
- Unlabeled uses: treatment of several malignant and viral conditions
- Orphan drug uses: chronic myelogenous leukemia, metastatic renal cell carcinoma, ovarian carcinoma, invasive carcinoma of cervix, primary malignant brain tumors, laryngeal papillomatosis, carcinoma in situ of urinary bladder, chronic delta hepatitis, acute hepatitis B

Contraindications/cautions
- Contraindicated in the presence of allergy to interferon-α or any components of the product, lactation.
- Use caution in the presence of cardiac disease, pulmonary disease, diabetes mellitus prone to ketoacidosis, coagulation disorders, bone marrow depression, pregnancy.

Dosage
Adult
- ***Hairy cell leukemia:*** 2 million IU/m^2 SC or IM three times per week. Continue for several months, depending on clinical and hematologic response.
- ***Condylomata acuminata:*** 1 million IU/lesion three times per week for 3 wk intralesionally. Maximum response occurs 4–8 wk after initiation of therapy.
- ***Chronic hepatitis, non-A, non B/C:*** 3 million IU SC or IM, three times per week.
- ***AIDS-related Kaposi's sarcoma:*** 30 million IU/m^2 three times per week SC or IM. Maintain dosage until disease progresses rapidly or severe intolerance occurs.
- ***Chronic hepatitis B:*** 30–35 million IU/wk SC or IM either as 5 million IU

dialy or 10 million IU three times per week for 16 wk.
Pediatric: Safety and efficacy not established in children younger than 18 y.

Pharmacokinetics

Route	Onset	Peak
IM/SC	Rapid	3–12 h

Metabolism: Renal; $T_{1/2}$: 2–3 h
Distribution: Crosses placenta; may enter breast milk
Excretion: Unknown

Adverse effects

- CNS: *Dizziness, confusion,* paresthesias, numbness, lethargy, decreased mental status, depression, visual disturbances, sleep disturbances, nervousness
- GI: *Anorexia, nausea,* diarrhea, vomiting, change in taste
- CV: Hypotension, edema, hypertension, chest pain, arrhythmias, palpitations
- Hematologic: Leukopenia, neutropenia, thrombocytopenia, anemia, decreased hemoglobin; increased levels of SGOT, LDH, alkaline phosphatase, bilirubin, uric acid, serum creatinine, BUN, blood sugar, serum phosphorus, neutralizing antibodies; hypocalcemia
- GU: Impairment of fertility in women, transient impotence
- Dermatologic: *Rash,* dryness or inflammation of the oropharnyx, *dry skin, pruritus,* partial alopecia
- General: *Flulike syndrome,* weight loss, diaphoresis, arthralgia

■ Nursing Considerations

Assessment
- *History:* Allergy to interferon-α or any components of the product, cardiac or pulmonary disease, diabetes mellitus prone to ketoacidosis, coagulation disorders, bone marrow depression, pregnancy, lactation
- *Physical:* Weight; temperature; skin—color, lesions; orientation, reflexes; P, BP, edema, ECG; liver evaluation; CBC, blood glucose, liver and renal function tests, urinalysis

Implementation
- Arrange for laboratory tests (CBC, differential, granulocytes and hairy cells, bone marrow and hairy cells) before beginning therapy and monthly during therapy.
- Prepare solution as follows:

Vial Strength in million IU	Amount of Diluent in ml	Final Conc in million IU/ml
3	1	3
5	1	5
10	2	5
25	5	5
10	1	10
50	1	50

- Use Bacteriostatic Water for Injection as diluent. Agitate gently. After reconstitution, stable for 1 mo if refrigerated.
- Administer IM or SC.
- Monitor for severe reactions of any kind, including hypersensitivity reactions; notify physician immediately; dosage reduction or discontinuation of drug may be necessary.
- Ensure that patient is well hydrated, especially during initiation of treatment.

Drug-specific teaching points
- Prepare a calendar to check off as drug is given. You and a significant other should learn the proper technique for SC or IM injection for outpatient use. Do not change brands of interferon without consulting with physician.
- Know that the following side effects may occur: loss of appetite, nausea, vomiting (frequent mouth care, small frequent meals may help; you will need to try to maintain good nutrition if at all possible; a dietician may be able to help; an antiemetic also may be ordered); fatigue, confusion, dizziness, numbness, visual disturbances, depression (it may help to know that these are drug effects; use special precautions to avoid injury if these occur; avoid driving a car or using dangerous machinery if these effects occur); flulike syndrome (taking the drug at bedtime may help; ensure rest periods

Adverse effects in *Italics* are most common; those in **Bold** are life-threatening.

for yourself; a medication may be ordered for fever).
- Arrange for regular blood tests to monitor the drug's effects.
- Report fever, chills, sore throat, unusual bleeding or bruising, chest pain, palpitations, dizziness, changes in mental status.

☐ interferon alfa-n3

(in ter feer' on)
Alferon N

Pregnancy Category C

Drug classes
Antineoplastic agent
Interferon

Therapeutic actions
Inhibits viral replication and suppresses cell proliferation; mechanism of action not completely understood. Interferons are produced by human leukocytes in response to viral infections and other stimuli. Interferon alfa-n3 is produced by harvesting human leukocytes.

Indications
- Intralesional treatment of refractory and recurring condylomata acuminata
- Unlabeled uses: treatment of a variety of cancers and viral infections, including AIDS-related diseases

Contraindications/cautions
- Contraindicated in the presence of allergy to interferon-α or any components of the product, egg protein or neomycin, pregnancy, lactation.
- Use caution in the presence of debilitating medical conditions.

Dosage
Adult
- **Condylomata acuminata:** 0.05 ml (250,000 U) per wart. Administer twice weekly for up to 8 wk. Maximum recommended dose per treatment session is 0.5 ml (2.5 million U). Inject into the base of each wart, preferably using a 30-gauge needle. For large warts, it may be injected at several points around the periphery of the wart, using a total dose of 0.05 ml per wart.

Pediatric (younger than 18 y): Safety and efficacy not established.

Pharmacokinetics
Not generally absorbed systemically.

Adverse effects
Adverse effects are possible if drug is absorbed.
- **CNS:** *Dizziness, confusion,* paresthesias, numbness, lethargy, decreased mental status, depression, visual disturbances, sleep disturbances, nervousness
- **GI:** *Anorexia, nausea,* diarrhea, vomiting, change in taste
- **CV:** Hypotension, edema, hypertension, chest pain, arrhythmias, palpitations
- **Hematologic:** Leukopenia, neutropenia, thrombocytopenia, anemia, decreased hemoglobin; increased levels of SGOT, LDH, alkaline phosphatase
- **GU:** Impairment of fertility in women, transient impotence
- **Dermatologic:** Rash, dryness or inflammation of the oropharnyx, dry skin, pruritus
- **General:** *Flulike syndrome,* weight loss, diaphoresis, arthralgia

■ Nursing Considerations

Assessment
- *History:* Allergy to interferon-α or any components of the product, egg protein or neomycin, debilitating medical conditions, pregnancy, lactation
- *Physical:* Weight; temperature; skin—color, lesions; orientation, reflexes; P, BP, edema; liver evaluation; CBC, blood glucose, liver function tests, renal function tests, urinalysis

Implementation
- Arrange for laboratory tests (CBC, differential) before beginning therapy and monthly during therapy.
- Monitor for severe reactions of any kind; notify physician immediately; dosage re-

Adverse effects in *Italics* are most common; those in **Bold** are life-threatening.

duction or discontinuation of drug may be necessary.
- Finish the full 8-wk course of therapy; most warts will resolve by this time. If a second course of therapy is needed, wait 3 mo before beginning.
- Assure patient that all steps possible are taken to ensure that there is little risk of hepatitis, AIDS from use of human blood products.

Drug-specific teaching points
- Prepare a calendar to check off as drug is given. You and a significant other should learn the proper technique for injection for outpatient use. Do not change brands of interferon without consulting with physician.
- Know that the following side effects may occur: loss of appetite, nausea, vomiting (frequent mouth care, small frequent meals may help; try to maintain good nutrition if at all possible; a dietician may be able to help; an antiemetic also may be ordered); fatigue, confusion, dizziness, numbness, visual disturbances, depression (it may help to know that these are drug effects; use special precautions to avoid injury if these occur; avoid driving a car or using dangerous machinery if these effects occur); impotence (usually transient and will pass when the drug is discontinued).
- Report hives, tightness of the chest, wheezing, fainting, dizziness, failure of warts to respond to treatment.

interferon beta-1b

(in ter feer' on)

rIFN-B

Betaseron

Pregnancy Category C

Drug classes
Interferon

Therapeutic actions
Interferons are produced by human leukocytes in response to viral infections and other stimuli; interferon beta-1b block replication of viruses and stimulate the host immunoregulatory activities. Interferon beta 1-b is produced by recombinant DNA technology using *E. coli.*

Indications
- Reduce the frequency of clinical exacerbations in relapsing, remitting multiple sclerosis (MS)
- Unlabeled uses: treatment of AIDS, AIDS-related Kaposi's sarcoma, metastatic renal cell carcinoma, malignant melanoma, cutaneous T-cell lymphoma, acute non-A, non-B hepatitis

Contraindications/cautions
- Contraindicated in the presence of allergy to beta interferon, human albumin, or any components of the product, pregnancy, lactation.
- Use caution in the presence of chronic progressive MS, suicidal tendencies, or mental disorders.

Dosage
Adult: 0.25 mg (8 ml IU) SC qod; discontinue use if disease is unremitting > 6 mo.
Pediatric (younger than 18 y): Safety and efficacy not established.

Pharmacokinetics

Route	Onset	Peak
SC	Slow	1–8 h

Metabolism: Hepatic and renal; $T_{1/2}$: 8 min–4.3 h
Distribution: Crosses placenta; may enter breast milk
Excretion: Urine

Adverse effects
- **CNS:** *Dizziness, confusion,* paresthesias, numbness, lethargy, decreased mental status, depression, visual disturbances, sleep disturbances, nervousness
- **GI:** *Anorexia, nausea,* diarrhea, vomiting, change in taste

Adverse effects in *Italics* are most common; those in **Bold** are life-threatening.

interferon beta-1b ■ 595

- **CV:** Hypotension, edema, hypertension, chest pain, arrhythmias, palpitations
- **Hematologic:** Leukopenia, neutropenia, thrombocytopenia, anemia, decreased hemoglobin; increased levels of SGOT, LDH, alkaline phosphatase, bilirubin, uric acid, serum creatinine, BUN, blood sugar, serum phosphorus, neutralizing antibodies; hypocalcemia
- **GU:** Impairment of fertility in women, transient impotence
- **Dermatologic:** *Photosensitivity*, rash, alopecia, sweating
- **General:** *Flulike syndrome*, weight loss, diaphoresis, arthralgia, injection site reaction

■ Nursing Considerations

Assessment
- *History:* Allergy to interferon beta or any components of the product, mental disorders, suicidal tendencies, pregnancy, lactation
- *Physical:* Weight; temperature; skin—color, lesions; orientation, reflexes; P, BP, edema, ECG; liver evaluation; CBC, blood glucose, liver and renal function tests, urinalysis

Implementation
- Arrange for laboratory tests (CBC, differential, granulocytes and hairy cells, bone marrow hairy cells, and liver function tests) before beginning therapy and monthly during therapy.
- Monitor for severe reactions of any kind; notify physician immediately; dosage reduction or discontinuation of drug may be necessary.
- Reconstitute by using a sterile syringe and needle to inject 1.2 ml supplied diluent into vial; gently swirl the vial to dissolve the drug completely; do not shake. Discard if any particulate matter or discoloration has occurred. After reconstitution, vial contains 0.25 mg/ml solution. Withdraw 1 ml of reconstituted solution with a sterile syringe fitted with a 27-gauge needle. Inject SC into arms, abdomen, hips, thighs. Vial is for single use only. Discard any unused portions. Refrigerate. Use reconstituted solution within 3 h.
- Ensure that patient is well hydrated, especially during initiation of treatment.
- Assure regular follow-up and treatment of MS; this drug is not a cure.
- Monitor patients with any history of mental disorders or suicidal tendencies carefully.
- Counsel female patients to use some form of birth control while on this drug. Drug is contraindicated in pregnancy.

Drug-specific teaching points
- Reconstitute by using a sterile syringe and needle to inject 1.2 ml supplied diluent into vial; gently swirl the vial to dissolve the drug completely; do not shake. Discard if any particulate matter or discoloration has occurred. After reconstitution, vial contains 0.25 mg/ml solution. Withdraw 1 ml of reconstituted solution with a sterile syringe fitted with a 27-gauge needle. Inject SC into arms, abdomen, hips, thighs. Vial is for single use only. Discard any unused portions. Refrigerate. Use reconstituted solution within 3 h.
- Keep a chart of injection sites to prevent overuse of one area.
- Know that the following side effects may occur: loss of appetite, nausea, vomiting (frequent mouth care, small frequent meals may help; try to maintain good nutrition if at all possible; a dietician may be able to help; an antiemetic also may be ordered); fatigue, confusion, dizziness, numbness, visual disturbances, depression (it may help to know that these are drug effects; use special precautions to avoid injury if these occur; avoid driving a car or using dangerous machinery if these effects occur); impotence (usually transient and will pass when the drug is discontinued); sensitivity to the sun (use a sunscreen and wear protective clothing if exposure to sun cannot be prevented).

Adverse effects in *Italics* are most common; those in **Bold** are life-threatening.

- Arrange for regular treatment and follow-up of MS; this drug is not a cure.
- Report fever, chills, sore throat, unusual bleeding or bruising, chest pain, palpitations, dizziness, changes in mental status.

☐ interferon gamma-1b

(in ter feer' on)
Actimmune

Pregnancy Category C

Drug classes
Interferon

Therapeutic actions
Interferons are produced by human leukocytes in response to viral infections and other stimuli; interferon gamma-1b block has potent phagocyte-activating effects; acts as an interleukin; produced by *E. coli* bacteria.

Indications
- For reducing the frequency and severity of serious infections associated with chronic granulomatous disease

Contraindications/cautions
- Contraindicated in the presence of allergy to interferon gamma, *E. coli*, or any components of the product, pregnancy, lactation.
- Use caution in the presence of seizure disorders, compromised CNS function, cardiac disease, myelosuppression.

Dosage
Adult: 50 $\mu g/m^2$ (1.5 million U/m^2) SC three times per week in patients with body surface area > 0.5 m^2; 1.5 $\mu g/kg$ per dose in patients with body surface area < 0.5 m^2.
Pediatric (younger than 18 y): Safety and efficacy not established.

Pharmacokinetics

Route	Onset	Peak
SC	Slow	7 h

Metabolism: Hepatic and renal; $T_{1/2}$: 2.9–5.9 h
Distribution: Crosses placenta; may enter breast milk
Excretion: Urine

Adverse effects
- **CNS:** *Dizziness, confusion,* paresthesias, numbness, lethargy, decreased mental status, depression, visual disturbances, sleep disturbances, nervousness
- **GI:** *Anorexia, nausea,* diarrhea, vomiting, change in taste, pancreatitis
- **CV:** Hypotension, edema, hypertension, chest pain, arrhythmias, palpitations
- **General:** *Flulike syndrome,* weight loss, diaphoresis, arthralgia, injection site reaction

■ Nursing Considerations

Assessment
- *History:* Allergy to interferon gamma, *E. coli,* or any components of the product, pregnancy, lactation, seizure disorders, compromised CNS function, cardiac disease, myelosuppression
- *Physical:* Weight; temperature; skin—color, lesions; orientation, reflexes; P, BP, edema, ECG; liver evaluation; CBC, blood glucose, liver function tests, renal function tests, urinalysis

Implementation
- Arrange for laboratory tests (CBC, differential, granulocytes and hairy cells, bone marrow and hairy cells, and liver function tests) before beginning therapy and monthly during therapy.
- Monitor for severe reactions of any kind; notify physician immediately; dosage reduction or discontinuation of drug may be necessary.
- Store in refrigerator; each vial is for one use only, discard after that time. Discard any vial that has been unrefrigerated for 12 h.
- Administer drug at bedtime if flulike symptoms become a problem.

Drug-specific teaching points
- Store in refrigerator; each vial is for one use only; discard after that time. Discard

Adverse effects in *Italics* are most common; those in **Bold** are life-threatening.

any vial that has been unrefrigerated for 12 h. You and a significant other should learn the proper technique for SC injections.
- Keep a chart of injection sites to prevent overuse of one area.
- Know that the following side effects may occur: loss of appetite, nausea, vomiting (frequent mouth care, small frequent meals may help; try to maintain good nutrition if at all possible; a dietician may be able to help; an antiemetic also may be ordered); fatigue, confusion, dizziness, numbness, visual disturbances, depression (it may help to know that these are drug effects; use special precautions to avoid injury if these occur; avoid driving a car or using dangerous machinery if these effects occur); flulike symptoms (eg, fever, chills, aches, pains; rest, acetaminophen for fever and headache; taking the drug at bedtime also may help).
- Report fever, chills, sore throat, unusual bleeding or bruising, chest pain, palpitations, dizziness, changes in mental status.

▢ iodine thyroid products

(eye' oh dine)
Lugol's Solution

potassium iodide, sodium iodide, strong iodine solution
Thyro-Block

Pregnancy Category C

Drug classes
Thyroid suppressant

Therapeutic actions
Inhibits synthesis of the active thyroid hormones T_3 and T_4 and inhibits the release of these hormones into circulation.

Indications
- Hyperthyroidism: adjunctive therapy with antithyroid drugs in preparation for thyroidectomy, treatment of thyrotoxic crisis or neonatal thyrotoxicosis
- Thyroid blocking in a radiation emergency
- Unlabeled uses: potassium iodide has been used effectively in patients with Sweet's syndrome, treatment of lymphocutaneous sporotrichosis

Contraindications/cautions
- Allergy to iodides; pulmonary edema, pulmonary tuberculosis (sodium iodide); pregnancy; lactation.

Dosage
Adult
- **RDA:** 150 μg PO.
- **Preparation for thyroidectomy:** 2–6 drops strong iodine solution tid PO for 10 d prior to surgery.
- **Thyroid blocking in a radiation emergency:** One tablet (130 mg potassium iodide) PO or 6 drops (21 mg potassium iodide/drop) added to half glass of liquid per day for 10 d.

Pediatric
- **Thyroid blocking in a radiation emergency:** *Children older than 1 y:* adult dose. *Younger than 1 y:* ½ crushed tablet or 3 drops in a small amount of liquid per day for 10 d. *Note:* Potassium iodide tablets and drops are available only to State and Federal agencies.

Pharmacokinetics

Route	Onset	Peak	Duration
Oral	24 h	10–15 d	6 wk

Metabolism: Hepatic; $T_{1/2}$: unknown
Distribution: Crosses placenta; may enter breast milk
Excretion: Urine

Adverse effects
- GI: *Swelling of the salivary glands, iodism* (metallic taste, burning mouth and throat, sore teeth and gums, head cold symptoms, stomach upset, diarrhea)
- Dermatologic: *Skin rash*
- Hypersensitivity: Allergic reactions-fever, joint pains, swelling of the face or body, shortness of breath

Adverse effects in *Italics* are most common; those in **Bold** are life-threatening.

598 ■ iodoquinol

- **Endocrine:** Hypothyroidism, hyperthyroidism, goiter

Clinically important drug-drug interactions
- Increased risk of hypothyroidism if taken concurrently with lithium

■ Nursing Considerations
Assessment
- *History:* Allergy to iodides, pulmonary edema, pulmonary tuberculosis, lactation
- *Physical:* Skin—color, lesions, edema; R, adventitious sounds; gums, mucous membranes; T_3, T_4

Implementation
- Arrange for skin testing for idiosyncrasy to iodine before administering parenteral doses.
- Dilute strong iodine solution with fruit juice or water to improve taste.
- Crush tablets for small children.
- Arrange for discontinuation of drug if symptoms of acute iodine toxicity occur: vomiting, abdominal pain, diarrhea, circulatory collapse.

Drug-specific teaching points
- Know that the drops may be diluted in fruit juice or water. Tablets may be crushed.
- Discontinue use and report fever, skin rash, swelling of the throat, metallic taste, sore teeth and gums, head cold symptoms, severe GI distress, enlargement of the thyroid gland.

❒ iodoquinol

*(eye oh doe **kwin'** ole)*

diiodohydroxyquinoline
Diodoquin (CAN), Yodoxin

Pregnancy Category C

Drug classes
Amebicide

Therapeutic actions
Direct amebicidal by an unknown mechanism; is poorly absorbed in the GI tract and is able to exert its amebicidal action directly in the large intestine.

Indications
- Acute or chronic intestinal amebiasis

Contraindications/cautions
- Contraindicated in the presence of hepatic failure, allergy to iodine preparations or 8-hydroxyquinolines.
- Use caution in the presence of thyroid disease, pregnancy, lactation.

Dosage
Adult: 650 mg tid PO after meals for 20 d.
Pediatric: 40 mg/kg per day PO, in three divided doses for 20 d. Maximum dose: 650 mg/dose. Do not exceed 1.95 g in 24 h for 20 d.

Pharmacokinetics

Route	Onset
Oral	Slow

Very poorly absorbed; exerts effects locally in the intestine.

Adverse effects
- **CNS:** Blurring of vision, weakness, fatigue, numbness, headache
- **GI:** *Nausea, vomiting, diarrhea,* anorexia
- **Dermatologic:** *Skin rash, pruritus*
- **General:** Fever, chills
- **Other:** Thyroid enlargement

Drug-lab test interferences
- Interferes with many tests of thyroid function; interference may last up to 6 mo after drug is discontinued.

■ Nursing Considerations
Assessment
- *History:* Hepatic failure, allergy to iodine preparations or 8-hydroxyquinolines, thyroid disease, lactation
- *Physical:* Skin—rashes, lesions; check reflexes, ophthalmologic exam; BP, P, R; liver and thyroid function tests (PBI, T_3, T_4)

Adverse effects in *Italics* are most common; those in **Bold** are life-threatening.

ipecac syrup

Implementation
- Administer drug after meals.
- Administer for full course of therapy.
- Maintain patient's nutrition.

Drug-specific teaching points
- Take drug after meals.
- Know that the following side effects often occur: GI upset, nausea, vomiting, diarrhea (small frequent meals, frequent mouth care often help).
- Report severe GI upset, skin rash, blurring of vision, unusual fatigue, fever.

❒ ipecac syrup

(ip' e kak)

Pregnancy Category C

Drug classes
Emetic

Therapeutic actions
Produces vomiting by a local GI mucosa irritant effect and a central medullary effect (CTZ stimulation).

Indications
- Treatment of drug overdose and certain poisonings

Contraindications/cautions
- Unconscious, semiconscious, convulsing states; poisoning with corrosives, such as alkalies, strong acids, petroleum distillates.

Dosage
Adult: 15–30 ml PO followed by 3–4 glasses of water.
Children younger than 1 y: 15 ml PO followed by 1–2 glasses of water.
Children older than 1 y: 5–10 ml PO followed by ½–1 glass of water. Repeat dosage if vomiting does not occur within 20 min. If vomiting does not occur within 30 min of second dose, perform gastric lavage.

Pharmacokinetics

Route	Onset	Peak
Oral	Varies	20–30 min

Minimal systemic absorption occurs if taken correctly.

Adverse effects
- CNS: *Mild CNS depression*
- GI: *Diarrhea, mild GI upset*
- CV: Heart conduction disturbances, atrial fibrillation, **fatal myocarditis** if drug is not vomited

■ Nursing Considerations

Assessment
- *History:* Unconscious, semiconscious, convulsing states; poisoning with corrosives; lactation
- *Physical:* Orientation, affect; P, baseline ECG, auscultation; stools, bowel sounds

Implementation
- Administer drug to conscious patients only.
- Administer drug as soon after poisoning as possible.
- Use caution to differentiate ipecac syrup from ipecac fluid extract, which is 14 times stronger and has caused some deaths.
- Consult with a Poison Control Center if in doubt and if vomiting does not occur within 20 min of second dose.
- Administer with adequate amounts of water.
- Maintain life support equipment on standby for poisoning and overdose; cardiac support will be needed if vomiting of ipecac does not occur.
- Arrange for use of activated charcoal if vomiting of ipecac does not occur or if overdose of ipecac occurs.

Drug-specific teaching points
- Drug is available in premeasured doses for emergency home use.
- Call physician, poison control center, or emergency room in cases of accidental ingestion.

Adverse effects in *Italics* are most common; those in **Bold** are life-threatening.

- Administer drug with adequate amounts of water. Do not exceed recommended dose.
- Know that the following side effects may occur: diarrhea, GI upset, drowsiness and lethargy.

ipratropium bromide

*(i pra **troe**' pee um)*
Atrovent

Pregnancy Category B

Drug classes
Anticholinergic
Antimuscarinic
Parasympatholytic

Therapeutic actions
Anticholinergic, chemically related to atropine, which blocks vagally mediated reflexes by antagonizing the action of acetylcholine.

Indications
- Bronchodilator for maintenance treatment of bronchospasm associated with COPD

Contraindications/cautions
- Contraindicated in the presence of hypersensitivity to atropine or its derivatives, acute episodes of bronchospasm.
- Use caution in the presence of narrow-angle glaucoma, prostatic hypertrophy, bladder neck obstruction, pregnancy, lactation.

Dosage
Adult: The usual dosage is 2 inhalations (36 μg) four times per day. Patients may take additional inhalations as required. Do not exceed 12 inhalations/24 h. *Solution for inhalation:* 500 mcg, 3–4 times/day with doses 6–8 h apart.
Pediatric: Safety and efficacy in children younger than 12 y not established.

Pharmacokinetics

Route	Onset	Peak	Duration
Inhalation	15 min	1–2 h	3–4 h

Adverse effects
- CNS: *Nervousness, dizziness, headache,* fatigue, insomnia, *blurred vision*
- GI: *Nausea,* GI distress, dry mouth
- Respiratory: *Cough,* exacerbation of symptoms, hoarseness
- Other: Palpitations, rash

Nursing Considerations

Assessment
- *History:* Hypersensitivity to atropine; acute bronchospasm, narrow-angle glaucoma, prostatic hypertrophy, bladder neck obstruction, pregnancy, lactation
- *Physical:* Skin—color, lesions, texture; body temperature; orientation, reflexes, bilateral grip strength; affect; ophthalmic exam; P, BP; R, adventitious sounds; bowel sounds, normal output; normal urinary output; prostate palpation

Implementation
- Protect solution for inhalation from light.
- Ensure adequate hydration, provide environmental control (temperature) to prevent hyperpyrexia.
- Encourage patient to void before taking medication if urinary retention could be a problem.
- Teach patient proper administration of inhalator.

Drug-specific teaching points
- Use this drug as an inhalation product. Review the proper use of inhalator.
- Know that the following side effects may occur: dizziness, headache, blurred vision (avoid driving a car or performing hazardous tasks); nausea, vomiting, GI upset (proper nutrition is important; consult with your dietician to maintain nutrition); cough.
- Report rash, eye pain, difficulty voiding, palpitations, vision changes.

iron dextran

InFeD

Pregnancy Category B

Drug classes
Iron preparation

Adverse effects in *Italics* are most common; those in **Bold** are life-threatening.

Therapeutic actions
Elevates the serum iron concentration and is then converted to hemoglobin or trapped in the reticuloendothelial cells for storage and eventual conversion to usable form of iron.

Indications
- Treatment of iron deficiency anemia only when oral administration of iron is unsatisfactory or impossible

Contraindications/cautions
- Contraindicated in the presence of allergy to iron dextran, anemias other than iron deficiency anemia, pregnancy.
- Use caution in the presence of impaired liver function, rheumatoid arthritis, allergies, asthma, lactation.

Dosage
Adult or Pediatric
- ***Iron deficiency anemia:*** Administer a 0.5 ml IM or IV test dose before beginning therapy. Base dosage on hematologic response with frequent hemoglobin determinations:

$$\text{mg iron} = \frac{0.3 \times (\text{weight in lbs}) \times [100 - (\text{hemoglobin in g\%}) \times 100]}{14.8}$$

To determine dose in ml, divide the result by 50. For patients < 30 lb (14 kg), give 80% the dose calculated from the formula.

- ***Iron replacement for blood loss:*** Determine dosage by the following formula:

$$\text{replacement iron (in mg)} = \text{blood loss (in ml)} \times \text{Hct}$$

- *IM:* Inject only into the upper outer quadrant of the buttocks. Do not exceed: 25 mg/d if < 4.5 kg; 50 mg/d if < 9 kg; 100 mg/d if < 50 kg; or 250 mg/d for all others.

Pharmacokinetics

Route	Onset	Peak
IM	Slow	1–2 wk

Metabolism: $T_{1/2}$: 6 h

Distribution: Crosses placenta; enters breast milk
Excretion: Blood loss

IV facts
Preparation: Intermittent IV: Calculate dose from formula. Individual doses of 2 ml or less per day may be given. Use single dose ampules without preservatives. IV infusion: dilute the needed dose in 200–250 ml of Normal Saline.

Infusion: Intermittent IV: give undiluted and slowly—1 ml or less/min. IV infusion (method is not approved by the FDA): infuse over 1–2 h after a test dose of 25 ml.

Adverse effects
- **CNS:** Headache, backache, dizziness, malaise, transitory paresthesias
- **GI:** *Nausea, vomiting*
- **CV:** Hypotension, chest pain, shock, tachycardia
- **Hypersensitivity:** Hypersensitivity reactions including fatal anaphylaxis; dyspnea, urticaria, rash and itching, arthralgia and myalgia, fever, sweating, purpura
- **Local:** *Pain, inflammation and sterile abscesses at injection site, brown skin discoloration* (IM use); *lymphadenopathy, local phlebitis, peripheral vascular flushing* (IV administration)
- **Other:** *Arthritic reactivation*, fever, shivering, cancer

Clinically important drug-drug interactions
- Delayed response to iron dextran therapy in patients taking chloramphenicol.

Drug-lab test interferences
- Use caution when interpreting serum iron levels when done within 1–2 wk of iron dextran injection • Serum may be discolored to a brownish color following IV injection • Bone scans using Tc-99m diphosphonate may have abnormal areas following IM injection

■ Nursing Considerations
Assessment
- *History:* Allergy to iron dextran, anemias other than iron deficiency anemia, im-

paired liver function, rheumatoid arthritis, allergies or asthma, lactation
- *Physical:* Skin—lesions, color; body temperature; injection site exam; range of motion, joints; R, adventitious sounds; liver evaluation; CBC, hemoglobin, hematocrit, serum ferritin assays, liver function tests

Implementation
- Ensure that patient does have iron deficiency anemia before treatment.
- Arrange for treatment of underlying cause of iron deficiency anemia whenever possible.
- Administer IM injections using the Z-track technique (displace skin laterally before injection) to avoid injection into the tissue and tissue staining. Use a large-gauge needle; if patient is standing, have him or her support himself or herself on the leg not receiving the injection. If lying, have the injection site uppermost.
- Monitor patient for hypersensitivity reactions, test dose is highly recommended. Maintain epinephrine on standby in case severe hypersensitivity reaction occurs.
- Monitor patient's serum ferritin levels periodically; these correlate well with iron stores. Do not administer with oral iron preparations.
- Caution patients with rheumatoid arthritis that acute exacerbation of joint pain and swelling may occur; provide appropriate comfort measures.

Drug-specific teaching points
- Know that treatment may no longer be necessary if cause of anemia can be corrected.
- Arrange for periodic blood tests during therapy to follow your response to the drug and determine the appropriate dosage for you.
- Do not take oral iron products or vitamins with iron added while on this drug.
- Know that the following side effects may occur: pain at injection site, headache, joint and muscle aches, GI upset.
- Report difficulty breathing, pain at injection site, rash, itching.

isoetharine hydrochloride

(eye soe eth' a reen)
Arm-a-Med Isoetharine HCl, Beta-2, Bronkosol

isoetharine mesylate
Bronkometer

Pregnancy Category C

Drug classes
Sympathomimetic drug
Beta-2 selective adrenergic agonist
Bronchodilator
Antiasthmatic drug

Therapeutic actions
In low doses, acts relatively selectively at beta-2 adrenergic receptors to cause bronchodilation; at higher doses, beta-2 selectivity is lost, and the drug acts at beta-1 receptors to cause typical sympathomimetic cardiac effects.

Indications
- Prophylaxis and treatment of bronchial asthma and reversible bronchospasm that may occur with bronchitis and emphysema

Contraindications/cautions
- Contraindicated in the presence of hypersensitivity to isoetharine; allergy to sulfites; tachyarrhythmias, tachycardia caused by digitalis intoxication; general anesthesia with halogenated hydrocarbons or cyclopropane (sensitize the myocardium to catecholamines); unstable vasomotor system disorders.
- Use caution in the presence of hypertension, coronary insufficiency, coronary artery disease, history of stroke, COPD patients who have developed degenerative heart disease, hyperthyroidism, history of seizure disorders, psychoneurotic individuals, labor and delivery (may inhibit labor; parenteral use of β_2-adrenergic agonists can accelerate fetal heart beat, cause hypoglycemia, hypokalemia, and pulmonary edema in the mother and hypoglycemia in the neonate); lactation.

isoetharine hydrochloride ■ 603

Dosage
Adult
- **Inhalation, metered-dose inhaler:** Each actuation of aerosol dispenser delivers 340 μg isoetharine. Dose is 1 or 2 inhalations. Occasionally more may be required; however, wait 1 full min after the initial dose. Treatment usually need not be repeated more than every 4 h.
- **Inhalant solutions:** Administer from hand bulb nebulizer (3–7 inhalations), with oxygen aerosolization, or using an IPPB device, following manufacturer's instructions.

Pediatric: Dosage not established.
Geriatric: Patients older than 60 y are more likely to develop adverse effects; use with extreme caution.

Pharmacokinetics

Route	Onset	Duration
Inhalation	5 min	1–3 h

Metabolism: Tissue
Distribution: Crosses placenta; may enter breast milk
Excretion: Urine

Adverse effects
- CNS: *Restlessness, apprehension, anxiety, fear,* CNS stimulation, hyperkinesia, insomnia, tremor, drowsiness, irritability, weakness, vertigo, headache
- GI: *Nausea,* vomiting, heartburn, unusual or bad taste
- CV: *Cardiac arrhythmias, tachycardia, palpitations,* PVCs, anginal pain
- Respiratory: *Respiratory difficulties, pulmonary edema, coughing,* bronchospasm, paradoxical airway resistance with repeated, excessive use of inhalation preparations
- Other: Sweating, pallor, flushing

Clinically important drug-drug interactions
- Increased likelihood of cardiac arrhythmias when given with halogenated hydrocarbon anesthetics (halothane), cyclopropane

■ Nursing Considerations
Assessment
- *History:* Hypersensitivity to isoetharine, allergy to sulfites, tachyarrhythmias, general anesthesia with halogenated hydrocarbons or cyclopropane, unstable vasomotor system disorders, hypertension, coronary insufficiency, history of stroke, COPD patients who have developed degenerative heart disease, hyperthyroidism, history of seizure disorders, psychoneuroses
- *Physical:* Body weight, skin—color, temperature, turgor; orientation, reflexes; P, BP; R, adventitious sounds; blood and urine glucose, serum electrolytes, thyroid function tests, ECG

Implementation
- Use minimal doses for minimal periods of time; drug tolerance can occur with prolonged use.
- Maintain a beta-adrenergic blocker (a cardioselective beta-blocker, such as atenolol, should be used in patients with respiratory distress) on standby in case cardiac arrhythmias occur.
- Do not exceed recommended dosage; administer aerosol during second half of inspiration, because the airways are open wider, and the aerosol distribution is more extensive.

Drug-specific teaching points
- Do not exceed recommended dosage; adverse effects or loss of effectiveness may result. Read the instructions that come with the aerosol product, and ask your health care provider or pharmacist if you have any questions.
- Know that the following side effects may occur: dizziness, drowsiness, fatigue, apprehension (use caution if driving or performing tasks that require alertness if these effects occur); nausea, heartburn, unusual taste (small, frequent meals may help); fast heart rate, anxiety, changes in breathing.

Adverse effects in *Italics* are most common; those in **Bold** are life-threatening.

isoniazid

(eye soe nye' a zid)
isonicotinic acid hydrazide, INH
Isotamine (CAN), Laniazid, Nydrazid, Rimifon (CAN)

Pregnancy Category C

Drug classes
Antituberculous agent ("first line")

Therapeutic actions
Bactericidal: interferes with lipid and nucleic acid biosynthesis in actively growing tubercle bacilli.

Indications
- Tuberculosis, all forms in which organisms are susceptible
- Prophylaxis in specific patients who are tuberculin reactors or household members of recently diagnosed tuberculars
- Unlabeled use of 300–400 mg/d, increased over 2 wk to 20 mg/kg per day for improvement of severe tremor in patients with multiple sclerosis

Contraindications/cautions
- Contraindicated in the presence of allergy to isoniazid, isoniazid-associated hepatic injury or other severe adverse reactions to isoniazid, acute hepatic disease, pregnancy.
- Use caution in the presence of renal dysfunction, lactation.

Dosage
Adult
- ***Treatment of active TB:*** 5 mg/kg per day (up to 300 mg) PO in a single dose, with other effective agents. "First-line treatment" is considered to be 300 mg INH plus 600 mg rifampin, each given in a single daily oral dose.
- ***Prophylaxis for TB:*** 300 mg/d PO in a single dose.

Pediatric
- ***Treatment of active TB:*** 10–20 mg/kg per day (up to 300–500 mg) PO in a single dose, with other effective agents.
- ***Prophylaxis for TB:*** 10 mg/kg per day (up to 300 mg) in a single dose. Continuous treatment for a sufficient period of time is needed to prevent relapse. Concomitant administration of 6–50 mg/d of pyridoxine is recommended for those who are malnourished or predisposed to neuropathy (alcoholics, diabetics).

Pharmacokinetics

Route	Onset	Peak	Duration
Oral	Varies	1–2 h	24 h
IM	Rapid	1–2 h	24 h

Metabolism: Hepatic; $T_{1/2}$: 1–4 h
Distribution: Crosses placenta; enters breast milk
Excretion: Urine

Adverse effects
- **CNS:** *Peripheral neuropathy*, convulsions, toxic encephalopathy, optic neuritis and atrophy, memory impairment, toxic psychosis
- **GI:** *Nausea, vomiting, epigastric distress,* bilirubinemia, bilirubinuria, *elevated AST,* ALT levels, jaundice, **hepatitis**
- **Hematologic:** Agranulocytosis, hemolytic or aplastic anemia, thrombocytopenia, eosinophilia, pyridoxine deficiency, pellagra, hyperglycemia, metabolic acidosis, hypocalcemia, hypophosphatemia due to altered vitamin D metabolism
- **Hypersensitivity:** Fever, skin eruptions, lymphadenopathy, vasculitis
- **Local:** *Local irritation at IM injection site*
- **Other:** Gynecomastia, rheumatic syndrome, systemic lupus erythematous syndrome

Clinically important drug-drug interactions

• Increased incidence of isoniazid-related hepatitis if taken with alcohol and possibly if taken in high doses with rifampin • Increased serum levels of phenytoin if given concurrently with isoniazid • Increased effectiveness and risk of toxicity of carbamazepine, if taken concurrently with isoniazid • Risk of high output renal failure in fast INH acetylators if taken concurrently with enflurane

Clinically important drug-food interactions

• Risk of sympathetic-type reactions with tyramine-containing foods and exaggerated response (headache, palpitations, sweating, hypotension, flushing, diarrhea, itching) to histamine-containing food (fish—skipjack, tuna—sauerkraut juice, yeast extracts)

■ Nursing Considerations

Assessment

- *History:* Allergy to isoniazid, isoniazid-associated adverse reactions; acute hepatic disease; renal dysfunction; lactation
- *Physical:* Skin—color, lesions; temperature; orientation, reflexes, peripheral sensitivity, bilateral grip strength; ophthalmologic examination; R, adventitious sounds; liver evaluation; CBC, liver and kidney function tests, blood glucose

Implementation

- Administer on an empty stomach, 1 h before or 2 h after meals; may be given with food if GI upset occurs.
- Administer in a single daily dose.
- Arrange for a diet that is low in tyramine-containing and histamine-containing food.
- Consult with physician and arrange for daily pyridoxine in diabetic, alcoholic, or malnourished patients; also for patients who develop peripheral neuritis.
- Discontinue drug, and consult with physician if any signs of hypersensitivity occur.

Drug-specific teaching points

- Take this drug in a single daily dose. Take on an empty stomach, 1 h before or 2 h after meals. If GI distress occurs, may be taken with food.
- Take this drug regularly; avoid missing doses; do not discontinue this drug without first consulting with your prescriber.
- Do not drink alcohol, or if you must drink alcohol, drink as little as possible while you are on this drug. There is an increased risk of hepatitis if these two drugs are combined.
- Avoid tyramine-containing foods while you are on this drug; speak with a dietician to obtain a list of tyramine-containing and histamine-containing foods.
- Know that the following side effects may occur: nausea, vomiting, epigastric distress (taking the drug with meals may help); skin rashes or lesions; numbness, tingling, loss of sensation (use caution if these occur to prevent injury or burns).
- Arrange to have periodic medical checkups, which will include an eye examination and blood tests to evaluate the drug effects.
- Report weakness, fatigue, loss of appetite, nausea, vomiting, yellowing of skin or eyes, darkening of the urine, numbness or tingling in hands or feet.

⬚ isoproterenol hydrochloride

*(eye soe proe **ter'** e nole)*

Dey-Dose Isoproterenol HCl, Dispos-a-Med Isoproterenol HCl, Isuprel

isoproterenol sulfate

Medihaler-Iso

Pregnancy Category C

Drug classes

Sympathomimetic drug
Beta-1 and beta-2 adrenergic agonist
Bronchodilator
Antiasthmatic drug
Drug used in shock

Therapeutic actions

Effects are mediated by beta-1 and beta-2 adrenergic receptors; acts on beta-1 receptors in the heart to produce positive chronotropic and positive inotropic effects and to increase automaticity; acts on beta-2 receptors in the bronchi to cause bronchodilation; acts on beta-2 receptors in smooth muscle in the walls of blood vessels in skeletal muscle and splanchnic beds to cause dilation (cardiac stimulation, vasodilation may be adverse effects when drug is used as bronchodilator).

Indications

- Inhalation: treatment of bronchospasm associated with acute and chronic bronchial asthma, pulmonary emphysema, bronchitis, bronchiectasis
- Injection: management of bronchospasm during anesthesia
- Adjunct in the management of shock (hypoperfusion syndrome) and in the treatment of cardiac standstill or arrest; carotid sinus hypersensitivity; Stokes-Adams syndrome; ventricular tachycardia and ventricular arrhythmias that require increased inotropic activity for therapy
- Sublingual: management of patients with bronchopulmonary disease; Stokes-Adams syndrome and AV heart block
- Rectal: Stokes-Adams syndrome and AV heart block

Contraindications/cautions

- Contraindicated in the presence of hypersensitivity to isoproterenol; tachyarrhythmias, tachycardia caused by digitalis intoxication; general anesthesia with halogenated hydrocarbons or cyclopropane (sensitize the myocardium to catecholamines); labor and delivery (may delay second stage of labor; can accelerate fetal heart beat; may cause hypoglycemia, hypokalemia, pulmonary edema in the mother and hypoglycemia in the neonate); lactation.
- Use caution in the presence of unstable vasomotor system disorders, hypertension, coronary insufficiency, history of stroke, COPD patients who have developed degenerative heart disease, diabetes mellitus, hyperthyroidism, history of seizure disorders, psychoneuroses.

Dosage

Adult

- **Injection**
  - *Bronchospasm during anesthesia:* 0.01–0.02 mg of diluted solution IV; repeat when necessary.
  - *Shock:* Dilute to 2 μg/ml and infuse IV at a rate adjusted on the basis of HR, central venous pressure, systemic BP, and urine flow.
  - *Cardiac standstill and arrhythmias: IV injection:* 0.02–0.06 mg of diluted solution. *IV infusion:* 5 μg/min of diluted solution. *IM, SC:* 0.2 mg of undiluted 1:5,000 solution. Intracardiac: 0.02 mg of undiluted 1:5,000 solution
- **Sublingual**
  - *Bronchospasm:* 10 mg average dose SL (15–20 mg may be required). Do not repeat more often than every 3 or 4 h or more than tid. Do not exceed a total dose of 60 mg/d.
  - *Heart block, certain ventricular arrhythmias:* Administer glossets sublingually or rectally for maintenance after stabilization with other therapy; 10–30 mg sublingually four to six times a day to prevent heart block in carotid sinus hypersensitivity; 5–15 mg rectally to treat heart block.
  - *Acute bronchial asthma: Hand bulb nebulizer:* Administer the 1:200 solution in a dosage of 5–15 deep inhalations. If desired, administer the 1:100 solution in 3–7 deep inhalations. If no relief after 5–10 min, repeat doses once more. If acute attack recurs, may repeat treatment up to five times per day. *Metered-dose inhaler:* Start with one inhalation; if no relief after 2–5 min, repeat. *Daily maintenance:* 1–2 inhalations four to six times per day. Do not take more than 2 inhalations at any one time. Do not take more than 6 inhalations per hour.
  - *Bronchospasm in COPD: Hand bulb nebulizer:* 5–15 inhalations using the 1:200 solution. Patients with severe attacks may require 3–7 inhalations using the 1:100 solution. Do not use at less than 3- to 4-h intervals. *Nebulization by compressed air or O_2, IPPB:* 0.5 ml of a 1:200 solution is diluted to 2–2.5

isoproterenol hydrochloride

ml with appropriate diluent for a concentration of 1:800 to 1:1,000 and delivered over 10–20 min. May repeat up to five times per day. *Metered-dose inhaler*: 1 or 2 inhalations; repeat at no less than 3- to 4-h intervals.

Pediatric
- **Sublingual glossets**
  - *Bronchospasm:* 5–10 mg sublingually. Do not repeat treatment more often than q3–4h or more often than tid. Do not exceed a total dose of 30 mg/d.
  - *Heart block:* 5 mg sublingually, 2.5 mg rectally; base subsequent doses on patient response.
  - *Nebulization (bronchospasm):* Administration is similar to that of adults; children's smaller ventilatory exchange capacity provides smaller aerosol intake. Use the 1:200 solution for an acute attack; do not use more than 0.25 ml of the 1:200 solution for each 10- to 15-min programmed treatment.

Geriatric: Patients older than 60 y are more likely to experience adverse effects; use with extreme caution.

Pharmacokinetics

Route	Onset	Duration
Inhalation	Rapid	50–60 min
IV	Immediate	1–2 min
SL	Rapid	2 h
PR	Slow	2–4 h

Metabolism: Tissue; $T_{1/2}$: unknown
Distribution: Crosses placenta; enters breast milk
Excretion: Urine

IV facts
Preparation: Dilute the 1:5,000 solutions for IV injection or infusion with 5% Dextrose Injection; a convenient dilution is 1 mg isoproterenol (5 ml) in 500 ml diluent (final concentration 1:500,000 or 2 μg/ml).

Infusion: Dosage of 5 μg/min is provided by infusing 2.5 ml/min.

Adverse effects
- **CNS:** *Restlessness, apprehension, anxiety, fear,* CNS stimulation, hyperkinesia, insomnia, tremor, drowsiness, irritability, weakness, vertigo, headache
- **GI:** *Nausea, vomiting, heartburn,* unusual or bad taste, swelling of the parotid glands
- **CV:** *Cardiac arrhythmias, tachycardia, palpitations,* anginal pain, changes in BP, paradoxical precipitation of Stokes-Adams seizures during normal sinus rhythm or transient heart block
- **Respiratory:** *Respiratory difficulties,* **pulmonary edema,** coughing, bronchospasm, paradoxical airway resistance with repeated, excessive use
- **Other:** *sweating, pallor,* flushing, muscle cramps

■ Nursing Considerations
Assessment
- *History:* Hypersensitivity to isoproterenol; tachyarrhythmias; general anesthesia with halogenated hydrocarbons or cyclopropane; unstable vasomotor system disorders; hypertension; coronary artery disease; history of stroke; COPD patients who have developed degenerative heart disease; diabetes mellitus; hyperthyroidism; history of seizure disorders; psychoneurotic individuals; labor and delivery; lactation
- *Physical:* Body weight; skin—color, temperature, turgor; orientation, reflexes; P, BP, R, adventitious sounds; blood and urine glucose, serum electrolytes, thyroid function tests, ECG

Implementation
- Use minimal doses for minimal periods of time; drug tolerance can occur with prolonged use.
- Maintain a beta-adrenergic blocker (a cardioselective beta-blocker, such as atenolol, should be used in patients with respiratory distress) on standby in case cardiac arrhythmias occur.
- Do not exceed recommended dosage of inhalation products; administer pressurized inhalation drug forms during second

Adverse effects in *Italics* are most common; those in **Bold** are life-threatening.

half of inspiration, because the airways are open wider and the aerosol distribution is more extensive. If a second inhalation is needed, administer at peak effect of previous dose, 3–5 min.

Drug-specific teaching points
- Do not exceed recommended dosage; adverse effects or loss of effectiveness may result. Read the instructions for use that come with the product (respiratory inhalant products), and ask your health care provider or pharmacist if you have any questions. Proper use of the inhalator is important for getting the best results and avoiding adverse effects.
- Do not swallow or chew sublingual tablets; allow to dissolve under the tongue.
- Know that the following side effects may occur: drowsiness, dizziness, inability to sleep (use caution if driving or performing tasks that require alertness if these effects occur); nausea, vomiting (small, frequent meals may help); anxiety; rapid heart rate.
- Report chest pain, dizziness, insomnia, weakness, tremor or irregular heart beat, failure to respond to usual dosage.

☐ isosorbide

*(eye soe **sor**' bide)*
Ismotic

Pregnancy Category C

Drug classes
Osmotic diuretic

Therapeutic actions
Elevates the osmolarity of the glomerular filtrate, hindering the reabsorption of water and leading to a loss of water, sodium, and chloride; creates an osmotic gradient in the eye between plasma and ocular fluids, reducing intraocular pressure.

Indications
- Glaucoma: to interrupt acute attacks, especially when a drug with less risk of nausea and vomiting than that posed by other oral osmotic agents is needed
- Short-term reduction of intraocular pressure prior to and after ocular surgery

Contraindications/cautions
- Allergy to isosorbide, anuria due to severe renal disease, severe dehydration, pulmonary edema, CHF, diseases associated with salt retention.

Dosage
Adult: PO use only. 1.5 g/kg (range 1–3 mg/kg) bid–qid as needed.

Pharmacokinetics

Route	Onset	Peak	Duration
Oral	10–30 min	1–1½ h	5–6 h

Metabolism: $T_{1/2}$: 5–9.5 h
Distribution: Crosses placenta
Excretion: Urine

Adverse effects
- **CNS:** *Headache, confusion, disorientation, dizziness,* lightheadedness, syncope, vertigo, irritability
- **GI:** Nausea, vomiting, GI discomfort, thirst, hiccoughs
- **Hematologic:** Hypernatremia, hyperosmolarity
- **Other:** Rash

■ Nursing Considerations
Assessment
- *History:* Allergy to isosorbide, anuria due to severe renal disease, severe dehydration, pulmonary edema, CHF, diseases associated with salt retention
- *Physical:* Skin—color, edema; orientation, reflexes, muscle strength, pupillary reflexes; pulses, BP, perfusion; R, pattern, adventitious sounds; urinary output patterns; serum electrolytes, urinalysis

Implementation
- Administer by oral route only, not for injection.
- Pour over cracked ice, and have patient sip drug to improve palatability.
- Monitor urinary output carefully.
- Monitor BP regularly and carefully.

Drug-specific teaching points
- Pour the drug over cracked ice to make it easier to take.

Adverse effects in *Italics* are most common; those in **Bold** are life-threatening.

- Know that the following side effects may occur: increased urination (bathroom facilities will be made readily available); GI upset (small, frequent meals may help); dry mouth (sugarless lozenges to suck may help this problem); headache, blurred vision, feelings of irritability (use caution when moving around; ask for assistance)
- Report severe headache, confusion, dizziness.

isosorbide dinitrate

(eye soe sor' bide)

Iso-Bid, Isordil, Isotrate Timecelles, Sorbitrate

Pregnancy Category C

Drug classes
Antianginal drug
Nitrate

Therapeutic actions
Relaxes vascular smooth muscle with a resultant decrease in venous return and decrease in arterial blood pressure, which reduces left ventricular workload and decreases myocardial oxygen consumption.

Indications
- Treatment and prevention of angina pectoris

Contraindications/cautions
- Allergy to nitrates, severe anemia, GI hypermobility (sustained-release tablets), head trauma, cerebral hemorrhage, hypertrophic cardiomyopathy, pregnancy, lactation.

Dosage
Adult
- ***Angina pectoris:*** *Starting dose:* 2.5–5 mg sublingual, 5-mg chewable tablets, 5- to 20-mg oral tablets or capsules, 40-mg sustained-release. *Maintenance:* 10–40 mg q6h oral tablets or capsules, 40–80 mg sustained-release, q8–12h.
- ***Acute prophylaxis:*** Initial dosage: 5–10 mg sublingual or chewable tablets q2–3h.

Pediatric: Safety and efficicacy not established.

Pharmacokinetics

Route	Onset	Duration
Oral	15–45 min	4 h
SL	2–5 min	1–2 h
Slow release	30–45 min	12 h

Metabolism: Hepatic; $T_{1/2}$: 5 min, then 2–5 h
Distribution: May cross placenta; may enter breast milk
Excretion: Urine

Adverse effects
- CNS: *Headache, apprehension, restlessness, weakness,* vertigo, dizziness, faintness
- GI: *Nausea,* vomiting, incontinence or urine and feces, abdominal pain
- CV: *Tachycardia, retrosternal discomfort, palpitations, hypotension,* **syncope,** collapse, postural hypotension, angina
- Dermatologic: Rash, exfoliative dermatitis, cutaneous vasodilation with flushing
- Other: Muscle twitching, pallor, perspiration, cold sweat

Clinically important drug-drug interactions
- Increased systolic blood pressure and decreased antianginal effect if taken concurrently with ergot alkaloids

Drug-lab test interferences
- False report of decreased serum cholesterol if done by Zlatkis-Zak color reaction

■ Nursing Considerations

Assessment
- *History:* Allergy to nitrates, severe anemia, GI hypermobility, head trauma, cerebral hemorrhage, hypertrophic cardiomyopathy, pregnancy, lactation
- *Physical:* Skin—color, temperature, lesions; orientation, reflexes, affect; P, BP, orthostatic BP, baseline ECG, peripheral perfusion; R, adventitious sounds; liver evaluation, normal output; CBC, hemoglobin

Adverse effects in *Italics* are most common; those in **Bold** are life-threatening.

Implementation

- Administer sublingual preparations under the tongue or in the buccal pouch; encourage the patient not to swallow.
- Administer chewable tablets slowly, only 5 mg initially because severe hypotension can occur.
- Administer oral preparations on an empty stomach, 1 h before or 2 h after meals; dosage may be taken with meals if headache becomes so severe that it cannot be effectively controlled.
- Maintain life support equipment on standby if overdose occurs or cardiac condition worsens.
- Arrange for gradual reduction in dose if anginal treatment is being terminated; rapid discontinuation can lead to problems of withdrawal.

Drug-specific teaching points

- Place sublingual tablets under your tongue or in your cheek; do not chew or swallow the tablet. Take the isosorbide before chest pain begins, when you anticipate that your activities or situation may precipitate an attack. Take oral isosorbide dinitrate on an empty stomach, 1 h before or 2 h after meals.
- Know that the following side effects may occur: dizziness, lightheadedness (this may pass as you adjust to the drug; use care to change positions slowly); headache (lying down in a cool environment and resting may help; OTC preparations may not help; taking the drug with meals also may help); flushing of the neck or face (this usually passes as the drug's effects pass).
- Report blurred vision, persistent or severe headache, skin rash, more frequent or more severe angina attacks, fainting.

◻ isotretinoin

*(eye so **tret'** i noyn)*
13-*cis*-retinoic acid, vitamin A metabolite

Accutane

Pregnancy Category X

Drug classes
Vitamin metabolite
Acne product

Therapeutic actions
Decreases sebaceous gland size and inhibits sebaceous gland differentiation, resulting in a reduction in sebum secretion; inhibits follicular keratinization; exact mechanism of action is not known.

Indications
- Treatment of severe recalcitrant cystic acne in patients who are unresponsive to conventional treatments
- Unlabeled uses: treatment of cutaneous disorders of keratinization; cutaneous T-cell lymphoma and leukoplakia

Contraindications/cautions
- Contraindicated in the presence of allergy to isotretinoin, parabens, or any component of the product; pregnancy (has caused severe fetal malformations and spontaneous abortions); lactation.
- Use caution in the presence of diabetes mellitus.

Dosage
Individualize dosage based on side effects and disease response.
Initial dose: 0.5–1 mg/kg per day PO; usual dosage range is 0.5–2 mg/kg per day divided into two doses for 15–20 wk.
Maximum daily dose: 2 mg/kg. If a second course of therapy is needed, allow a rest period of at least 8 wk between courses.

Pharmacokinetics

Route	Onset	Peak	Duration
Oral	Varies	2.9–3.2 h	6–20 h

Metabolism: Hepatic; $T_{1/2}$: 10–20 h
Distribution: Crosses placenta; may enter breast milk
Excretion: Urine

Adverse effects
- CNS: *Lethargy, insomnia, fatigue, headache,* pseudotumor cerebri (papilledema, headache, nausea, vomiting, visual disturbances)

Adverse effects in *Italics* are most common; those in **Bold** are life-threatening.

- **GI:** *Nausea, vomiting, abdominal pain,* anorexia, inflammatory bowel disease
- **Respiratory:** *Epistaxis, dry nose, dry mouth*
- **Hematologic:** *Elevated sedimentation rate, hypertriglyceridemia,* abnormal liver function tests, increased fasting serum glucose
- **GU:** *White cells in the urine, proteinuria, hematuria*
- **MS:** Skeletal hyperostosis, arthralgia, bone and joint pain and stiffness
- **EENT:** *Cheilitis, eye irritation, conjunctivitis,* corneal opacities
- **Dermatologic:** *Skin fragility, dry skin, pruritus, rash,* thinning of hair, peeling of palms and soles, skin infections, photosensitivity, nail brittleness, petechiae

■ Nursing Considerations

Assessment
- *History:* Allergy to isotretinoin, parabens or any component of the product; diabetes mellitus; pregnancy; lactation
- *Physical:* Skin—color, lesions, turgor, texture; joints—range of motion; orientation, reflexes, affect, ophthalmologic exam; mucous membranes, bowel sounds; serum triglycerides, HDL, sedimentation rate, CBC and differential, urinalysis, pregnancy test

Implementation
- Ensure that patient is not pregnant before administering; arrange for a pregnancy test within 2 wk of beginning therapy. Advise patient to use contraceptive measures during treatment and for 1 mo after treatment is discontinued.
- Do not administer a second course of therapy within 8 wk of a course of isotretinoin.
- Administer drug with meals; do not crush capsules.
- Do not administer vitamin supplements that contain vitamin A.
- Discontinue drug if signs of papilledema occur, and consult with a neurologist for further care.
- Discontinue drug if visual disturbances occur, and arrange for an ophthalmologic exam.
- Discontinue drug if abdominal pain, rectal bleeding, or severe diarrhea occurs, and consult with physician.
- Monitor triglycerides during therapy; if elevations occur, institute other measures to lower serum triglycerides: weight reduction, reduction in dietary fat, exercise, increased intake of insoluble fiber, decreased alcohol consumption.
- Monitor diabetic patients with frequent bood glucose determinations.
- Do not allow blood donation from patients taking isotretinoin due to the teratogenic effects of the drug.

Drug-specific teaching points
- Take drug with meals; do not crush capsules.
- Be aware that a transient flare-up of the acne may occur during the beginning of therapy.
- Use contraceptive measures during treatment and for 1 mo after treatment is discontinued. This drug has been associated with severe birth defects and miscarriages; it is contraindicated in pregnant women. It is important to use contraceptive measures while on this drug. If you think that you have become pregnant, consult with your physician immediately.
- Know that you will not be permitted to donate blood while on this drug because of its possible effects on the fetus of a blood recipient.
- Know that the following side effects may occur: dizziness, lethargy, headache, visual changes (avoid driving or performing tasks that require alertness if these occur); sensitivity to the sun (avoid sunlamps, exposure to the sun; use sunscreens, protective clothing if it cannot be avoided); diarrhea, abdominal pain, loss of appetite (taking the drug with meals may help); dry mouth (sucking sugarless lozenges is often helpful); eye irritation and redness, inability to wear contact lenses; dry skin, itching, redness.

Adverse effects in *Italics* are most common; those in **Bold** are life-threatening.

- Avoid the use of vitamin supplements containing vitamin A while you are on this drug; serious toxic effects may occur. Limit your consumption of alcohol while on this drug. You also may need to limit your intake of fats and increase exercise to limit effects this drug has on blood triglyceride levels.
- Report headache with nausea and vomiting, severe diarrhea or rectal bleeding, visual difficulties.

☐ isradipine

*(eyes **rad'** i peen)*
DynaCirc

Pregnancy Category C

Drug classes
Calcium channel-blocker
Antihypertensive

Therapeutic actions
Inhibits the movement of calcium ions across the membranes of cardiac and arterial muscle cells; calcium is involved in the generation of the action potential in specialized automatic and conducting cells in the heart and in arterial smooth muscle and excitation-contraction coupling in cardiac muscle cells; inhibition of transmembrane calcium flow results in the depression of impulse formation in specialized cardiac pacemaker cells, slowing of the velocity of conduction of the cardiac impulse, the depression of myocardial contractility, and the dilation of coronary arteries and arterioles and peripheral arterioles. These effects lead to decreased cardiac work, cardiac energy consumption, and blood pressure.

Indications
- Management of hypertension alone or in combination with thiazide-type diuretics

Contraindications/cautions
- Contraindicated in the presence of allergy to isradipine; sick sinus syndrome, except in presence of ventricular pacemaker; heart block (second or third degree); IHSS; cardiogenic shock, severe CHF; pregnancy; lactation.
- Use caution in the presence of hypotension, impaired hepatic or renal function (repeated doses may accumulate).

Dosage
Adult: Initial dose of 2.5 mg PO bid. An antihypertensive effect is usually seen within 2–3h; maximal response may require 2–4 wk. Dosage may be increased in increments of 5 mg/d at 2- to 4-wk intervals. *Maximum dose:* 20 mg/d.

Pharmacokinetics

Route	Onset	Peak
Oral	120 min	1½ h

Metabolism: Hepatic; $T_{1/2}$: 8 h
Distribution: Crosses placenta; enters breast milk
Excretion: Urine

Adverse effects
- CNS: *Dizziness,* vertigo, emotional depression, sleepiness, **headache**
- GI: *Nausea,* constipation
- CV: *Peripheral edema, hypotension,* arrhythmias, bradycardia, **AV heart block**
- Other: Muscle fatigue, diaphoresis

Clinically important drug-drug interactions
- Increased cardiac depression if taken concurrently with beta-adrenergic blocking agents • Increased serum levels of digoxin, carbamazepine, prazosin, quinidine if given concurrently with isradipine • Increased respiratory depression if given to patients receiving atracurium, gallamine, metocurine, pancuronium, tubocurarine, vecuronium • Decreased effects of isradipine if taken with calcium, rifampin

■ Nursing Considerations

Assessment
- *History:* Allergy to isradipine; sick sinus syndrome, heart block; IHSS; cardiogenic shock, severe CHF; hypotension; impaired

Adverse effects in *Italics* are most common; those in **Bold** are life-threatening.

hepatic or renal function; pregnancy; lactation
- *Physical:* Skin—color, edema; orientation, reflexes; P, BP, baseline ECG, peripheral perfusion, auscultation; R, adventitious sounds; liver evaluation, normal output; liver and renal function tests, urinalysis

Implementation
- Monitor patient carefully (BP, cardiac rhythm, and output) while drug is being titrated to therapeutic dose.
- Monitor BP very carefully if patient is on concurrent doses of any other antihypertensive drugs.
- Monitor cardiac rhythm regularly during stabilization of dosage and periodically during long-term therapy.
- Monitor patients with renal or hepatic impairment very carefully for possible drug accumulation and adverse reactions.

Drug-specific teaching points
- Know that the following side effects may occur: nausea, vomiting (small, frequent meals may help); headache (monitor the lighting, noise, and temperature; medication may be ordered if this becomes severe); dizziness, sleepiness (avoid driving or operating dangerous equipment while on this drug); emotional depression (it may help to know that this is a drug effect and should pass when the drug is stopped); constipation (measures may need to be taken to alleviate this problem).
- Report irregular heart beat, shortness of breath, swelling of the hands or feet, pronounced dizziness, constipation.

▯ itraconazole

*(eye tra **kon**' a zole)*
Sporanox

Pregnancy Category C

Drug classes
Antifungal agent

Therapeutic actions
Binds to sterols in the fungal cell membrane, changing membrane permeability; fungicidal or fungistatic depending on concentration and organism.

Indications
- Treatment of blastomycosis, histoplasmosis in immunocompromised and non-immunocompromised patients
- Unlabeled uses: treatment of superficial and systemic mycoses, fungal keratitis, cutaneous leishmaniasis

Contraindications/cautions
- Contraindicated in the presence of hypersensitivity to itraconazole or other azoles, lactation.
- Use caution in the presence of hepatic impairment.

Dosage
Adult: 200 mg PO qd. If no obvious improvement, increase dose in 100-mg increments to a maximum of 400 mg qd. Give doses > 200 mg/d in divided doses.
- *Life-threatening infections:* Loading dose of 200 mg PO tid for the first 3 d. Continue treatment for a minimum of 3 mo and until clinical parameters and laboratory tests indicate that the active fungal infection has subsided.

Pediatric: Safety and efficacy not established.

Pharmacokinetics

Route	Onset	Peak	Duration
Oral	Slow	4.6 h	4–6 d

Metabolism: Hepatic; $T_{1/2}$: 21 h, then 64 h
Distribution: Crosses placenta; may enter breast milk
Excretion: Urine

Adverse effects
- CNS: *Headache,* dizziness
- GI: *Nausea, vomiting, diarrhea, abdominal pain,* abdominal pain, anorexia
- Other: *Skin rash, edema,* fever, malaise

Adverse effects in *Italics* are most common; those in **Bold** are life-threatening.

Clinically important drug-drug interactions

• Increased serum levels and therefore therapeutic and toxic effects of cyclosporine, digoxin, oral hypoglycemics, warfarin anticoagulants, terfenadine, phenytoin if taken concurrently with itraconazole • Decreased serum levels of itraconazole if taken concurrently with H_2 antagonists, isoniazid, phenytoin, rifampin

■ Nursing Considerations

Assessment

- *History:* Hypersensitivity to itraconazole, hepatic impairment, lactation
- *Physical:* Skin—color, lesions; body temperature; orientation, reflexes, affect; bowel sounds; hepatic function tests; culture of area involved

Implementation

- Arrange for appropriate culture of infection before beginning therapy; treatment should begin, however, before laboratory results are returned.
- Arrange for decreased dosage in cases of hepatic failure.
- Administer drug with meals to facilitate absorption.
- Monitor hepatic function tests regularly in patients with a history of hepatic dysfunction; discontinue or decrease dosage of drug at any sign of increased renal toxicity.

Drug-specific teaching points

- Take the full course of drug therapy that has been prescribed. Therapy may need to be long term.
- Take drug with food.
- Be aware that hygiene measures will be needed to prevent reinfection or spread of infection.
- Arrange for frequent follow-up while you are on this drug. Be sure to keep all appointments, which may include blood tests.
- Know that the following side effects may occur: nausea, vomiting, diarrhea (small frequent meals may help); headache (analgesics may be ordered); rash, itching (appropriate medication may help).
- Report unusual fatigue, anorexia, vomiting, jaundice, dark urine, pale stool.

☐ kanamycin sulfate

(kan a mye' sin)
Anamid (CAN), Kantrex

Pregnancy Category C

Drug classes
Aminoglycoside antibiotic

Therapeutic actions
Bactericidal: inhibits protein synthesis in susceptible strains of gram-negative bacteria; functional integrity of cell membrane appears to be disrupted, causing cell death.

Indications

- Infections caused by susceptible strains of *E. coli, Proteus, Enterobacter aerogenes, Klebsiella pneumoniae, Serratia marcescens, Acinetobacter*
- May be used for treatment of severe infections due to susceptible strains of staphylococci in patients allergic to other antibiotics
- Suppression of GI bacterial flora (oral, adjunctive therapy)
- Hepatic coma, to reduce ammonia-forming bacteria in the GI tract (oral)

Contraindications/cautions

- Contraindicated in the presence of allergy to aminoglycosides; intestinal obstruction, pregnancy, lactation.
- Use caution if administering this drug to the elderly or to any patient with diminished hearing, decreased renal function, dehydration, neuromuscular disorders.

Dosage
Adult or Pediatric

- *IM:* 7.5 mg/kg q12h or 15 mg/kg per day in equally divided doses q6–8h. Usual duration is 7–10 d. If no effect in 3–5 d, discontinue therapy. *Do not exceed 1.5 g/d.*
- *IV:* 15 mg/kg per day divided into two to three equal doses, administered slowly.

kanamycin sulfate ■ 615

- ***Intraperitoneal:*** 500 mg diluted in 20 ml sterile water instilled into the wound closure.
- ***Aerosol:*** 250 mg bid–qid, nebulized.
- ***Oral suppression of intestinal bacteria:*** 1 g every hour for 4 h followed by 1 g q6h for 36–72 h.
- ***Hepatic coma:*** 8–12 g/d in divided doses PO.

Geriatric or renal failure patients: Reduce dosage, and carefully monitor serum drug levels and renal function tests throughout treatment. If this is not possible, reduce frequency of administration. Calculate dosage formula from the following formula: dosage interval in h = serum creatinine (mg/100 ml) × 9.

Pharmacokinetics

Route	Onset	Peak
IM/IV	Rapid	30–120 min
PO	Slow; not absorbed systemically	

Metabolism: $T_{1/2}$: 2–3 h
Distribution: Crosses placenta; enters breast milk
Excretion: Urine

IV facts

Preparation: Do not mix with any other antibacterial agents; administer seperately; dilute contents of 500-mg vial with 100–200 ml of Normal Saline or 5% Dextrose in Water; dilute 1 g-vial with 200–400 ml of diluent; vials may darken during storage with no effect on potency.

Infusion: Administer dose slowly over 30–60 min (especially important in children).

Adverse effects

Although oral kanamycin is only negligibly absorbed from the intact GI mucosa, there is a risk of absorption from ulcerated areas or when used as an irrigant or aerosol.

- CNS: *Ototoxicity—tinnitus, dizziness, ringing in the ears, vertigo, deafness (partially reversible to irreversible),* confusion, disorientation, depression, lethargy, nystagmus, visual disturbances, headache, fever, numbness, tingling, tremor, paresthesias, muscle twitching, **convulsions,** muscular weakness, **neuromuscular blockade, apnea**
- GI: *Nausea, vomiting, anorexia, diarrhea,* weight loss, stomatitis, increased salivation, splenomegaly, malabsorption syndrome
- CV: Palpitations, hypotension, hypertension
- Hematologic: Leukemoid reaction, agranulocytosis, granulocytosis, leukopenia, leukocytosis, thrombocytopenia, eosinophilia, pancytopenia, anemia, hemolytic anemia, increased or decreased reticulocyte count, electrolyte disturbances
- GU: *Nephrotoxicity*
- Hypersensitivity: Purpura, rash, urticaria, exfoliative dermatitis, itching
- Hepatic: Hepatic toxicity; hepatomegaly
- Other: *Superinfections, pain and irritation at IM injection sites*

Clinically important drug-drug interactions

- Increased ototoxic and nephrotoxic effects if taken with potent diuretics and other ototoxic and nephrotoxic drugs (cephalosporins, penicillins) • Increased likelihood of neuromuscular blockade if given shortly after general anesthetics, depolarizing and nondepolarizing neuromuscular junction blockers, succinylcholine • Decreased absorption and therapeutic levels of digoxin if taken concurrently with kanamycin

■ Nursing Considerations

Assessment

- *History:* Allergy to aminoglycosides; intestinal obstruction, lactation, diminished hearing, decreased renal function, dehydration, neuromuscular disorders
- *Physical:* Site of infection, skin—color, lesions; orientation, reflexes, eighth cranial nerve function; P, BP; R, adventitious sounds; bowel sounds, liver evaluation; urinalysis, BUN, serum creatinine, serum electrolytes, liver function tests, CBC

Adverse effects in *Italics* are most common; those in **Bold** are life-threatening.

Implementation
- Arrange culture and sensitivity tests on infection before beginning therapy.
- Monitor duration of treatment: usual duration of treatment is 7–10 d. If clinical response does not occur within 3–5 d, stop therapy. Prolonged treatment leads to increased risk of toxicity. If drug is used longer than 10 d, monitor auditory and renal function daily.
- Administer IM dosage by deep intramuscular injection into upper outer quadrant of the gluteal muscle.
- Ensure that patient is well hydrated before and during therapy.

Drug-specific teaching points
- Complete the full course of drug therapy.
- Know that the following side effects may occur: ringing in the ears, headache, dizziness (these effects are reversible; safety measures may need to be taken if these become severe); nausea, vomiting, loss of appetite (small frequent meals, frequent mouth care may help).
- Report severe headache, dizziness, loss of hearing, severe diarrhea.

ketoconazole

*(kee toe **koe'** na zole)*
Nizoral

Pregnancy Category C

Drug classes
Antifungal

Therapeutic actions
Impairs the synthesis of ergosterol, the main sterol of fungal cell membranes, allowing increased permeability and leakage of cellular components and causing cell death.

Indications
- Treatment of systemic fungal infections: candidiasis, chronic mucocutaneous candidiasis, oral thrush, candiduria, blastomycosis, coccidioidomycosis, histoplasmosis, chromomycosis, paracoccidioidomycosis
- Treatment of dermatophytosis (recalcitrant infections not responding to topical or griseofulvin therapy)
- Unlabeled uses: treatment of onychomycosis, pityriasis versicolor, vaginal candidiasis; CNS fungal infections at high doses (800–1,200 mg/d); treatment of advanced prostate cancer at doses of 400 mg q8h
- Topical treatment of tinea corporis and tinea cruris caused by *Trichophyton rubrum*, *Trichophyton mentagrophytes*, and *Epidermophyton floccosum* and the treatment of tinea versicolor caused by *Malassezia furfur* (topical administration)
- Reduction of scaling due to dandruff (shampoo)
- Orphan drug use: with cyclosporine to diminish cyclosporine-induced nephrotoxicity in organ transplant

Contraindications/cautions
- Contraindicated in the presence of allergy to ketoconazole; fungal meningitis; pregnancy; lactation.
- Use caution in the presence of hepatocellular failure (increased risk of hepatocellular necrosis).

Dosage
Adult: 200 mg PO, qd. Up to 400 mg/d may be needed in severe infections. Period of treatment must be long enough to prevent recurrence, 3 wk–6 mo, depending on infecting organism and site.
- ***Topical cream:*** Apply once daily to affected area and immediate surrounding area. Severe cases may be treated twice daily. Continue treatment for at least 2 wk.
- ***Shampoo:*** Moisten hair and scalp thoroughly with water; apply sufficient shampoo to produce a lather; gently massage for 1 min; rinse hair with warm water; repeat, leaving on hair for 3 min. Shampoo twice a week for 4 wk with at least 3 d between shampooing.

Pediatric: Older than 2 y: 3.3–6.6 mg/kg per day PO as a single dose. Apply topical cream once daily to affected area and immediate surrounding area. Severe cases may be treated twice daily. Continue treatment for at least 2 wk. *Older than 2 y:* Safety and efficacy not established.

Pharmacokinetics

Route	Onset	Peak
Oral	Varies	1–4 h
Topical	Slow; not appreciably systemically absorbed	

Metabolism: Hepatic; $T_{1/2}$: 8 h
Distribution: Crosses placenta; enters breast milk
Excretion: Bile

Adverse effects

- **CNS:** Headache, dizziness, somnolence, photophobia
- **GI:** Hepatotoxicity, *nausea, vomiting,* abdominal pain
- **GU:** Impotence, oligospermia (with very high doses)
- **Hematologic:** Thrombocytopenia, leudopenia, hemolytic anemia
- **Hypersensitivity:** Urticaria to anaphylaxis
- **General:** *Pruritus,* fever, chills, gynecomastia
- **Local:** *Severe irritation, pruritus, stinging* with topical application

Clinically important drug-drug interactions

- Decreased blood levels of ketoconazole if taken with rifampin • Increased blood levels of cyclosporine and risk of toxicity when taken with ketoconazole • Increased duration of adrenal suppression when methylprednisolone, corticosteroids are taken with ketoconazole

■ Nursing Considerations

Assessment

- *History:* Allergy to ketoconazole, fungal meningitis, hepatocellular failure, pregnancy, lactation
- *Physical:* Skin—color, lesions; orientation, reflexes, affect; bowel sounds, liver evaluation; liver function tests; CBC and differential; culture of area involved

Implementation

- Arrange for culture of fungus involved before beginning therapy; treatment should begin, however, before laboratory results are returned.
- Maintain epinephrine on standby in case of severe anaphylaxis after first dose.
- Administer oral drug with food to decrease GI upset.
- Do not administer with antacids; ketoconazole requires an acid environment for absorption; if antacids are required, administer at least 2 h apart.
- Continue administration for long-term therapy until infection is eradicated: candidiasis, 1–2 wk; other systemic mycoses, 6 mo; chronic mucocutaneous candidiasis, often requires maintainance therapy; tinea veriscolor, 2 wk of topical application.
- Discontinue treatment, and consult physician about actual diagnosis if no improvement is seen within 2 wk of topical application.
- Discontinue topical applications if sensitivity or chemical reaction occurs.
- Administer shampoo as follows: moisten hair and scalp thoroughly with water; apply sufficient shampoo to produce a lather; gently massage for 1 min; rinse hair with warm water; repeat, leaving on hair for 3 min.
- Arrange to monitor hepatic function tests before beginning therapy and monthly or more frequently throughout treatment.

Drug-specific teaching points

- Take the full course of drug therapy. Long-term use of the drug will be needed; beneficial effects may not be seen for several weeks. Take oral drug with meals to decrease GI upset. Apply topical drug to affected area and immediate surrounding area. If using shampoo, moisten hair and scalp thoroughly with water; apply sufficient shampoo to produce a lather; gently massage for 1 min; rinse hair with warm water; repeat, leaving on hair for 3 min. Shampoo twice a week for 4 wk with at least 3 d between shampooing.
- Use appropriate hygiene measures to prevent reinfection or spread of infection.

Adverse effects in *Italics* are most common; those in **Bold** are life-threatening.

- Know that the following side effects may occur: nausea, vomiting, diarrhea (taking the drug with food may help); sedation, dizziness, confusion (avoid driving or performing tasks that require alertness if these occur); stinging, irritation (with local application).
- Do not take antacids with this drug; if they are needed, take this drug at least 2 h after their administration.
- Report skin rash, severe nausea, vomiting, diarrhea, fever, sore throat, unusual bleeding or bruising, yellow skin or eyes, dark urine or pale stools, severe irritation (local application).

☐ ketoprofen

*(kee toe **proe' fen**)*
Orudis, Oruvail (SR)

Pregnancy Category B

Drug classes
NSAID
Non-narcotic analgesic

Therapeutic actions
Anti-inflammatory and analgesic activity; inhibits prostaglandin and leukotriene synthesis and has antibradykinin and lysosomal membrane-stabilizing actions.

Indications
- Acute and long-term treatment of signs and symptoms of rheumatoid arthritis and osteoarthritis (capsules or sustained release—Oruvail)
- Relief of mild to moderate pain
- Treatment of dysmenorrhea
- Reduction of fever

Contraindications/cautions
- Contraindicated in the presence of significant renal impairment, pregnancy, lactation.
- Use caution in the presence of impaired hearing, allergies, hepatic, cardiovascular, and GI conditions

Dosage
Do not exceed 300 mg/d.
Adult
- ***Rheumatoid arthritis, osteoarthritis:*** Starting dose: 75 mg tid or 50 mg qid PO. Maintenance dose: 150–300 mg PO in three to four divided doses. Oruvail, 200 mg PO qd.
- ***Mild to moderate pain, primary dysmenorrhea:*** 25–50 mg PO q6–8h as needed. Do not use Oruvail.

Pediatric: Safety and efficacy not established.
Geriatric or hepatic or renal impaired: Reduce starting dose by one-half or one-third. Do not use Oruvail.

Pharmacokinetics

Route	Onset	Peak
Oral	30–60 min	0.5–2 h

Metabolism: Hepatic; $T_{1/2}$: 2–4 h
Distribution: Crosses placenta; enters breast milk
Excretion: Urine.

Adverse effects
NSAIDs
- CNS: *Headache, dizziness, somnolence, insomnia,* fatigue, tiredness, dizziness, tinnitus, ophthalmologic effects
- GI: *Nausea, dyspepsia, GI pain,* diarrhea, vomiting, *constipation,* flatulence
- Respiratory: Dyspnea, hemoptysis, pharyngitis, bronchospasm, rhinitis
- Hematologic: Bleeding, platelet inhibition with higher doses, neutropenia, eosinophilia, leukopenia, pancytopenia, thrombocytopenia, agranulocytosis, granulocytopenia, aplastic anemia, decreased hemoglobin or hematocrit, bone marrow depression, menorrhagia
- GU: Dysuria, **renal impairment**
- Dermatologic: *Rash,* pruritus, sweating, dry mucous membranes, stomatitis
- Other: Peripheral edema, **anaphylactoid reactions to fatal anaphylactic shock**

Adverse effects in *Italics* are most common; those in **Bold** are life-threatening.

Nursing Considerations

Assessment
- *History:* Renal impairment, impaired hearing, allergies, hepatic, cardiovascular, and GI conditions, lactation
- *Physical:* Skin color and lesions; orientation, reflexes, ophthalmologic and audiometric evaluation, peripheral sensation; P, edema; R, adventitious sounds; liver evaluation; CBC, clotting times, renal and liver function tests; serum electrolytes, stool guaiac

Implementation
- Administer drug with food or after meals if GI upset occurs.
- Arrange for periodic ophthalmologic examination during long-term therapy.
- Institute emergency procedures if overdose occurs: gastric lavage, induction of emesis, supportive therapy.

Drug-specific teaching points
- Take drug with food or meals if GI upset occurs; take only the prescribed dosage.
- Know that dizziness, drowsiness can occur (avoid driving or the use of dangerous machinery while on this drug).
- Report sore throat, fever, rash, itching, weight gain, swelling in ankles or fingers; changes in vision; black, tarry stools.

☐ ketorolac tromethamine

(kee' toe role ak)
Acular (ophthalmic), Toradol

Pregnancy Category B

Drug classes
NSAID
Non-narcotic analgesic

Therapeutic actions
Anti-inflammatory and analgesic activity; inhibits prostaglandins and leukotriene synthesis.

Indications
- Short-term management of pain, up to only 5 days
- Relief of ocular itching due to seasonal conjunctivitis (ophthalmic)

Contraindications/cautions
- Contraindicated in the presence of significant renal impairment, pregnancy, lactation; patients wearing soft contact lenses (ophthalmic); GI bleed (risk of bleeding intraoperatively, postoperatively).
- Use caution in the presence of impaired hearing, allergies, hepatic, cardiovascular, and GI conditions.

Dosage
Adult: Initial dosage: 30–60 mg IM, as a loading dose, followed by half of the loading dose q6h as long as needed to control pain. *Maximum total dose:* 150 mg for the first day and 120 mg qd thereafter.
- **Oral:** 10 mg PO q4–6h as needed; *maximum daily dose:* 40 mg.
- **Transition from IM to oral:** Do not exceed total combined dose of 120 mg on day of transition.
- **Ophthalmic:** 1 drop (0.25 mg) qid. Do not use longer than 1 wk.

Pediatric: Safety and efficacy not established.
Geriatric: Use the lower recommended dosage range for patients < 110 lb, older than 65 y, or with reduced renal function.

Pharmacokinetics

Route	Onset	Peak	Duration
Oral	Varies	½–1 h	6 h
IM	10 min	30–60 min	6 h

Metabolism: Hepatic; $T_{1/2}$: 2.4–8.6 h
Distribution: Crosses placenta; enters breast milk
Excretion: Urine

Adverse effects
NSAIDs:
- CNS: *Headache, dizziness, somnolence, insomnia,* fatigue, tiredness, dizziness, tinnitus, ophthamological effects

---
Adverse effects in *Italics* are most common; those in **Bold** are life-threatening.

- **GI:** *Nausea, dyspepsia, GI pain,* diarrhea, vomiting, *constipation,* flatulence
- **Respiratory:** Dyspnea, hemoptysis, pharyngitis, bronchospasm, rhinitis
- **Hematologic:** Bleeding, platelet inhibition with higher doses, neutropenia, eosinophilia, leukopenia, pancytopenia, thrombocytopenia, agranulocytosis, granulocytopenia, aplastic anemia, decreased hemoglobin or hematocrit, bone marrow depression, menorrhagia
- **GU:** Dysuria, **renal impairment**
- **Dermatologic:** *Rash,* pruritus, sweating, dry mucous membranes, stomatitis
- **Other:** Peripheral edema, **anaphylactoid reactions to fatal anaphylactic shock**, *local burning, stinging* (ophthalmic)

■ Nursing Considerations

Assessment
- *History:* Renal impairment; impaired hearing; allergies; hepatic, cardiovascular, and GI conditions; lactation
- *Physical:* Skin—color and lesions; orientation, reflexes, ophthalmologic and audiometric evaluation, peripheral sensation; P, edema; R, adventitious sounds; liver evaluation; CBC, clotting times, renal and liver function tests; serum electrolytes, stool guaiac

Implementation
- Maintain emergency equipment on standby at time of initial dose, in case of severe hypersensitivity reaction.
- Protect drug vials from light.
- Administer every 6 h to maintain serum levels and control pain.

Drug-specific teaching points
- Know that every effort will be made to administer the drug on time to control pain; dizziness, drowsiness can occur (avoid driving or the use of dangerous machinery while on this drug); burning and stinging on application (ophthalmic).
- Report sore throat, fever, rash, itching, weight gain, swelling in ankles or fingers; changes in vision; black, tarry stools.

☐ labetalol hydrochloride

*(la **bet**' a lol)*
Normodyne, Trandate

Pregnancy Category C

Drug classes
Alpha-/beta-adrenergic blocking agent (α_1-blocker, nonselective beta-blocker)
Antihypertensive drug

Therapeutic actions
Competetively blocks α_1 and β_1- and β_2-adrenergic receptors, and has some sympathomimetic activity at β_2-receptors. Alpha- and beta-blocking actions contribute to the blood pressure-lowering effect; beta blockade prevents the reflex tachycardia seen with most alpha-blocking drugs and decreases plasma renin activity.

Indications
- Hypertension, alone or with other oral drugs, especially diuretics
- Severe hypertension (parenteral preparations)

Contraindications/cautions
- Contraindicated in the presence of sinus bradycardia, second- or third-degree heart block, cardiogenic shock, CHF, asthma, pregnancy, lactation.
- Use caution in the presence of diabetes or hypoglycemia (can mask usual cardiac signs of hypoglycemia), nonallergic bronchospasm (use only oral drug—IV drug is absolutely contraindicated), pheochromocytoma (paradoxical increases in BP have occurred).

Dosage
Adult
- **Oral:** Initial dose 100 mg bid. After 2–3 d, using standing BP as indicator, titrate dosage in increments of 100 mg bid q2–3 d. *Maintenance:* 200 to 400 mg bid. Up to 2,400 mg/d may be required; to

Adverse effects in *Italics* are most common; those in **Bold** are life-threatening.

labetalol hydrochloride ■ 621

- improve tolerance, divide total daily dose and give tid.
- ***Parenteral (severe hypertension):*** *Repeated IV injection:* 20 mg (0.25 mg/kg) slowly over 2 min. Individualize dosage using supine BP; additional doses of 40 or 80 mg can be given at 10-min intervals until desired BP is achieved or until a dose of 300 mg has been injected. *Continuous IV infusion:* Dilute ampule as described below and infuse at the rate of 2 mg/min with adjustments made according to BP response up to 300 mg total dose. Transfer to oral therapy as soon as possible.

Pediatric: Safety and efficacy not established.

Pharmacokinetics

Route	Onset	Peak	Duration
Oral	Varies	1–2 h	8–12 h
IV	Immediate	5 min	5.5 h

Metabolism: Hepatic, $T_{1/2}$: 6–8 h
Distribution: Crosses placenta; enters breast milk
Excretion: Urine

IV facts

Preparation: Add 2 mg (2 ampuls) to 160 ml of a compatible IV fluid to make a 1 mg/ml solution; infuse at 2 ml/min, or add 200 mg (2 ampuls) to 250 ml of IV fluid. Compatible IV fluids include Ringer's, Lactated Ringer's, 0.9% Sodium Chloride, 2.5% Dextrose and 0.45% Sodium Chloride, 5% Dextrose, 5% Dextrose and Ringer's, 5% Dextrose and 5% Lactated Ringer's, and 5% Dextrose and 0.2%, 0.33%, or 0.9% Sodium Chloride. Stable for 24 h in these solutions at concentrations between 1.25 and 3.75 mg/ml.
Infusion: Administer at 3 ml/min.
Compatibilities: Do not dilute drug in 5% Sodium Bicarbonate Injection.

Adverse effects

- CNS: *Dizziness, vertigo, tinnitus, fatigue,* emotional depression, paresthesias, sleep disturbances, hallucinations, disorientation, memory loss, slurred speech
- GI: *Gastric pain, flatulence, constipation, diarrhea, nausea, vomiting,* anorexia, ischemic colitis, renal and mesenteric arterial thrombosis, retroperitoneal fibrosis, hepatomegaly, acute pancreatitis
- CV: CHF, cardiac arrhythmias, peripheral vascular insufficiency, claudication, cerebrovascular accident, pulmonary edema, hypotension
- Respiratory: *Bronchospasm, dyspnea, cough,* bronchial obstruction, nasal stuffiness, rhinitis, pharyngitis
- GU: *Impotence, decreased libido,* Peyronie's disease, dysuria, nocturia, polyuria
- EENT: Eye irritation, dry eyes, conjunctivitis, blurred vision
- Dermatologic: Rash, pruritus, sweating, dry skin
- Other: *Decreased exercise tolerance,* development of antinuclear antibodies, hyperglycemia or hypoglycemia, elevated liver enzymes

Clinically important drug-drug interactions

- Risk of excessive hypotension if taken concurrently with enflurane, halothane, or isoflurane

Drug-lab test interferences

- Possible falsely elevated urinary catecholamines in lab tests using a trihydroxyindole reaction

■ Nursing Considerations

Assessment

- *History:* Sinus bradycardia, second- or third-degree heart block, cardiogenic shock, CHF, asthma, pregnancy, lactation, diabetes or hypoglycemia, nonallergic bronchospasm, pheochromocytoma
- *Physical:* Baseline body weight, skin condition, neurologic status, P, BP, ECG, respiratory status, kidney and thyroid function, blood and urine glucose

Adverse effects in *Italics* are most common; those in **Bold** are life-threatening.

Implementation
- Do not discontinue drug abruptly after chronic therapy. (Hypersensitivity to catecholamines may have developed, causing exacerbation of angina, MI and ventricular dysrhythmias; taper drug gradually over 2 wk with monitoring.)
- Consult with physician about withdrawing the drug if the patient is to undergo surgery (withdrawal is controversial).
- Keep patient supine during parenteral therapy, and assist initial ambulation.
- Position patient to decrease effects of edema.
- Provide support and encouragement to deal with drug effects and disease.

Drug-specific teaching points
- Take drug with meals.
- Do not stop taking this drug unless instructed to do so by a health care provider.
- Know that the following side effects may occur: dizziness, lightheadedness, loss of appetite, nightmares, depression, sexual impotence.
- Report difficulty breathing, night cough, swelling of extremities, slow pulse, confusion, depression, rash, fever, sore throat.

☐ lactulose

(lak' tyoo lose)
Laxative: Chronulac, Constilac, Duphalac
Ammonia-reducing agent: Cephulac, Cholac, Enulose
Pregnancy Category C

Drug classes
Laxative
Ammonia-reducing agent

Therapeutic actions
The drug passes unchanged into the colon where bacteria break it down to organic acids that increase the osmotic pressure in the colon and slightly acidify the colonic contents, resulting in an increase in stool water content, stool softening, laxative action, and migration of blood ammonia into the colon contents with subsequent trapping and expulsion in the feces.

Indications
- Treatment of constipation
- Prevention and treatment of portal-systemic encephalopathy

Contraindications/cautions
- Contraindicated in the presence of allergy to lactulose and with a low-galactose diet.
- Use caution in the presence of diabetes and lactation.

Dosage
Adult
- ***Laxative:*** 15–30 ml/d PO; may be increased to 60 ml/d as needed.
- ***Portal-systemic encephalopathy***
  – *Oral:* 30–45 ml tid or qid. Adjust dosage every day or two to produce 2–3 soft stools/day. 30–45 ml/h may be used if necessary. Return to standard dose as soon as possible.
  – *Rectal:* 300 ml lactulose mixed with 700 ml water or physiologic saline as a retention enema, retained for 30–60 min. May be repeated q4–6h. Start oral drug as soon as feasible and before stopping enemas.

Pediatric
- ***Laxative:*** Safety and efficacy not established.
- ***Portal-systemic encephalopathy***
  – *Oral:* Standards not clearly established. Initial dose of 2.5–10 ml/d in divided dose for small children or 40–90 ml/d for older children is suggested. Attempt to produce 2–3 soft stools daily.

Pharmacokinetics

Route	Onset	Peak	Duration
Oral	Varies	20 h	24–48 h

Very minimally absorbed systemically

Adverse effects
- GI: *Transient flatulence, distension, intestinal cramps, belching,* diarrhea, nausea
- Hematologic: Acid–base imbalances

lamotrigine ■ 623

Nursing Considerations

Assessment
- *History:* Allergy to lactulose, low-galactose diet, diabetes, lactation
- *Physical:* Abdominal exam, bowel sounds, serum electrolytes, serum ammonia levels

Implementation
- Do not freeze laxative form. Extremely dark or cloudy syrup may be unsafe; do not use.
- Administer laxative syrup orally with fruit juice, water, or milk to increase palatability.
- Administer retention enema using a rectal balloon catheter. Do not use cleansing enemas containing soap suds or other alkaline agents that counteract the effects of lactulose.
- Do not administer other laxatives while using lactulose.
- Monitor serum ammonia levels as appropriate.
- Monitor patients on long-term therapy for potential electrolyte and acid–base imbalances.

Drug-specific teaching points
- Do not use other laxatives while taking this drug. The drug may be mixed in water, juice, or milk to make it more tolerable.
- Know that the following side effects may occur: abdominal fullness, flatulence, belching.
- Assure ready access to bathroom facilities; bowel movements will be increased to 2–3 per day.
- Report diarrhea, severe belching, abdominal fullness.

▢ lamotrigine

(la mo' tri geen)
Lamictal

Pregnancy Category C

Drug classes
Antiepileptic

Therapeutic actions
Mechanism of action not understood; may inhibit voltage-sensitive sodium channels, stabilizing the neuronal membrane and modulating calcium-dependent presynaptic release of excitatory amino acids.

Indications
- Adjuvant therapy in the treatment of partial seizures in adults with epilepsy

Contraindications/cautions
- Contraindicated in lactation.
- Use caution in the presence of impaired hepatic, renal or cardiac function.

Dosage
Adult
- ***Patients taking enzyme inducing antiepileptic drugs:*** 50 mg PO qd for 2 wk; then 100 mg PO qd in 2 divided doses for 2 wks; may increase by 100 mg/d every wk up to a maintenance dose of 300–500 mg/d in 2 divided doses. *If valproic acid is also being taken*: 25 mg PO every other d for 2 wk; then 25 mg PO qd for 2 wk, then may increase by 25–50 mg every 1-2 wk up to a maintenance dose of 100-150 mg/d PO in 2 divided doses.

Pediatric: Not recommended in children <16 yr.

Pharmacokinetics

Route	Onset	Peak
Oral	Rapid	2–5 h

Metabolism: Hepatic metabolism; $T_{1/2}$: 29 h
Distribution: Crosses placenta; may pass into breast milk
Excretion: Urine

Adverse effects
- CNS: *dizziness*, insomnia, headache, somnolence, *ataxia*, diplopia, blurred vision
- GI:*nausea*, vomiting
- Dermatologic: *rash*

Clinically important drug-drug interactions
- Rapid elimination of lamotrigine if taken with enzyme-inducing antipiletic agents:

Adverse effects in *Italics* are most common; those in **Bold** are life-threatening.

carbamazepine, phenytoin, phenobarbital, primidone • Decreased clearance of lamotrigine, requiring a lower dose, if taken with valproic acid

■ Nursing Considerations

Assessment
- *History*: Lactation; impaired hepatic, renal or cardiac function
- *Physical:* Body weight; body temperature; skin— color, lesions; orientation, affect, reflexes; P, BP, perfusion; bowel sounds, normal output; liver and renal function tests

Implementation
- Monitor renal and hepatic function before and periodically during therapy; abnormal findings are an indication to reevaluate therapy.
- Monitor drug doses carefully when starting therapy and with each increase in dose; special care will need to be taken when changing the dose or frequency of any other antiepiletic.
- Taper drug slowly over a 2 wk period when discontinuing.

Drug specific teaching points
- Take this drug exactly as prescribed.
- Do not discontinue this drug abruptly or change dosage, except on the advice of your physician.
- Know that the following side effects may occur: dizziness, drowsiness (avoid driving a car or performing other tasks requiring alertness or visual acuity if this occurs); GI upset (taking the drug with food or milk and eating frequent small meals may help); headache (medication can be ordered).
- You should wear a medical alert tag at all times so that any emergency medical personnel taking care of you will know that you are an epileptic taking antiepileptic medication.
- Report yellowing of skin, abdominal pain, changes in color of urine or stools, fever, sore throat, mouth sores, unusual bleeding or bruising, skin rash.

▢ leucovorin calcium

(loo koe vor' in)

citrovorum factor, folinic acid
Wellcovorin

Pregnancy Category C

Drug classes
Folic acid derivative

Therapeutic actions
Active reduced form of folic acid; required for nucleoprotein synthesis and maintenance of normal erythropoiesis.

Indications
- "Leucovorin rescue"—after high-dose methotrexate therapy in osteosarcoma
- Treatment of megaloblastic anemias due to sprue, nutritional deficiency, pregnancy, and infancy when oral folic acid therapy is not feasible—parenteral form
- With 5-fluorouracil for palliative treatment of metastatic colorectal cancer

Contraindications/cautions
- Allergy to leucovorin on previous exposure, pernicious anemia or other megaloblastic anemias in which vitamin B_{12} is deficient, lactation

Dosage
Adult
- *Rescue after methotrexate therapy:* Give 12–15 g/m^2 PO or parenterally, followed by 10 mg/m^2 PO q6h for 72 h. If at 24 h following methotrexate administration, the serum creatinine is 50% greater than the pretreatment level, increase the leucovorin dose to 100 mg/m^2 q3h until the serum methotrexate level is $< 5 \times 10^{-8}$ M. For drugs with less affinity for mammalian dihydrofolate reductase, 5 to 15 mg/d has been used.
- *Megaloblastic anemia:* Up to 1 mg/d IM may be used. Do not exceed 1 mg/d.
- *Metastatic colon cancer:* Give 200 mg/m^2 by slow IV injection over 3 min, followed by 5-FU 370 mg/m^2 IV *or* 20 mg/m^2 IV, followed by 5-FU 425 mg/m^2

leuprolide acetate ■ 625

IV. Repeat daily for 5 d; may be repeated at 4-wk intervals.

Pharmacokinetics

Route	Onset	Peak	Duration
Oral	30 min	2.4 h	3–6 h
IM	Rapid	52 min	3–6 h
IV	Immediate	10 min	3–6 h

Metabolism: Hepatic, $T_{1/2}$: unknown
Distribution: Crosses placenta; enters breast milk
Excretion: Urine and feces

IV facts

Preparation: Prepare solution by diluting a 50-mg vial of powder with 5 ml Bacteriostatic Water for Injection, which contains benzyl alcohol, and use within 7 d, or reconstitute with Water for Injection, and use immediately. Protect from light.
Infusion: Infuse slowly over 3–5 min.

Adverse effects

- Hypersensitivity: Allergic reactions
- Local: *Pain and discomfort at injection site*

■ Nursing Considerations

Assessment

- *History:* Allergy to leucovorin on previous exposure, pernicious anemia or other megaloblastic anemias, lactation
- *Physical:* Skin—lesions, color; R, adventitious sounds; CBC, hemoglobin, Hct, serum folate levels

Implementation

- Do not use solutions with benzyl alcohol when administering leucovorin to premature infants; a fatal gasping syndrome has occurred.
- Begin leucovorin rescue within 24 h of methotrexate administration. Arrange for fluid loading and urine alkalinization during this procedure to decrease methotrexate nephrotoxicity.
- Administer drug orally unless patient is unable to tolerate the oral route due to nausea and vomiting associated with chemotherapy or the clinical condition. Switch to oral drug whenever feasible.
- Monitor patient for hypersensitivity reactions, especially if patient has received the drug before. Maintain supportive equipment and emergency drugs on standby in case of serious allergic response.

Drug-specific teaching points

- Know that the action of leucovorin "rescues" normal cells from the effects of chemotherapy and allows them to survive.
- Report rash, difficulty breathing, pain, or discomfort at injection site.

☐ leuprolide acetate

(loo proe' lide)
Lupron, Lupron Depot, Lupron Depot-Ped

Pregnancy Category X

Drug classes

Antineoplastic agent
Hormone

Therapeutic actions

An LH-RH agonist that occupies pituitary gonadotropin-releasing hormone receptors and desensitizes them; inhibits gonadotropin secretion when given continuously.

Indications

- Advanced prostatic cancer—palliative treatment as an alternative to orchiectomy or estrogen therapy
- Endometriosis
- Central precocious puberty
- Unlabeled uses—treatment of breast, ovarian, and endometrial cancer; leiomyoma uteri; infertility; prostatic hypertrophy

Contraindications/cautions

- Allergy to leuprolide, pregnancy

Adverse effects in *Italics* are most common; those in **Bold** are life-threatening.

Dosage
Adult
- **Advanced prostate cancer:** 1 mg/d SC; use only the syringes that come with the drug.
- *Depot:* 7.5 mg IM moly (q28–33 d). Do not use needles smaller than 22 gauge.
- **Central precocious puberty:** 50 μg/kg per d SC; may be titrated up to 10 μg/kg per d. *Depot:* 0.3 mg/kg IM moly every 4 wk.
- **Endometriosis:** 3.75 mg as a single moly IM injection. Continue for 6 mo.

Adverse effects
- CNS: *Dizziness, headache, pain*, paresthesia, blurred vision, lethargy, fatigue, insomnia, memory disorder
- GI: GI bleeding, *nausea, vomiting, anorexia*, sour taste, *constipation*
- CV: *Peripheral edema, cardiac arrhythmias*, thrombophlebitis, CHF, myocardial infarction
- Respiratory: Difficulty breathing, pleural rub, worsening of pulmonary fibrosis
- GU: *Frequency, hematuria*, decrease in size of testes, increased BUN and creatinine
- Dermatologic: Skin rash, hair loss, itching, erythema
- General: *Hot flashes, sweats*, bone pain
- Local: Ecchymosis at injection site

■ Nursing Considerations

Assessment
- *History:* Allergy to leuprolide, pregnancy
- *Physical:* Skin—lesions, color, turgor; testes; injection sites; orientation, affect, reflexes, peripheral sensation; peripheral pulses, edema, P; R, adventitious sounds; serum testosterone and acid phosphatase

Implementation
- Administer only with the syringes provided with the drug.
- Administer SC; monitor injection sites for bruising and rash; rotate injection sites to decrease local reaction.
- Administer depot injection deep into muscle. Prepare a calendar for patient to return each mo (28–33 d) for new injection.
- Refrigerate the vials until dispensed; must be stored below 30°C if unrefrigerated.
- Arrange for periodic serum testosterone and acid phosphatase determinations.
- Teach patient and significant other the proper technique for SC injection, and observe their administration of the drug before home administration.

Drug-specific teaching points
- Administer SC only, using the syringes that come with the drug. If depot route is used, prepare calendar for return dates, stressing the importance of receiving the injection each mo.
- Do not stop taking this drug without first consulting the health care provider.
- Know that the following side effects may occur: bone pain, difficulty urinating (these usually occur only during the first few weeks of treatment); hot flashes (staying in cool temperatures may help); nausea, vomiting (small, frequent meals may help); dizziness, headache, lightheadedness (use caution when driving or performing tasks that require alertness if these occur).
- Report injection site pain, burning, itching, swelling, numbness, tingling, severe GI upset, pronounced hot flashes.

☐ levamisole hydrochloride

(lev am' ib sole)
Ergamisol

Pregnancy Category C

Drug classes
Antineoplastic

Therapeutic actions
Immunomodulator: appears to restore depressed immune function, stimulates formation of antibodies, enhances T cell response, potentiates monocyte and macrophage activity

Adverse effects in *Italics* are most common; those in **Bold** are life-threatening.

Indications
- Adjunctive treatment in combination with fluorouracil after surgical resection in patients with Dukes' stage C colon cancer

Contraindications/cautions
- Allergy to levamisole or any of its components, pregnancy, lactation

Dosage
Adult
- ***Initial therapy:*** 50 mg PO q8h for 3 d starting 7–30 d after surgery with fluorouracil 450 mg/m^2 per day IV for 5 d concomitant with a 3-day course of levamisole starting 21–34 d after surgery.
- ***Maintenance therapy:*** 50 mg PO q8h for 3 d every 2 wk with fluorouracil 450 mg/m^2 per day IV once a wk beginning 28 d after the initiation of the 5-day course.

Pharmacokinetics

Route	Onset	Peak
Oral	Varies	1.5–2 h

Metabolism: Hepatic, $T_{1/2}$: 3–4 h
Distribution: Crosses placenta; may enter breast milk
Excretion: Urine

Adverse effects
- **CNS:** *Taste perversion*, dizziness, headache, paresthesia, somnolence, depression
- **GI:** *Nausea, diarrhea*, stomatitis, anorexia, abdominal pain, constipation
- **Hematologic:** Bone marrow depression
- **Dermatologic:** Dermatitis, alopecia
- **General:** *Fatigue*, fever, rigors, *arthralgia*, myalgia, infection

Clinically important drug-drug interactions
- Disulfiram-like reaction possible if taken concurrently with alcohol • Increased phenytoin levels and possible toxicity if taken with levamisole

■ Nursing Considerations
Assessment
- *History:* Allergy to levamisole, lactation
- *Physical:* Body temperature; skin—lesions, color; R, adventitious sounds; orientation, reflexes; CBC, hemoglobin, Hct, liver function tests, electrolytes

Implementation
- Initiate levamisole therapy no earlier than 7 and no later than 30 d after surgery. Initiate fluorouracil no earlier than 21 d and no later than 35 d after surgery.
- Do not exceed recommended dosage. Monitor CBC before, during, and after therapy. Defer administration of fluorouracil until WBC is > 3,500/mm^3.
- Advise patient to use birth control measures while on this drug; drug causes fetal toxicity.

Drug-specific teaching points
- Avoid crowded areas and exposure to any infection while on this drug.
- Know that the following side effects may occur: nausea, vomiting (small, frequent meals may help); diarrhea; skin rash (appropriate medication may be available to help, avoid exposure to the sun or extremes of temperature if rash occurs).
- Do not become pregnant while on this drug; use of some form of birth control is advised.
- Report fever, chills, muscle aches, extreme vomiting, or diarrhea.

☐ levodopa

*(lee voe **doe'** pa)*
Dopar, Larodopa

Pregnancy Category C

Drug classes
Antiparkinsonism drug

Therapeutic actions
Biochemical precursor of the neurotransmitter dopamine, which is deficient in the basal ganglia of parkinsonism pa-

Adverse effects in *Italics* are most common; those in **Bold** are life-threatening.

tients; unlike dopamine, levodopa penetrates the blood–brain barrier. It is transformed in the brain to dopamine; thus, levodopa is a form of replacement therapy. It is efficacious for 2–5 y in relieving the symptoms of parkinsonism but not drug-induced extrapyramidal disorders.

Indications
- Treatment of parkinsonism (postencephalitic, arteriosclerotic, and idiopathic types) and symptomatic parkinsonism, which may follow injury to the nervous system by carbon monoxide or manganese intoxication
- Given with carbidopa (*Lodosyn;* fixed combinations, Sinemet), an enzyme inhibitor that decreases the activity of dopa decarboxylase in the periphery, thus reducing blood levels of levodopa and decreasing the intensity and incidence of many of the adverse effects of levodopa
- Unlabeled use: relief of herpes zoster (shingles) pain

Contraindications/cautions
- Contraindicated in the presence of hypersensitivity to levodopa; allergy to tartrazine (in preparations marketed as Dopar); glaucoma, especially angle-closure glaucoma; history of melanoma; suspicious or undiagnosed skin lesions; lactation.
- Use caution in the presence of severe cardiovascular or pulmonary disease; occlusive cerebrovascular disease; history of MI with residual arrhythmias; bronchial asthma; renal, hepatic, endocrine disease; history of peptic ulcer; psychiatric patients, especially those who are depressed or psychotic; pregnancy.

Dosage
Adult: Individualize dosage. Increase dosage gradually to minimize side effects; titrate dosage carefully to optimize benefits and minimize side effects. Initially, 0.5–1 g PO daily divided into 2 or more doses given with food. Increase gradually in increments not exceeding 0.75 g/d q3–7 d as tolerated. Do not exceed 8 g/d, except for exceptional patients. A significant therapeutic response may not be obtained for 6 mo.
Pediatric: Safety for use in children < 12 y not established.

Pharmacokinetics

Route	Onset	Peak
Oral	Varies	0.5–2 h

Metabolism: Hepatic metabolism, $T_{1/2}$: 1–3 h
Distribution: Crosses placenta; enters breast milk
Excretion: Urine

Adverse effects
- **CNS:** *Adventitious movements, ataxia, increased hand tremor, headache, dizziness, numbness, weakness and faintness,* bruxism, confusion, insomnia, nightmares, hallucinations and delusions, *agitation and anxiety, malaise, fatigue, euphoria,* mental changes (including paranoid ideation), psychotic episodes, depression with or without suicidal tendencies, dementia, bradykinesia ("on-off" phenomenon), muscle twitching and blepharospasm, diplopia, blurred vision, dilated pupils
- **GI:** *Anorexia, nausea, vomiting, abdominal pain or distress, dry mouth, dysphagia, dysgeusia,* bitter taste, sialorrhea, trismus, burning sensation of the tongue, diarrhea, constipation, flatulence, weight gain or loss, upper GI hemorrhage in patients with history of peptic ulcer
- **CV:** Cardiac irregularities, palpitations, orthostatic hypotension
- **Respiratory:** Bizarre breathing patterns
- **Hematologic:** Leukopenia, decreased hemoglobin and hematocrit, elevated BUN, SGOT, SGPT, LDH, bilirubin, alkaline phosphatase, protein-bound iodine
- **GU:** Urinary retention, urinary incontinence
- **Dermatologic:** Flushing, hot flashes, increased sweating, skin rash

Adverse effects in *Italics* are most common; those in **Bold** are life-threatening.

levomethadyl acetate hydrochloride ■ 629

Clinically important drug-drug interactions
• Increased therapeutic effects and possible hypertensive crisis when levodopa is given with monoamine oxidase inhibitors (MAOIs); withdraw MAOIs at least 14 d before starting levodopa therapy • Decreased efficacy of levodopa given with pyridoxine (vitamin B_6) and phenytoin

Drug-lab test interferences
• May interfere with urine tests for sugar or ketones • False Coombs' test results • False elevations of uric acid when using colorimetric method

■ Nursing Considerations

Assessment
- *History:* Hypersensitivity to levodopa, tartrazine; glaucoma; history of melanoma; suspicious or undiagnosed skin lesions; severe cardiovascular or pulmonary disease; occlusive cerebrovascular disease; history of MI with residual arrhythmias; bronchial asthma; renal, hepatic, endocrine disease; history of peptic ulcer; psychiatric disorders; lactation
- *Physical:* Body weight; body temperature; skin—color, lesions; orientation, affect, reflexes, bilateral grip strength, vision exam; P, BP, orthostatic BP, auscultation; R, depth, adventitious sounds; bowel sounds, normal output, liver evaluation; voiding pattern, normal output, prostate palpation; liver and kidney function tests; CBC with differential

Implementation
- Arrange to decrease dosage if therapy has been interrupted for any reason; observe all patients for the development of suicidal tendencies.
- Give with meals if GI upset occurs.
- Ensure that patient voids just before receiving each dose of drug if urinary retention is a problem.
- Monitor hepatic, renal, hematopoietic, and cardiovascular function periodically during therapy.
- Arrange for patients who feel the need to take a multivitamin preparation to use Larobec, a preparation without pyridoxine.

Drug-specific teaching points
- Take this drug exactly as prescribed.
- Do not take multivitamin preparations containing pyridoxine. These could prevent any therapeutic effect of levodopa. Notify your nurse or physician if you feel the need for a vitamin preparation.
- Know that the following side effects may occur: drowsiness, dizziness, confusion, blurred vision (avoid driving a car or engaging in activities that require alertness and visual acuity if these occur); nausea (taking the drug with meals, eating frequent small meals may help); dry mouth (sucking sugarless lozenges or ice chips may help); painful or difficult urination (emptying the bladder immediately before each dose may help); constipation (if maintaining adequate fluid intake and exercising regularly do not help, consult your nurse or physician); dark sweat or urine (these effects are not harmful and should not worry you); dizziness or faintness when you get up (change position slowly and use caution when climbing stairs).
- Report fainting, lightheadedness, dizziness; uncontrollable movements of the face, eyelids, mouth, tongue, neck, arms, hands, or legs; mental changes; irregular heartbeat or palpitations; difficult urination; severe or persistent nausea or vomiting.

❒ levomethadyl acetate hydrochloride

(lev oh meth' a dil)
ORLAAM

Pregnancy Category B
C-II Controlled Substance

Drug classes
Narcotic agonist analgesic

Therapeutic actions
Acts at specific opioid receptors, causing analgesia, respiratory depression, physical depression, euphoria.

Indications
- Management of opiate dependence

Contraindications/cautions
- Contraindicated in the presence of hypersensitivity to narcotics, diarrhea caused by poisoning, acute bronchial asthma, upper airway obstruction, pregnancy.
- Use caution in the presence of bradycardia, history of seizures, lactation.

Dosage
Must be administered in an opiate withdrawal clinic, which maintains control over drug delivery.

Adult
- ***Usual induction dose:*** 20–40 mg PO, increase in increments of 5–10 mg every 48–72 h as tolerated.
- ***Maintenance:*** 60–90 mg PO 3 times a wk.
- ***Transfer from methadone:*** Higher initial doses of levomethadyl may be needed.
- ***Transfer from levomethadyl to methadone:*** Start methadone at 80% of the usual dose, giving the initial methadone dose no sooner than 48 h after the last levomethadyl dose.

Pediatric: Safety and efficacy not established.

Pharmacokinetics

Route	Onset	Duration
PO	Varies	up to 72 h

Metabolism: Plasma, $T_{1/2}$: 15–40 h
Distribution: Crosses placenta; enters breast milk

Adverse effects
- CNS: *Sedation, clamminess, sweating, headache, vertigo, floating feeling, dizziness, lethary, confusion, lightheadedness,* nervousness, unusual dreams, agitation, euphoria, hallucinations, delirium, insomnia, anxiety, fear, disorientation, impaired mental and physical performance, coma, mood changes, weakness, headache, tremor, convulsions
- GI: *Nausea, vomiting,* dry mouth, anorexia, constipation, biliary tract spasm
- CV: Palpitation, increase or decrease in BP, circulatory depression, **cardiac arrest**, **shock**, arrhythmia, palpitations
- Respiratory: Slow, shallow respiration; apnea; suppression of cough reflex; laryngospasm; bronchospasm
- EENT: Diplopia, blurred vision
- Dermatologic: Rash, hives, pruritus, flushing, warmth, sensitivity to cold
- Other: Physical tolerance and dependence, psychological dependence

Clinically important drug-drug interactions
- Potentiation of effects of levomethadyl when given with barbiturate anesthetics

Drug-lab test interferences
- Elevated biliary tract pressure may cause increases in plasma amylase and lipase; determinations of these levels may be unreliable for 24 h after administration of narcotics.

■ Nursing Considerations

Assessment
- *History:* Hypersensitivity to narcotics, physical dependence on a narcotic analgesic, pregnancy, labor, lactation, bronchial asthma, COPD, respiratory depression, anoxia, increased intracranial pressure, acute MI, ventricular failure, coronary insufficiency, hypertension, biliary tract surgery, and renal or hepatic dysfunction
- *Physical:* Orientation, reflexes, bilateral grip strength, affect; pupil size, vision; P, auscultation, BP; R, adventitious sounds; bowel sounds, normal output; liver and kidney function tests

Implementation
- Administer to women who are lactating 4–6 h before the next scheduled feeding to minimize the amount in milk.
- Provide narcotic antagonist, and have facilities for assisted or controlled respiration on standby during parenteral administration.
- Caution patient that clinic visits must be kept; use of street drugs can cause serious complications and even death while on this drug.

Adverse effects in *Italics* are most common; those in **Bold** are life-threatening.

Drug-specific teaching points
- Return to the clinic for scheduled dosing; skipping doses can cause serious side effects. Use of street drugs while on this drug can cause serious complications.
- Know that the following side effects may occur: dizziness, sedation, drowsiness, impaired visual acuity (ask for assistance if you need to move); nausea, loss of appetite (lying quietly and eating frequent, small meals should minimize these effects); constipation (notify your nurse or physician if this is severe; a laxative may help).
- Report severe nausea, vomiting, palpitations, shortness of breath, or difficulty breathing.

▢ levonorgestrel

(lee' voe nor jess trel)
Norplant System

Pregnancy Category X

Drug classes
Hormonal agent
Progestin
Contraceptive

Therapeutic actions
Synthetic progestational agent. The endogenous female progestin, progesterone, transforms proliferative endometrium into secretory endometrium; inhibits the secretion of pituitary gonadotropins, which prevents follicular maturation and ovulation; and inhibits spontaneous uterine contractions. The primary mechanism by which norgestrel prevents conception is not known, but progestin-only oral contraceptives are known to alter the cervical mucus, exert a progestional effect on the endometrium that interferes with implantation, and in some patients, suppress ovulation.

Indications
- Prevention of pregnancy

Contraindications/cautions
- Contraindicated in the presence of allergy to progestins; thrombophlebitis, thromboembolic disorders, cerebral hemorrhage, or history of these conditions; CAD; hepatic disease, carcinoma of the breast or genital organs, undiagnosed vaginal bleeding, missed abortion; lactation; pregnancy.
- Use caution in the presence of epilepsy, migraine, asthma, and cardiac or renal dysfunction.

Dosage
Adult: Six Silastic capsules, each containing 36 mg of levonorgestrel implanted, for a total dose of 216 mg. All 6 capsules should be inserted during the first 7 d of the onset of menses by a health care professional instructed in the insertion technique. Capsules are effective for 5 y.
Pediatric: Safety and efficacy not established.

Pharmacokinetics

Route	Onset	Peak
Implant	Slow	24 h

Metabolism: Hepatic and cellular, $T_{1/2}$: unknown
Distribution: Crosses placenta; enters breast milk
Excretion: Urine

Adverse effects
- **CNS**: Neuro-ocular lesions, mental depression, migraine, *headache, changes in corneal curvature,* contact lens intolerance
- **GI**: Gallbladder disease, liver tumors, hepatic lesions, *nausea,* vomiting, *abdominal cramps,* bloating, cholestatic jaundice, *change in appetite*
- **CV**: Thrombophlebitis, thrombosis, pulmonary embolism, coronary thrombosis, MI, cerebral thrombosis, Raynaud's disease, arterial thromboembolism, renal artery thrombosis, cerebral hemorrhage, hypertension
- **GU**: *Breakthrough bleeding, spotting, change in menstrual flow, amenorrhea,* changes in cervical erosion and cervical secretions, endocervical hyperplasia, vaginal candidiasis, *vaginitis*

Adverse effects in *Italics* are most common; those in **Bold** are life-threatening.

- **Dermatologic:** Rash with or without pruritus, *dermatitis, hirsutism, hypertrichosis, scalp hair loss, acne,* melasma
- **Local:** Pain or itching at insertion site, removal difficulties, infection at insertion site
- **Other:** *Breast tenderness and secretion, enlargement;* fluid retention; edema; *increase in weight; musculoskeletal pain*

Clinically important drug-drug interactions
- Pregnancy has occurred when users of levonorgestrel took carbamazepine and phenytoin.

Drug-lab test interferences
- Abnormal tests of endocrine function while levonorgestrel is used

■ Nursing Considerations

Assessment
- *History:* Allergy to progestins, thrombophlebitis, thromboembolic disorders, cerebral hemorrhage, CAD, hepatic disease, carcinoma of the breast or genital organs, undiagnosed vaginal bleeding, missed abortion, epilepsy, migraine, asthma, cardiac or renal dysfunction, pregnancy, lactation
- *Physical:* Skin—color, lesions, turgor; hair; breasts; pelvic exam; insertion site; orientation, affect; ophthalmologic exam; P, auscultation, peripheral perfusion, edema; R, adventitious sounds; liver evaluation; liver and renal function tests, glucose tolerance, Pap smear, pregnancy test if appropriate

Implementation
- Arrange for pretreatment and periodic (at least annual) history and physical exam, which should include BP, breasts, abdomen, pelvic organs, and a Pap smear.
- Arrange for insertion of capsules during the first 7 d of the menstrual cycle. Insertion is made in the midportion of the upper arm about 8–10 cm above the elbow crease. Distribution is in a fanlike pattern about 15 degrees apart, for a total area of 75 degrees. Insertion area is closed using a skin closure; cover the area with a dry compress and gauze wrap. Sterile technique should be observed.
- Monitor insertion site for signs of bleeding, infection, and irritation.
- Be aware that capsules are removed using a local anesthetic, aseptic technique, and small incision in the area. Capsules should be removed at the end of 5 y or if the patient desires to become pregnant.

Drug-specific teaching points
- Be aware that the drug must be inserted using a local anesthetic, and six capsules are inserted into the mid-upper arm, just above the elbow crease. The procedure takes 15–20 min and should not be too uncomfortable. The drug is slowly released from the capsules, and the capsules are effective for 5 y. If you decide to become pregnant before that time, the capsules can be removed in a procedure similar to the insertion. If you keep the capsules in place for 5 y, you can then have them replaced.
- Arrange for annual medical exams, including Pap smear, while these capsules are in place. It is important to monitor the effect of this drug on your body.
- Know that the following side effects may occur: sensitivity to light (avoid exposure to the sun, use sunscreen and protective clothing if exposure is necessary); dizziness, sleeplessness, depression (use caution if driving or performing tasks that require alertness if these occur); skin rash, skin color changes, loss of hair; fever; nausea; breakthrough bleeding or spotting (this may occur during the first month of therapy; if it continues into the second month, consult your nurse or physician); intolerance to contact lenses due to corneal changes.
- Do not take this drug during pregnancy—serious fetal abnormalities have been reported. If you think that you have become pregnant, consult physician immediately.

- Report pain or swelling and warmth in the calves, acute chest pain or shortness of breath, sudden severe headache or vomiting, dizziness or fainting, visual disturbances, numbness or tingling in the arm or leg, breakthrough bleeding or spotting, pain or irritation at insertion site.

☐ levorphanol sulfate

(lee vor' fa nole)
Levo-Dromoran

Pregnancy Category C
C-II controlled substance

Drug classes
Narcotic agonist analgesic

Therapeutic actions
Acts as agonist at specific opioid receptors in the CNS to produce analgesia, euphoria, sedation; the receptors are thought to be the same as those mediating the effects of endogenous opioids (enkephalins, endorphins).

Indications
- Relief of moderate to severe acute and chronic pain
- Preoperative medication to allay apprehension, provide prolonged analgesia, reduce thiopental requirements, and shorten recovery time

Contraindications/cautions
- Contraindicated in the presence of hypersensitivity to narcotics, diarrhea caused by poisoning (before toxins are eliminated), pregnancy (neonatal withdrawal has occurred in infants born to mothers who used narcotics during pregnancy), labor or delivery (administration of narcotics to the mother can cause respiratory depression of neonate—premature infants are especially at risk; may prolong labor), bronchial asthma, acute alcoholism, increased intracranial pressure, respiratory depression, anoxia.
- Use caution in the presence of COPD, cor pulmonale, acute abdominal conditions, cardiovascular disease, supraventricular tachycardias, myxedema, convulsive disorders, delirium tremens, cerebral arteriosclerosis, ulcerative colitis, fever, kyphoscoliosis, Addison's disease, prostatic hypertrophy, urethral stricture, recent GI or GU surgery, toxic psychosis, and renal or hepatic dysfunction.

Dosage
Adult: Average dose is 2 mg PO or SC. Increase to 3 mg if necessary. Has been given by slow IV injection.
Geriatric or impaired adult: Use caution—respiratory depression may occur in the elderly, the very ill, and those with respiratory problems. Reduced dosage may be necessary.

Pharmacokinetics

Route	Onset	Peak	Duration
Oral/SC	30–90 min	0.5–1 h	6–8 h

Metabolism: Hepatic, $T_{1/2}$: 12–16 h
Distribution: Crosses placenta; enters breast milk
Excretion: Urine

Adverse effects
- **CNS**: *Lightheadedness, dizziness, sedation,* euphoria, dysphoria, delirium, insomnia, agitation, anxiety, fear, hallucinations, disorientation, drowsiness, lethargy, impaired mental and physical performance, coma, mood changes, weakness, headache, tremor, convulsions, miosis, visual disturbances, suppression of cough reflex
- **GI**: *Nausea, vomiting,* dry mouth, anorexia, constipation, biliary tract spasm, increased colonic motility in patients with chronic ulcerative colitis
- **CV**: Facial flushing, peripheral circulatory collapse, tachycardia, bradycardia, arrhythmia, palpitations, chest wall rigidity, hypertension, hypotension, orthostatic hypotension, syncope

Adverse effects in *Italics* are most common; those in **Bold** are life-threatening.

634 ■ levothyroxine sodium

- GU: Ureteral spasm, spasm of vesicle sphincters, urinary retention or hesitancy, oliguria, antidiuretic effect, reduced libido or potency
- Dermatologic: Pruritus, urticaria, laryngospasm, bronchospasm, edema, hemorrhagic urticaria (rare)
- Local: Tissue irritation and induration (SC injection)
- Major hazards: Respiratory depression, apnea, circulatory depression, respiratory arrest, shock, cardiac arrest
- Other: *Sweating* (more common in ambulatory patients and those without severe pain), physical tolerance and dependence, psychological dependence

Clinically important drug-drug interactions
- Potentiation of effects of levorphanol when given with barbiturate anesthetics; decrease dose of levorphanol when coadministering.

Drug-lab test interferences
- Elevated biliary tract pressure may cause increases in plasma amylase and lipase; determinations of these levels may be unreliable for 24 h after administration of narcotics.

■ Nursing Considerations

Assessment
- *History:* Hypersensitivity to narcotics, diarrhea caused by poisoning, labor or delivery, bronchial asthma, acute alcoholism, increased intracranial pressure, respiratory depression, cor pulmonale, acute abdominal conditions, cardiovascular disease, myxedema, convulsive disorders, delirium tremens, cerebral arteriosclerosis, ulcerative colitis, fever, kyphoscoliosis, Addison's disease, prostatic hypertrophy, urethral stricture, recent GI or GU surgery, toxic psychosis, renal or hepatic dysfunction
- *Physical:* Body temperature; skin—color, texture, lesions; orientation, reflexes, pupil size, bilateral grip strength, affect; P, auscultation, BP, orthostatic BP, perfusion; respiratory rate, adventious sounds; bowel sounds, normal output; frequency and pattern of voiding, normal output; ECG; EEG; thyroid, liver, kidney function tests

Implementation
- Administer to women who are lactating 4–6 h before the next scheduled feeding to minimize the amount in milk.
- Provide narcotic antagonist and have facilities for assisted or controlled respiration on standby during parenteral administration.
- Use caution when injecting SC into chilled areas or in patients with hypotension or in shock; impaired perfusion may delay absorption. With repeated doses, an excessive amount may be absorbed when circulation is restored.
- Reassure patient about addiction liability; most patients who receive opiates for medical reasons do not develop dependence syndromes.

Drug-specific teaching points
- Take drug exactly as prescribed.
- Know that the following side effects may occur: nausea, loss of appetite (taking the drug with food and lying quietly and eating frequent, small meals should minimize these effects); constipation (a laxative may help); dizziness, sedation, drowsiness, impaired visual acuity (avoid driving a car, performing other tasks that require alertness, visual acuity).
- Do not take any leftover medication for other disorders, and do not let anyone else take your prescription.
- Report severe nausea, vomiting, constipation, shortness of breath, or difficulty breathing.

☐ levothyroxine sodium

*(lee voe thye **rox'** een)*

L-thyroxine, T_4

Eltroxin (CAN), Levothroid, Synthroid

Pregnancy Category A

Adverse effects in *Italics* are most common; those in **Bold** are life-threatening.

levothyroxine sodium

Drug classes
Thyroid hormone

Therapeutic actions
Increases the metabolic rate of body tissues, thereby increasing oxygen consumption; R and heart rate; rate of fat, protein, and carbohydrate metabolism; and growth and maturation.

Indications
- Replacement therapy in hypothyroidism
- Pituitary TSH suppression in the treatment and prevention of euthyroid goiters and in the management of thyroid cancer
- Thyrotoxicosis in conjunction with antithyroid drugs and to prevent goitrogenesis, hypothyroidism, and thyrotoxicosis during pregnancy
- Treatment of myxedema coma

Contraindications/cautions
- Contraindicated in the presence of allergy to active or extraneous constituents of drug, thyrotoxicosis, and acute MI uncomplicated by hypothyroidism.
- Use caution in the presence of Addison's disease (treatment of hypoadrenalism with corticosteroids should precede thyroid therapy) and lactation.

Dosage
0.1 mg equals approximately 65 mg (1 grain) thyroid.

Adult
- **Hypothyroidism:** Initial dose: 0.05 mg PO, with increasing increments of 0.025 mg PO q2–3 wk; maintenance of 0.2 mg/d IV or IM injection can be substituted for the oral dosage form when oral ingestion is not possible.
- **Myxedema coma without severe heart disease:** 0.4 mg IV as initial dose, then 0.1 to 0.2 mg IV as a solution containing 0.1 mg/ml; daily maintenance of 0.05 to 0.1 mg.
- **TSH suppression in thyroid cancer, nodules, and euthyroid goiters:** Larger amounts than used for normal suppression.
- **Thyroid suppression therapy:** 2.6 μg/kg per d PO for 7–10 d.

Pediatric
- **Cretinism:** Infants require replacement therapy from birth. Starting dose is 0.025 to 0.05 mg/d PO with 0.05–0.1-mg increments at weekly intervals until the child is euthyroid. Usual maintenance dose may be as high as 0.3–0.4 mg/d PO.

Pharmacokinetics

Route	Onset	Peak
Oral	Slow	1–3 wk
IV	6–8 h	24–48 h

Metabolism: Hepatic, $T_{1/2}$: 6–7 d
Distribution: Crosses placenta; enters breast milk
Excretion: Bile

IV facts
Preparation: Add 5 ml 0.9% Sodium Chloride Injection, USP or Bacteriostatic Sodium Chloride Injection, USP with benzyl alcohol. Shake the vial to assure complete mixing. Use immediately after reconstitution. Discard any unused portion.
Infusion: Inject directly and rapidly.
Incompatabilities: Do not mix with any other IV fluids.

Adverse effects
- Endocrine: Symptoms of hyperthyroidism
- Dermatologic: Allergic skin reactions, partial loss of hair in first few months of therapy in children

Clinically important drug-drug interactions
- Decreased absorption of oral thyroid preparation if taken concurrently with cholestyramine • Increased risk of bleeding if taken with warfarin, dicumarol, anisindione—reduce dosage of anticoagulant when T_4 is begun • Decreased effectiveness of digitalis glycosides if taken with thyroid replacement • Decreased theophylline clearance when patient is in hypothyroid state; monitor levels and patient response as euthyroid state is achieved

Adverse effects in *italics* are most common; those in **Bold** are life-threatening.

lidocaine hydrochloride

■ Nursing Considerations

Assessment
- *History:* Allergy to active or extraneous constituents of drug, thyrotoxicosis, acute MI uncomplicated by hypothyroidism, Addison's disease, lactation
- *Physical:* Skin—lesions, color, temperature, texture; body temperature; muscle tone, orientation, reflexes; P, auscultation, baseline ECG, BP; R, adventitious sounds; thyroid function tests

Implementation
- Monitor patient response carefully when beginning therapy, and adjust dosage accordingly.
- Do not change brands of T_4 products—bioequivalence problems have been documented.
- Do not add IV doses to other IV fluids; full therapeutic effect may not be seen until the second day; use caution in patients with cardiovascular disease.
- Administer oral drug as a single daily dose before breakfast.
- Arrange for regular, periodic blood tests of thyroid function.
- Monitor cardiac response throughout therapy.

Drug-specific teaching points
- Take as a single dose before breakfast.
- Be aware that this drug replaces an important hormone and will need to be taken for life. Do not discontinue this drug for any reason without consulting your nurse or physician; serious problems can occur.
- Consider wearing or carrying a medical alert tag to alert medical personnel who may take care of you in an emergency that you are on this drug.
- Arrange to have periodic blood tests and medical evaluations while you are on this drug. It is important to keep your scheduled appointments.
- Report headache, chest pain, palpitations, fever, weight loss, sleeplessness, nervousness, irritability, unusual sweating, intolerance to heat, diarrhea.

▢ lidocaine hydrochloride

(lye' doe kane)

lidocaine HCl in 5% dextrose, lidocaine HCl without preservatives

Antiarrhythmic Preparations: Xylocaine HCl IV for Cardiac Arrhythmias, LidoPen Auto-Injector, Xylocaine HCl IM for Cardiac Arrhythmias

Local Anesthetic Preparations: Baylocaine, Dalcaine, Dilocaine, Duo-Trach Kit, L-Caine, Lidoject, Nervocaine, Xylocaine HCL (injectable)

Topical for Mucous Membranes: Anestacon, Baylocaine, L-Caine, Xylocaine

Topical Dermatologic: Xylocaine

Pregnancy Category B

Drug classes
Antiarrhythmic
Local anesthetic

Therapeutic actions
Type 1 antiarrhythmic: decreases diastolic depolarization, decreasing automaticity of ventricular cells; increases ventricular fibrillation threshold.

Local anesthetic: blocks the generation and conduction of action potentials in sensory nerves by reducing sodium permeability, reducing height and rate of rise of the action potential, increasing excitation threshold, and slowing conduction velocity.

Indications
- As antiarrhythmic: Management of acute ventricular arrhythmias during cardiac surgery and MI (IV use). Use IM when IV administration is not possible or when ECG monitoring is not available and the danger of ventricular arrhythmias is

great (single-dose IM use, for example, by paramedics in a mobile coronary care unit).
- As anesthetic: Infiltration anesthesia, peripheral and sympathetic nerve blocks, central nerve blocks, spinal and caudal anesthesia, retrobulbar and transtracheal injection; topical anesthetic for skin disorders and accessible mucous membranes

Contraindications/cautions
- Contraindicated in the presence of allergy to lidocaine or amide-type local anesthetics, CHF, cardiogenic shock, second- or third-degree heart block (if no artificial pacemaker), Wolff-Parkinson-White syndrome, Stokes-Adams syndrome.
- Use caution in the presence of hepatic or renal disease, inflammation or sepsis in the region of injection (local anesthetic), labor and delivery (epidural anesthesia may prolong the second stage of labor; monitor for fetal and neonatal CVS and CNS toxicity), and lactation.

Dosage
Adult
- ***IM:*** Use only the 10% solution for IM injection. 300 mg in deltoid or thigh muscle. Switch to IV lidocaine or oral antiarrhythmic as soon as possible.
- ***IV bolus:*** Use only lidocaine injection labeled for IV use and without preservatives or catecholamines. Give 50 to 100 mg at rate of 20–50 mg/min. One-third to one-half the initial dose may be given after 5 min if needed. *Do not exceed 200–300 mg in 1 h.*
- ***IV continuous infusion:*** Give 1–4 mg/min. Titrate the dose down as soon as the cardiac rhythm stabilizes.

Pediatric: Safety and efficacy have not been established. American Heart Association recommends bolus of 1 mg/kg IV, followed by 30 μg/kg per min with caution. The IM auto-injector device is not recommended.

As local anesthetic: Preparations containing preservatives should not be used for spinal or epidural anesthesia. Drug concentration and diluent should be appropriate to particular local anesthetic use: 5% solution with glucose is used for spinal anesthesia, 1.5% solution with dextrose for low spinal or "saddle block" anesthesia. Dosage varies with the area to be anesthetized and the reason for the anesthesia; use the lowest dose possible to achieve results. Caution: Use lower concentrations in debilitated, elderly, and pediatric patients.

Pharmacokinetics

Route	Onset	Peak	Duration
IM	5–10 min	5–15 min	2 h
IV	Immediate	Immediate	10–20 min
Topical	Minimally absorbed systemically		

Metabolism: Hepatic, $T_{1/2}$: 10 min, then 1.5 to 3 h
Distribution: Crosses placenta; enters breast milk
Excretion: Urine

IV facts
Preparation: Prepare solution for IV infusion as follows: 1–2 g lidocaine to 1 L 5% Dextrose in Water = 0.1%–0.2% solution; 1–2 mg lidocaine/ml. Stable for 24 h after dilution.

Infusion: An infusion rate of 1–4 ml/min will provide 1–4 mg lidocaine/min. Use only preparations of lidocaine specifically labeled for IV infusion.

Adverse effects
Lidocaine as Antiarrhythmic—Systemic Administration
- CNS: *Dizziness/lightheadedness, fatigue, drowsiness*, unconsciousness, tremors, twitching, vision changes, may progress to seizures, convulsions
- GI: *Nausea*, vomiting
- CV: *Cardiac arrhythmias,* **cardiac arrest,** vasodilation, *hypotension*
- Respiratory: **Respiratory depression and arrest**
- Hypersensitivity: Rash, anaphylactoid reactions
- Other: **Malignant hyperthermia**

Adverse effects in *Italics* are most common; those in **Bold** are life-threatening.

Lidocaine as Injectable Local Anesthetic for Epidural or Caudal Anesthesia

- CNS: *Headache, backache*, septic meningitis, persistent sensory, motor, or autonomic deficit of lower spinal segments, sometimes with incomplete recovery
- CV: *Hypotension* due to sympathetic block
- GU: *Urinary retention, urinary or fecal incontinence*

Lidocaine as Topical Local Anesthetic

- Dermatologic: Contact dermatitis, urticaria, cutaneous lesions
- Hypersensitivity: Anaphylactoid reactions
- Local: *Burning, stinging, tenderness, swelling, tissue irritation*, tissue sloughing and necrosis
- Other: Methemoglobinemia, seizures

Clinically important drug-drug interactions

- Increased lidocaine levels if given with beta-blockers (propranolol, metoprolol, nadolol, pindolol, atenolol), cimetidine, ranitidine • Prolonged apnea when given with succinlycholine

Drug-lab test interferences

- Increased CPK if given IM

■ Nursing Considerations

Assessment

- *History:* Allergy to lidocaine or amide-type local anesthetics, CHF, cardiogenic shock, second- or third-degree heart block, Wolff-Parkinson-White syndrome, Stokes-Adams syndrome, hepatic or renal disease, inflammation or sepsis in region of injection, lactation
- *Physical:* Temperature; skin—color, rashes, lesions; orientation, speech, reflexes, sensation and movement (local anesthetic); P, BP, auscultation, continuous ECG monitoring during use as antiarrhythmic, edema; R, adventitious sounds; bowel sounds, liver evaluation; urine output; serum electrolytes, liver and renal function tests

Implementation

- Check drug concentration carefully; many different concentrations are available.
- Arrange for reduced dosage in patients with hepatic or renal failure.
- Continuously monitor patient response when used as antiarrhythmic or injected as local anesthetic.
- Maintain life-support equipment, and have vasopressors on standby in case severe adverse reaction (CNS, CVS, or respiratory) occurs when lidocaine is injected.
- Establish safety precautions if CNS changes occur; have IV diazepam or short-acting barbiturate (thiopental, thiamylal) on standby in case convulsions occur.
- Monitor for malignant hyperthermia (jaw muscle spasm, rigidity); have life-support equipment and IV dantrolene on standby.
- Titrate dose to minimum needed for cardiac stability, when using lidocaine as antiarrhythmic, .
- Arrange for reduced dosage when treating arrhythmias in CHF, digitalis toxicity with AV block, and geriatric patients.
- Monitor fluid load carefully; more concentrated solutions can be used to treat arrhythmias in patients on fluid restrictions.
- Have patients who have received lidocaine as a spinal anesthetic remain lying flat for 6–12 h afterward, and ensure that they are adequately hydrated to minimize risk of headache.
- Check lidocaine preparation carefully; epinephrine is added to solutions of lidocaine to retard the absorption of the local anesthetic from the injection site. Be sure that such solutions are used *only* to produce local anesthesia. These solutions should be injected cautiously in body areas supplied by end arteries and used cautiously in patients with peripheral vascular disease, hypertension, thyrotoxicosis, or diabetes.

Adverse effects in *Italics* are most common; those in **Bold** are life-threatening.

lincomycin hydrochloride ■ 639

- Use caution to prevent choking. Patient may have difficulty swallowing following use of oral topical anesthetic. Do not give patient food or drink for 1 h after use of oral anesthetic.
- Treat methemoglobinemia with 1% methylene blue, 0.1 mg/kg, IV over 10 min.
- Apply lidocaine ointments or creams to a gauze or bandage before applying to the skin.
- Monitor for safe and effective serum drug concentrations (antiarrhythmic use; 1–5 μg/ml).

Drug-specific teaching points
- Be aware that drug dosage is changed frequently in response to cardiac rhythm on monitor.
- Know that the following side effects may occur: drowsiness, dizziness, numbness, double vision; nausea, vomiting; stinging, burning, local irritation (local anesthetic).
- Be aware that oral lidocaine can cause numbness of the tongue, cheeks, and throat. Do not eat or drink for 1 h after using oral lidocaine to prevent biting cheeks or tongue and choking.
- Report difficulty speaking, "thick" tongue, numbness, tingling, difficulty breathing, pain or numbness at IV site, swelling, or pain at site of local anesthetic use.

☐ lincomycin hydrochloride

(lin koe mye' sin)
Lincocin, Lincorex

Pregnancy Category B

Drug classes
Lincosamide antibiotic

Therapeutic actions
Inhibits protein synthesis in susceptible bacteria, causing cell death.

Indications
- Treatment of some staphylococcal, streptococcal, and pneumococcal infections resistant to other antibiotics in penicillin-allergic patients or when penicillin is inappropriate. Less toxic antibiotics (erythromycin) should be considered.

Contraindications/cautions
- Contraindicated in the presence of allergy to lincomycin, history of asthma or other allergies, and lactation.
- Use caution in the presence of hepatic or renal dysfunction.

Dosage
Adult
- **Oral:** 500 mg q6–8h, depending on severity of infection.
- **IM:** 600 mg q12–24h, depending on severity of infection.
- **IV:** 600 mg–1 g q8–12h, up to 8 g/d in severe infections.

Pediatric (> 1 mo)
- **Oral:** 30–60 mg/kg per d in 3–4 equally divided doses.
- **IM:** 10 mg/kg q12–24h, depending on severity of infection.
- **IV:** 10–20 mg/kg per d in divided doses, depending on severity of infection.

Newborns: Not indicated for use in newborns.

Geriatric or renal failure patients: Reduce dose to 25% to 30% of that normally recommended.

Pharmacokinetics

Route	Onset	Peak	Duration
Oral	Varies	2–4 h	6–8 h
IM	20–30 min	0.5 h	24 h
IV	Immediate	Immediate	14 h

Metabolism: Hepatic, $T_{1/2}$: 5 h
Distribution: Crosses placenta; enters breast milk
Excretion: Urine and feces

IV facts
Preparation: Dilute to a concentration of 1 g/100 ml. Severe cardiopulmonary reactions have occurred when given at greater than recommended concentrations and rate. IV administration in 250–500 ml of 5% Dextrose in Water or Normal Saline produces no local irritation or phlebitis. Use with 5% Dextrose in Water or in Saline.

Infusion: *Do not* inject as a bolus, infuse over 10–60 min.
Incompatibilities: Lincomycin is *not* compatible in solution with novobiocin, kanamycin, or phenytoin sodium.

Adverse effects
- CNS: Tinnitus, vertigo
- GI: Severe colitis, including **pseudomembranous colitis** (fatal in some instances), *nausea, vomiting, diarrhea, stomatitis, glossitis, pruritus ani,* jaundice, liver function changes
- Hematologic: *Neutropenia,* leukopenia, agranulocytosis, thrombocytopenia, aplastic anemia
- GU: Vaginitis, kidney function changes
- Dermatologic: Skin rashes, urticaria to anaphylactoid reactions, angioneurotic edema
- Local: *Pain following injection*
- Other: Serum sickness

Clinically important drug-drug interactions
- Increased neuromuscular blockade if taken with neuromuscular blocking agents
- Decreased GI absorption if taken with kaolin, aluminum salts, magaldrate

■ Nursing Considerations

Assessment
- *History:* Allergy to lincomycin, history of asthma or other allergies, hepatic or renal dysfunction, lactation
- *Physical:* Site of infection, skin color, lesions; orientation, reflexes, auditory function; BP; R, adventitious sounds; bowel sounds, output, liver evaluation; CBC, renal and liver function tests

Implementation
- Administer oral drug on an empty stomach, 1 h before or 2–3 h after meals. Give with a full glass of water.
- Culture site of infection before beginning therapy.
- Do not use for minor bacterial or viral infections.
- Monitor renal function tests with prolonged therapy.
- Arrange for vancomycin and corticosteroids to be available for serious colitis.

Drug-specific teaching points
- Take drug on an empty stomach, 1 h before or 2–3 h after meals. Take the drug with a full glass of water.
- Take the full prescribed course of this drug. Do not stop taking this drug without notifying your nurse or physician.
- Know that the following side effects may occur: nausea, vomiting (small frequent meals may help); superinfections in the mouth, vagina (frequent hygiene measures will help, ask your health care provider for appropriate treatment if it becomes severe); rash, flulike sickness (report this if it becomes severe).
- Report severe or watery diarrhea, inflamed mouth or vagina, skin rash or lesions.

☐ liothyronine sodium

(lye' oh thye' roe neen)

T_3, triiodithyronine
Cytomel, Triostat

Pregnancy Category A

Drug classes
Thyroid hormone

Therapeutic actions
Increases the metabolic rate of body tissues, thereby increasing oxygen consumption; respiratory and heart rate; rate of fat, protein, and carbohydrate metabolism; and growth and maturation.

Indications
- Replacement therapy in hypothyroidism
- Pituitary TSH suppression in the treatment and prevention of euthyroid goiters and in the management of thyroid cancer
- Thyrotoxicosis in conjunction with antithyroid drugs and to prevent goitrogenesis, hypothyroidism, and thyrotoxicosis during pregnancy

Adverse effects in *Italics* are most common; those in **Bold** are life-threatening.

liothyronine sodium

- Synthetic hormone that can be used in patients who are allergic to desiccated thyroid or thyroid extract derived from pork or beef
- Diagnostic use: T_3 suppression test to differentiate suspected hyperthyroidism from euthyroidism
- Orphan drug use—treatment of myxedema coma and precoma

Contraindications/cautions
- Contraindicated in the presence of allergy to active or extraneous constituents of drug, thyrotoxicosis, and acute MI uncomplicated by hypothyroidism.
- Use caution in the presence of Addison's disease (treatment of hypoadrenalism with corticosteroids should precede thyroid therapy) and lactation.

Dosage
Drug is given only PO. 25 µg equals approximately 65 mg (1 grain) thyroid.
Adult
- *Hypothyroidism:* Initial dosage: 25 µg/d PO. May be increased every 1–2 wk in 12.5- to 25-µg increments. Maintenance: 25 to 75 µg/d.
- *Myxedema:* Initial dosage: 5 µg/d PO. Increase in 5- to 10-µg increments every 1–2 wk. Maintenance: 50 to 100 µg/d.
- *Myxedema coma and precoma:* 25 to 50 µg IV q4–12h; do not give IM or SC.
- *Simple goiter:* Initial dosage: 5 µg/d PO. May be increased by 5- to 10-µg increments every 1–2 wk. Maintenance: 75 µg/d.
- *T_3 suppression test:* 75 to 100 µg/d PO for 7 d, then repeat I-131 uptake test. I-131 uptake will be unaffected in the hyperthyroid patient but will be decreased by 50% or more in the euthyroid patient.

Pediatric
- *Cretinism:* Infants require replacement therapy from birth. Starting dose is 5 µg/d PO with 5-µg increments q3–4 d until the desired dosage is reached. Usual maintenance dosage: 20 µg/d PO up to 1 y of age; 50 µg/d for 1–3 y of age. Adult dosage after 3 y.

Geriatric: Start therapy with 5 µg/d PO. Increase by only 5-µg increments, and monitor patient response.

Pharmacokinetics

Route	Onset	Peak	Duration
Oral	Varies	2–3 d	3–4 d

Metabolism: Hepatic, $T_{1/2}$: 1–2 d
Distribution: Does not cross placenta; enters breast milk
Excretion: Urine

Adverse effects
- **Dermatologic:** Allergic skin reactions, partial loss of hair in first few months of therapy in children
- **Endocrine:** Mainly symptoms of hyperthyroidism: *palpitations, elevated P pressure, tachycardia, arrhythmias*, angina pectoris, cardiac arrest; tremors, *headache, nervousness, insomnia; nausea,* diarrhea, changes in appetite; weight loss, menstrual irregularities, sweating, heat intolerance, fever

Clinically important drug-drug interactions
- Decreased absorption of oral thyroid preparation if taken concurrently with cholestyramine • Increased risk of bleeding if taken with warfarin or dicumarol—reduce dosage of anticoagulant when T_4 is begun • Decreased effectiveness of digitalis glycosides if taken with thyroid replacement • Decreased clearance of theophyllines if patient is in hypothyroid state; monitor response and adjust dosage accordingly as patient approaches euthyroid state

■ Nursing Considerations
Assessment
- *History:* Allergy to active or extraneous constituents of drug, thyrotoxicosis, acute MI uncomplicated by hypothyroidism, Addison's disease, lactation
- *Physical:* Skin—lesions, color, temperature, texture; temperature; muscle tone, orientation, reflexes; P, auscultation,

Adverse effects in *Italics* are most common; those in **Bold** are life-threatening.

baseline ECG, BP; R, adventitious sounds; thyroid function tests

Implementation
- Monitor patient response carefully when beginning therapy, and adjust dosage accordingly.
- Monitor exchange from one form of thyroid replacement to T_3. Discontinue the other medication, then begin this drug at a low dose with gradual increases based on the patient's response.
- Administer as a single daily dose before breakfast.
- Arrange for regular, periodic blood tests of thyroid function.
- Monitor cardiac response throughout therapy.

Drug-specific teaching points
- Take as a single dose before breakfast.
- Be aware that this drug replaces an important hormone and will need to be taken for life. Do not discontinue this drug for any reason without consulting your nurse or physician; serious problems can occur.
- Consider wearing or carrying a medical alert tag to alert medical personnel who may take care of you in an emergency that you are on this drug.
- Know that nausea and diarrhea may occur (dividing the dose may help).
- Have periodic blood tests and medical evaluations while you are on this drug.
- Report headache, chest pain, palpitations, fever, weight loss, sleeplessness, nervousness, irritability, unusual sweating, intolerance to heat, diarrhea.

☐ liotrix

(lye' oh trix)
Thyrolar

Pregnancy Category A

Drug classes
Thyroid hormone (contains synthetic T_3 and T_4 in a ratio of 1 to 4 by weight)

Therapeutic actions
Increases the metabolic rate of body tissues, thereby increasing oxygen consumption; respiratory and heart rate; rate of fat, protein, and carbohydrate metabolism; and growth and maturation.

Indications
- Replacement therapy in hypothyroidism
- Pituitary TSH suppression in the treatment and prevention of euthyroid goiters and in the management of thyroid cancer
- Thyrotoxicosis in conjunction with antithyroid drugs and to prevent goitrogenesis, hypothyroidism, and thyrotoxicosis during pregnancy

Contraindications/cautions
- Contraindicated in the presence of allergy to active or extraneous constituents of drug, thyrotoxicosis, and acute MI uncomplicated by hypothyroidism.
- Use caution in the presence of Addison's disease (treatment of hypoadrenalism with corticosteroids should precede thyroid therapy) and lactation.

Dosage
60 mg equals 65 mg (1 grain) thyroid; administered only PO.
Adult
- ***Hypothyroidism:*** Initial dosage: 15–30 mg/d PO. Increase gradually every 1–2 wk in 15-mg increments (2 wk in children).
- ***Maintenance dose:*** 60 to 120 mg/d PO.

Pediatric: 0–6 mo: 25–50 μg/d (8–10 μg/kg/d PO); *6–12 mo:* 50–75 μg/d (6–8 μg/kg/d PO); *1–5 y:* 75–100 μg/d (5–6 μg/kg/d PO); *6–12 y:* 100–150 μg/d (4–5 μg/kg/d PO); *> 12 y:* more than 150 μg/d (2–3 μg/kg/d) PO.

Pharmacokinetics

Route	Onset	Peak	Duration
Oral	Varies	2–3 d	3 d

Metabolism: Hepatic, $T_{1/2}$: 1–6 d
Distribution: Does not cross placenta; enters breast milk
Excretion: Urine

Adverse effects
- **Dermatologic:** Allergic skin reactions, partial loss of hair in first few months of therapy in children
- **Endocrine:** Mainly symptoms of hyperthyroidism: *palpitations, elevated P pressure, tachycardia, arrhythmias,* angina pectoris, cardiac arrest; tremors, *headache, nervousness, insomnia; nausea,* diarrhea, changes in appetite; weight loss, menstrual irregularities, sweating, heat intolerance, fever

Clinically important drug-drug interactions
- Decreased absorption of oral thyroid preparation if taken concurrently with cholestyramine • Increased risk of bleeding if taken with warfarin or dicumarol—reduce dosage of anticoagulant when T_4 is begun • Decreased effectiveness of digitalis glycosides if taken with thyroid replacement • Decreased clearance of theophyllines if patient is in hypothyroid state; monitor response and adjust dosage accordingly as patient approaches euthyroid state

■ Nursing Considerations

Assessment
- *History:* Allergy to active or extraneous constituents of drug, thyrotoxicosis, acute MI uncomplicated by hypothyroidism, Addison's disease, lactation
- *Physical:* Skin—lesions, color, temperature, texture; temperature; muscle tone, orientation, reflexes; P, auscultation, baseline ECG, BP; R, adventitious sounds; thyroid function tests

Implementation
- Monitor patient response carefully when beginning therapy, and adjust dosage accordingly.
- Administer as a single daily dose before breakfast.
- Arrange for regular, periodic blood tests of thyroid function.
- Monitor cardiac response throughout therapy.

Drug-specific teaching points
- Take as a single dose before breakfast.
- Be aware that this drug replaces an important hormone and will need to be taken for life. Do not discontinue this drug for any reason without consulting your nurse or physician; serious problems can occur.
- Consider wearing or carrying a medical alert tag to alert medical personnel who may take care of you in an emergency that you are on this drug.
- Know that nausea and diarrhea may occur (dividing the dose may help).
- Have periodic blood tests and medical evaluations while you are on this drug.
- Report headache, chest pain, palpitations, fever, weight loss, sleeplessness, nervousness, irritability, unusual sweating, intolerance to heat, diarrhea.

❒ lisinopril

*(lyse **in'** ob pril)*
Prinivil, Zestril

Pregnancy Category C

Drug classes
Antihypertensive
Angiotensin-converting enzyme inhibitor

Therapeutic actions
Renin, synthesized by the kidneys, is released into the circulation where it acts on a plasma precursor to produce angiotensin I, which is converted by angiotensin-converting enzyme to angiotensin II, a potent vasoconstrictor that also causes release of aldosterone from the adrenals. Lisinopril blocks the conversion of angiotensin I to angiotensin II, leading to decreased BP, decreased aldosterone secretion, a small increase in serum potassium levels, and sodium and fluid loss.

Indications
- Treatment of hypertension alone or in combination with thiazide-type diuretics

Adverse effects in *Italics* are most common; those in **Bold** are life-threatening.

- Adjunctive therapy in CHF for patients not responding adequately to diuretics and digitalis

Contraindications/cautions
- Contraindicated in the presence of allergy to lisinopril or enalapril.
- Use caution in the presence of impaired renal function, CHF, salt or volume depletion, and lactation.

Dosage
Adult
- ***Patients not taking diuretics:*** Initial dose: 10 mg/d PO. Adjust dosage based on patient response. Usual range is 20–40 mg/d as a single dose.
- ***Patients taking diuretics:*** Discontinue diuretic for 2–3 d if possible. If it is not possible to discontinue diuretic, give initial dose of 5 mg, and monitor for excessive hypotension.
- ***CHF:*** 5 mg PO qd with diuretics and digitalis. Effective range: 5 to 20 mg/d.

Pediatric: Safety and efficacy not established.

Geriatric and renal impaired: Excretion is reduced in renal failure. Use smaller initial dose, and titrate upward to a maximum of 40 mg/d PO. Creatine clearance >30: 10 mg/d; ≥10≤30, 5mg/d; <10, 2.5 mg/d.

Creatinine Clearance (ml/min)	Initial Dose
>30	10 mg/d
≥10 ≤30	5 mg/d (2.5 mg for CHF)
Dialysis	2.5 mg on dialysis d

Pharmacokinetics

Route	Onset	Peak	Duration
Oral	1 h	7 h	24 h

Metabolism: Hepatic, $T_{1/2}$ 12 h
Distribution: Crosses placenta; enters breast milk
Excretion: Urine

Adverse effects
- CNS: *Headache, dizziness, insomnia, fatigue,* paresthesias
- GI: *Gastric irritation, nausea, diarrhea,* aphthous ulcers, peptic ulcers, dysgeusia, cholestatic jaundice, hepatocellular injury, anorexia, constipation
- CV: *Orthostatic hypotension,* tachycardia, angina pectoris, MI, Raynaud's syndrome, CHF, severe hypotension in salt or volume depleted patients
- Hematologic: Neutropenia, agranulocytosis, thrombocytopenia, hemolytic anemia, **fatal pancytopenia**
- GU: *Proteinuria,* renal insufficiency, renal failure, polyuria, oliguria, frequency
- Other: *Angioedema* (particularly of the face, extremities, lips, tongue, larnyx; death has been reported with **airway obstruction**); *cough,* muscle cramps, impotence

Clinically important drug-drug interactions
- Decreased antihypertensive effects if taken with indomethacin

■ Nursing Considerations

Assessment
- *History:* Allergy to lisinopril or enalapril, impaired renal function, CHF, salt or volume depletion, lactation
- *Physical:* Skin—color, lesions, turgor; body temperature; P, BP, peripheral perfusion; mucous membranes, bowel sounds, liver evaluation; urinalysis, renal and liver function tests, CBC and differential

Implementation
- Maintain epinephrine on standby in case of angioedema of the face or neck region; if breathing difficulty occurs, consult with physician, and administer epinephrine as appropriate.
- Alert surgeon, and mark patient's chart with notice that lisinopril is being taken. The angiotensin II formation subsequent to compensatory renin release during surgery will be blocked. Hypotension may be reversed with volume expansion.
- Monitor patients on diuretic therapy for excessive hypotension following the first few doses of lisinopril.

Adverse effects in *Italics* are most common; those in **Bold** are life-threatening.

- Monitor patients closely in any situation that may lead to a decrease in BP secondary to reduction in fluid volume—excessive perspiration and dehydration, vomiting, diarrhea—because excessive hypotension may occur.
- Arrange for reduced dosage in patients with impaired renal function.

Drug-specific teaching points
- Take this drug once a day. It may be taken with meals. Do not stop taking the medication without consulting your prescriber.
- Know that the following side effects may occur: GI upset, loss of appetite, change in taste perception (these may be limited effects that will pass with time; taking the drug with meals may help); mouth sores (frequent mouth care may help); skin rash; fast heart rate; dizziness, lightheadedness (this usually passes after the first few days of therapy; if it occurs, change position slowly, and limit your activities to those that do not require alertness and precision); headache, fatigue, sleeplessness.
- Be careful in any situation that may lead to a drop in BP—diarrhea, sweating, vomiting, dehydration. If lightheadedness or dizziness occurs, consult your nurse or physician.
- Report mouth sores; sore throat; fever; chills; swelling of the hands or feet; irregular heartbeat; chest pains; swelling of the face, eyes, lips, or tongue; and difficulty breathing.

◻ lithium carbonate

(lith' ee um)
Carbolith (CAN), Duralith (CAN), Eskalith, Lithane, Lithizine (CAN), Lithonate, Lithotabs

lithium citrate

Pregnancy Category D

Drug classes
Antimanic agent

Therapeutic actions
Mechanism of action is not known; alters sodium transport in nerve and muscle cells; inhibits release of norepinephrine and dopamine, but not serotonin, from stimulated neurons; slightly increases intraneuronal stores of catecholamines; decreases intraneuronal content of second messengers and may thereby selectively modulate the responsiveness of hyperactive neurons that might contribute to the manic state.

Indications
- Treatment of manic episodes of manic-depressive illness; maintenance therapy to prevent or diminish the frequency and intensity of subsequent manic episodes
- Unlabeled use—improvement of neutrophil counts in patients with cancer chemotherapy-induced neutropenia and in children with chronic neutropenia (doses of 300–1000 mg/d, serum levels of 0.5 and 1.0 mEq/L); prophylaxis of cluster headache and cyclic migraine headache (doses of 600–900 mg/d)

Contraindications/cautions
- Contraindicated in the presence of hypersensitivity to tartrazine (in tablets marketed as *Lithane*); significant renal or cardiovascular disease; severe debilitation, dehydration; sodium depletion, patients on diuretics (lithium decreases sodium reabsorption, and hyponatremia increases lithium retention); pregnancy; lactation.
- Use caution in the presence of protracted sweating and diarrhea; suicidal or impulsive patients; infection with fever.

Dosage
Individualize dosage according to serum levels and clinical response.
Adult
- ***Acute mania:*** 600 mg PO tid or 900 mg slow-release form PO bid to produce effective serum levels between 1 and 1.5 mEq/L. Serum levels should be determined twice wkly in samples drawn immediately before a dose and 8–12 h after the previous dose.
- ***Long-term use:*** 300 mg PO tid to qid to produce a serum level of 0.6 to

1.2 mEq/L. Serum levels should be determined at least every 2 mo in samples drawn immediately before a dose and 8 to 12 h after the previous dose.
- *Conversion from conventional to slow-release dosage forms:* Give the same total daily dose divided into 2 or 3 doses.

Pediatric: Safety and efficacy for children < 12 y not established.

Geriatric and renal impaired: Reduced dosage may be necessary. Elderly patients often respond to reduced dosage and may exhibit signs of toxicity at serum levels tolerated by other patients. Plasma half-life is prolonged in renal impairment.

Pharmacokinetics

Route	Onset	Peak
Oral	5–7 d	10–21 d

Metabolism: Hepatic, $T_{1/2}$: 17–36 h
Distribution: Crosses placenta; enters breast milk
Excretion: Urine

Adverse effects
Reactions are related to serum lithium levels (toxic lithium levels are close to therapeutic levels: therapeutic levels in acute mania range between 1 and 1.5 mEq/L; therapeutic levels for maintenance are 0.6 to 1.2 mEq/L).

< 1.5 mEq/L
- CNS: *Lethargy, slurred speech, muscle weakness, fine hand tremor*
- GI: *Nausea, vomiting, diarrhea, thirst*
- GU: *Polyuria*

1.5–2.0 mEq/L (mild to moderate toxic reactions)
- CNS: Coarse hand tremor, mental confusion, hyperirritability of muscles, drowsiness, incoordination
- GI: Persistent GI upset, gastritis, salivary gland swelling, abdominal pain, excessive salivation, flatulence, indigestion
- CV: ECG changes

2.0–2.5 mEq/L (moderate to severe toxic reactions)
- CNS: Ataxia, giddiness, fasciculations, tinnitus, blurred vision, clonic movements, seizures, stupor, coma

- CV: Serious ECG changes, severe hypotension
- **Respiratory**: Fatalities secondary to pulmonary complications
- GU: Large output of dilute urine

> 2.5 mEq/L (life-threatening toxicity)
- **General**: Complex involvement of multiple organ systems

Reactions unrelated to serum levels
- CNS: Headache, worsening of organic brain syndromes, fever, reversible short-term memory impairment, dyspraxia
- GI: Dysgeusia/taste distortion, salty taste; swollen lips; dental caries
- CV: ECG changes; hyperkalemia associated with ECG changes; syncope; tachycardia-bradycardia syndrome; rarely, arrhythmias, CHF, diffuse myocarditis, death
- Dermatologic: Pruritus with or without rash; maculopapular, acneiform, and follicular eruptions; cutaneous ulcers; edema of ankles or wrists
- Endocrine: diffuse nontoxic goiter; hypercalcemia associated with hyperparathyroidism; transient hyperglycemia; irreversible nephrogenic diabetes insipidus, which improves with diuretic therapy; impotence or sexual dysfunction
- Miscellaneous: Weight gain (5–10 kg); chest tightness; reversible respiratory failure; swollen or painful joints, eye irritation, worsening of cataracts, disturbance of visual accommodation

Clinically important drug-drug interactions
- Increased risk of toxicity when given with thiazide diuretics due to decreased renal clearance of lithium—reduced lithium dosage may be necessary • Increased plasma lithium levels with indomethacin and some other NSAIDs—phenylbutazone, piroxicam, ibuprofen • Increased CNS toxicity of lithium when given with carbamazepine • Encephalopathic syndrome (weakness, lethargy, fever, tremulousness, confusion, extrapyramidal symptoms, leu-

Adverse effects in *Italics* are most common; those in **Bold** are life-threatening.

kocytosis, elevated serum enzymes) with irreversible brain damage when taken with haloperidol • Greater risk of hypothyroidsim when given with iodide salts • Decreased effectiveness of lithium due to increased excretion of lithium when given with urinary alkalinizers, including antacids, tromethamine

■ Nursing Considerations

Assessment
- *History:* Hypersensitivity to tartrazine; significant renal or cardiovascular disease; severe debilitation, dehydration; sodium depletion, patients on diuretics; protracted sweating, diarrhea; suicidal or impulsive patients; infection with fever; pregnancy; lactation
- *Physical:* Body weight and temperature; skin—color, lesions; orientation, affect, reflexes; ophthalmic exam; P, BP, R, adventitious sounds; bowel sounds, normal fluid intake, normal output, voiding pattern; thyroid, renal glomerular and tubular function tests, urinalysis, CBC and differential, baseline ECG

Implementation
- Give with caution and daily monitoring of serum lithium levels to patients with renal or cardiovascular disease, debilitation, or dehydration who have life-threatening psychiatric disorders.
- Give drug with food or milk or after meals.
- Monitor patient's clinical status closely, especially during the initial stages of therapy.
- Be aware that individual patients vary in their reponse to this drug; in particular, some patients may exhibit toxic signs at serum lithium levels that are usually considered within the therapeutic range.
- Decrease dosage after the acute manic episode is controlled; lithium tolerance is greater during the acute manic phase and decreases when manic symptoms subside.
- Ensure that patient maintains adequate intake of salt and adequate intake of fluid (2,500–3,000 ml/d).

Drug-specific teaching points
- Take this drug exactly as prescribed, after meals or with food or milk.
- Eat a normal diet with normal salt intake; maintain adequate fluid intake (at least $2\frac{1}{2}$ quarts/d).
- Arrange for frequent checkups, including blood tests, while you are taking this drug. It is important that you keep all appointments for these checkups so that you can receive the maximum benefit with the least risk of toxicity from this drug therapy.
- Know that the following side effects may occur: drowsiness, dizziness (avoid driving a car or performing other tasks that require alertness if this occurs); GI upset (frequent small meals may help); mild thirst, greater than usual urine volume, fine hand tremor (these drug effects may persist throughout therapy; notify your nurse or physician if these are severe or a problem).
- Use contraceptive measures to avoid becoming pregnant while you are taking this drug. If you wish to become pregnant or believe that you have become pregnant, consult your nurse or physician.
- Discontinue drug, and notify your nurse or physician if signs of toxicity occur: diarrhea, vomiting, ataxia, tremor, drowsiness, lack of coordination or muscular weakness.
- Report diarrhea or fever.

▢ lomefloxacin hydrochloride

(low ma flox' a sin)
Maxaquin

Pregnancy Category C

Drug classes
Antibacterial drug

Therapeutic actions
Bactericidal: interferes with DNA replication in susceptible gram-negative bacteria, preventing cell reproduction and causing cell death.

lomefloxacin hydrochloride

Indications
- For the treatment of infections in adults caused by susceptible organisms: lower respiratory tract infections caused by *Haemophilus influenzae, Moraxella catarrhalis*; urinary tract infections due to *Escherichia coli, Klebsiella pneumoniae, Proteus mirabilis, Staphylococcus epidermidis, Enterobacter cloacae, Citrobacter diversus, Pseudomonas aeruginosa*
- Prophylaxis: preoperatively to reduce the incidence of urinary tract infections in early postoperative period in patients undergoing transurethral procedures

Contraindications/cautions
- Contraindicated in presence of allergy to lomefloxacin, norfloxacin, syphilis, pregnancy, lactation.
- Use caution in the presence of renal dysfunction and seizures.

Dosage
Adult
- ***Lower respiratory tract infection:*** 400 mg qd PO for 10 d.
- ***UTIs:*** 400 mg qd PO for 10 d.
- ***Complicated UTIs:*** 400 mg qd PO for 14 d.
- ***Prophylaxis:*** Single dose of 400 mg PO 2–6 h prior to surgery when oral preoperative medication is appropriate.

Pediatric: Not recommended for children > 18 y; produced lesions of joint cartilage in immature experimental animals.

Impaired renal function: Creatinine clearance > 10 but < 30 ml/min per 1.73 m^2 initial dose of 400 mg followed by 200 mg qd for the rest of the course.

Pharmacokinetics

Route	Onset	Peak	Duration
Oral	Varies	1–1.5 h	8–10 h

Metabolism: Hepatic, T$_{1/2}$: 8 h
Distribution: Crosses placenta; enters breast milk
Excretion: Urine and feces

Adverse effects
- **CNS:** *Headache, dizziness,* insomnia, fatigue, somnolence, depression, blurred vision
- **GI:** *Nausea, vomiting,* dry mouth, diarrhea, abdominal pain
- **Hematologic:** Elevated BUN, SGOT, SGPT, serum creatinine, and alkaline phosphatase; decreased WBC, neutrophil count, hematocrit
- **Other:** Fever, rash, photosensitivity

Clinically important drug-drug interactions
- Decreased therapetic effect of enoxacin if taken concurrently with iron salts • Decreased absorption of enoxacin if taken with antacids • Increased serum levels and toxic effects of theophyllines if taken concurrently with enoxacin

■ Nursing Considerations

Assessment
- *History:* Allergy to lomefloxacin, ciprofloxacin, norfloxacin; renal dysfunction; seizures; lactation
- *Physical:* Skin—color, lesions; body temperature; orientation, reflexes, affect; mucous membranes, bowel sounds; renal and liver function tests

Implementation
- Arrange for culture and sensitivity tests before beginning therapy.
- Continue therapy for 2 d after the signs and symptoms of infection have disappeared.
- Administer oral drug without regard to meals.
- Ensure that patient is well hydrated during course of drug therapy.
- Administer antacids if needed at least 2 h after dosing.
- Monitor clinical response; if no improvement is seen or a relapse occurs, repeat culture and sensitivity.

Drug-specific teaching points
- Take oral drug without regard to meals. If an antacid is needed, do not take it within 2 h of lomefloxacin dose.

Adverse effects in *Italics* are most common; those in **Bold** are life-threatening.

- Drink plenty of fluids while you are taking this drug.
- Know that the following side effects may occur: nausea, vomiting, abdominal pain (small, frequent meals may help); drowsiness, blurred vision, dizziness (observe caution if driving or using dangerous equipment).
- Report rash, visual changes, severe GI problems, weakness, tremors.

☐ lomustine

(loe mus' teen)
CCNU, CeeNu

Pregnancy Category D

Drug classes
Alkylating agent, nitrosourea
Antineoplastic drug

Therapeutic actions
Cytotoxic: exact mechanism of action is not known, but it alkylates DNA and RNA, thus inhibiting DNA, RNA, and protein synthesis.

Indications
- Palliative therapy in combination with other agents for primary and metastatic brain tumors and Hodgkin's disease

Contraindications/cautions
- Contraindicated in the presence of allergy to lomustine, radiation therapy, chemotherapy, hematopoietic depression, pregnancy (teratogenic and embryotoxic in preclinical studies), and lactation.
- Use caution in the presence of impaired renal or hepatic function.

Dosage
Adult and Pediatric: 130 mg/m^2 PO as a single dose every 6 wk. Adjustments must be made in patients with bone marrow suppression; initially reduce the dose to 100 mg/m^2 PO every 6 wk; do not give a repeat dose until platelets are > 100,000/mm^3 and leukocytes are > 4,000/mm^3; adjust dosage after initial dose based on hematologic response as follows:

- Minimum count after prior dose:

Leukocytes	Platelets	Percentage of Prior Dose to Give
>4,000	>100,000	100%
3,000–3,999	75,000–99,999	100%
2,000–2,999	25,000–74,999	70%
<2,000	<25,000	50%

Pharmacokinetics

Route	Onset	Peak	Duration
Oral	10 min	3 h	48 h

Metabolism: Hepatic, T$_{1/2}$: 16 to 72 h
Distribution: Crosses placenta; enters breast milk
Excretion: Urine

Adverse effects
- **GI:** *Nausea, vomiting,* stomatitis, hepatotoxicity
- **Hematologic:** *Leukopenia; thrombocytopenia; anemia,* delayed for 4 to 6 wk; immunosuppression
- **GU:** Renal toxicity
- **Other:** Cancer

■ Nursing Considerations

Assessment
- *History:* Allergy to lomustine, radiation therapy, chemotherapy, hematopoietic depression, impaired renal or hepatic function, pregnancy, lactation
- *Physical:* Temperature; weight; mucous membranes, liver evaluation; CBC, differential; urinalysis, liver and renal function tests

Implementation
- Arrange for blood tests to evaluate hematopoietic function before beginning therapy and wkly for at least 6 wk after therapy.
- Do not give full dosage within 2–3 wk after a full course of radiation therapy or chemotherapy because of the risk of severe bone marrow depression; reduced dosage may be needed.
- Arrange for reduced dosage in patients with depressed bone marrow function.

Adverse effects in *Italics* are most common; those in **Bold** are life-threatening.

- Administer tablets on an empty stomach to decrease GI upset; antiemetics may be needed for nausea and vomiting.

Drug-specific teaching points
- Take this drug on an empty stomach.
- Know that the following side effects may occur: nausea, vomiting, loss of appetite (taking the drug on an empty stomach may help, an antiemetic also may be ordered for you; small frequent meals also may help).
- Maintain your fluid intake and nutrition while on this drug.
- Consider the use of birth control methods while on this drug; this drug can cause severe birth defects.
- Report unusual bleeding or bruising, fever, chills, sore throat, stomach or flank pain, sores on your mouth or lips, unusual tiredness, confusion.

◻ loperamide hydrochloride

*(loe **per'** a mide)*
Prescription: Imodium
OTC: Imodium A-D, Kaopectate II, Maalox Anti-Diarrheal Caplets, Pepto-Bismol
Pregnancy Category B

Drug classes
Antidiarrheal agent

Therapeutic actions
Slows intestinal motility and affects water and electrolyte movement through the bowel by inhibiting peristalsis through direct effects on the circular and longitudinal muscles of the intestinal wall.

Indications
- Control and symptomatic relief of acute nonspecific diarrhea and chronic diarrhea associated with inflammatory bowel disease
- Reduction of volume of discharge from ileostomies
- OTC use: control of diarrhea, including traveler's diarrhea

Contraindications/cautions
- Contraindicated in the presence of allergy to loperamide, patients who must avoid constipation, diarrhea associated with organisms that penetrate the intestinal mucosa (*E. coli, Salmonella, Shigella*).
- Use caution in the presence of hepatic dysfunction, acute ulcerative colitis, pregnancy, and lactation.

Dosage
Adult
- ***Acute diarrhea:*** Initial dose of 4 mg PO followed by 2 mg after each unformed stool. Do not exceed 16 mg/d. Clinical improvement is usually seen within 48 h.
- ***Chronic diarrhea:*** Initial dose of 4 mg PO followed by 2 mg after each unformed stool until diarrhea is controlled. Individualize dose based on patient response. Optimal daily dose is 4–8 mg. If no clinical improvement is seen with dosage of 16 mg/d for 10 d, further treatment will probably not be effective.
- ***OTC—traveler's diarrhea:*** 4 mg PO after first loose stool, followed by 2 mg after each subsequent stool; do not exceed 8 mg/d for more than 2 d.

Pediatric: Avoid use in children < 2 y, and use extreme caution in younger children. The OTC product should not be used with children.
- ***Acute diarrhea:*** First-day dosage schedule:

Age	Weight	Dose Form	Amount
2–5 y	13–20 kg	Liquid	1 mg tid
5–8 y	20–30 kg	Liquid or capsule	2 mg bid
8–12 y	>30 kg	Liquid or capsule	2 mg tid

- Subsequent doses: Administer 1 mg/10 kg PO only after a loose stool. Do not exceed daily dosage of the recommended dosage for the first day.
- ***Chronic diarrhea:*** Dosage schedule has not been established.
- ***OTC—traveler's diarrhea:*** *9–11 y:* 2 mg PO after first loose stool followed by 1 mg after each subsequent stool; *6–8 y:* 1 mg PO after first loose stool,

followed by 1 mg after each subsequent loose stool—do not exceed 4 mg/d; *< 6 y:* consult with physician; not recommended.

Pharmacokinetics

Route	Onset	Peak
Oral	Varies	5 h

Metabolism: Hepatic, $T_{1/2}$: 10.8 h
Distribution: May cross placenta and enter breast milk
Excretion: Urine and feces

Adverse effects

- CNS: Tiredness, drowsiness, or dizziness
- GI: Toxic megacolon (in patients with ulcerative colitis), *abdominal pain, distention or discomfort, constipation, dry mouth, nausea,* vomiting
- Hypersensitivity: Skin rash

■ Nursing Considerations

Assessment

- *History:* Allergy to loperamide, patients who must avoid constipation, diarrhea associated with organisms that penetrate the intestinal mucosa (*E. coli, Salmonella, Shigella*); hepatic dysfunction, acute ulcerative colitis, lactation
- *Physical:* Skin—color, lesions; orientation, reflexes; abdominal exam, bowel sounds, liver evaluation; serum electrolytes (with extended use)

Implementation

- Monitor patient for response. If improvement is not seen within 48 h, discontinue treatment and notify physician.
- Administer drug after each unformed stool. Keep track of amount given to avoid exceeding the recommended daily dosage.
- Have the narcotic antagonist naloxone on standby in case of overdose and CNS depression.

Drug-specific teaching points

- Take drug as prescribed. Do not exceed prescribed dosage or recommended daily dosage (as appropriate).
- Know that the following side effects may occur: abdominal fullness, nausea, vomiting; dry mouth (sucking on sugarless lozenges may help); dizziness.
- Report abdominal pain or distention, fever, and diarrhea that does not stop after a few days.

▢ loracarbef

*(lor ah **kar'** bef)*
Lorabid

Pregnancy Category B

Drug classes
Antibiotic
Cephalosporin (second generation)

Therapeutic actions
Bactericidal: inhibits synthesis of bacterial cell wall, causing cell death.

Indications

- Pharyngitis/tonsillitis caused by *Streptococcus pyogenes*
- Secondary bacterial infection of acute bronchitis and exacerabation of chronic bronchitis caused by *S. pneumoniae, H. influenzae, M. catarrhalis*
- Pneumonia caused by *S. pneumoniae, H. influenzae*
- Dermatologic infections caused by *Staphylococcus aureus, S. pyogenes*
- Urinary tract infections caused by *E. coli, Staphylococcus saprophyticus*
- Otitis media caused by *S. pneumoniae, H. influenzae, M. catarrhalis, S. pyogenes*

Contraindications/cautions

- Allergy to cephalosporins or penicillins, renal failure, lactation

Dosage
Adult: 200 to 400 mg PO q12h. Continue treatment for 7 to 14 d, depending on the severity of the infection.
Pediatric: 15 to 30 mg/kg per d in divided doses q12h PO. Continue treatment for 7 to 10 d.

Adverse effects in *Italics* are most common; those in **Bold** are life-threatening.

652 ■ loratidine

Geriatric or renal impaired
- **Creatinine clearance > 50 ml/min:** Use standard dose.
- **Creatinine clearance 10 to 49 ml/min:** Use 50% of standard dose.

Pharmacokinetics

Route	Peak
PO	90 min

Metabolism: Hepatic, $T_{1/2}$: 60 min
Distribution: Crosses the placenta, enters breast milk
Excretion: Renal, unchanged

Adverse effects
- CNS: Headache, dizziness, lethargy, paresthesias
- GI: *Nausea, vomiting, diarrhea, anorexia, abdominal pain, flatulence,* **pseudomembranous colitis,** liver toxicity
- Hematologic: Bone marrow depression
- GU: Nephrotoxicity
- Hypersensitivity: *Ranges from rash to fever* to **anaphylaxis;** serum sickness reaction
- Other: *Superinfections*

Clinically important drug-drug interactions
- Increased nephrotoxicity with aminoglycosides • Increased bleeding effects if taken with oral anticoagulants • Disulfiram-like reaction if alcohol is taken within 72 h after loracarbef administration

Drug-lab test interferences
- Possibility of false results on tests of urine glucose using Benedict's solution, Fehling's solution, Clinitest tablets, urinary 17-ketosteroids, direct Coombs' test

■ Nursing Considerations

Assessment
- *History:* Penicillin or cephalosporin allergy, pregnancy or lactation
- *Physical:* Kidney function, respiratory status, skin status; culture and sensitivity tests of infected area

Implementation
- Culture infected area before beginning drug therapy.
- Give drug on an empty stomach, 1 h before or 2 h after meals.
- Reconstitute solution by adding 30–60 ml water in two portions to the dry mixture in the 50- or 100-ml bottle, respectively.
- Keep suspension at room temperature after reconstitution, and discard after 14 d.
- Discontinue drug if hypersensitivy reaction occurs.
- Arrange for oral vancomycin for serious colitis that fails to respond to discontinuation.
- Reculture infected area if infection fails to respond.

Drug-specific teaching points
- Take this drug on an empty stomach, 1 h before or 2 h after meals. Store suspension at room temperature, and discard any unused portions after 14 d.
- Complete the full course of this drug, even if you feel better before the course of treatment is over.
- Be aware that this drug is prescribed for this particular infection; do not self-treat any other infection with this drug.
- Know that the following side effects may occur: stomach upset, loss of appetite, nausea (taking the drug with food may help); diarrhea (stay near bathroom facilities); headache, dizziness.
- Report severe diarrhea with blood, pus, or mucus; rash or hives; difficulty breathing; unusual tiredness or fatigue; unusual bleeding or bruising.

☐ loratidine

(lor at' a deen)
Claritin

Pregnancy Category C

Drug classes
Antihistamine (nonsedating type)

Adverse effects in *Italics* are most common; those in **Bold** are life-threatening.

Therapeutic actions
Competitively blocks the effects of histamine at peripheral H_1 receptor sites; has anticholinergic (atropine-like) and antipruritic effects.

Indications
- Symptomatic relief of symptoms associated with perennial and seasonal allergic rhinitis, vasomotor rhinitis, allergic conjunctivitis, and mild, uncomplicated urticaria and angioedema
- Amelioraton of allergic reactions to blood or plasma
- Dermatographism
- Adjunctive therapy in anaphylactic reactions

Contraindications/cautions
- Allergy to any antihistamines; narrow-angle glaucoma, stenosing peptic ulcer, symptomatic prostatic hypertrophy, asthmatic attack, bladder neck obstruction, pyloroduodenal obstruction (avoid use or use with caution as condition may be exacerbated by drug effects); lactation

Dosage
Adult and children > 12 y: 10 mg qd PO on an empty stomach.
Pediatric < 12 y: Safety and efficacy not established.
Geriatric or hepatic impairment: 10 mg PO qod.

Pharmacokinetics

Route	Onset	Peak	Duration
Oral	1–3 h	8–12 h	24 h

Metabolism: Hepatic, $T_{1/2}$: 8.4 h
Distribution: Crosses placenta; enters breast milk
Excretion: Urine and feces

Adverse effects
- **CNS:** *Headache, nervousness, dizziness,* depression
- **GI:** *Appetite increase,* nausea, diarrhea, abdominal pain
- **CV:** Palpitation, edema
- **Respiratory:** Bronchospasm, pharyngitis
- **General:** *Weight gain*
- **Other:** Fever, photosensitivity, rash, myalgia, arthralgia, angioedema

Clinically important drug-drug interactions
- Additive CNS depressant effects if taken with alcohol or other CNS depressants • Increased and prolonged anticholinergic (drying) effects if taken with MAO inhibitors; avoid this combination.

Drug-lab test interferences
- False skin testing procedures if done while patient is on antihistamines.

■ Nursing Considerations

Assessment
- *History:* Allergy to any antihistamines; narrow-angle glaucoma, stenosing peptic ulcer, symptomatic prostatic hypertrophy, asthmatic attack, bladder neck obstruction, pyloroduodenal obstruction; lactation
- *Physical:* Skin—color, lesions, texture; orientation, reflexes, affect; vision exams; R, adventitious sounds; prostate palpation; serum transaminase levels

Implementation
- Administer on an empty stomach 1 h before or 2 h after meals.

Drug-specific teaching points
- Take this drug on an empty stomach 1 h before or 2 h after meals or food of any kind.
- Know that the following side effects may occur: dizziness, sedation, drowsiness (use caution if driving or performing tasks that require alertness if these occur); headache; thickening of bronchial secretions, dryness of nasal mucosa (use of a humidifier may help if this becomes a problem).
- Avoid the use of alcohol while on this drug; serious sedation could occur.
- Report difficulty breathing, hallucinations, tremors, loss of coordination, irregular heartbeat.

Adverse effects in *Italics* are most common; those in **Bold** are life-threatening.

lorazepam

(lor a' ze pam)
Apo-Lorazepam (CAN),
Ativan, Novolorazem (CAN)

Pregnancy Category D
C-IV controlled substance

Drug classes
Benzodiazepine
Antianxiety drug
Sedative/hypnotic

Therapeutic actions
Exact mechanisms of action are not understood; acts mainly at subcortical levels of the CNS, leaving the cortex relatively unaffected. Main sites of action may be the limbic system and reticular formation; benzodiazepines potentiate the effects of GABA, an inhibitory neurotransmitter; anxiolytic effects occur at doses well below those necessary to cause sedation and ataxia.

Indications
- Management of anxiety disorders or for short-term relief of symptoms of anxiety or anxiety associated with depression (oral)
- Preanesthetic medication in adults to produce sedation, relieve anxiety, and decrease recall of events related to surgery (parenteral)
- Unlabeled parenteral use—management of status epilepticus, chemotherapy induced nausea and vomiting, acute alcohol withdrawal

Contraindications/cautions
- Contraindicated in the presence of hypersensitivity to benzodiazepines, propylene glycol, polyethylene glycol or benzyl alcohol (parenteral lorazepam); psychoses; acute narrow-angle glaucoma; shock; coma; acute alcoholic intoxication with depression of vital signs; pregnancy (crosses the placenta; risk of congenital malformations and neonatal withdrawal syndrome); labor and delivery ("floppy infant" syndrome reported when mothers were given benzodiazepines during labor); and lactation.
- Use caution in the presence of impaired liver or kidney function or debilitation.

Dosage
Adult
- **Oral:** Usual dose is 2–6 mg/d; range 1–10 mg/d given in divided doses with largest dose at bedtime. Insomnia due to transient stress: 2–4 mg given at bedtime.
- **IM:** 0.05 mg/kg up to a maximum of 4 mg administered at least 2 h before operative procedure.
- **IV:** Initial dose is 2 mg total or 0.044 mg/kg, whichever is smaller. Do not exceed this dose in patients older than 50 y. Doses as high as 0.05 mg/kg up to a total of 4 mg may be given 15 to 20 min before the procedure to other patients in whom a greater lack of recall would be beneficial.

Pediatric: Drug should not be used in children < 12 y.

Geriatric patients or those with debilitating disease: Initially, 1 to 2 mg/d in divided doses. Adjust as needed and tolerated.

Pharmacokinetics

Route	Onset	Peak	Duration
Oral	Intermed.	1–6 h	12–24 h
IM	15–30 min	60–90 min	12-24 h
IV	1–5 min	10–15 min	12–24 h

Metabolism: Hepatic, $T_{1/2}$: 10–20 h
Distribution: Crosses placenta; enters breast milk
Excretion: Urine

IV facts
Preparation: Dilute lorazepam immediately prior to IV use. For direct IV injection or injection into IV line, dilute with an equal volume of compatible solution (Sterile Water for Injection, Sodium Chloride Injection or 5% Dextrose Injection); do not use if solution is discolored or contains a precipitate. Protect from light; refrigerate.
Infusion: Direct inject slowly, or infuse at maximum rate of 2 mg/min.

Adverse effects
- **CNS:** *Transient, mild drowsiness initially; sedation, depression, lethargy, apathy, fatigue, lightheadedness, disorientation, anger, hostility,* episodes of mania and hypomania, *restlessness, confusion, crying,* delirium, *headache,* slurred speech, dysarthria, stupor, rigidity, tremor, dystonia, vertigo, euphoria, nervousness, difficulty concentrating, vivid dreams, psychomotor retardation, extrapyramidal symptoms; *mild paradoxical excitatory reactions during first 2 wk of treatment*
- **GI:** *Constipation, diarrhea, dry mouth,* salivation, *nausea,* anorexia, vomiting, difficulty in swallowing, gastric disorders, hepatic dysfunction
- **CV:** Bradycardia, tachycardia, cardiovascular collapse, hypertension and hypotension, palpitations, edema
- **Hematologic:** Elevations of blood enzymes: LDH, alkaline phosphatase, SGOT, SGPT; blood dyscrasias: **agranulocytosis**, leukopenia
- **GU:** Incontinence, urinary retention, changes in libido, menstrual irregularities
- **EENT:** Visual and auditory disturbances, diplopia, nystagmus, depressed hearing, nasal congestion
- **Dermatologic:** Urticaria, pruritus, skin rash, dermatitis
- **Other:** Hiccups, fever, diaphoresis, paresthesias, muscular disturbances, gynecomastia. *Drug dependence with withdrawal syndrome when drug is discontinued; more common with abrupt discontinuation of higher dosage used for longer than 4 mo.*

Clinically important drug-drug interactions
- Increased CNS depression when taken with alcohol • Decreased effectiveness of lorazepam if taken concurrently with theophyllines

■ Nursing Considerations
Assessment
- ***History:*** Hypersensitivity to benzodiazepines, propylene glycol, polyethylene glycol or benzyl alcohol; psychoses; acute narrow-angle glaucoma; shock; coma; acute alcoholic intoxication with depression of vital signs; pregnancy; lactation; impaired liver or kidney function, debilitation
- ***Physical:*** Skin—color, lesions; body temperature; orientation, reflexes, affect, ophthalmologic exam; P, BP; R, adventitious sounds; liver evaluation, abdominal exam, bowel sounds, normal output; CBC, liver and renal function tests

Implementation
- Do not administer intra-arterially; arteriospasm, gangrene may result.
- Give IM injections of undiluted drug deep into muscle mass, monitor injection sites.
- Do not use solutions that are discolored or contain a precipitate. Protect drug from light, and refrigerate solution.
- Keep equipment to maintain a patent airway on standby whenever drug is given IV.
- Reduce dose of narcotic analgesics by at least half in patients who have received parenteral lorazepam.
- Keep patients who have received parenteral doses of lorazepam under close observation, preferably in bed, for up to 3 h. Do not permit ambulatory patients to drive following an injection.
- Taper dosage gradually after long-term therapy, especially in epileptic patients.

Drug-specific teaching points
- Take drug exactly as prescribed; do not stop taking drug (long-term therapy) without consulting health care provider.
- Know that the following side effects may occur: drowsiness, dizziness (these may become less pronounced after a few days; avoid driving a car or engaging in other dangerous activities if these occur); GI upset (taking the drug with food may help); nocturnal sleep disturbances for several nights after discontinuing the drug when it has been used as a sedative/hypnotic; depression, dreams, emotional upset, crying.

Adverse effects in *Italics* are most common; those in **Bold** are life-threatening.

- Report severe dizziness, weakness, drowsiness that persists, rash or skin lesions, palpitations, edema of the extremities; visual changes; difficulty voiding.

☐ lovastatin

(loe va sta' tin)

mevinolin
Mevacor

Pregnancy Category X

Drug classes
Antihyperlipidemic agent

Therapeutic actions
Inhibits the enzyme that catalyzes the rate-limiting step in the cholesterol synthesis pathway, resulting in a decrease in serum cholesterol, serum LDL's (the lipids associated with the development of coronary artery disease), and either an increase or no change in serum HDL's (the lipids associated with decreased risk of CAD).

Indications
- Treatment of familial hypercholesterolemia
- Adjunctive treatment of type II hyperlipidemia
- Unlabeled use—diabetic dyslipidemia, nephrotic hyperlipidemia

Contraindications/cautions
- Contraindicated in the presence of allergy to lovastatin, fungal byproducts, pregnancy.
- Use caution in the presence of impaired hepatic function, cataracts, and lactation.

Dosage
Adult: Initial 20 mg/d PO administered in the evening. Maintenance doses range from 20 to 80 mg/d PO. Do not exceed 80 mg/d. Adjust at intervals of 4 wk or more. Patients receiving immunosuppressive drugs should receive a maximum of 20 mg/d PO.

Pediatric: Safety and efficacy not established.

Pharmacokinetics

Route	Onset	Peak
Oral	2 wk	4–6 wk

Metabolism: Hepatic, $T_{1/2}$: unknown
Distribution: Crosses placenta; enters breast milk
Excretion: Bile and feces

Adverse effects
- **CNS:** *Headache, blurred vision*, dizziness, insomnia, fatigue, muscle cramps, cataracts
- **GI:** *Flatulence, abdominal pain, cramps, constipation, nausea*, dyspepsia, heartburn
- **Hematologic:** Elevations of creatinine phosphokinase, alkaline phosphatase, and transaminases

Clinically important drug-drug interactions
- Possibility of severe myopathy or rhabdomyolysis if taken with cyclosporine or gemfibrozil

■ Nursing Considerations

Assessment
- *History:* Allergy to lovastatin, fungal byproducts; impaired hepatic function; cataracts; pregnancy; lactation
- *Physical:* Orientation, affect, ophthalmologic exam; liver evaluation; lipid studies, liver function tests

Implementation
- Administer drug in the evening; highest rates of cholesterol synthesis are between midnight and 5 AM.
- Arrange for regular follow-up during long-term therapy.
- Arrange for periodic ophthalmologic exams to check for cataract development, and liver function studies q 4–6 wk during first 15 mo and then periodically.

Drug-specific teaching points
- Take drug in the evening.
- Know that the following side effects may occur: nausea (small frequent meals may

loxapine hydrochloride ■ 657

help), headache, muscle and joint aches and pains (these may lessen with time).
- Arrange to have periodic ophthalmic exams while you are on this drug.
- Report severe GI upset, changes in vision, unusual bleeding or bruising, dark urine, or light colored stools.

❐ loxapine hydrochloride

(lox' a peen)
Oral concentrate: Loxitane-C
IM injection: Loxitane

loxapine succinate
Oral capsules: Loxapac (CAN), Loxitane

Pregnancy Category C

Drug classes
Dopaminergic blocking drug
Antipsychotic drug

Therapeutic actions
Mechanism of action is not fully understood: antipsychotic drugs block postsynaptic dopamine receptors in the brain, but this may not be necessary and sufficient for antipsychotic activity.

Indications
- Management of manifestations of psychotic disorders

Contraindications/cautions
- Contraindicated in the presence of coma or severe CNS depression; bone marrow depression; blood dyscrasia; circulatory collapse; subcortical brain damage; Parkinson's disease; liver damage; cerebral arteriosclerosis; coronary disease; severe hypotension or hypertension.
- Use caution in the presence of respiratory disorders ("silent pneumonia" may develop); glaucoma, prostatic hypertrophy; epilepsy or history of epilepsy; breast cancer (elevations in prolactin may stimulate a prolactin-dependent tumor); thyrotoxicosis; peptic ulcer, decreased renal function; myelography within previous 24 h or myelography scheduled within 48 h; exposure to heat or phosphorus insecticides; pregnancy; and lactation.

Dosage
Adult
- *Oral:* Individualize dosage, and administer in divided doses bid to qid, initially 10 mg bid. Severely disturbed patients may need up to 50 mg/d. Increase dosage fairly rapidly over the first 7–10 d until symptoms are controlled. Usual dosage range is 60–100 mg/d; dosage greater than 250 mg/d is not recommended. Maintenance: reduce dosage to minimum compatible with symptom control. Usual range is 20–60 mg/d.
- *IM:* For prompt control of symptoms in acutely agitated patients, 12.5 to 50 mg q4–6h or longer, depending on response. Once symptoms are controlled (usually within 5 d), change to oral medication.

Pediatric: Not recommended for children < 16 y.
Geriatric: Use lower doses, and increase dosage more gradually than in younger patients.

Pharmacokinetics

Route	Onset	Peak	Duration
Oral	30 min	1.5–3 h	12 h
IM	Rapid		

Metabolism: Hepatic, $T_{1/2}$: 19 h
Distribution: Not known
Excretion: Urine

Adverse effects
- CNS: *Drowsiness*, insomnia, vertigo, headache, weakness, tremor, ataxia, slurring, cerebral edema, seizures, exacerbation of psychotic symptoms, extrapyramidal syndromes—*pseudoparkinsonism; dystonias; akathisia*, tardive dyskinesias, potentially irreversible, **neuroleptic malignant syndrome**
- CV: Hypotension, orthostatic hypotension, hypertension, tachycardia, bradycardia, cardiac arrest, CHF, cardiomeg-

Adverse effects in *Italics* are most common; those in **Bold** are life-threatening.

aly, **refractory arrhythmias** (some fatal), pulmonary edema
- **Respiratory:** Bronchospasm, laryngospasm, dyspnea; suppression of cough reflex and potential for aspiration
- **Hematologic:** Eosinophilia, leukopenia, leukocytosis, anemia; aplastic anemia; hemolytic anemia; thrombocytopenic, or nonthrombocytopenic purpura; pancytopenia
- **Autonomic:** Dry mouth, salivation, nasal congestion, nausea, vomiting, anorexia, fever, pallor, flushed facies, sweating, constipation, paralytic ileus, urinary retention, incontinence, polyuria, enuresis, priapism, ejaculation inhibition, male impotence
- **Endocrine:** Lactation, breast engorgement in females, galactorrhea; syndrome of inappropriate ADH secretion; amenorrhea, menstrual irregularities; gynecomastia in males; changes in libido; hyperglycemia or hypoglycemia; glycosuria; hyponatremia; pituitary tumor with hyperprolactinemia; inhibition of ovulation, infertility, pseudopregnancy; reduced urinary levels of gonadotropins, estrogens, progestins
- **Hypersensitivity:** Jaundice, urticaria, angioneurotic edema, laryngeal edema, photosensitivity, eczema, asthma, anaphylactoid reactions, exfoliative dermatitis

■ Nursing Considerations

Assessment
- *History:* Coma or severe CNS depression; blood dyscrasia; circulatory collapse; subcortical brain damage; Parkinson's disease; liver damage; cerebral arteriosclerosis; coronary disease; severe hypotension or hypertension; respiratory disorders; glaucoma, prostatic hypertrophy; epilepsy; breast cancer; thyrotoxicosis; peptic ulcer, decreased renal function; myelography within previous 24 h or myelography scheduled within 48 h; exposure to heat or phosphorus insecticides; pregnancy
- *Physical:* Body weight, temperature; reflexes, orientation, intraocular pressure; P, BP, orthostatic BP; R, adventitious sounds; bowel sounds and normal output, liver evaluation; urinary output, prostate size; CBC, urinalysis, thyroid, liver, and kidney function tests

Implementation
- Mix the oral concentrate with orange or grapefruit juice shortly before administration.
- Do not give *Loxitane IM* intravenously.
- Arrange for discontinuation of drug if serum creatinine or BUN become abnormal or if WBC count is depressed.
- Monitor elderly patients for dehydration, and institute remedial measures promptly; sedation and decreased sensation of thirst related to CNS effects of drug can lead to severe dehydration.
- Consult physician regarding appropriate warning of patient or patient's guardian about tardive dyskinesias.
- Consult physician about dosage reduction and use of anticholinergic antiparkinsonian drugs (controversial) if extrapyramidal effects occur.

Drug-specific teaching points
- Take drug exactly as prescribed.
- Avoid driving a car or engaging in other dangerous activities if CNS or vision changes occur.
- Avoid prolonged exposure to sun or use a sunscreen or covering garments if sensitivity to the sun occurs.
- Maintain fluid intake, and use precautions against heat stroke in hot weather.
- Report sore throat, fever, unusual bleeding or bruising, rash, weakness, tremors, impaired vision, dark urine, pale stools, and yellowing of the skin or eyes.

❒ lypressin

(lye press' in)

8-lysine vasopressin
Diapid

Pregnancy Category C

Adverse effects in *Italics* are most common; those in **Bold** are life-threatening.

lypressin

Drug classes
Hormonal agent

Therapeutic actions
Synthetic vasopressin analog with antidiuretic hormone activity and relatively little oxytocic or vasopressor activity; promotes resorption of water in the renal tubular epithelium.

Indications
- Control or prevention of symptoms and complications of neurogenic diabetes insipidus, especially in patients who are unresponsive to other therapy or sensitive to antidiuretic preparations of animal origin

Contraindications/cautions
- Contraindicated in the presence of allergy to lypression or antidiuretic hormone.
- Use caution in the presence of vascular disease (large doses can cause coronary vasoconstriction) and pregnancy.

Dosage
Administer 1–2 sprays to one or both nostrils whenever frequency of urination increases or significant thirst develops. Usual dosage is 1–2 sprays into each nostril qid. An additional bedtime dose helps to eliminate nocturia not controlled with regular daily dosage. If more drug is needed, decrease the interval between doses, not the number of sprays per dose (more than 2–3 sprays in each nostril is wasteful); drug will not be absorbed and will drain into the nasopharnyx and digestive tract and be digested.

Pharmacokinetics

Route	Onset	Peak	Duration
Intranasal	Prompt	30–120 min	3–8 h

Metabolism: Hepatic and renal, $T_{1/2}$: 15 min
Distribution: Crosses placenta; enters breast milk
Excretion: Urine

Adverse effects
- CNS: *Headache*, conjunctivitis, periorbital edema with itching
- GI: Heartburn secondary to excessive intranasal administration with drippage into the pharynx, abdominal cramps, diarrhea
- **Respiratory**: *Rhinorrhea, nasal congestion*, irritation and pruritus of the nasal passages, nasal ulceration, substernal tightness, coughing, transient dyspnea with inadvertent inhalation

Clinically important drug-drug interactions
- Possibly increased antidiuretic effect if taken concurrently with carbamazepine, chlorpropamide

■ Nursing Considerations

Assessment
- *History:* Allergy to lypression or antidiuretic hormone, vascular disease, pregnancy
- *Physical:* Nasal mucous membranes; P, BP, edema; R, adventitous sounds; bowel sounds, abdominal exam

Implementation
- Administer intranasally only: Hold bottle upright with patient in a vertical position with head upright; spray only 2 to 3 sprays at any given dose.
- Monitor therapeutic effects if patient has nasal congestion, allergic rhinitis, or upper respiratory infections; larger doses or adjunctive therapy may be needed because of decreased nasal absorption.
- Monitor condition of nasal passages during long-term therapy; inappropriate administration can lead to nasal ulcerations.
- Monitor patients with cardiovascular diseases carefully for cardiac reactions.

Drug-specific teaching points
- Learn proper administration technique for nasal use (see above). Watch patient administer drug, and review administration technique periodically with patient.
- Know that the following side effects may occur: GI cramping, passing of gas, diarrhea; nasal irritation (proper administration may decrease these problems).

Adverse effects in *Italics* are most common; those in **Bold** are life-threatening.

- Report drowsiness, listlessness, headache, shortness of breath, heartburn, abdominal cramps, severe nasal congestion or irritation.

☐ magaldrate

(mag' al drate)

hydroxymagnesium aluminate
Lowsium, Riopan

Pregnancy Category C

Drug classes
Antacid

Therapeutic actions
Neutralizes or reduces gastric acidity, resulting in an increase in the pH of the stomach and duodenal bulb and inhibiting the proteolytic activity of pepsin; the combination of magnesium (causes diarrhea when administered alone) and aluminum (constipating when administered alone) salts usually minimizes adverse GI effects.

Indications
- Symptomatic relief of upset stomach associated with hyperacidity
- Hyperacidity associated with peptic ulcer, gastritis, peptic esophagitis, gastric hyperacidity, and hiatal hernia

Contraindications/cautions
- Contraindicated in the presence of allergy to magnesium or aluminum products.
- Use caution in the presence of renal insufficiency, gastric outlet obstruction (aluminum salt may inhibit gastric emptying).

Dosage
Adult: 480–1,080 mg PO 1 and 3 h after meals and at bedtime.

Pharmacokinetics

Route	Onset	Peak
Oral	30 min	30–60 min

Not generally absorbed systemically.

Adverse effects
- **GI:** *Rebound hyperacidity*
- **Metabolic:** Decreased absorption of fluoride and accumulation of aluminum in serum, bone, CNS (aluminum may be neurotoxic), *alkalosis,* hypermagnesemia and toxicity in renal failure patients

Clinically important drug-drug interactions
- Do not administer other oral drugs within 1–2 h of antacid administration; change in gastric pH may interfere with absorption of oral drugs • Decreased pharmacologic effect of tetracyclines, penicillamine, nitrofurantoin • Decreased absorption and therapeutic effects of clindamycin and lincomycin if taken concurrently with magaldrate

■ Nursing Considerations

Assessment
- *History:* Allergy to magnesium or aluminum products, renal insufficiency, gastric outlet obstruction
- *Physical:* Bone and muscle strength; abdominal exam, bowel sounds; renal function tests, serum magnesium as appropriate

Implementation
- Do not administer oral drugs within 1–2 h of antacid administration.
- Have patient chew tablets thoroughly before swallowing; follow with a glass of water or milk.
- Administer drug between meals and at bedtime.
- Monitor patients on long-term therapy for signs of aluminum accumulation: bone pain, muscle weakness, malaise. Discontinue drug as needed.

Drug-specific teaching points
- Take between meals and at bedtime. If tablets are being used, chew thoroughly before swallowing, and follow with a glass of water.
- Do not take with any other oral medications; absorption of those medications can be inhibited. Take other oral medications at least 1–2 h after aluminum salt.

Adverse effects in *Italics* are most common; those in **Bold** are life-threatening.

- Report bone pain, muscle weakness, coffee ground vomitus, black tarry stools, no relief from symptoms being treated.

magnesium citrate

Citrate of Magnesia

magnesium hydroxide
magnesia, *Milk of Magnesia*

magnesium oxide
Maox, Mag-Ox, Uro-mag

Pregnancy Category C

Drug classes
Antacid
Laxative

Therapeutic actions
Antacid (magnesium hydroxide, magnesium oxide): neutralizes or reduces gastric acidity, resulting in an increase in the pH of the stomach and duodenal bulb and inhibition of the proteolytic activity of pepsin. Laxative (magnesium citrate, magnesium hydroxide): attracts/retains water in intestinal lumen and distends bowel; causes the duodenal secretion of cholecystokinin, which stimulates fluid secretion and intestinal motility.

Indications
- Symptomatic relief of upset stomach associated with hyperacidity
- Hyperacidity associated with peptic ulcer, gastritis, peptic esophagitis, gastric hyperacidity, and hiatal hernia
- Prophylaxis of GI bleeding, stress ulcers, aspiration pneumonia
- Short-term relief of constipation; evacuation of the colon for rectal and bowel examination

Contraindications/cautions
- Contraindicated in the presence of allergy to magnesium products.
- Use caution in the presence of renal insufficiency.

Dosage
Adult
- ***Magnesium citrate:*** 1 glassful (240 ml) PO as needed.
- ***Magnesium hydroxide:*** Antacid: 5–15 ml liquid or 650 mg to 1.3 g tablets PO qid (adult and children older than 12 y). Laxative: 15–60 ml PO taken with liquid.
- ***Magnesium oxide:*** Capsules: 280 mg–1.5 g PO taken with water or milk, qid. Tablets: 400–820 mg/d PO.

Pediatric
- ***Magnesium citrate:*** Half the adult dose; repeat as needed.
- ***Magnesium hydroxide as laxative:*** One-fourth to one-half the adult dose, depending on age.

Pharmacokinetics

Onset

3–6 h
Minimally absorbed systemically

Excretion: Renal

Adverse effects
- **CNS:** Dizziness, fainting, sweating
- **GI:** *Diarrhea, nausea, perianal irritation*
- **Metabolic:** Hypermagnesemia and toxicity in renal failure patients

Clinically important drug-drug interactions
- Do not administer other oral drugs within 1–2h of antacid administration; change in gastric pH may interfere with absorption of oral drugs • Decreased pharmacologic effect of tetracyclines, penicillamine, nitrofurantoin

■ Nursing Considerations

Assessment
- *History:* Allergy to magnesium products; renal insufficiency
- *Physical:* Abdominal exam, bowel sounds; renal function tests, serum magnesium

Implementation
- Do not administer oral drugs within 1–2 h of antacid administration.

Adverse effects in *Italics* are most common; those in **Bold** are life-threatening.

- Have patient chew antacid tablets thoroughly before swallowing; follow with a glass of water.
- Administer antacid between meals and at bedtime.

Drug-specific teaching points
- Take antacid between meals and at bedtime. If tablets are being used, chew thoroughly before swallowing, and follow with a glass of water.
- Do not use laxatives in the presence of abdominal pain, nausea, or vomiting.
- Refrigerate magnesium citrate solutions to retain potency and increase palatability.
- Do not take with any other oral medications; absorption of those medications can be inhibited. Take other oral medications at least 1–2 h after aluminum salt.
- Know that diarrhea may occur with antacid therapy.
- Know that the following side effects may occur as a result of laxative therapy: excessive bowel activity, gripping, diarrhea, nausea, dizziness (ensure ready access to bathroom facilities; exercise precaution not to fall).
- Do not use laxatives chronically. Prolonged or excessive use can lead to serious problems. You should increase your intake of water (6–8 glasses/d) and fiber, and exercise regularly.
- Report: Antacid use—diarrhea; coffee ground vomitus; black, tarry stools; no relief from symptoms being treated. Report: Laxative use—rectal bleeding, muscle cramps or pain, weakness, dizziness (not related to abdominal cramps and bowel movement), unrelieved constipation.

☐ magnesium sulfate

*(mag **nee'** zhum)*

epsom salt granules

Pregnancy Category A

Drug classes
Electrolyte
Anticonvulsant
Laxative

Therapeutic actions
Cofactor of many enzyme systems involved in neurochemical transmission and muscular excitability; prevents or controls convulsions by blocking neuromuscular transmission; attracts/retains water in the intestinal lumen and distends the bowel to promote mass movement and relieve constipation.

Indications
- Hypomagnesemia, replacement therapy (IV)
- Toxemia/eclampsia/nephritis (IV, IM)
- Short-term treatment of constipation (PO)
- Evacuation of the colon for rectal and bowel examinations (PO)
- Unlabeled use: inhibition of premature labor (parenteral)

Contraindications/cautions
- Contraindicated in the presence of allergy to magnesium products; heart block, myocardial damage; abdominal pain, nausea, vomiting or other symptoms of appendicitis; acute surgical abdomen, fecal impaction, intestinal and biliary tract obstruction, hepatitis. Do not give during 2 h preceding delivery because of risk of magnesium toxicity in the neonate.
- Use caution in the presence of renal insufficiency.

Dosage
Adult
- ***Hyperalimentation:*** 8–24 mEq/d IV.
- ***Mild magnesium deficiency:*** 1 g IM q6h for four doses (32.5 mEq/24 h).
- ***Severe hypomagnesemia:*** Up to 2 mEq/kg IM within 4 h or 5 g (40 mEq)/1,000 ml D_5W IV infused over 3 h.
- ***Toxemia/eclampsia/nephritis***
  - *IM:* 4–5 g of a 50% solution q4h as necessary.
  - *IV:* 1–4 g of a 10%–20% solution. Do not exceed 1.5 ml/min of a 10% solution.
  - *IV infusion:* 4–5 g in 250 ml of 5% dextrose. Do not exceed 3 ml/min.
- ***Laxative:*** 10–15 g PO epsom salt in glass of water.

magnesium sulfate ■ 663

Pediatric
- ***Hyperalimentation (infants):*** 2–10 mEq/d IV.
- ***Anticonvulsant:*** 20–40 mg/kg in a 20% solution, IM. Repeat as necessary.
- ***Laxative:*** 5–10 g PO epsom salt in glass of water.

Pharmacokinetics

Route	Onset	Peak
IV	Immediate	30 min
IM	60 min	3–4 h
PO	1–2 h	3–4 h

Metabolism: T$_{1/2}$: unknown
Distribution: Crosses placenta, enters breast milk
Excretion: Urine

IV facts
Preparation: Dilute IV infusion to a concentration of 20% or less prior to IV administration; dilute 4–5 g in 250 ml D$_5$W or Sodium Chloride Solution.
Infusion: Do not exceed 1.5 ml of a 10% solution per minute IV or 3 ml/min IV infusion.

Adverse effects
- CNS: *Weakness, dizziness,* fainting, sweating (PO)
- GI: *Excessive bowel activity, perianal irritation* (PO)
- CV: Palpitations (PO)
- Metabolic: *Magnesium intoxication* (flushing, sweating, hypotension, depressed relfexes, flaccid paralysis,hypothermia, circulatory collapse, cardiac and CNS depression—parenteral); hypocalcemia with tetany (secondary to treatment of eclampsia—parenteral)

Clinically important drug-drug interactions
- Potentiation of neuromuscular blockade produced by nondepolarizing neuromuscular relaxants (tubocurarine, atracurium, gallamine, metocurine iodide, pancuronium, vecuronium)

■ Nursing Considerations
Assessment
- *History:* Allergy to magnesium products; renal insufficiency; heart block, myocardial damage; symptoms of appendicitis; acute surgical abdomen, fecal impaction, intestinal and biliary tract obstruction, hepatitis
- *Physical:* Skin—color, texture; muscle tone; body temperature; orientation, affect, reflexes, peripheral sensation; P, auscultation, BP, rhythm strip; abdominal exam, bowel sounds; renal function tests, serum magnesium and calcium, liver function tests (oral use)

Implementation
- Reserve IV use in eclampsia for immediate life threatening situations.
- Administer IM route by deep IM injection of the undiluted (50%) solution for adults; dilute to a 20% solution for children.
- Monitor serum magnesium levels during parenteral therapy. Arrange to discontinue administration as soon as levels are within normal limits (1.5–3 mEq/L) and desired clinical response is obtained.
- Monitor knee-jerk reflex before repeated parenteral administration. If knee-jerk reflexes are suppressed, do not administer magnesium because respiratory center failure may occur.
- Administer oral magnesium sulfate as a laxative only as a temporary measure. Arrange for appropriate dietary measures (fiber, fluids) and exercise, environmental control to encourage return to normal bowel activity.
- Do not administer oral magnesium sulfate in presence of abdominal pain, nausea, vomiting.
- Monitor bowel function; if diarrhea and cramping occur, discontinue oral drug.
- Maintain urine output at a level of 100 ml q4h during parenteral administration.

Drug-specific teaching points
- Use only as a temporary measure to relieve constipation. Do not take if ab-

Adverse effects in *Italics* are most common; those in **Bold** are life-threatening.

dominal pain, nausea, or vomiting occur.
- Know that the following side effects may occur: diarrhea (discontinue drug and consult physician or nurse—oral use).
- Report sweating, flushing, muscle tremors, or twitching, inability to move extremities.

mannitol

(man' i tole)

Osmitrol, Resectisol (urinary irrigant)

Pregnancy Category C

Drug classes
Osmotic diuretic
Diagnostic Agent
Urinary Irrigant

Therapeutic actions
Elevates the osmolarity of the glomerular filtrate, thereby hindering the reabsorption of water and leading to a loss of water, sodium, chloride (used for diagnosis of glomerular filtration rate); creates an osmotic gradient in the eye between plasma and ocular fluids, thereby reducing intraocular pressure; creates an osmotic effect, leading to decreased swelling in posttransurethral prostatic resection.

Indications
- Prevention and treatment of the oliguric phase of renal failure
- Reduction of intracranial pressure and treatment of cerebral edema; of elevated intraocular pressure when the pressure cannot be lowered by other means
- Promotion of the urinary excretion of toxic substances
- Measurement of glomerular filtration rate (diagnostic use)
- Irrigant in transurethral prostatic resection or other transurethral procedures

Contraindications/cautions
- Anuria due to severe renal disease, pulmonary congestion, active intracranial bleeding (except during craniotomy), dehydration, renal disease, CHF

Dosage
Adult: IV infusion only; individualize concentration and rate of administration. Dosage is 50–200 g/d. Adjust dosage to maintain urine flow of 30–50 ml/h.
- ***Prevention of oliguria:*** 50–100 g IV as a 5%–25% solution.
- ***Treatment of oliguria:*** 50–100 g IV of a 15%–25% solution.
- ***Reduction of intracranial pressure and brain mass:*** 1.5–2 g/kg IV as a 15%–25% solution over 30–60 min. Evidence of reduced pressure should be seen in 15 min.
- ***Reduction of intraocular pressure:*** Infuse 1.5–2 g/kg IV as a 25% solution, 20% solution, or 15% solution over 30 min. If used preoperatively, use 1–1$\frac{1}{2}$ h before surgery.
- ***Adjunctive therapy to promote diuresis in intoxications:*** Maximum of 200 g IV of mannitol with other fluids and electrolytes.
- ***Measurement of glomerular filtration rate:*** Dilute 100 ml of a 20% solution with 180 ml of sodium chloride injection. Infuse this 280 ml of 7.2% solution IV at a rate of 20 ml/min. Collect urine with a catheter for the specified time for measurement of mannitol excreted in mg/min. Draw blood at the start and at the end of the time for measurement of mannitol in mg/ml plasma.
- ***Test dose of mannitol:*** Infuse 0.2 g/kg IV (about 60 ml of a 25% solution, 75 ml of a 20% solution, or 100 ml of a 15% solution) in 3–5 min to produce a urine flow of 30–50 ml/h. If urine flow does not increase, repeat dose. If no response to second dose, reevaluate patient situation.

Urologic irrigation: Add contents of two 50-ml vials (25%) to 900 ml sterile water for injection; irrigate as needed.
Pediatric: Dosage for children younger than 12 y not established.

Pharmacokinetics
Metabolism: $T_{1/2}$: 15–100 min

maprotiline hydrochloride ■ 665

Distribution: Crosses placenta; may enter breast milk
Excretion: Urine

Route	Onset	Peak	Duration
IV	30–60 min	1 h	6–8 h
Irrigant	Rapid	Rapid	Short

IV facts
Preparation: Prepare as listed under each indication.
Infusion: Infuse as rates listed under each indication.

Adverse effects
- CNS: *Dizziness,* headache, blurred vision, convulsion
- GI: *Nausea, anorexia, dry mouth, thirst*
- CV: Hypotension, hypertension, edema, thrombophlebitis, tachycardia, chest pain
- **Respiratory:** Pulmonary congestion, rhinitis
- **Hematologic:** Fluid and electrolyte imbalances
- GU: *Diuresis,* urinary retention
- **Dermatologic:** Uriticaria, skin necrosis

■ Nursing Considerations

Assessment
- *History:* Pulmonary congestion, active intracranial bleeding, dehydration, renal disease, CHF
- *Physical:* Skin color, lesions, edema, hydration; orientation, reflexes, muscle strength, pupils; pulses, BP, perfusion; R, pattern, adventitious sounds; urinary output patterns; CBC, serum electrolytes, urinalysis, renal function tests

Implementation
- Do not give electrolyte-free mannitol with blood. If blood must be given, add at least 20 mEq of sodium chloride to each liter of mannitol solution.
- Do not expose solutions to low temperatures; crystallization may occur. If crystals are seen, warm the bottle in a hot water bath, then cool to body temperature before administering.
- Make sure the infusion set contains a filter if giving concentrated mannitol.
- Monitor serum electrolytes periodically with prolonged therapy.

Drug-specific teaching points
- Know that the following side effects may occur: increased urination; GI upset (small, frequent meals may help); dry mouth (sugarless lozenges to suck may help this problem); headache, blurred vision (use caution when moving around, ask for assistance).
- Report difficulty breathing, pain at the IV site, chest pain.

❒ maprotiline hydrochloride

(ma proe' ti leen)
Ludiomil

Pregnancy Category B

Drug classes
Antidepressant (tetracyclic)

Therapeutic actions
Mechanism of action unknown; appears to act similarly to the tricyclic antidepressants (TCAs); the TCAs act to inhibit the presynaptic reuptake of the neurotransmitters norepinephrine and serotonin; anticholinergic at CNS and peripheral receptors; sedating; the relation of these effects to clinical efficacy is unknown.

Indications
- Relief of symptoms of depression (endogenous depression most responsive)
- Treatment of depression in patients with manic-depressive illness
- Treatment of anxiety associated with depression

Contraindications/cautions
- Contraindicated in the presence of hypersensitivity to any tricyclic drug, concomitant therapy with an MAO inhibitor, recent MI, myelography within previous 24 h or scheduled within 48 h, pregnancy

Adverse effects in *Italics* are most common; those in **Bold** are life-threatening.

(limb reduction abnormalities reported), lactation.
- Use caution in the presence of electroshock therapy; preexisting cardiovascular disorders (possibly increased risk of serious CVS toxicity with TCAs); angle-closure glaucoma, increased intraocular pressure, urinary retention, ureteral or urethral spasm; seizure disorders (TCAs lower the seizure threshold); hyperthyroidism (predisposes to CVS toxicity, including cardiac arrhythmias); impaired hepatic, renal function; psychiatric patients (schizophrenic or paranoid patients may exhibit a worsening of psychosis with TCA therapy); manic-depressive patients (may shift to hypomanic or manic phase); elective surgery (TCAs should be discontinued as long as possible before surgery).

Dosage
Adult
- ***Mild to moderate depression:*** Initially, 75 mg/d PO in outpatients. Maintain initial dosage for 2 wk because of long drug half-life. Dosage may then be increased gradually in 25-mg increments. Most patients respond to 150 mg/d, but some may require 225 mg/d.
- ***More severe depression:*** Initially, 100–150 mg/d PO in hospitalized patients. If needed, may gradually increase to 300 mg/d.
- ***Maintenance:*** Reduce dosage to lowest effective level, usually 75–150 mg/d PO.

Pediatric: Not recommended in children younger than 18 y.
Geriatric: Give lower doses to patients older than 60 y; use 50–75 mg/d PO for maintenance.

Pharmacokinetics

Route	Onset	Peak	Duration
Oral	Slow	2–4 h	2–4 wk

Metabolism: Hepatic, $T_{1/2}$: 51 h
Distribution: Crosses placenta; enters breast milk
Excretion: Urine and feces

Adverse effects
- **CNS:** *Sedation and anticholinergic (atropine-like) effects; confusion* (especially in elderly), *disturbed concentration,* hallucinations, disorientation, decreased memory, feelings of unreality, delusions, anxiety, nervousness, restlessness, agitation, panic, insomnia, nightmares, hypomania, mania, exacerbation of psychosis, drowsiness, weakness, fatigue, headache, numbness, tingling, paresthesias of extremities, incoordination, motor hyperactivity, akathisia, ataxia, tremors, peripheral neuropathy, extrapyramidal symptoms, *seizures,* speech blockage, dysarthria, tinnitus, altered EEG
- **GI:** *Dry mouth, constipation,* paralytic ileus, *nausea,* vomiting, anorexia, epigastric distress, diarrhea, flatulence, dysphagia, peculiar taste, increased salivation, stomatitis, glossitis, parotid swelling, abdominal cramps, black tongue, hepatitis, jaundice (rare), elevated transaminase, altered alkaline phosphatase
- **CV:** *Orthostatic hypotension,* hypertension, syncope, tachycardia, palpitations, MI, arrhythmias, heart block, precipitation of CHF, stroke
- **Hematologic:** Bone marrow depression, eosinophila, purpura, thrombocytopenia, leukopenia
- **GU:** Urinary retention, delayed micturition, dilation of the urinary tract, gynecomastia, testicular swelling in men; breast enlargement, menstrual irregularity and galactorrhea in women; increased or decreased libido; impotence
- **Hypersensitivity:** Skin rash, pruritus, vasculitis, petechiae, photosensitization, edema
- **Endocrine:** Elevated or depressed blood sugar, elevated prolactin levels, inappropriate ADH secretion
- **Withdrawal:** Symptoms with abrupt discontinuation of prolonged therapy: nausea, headache, vertigo, nightmares, malaise

Adverse effects in *Italics* are most common; those in **Bold** are life-threatening.

- **Other:** Nasal congestion, excessive appetite, weight gain or loss; sweating (paradoxical effect in a drug with prominent anticholinergic effects), alopecia, lacrimation, hyperthermia, flushing, chills

Nursing Considerations
Assessment
- *History:* Hypersensitivity to any tricyclic drug; concomitant therapy with an MAO inhibitor; recent MI; myelography within previous 24 h or scheduled within 48 h; lactation; electroshock therapy; preexisting cardiovascular disorders; angle-closure glaucoma, increased intraocular pressure, urinary retention, ureteral or urethral spasm; seizure disorders; hyperthyroidism; impaired hepatic, renal function; psychiatric problems; manic-depressive patients; elective surgery
- *Physical:* Body weight; temperature; skin—color, lesions; orientation, affect, reflexes, vision and hearing; P, BP, orthostatic BP, perfusion; bowel sounds, normal output, liver evaluation; urine flow, normal output; usual sexual function, frequency of menses, breast and scrotal examination; liver function tests, urinalysis, CBC, ECG

Implementation
- Ensure that depressed and potentially suicidal patients have access to only limited quantities of the drug.
- Expect clinical response in 3–7 d up to 2–3 wk (the latter is more usual).
- Administer major portion of dose at bedtime if drowsiness, severe anticholinergic effects occur.
- Arrange to reduce dosage if minor side effects develop; arrange to discontinue the drug if serious side effects occur.
- Arrange for CBC if patient develops fever, sore throat, or other sign of infection during therapy.

Drug-specific teaching points
- Take drug exactly as prescribed, and do not to stop taking this drug abruptly or without consulting the physician or nurse.
- Avoid alcohol, other sleep-inducing drugs, OTC drugs while on this drug.
- Avoid prolonged exposure to sunlight or sunlamps, and use a sunscreen or protective garments if long exposure to sunlight is unavoidable.
- Know that the following side effects may occur: headache, dizziness, drowsiness, weakness, blurred vision (these effects are reversible; safety measures may need to be taken if these become severe, and you should avoid driving an automobile or performing tasks that require alertness while these persist); nausea, vomiting, loss of appetite, dry mouth (small frequent meals, frequent mouth care and sucking sugarless candies may help); nightmares, inability to concentrate, confusion; changes in sexual function.
- Report dry mouth, difficulty in urination, excessive sedation

☐ mebendazole
*(me **ben'** da zole)*
Vermox

Pregnancy Category C

Drug classes
Anthelmintic

Therapeutic actions
Irreversibly blocks glucose uptake by susceptible helminths, depleting glycogen stores needed for survival and reproduction of the helminths, causing death.

Indications
- Treatment of *Trichuris trichiura* (whipworm), *Enterobius vermicularis* (pinworm), *Ascaris lumbricoides* (roundworm), *Ancylostoma duodenale* (common hookworm), *Necator americanus* (American hookworm)

Contraindications/cautions
- Allergy to mebendazole, pregnancy (embryotoxic and teratogenic in preclinical studies; avoid use in pregnancy, especially during first trimester), lactation.

Adverse effects in *Italics* are most common; those in **Bold** are life-threatening.

mecamylamine hydrochloride

Dosage
Adult
- **Trichuriasis, ascariasis, hookworm infections:** 1 tablet PO morning and evening on 3 consecutive d.
- **Enterobiasis:** 1 tablet given once PO. If patient is not cured 3 wk after treatment, a second treatment course is advised.

Pediatric: Safety and efficacy for use in children younger than 2 y not established.

Pharmacokinetics

Route	Onset	Peak
Oral	Slow	2–4 h

Metabolism: Hepatic, $T_{1/2}$: $2\frac{1}{2}$–9 h
Distribution: Crosses placenta; may enter breast milk
Excretion: Feces and urine

Adverse effects
- **GI:** *Transient abdominal pain, diarrhea*
- **General:** Fever

■ Nursing Considerations

Assessment
- *History:* Allergy to mebendazole, pregnancy, lactation
- *Physical:* Temperature; bowel sounds, output

Implementation
- Culture for ova and parasites.
- Administer drug with food; tablets may be chewed, swallowed whole, or crushed and mixed with food if desired.
- Arrange for second course of treatment if patient is not cured 3 wk after treatment.
- Arrange for treatment of all family members when pinworm infestation is involved.
- Arrange for disinfection of toilet facilities after patient use (pinworms).
- Arrange for daily laundry of bed linens, towels, nightclothes, and undergarments (pinworms).

Drug-specific teaching points
- Chew or swallow whole or crushed and mixed with food.
- Be aware that pinworms are easily transmitted; all family members should be treated for complete eradication.
- Use strict handwashing and hygiene measures. Launder undergarments, bedlinens, nightclothes daily. Disinfect toilet facilities daily and bathroom floors periodically (pinworms).
- Know that the following side effects may occur: nausea, abdominal pain, diarrhea (small, frequent meals may help).
- Report fever, return of symptoms, severe diarrhea.

☐ mecamylamine hydrochloride

*(mek a **mill'** a meen)*
Inversine
Pregnancy Category C

Drug classes
Antihypertensive drug
Ganglionic blocker

Therapeutic actions
Occupies cholinergic receptors of autonomic postganglionic neurons, blocking the effects of acetylcholine released from preganglionic nerve terminals, decreasing the effects of the sympathetic (and parasympathetic) nervous systems on effector organs; reduces sympathetic tone on the vasculature, causing vasodilation and decreased BP; decreases sympathetic impulses to the heart; and decreases the release of catecholamines from the adrenal medulla.

Indications
- Moderately severe to severe hypertension
- Uncomplicated malignant hypertension

Contraindications/cautions
- Contraindicated in the presence of hypersensitivity to mecamylamine; coronary insufficiency, recent MI; uncooperative patients; uremia; chronic pyelonephritis when patient is receiving antibiotics and

sulfonamides; glaucoma; organic pyloric stenosis; lactation.
- Use caution in the presence of prostatic hypertrophy, bladder neck obstruction, urethral stricture (urinary retention, which may be more serious in patients with these disorders); cerebral or renal insufficiency; high ambient temperature, fever, infection, hemorrhage, surgery, vigorous exercise, salt depletion resulting from diminished intake or increased excretion due to diarrhea, vomiting, sweating or diuretics; pregnancy.

Dosage
Adult: Initially 2.5 mg PO bid. Adjust dosage in increments of 2.5 mg at intervals of not less than 2 d until the desired BP response occurs (a dosage just under that which causes signs of mild postural hypotension). Average total daily dosage is 25 mg, usually in three divided doses. Partial tolerance may develop, necessitating increased dosage. When given with other antihypertensives, reduce the dosage of the other agents and that of mecamylamine; however, continue thiazides at usual dosage while decreasing mecamylamine dosage by at least 50%.

Pharmacokinetics

Route	Onset	Peak	Duration
Oral	½–2 h	3–5 h	6–12 h

Metabolism: $T_{1/2}$: 4–6 h
Distribution: Crosses placenta; enters breast milk
Excretion: Urine

Adverse effects
- CNS: Syncope, paresthesia, *weakness, fatigue, sedation,* dilated pupils and blurred vision, tremor, choreiform movements, mental aberrations, convulsions
- GI: *Anorexia, dry mouth, glossitis, nausea,* vomiting, constipation and ileus
- CV: *Orthostatic hypotension* and dizziness
- Respiratory: Interstitial pulmonary edema and fibrosis
- GU: *Decreased libido, impotence, urinary retention*

■ Nursing Considerations
Assessment
- *History:* Hypersensitivity to mecamylamine; coronary insufficiency, recent MI; uremia; chronic pyelonephritis; glaucoma; organic pyloric stenosis; prostatic hypertrophy, bladder neck obstruction, urethral stricture; cerebral or renal insufficiency; high ambient temperature, fever, infection, hemorrhage, surgery, vigorous exercise, salt depletion, vomiting, sweating, or diuretics; lactation
- *Physical:* Body temperature; orientation, affect, reflexes; ophthalmic exam, including tonometry; P, BP, orthostatic BP, supine BP, perfusion, edema, auscultation; bowel sounds, normal output; normal urinary output, voiding pattern, prostate palpation; renal, hepatic function tests

Implementation
- Administer drug after meals for more gradual absorption and smoother control of blood pressure; timing of doses with regard to meals should be consistent.
- Consider giving larger doses at noontime and in the evening rather than in the morning; the response is greater in the morning. The morning dose should be relatively small or may be omitted, based on the adequacy of patient's BP response, whether there are symptoms of faintness, lightheadedness.
- Determine the initial and maintenance dosage by BP readings in the erect position at the time of maximal drug effect and by other signs and symptoms of orthostatic hypotension.
- Arrange to discontinue drug gradually, substituting another antihypertensive drug as mecamylamine is withdrawn. Abrupt discontinuation of mecamylamine in patients with malignant hypertension may cause return of hypertension and fatal cerebral vascular accidents or acute CHF.

Adverse effects in *Italics* are most common; those in **Bold** are life-threatening.

- Arrange to decrease dosage in the presence of fever, infection, salt depletion, which decrease drug requirements.
- Monitor patient for orthostatic hypotension, which is most marked in the morning and is accentuated by hot weather, alcohol, exercise.
- Ensure adequate salt intake, especially when factors that predispose to sodium loss are present.
- Monitor bowel function carefully; paralytic ileus has occurred. Constipation may be prevented by giving pilocarpine or neostigmine with each dose. Treat constipation with *Milk of Magnesia* or similar laxative; do not use bulk laxatives.
- Discontinue drug immediately, and arrange for remedial steps at the first signs of paralytic ileus: frequent loose bowel movements with abdominal distention and decreased borborygmi.

Drug-specific teaching points
- Take drug after meals and in a consistent relation to meals. Do not stop taking this drug without consulting your nurse or physician.
- Learn, with a significant other if possible, to monitor your blood pressure, and check your blood pressure frequently for the safest, most efficacious therapy (if this is possible, patient may be given instructions to reduce or omit a dose if readings fall below a designated level or if faintness or lightheadedness occurs).
- Ensure an adequate intake of salt, especially in hot weather, if you are exercising a lot, or if you are sweating excessively.
- Know that the following side effects may occur: dizziness, weakness (these are more likely to occur when you change position, in the early morning, after exercise, in hot weather, and when you have consumed alcohol; some tolerance may occur after you have taken the drug for a while; avoid driving a car or engaging in tasks that require alertness while you are experiencing these symptoms, and remember to change position slowly; use caution in climbing stairs); blurred vision, dilated pupils, sensitivity to bright light (a different eyeglass prescription, wearing sunglasses in bright light may help); constipation (it may be necessary for you to take a laxative or GI stimulant while you are taking mecamylamine); dry mouth (sucking sugarless lozenges, ice chips may help); GI upset (frequent, small meals may help); impotence, decreased libido.
- Report tremor, seizure, frequent dizziness or fainting, severe or persistent constipation, or frequent loose stools with abdominal distention.

▢ mechlorethamine hydrochloride

(me klor eth' a meen)

HN_2, nitrogen mustard
Mustargen

Pregnancy Category D

Drug classes
Alkylating agent, nitrogen mustard
Antineoplastic drug

Therapeutic actions
Cytotoxic: reacts chemically with DNA, RNA, other proteins to prevent replication and function of susceptible cells, causing cell death; cell cycle nonspecific.

Indications
- Palliative treatment of Hodgkin's disease, lymphosarcoma, chronic myelocytic or chronic lymphocytic leukemia, polycythemia vera, mycosis fungoides, bronchogenic carcinoma (IV use)
- Palliative treatment of effusion secondary to metastatic carcinoma (intrapleural, intraperitoneal, intrapericardial use)
- Unlabeled use: topical treatment of cutaneous mycosis fungoides

Contraindications/cautions
- Contraindicated in the presence of allergy to mechlorethamine, infectious disease, pregnancy, lactation.
- Use caution in the presence of amyloidosis, hematopoietic depression,

mechlorethamine hydrochloride

chronic lymphatic leukemia, concomitant steroid therapy.

Dosage
Individualize dosage based on hematologic profile and response.
Adult: Usual dose: total of 0.4 mg/kg IV for each course of therapy as a single dose *or* in two to four divided doses of 0.1–0.2 mg/kg per day. Give preferably at night in case sedation is required for side effects. Interval between courses of therapy is usually 3–6 wk.
- *Intracavitary administration:* Dose and preparation vary considerably with cavity and disease being treated: consult manufacturer's label.

Pharmacokinetics

Route	Onset	Peak	Duration
IV	Immediate	Seconds	Minutes

Metabolism: $T_{1/2}$: minutes
Distribution: Crosses placenta; may enter breast milk
Excretion: Urine

IV facts
Preparations: Reconstitute vial with 10 ml of Sterile Water for Injection or Sodium Chloride Injection; resultant solution contains 1 mg/ml of mechlorethamine HCl. Prepare solution immediately before use; decomposes on standing.
Infusion: Inject into tubing of a flowing IV infusion.

Adverse effects
- CNS: *Weakness, vertigo,* tinnitus, diminished hearing
- Local: *Vesicant thrombosis, thrombophlebitis,* tissue necrosis if extravasation occurs
- GI: *Nausea, vomiting, anorexia,* diarrhea, jaundice
- Hematologic: **Bone marrow depression,** immunosuppression, hyperuricemia
- GU: *Impaired fertility*
- Dermatologic: Maculopapular skin rash, alopecia (infrequently)

■ Nursing Considerations

Assessment
- *History:* Allergy to mechlorethamine, infectious disease, amyloidosis, hematopoietic depression, chronic lymphatic leukemia, concomitant steroid therapy, pregnancy, lactation
- *Physical:* Temperature; weight; skin—color, lesions; injection site; orientation, reflexes, hearing evaluation; CBC, differential, uric acid

Implementation
- Arrange for blood tests to evaluate hematopoietic function before beginning therapy and periodically during therapy.
- Use caution when preparing drug for administration; use rubber gloves for handling drug; drug is highly toxic and a vesicant. Avoid inhalation of dust or vapors and contact with skin or mucous membranes (especially the eyes). If eye contact occurs, immediately irrigate with copious amount of ophthalmic irrigating solution, and obtain an ophthalmologic consultation. If skin contact occurs, irrigate with copious amount of water for 15 min, followed by application of 2% sodium thiosulfate.
- *Use caution when determining correct amount of drug for injection.* The margin of safety is very small; double check dosage before administration.
- Monitor injection site for any sign of extravasation. Painful inflammation and induration or sloughing of skin may occur. If leakage is noted, promptly infiltrate with sterile isotonic sodium thiosulfate ($1/6$ molar), and apply an ice compress for 6–12 h. Notify physician.
- Consult physician for premedication with antiemetics or sedatives to prevent severe nausea and vomiting. Administration at night also may help alleviate this problem.
- Ensure that patient is well hydrated before treatment.

Adverse effects in *Italics* are most common; those in **Bold** are life-threatening.

- Monitor uric acid levels; ensure adequate fluid intake, and prepare for appropriate treatment if hyperuricemia occurs.

Drug-specific teaching points
- Be aware that this drug must be given IV or directly into a body cavity.
- Know that the following side effects may occur: nausea, vomiting, loss of appetite (an antiemetic or sedative may be ordered to help alleviate this problem; the drug may be given at night; it is important that you try to maintain your fluid intake and nutrition while on this drug); weakness, dizziness, ringing in the ears or loss of hearing (use special precautions to avoid injury); infertility, from irregular menses to complete amenorrhea; men may stop producing sperm (this may be an irreversible problem).
- Use birth control measures while you are taking this drug. This drug cannot be taken during pregnancy; serious fetal effects can occur. If you think you are pregnant or wish to become pregnant, consult your prescriber.
- Report pain, burning at IV site, severe GI distress, sore throat, rash, joint pain.

▢ meclizine hydrochloride

(mek' li zeen)
Bonamine (CAN), Bonine, Dizmiss

Oral prescription tablets:
Antivert, Antrizine, Ru-Vert M

Pregnancy Category B

Drug classes
Antiemetic
Anti-motion sickness drug
Antihistamine
Anticholinergic drug

Therapeutic actions
Reduces sensitivity of the labyrinthine apparatus; probably acts at least partly by blocking cholinergic synapses in the vomiting center, which receives input from the chemoreceptor trigger zone and from peripheral nerve pathways; peripheral anticholinergic effects may contribute to efficacy.

Indications
- Prevention and treatment of nausea, vomiting, motion sickness
- "Possibly effective" for the management of vertigo associated with diseases affecting the vestibular system

Contraindications/cautions
- Contraindicated in the presence of allergy to meclizine or cyclizine, pregnancy.
- Use caution in the presence of lactation, narrow-angle glaucoma, stenosing peptic ulcer, symptomatic prostatic hypertrophy, bronchial asthma, bladder neck obstruction, pyloroduodenal obstruction, cardiac arrhythmias, postoperative state (hypotensive effects of drug may be confusing and dangerous).

Dosage
Adult
- ***Motion sickness:*** 25–50 mg PO 1 h prior to travel. May repeat dose every 24 h for the duration of the journey.
- ***Vertigo:*** 25–100 mg PO daily in divided doses.

Pediatric: Not recommended for use in children younger than 12 y.
Geriatric: More likely to cause dizziness, sedation, syncope, toxic confusional states and hypotension in elderly patients; use with caution.

Pharmacokinetics

Route	Onset	Peak	Duration
Oral	1 h	1–2 h	12–24 h

Metabolism: $T_{1/2}$: 6 h
Distribution: Crosses placenta; may enter breast milk
Excretion: Feces

Adverse effects
- CNS: *Drowsiness, confusion,* euphoria, nervousness, restlessness, insomnia and excitement, convulsions, vertigo, tinni-

tus, blurred vision, diplopia, auditory and visual hallucinations
- GI: *Dry mouth, anorexia, nausea,* vomiting, diarrhea or constipation
- CV: Hypotension, palpitations, tachycardia
- Respiratory: **Respiratory depression, death** (overdose, especially in young children), dry nose and throat
- GU: *Urinary frequency, difficult urination,* urinary retention
- Dermatologic: Urticaria, drug rash

■ Nursing Considerations

Assessment
- *History:* Allergy to meclizine or cyclizine, pregnancy, narrow-angle glaucoma, stenosing peptic ulcer, symptomatic prostatic hypertrophy, bronchial asthma, bladder neck obstruction, pyloroduodenal obstruction, cardiac arrhythmias, postoperative patients, lactation
- *Physical:* Skin—color, lesions, texture; orientation, reflexes, affect; ophthalmic exam; P, BP; R, adventitious sounds; bowel sounds, normal output, status of mucous membranes; prostate palpation, normal output

Implementation
- Monitor I&O, and take appropriate measures if urinary retention becomes a problem.

Drug-specific teaching points
- Take as prescribed. Avoid excessive dosage. Chew the chewable tablets carefully before swallowing.
- Be aware that anti-motion sickness drugs work best if used prophylactically.
- Know that the following side effects may occur: dizziness, sedation, drowsiness (use caution if driving or performing tasks that require alertness if these occur); epigastric distress, diarrhea, or constipation (taking the drug with food may help); dry mouth (frequent mouth care, sucking sugarless lozenges may help); dryness of nasal mucosa (another type of motion sickness, antivertigo remedy may be available).

- Avoid alcohol while taking this drug; serious sedation could occur.
- Report difficulty breathing, hallucinations, tremors, loss of coordination, visual disturbances, irregular heartbeat.

❐ meclofenamate sodium

(me kloe fen am' ate)
Meclomen

Pregnancy Category C

Drug classes
NSAID

Therapeutic actions
Anti-inflammatory, analgesic, and antipyretic activities related to inhibition of prostaglandin synthesis; exact mechanisms of action are not known.

Indications
- Acute and chronic rheumatoid arthritis and osteoarthritis (not recommended as initial therapy because of GI adverse effects, including severe diarrhea)
- Relief of mild to moderate pain
- Treatment of idiopathic heavy menstrual blood loss
- Treatment of primary dysmenorrhea

Contraindications/cautions
- Contraindicated in the presence of pregnancy and lactation.
- Use caution in the presence of allergies, renal, hepatic, cardiovascular, and GI dysfunction.

Dosage
Adult
- **Rheumatoid arthritis:** Usual dosage 200–400 mg/d PO in three to four equal doses. Initiate therapy with a lower dose, and increase as needed. Do not exceed 400 mg/d. 2–3 wk may be needed to achieve optimum therapeutic effect.
- **Mild to moderate pain:** 50 mg PO q4–6h. Doses of 100 mg may be required for optimal pain relief. Do not exceed 400 mg/d.

674 ■ medroxyprogesterone acetate

- ***Excessive menstrual blood loss and primary dysmenorrhea:*** 100 mg PO tid for up to 6 d, starting at the onset of menstrual flow.

Pediatric: Safety and efficacy in children younger than 14 y not established.

Pharmacokinetics

Route	Onset	Peak
Oral	Varies	30–60 min

Metabolism: Hepatic, $T_{1/2}$: 2–4 h
Distribution: Crosses placenta; enters breast milk
Excretion: Urine

Adverse effects
NSAIDs
- CNS: *Headache, dizziness, somnolence, insomnia,* fatigue, tiredness, dizziness, tinnitus, ophthalmologic effects
- GI: *Nausea, dyspepsia, GI pain,* diarrhea, vomiting, *constipation*, flatulence
- Respiratory: Dyspnea, hemoptysis, pharyngitis, bronchospasm, rhinitis
- GU: Dysuria, renal impairment
- Hematologic: Bleeding, platelet inhibition with higher doses, neutropenia, eosinophilia, leukopenia, pancytopenia, thrombocytopenia, agranulocytosis, granulocytopenia, aplastic anemia, decreased hemoglobin or Hct, bone marrow depression, mennorrhagia
- Dermatologic: *Rash*, pruritus, sweating, dry mucous membranes, stomatitis
- Other: Peripheral edema, **anaphylactoid reactions to fatal anaphylactic shock**

■ Nursing Considerations

Assessment
- *History:* Renal, hepatic, cardiovascular, and GI conditions, pregnancy, lactation
- *Physical:* Skin—color and lesions; orientation, reflexes, ophthalmologic and audiometric evaluation, peripheral sensation; P, edema; R, adventitious sounds; liver evaluation; CBC, clotting times, renal and liver function tests; serum electrolytes, stool guaiac.

Implementation
- Administer with milk or food to decrease GI upset.
- Arrange for periodic ophthalmologic examination during long-term therapy.
- Institute emergency procedures if overdose occurs: gastric lavage, induction of emesis, supportive therapy.

Drug-specific teaching points
- Take drug with food; take only the prescribed dosage.
- Know that dizziness, drowsiness can occur (avoid driving or the use of dangerous machinery while on this drug).
- Report sore throat, fever, rash, itching, weight gain, swelling in ankles or fingers; changes in vision; black, tarry stools; severe diarrhea.

☐ medroxyprogesterone acetate

*(me **drox'** ee proe jess' te rone)*
Oral: Amen, Curretab, Provera
Parenteral, antineoplastic: Depo-Provera
Pregnancy Category X

Drug classes
Hormonal agent
Progestin
Antineoplastic

Therapeutic actions
Progesterone derivative; endogenous progesterone transforms proliferative endometrium into secretory endometrium; inhibits the secretion of pituitary gonadotropins, which prevents follicular maturation and ovulation; inhibits spontaneous uterine contraction.

Indications
- Treatment of secondary amenorrhea (oral)
- Abnormal uterine bleeding due to hormonal imbalance in the absence of organic pathology (oral)

Adverse effects in *Italics* are most common; those in **Bold** are life-threatening.

- Adjunctive therapy and palliative treatment of inoperable, recurrent, and metastatic endometrial carcinoma or renal carcinoma (parenteral)
- Unlabeled use for depot form: long-acting contraceptive, treatment of breast cancer

Contraindications/cautions
- Contraindicated in the presence of allergy to progestins; thrombophlebitis, thromboembolic disorders, cerebral hemorrhage or history of these conditions; hepatic disease, carcinoma of the breast or genital organs, undiagnosed vaginal bleeding, missed abortion; pregnancy (fetal abnormalities, including masculinization of the female fetus have been reported); lactation.
- Use caution in the presence of epilepsy, migraine, asthma, cardiac or renal dysfunction.

Dosage
Adult
- ***Secondary amenorrhea:*** 5–10 mg/d PO for 5–10 d. A dose for inducing an optimum secretory transformation of an endometrium that has been primed with exogenous or endogenous estrogen is 10 mg/d for 10 d. Start therapy at any time; withdrawal bleeding usually occurs 3–7 d after therapy ends.
- ***Abnormal uterine bleeding:*** 5–10 mg/d PO for 5–10 d, beginning on the 16th or 21st day of the menstrual cycle. To produce an optimum secretory transformation of an endometrium that has been primed with estrogen, give 10 mg/d PO for 10 d, beginning on the 16th day of the cycle. Withdrawal bleeding usually occurs 3–7 d after discontinuing therapy. If bleeding is controlled, administer two subsequent cycles.
- ***Endometrial or renal carcinoma:*** 400–1,000 mg/wk IM. If improvement occurs within a few weeks or months and the disease appears stabilized, it may be possible to maintain improvement with as little as 400 mg/mo IM.

Pharmacokinetics

Route	Onset	Peak
Oral	Slow	Unknown
IM	Weeks	Months

Metabolism: Hepatic, $T_{1/2}$: unknown
Distribution: Crosses placenta; enters breast milk
Excretion: Unknown

Adverse effects
- **CNS:** Sudden, partial, or complete loss of vision; proptosis, diplopia, migraine, precipitation of acute intermittent porphyria, mental depression, pyrexia, insomnia, somnolence
- **GI:** Cholestatic jaundice, nausea
- **CV:** Thrombophlebitis, cerebrovascular disorders, retinal thrombosis, pulmonary embolism, thromboembolic and thrombotic disease, increased blood pressure
- **GU:** *Breakthrough bleeding, spotting, change in menstrual flow, amenorrhea,* changes in cervical erosion and cervical secretions, breast tenderness and secretion
- **Dermatologic:** *Rash with or without pruritus, acne,* melasma or chloasma, alopecia, hirsutism, photosensitivity
- **General:** *Fluid retention, edema, increase or decrease in weight*
- **Other:** Decreased glucose tolerance

Drug-lab test interferences
- Inaccurate tests of hepatic and endocrine function

■ Nursing Considerations

Assessment
- *History:* Allergy to progestins; thrombophlebitis, thromboembolic disorders, cerebral hemorrhage; hepatic disease, carcinoma of the breast or genital organs, undiagnosed vaginal bleeding, missed abortion; epilepsy, migraine, asthma, cardiac or renal dysfunction; pregnancy; lactation
- *Physical:* Skin—color, lesions, turgor; hair; breasts; pelvic exam; orientation, affect; ophthalmologic exam; P, auscultation, peripheral perfusion, edema; R,

adventitious sounds; liver evaluation; liver and renal function tests, glucose tolerance, Pap smear

Implementation
- Arrange for pretreatment and periodic (at least annual) history and physical, which should include BP, breasts, abdomen, pelvic organs and a Pap smear.
- Caution patient before beginning therapy of the need to prevent pregnancy during treatment, the need for frequent medical follow-up.
- Arrange to discontinue medication and consult physician if sudden partial or complete loss of vision occurs; if papilledema or retinal vascular lesions are present on exam, the drug should be discontinued.
- Arrange to discontinue medication and consult physician at the first sign of thromboembolic disease (leg pain, swelling, peripheral perfusion changes, shortness of breath).

Drug-specific teaching points
- Prepare a calendar, marking drug days (PO drug).
- Know that the following side effects may occur: sensitivity to light (avoid exposure to the sun; use sunscreen and protective clothing if exposure is necessary); dizziness, sleeplessness, depression (use caution if driving or performing tasks that require alertness if these occur); skin rash, color changes, loss of hair; fever; nausea.
- Be aware that this drug should not be taken during pregnancy; serious fetal abnormalities have been reported.
- Report pain or swelling and warmth in the calves, acute chest pain or shortness of breath, sudden severe headache or vomiting, dizziness or fainting, visual disturbances, numbness or tingling in the arm or leg.

☐ mefenamic acid

*(me fe **nam'** ik)*
Ponstan (CAN), Ponstel
Pregnancy Category C

Drug classes
NSAID (fenamate derivative)
Non-narcotic analgesic

Therapeutic actions
Anti-inflammatory, analgesic, and antipyretic activities related to inhibition of prostaglandin synthesis; exact mechanisms of action are not known.

Indications
- Relief of moderate pain when therapy will not exceed 1 wk
- Treatment of primary dysmenorrhea

Contraindications/cautions
- Contraindicated in the presence of pregnancy, lactation.
- Use caution in the presence of allergies; renal, hepatic, cardiovascular, and GI conditions.

Dosage
Adult
- ***Acute pain:*** Initially 500 mg PO followed by 250 mg q6h as needed. Do not exceed 1 wk of therapy.
- ***Primary dysmenorrhea:*** Initially 500 mg PO then 250 mg q6h starting with the onset of bleeding. Can be initiated with the start of menses and should not be necessary for longer than 2–3 d.

Pediatric: Safety and efficacy for children younger than 14 y not established; use adult dosage for children older than 14 y.

Pharmacokinetics

Route	Onset	Peak	Duration
Oral	Varies	2–4 h	6 h

Metabolism: Hepatic, $T_{1/2}$: 2–4 h
Distribution: Crosses placenta; enters breast milk
Excretion: Urine and feces

Adverse effects
NSAIDs
- CNS: *Headache, dizziness, somnolence, insomnia,* fatigue, tiredness, dizziness, tinnitus, ophthalmologic effects
- GI: *Nausea, dyspepsia, GI pain,* diarrhea, vomiting, *constipation,* flatulence

Adverse effects in *Italics* are most common; those in **Bold** are life-threatening.

mefloquine hydrochloride ■ 677

- **Respiratory**: Dyspnea, hemoptysis, pharyngitis, bronchospasm, rhinitis
- **Hematologic**: Bleeding, platelet inhibition with higher doses, neutropenia, eosinophilia, leukopenia, pancytopenia, thrombocytopenia, agranulocytosis, granulocytopenia, aplastic anemia, decreased hemoglobin or hematocrit, bone marrow depression, mennorhagia
- **GU**: Dysuria, **renal impairment**
- **Dermatologic**: *Rash,* pruritus, sweating, dry mucous membranes, stomatitis
- **Other**: Peripheral edema, anaphylactoid reactions to fatal anaphylactic shock

Drug-lab test interferences
- False-positive reaction for urinary bile using the diazo tablet test

■ Nursing Considerations

Assessment
- *History:* Allergies; renal, hepatic, cardiovascular, GI conditions; pregnancy; lactation
- *Physical:* Skin—color and lesions; orientation, reflexes, ophthalmologic and audiometric evaluation, peripheral sensation; P, edema; R, adventitious sounds; liver evaluation; CBC, clotting times, renal and liver function tests; serum electrolytes, stool guaiac

Implementation
- Administer with milk or food to decrease GI upset.
- Arrange for periodic ophthalmologic examination during long-term therapy.
- Institute emergency procedures if overdose occurs: gastric lavage, induction of emesis, supportive therapy.

Drug-specific teaching points
- Take drug with food; take only the prescribed dosage; do not take the drug longer than 1 wk.
- Know that dizziness, drowsiness can occur (avoid driving or the use of dangerous machinery while on this drug).
- Discontinue drug and consult the nurse or physician if rash, diarrhea, or digestive problems occur.
- Report sore throat, fever, rash, itching, weight gain, swelling in ankles or fingers; changes in vision; black, tarry stools; severe diarrhea.

❏ mefloquine hydrochloride

(me' floe kwin)
Lariam, Mephaquin

Pregnancy Category C

Drug classes
Antimalarial

Therapeutic actions
Acts as a blood schizonticide; exact mechanism of action is not known, but may act by raising intravesicular pH in parasite acid vesicles, causing death; is structurally related to quinine.

Indications
- Treatment of acute malaria infections
- Prophylaxis of *Plasmodium falciparum* and *Plasmodium vivax* malaria infections, including prophylaxis of chloroquine-resistant *P. falciparum.* Recommended by the CDC for use in travel to areas of risk where chloroquine-resistant *P. falciparum* exists.

Contraindications/cautions
- Contraindicated in the presence of allergy to mefloquine or related compounds; life threatening or overwhelming infection with *P. falciparum* (IV malarial drug should be used for treatment; mefloquine may be given orally following completion of the IV treatment); pregnancy (teratogenic and embryotoxic in preclinical studies; warn women not to travel to malaria-endemic areas while they are pregnant and to use contraceptive methods during and 2 mo before and after travel to such areas).
- Use caution in lactation.

Dosage
Adult
- ***Treatment of mild to moderate malaria:*** 5 tablets (1,250 mg) PO as

Adverse effects in *Italics* are most common; those in **Bold** are life-threatening.

a single dose. Do not administer on an empty stomach. Administer with at least 240 mg (8 oz) water.
- **Prophylaxis:** 250 mg PO once weekly for 4 wk, then 250 mg PO every other week. CDC recommends a single dose taken weekly starting 1 wk before travel and for 4 wk after leaving the area. For prolonged stays in endemic area, take weekly for 4 wk, then every other week until the traveler has taken three doses after return to a malaria-free area. Do not administer on an empty stomach. Administer with at least 240 mg (8 oz) water.

Pediatric
- **Prophylaxis:** Starting 1 wk before travel and continued weekly during travel and for 4 wk after leaving such areas: 15–19 kg: ¼ tablet PO. 20–30 kg: ½ tablet PO. 31–45 kg: ¾ tablet PO. > 45 kg: 1 tablet PO.

Pharmacokinetics

Route	Onset	Peak
Oral	Varies	Days

Metabolism: Hepatic, $T_{1/2}$: 13–24 d
Distribution: Crosses placenta; may enter breast milk
Excretion: Unknown

Adverse effects
Prophylaxis
- CNS: Dizziness, encephalopathy, syncope
- GI: *Vomiting*
- Hematologic: Elevations of transaminases, leukocytosis, thrombocytopenia

Treatment
- CNS: *Dizziness, myalgia, headache,* fatigue, tinnitus, vertigo, visual disturbances, psychotic manifestations, hallucinations, confusion, anxiety, depression, convulsions, ocular lesions
- GI: *Nausea, vomiting, diarrhea,* abdominal pain, anorexia
- CV: Bradycardia
- Dermatologic: Rash, loss of hair, pruritus
- Hematologic: Decreased Hct, elevation of transaminases, leukopenia, thrombocytopenia
- Other: *Fever*

Clinically important drug-drug interactions
- Increased risk of convulsions if taken concurrently with chloroquine • Increased risk of cardiac toxicity and convulsions if taken concurrently with quinine, quinidine; do not give these drugs concurrently; delay use of mefloquine for at least 12 h after the last dose of quinine or quinidine

■ Nursing Considerations
Assessment
- *History:* Allergy to mefloquine or related compounds; life threatening or overwhelming infection with *P. falciparum*; lactation
- *Physical:* Skin—lesions; temperature; reflexes, affect, ophthalmic exam; P; CBC, Hct, transaminase levels

Implementation
- Obtain cultures to determine sensitivity to mefloquine in acute treatment.
- Arrange for subsequent treatment with an 8-aminoquinolone (eg, primaquine) for patients with acute *P. vivax* infection; mefloquine does not eliminate the exoerythrocytic parasites, and subsequent relapse may occur.
- Do not administer on an empty stomach; always administer with at least 8 oz (240 ml) of water.
- Administer prophylactic drug 1 wk prior to departure to endemic area; prepare a calendar for the patient noting weekly drug days: the same day each wk for 4 wk and every other week until traveler has taken three doses after return to malaria-free area.
- Arrange for periodic ophthalmic examinations for patients on long-term therapy.

Drug-specific teaching points
- Take the drug weekly, on the same day of the week, for 4 wk, beginning 1 wk before traveling to an endemic area. If

staying in the area longer, the drug should be taken every other week; continue the drug for three doses after returning to a malaria-free area (prophylaxis). Prepare a calendar for the patient marking these dates. Treatment of malaria will consist of 5 tablets taken as one dose. Do not take this drug on an empty stomach. Always take the drug with at least 8 oz of water.
- Be aware that periodic physical exams, including ophthalmic examinations, will be needed if the drug is taken for a prolonged period.
- Know that the following side effects may occur: dizziness, visual disturbances (avoid driving a car or performing hazardous tasks); headache, fatigue, joint pain (medications may be available to help); nausea, vomiting, diarrhea (proper nutrition is important).
- Be aware that this drug should not be taken during pregnancy. It is advisable to use contraceptive measures before, during, and for 2 mo after travel to a malaria-endemic area.
- Report anxiety, depression, restlessness, confusion, palpitations.

☐ megestrol acetate

(me jess' trole)
Megace

Pregnancy Category X

Drug classes
Hormonal agent
Progestin
Antineoplastic agent

Therapeutic actions
Synthetic progestational agent; mechanism of antineoplastic activity is unknown but may be due to a pituitary-mediated antileutinizing effect.

Indications
- Palliative treatment of advanced carcinoma of the breast or endometrium; not for use instead of surgery, radiation, or chemotherapy
- Orphan drug use: appetite stimulant in HIV-related cachexia

Contraindications/cautions
- Contraindicated in the presence of allergy to progestins; thrombophlebitis, thromboembolic disorders, cerebral hemorrhage or history of these conditions; hepatic disease, carcinoma of the breast or genital organs, undiagnosed vaginal bleeding, missed abortion; pregnancy (masculinization of the female fetus has been reported); lactation.
- Use caution in the presence of epilepsy, migraine, asthma, cardiac or renal dysfunction.

Dosage
Adult
- **Breast cancer:** 160 mg/d PO (40 mg qid).
- **Endometrial cancer:** 40–320 mg/d PO in divided doses.
- **Cachexia:** 80 mg PO four times per day.

Pharmacokinetics

Route	Onset	Peak
Oral	Slow	Weeks

Metabolism: Hepatic, $T_{1/2}$: unknown
Distribution: Crosses placenta; enters breast milk
Excretion: Urine

Adverse effects
- CNS: Sudden, partial, or complete loss of vision; proptosis; diplopia; migraine; precipitation of acute intermittent porphyria; mental depression; pyrexia; insomnia; somnolence
- GI: Cholestatic jaundice, nausea
- CV: Thrombophlebitis, cerebrovascular disorders, retinal thrombosis, pulmonary embolism, thromboembolic and thrombotic disease, increased blood pressure
- GU: *Breakthrough bleeding, spotting, change in menstrual flow, amenorrhea*, changes in cervical erosion and

cervical secretions, breast tenderness and secretion
- **Dermatologic:** *Rash with or without pruritus, acne*, melasma or chloasma, alopecia, hirsutism, photosensitivity
- **General:** *Fluid retention, edema, increase in weight*
- **Other:** Decreased glucose tolerance

Drug-lab test interferences
- Inaccurate tests of hepatic and endocrine function

Nursing Considerations

Assessment
- *History:* Allergy to progestins; thrombophlebitis, thromboembolic disorders, cerebral hemorrhage; hepatic disease, carcinoma of the breast or genital organs, undiagnosed vaginal bleeding, missed abortion; epilepsy, migraine, asthma, cardiac or renal dysfunction; pregnancy; lactation
- *Physical:* Skin—color, lesions, turgor; hair; breasts; pelvic exam; orientation, affect; ophthalmologic exam; P, auscultation, peripheral perfusion, edema; R, adventitious sounds; liver evaluation; liver and renal function tests, glucose tolerance, Pap smear

Implementation
- Arrange to discontinue medication and consult physician at the first sign of thromboembolic disease: leg pain, swelling, peripheral perfusion changes, shortness of breath.

Drug-specific teaching points
- Know that the following side effects may occur: sensitivity to light (avoid exposure to the sun; use sunscreen and protective clothing if exposure is necessary); dizziness, sleeplessness, depression (use caution if driving or performing tasks that require alertness if these occur); skin rash, color changes, loss of hair; fever; nausea.
- Be aware that this drug causes serious fetal abnormalities or fetal death; avoid pregnancy while on this drug.
- Report pain or swelling and warmth in the calves, acute chest pain or shortness of breath, sudden severe headache or vomiting, dizziness or fainting, numbness or tingling in the arm or leg.

melphalan

(mel' fa lan)
Alkeran, L-PAM, L-sarcolysin, PAM, Phenylalanine Mustard

Pregnancy Category D

Drug classes
Alkylating agent, nitrogen mustard
Antineoplastic drug

Therapeutic actions
Cytotoxic: alkylates cellular DNA, thus interfering with the replication of susceptible cells, causing cell death.

Indications
- Palliative treatment of multiple myeloma, nonresectable epthelial ovarian carcinoma
- IV use is reserved for patients in whom oral therapy is not possible

Contraindications/cautions
- Allergy to melphalan or chlorambucil, radiation therapy, chemotherapy, pregnancy (potentially mutagenic and teratogenic; avoid use in the first trimester), lactation.

Dosage
Individualize dosage based on hematologic profile and response.
Adult
- ***Multiple myeloma:*** 6 mg/d PO. After 2–3 wk, stop drug for up to 4 wk, and monitor blood counts. When blood counts are rising, institute maintenance dose of 2 mg/d PO. Response may occur gradually over many months (many alternative regimens, some including predinisone, are used).
- ***Epithelial ovarian carcinoma:*** 0.2 mg/kg per day PO for 5 d as a single

course. Repeat courses every 4–5 wk, depending on hematologic response.
- *IV:* 16 mg/m^2 administered as a single infusion over 15–20 min; administered at 2-wk intervals for four doses, then at 4-wk intervals

Pharmacokinetics

Route	Onset	Peak
Oral	Varies	2 h
IV	Rapid	1 h

Metabolism: T$_{1/2}$: 90 min
Distribution: Crosses placenta; enters breast milk
Excretion: Urine

IV facts

Preparation: Reconstitute with 10 ml of supplied diluent, and shake vigorously until a clear solution is obtained; this provides 5 mg/ml solution. Immediately dilute in 0.9% Sodium Chloride Injection to a dilution of < 0.45 mg/ml. Complete infusion within 60 min of reconstitution. Protect from light. Dispense in glass containers. Do not refrigerate reconstituted solution.

Infusion: Administer dilute product over a minimum of 15 min; complete within 60 min of reconstitution.

Adverse effects

- **GI:** *Nausea, vomiting,* oral ulceration
- **Respiratory:** Bronchopulmonary dysplasia, **pulmonary fibrosis**
- **Hematologic:** *Bone marrow depression*, hyperuricemia
- **Dermatologic:** Maculopapular skin rash, urticaria, *alopecia*
- **Other:** *Amenorrhea*, cancer, acute leukemia

Drug-lab test interferences

- Increased urinary 5-hydroxyindole acetic acid levels (5-HIAA) due to tumor cell destruction

■ Nursing Considerations

Assessment

- *History:* Allergy to melphalan or chlorambucil, radiation therapy, chemotherapy, pregnancy, lactation
- *Physical:* temperature; weight; skin—color, lesions; R, adventitious sounds; liver evaluation; CBC, differential, hemoglobin, uric acid, renal function tests

Implementation

- Arrange for blood tests to evaluate hematopoietic function before beginning therapy and weekly during therapy.
- Do not give full dosage within 4 wk after a full course of radiation therapy or chemotherapy because of the risk of severe bone marrow depression.
- Arrange for reduced dosage in patients with impaired renal function.
- Ensure that patient is well hydrated before treatment.
- Monitor uric acid levels; ensure adequate fluid intake, and prepare for appropriate treatment if hyperuricemia occurs.
- Arrange to divide single daily dose if nausea and vomiting occur with large single dose.

Drug-specific teaching points

- Take drug once a day. If nausea and vomiting occur, consult with nurse or physician about dividing the dose.
- Know that the following side effects may occur: nausea, vomiting, loss of appetite (dividing the dose may help, small frequent meals also may help; it is important that you try to maintain your fluid intake and nutrition while on this drug; drink at least 10–12 glassses of fluid each day); skin rash, loss of hair (you may wish to arrange for a wig if hair loss occurs; head should be covered at extremes of temperature).
- Be aware that this drug can cause severe birth defects; it is advisable to use birth control methods while on this drug.
- Report unusual bleeding or bruising, fever, chills, sore throat, cough, shortness of breath, black, tarry stools, flank or stomach pain, joint pain.

☐ menotropins

*(men oh **troe**′ pins)*
Pergonal
Pregnancy Category C

Adverse effects in *Italics* are most common; those in **Bold** are life-threatening.

menotropins

Drug classes
Hormonal agent
Fertility drug

Therapeutic actions
A purified preparation of human gonadotropins; in women, produces ovarian follicular growth; when followed by administration of HCG, produces ovulation; used with HCG for at least 3 mo to induce spermatogenesis in men with primary or secondary pituitary hypofunction who have previously achieved adequate masculinization with HCG administration.

Indications
- Women: Given with HCG sequentially to induce ovulation and pregnancy in anovulatory infertile patients without primary ovarian failure
- Men: With concomitant HCG therapy to stimulate spermatogenesis in men with primary hypogonadotropic hypogonadism due to a congenital factor or prepubertal hypophysectomy and in men with secondary hypogonadotropic hypogonadism due to hypophysectomy, craniopharyngioma, cerebral aneurysm, or chromophobe adenoma

Contraindications/cautions
- Known sensitivity to menotropins; high gonadotropin levels, indicating primary ovarian failure; overt thyroid or adrenal dysfunction, abnormal bleeding of undetermined origin, ovarian cysts or enlargement not due to polycystic ovary syndrome, intracranial lesion, such as pituitary tumor, pregnancy (women); normal gonadotropin levels, indicating pituitary function; elevated gonadotropin levels, indicating primary testicular failure; infertility disorders other than hypogonadotropic hypogonadism (men).

Dosage
Women: To achieve ovulation, HCG must be given following menotropins when clinical assessment indicates sufficient follicular maturation as indicated by urinary excretion of estrogens; initial dose is 5 IU FSH/75 IU LH/d IM for 9–12 d. Follow administration with 10,000 IU HCG 1 d after the last dose of menotropins. Do not administer for longer than 12 d. Treat until estrogen levels are normal or slightly higher than normal. When urinary estrogen excretion is < 100 μg/24 h, and urinary estriol excretion is < 50 μg/24 h prior to HCG administration, there is less risk of ovarian overstimulation. Do not administer if urinary excretion exceeds these values. Couple should engage in intercourse daily beginning on the day prior to the HCG administration and until ovulation occurs. If there is evidence of ovulation but pregnancy does not occur, repeat regimen for at least 2 more courses before increasing dose to 150 IU FSH/150 IU LH/d IM for 9–12 d followed by 10,000 IU HCG 1 d after the last dose of menotropins. If there is evidence of ovulation but pregnancy does not occur, repeat this regimen twice more. Larger doses are not recommended.

Men: Pretreat with HCG (5,000 IU three times per week) until serum testosterone levels are within a normal range and masculinization has occurred. Pretreatment may take 4–6 mo. Then give 1 amp (75 IU FSH/75 IU LH) menotropins IM three times per week and HCG 2,000 IU twice a wk. Continue for a minimum of 4 mo. If increased spermatogenesis has not occurred at the end of 4 mo, continue treatment with 1 amp menotropins three times per week or 2 amps (dose of 150 IU FSH/150 IU LH) menotropins three times per week with the HCG dose unchanged.

Pharmacokinetics

Route	Onset	Peak	Duration
IM	Slow	Weeks	Months

Metabolism: $T_{1/2}$: unknown
Distribution: Crosses placenta
Excretion: Urine

Adverse effects
Women
- CV: Arterial thromboembolism
- GU: *Ovarian enlargement,* hyperstimulation syndrome, hemoperitoneum

Adverse effects in *Italics* are most common; those in **Bold** are life-threatening.

- **Hypersensitivity:** Hypersensitivity reactions
- **Other:** *Febrile reactions;* birth defects in resulting pregnancies, *multiple pregnancies*

Men
- **Endocrine:** Gynecomastia

■ Nursing Considerations

Assessment
- *History:* Sensitivity to menotropins; high gonadotropin levels; overt thyroid or adrenal dysfunction, abnormal bleeding of undetermined origin, ovarian cysts or enlargement not due to polycystic ovary syndrome, intracranial lesion (women); normal gonadotropin levels; elevated gonadotropin levels; infertility disorders other than hypogonadotropin hypogonadism (men)
- *Physical:* Body temperature; masculinization (men); abdominal exam, pelvic exam; testicular exam; serum gonadotropin levels; 24 h urinary estrogens and estriol excretion (women); serum testosterone levels (men)

Implementation
- Dissolve contents of 1 amp in 1–2 ml of Sterile Saline. Administer IM immediately. Discard any unused portion.
- Store ampules at room temperature or in refrigerator; do not freeze.
- Monitor women at least every other day during treatment and for 2 wk after treatment for any sign of ovarian enlargement.
- Discontinue drug at any sign of ovarian overstimulation, and arrange to have patient admitted to the hospital for observation and supportive measures. Do not attempt to remove ascitic fluid because of the risk of injury to the ovaries. Have the patient refrain from intercourse if ovarian enlargement occurs.
- Provide women with calendar of treatment days and explanations about what signs of estrogen and progesterone activity to watch for. Caution patient that 24-h urine collections will be needed periodically, that HCG also must be given to induce ovulation, and that daily intercourse should begin 1 d prior to HCG administration and until ovulation occurs.
- Caution patient about the risks and hazards of multiple births.
- Provide support and encouragement to the male patient, explaining the need for long-term treatment, regular sperm counts, and masculinizing effects of HCG.

Drug-specific teaching points
- Prepare a calendar showing the treatment schedule; drug can only be given IM and must be used with HCG to achieve the desired effects.
- Have intercourse daily beginning on the day prior to HCG therapy until ovulation occurs.
- Know that the following may occur: breast enlargement (men); ovarian enlargement, abdominal discomfort, fever, multiple births (women).
- Report pain at injection site, severe abdominal or lower back pain, fever, fluid in the abdomen.

▢ meperidine hydrochloride

(me per' i deen)

pethidine

Demer-Idine (CAN), Demerol HCl

Pregnancy Category C
C-II controlled substance

Drug classes
Narcotic agonist analgesic

Therapeutic actions
Acts as agonist at specific opioid receptors in the CNS to produce analgesia, euphoria, sedation; the receptors mediating these effects are thought to be the same as those mediating the effects of endogenous opioids (enkephalins, endorphins).

Adverse effects in *Italics* are most common; those in **Bold** are life-threatening.

meperidine hydrochloride

Indications
- Relief of moderate to severe pain (oral, parenteral)
- Preoperative medication, support of anesthesia, and obstetric analgesia (parenteral)

Contraindications/cautions
- Contraindicated in the presence of hypersensitivity to narcotics, diarrhea caused by poisoning (before toxins are eliminated), bronchial asthma, COPD, cor pulmonale, respiratory depression, anoxia, kyphoscoliosis, acute alcoholism, increased intracranial pressure, pregnancy.
- Use caution in the presence of acute abdominal conditions, cardiovascular disease, supraventricular tachycardias, myxedema, convulsive disorders, delirium tremens, cerebral arteriosclerosis, ulcerative colitis, fever, Addison's disease, prostatic hypertrophy, urethral stricture, recent GI or GU surgery, toxic psychosis, labor or delivery (administration of narcotics, including meperidine, to the mother can cause respiratory depression of neonate; premature infants are especially at risk), renal or hepatic dysfunction.

Dosage
Adult
- ***Relief of pain:*** Individualize dosage; 50–150 mg IM, SC, or PO q3–4h as necessary. Diluted solution may be given by slow IV injection if necessary. IM route is preferred for repeated injections.
- ***Preoperative medication:*** 50–100 mg IM or SC, 30–90 min before beginning anesthesia.
- ***Support of anesthesia:*** Dilute to 10 mg/ml, and give repeated doses by slow IV injection, or dilute to 1 mg/ml and infuse continuously. Individualize dosage.
- ***Obstetric analgesia:*** When pains become regular 50–100 mg IM or SC; repeat q1–3h.

Pediatric: Contraindicated in premature infants.
- ***Relief of pain:*** 0.5–0.8 mg/lb (1–1.8 mg/kg) IM, SC, or PO up to adult dose q3–4h as necessary.
- ***Preoperative medication:*** 0.5–1 mg/lb (1–2 mg/kg) IM or SC, up to adult dose, 30–90 min before beginning anesthesia.

Geriatric or impaired adult: Use caution; respiratory depression may occur in elderly, the very ill, those with respiratory problems. Reduced dosage may be necessary.

Pharmacokinetics

Route	Onset	Peak	Duration
Oral	15 min	60 min	2–4 h
IM, SC	10–15 min	30–60 min	2–4 h
IV	Immediate	5–7 min	2–4 h

Metabolism: Hepatic, $T_{1/2}$: 3–8 h
Distribution: Crosses placenta; enters breast milk
Excretion: Urine

IV facts
Preparation: Dilute parenteral solution prior to IV injection using 5% Dextrose and Lactated Ringer's; Dextrose-Saline combinations; 2.5%, 5%, or 10% Dextrose in Water, Ringer's, or Lactated Ringer's; 0.45% or 0.9% Sodium Chloride; 1/6 Molar Sodium Lactate.

Infusion: Administer by slow IV injection or by continuous infusion when diluted to 1 mg/ml.

Incompatibilities: Do *not* mix meperidine solutions with solutions of barbiturates, aminophylline, heparin, morphine sulfate, methicillin, phenytoin, sodium bicarbonate, iodide, sulfadiazine, sulfisoxazole.

Adverse effects
May produce less intense smooth muscle spasm, less constipation, less cough reflex suppression than equianalgesic doses of morphine.

Adverse effects in *Italics* are most common; those in **Bold** are life-threatening.

- CNS: *Lightheadedness, dizziness, sedation,* euphoria, dysphoria, delirium, insomnia, agitation, anxiety, fear, hallucinations, disorientation, drowsiness, lethargy, impaired mental and physical performance, coma, mood changes, weakness, headache, tremor, convulsions, miosis, visual disturbances, suppression of cough reflex
- GI: *Nausea, vomiting,* dry mouth, anorexia, constipation, biliary tract spasm, increased colonic motility in patients with chronic ulcerative colitis
- CV: Facial flushing, peripheral circulatory collapse, tachycardia, bradycardia, arrhythmia, palpitations, chest wall rigidity, hypertension, hypotension, orthostatic hypotension, syncope
- GU: Ureteral spasm, spasm of vesical sphincters, urinary retention or hesitancy, oliguria, antidiuretic effect, reduced libido or potency
- Dermatologic: Pruritus, urticaria, laryngospasm, bronchospasm, edema
- Local: tissue irritation and induration (SC injection)
- Major hazards: **Respiratory depression, apnea, circulatory depression, respiratory arrest, shock, cardiac arrest**
- Other: *Sweating,* physical tolerance and dependence, psychological dependence

Clinically important drug-drug interactions
- Potentiation of effects of meperidine when given with barbiturate anesthetics; decrease dose of meperidine when coadministering • Severe and sometimes fatal reactions (resembling narcotic overdose in some patients; characterized by convulsions, hypertension, hyperpyrexia in others) when given to patients who are receiving or who have recently received monoamine oxidase inhibitors (MAOIs); do not give meperidine to patients on MAO inhibitors. • Increased likelihood of respiratory depression, hypotension, profound sedation, or coma in patients receiving phenothiazines

Drug-lab test interferences
- Elevated biliary tract pressure may cause increases in plasma amylase, lipase; determinations of these levels may be unreliable for 24 h after administration of narcotics.

■ Nursing Considerations
Assessment
- *History:* Hypersensitivity to narcotics, diarrhea caused by poisoning, bronchial asthma, COPD, cor pulmonale, respiratory depression, anoxia, kyphoscoliosis, acute alcoholism, increased intracranial pressure; acute abdominal conditions, cardiovascular disease, supraventricular tachycardias, myxedema, convulsive disorders, delirium tremens, cerebral arteriosclerosis, ulcerative colitis, fever, Addison's disease, prostatic hypertrophy, urethral stricture, recent GI or GU surgery, toxic psychosis, renal or hepatic dysfunction, pregnancy
- *Physical:* Body temperature; skin—color, texture, lesions; orientation, reflexes, bilateral grip strength, affect, pupil size; P, auscultation, BP, orthostatic BP, perfusion; R, adventious sounds; bowel sounds, normal output; frequency and pattern of voiding, normal output; ECG; EEG; thyroid, liver, kidney function tests

Implementation
- Administer to women who are lactating 4–6 h before the next scheduled feeding to minimize the amount in milk.
- Provide narcotic antagonist, facilities for assisted or controlled respiration on standby during parenteral administration.
- Use caution when injecting SC into chilled areas or in patients with hypotension or in shock; impaired perfusion may delay absorption; with repeated doses, an excessive amount may be absorbed when circulation is restored.
- Arrange to reduce dosage of meperidine by 25%–50% in patients who are receiving phenothiazines or other tranquilizers.

Adverse effects in *Italics* are most common; those in **Bold** are life-threatening.

- Give each dose of the oral syrup in half glass of water. If taken undiluted, it may exert a slight local anesthetic effect on mucous membranes.
- Reassure patient about addiction liability; most patients who receive opiates for medical reasons do not develop dependence syndromes.

Drug-specific teaching points
- Take drug exactly as prescribed.
- Avoid alcohol, antihistamines, sedatives, tranquilizers, OTC drugs while taking this drug.
- Know that the following side effects may occur: nausea, loss of appetite (taking the drug with food and lying quietly, eating frequent small meals should minimize these effects); constipation (notify your nurse or physician if this is severe; a laxative may help); dizziness, sedation, drowsiness, impaired visual acuity (avoid driving a car, performing other tasks that require alertness, visual acuity).
- Do not take any leftover medication for other disorders, and do not let anyone else take the prescription.
- Report severe nausea, vomiting, constipation, shortness of breath, or difficulty breathing.

❏ mephentermine sulfate

(me fen' ter meen)

Wyamine

Pregnancy Category D

Drug classes
Sympathomimetic

Therapeutic actions
Sympathomimetic amine that acts directly and indirectly (causes norepinephrine release); increases cardiac output, increases peripheral resistance.

Indications
- Treatment of hypotension secondary to ganglionic blockade, spinal anesthesia
- Emergency maintenance of blood pressure until blood or blood substitute is available

Contraindications/cautions
- Contraindicated in the presence of hypotension induced by chlorpromazine (drug interaction will potentiate hypotension); use of MAO inhibitors.
- Use caution in the presence of cardivascular disease, chronic illness, pregnancy, lactation.

Dosage
Adult
- ***Prevention of hypotension attendant to spinal anesthesia:*** 30–45 mg IM, 10–20 min prior to procedure.
- ***Hypotension following spinal anesthesia:*** 30–45 mg IV as a single injection. Repeat doses of 30 mg as necessary.
- ***Hypotension following spinal anesthesia in obstetric patients:*** Initial dose of 15 mg IV; repeat as needed.
- ***Treatment of shock following hemorrhage:*** Continuous IV infusion of 0.1% solution in 5% dextrose in water just until blood replacement can be achieved.

Pharmacokinetics

Route	Onset	Peak	Duration
IM	10–15 min	30–60 min	1–2 h
IV	Immediate	15–30 min	

Metabolism: Hepatic, $T_{1/2}$: 15–20 min
Distribution: Crosses placenta; may enter breast milk
Excretion: Urine

IV facts
Preparation: Prepare 0.1% solution by adding 10 or 20 ml mephenterine, 30 mg/ml, to 250 or 500 ml of 5% Dextrose in Water, respectively.

Infusion: Administer as a single IV injection or by continuous infusion of 0.1% solution; regulate dose based on blood pressure response.

Adverse effects
- CNS: *Anxiety,* fear, hallucinations
- CV: *BP changes,* arrhythmias (more likely in patients with heart disease)

Clinically important drug-drug interactions
- Decreased effects of guanethidine if taken with mephentermine • Severe and sometimes fatal reactions (including hypertensive crisis and intracranial hemorrhage) in patients also taking MAOIs, furazolidone • Increased likelihood of serious arrhythmias if given with halogenated hydrocarbon anesthetics

■ Nursing Considerations
Assessment
- *History:* Hypotension induced by chlorpromazine; use of MAOIs, cardiovascular disease, chronic illness, pregnancy, lactation
- *Physical:* Body temperature; skin—color, texture, lesions; orientation; P, auscultation, BP, orthostatic BP, perfusion; R, adventious sounds; liver, kidney function tests

Implementation
- Monitor blood pressure continously during and after administration.
- Arrange for immediate replacement with blood or blood products if used in emergency situation for shock.

Drug-specific teaching points
Drug teaching should be incorporated into total teaching plan of patient receiving spinal anesthesia.
- Know that you may experience a feeling of anxiety while receiving this drug.
- Report difficulty breathing, numbness of tingling, palpitations.

☐ mephenytoin

(me fen' i toyn)
Mesantoin
Pregnancy Category C

Drug classes
Antiepileptic
Hydantoin

Therapeutic actions
Has antiepileptic activity without causing general CNS depression; stabilizes neuronal membranes and prevents hyperexcitability caused by excessive stimulation; limits the spread of seizure activity from an active focus.

Indications
- Control of grand mal (tonic-clonic), psychomotor, focal, and Jacksonian seizures in patients refractory to less toxic antiepileptic drugs

Contraindications/cautions
- Contraindicated in the presence of hypersensitivity to hydantoins; pregnancy; lactation; hepatic abnormalities; hematologic disorders.
- Use caution in the presence of acute intermittent porphyria; hypotension, severe myocardial insufficiency; diabetes mellitus, hyperglycemia.

Dosage
Adult: Start with 50–100 mg/d PO during the first week. Thereafter increase the daily dose by 50–100 mg at weekly intervals. No dose should be increased until it has been taken for at least 1 wk. Average dose ranges from 200–600 mg/d PO. Up to 800 mg/d may be needed for full seizure control.
- ***Replacement therapy:*** 50–100 mg/d PO during the first week. Gradually increase, as described above, while decreasing the dose of the drug being discontinued, over 3–6 wk. If patient also has been receiving phenobarbital, continue it until the transition is completed, at which time gradual withdrawal of the phenobarbital may be attempted.

Pediatric: Usual dose is 100–400 mg/d PO.

Geriatric and hepatic impairment: Use caution and monitor for early signs of toxicity; mephenytoin is metabolized in the liver.

Adverse effects in *Italics* are most common; those in **Bold** are life-threatening.

Pharmacokinetics

Route	Onset	Peak	Duration
Oral	30 min	1–3 h	24–48 h

Metabolism: Hepatic, $T_{1/2}$: 144 h
Distribution: Crosses placenta; enters breast milk
Excretion: Urine

Adverse effects

- **CNS:** *Nystagmus, ataxia, dysarthria, slurred speech, mental confusion, dizziness, drowsiness, insomnia, transient nervousness, motor twitchings, fatigue, irritability, depression, numbness, tremor, headache,* photophobia, diplopia, conjunctivitis
- **GI:** *Nausea,* vomiting, diarrhea, constipation, *gingival hyperplasia*, **toxic hepatitis, liver damage, sometimes fatal; hypersensitivity reactions with hepatic involvement, including hepatocellular degeneration and fatal hepatocellular necrosis**
- **Respiratory:** **Pulmonary fibrosis, acute pneumonitis**
- **Hematologic:** **Hematopoietic complications, sometimes fatal: thrombocytopenia, leukopenia, granulocytopenia, agranulocytosis, pancytopenia;** macrocytosis and megaloblastic anemia that usually respond to folic acid therapy; eosinophilia, monocytosis, leukocytosis, simple anemia, hemolytic anemia, aplastic anemia, hyperglycemia
- **GU:** Nephrosis
- **Dermatologic:** Scarlatiniform, morbilliform, maculopapular, urticarial and nonspecific rashes; also serious and sometimes fatal dermatologic reactions: **bullous, exfoliative, or purpuric dermatitis, lupus erythematosus, and Stevens-Johnson syndrome; toxic epidermal necrolysis,** hirsutism, alopecia, coarsening of the facial features, enlargement of the lips, Peyronie's disease
- **Other:** lymph node hyperplasia, sometimes progressing to frank malignant lymphoma; monoclonal gammopathy and multiple myeloma (prolonged therapy); polyarthropathy; osteomalacia; weight gain; chest pain; periarteritis nodosa

Clinically important drug-drug interactions

- Increased pharmacologic effects of hydantoins when given with: chloramphenicol, cimetidine, disulfiram, isoniazid, phenacemide, phenylbutazone, sulfonamides, trimethoprim • Complex interactions and effects when hydantoins and valproic acid are given together: toxicity with apparently normal serum ethotoin levels; decreased plasma levels of valproic acid given with hydantoins; breakthrough seizures when the two drugs are given together • Decreased pharmacologic effects of hydantoins when given with antineoplastics, diazoxide, folic acid, rifampin, theophyllines • Increased pharmacologic effects and toxicity when primidone, oxyphenbutazone, fluconazole, amiodarone are given concurrently with hydantoins • Increased hepatotoxicity if given concurrently with acetaminophen • Decreased pharmacologic effects of the following drugs when given with hydantoins: corticosteroids, cyclosporine, dicumarol, disopyramide, doxycycline, estrogens, levodopa, methadone, metyrapone, mexiletine, oral contraceptives, quinestrol, carbamazepine

Drug-lab test interferences

- Interference with the metyrapone and the 1-mg dexamethasone tests; avoid hydantoins for at least 7 d prior to metyrapone testing

■ Nursing Considerations

Assessment

- *History:* Hypersensitivity to hydantoins; hepatic abnormalities; hematologic disorders; acute intermittent porphyria; hypotension, severe myocardial insufficiency; diabetes mellitus, hyperglycemia; pregnancy; lactation
- *Physical:* Body temperature; skin—color, lesions; lymph node palpation; orientation, affect, reflexes, vision exam; P, BP; R, adventitious sounds; bowel sounds,

Adverse effects in *Italics* are most common; those in **Bold** are life-threatening.

normal output, liver evaluation; periodontal exam; liver function tests, urinalysis, CBC and differential, blood proteins, blood and urine glucose, EEG and ECG

Implementation
- Give drug with food to enhance absorption and reduce GI upset.
- Arrange to reduce dosage, discontinue mephenytoin, or substitute other antiepileptic medication gradually; abrupt discontinuation may precipitate status epilepticus.
- Be aware that mephenytoin is ineffective in controlling absence (petit mal) seizures; patients with combined seizures will need other medication for their absence seizures.
- Arrange to discontinue drug if skin rash, depression of blood count, enlarged lymph nodes, hypersensitivity reaction, signs of liver damage, or Peyronie's disease (induration of the corpora cavernosa of the penis) occurs; arrange to institute another antiepileptic drug promptly.
- Monitor CBC and differential before therapy is instituted, at 2 wk, 4 wk, and monthly thereafter for the first year, then every 3 mo. If neutrophils drop to between 2,500 and 1,600/mm^3, counts should be made every 2 wk. If neutrophils drop to < 1,600/mm^3, discontinue drug.
- Monitor hepatic function periodically during chronic therapy.
- Arrange to have lymph node enlargement occurring during therapy evaluated carefully lymphadenopathy that simulates Hodgkin's disease has occurred; lymph node hyperplasia may progress to lymphoma.
- Arrange dental consultation to instruct patients receiving long-term hydantoin therapy in proper oral hygiene technique to prevent development of gum hyperplasia.
- Arrange for appropriate counseling for women of childbearing age who need chronic maintenance therapy with antiepileptic drugs and who wish to become pregnant.

Drug-specific teaching points
- Take this drug exactly as prescribed, with food to enhance absorption and reduce GI upset. Do not discontinue this drug abruptly or change dosage, except on the advice of your health care provider.
- Be especially careful not to miss a dose if you are on once-a-day therapy.
- Maintain good oral hygiene (regular brushing and flossing) while you are taking this drug to prevent gum disease; arrange frequent dental checkups to prevent serious gum disease.
- Arrange for frequent checkups to monitor your response to this drug. It is important that you keep all appointments.
- Know that the following side effects may occur: drowsiness, dizziness, confusion, blurred vision (avoid driving a car or performing other tasks requiring alertness or visual acuity if these occur); GI upset (taking the drug with food and eating frequent, small meals may help).
- Wear a medical alert tag at all times so that any emergency medical personnel taking care of you will know that you are an epileptic taking antiepileptic medication.
- Report skin rash, severe nausea or vomiting, drowsiness, slurred speech, impaired coordination (ataxia), swollen glands, bleeding, swollen or tender gums, yellowish discoloration of the skin or eyes, joint pain, unexplained fever, sore throat, unusual bleeding or bruising, persistent headache, malaise, any indication of an infection or bleeding tendency, abnormal erection, pregnancy.

mephobarbital

(me foe bar' bi tal)
Mebaral

Pregnancy Category D
C-IV controlled substance

Drug classes
Barbiturate (long-acting)
Sedative
Antiepileptic

Therapeutic actions
General CNS depressant; barbiturates inhibit impulse conduction in the ascending reticular activating system, depress the cerebral cortex, alter cerebellar function, depress motor output, and can produce excitation (especially with subanesthetic doses in the presence of pain), sedation, hypnosis, anesthesia, and deep coma.

Indications
- Sedative for the relief of anxiety, tension, and apprehension
- Antiepileptic for the treatment of grand mal and petit mal epilepsy

Contraindications/cautions
- Contraindicated in the presence of hypersensitivity to barbiturates; manifest or latent porphyria; marked liver impairment; nephritis; severe respiratory distress; previous addiction to sedative/hypnotic drugs; pregnancy.
- Use caution in the presence of acute or chronic pain (drug may cause paradoxical excitement or mask important symptoms); seizure disorders (abrupt discontinuation of daily doses of drug can result in status epilepticus); lactation (secreted in breast milk; has caused drowsiness in nursing infants); fever, hyperthyroidism, diabetes mellitus, severe anemia, pulmonary or cardiac disease, status asthmaticus, shock, uremia; impaired liver or kidney function, debilitation.

Dosage
Adult
- ***Daytime sedation:*** 32–100 mg PO tid–qid. Optimum dose is 50 mg tid–qid PO.
- ***Epilepsy:*** Average dose is 400–600 mg/d PO. Start treatment with a low dose and gradually increase over 4–5 d until optimum dosage is determined. Give at bedtime if seizures occur at night, during the day if attacks are diurnal. May be given with phenobarbital or with phenytoin; decrease dose of mephobarbital and phenobarbital to about half that when drug is used alone. Decrease dose of phenytoin, but not mephobarbital, when phenytoin is given with mephobarbital. Satisfactory results have been obtained with an average daily dose of 230 mg phenytoin and 600 mg mephobarbital.

Pediatric: Use caution: barbiturates may produce irritability, excitability, inappropriate tearfulness, and aggression. Base dosage on body weight, age (see Appendix C), and response.
- ***Sedative:*** 16–32 mg PO tid–qid.
- ***Epilepsy:*** Younger than 5 y: 16–32 mg tid–qid PO. Older than 5 y: 32–64 mg tid–qid PO.

Geriatric patients or those with debilitating disease: Reduce dosage and monitor closely; may produce excitement, depression, confusion.

Pharmacokinetics

Route	Onset	Peak	Duration
Oral	30–60 min	3–4 h	10–16 h

Metabolism: Hepatic, $T_{1/2}$: 11–67 h
Distribution: Crosses placenta; enters breast milk
Excretion: Urine

Adverse effects
- **CNS:** *Somnolence, agitation, confusion, hyperkinesia, ataxia, vertigo, CNS depression, nightmares, lethargy, residual sedation (hangover), paradoxical excitement, nervousness, psychiatric disturbance, hallucinations, insomnia, anxiety, dizziness, thinking abnormality*
- **GI:** *Nausea, vomiting, constipation, diarrhea, epigastric pain*
- **CV:** *Bradycardia, hypotension, syncope*
- **Respiratory:** *Hypoventilation, apnea, respiratory depression,* laryngospasm, bronchospasm, **circulatory collapse**
- **Hypersensitivity:** Skin rashes, angioneurotic edema, serum sickness, morbiliform rash, urticaria; rarely, exfoliative dermatitis, **Stevens-Johnson syndrome, sometimes fatal**
- **Other:** Tolerance, psychological and physical dependence; **withdrawal syndrome** (sometimes fatal)

Adverse effects in *Italics* are most common; those in **Bold** are life-threatening.

meprobamate ■ 691

Clinically important drug-drug interactions
- Increased CNS depression when taken with alcohol • Increased risk of nephrotoxicity if taken with methoxyflurane • Decreased effects of the following drugs given with barbiturates: theophyllines, oral anticoagulants, beta-blockers, doxycycline, griseofulvin corticosteroids, oral contraceptives and estrogens, metronidazole, phenylbutazones, quinidine, carbamazepine

■ Nursing Considerations
Assessment
- *History:* Hypersensitivity to barbiturates, manifest or latent porphyria; marked liver impairment, nephritis, severe respiratory distress; previous addiction to sedative-hypnotic drugs, acute or chronic pain, seizure disorders, fever, hyperthyroidism, diabetes mellitus, severe anemia, pulmonary or cardiac disease, shock, uremia, debilitation, pregnancy, lactation
- *Physical:* Body weight; body temperature; skin—color, lesions; orientation, affect, reflexes; P, BP, orthostatic BP; R, adventitious sounds; bowel sounds, normal output, liver evaluation; liver and kidney function tests, blood and urine glucose, BUN

Implementation
- Monitor patient responses, blood levels (as appropriate) if any of the above interacting drugs are given with mephobarbital; suggest alternate means of contraception to women on oral contraceptives for whom mephobarbital is prescribed.
- Provide resuscitative facilities on standby in case of respiratory depression, hypersensitivity reaction.
- Arrange to taper dosage gradually after repeated use, especially in epileptic patients. When changing from one antiepileptic medication to another, arrange to taper dosage of the drug being discontinued as the dosage of the replacement drug is increased.

Drug-specific teaching points
- Take this drug exactly as prescribed; do not reduce the dosage or discontinue this drug (when used for epilepsy) without consulting the nurse or physician; the abrupt discontinuation of the drug could result in a serious increase in seizures.
- Be aware that this drug is habit forming.
- Avoid alcohol, sleep-inducing, or OTC drugs while on this drug because these could cause dangerous effects.
- Use a means of contraception other than oral contraceptive preparations while on mephobarbital; you should not become pregnant while taking this drug.
- Know that the following side effects may occur: drowsiness, dizziness, "hangover," impaired thinking (these effects may become less pronounced after a few days; avoid driving a car or engaging in dangerous activities if these occur); GI upset (taking the drug with food may help); dreams, nightmares, difficulty concentrating, fatigue, nervousness (it may help to know that these are effects of the drug that will go away when the drug is discontinued).
- Wear a medical alert tag so that emergency medical personnel would immediately know that you are an epileptic taking this medication.
- Report severe dizziness, weakness, drowsiness that persists, rash or skin lesions, fever, sore throat, mouth sores, easy bruising or bleeding, nosebleed, petechiae, pregnancy.

☐ meprobamate

*(me proe **ba'** mate)*

Apo-Meprobamate (CAN), Equanil, Meprospan, Miltown, Neo-Tran (CAN), Novomepro (CAN)

Pregnancy Category D
C-IV controlled substance

Drug classes
Antianxiety agent

Therapeutic actions
Has effects at many sites in the CNS, including the thalamus and limbic system; inhibits multineuronal spinal reflexes;

is mildly tranquilizing; has some anticonvulsant and central skeletal muscle relaxing properties.

Indications
- Management of anxiety disorders for the short-term relief of the symptoms of anxiety (anxiety or tension associated with the stress of everyday life usually does not require treatment with anxiolytic drugs); effectiveness for use longer than 4 mo not established.

Contraindications/cautions
- Contraindicated in the presence of hypersensitivity to meprobamate or to related drugs, such as carisoprodol; acute intermittent porphyria; hepatic or renal impairment; pregnancy; lactation.
- Use caution in the presence of epilepsy (drug may precipitate seizures).

Dosage
Adult: 1,200–1,600 mg/d PO in three to four divided doses. *Sustained release:* 400–800 mg PO in the morning and at bedtime. Do not exceed 2,400 mg/d.
Pediatric: 6–12 y: 100–200 mg PO bid–tid. *Sustained release:* 200 mg PO in the morning and at bedtime. *Younger than 6 y:* Safety and efficacy not established.
Geriatric: Use lowest effective dose to avoid oversedation.

Pharmacokinetics

Route	Onset	Peak
Oral	Varies	1–3 h

Metabolism: Hepatic, $T_{1/2}$: 6–17 h
Distribution: Crosses placenta; enters breast milk
Excretion: Urine

Adverse effects
- CNS: *Drowsiness, ataxia, dizziness, slurred speech, headache, vertigo, weakness, impairment of visual accommodation,* euphoria, overstimulation, paradoxical excitement, paresthesias
- GI: *Nausea, vomiting, diarrhea*
- CV: *Palpitations, tachycardia,* various arrhythmias, syncope, **hypotensive crisis**
- Hematologic: Agranulocytosis, aplastic anemia; thrombocytopenic purpura; exacerbation of porphyric symptoms
- Hypersensitivity: Allergic or idiosyncratic reactions (usually seen between first and fourth doses in patients without previous drug exposure): *itchy, urticarial or erythematous maculopapular rash;* leukopenia, acute nonthromobocytopenic purpura, petechiae, ecchymoses, eosinophilia, peripheral edema, adenopathy, fever, fixed drug eruption; hyperpyrexia, chills, angioneurotic edema, bronchospasm, oliguria, anuria, anaphylaxis, erythema multiforme, exfoliative dermatitis, stomatitis, proctitis; Stevens-Johnson syndrome, bullous dermatitis
- Other: Physical, psychological dependence; withdrawal reaction

Clinically important drug-drug interactions
- Additive CNS depression when given with alcohol

■ Nursing Considerations

Assessment
- *History:* Hypersensitivity to meprobamate or to related drugs; acute intermittent porphyria; hepatic or renal impairment; epilepsy; pregnancy; lactation
- *Physical:* Body temperature; skin—color, lesions; orientation, affect, reflexes, vision exam; P, BP; R, adventitious sounds; bowel sounds, normal output, liver evaluation; liver and kidney function tests, CBC and differential, EEG and ECG

Implementation
- Supervise carefully dose and amount of drug prescribed in patients who are addiction prone or alcoholic.
- Dispense least amount of drug feasible to patients who are depressed or suicidal.
- Caution patient not to crush or chew sustained-release capsules.

- Withdraw gradually over 2 wk if patient has been maintained on high doses for weeks or months.
- Arrange to withdraw drug if allergic or idiosyncratic reactions occur.
- Provide epinephrine, antihistamines, corticosteroids, life support equipment on standby in case allergic or idiosyncratic reaction occurs.

Drug-specific teaching points
- Take this drug exactly as prescribed. This drug has not been assessed for effectiveness after several months of therapy; continue to see your health care provider as needed. Do not crush or chew sustained-release capsules.
- Avoid alcohol, sleep-inducing, or OTC drugs while you are on this drug; these could cause dangerous effects.
- Know that the following side effects may occur: drowsiness, dizziness, lightheadedness, blurred vision (avoid driving a car or performing other tasks requiring alertness or visual acuity if these occur); GI upset (frequent, small meals may help).
- Use some form of birth control while on this drug; it is not advisable to take this drug during pregnancy. Consult your physician immediately if you decide to become pregnant or find that you are pregnant.
- Report skin rash, sore throat, fever.

◻ mercaptopurine

*(mer kap toe **pyoor' een**)*

6-mercaptopurine, 6-MP
Purinethol

Pregnancy Category D

Drug classes
Antimetabolite
Antineoplastic drug

Therapeutic actions
Tumor-inhibiting properties, probably due to interference with purine nucleotide synthesis and hence with RNA and DNA synthesis, leading to cell death.

Indications
- Remission induction, remission consolidation, and maintenance therapy of acute leukemia (lymphatic, myelogenous and acute myelomonocytic)

Contraindications/cautions
- Contraindicated in the presence of allergy to mercaptopurine, prior resistance to mercaptopurine (cross-resistance with thioguanine is frequent), hematopoietic depression, pregnancy, lactation.
- Use caution in the presence of impaired renal function (slower drug elimination and greater accumulation; reduce dosage).

Dosage
Adult and Pediatric
- ***Induction therapy:*** Usual initial dose is 2.5 mg/kg per day PO (about 100–200 mg in adults, 50 mg in the average 5-year-old). Continue daily for several weeks. After 4 wk, if no clinical improvement or toxicity, increase to 5 mg/kg per day.
- ***Maintenance therapy after complete hematologic remission:*** 1.5–2.5 mg/kg per day PO as a single daily dose. Often effective in children with acute lymphatic leukemia, especially in combination with methotrexate. Effectiveness in adults has not been noted.

Pharmacokinetics

Route	Onset	Peak
Oral	Varies	2 h

Metabolism: Hepatic, $T_{1/2}$: 20–50 min
Distribution: Crosses placenta; enters breast milk
Excretion: Urine

Adverse effects
- **GI:** Hepatotoxicity; oral lesions—resemble thrush; nausea; vomiting; anorexia
- **Hematologic:** ***Bone marrow depression, immunosuppression,*** *hyperuri-*

Adverse effects in *Italics* are most common; those in **Bold** are life-threatening.

cemia as consequence of antineoplastic effect and cell lysis
- Other: Drug fever, cancer, chromosomal aberrations

Clinically important drug-drug interactions

- Increased risk of severe toxicity if mercaptopurine is taken concurrently with allopurinol; reduce dose of mercaptopurine to one-third to one-fourth the usual dose
- Decreased or reversed actions of nondepolarizing neuromuscular relaxants (atracurium, gallamine, metocurine iodide, pancuronium, tubocurarine, vecuronium) if taken concurrently with mercaptopurine

■ Nursing Considerations

Assessment

- *History:* Allergy to mercaptopurine; prior resistance to mercaptopurine; hematopoietic depression; impaired renal function; pregnancy; lactation
- *Physical:* Temperature; mucous membranes, liver evaluation, abdominal exam; CBC, differential, hemoglobin, platelet counts; renal and liver function tests; urinalysis; serum uric acid

Implementation

- Arrange for tests to evaluate hematopoietic status before beginning therapy and frequently during therapy.
- Ensure that patient is well hydrated before and during therapy to minimize adverse effects of hyperuricemia.
- Administer as a single daily dose.

Drug-specific teaching points

- Drink adequate fluids while you are on this drug; drink at least 8–10 glasses of fluid each day.
- Know that the following side effects may occur: mouth sores (frequent mouth care will be needed); miscarriages (it is advisable to use birth control while on this drug).
- Arrange to have frequent, regular medical follow-up, including frequent blood tests to follow the effects of the drug on your body.
- Report fever, chills, sore throat, unusual bleeding or bruising, yellow discoloration of the skin or eyes, abdominal pain, flank pain, joint pain, fever, weakness, diarrhea.

☐ mesalamine

*(me **sal'** a meen)*

5-aminosalicylic acid, 5-ASA
Asacol (oral), Rowasa

Pregnancy Category B

Drug classes
Anti-inflammatory

Therapeutic actions
Mechanism of action is unknown; thought to be a direct, local anti-inflammatory effect in the colon where mesalamine blocks cyclooxygenase and inhibits prostaglandin production in the colon.

Indications
- Treatment of active mild to moderate distal ulcerative colitis, proctosigmoiditis, or proctitis

Contraindications/cautions
- Contraindicated in the presence of hypersensitivity to mesalamine, salicylates, any component of the formulation.
- Use caution in the presence of renal impairment, pregnancy, lactation.

Dosage
Adult
- ***Suspension enema:*** 60 ml U in one rectal instillation (4 g) once a day, preferably at bedtime, and retained for approximately 8 h. Usual course of therapy is 3–6 wk. Effects may be seen within 3–21 d.
- *Rectal suppository:* 500 mg (1 suppository) bid. Retain suppository for 1–3 h or more. Usual course is 3–6 wk.
- *Oral:* 800 mg PO tid for 6 wk.

Pediatric: Safety and efficacy not established.

Adverse effects in *Italics* are most common; those in **Bold** are life-threatening.

Pharmacokinetics

Route	Onset	Peak
Oral	Varies	3–6 h
Rectal	Slow	3–6 h

Metabolism: $T_{1/2}$: 5–10 h
Distribution: Unknown
Excretion: Feces

Adverse effects

- CNS: *Headache, fatigue, malaise,* dizziness, asthenia, insomnia
- GI: *Abdominal pain, cramps, discomfort; gas; flatulence; nausea;* diarrhea, bloating, hemmorhoids, rectal pain, constipation
- GU: UTI, urinary burning
- Other: *Flulike symptoms, fever, cold,* rash, back pain, hair loss, peripheral edema

■ Nursing Considerations

Assessment

- *History:* Hypersensitivity to mesalamine, salicylates, any component of the formulation; renal impairment; lactation
- *Physical:* Temperature, hair status; reflexes, affect; abdominal exam, rectal exam; urinary output; renal function tests

Implementation

- Administer enemas as follows: Shake bottle well to ensure suspension is homogenous. Remove protective applicator sheath; hold bottle at the neck to ensure that none of the dose is lost. Have patient lie on the left side (to facilitate migration of drug into the sigmoid colon) with the lower leg extended and the upper leg flexed forward. Knee-chest position can be used if more acceptable to the patient. Gently insert the application tip into the rectum pointing toward the umbilicus; steadily squeeze the bottle to discharge the medication. Patient must retain medication for approximately 8 h.
- Administer rectal suppository as follows: remove the foil wrapper; avoid excessive handling (suppository will melt at body temperature); insert completely into the rectum with pointed end first; have patient retain for 3 h or more.
- Caution patient not to chew tablet; swallow whole. Notify physician if intact tablets are found in the stool.
- Monitor patients with renal impairment for possible adverse effects.

Drug-specific teaching points

- Be aware that if the drug is given as a suspension enema, so the medication must be retained for approximately 8 h; it is best given at bedtime to facilitate the retention; the effects of the drug are usually seen within 3–21 d, but a full course of therapy is about 6 wk. (Review administration with patient and significant other.)
- Administer rectal suppository as follows: remove the foil wrapper; avoid excessive handling (suppository will melt at body temperature); insert completely into the rectum with pointed end first; retain for 3 h or more.
- Do not chew oral tablets; swallow whole. If intact tablets are seen in the stool, notify physician.
- Know that the following side effects may occur: abdominal cramping, discomfort, pain, gas (relax; maintain the position used for insertion to relieve pressure on the abdomen); headache, fatigue, fever, flulike symptoms (medications may be available to help); hair loss (this is usually mild and transient; it may help to know that it is a drug effect).
- Report difficulty breathing, rash, severe abdominal pain, fever, headache.

❒ mesna

(mes' na)
Mesnex

Pregnancy Category B

Drug classes
Antidote

Therapeutic actions
Reacts chemically with the urotoxic ifosfamide metabolites to inhibit hemorrhagic cystitis induced by ifosfamide.

Adverse effects in *Italics* are most common; those in **Bold** are life-threatening.

Indications
- Prophylactic agent to reduce the incidence of ifosfamide-induced hemorrhagic cystitis
- Orphan drug use: reduction of the incidence of cyclophosphamide-induced hemorrhagic cystitis

Contraindications/cautions
- Hypersensitivity to mesna of thiol compounds, pregnancy, lactation.

Dosage
Dosage is equal to 20% of the ifosfamide dose, given as a single bolus IV injection at the time ifosfamide injection and at 4 and 8 h after each dose (eg, 1.2 g/m^2 ifosfmamide: mesna 240 mg/m^2 at time of dose, at 4 h, and at 8 h). Repeat each day that ifosfamide is given; if ifosfamide dose is adjusted, adjust mesna dose accordingly.

Pharmacokinetics

Route	Onset	Duration
IV	Rapid	Hours

Metabolism: T$_{1/2}$: 0.36–1.7 h
Distribution: Crosses placenta; may enter breast milk
Excretion: Urine

IV facts
Preparation: Dilute by adding the contents of a mesna ampule to obtain a final concentration of 20 mg mesna/ml fluid to 5% Dextrose Injection, 5% Dextrose and Sodium Chloride Injection, 0.9% Sodium Chloride Injection or Lactated Ringer's Injection. Refrigerate for use within 6 h of dilution; discard any unused drug in the ampule after opening.
Infusion: Administer as an IV bolus.
Incompatibilities: Do not mix with cisplatin.

Adverse effects
Because mesna is given in combination with other toxic drugs, seperate adverse effects are difficult to distinguish.
- GI: *Nausea, vomiting, diarrhea*

Drug-lab test interferences
- False-positive test for urinary ketones

■ Nursing Considerations
Assessment
- *History:* Hypersensitivity to mesna, thiol compounds, pregnancy, lactation
- *Physical:* Body temperature; skin—color, texture, lesions; orientation, frequency and pattern of voiding, normal output; kidney function tests

Implementation
- Prepare within 6 h of use; discard any unused drug in the ampule.
- Record timing of ifosfamide administration accurately to determine timing of mesna dose.
- Monitor patient for signs of bladder hemorrhage.

Drug-specific teaching points
- Be aware that this drug will be given IV to help prevent some of the side effects of your chemotherapy.

⬜ mesoridazine besylate

*(mez oh **rid**' a zeen)*
Serentil

Pregnancy Category C

Drug classes
Phenothiazine (piperidine)
Dopaminergic-blocking drug
Antipsychotic drug
Antianxiety drug

Therapeutic actions
Mechanism of action not fully understood: antipsychotic drugs block postsynaptic dopamine receptors in the brain, depressing the reticular activating system, including the parts of the brain involved with wakefulness and emesis; anticholinergic, antihistaminic (H$_1$), and alpha-adrenergic blocking activity also may contribute to some of its therapeutic (and adverse) actions.

Adverse effects in *Italics* are most common; those in **Bold** are life-threatening.

Indications
- Schizophrenia: reduces severity of symptoms
- Behavioral problems in mental deficiency and chronic brain syndrome: reduces hyperactivity and uncooperativeness
- Alcoholism: ameliorate anxiety, depression, nausea in acute and chronic alcoholics
- Psychoneurotic manifestations: reduces symptoms of anxiety and tension

Contraindications/cautions
- Contraindicated in the presence of coma or severe CNS depression; bone marrow depression; blood dyscrasia; circulatory collapse; subcortical brain damage; Parkinson's disease; liver damage; cerebral arteriosclerosis; coronary disease; severe hypotension or hypertension.
- Use caution in the presence of respiratory disorder ("silent pneumonia" may develop); glaucoma, prostatic hypertrophy, epilepsy or history of epilepsy, breast cancer, thyrotoxicosis, peptic ulcer, decreased renal function, myelography within previous 24 h or scheduled within 48 h, exposure to heat or phosphorous insecticides; pregnancy; lactation; children younger than 12 y, especially those with chickenpox, CNS infections (children are especially susceptible to dystonias that may confound the diagnosis of Reye's syndrome).

Dosage
Full clinical effects may require 6 wk–6 mo of therapy.
Adult
- ***Schizophrenia:*** Initial dosage 50 mg PO tid (optimal total dosage range 100–400 mg/d).
- ***Behavior problems in mental deficiency:*** Initial dosage 25 mg PO (optimal total dosage range 75–300 mg/d).
- ***Alcoholism:*** Initial dosage 25 mg PO bid (optimal total dosage range 50–200 mg/d).
- ***Psychoneurotic manifestations:*** Initial dosage 10 mg PO tid (optimal total dosage range 30–150 mg/d).
- ***IM administration:*** Initial dose 25 mg; may repeat in 30–60 min if necessary (usually optimum dosage range 25–500 mg/d).

Pediatric: Generally not recommended for children younger than 12 y.
Geriatric: Use lower doses, and increase dosage more gradually than in younger patients.

Pharmacokinetics

Route	Onset	Peak	Duration
Oral	Varies	2–4 h	4–6 h
IM	Rapid	30 min	6–8 h

Metabolism: Hepatic, $T_{1/2}$: 24–48 h
Distribution: Crosses placenta; enters breast milk
Excretion: Renal and bile

Adverse effects
Antipsychotic Drugs
- CNS: *Drowsiness,* insomnia, vertigo, headache, weakness, tremor, ataxia, slurring, cerebral edema, seizures, exacerbation of psychotic symptoms, extrapyramidal syndromes—*pseudoparkinsonism; dystonias; akathisia,* tardive dyskinesias, potentially irreversible (no known treatment), neuroleptic malignant syndrome (NMS)
- CV: Hypotension, orthostatic hypotension, hypertension, tachycardia, bradycardia, cardiac arrest, CHF, cardiomegaly, **refractory arrhythmias** (some fatal), pulmonary edema
- Respiratory: Bronchospasm, laryngospasm, dyspnea, suppression of cough reflex and potential for aspiration
- Hematologic: Eosinophilia, leukopenia, leukocytosis, anemia; aplastic anemia; hemolytic anemia; thrombocytopenic or nonthrombocytopenic purpura; pancytopenia
- Hypersensitivity: Jaundice, urticaria, angioneurotic edema, laryngeal edema, photosensitivity, eczema, asthma, ana-

Adverse effects in *Italics* are most common; those in **Bold** are life-threatening.

phylactoid reactions, exfoliative dermatitis
- **Endocrine:** Lactation, breast engorgement in females, galactorrhea; syndrome of inappropriate ADH secretion (SIADH); amenorrhea, menstrual irregularities; gynecomastia in males; changes in libido; hyperglycemia or hypoglycemia; glycosuria; hyponatremia; pituitary tumor with hyperprolactinemia; inhibition of ovulation, infertility, pseudopregnancy; reduced urinary levels of gonadotropins, estrogens, progestins
- **Autonomic:** Dry mouth, salivation, nasal congestion, nausea, vomiting, anorexia, fever, pallor, flushed facies, sweating, constipation, paralytic ileus, urinary retention, incontinence, polyuria, enuresis, priapism, ejaculation inhibition, male impotence

Clinically important drug-drug interactions
- Additive CNS depression with alcohol • Additive anticholinergic effects and possibly decreased antipsychotic efficacy with anticholinergic drugs • Increased likelihood of seizures with metrizamide (contrast agent used in myelography) • Decreased antihypertensive effect of guanethidine when taken with antipsychotic drugs

Drug-lab test interferences
- False-positive pregnancy tests (less likely if serum test is used) • Increase in protein-bound iodine, not attributable to an increase in thyroxine

■ Nursing Considerations

Assessment
- *History:* Coma or severe CNS depression, bone marrow depression, circulatory collapse, subcortical brain damage, Parkinson's disease, liver damage, cerebral arteriosclerosis, coronary disease, severe hypotension or hypertension, respiratory disorders, glaucoma, prostatic hypertrophy, epilepsy, breast cancer, thyrotoxicosis, peptic ulcer, decreased renal function, myelography within previous 24 h or scheduled within 48 h, exposure to heat or phosphorous insecticides, lactation, children younger than 12
- *Physical:* Body weight, temperature; reflexes, orientation, intraocular pressure; P, BP, orthostatic BP; R, adventitious sounds; bowel sounds and normal output, liver evaluation; urinary output, prostate size; CBC, urinalysis, thyroid, liver and kidney function tests

Implementation
- Do not change dosage in chronic therapy more often than weekly; drug requires 4–7 d to achieve steady state plasma levels.
- Avoid skin contact with oral solution; contact dermatitis has occurred.
- Arrange for discontinuation of drug if serum creatinine, BUN become abnormal or if WBC count is depressed.
- Monitor elderly patients for dehydration, and institute remedial measures promptly; sedation and decreased sensation of thirst related to CNS effects of drug can lead to severe dehydration.
- Consult physician regarding appropriate warning of patient or patient's guardian about tardive dyskinesias.
- Consult physician about dosage reduction; use of anticholinergic antiparkinsonian drugs (controversial) if extrapyramidal effects occur.

Drug-specific teaching points
- Take drug exactly as prescribed.
- Avoid skin contact with drug solutions.
- Avoid driving a car or engaging in other dangerous activities if CNS, vision changes occur.
- Avoid prolonged exposure to sun or to use a sunscreen or covering garments if this is necessary.
- Maintain fluid intake and use precautions against heatstroke in hot weather.
- Report sore throat, fever, unusual bleeding or bruising, rash, weakness, tremors, impaired vision, dark colored urine (pink or reddish brown urine is to be expected), pale stools, yellow of the skin or eyes.

Adverse effects in *Italics* are most common; those in **Bold** are life-threatening.

☐ metaproterenol sulfate

*(met a proe **ter'** e nole)*
Alupent, Metaprel

Pregnancy Category C

Drug classes
Sympathomimetic drug
β_2 selective adrenergic agonist
Bronchodilator
Antiasthmatic drug

Therapeutic actions
In low doses, acts relatively selectively at β_2 adrenergic receptors to cause bronchodilation; at higher doses, β_2 selectivity is lost and the drug also acts at β_1 receptors to cause typical sympathomimetic cardiac effects.

Indications
- Prophylaxis and treatment of bronchial asthma and reversible bronchospasm that may occur with bronchitis and emphysema

Contraindications/cautions
- Contraindicated in the presence of hypersensitivity to metaproterenol; tachyarrhythmias, tachycardia caused by digitalis intoxication; general anesthesia with halogenated hydrocarbons or cyclopropane, which sensitize the myocardium to catecholamines.
- Use caution in the presence of unstable vasomotor system disorders; hypertension; coronary artery disease; history of stroke; COPD patients who have developed degenerative heart disease; hyperthyroidism; history of seizure disorders; psychoneurotic individuals; pregnancy; labor and delivery (may inhibit labor; parenteral use of β_2-adrenergic agonists can accelerate fetal heart beat, cause hypoglycemia, hypokalemia, and pulmonary edema in the mother and hypoglycemia in the neonate); lactation.

Dosage
Adult
- ***Oral:*** 20 mg tid or qid.
- ***Inhalation—metered dose inhaler:*** Each actuation of aerosol dispenser delivers 0.65 micronized metaproterenol powder: 2–3 inhalations q3–4h. Do not exceed 12 inhalations/d.
- ***Inhalant solutions:*** Administer tid–qid from hand bulb nebulizer or using an IPPB device, following manufacturer's instructions.

Pediatric
- ***Oral:*** *9 y or 60 lbs:* 20 mg tid or qid.
 6-9 y or < 60 lbs: 10 mg tid or qid.
 < 6 y: doses of 1.3–2.6 mg/kg/d in divided doses of syrup have been well tolerated.
- ***Inhalation:*** *> 12 y:* same as adult.
 < 12 y: Not recommended.

Geriatric: Patients > 60 y are more likely to develop adverse effects, use extreme caution.

Pharmacokinetics

Route	Onset	Peak	Duration
PO	15 min	1 h	4 h
Inhal.	1–4 min	1 h	3–4 h

Metabolism: Liver and tissue; T1/2: unknown
Excretion: Bile and feces

Adverse effects
- **CNS:** *Restlessness, apprehension, anxiety, fear, CNS stimulation,* hyperkinesia, insomnia, tremor, drowsiness, irritability, weakness, vertigo, headache
- **GI:** *Nausea, vomiting, heartburn,* unusual or bad taste
- **CV:** *Cardiac arrhythmias, tachycardia,* palpitations, PVC's (rare), anginal pain—less likely with bronchodilator doses of this drug than with bronchodilator doses of a non-selective beta-agonist (isoproterenol), changes in BP (increases or decreases)
- **Respiratory:** Respiratory difficulties, pulmonary edema, coughing, bronchospasm, paradoxical airway resistance

---
Adverse effects in *Italics* are most common; those in **Bold** are life-threatening.

with repeated, excessive use of inhalation preparations
- Other: *Sweating, pallor, flushing*

■ Nursing Considerations
Assessment
- *History:* Hypersensitivity to metaproterenol; tachyarrhythmias; general anesthesia with halogenated hydrocarbons or cyclopropane; unstable vasomotor system disorders; hypertension; coronary artery disease; stroke; COPD patients who have developed degenerative heart disease; hyperthyroidism; seizure disorders; psychoneuroses; pregnancy; labor; lactation.
- *Physical:* Body weight, skin—color, temperature, turgor; orientation, reflexes; P, BP; R, adventitious sounds; blood and urine glucose, serum electrolytes, thyroid function tests, ECG

Implementation
- Use minimal doses for minimal periods of time–drug tolerance can occur with prolonged use.
- Maintain a beta-adrenergic blocker (a cardioselective beta blocker such as atenolol should be used in patients with respiratory distress) on standby in case cardiac arrhythmias occur.
- Do not exceed recommended dosage. Administer aerosol during second half of inspiration, as the airways are open wider and the aerosol distribution is more extensive.
- Consult manufacturer's instructions for use of aerosol delivery equipment; specifics of administration vary with each product.

Drug-specific teaching points
- Do not exceed recommended dosage; adverse effects or loss of effectiveness may result. Read the instructions for use that come with the aerosol product and ask your health care provider or pharmacist if you have any questions.
- Know that the following side effects may occur: nausea, vomiting, change in taste (small, frequent meals may help); dizziness, drowsiness, fatigue, weakness (use caution if driving or performing tasks that require alertness if these effects occur); irritability, apprehension, sweating, flushing.
- Report chest pain, dizziness, insomnia, weakness, tremor or irregular heart beat, difficulty breathing, productive cough, failure to respond to usual dosage.

☐ metaraminol bitartrate

*(met a **ram'** i nole)*
Aramine

Pregnancy Category D

Drug classes
Sympathomimetic drug
Alpha-adrenergic agonist
Vasopressor
Drug used in shock

Therapeutic actions
Vasopressor without cardiac stimulation; effects are mediated by alpha adrenergic receptors in the vasculature; potent vasoconstrictor.

Indications
- Prevention and treatment of acute hypotension with spinal anesthesia
- Adjunctive treatment of hypotension due to hemorrhage, drug reactions, surgical complications, shock associated with brain damage due to trauma or tumor
- 'Probably effective' as adjunct in treatment of hypotension due to cardiogenic or septicemic shock

Contraindications/cautions
- Contraindicated in the presence of cyclopropane or halothane anesthesia (cardiac arrhythmias may occur); hypovolemia (metaraminol is not a substitute for restoration of fluids, plasma, electrolytes, which should be replaced promptly when loss has occurred).
- Use caution in the presence of hyperthyroidism, severe hypertension, heart disease, diabetes mellitus, cirrhosis (restore

electrolytes lost in drug-induced diuresis), malaria, pregnancy, lactation.

Dosage
Individualize dosage on the basis of the patient's response. At least 10 min should be allowed between successive doses so that effects of previous dose are fully apparent.
Adult
- *IM or SC (prevention of hypotension):* 2–10 mg.
- *IV infusion (adjunctive therapy of hypotension):* 15–100 mg in 500 ml Sodium Chloride Injection or 5% Dextrose Injection. Adjust rate of infusion to maintain desired BP. Adjust drug concentration on the basis of the patient's need for fluid. Concentrations of 150–500 mg/500 ml of infusion fluid have been used.
- *Direct IV injection (severe shock):* 0.5–5 mg, followed by infusion of 15–100 mg in 500 ml IV fluid.

Pediatric: 0.01 mg/kg as a single dose or a solution of 1 mg/25 ml in dextrose or saline.

Pharmacokinetics

Route	Onset	Duration
SC	5–20 min	1 h
IM	10 min	1 h
IV	1–2 min	15–20 min

Metabolism: Tissue; $T_{1/2}$: unknown

IV facts
Preparation: Dilute 15–100 mg in 500 ml Sodium Chloride Injection or 5% Dextrose Injection for continuous infusion. Direct injection can be given undiluted, but follow with infusion of 15–100 mg in 500 ml of IV fluid. Use diluted solutions within 24 h.

Infusion: Rate of infusion in determined by patient response to drug.

Compatibilities: Compatible with Sodium Chloride Injection, 5% Dextrose Injection, Ringer's Injection, Lactated Ringer's Injection, 6% Dextran in Saline, *Normosol-R*, *Normosol-M* in D$_5$W.

Adverse effects
- **CNS:** *Headache, flushing*, sweating, tremors, dizziness, apprehension
- **CV:** *Sinus or ventricular tachycardia, other arrhythmias* (especially in MI patients), cardiac arrest, palpitation, hypertension; hypotension upon withdrawal
- **GI:** Nausea
- **Local:** Abscess formation, tissue necrosis, sloughing at injection site

Clinically important drug-drug interactions
- Increased hypertensive effects when given to patients receiving tricyclic antidepressants (imipramine, etc.), MAO inhibitors; guanethidine, reserpine (rauwolfia alkaloids), methyldopa, furazolidine.

■ Nursing Considerations
Assessment
- *History:* Cyclopropane or halothane anesthesia; hypovolemia; hyperthyroidism; severe hypertension; heart disease; diabetes mellitus; cirrhosis; malaria; pregnancy; lactation
- *Physical:* Body weight, skin—color, temperature, turgor; injection sites; orientation, reflexes, affect; P, BP; R, adventitious sounds; liver palpation; urine output; serum electrolytes, thyroid and liver function tests, blood and urine glucose, ECG

Implementation
- Administer IV infusions into a large vein, preferably of the antecubital fossa, to prevent extravasation.
- Do not infuse into veins of the ankle or dorsum of the hand in patients with peripheral vascular disease, diabetes mellitus, or hypercoagulability states.
- Monitor BP frequently; avoid excessive BP response—rapidly induced hypertensive responses have been reported to cause pulmonary edema, arrhythmias, cardiac arrest.
- Provide phentolamine on standby in case extravasation occurs (5–10 mg phentolamine in 10–15 ml saline should be used to infiltrate the affected area).

Drug-specific teaching points
- Since metaraminol is used mainly during anesthesia or acute emergency states, patient teaching will relate mainly to anesthesia, the procedure, and monitors rather than specifically to therapy with metaraminol. Points patient should be told include: this drug may cause dizziness, apprehension, sweating, flushing; report any pain at the injection site.

◻ metformin

(met fore' min)
Glucophage

Pregnancy Category C̆

Drug classes
Antidiabetic agent

Therapeutic actions
Exact mechanism of action is not understood; possibly increases peripheral utilization of glucose, increases production of insulin, decreases hepatic glucose production and alters intestinal absorption of glucose.

Indications
- Adjunct to diet to lower blood glucose in patients with non-insulin-dependent diabetes mellitus (type II)

Contraindications/cautions
- Allergy to metformin; diabetes complicated by fever, severe infections, severe trauma, major surgery, ketosis, acidosis, coma (insulin is indicated in these conditions); type I or juvenile diabetes, serious hepatic impairment, serious renal impairment, uremia, thyroid or endocrine impairment, glycosuria, hyperglycemia associated with primary renal disease; ; labor and delivery— if metformin is used during pregnancy, discontinue drug at least 1 mo before delivery; lactation, safety not established.

Dosage
Adult: 500 mg/d PO in divided doses to a maximum of 3000 mg/d. Dose should be titrated based on patient response and blood glucose level.
Pediatric: Safety and efficacy not established.
Geriatric and renal impaired: Smaller doses may be necessary; monitor closely and titrate slowly

Pharmacokinetics

Route	Peak	Duration
Oral	2–2.5 h	10–16 h

Metabolism: Hepatic metabolism; $T_{1/2}$: 1.5 and 4.9 hours
Distribution: Crosses placenta; passes into breast milk
Excretion: Urine

Adverse effects
- GI: *anorexia, nausea,* vomiting, *epigastric discomfort, heartburn , diarrhea*
- Endocrine: *hypoglycemia,* **lacticacidosis**
- Hypersensitivity: *allergic skin reactions*, eczema, pruritus, erythema, urticaria

Clinically important drug-drug interactions
- Increased risk of hypoglycemia if taken concurrently with cimetidine • Increased risk of lactic acidosis if taken with glucocorticoids or ethanol

■ Nursing Considerations
Assessment
- *History:* Allergy to metformin; diabetes complicated by fever, severe infections, severe trauma, major surgery, ketosis, acidosis, coma; type I or juvenile diabetes, serious hepatic or renal impairment, uremia, thyroid or endocrine impairment, glycosuria, hyperglycemia associated with primary renal disease.
- *Physical:* Skin—Color, lesions; body temperature orientation, reflexes, peripheral sensation; R, adventitious sounds; liver evaluation, bowel sounds; urinaly-

Adverse effects in *Italics* are most common; those in **Bold** are life-threatening.

sis, BUN, serum creatinine, liver function tests, blood glucose, CBC.

Implementation
- Monitor urine and serum glucose levels frequently to determine effectiveness of drug and dosage.
- Arrange for transfer to insulin therapy during periods of high stress (infections, surgery, trauma, and so forth).
- Arrange for use of IV glucose if severe hypoglycemia occurs as a result of overdose.

Drug-specific teaching points
- Do not discontinue this medication without consulting your physician.
- Monitor urine or blood for glucose and ketones as prescribed.
- Do not use this drug during pregnancy.
- Avoid the use of alcohol while on this drug.
- Report fever, sore throat, unusual bleeding or bruising, skin rash, dark urine, light-colored stools, hypo- or hyperglycemic reactions.

☐ methadone hydrochloride

(meth' a done)
Dolophine

Pregnancy Class C
C-II controlled substance

Drug classes
Narcotic agonist analgesic

Therapeutic actions
Acts as agonist at specific opioid receptors in the CNS to produce analgesia, euphoria, sedation; the receptors mediating these effects are thought to be the same as those mediating the effects of endogenous opioids (enkephalins, endorphins); when used in approved methadone maintenance programs, can substitute for heroin, other illicit narcotics in patients who want to terminate a drug-seeking way of life.

Indications
- Relief of severe pain
- Detoxification and temporary maintenance treatment of narcotic addiction (ineffective for relief of general anxiety)

Contraindications/cautions
- Contraindicated in the presence of hypersensitivity to narcotics, diarrhea caused by poisoning (before toxins are eliminated), bronchial asthma, COPD, cor pulmonale, respiratory depression, anoxia, kyphoscoliosis, acute alcoholism, increased intracranial pressure.
- Use caution in the presence of acute abdominal conditions, cardiovascular disease, supraventricular tachycardias, myxedema, convulsive disorders, delirium tremens, cerebral arteriosclerosis, ulcerative colitis, fever, Addison's disease, prostatic hypertrophy, urethral stricture, recent GI or GU surgery, toxic psychosis, pregnancy prior to labor (readily crosses placenta; neonatal withdrawal has occurred in infants born to mothers who used narcotics during pregnancy; safety for use in pregnancy before labor not established), labor or delivery (administration of narcotics, including meperidine, to the mother can cause respiratory depression of neonate—premature infants are especially at risk), renal or hepatic dysfunction, lactation.

Dosage
Oral methadone is approximately 1/2 as potent as parenteral methadone.
Adult
- ***Relief of pain:*** 2.5–10 mg IM, SC or PO q3–4 h as necessary. IM route is preferred to SC for repeated doses. Individualize dosage: patients with excessively severe pain and those who have become tolerant to the analgesic effect of narcotics may need higher dosage.
- ***Detoxification:*** Initially, 15–20 mg PO or parenteral–PO preferred. Increase dose to suppress withdrawal signs. 40 mg/d in single or divided doses is usually an adeqate stabilizing dose for patients who are physically dependent on high doses. Continue stabilizing doses for 2–3 d, then gradually decrease dosage every

d or every 2 d. A daily reduction of 20% of the total dose may be tolerated. Provide sufficient dosage to keep withdrawal symptoms at tolerable level. Treatment should not exceed 21 d and may not be repeated earlier than 4 wk after completion of previous course. Detoxification treatment continued longer than 21 d becomes maintenance treatment, which may be undertaken only by approved programs (except that addicts who are hospitalized for other medical conditions may receive methadone maintenance treatment).

- **Maintenance treatment:** For patients who are heavy heroin users up until hospital admission, initial dose of 20 mg q4-8 h or 40 mg in a single dose PO. For patients with little or no narcotic tolerance, half this dose may suffice. Dosage should suppress withdrawal symptoms but not produce acute narcotic effects of sedation, respiratory depression, etc.. Give additional 10 mg doses if needed to suppress withdrawal syndrome. Adjust dosage, up to 120 mg/d.

Pediatric: Not recommended for relief of pain in children due to insufficient documentation.

Geriatric or impaired adult: Use caution–respiratory depression may occur in the elderly, the very ill, those with respiratory problems. Reduced dosage may be necessary.

Pharmacokinetics

Route	Onset	Peak	Duration
PO	30–60 min	90–120 min	4–12 h
IM	10–20 min	1–2 h	4–6 h
SC	10–20 min	1–2 h	4–6 h

Metabolism: Liver; $T_{1/2}$: 25 h
Distribution: Crosses placenta and enters breast milk
Excretion: Bile and feces

Adverse effects

- CNS: *Lightheadedness, dizziness, sedation,* euphoria, dysphoria, delirium, insomnia, agitation, anxiety, fear, hallucinations, disorientation, drowsiness, lethargy, impaired mental and physical performance, coma, mood changes, weakness, headache, tremor, convulsions, miosis, visual disturbances, suppression of cough reflex
- GI: *Nausea, vomiting,* dry mouth, anorexia, constipation, biliary tract spasm; increased colonic motility in patients with chronic ulcerative colitis
- CV: Facial flushing, peripheral circulatory collapse, arrhythmia, palpitations, chest wall rigidity, hypertension, hypotension, orthostatic hypotension, syncope
- GU: Ureteral spasm, spasm of vesical sphincters, urinary retention or hesitancy, oliguria, antidiuretic effect, reduced libido or potency
- Dermatologic: Pruritus, urticaria, laryngospasm, bronchospasm, edema, hemorrhagic urticaria (rare)
- Local: Tissue irritation and induration (SC injection)
- Other: Sweating (more common in ambulatory patients and those without severe pain),physical tolerance and dependence, psychological dependence
- Major hazards: **Respiratory depression, apnea, circulatory depression, respiratory arrest, shock, cardiac arrest**

Clinically important drug-drug interactions

- Potentiation of effects of levorphanol when given with barbiturate anesthetics–decrease dose of meperidine when coadministering • Decreased effectiveness of methadone if taken concurrently with hydantoins, rifampin, urinary acidifiers (ammonium chloride, potassium acid phosphate, sodium acid phosphate) • Increased effects and toxicity of methadone if taken concurrently with cimetidine, ranitidine

Adverse effects in *Italics* are most common; those in **Bold** are life-threatening.

Drug-lab test interferences
- Elevated biliary tract pressure (an effect of narcotics) may cause increases in plasma amylase, lipase; determinations of these levels may be unreliable for 24 h after administration of narcotics.

■ Nursing Considerations
Assessment
- *History:* Hypersensitivity to narcotics, diarrhea caused by poisoning, bronchial asthma, COPD, cor pulmonale, respiratory depression, kyphoscoliosis, acute alcoholism, increased intracranial pressure; acute abdominal conditions, cardiovascular disease, supraventricular tachycardias, myxedema, convulsive disorders, delirium tremens, cerebral arteriosclerosis, ulcerative colitis, fever, Addison's disease, prostatic hypertrophy, urethral stricture, recent GI or GU surgery, toxic psychosis; pregnancy; labor; lactation.
- *Physical:* Body temperature; skin—color, texture, lesions; orientation, reflexes, bilateral grip strength, affect, pupil size; pulse, auscultation, BP, orthostatic BP, perfusion; R, adventious sounds; bowel sounds, normal output; frequency and pattern of voiding, normal output; ECG; EEG; thyroid, liver, kidney function tests.

Implementation
- Administer to women who are nursing a baby 4–6 h before the next scheduled feeding to minimize the amount in milk.
- Provide narcotic antagonist, facilities for assisted or controlled respiration on standby during parenteral administration.
- Use caution when injecting SC into chilled areas or in patients with hypotension or in shock—impaired perfusion may delay absorption; with repeated doses, an excessive amount may be absorbed when circulation is restored.

Drug-specific teaching points
- Take drug exactly as prescribed.
- Avoid the use of alcohol while taking this drug.
- Know that the following side effects may occur: nausea, loss of appetite (taking the drug with food and lying quietly, eating frequent small meals should minimize these effects); constipation (a laxative may help); dizziness, sedation, drowsiness, impaired visual acuity (avoid driving a car, performing other tasks that require alertness, visual acuity).
- Do not take any leftover medication for other disorders and do not let anyone else take the prescription.
- Report severe nausea, vomiting, constipation, shortness of breath or difficulty breathing.

▢ methazolamide

(meth a zoe' la mide)
Neptazane
Pregnancy Category C

Drug classes
Carbonic anhydrase inhibitor
Antiglaucoma agent
Diuretic
Sulfonamide (nonbacteriostatic)

Therapeutic actions
Inhibits the enzyme carbonic anhydrase, thereby: decreasing aqueous humor formation and hence decreasing intraocular pressure; decreasing hydrogen ion secretion by renal tubule cells and hence increasing sodium, potassium, bicarbonate, and water excretion by the kidney.

Indications
- Adjunctive treatment of chronic open-angle glaucoma, secondary glaucoma
- Preoperative use in acute angle-closure glaucoma where delay of surgery is desired to lower intraocular pressure
- Unlabeled uses: treatment of hyperkalemia and hypokalemia periodic paralysis

Contraindications/cautions
- Contraindicated in the presence of allergy to dichlorphenamide, sulfonamides.
- Use caution in the presence of renal or liver disease; adrenocortical insufficiency;

706 ■ methdilazine hydrochloride

respiratory acidosis; COPD; chronic noncongestive angle-closure glaucoma; decreased sodium, potassium; hyperchloremic acidosis; pregnancy; lactation.

Dosage
Adult: 50–100 mg PO bid or tid. Most effective if taken with other miotics.

Pharmacokinetics

Route	Onset	Peak	Duration
PO	2–4 h	6–8 h	10–18 h

Metabolism: Liver, $T_{1/2}$: 14 h
Distribution: Crosses placenta and enters breast milk
Excretion: Urine

Adverse effects
- **CNS:** *Photophobia,* weakness, fatigue, nervousness, sedation, drowsiness, dizziness, depression, tremor, ataxia, headache, paresthesias, convulsions, flaccid paralysis, transient myopia
- **GI:** *Anorexia, nausea, vomiting, constipation,* melena, hepatic insufficiency
- **Hematologic:** Bone marrow depression
- **GU:** Hematuria, glycosuria, urinary frequency, renal colic, renal calculi, crystalluria, polyuria
- **Dermatologic:** Urticaria, pruritus, rash, *photosensitivity,* erythema multiforme
- **Other:** Weight loss, fever, acidosis

Clinically important drug-drug interactions
- Increased risk of salicylate toxicity, due to metabolic acidosis when salicylates are taken concurrently.

Drug-lab test interferences
- False-positive results on tests for urinary protein.

■ Nursing Considerations

Assessment
- *History:* Allergy to dichlorphenamide, sulfonamides; renal or liver disease; adrenocortical insufficiency; respiratory acidosis; COPD; chronic noncongestive angle-closure glaucoma; pregnancy; lactation.
- *Physical:* Skin color and lesion; temperature; weight; orientation, reflexes, muscle strength, ocular pressure; R, pattern, adventitious sounds; liver evaluation and bowel sounds; CBC, serum electrolytes, liver and renal function tests, urinalysis.

Implementation
- Administer with food if GI upset occurs; provide small, frequent meals.

Drug-specific teaching points
- Arrange to have periodic checks of intraocular pressure.
- Provide protection from the sun—use a sunscreen or wear protective clothing, you may be very sensitive to the sun.
- Report loss or gain of more than 3 lbs/d, unusual bleeding or bruising, dizziness, muscle cramps or weakness, skin rash.

❒ methdilazine hydrochloride

(meth **dill'** a zeen)
Dilosyn (CAN), Tacaryl

Pregnancy Category C

Drug classes
Phenothiazine (piperidine)
Dopaminergic blocking drug
Antihistamine

Therapeutic actions
Selectively blocks H_1 receptors, thereby diminishing the effects of histamine on cells of the upper respiratory tract and eyes and decreasing the sneezing, mucus production, itching, and tearing that accompany allergic reactions in sensitized people exposed to antigens.

Indications
- Symptomatic relief of symptoms associated with perennial and seasonal allergic rhinitis, vasomotor rhinitis, allergic conjunctivitis
- Mild, uncomplicated urticaria and angioedema
- Amelioration of allergic reactions to blood or plasma

Adverse effects in *Italics* are most common; those in **Bold** are life-threatening.

methdilazine hydrochloride ■ 707

- Dermatographism, adjunctive therapy (with epinephrine and other measures) in anaphylactic reactions

Contraindications/cautions

- Contraindicated in the presence of hypersensitivity to antihistamines or phenothiazines, coma or severe CNS depression; bone marrow depression; vomiting of unknown cause; concomitant therapy with MAO inhibitors; lactation (lactation may be inhibited; drug may be secreted in breast milk; drug has higher risk of adverse effects in newborns and premature infants).
- Use caution in the presence of lower respiratory tract disorders (drug may cause thickening of secretions and impair expectoration); glaucoma, prostatic hypertrophy (anticholinergic effects may exacerbate glaucoma and urinary retention); cardiovascular disease or hypertension; breast cancer (elevations in prolactin may stimulate a prolactin-dependent tumor); thyrotoxicosis (severe neurotoxicity may develop); peptic ulcer; decreased renal function; pregnancy; lactation; children under 12 y of age, especially those with chicken pox, CNS infections (children are especially susceptible to dystonias that may confound the diagnosis of Reye's syndrome); the elderly (antihistamines are more likely to cause dizziness, sedation, syncope, toxic confusional states, hypotension, and extrapyramidal effects in the elderly).

Dosage

Adult: 8 mg PO bid–qid.
Pediatric: Children > 3 y: 4 mg PO bid–qid.
Geriatric: Use special caution, elderly patients are more susceptible to adverse effects, reduced dosage may be needed.

Pharmacokinetics

Route	Onset	Peak	Duration
PO	15–30 min	1–2 h	4–6 h

Metabolism: Liver; $T_{1/2}$: 18 h

Distribution: Crosses placenta and enters breast milk
Excretion: Urine

Adverse effects

- **CNS:** *Dizziness, drowsiness, poor coordination, confusion, restlessness, excitation,* convulsions, tremors, headache, blurred vision, diplopia, vertigo, tinnitus
- **GI:** *Epigastric distress,* nausea, vomiting, diarrhea, constipation
- **CV:** Hypotension, palpitations, bradycardia, tachycardia, extrasystoles
- **Respiratory:** **Thickening of bronchial secretions;** chest tightness; dry mouth, nose and throat; respiratory depression; suppression of cough reflex, potential for aspiration
- **Hematologic:** Hemolytic anemia, hypoplastic anemia, thrombocytopenia, leukopenia, agranulocytosis, pancytopenia
- **GU:** *Urinary frequency, dysuria,* urinary retention, decreased libido, impotence
- **Dermatologic:** Uritcaria, rash, photosensitivity, chills
- **Other:** Tingling, heaviness and wetness of the hands

Clinically important drug-drug interactions

- Additive anticholinergic effects when taken concurrently with anticholinergic drugs. Increased likelihood of seizures with metrizamide (contrast agent used in myelography) • Decreased antihypertensive effect of guanethidine when taken concurrently

■ Nursing Considerations

Assessment

- *History:* Hypersensitivity to antihistamines or phenothiazines, coma or severe CNS depression; bone marrow depression; vomiting of unknown cause; concomitant therapy with MAO inhibitors; lactation; lower respiratory tract disorders ; glaucoma, prostatic hypertrophy; cardiovascular disease or hypertension; breast cancer; thyrotoxicosis; peptic ulcer;

Adverse effects in *Italics* are most common; those in **Bold** are life-threatening.

chicken pox, CNS infections; pregnancy; lactation
- *Physical:* Body weight, temperature; reflexes, orientation, intraocular pressure; P, BP, orthostatic BP; R, adventitious sounds; bowel sounds and normal output, liver evaluation; urinary output, prostate size; CBC, urinalysis, thyroid, liver and kidney function tests

Implementation
- Monitor patient for adverse response to anticholinergic effects and provide supportive care as needed.

Drug-specific teaching points
- Take this drug exactly as prescribed.
- Avoid skin contact with drug solutions.
- Avoid driving a car or engaging in other dangerous activities if CNS, vision changes occur.
- Avoid prolonged exposure to sun or to use a sunscreen or covering garments if this is necessary.
- Maintain fluid intake and use precautions against heatstroke in hot weather.
- Report sore throat, fever, unusual bleeding or bruising, rash, weakness, tremors, impaired vision, dark-colored urine, pale stools, yellowing of the skin or eyes.

methenamine

(meth *en'* a meen)

methenamine hippurate
Hiprex, Hip-Rex (CAN), Urex

methenamine mandelate
Mandelamine, Sterine (CAN)

Pregnancy Category C

Drug classes
Urinary tract anti-infective
Antibacterial drug

Therapeutic actions
Hydrolyzed in acid urine to ammonia and formaldehyde, which is bactericidal; the hippurate and mandelate salts help to maintain an acid urine.

Indications
- Suppression or elimination of bacteriuria associated with pyelonephritis, cystitis, chronic urinary tract infections, residual urine (accompanying some neurologic disorders), and in anatomic abnormalities or the urinary tract

Contraindications/cautions
- Contraindicated in the presence of allergy to methenamine, tartrazine (in preparations of methenamine hippurate marketed as *Hiprex*), aspirin (often associated with tartrazine allergy), pregnancy, lactation.
- Use caution in the presence of hepatic or renal dysfunction. gout (may cause urate crystals to precipitate in the urine).

Dosage
Adult
- ***Methenamine:*** 1 g qid PO.
- ***Methenamine hippurate:*** 1 g bid PO.
- ***Methenamine mandelate:*** 1 g qid PO after meals and at bedtime.

Pediatric
- ***Methenamine:*** 6–12 y: 500 mg qid PO. Younger than 6 y: 50 mg/kg per day PO divided into three doses.
- ***Methenamine hippurate:*** 6–12 y: 0.5–1 g bid PO. Older than 12 y: 1 g bid PO.
- ***Methenamine mandelate:*** 6–12 y: 0.5 gm qid PO. Younger than 6 y: 0.25 g/14 kg qid PO.

Pharmacokinetics

Route	Onset	Peak
Oral	Rapid	2–3 h

Metabolism: Hepatic, $T_{1/2}$: 3–6 h
Distribution: Crosses placenta; enters breast milk
Excretion: Urine

Adverse effects
- **GI:** *Nausea, abdominal cramps, vomiting, diarrhea,* anorexia, stomatitis

Adverse effects in *Italics* are most common; those in **Bold** are life-threatening.

- **GU:** *Bladder irritation, dysuria,* proteinuria, hematuria, frequency, urgency, cystalluria
- **Dermatologic:** pruritus, urticaria, erythematous eruptions
- **Other:** Headache, dyspnea, generalized edema, elevated serum transaminase (with hippurate salt)

Drug-lab test interferences
- False increase in 17-hydroxycorticosteroids, catecholamines • False decrease in 5-hydroxyindoleacetic acid • Inaccurate measurement of urine estriol levels by acid hydrolysis procedures during pregnancy

■ Nursing Considerations
Assessment
- *History:* Allergy to methenamine, tartrazine, aspirin; renal or hepatic dysfunction; dehydration; gout; lactation
- *Physical:* Skin—color, lesions; hydration; ear lobes—tophi; joints; liver evaluation; urinalysis, liver function tests; serum uric acid

Implementation
- Arrange for culture and sensitivity tests before and during therapy.
- Administer drug with food or milk to prevent GI upset; give drug around the clock for best effects.
- Ensure that patient avoids an excessive intake of foods or medications that alkalinize the urine.
- Ensure adequate hydration for patient.
- Monitor clinical response; if no improvement is seen or a relapse occurs, send urine for repeat culture and sensitivity tests.
- Monitor liver function tests with methenamine hippurate.

Drug-specific teaching points
- Take drug with food. Complete the full course of drug therapy to resolve the infection. Take this drug at regular intervals around the clock; consult your nurse or pharmacist for help setting up a schedule that does not interfere with your usual activities.
- Avoid foods that are alkalinizing (citrus fruits, milk products) or alkalinizing medications (sodium bicarbonate). Check with your nurse or physician if you are taking any other medications while on this drug.
- Drink plenty of fluids while you are on this drug.
- Know that the following side effects may occur: nausea, vomiting, abdominal pain (small, frequent meals may help); diarrhea; painful urination, frequency, blood in urine (drink plenty of fluids).
- Report rash, painful urination, severe GI upset.

☐ methicillin sodium

*(meth i **sill'** in)*

Staphcillin

Pregnancy Category B

Drug classes
Antibiotic
Penicillinase-resistant pencillin

Therapeutic actions
Bactericidal: inhibits cell wall synthesis of sensitive organisms, causing cell death.

Indications
- Infections due to penicillinase-producing staphylococci
- Initiation of treatment in any infection suspected to be staphylococcal

Contraindications/cautions
- Contraindicated in the presence of allergies to penicillins, cephalosporins, or other allergens.
- Use caution in the presence of renal disorders, pregnancy, lactation (may cause diarrhea or candidiasis in the infant).

Dosage
Maximum recommended dosage: 4 g/d.
Adult: 4–12 g/d IM or IV in divided doses q4–6h.
Pediatric: 100–300 mg/kg per d IM or IV in divided doses q4–6h. Reduced dosage is necessary in newborn and premature babies. See manufacturer's instructions.

methicillin sodium

Geriatric or renal impaired: If creatinine clearance < 10 ml/min, do not exceed 2 g q2h IM or IV.

Pharmacokinetics

Route	Onset	Peak	Duration
IM	Rapid	30–60 min	4 h
IV	Immediate	15 min	2 h

Metabolism: Hepatic, $T_{1/2}$: 20–30 min
Distribution: Crosses placenta; enters breast milk
Excretion: Urine and feces

IV facts

Preparation: Reconstitute in 50 ml of Sodium Chloride Injection. Dilute each ml of reconstituted solution with 20–25 ml Sodium Chloride Injection or Sterile Water for Injection. Further dilute reconstituted IV infusion solution with compatible IV solution: 0.9% Sodium Chloride Injection, 5% Dextrose in Water or in Normal Saline, 10% D-Fructose in Water or in Normal Saline, M/6 Sodium Lactate Solution, Lactated Ringer's Injection, Lactated Potassic Saline Injection, 5% Plasma Hydrolysate in Water, 10% Invert Sugar in Water or in Normal Saline, 10% Invert Sugar plus 0.3% Potassium Chloride in Water, Travert 10% Electrolyte #1, #2, or #3.
Infusion: Administer at rate of 10 ml/min.
Incompatibilities: Do not mix other agents with methicillin; give separately.

Adverse effects

- CNS: Lethargy, hallucinations, seizures
- GI: *Glossitis, stomatitis, gastritis, sore mouth,* furry tongue, black "hairy" tongue, *nausea, vomiting, diarrhea,* abdominal pain, bloody diarrhea, enterocolitis, pseudomembranous colitis, nonspecific hepatitis
- Hematologic: Anemia, thrombocytopenia, leukopenia, neutropenia, prolonged bleeding time
- GU: Nephritis (more common with this drug than with other penicillins)
- **Hypersensitivity reactions:** *Rash, fever, wheezing,* anaphylaxis
- Local: Pain, phlebitis, thrombosis at injection site
- Other: *Superinfections*—oral and rectal moniliasis, vaginitis

Clinically important drug-drug interactions

- Decreased effectiveness of methicillin if taken concurrently with tetracyclines
- Inactivation of parenteral aminoglycosides (amikacin, gentamicin, kanamycin, neomycin, metilmicin, streptomycin, tobramycin) if taken concurrently

Drug-lab test interferences

- Monitor for false-positive Coombs' test with IV use.

■ Nursing Considerations

Assessment

- *History:* Allergies to penicillins, cephalosporins, or other allergens; renal disorders; lactation.
- *Physical:* Culture infected area; skin—color, lesion; R, adventitious sounds; bowel sounds; CBC, liver and renal function tests, serum electrolytes, Hct, urinalysis.

Implementation

- Culture infected area before beginning treatment; reculture area if response is not as expected.
- Administer by IV and IM routes only.
- Reconstitute powder with Sterile Water for Injection or Sodium Chloride Injection.
- Dilute for IM injection as follows: 1-g vial, 1.5 ml of diluent; 4-g vial, 5.7 ml of diluent; 6-g vial, 8.6 ml of diluent. Each ml of reconstituted solution contains 500 mg of methicillin.
- Date reconstituted solution; stable for 8 h except for 2 mg/ml solutions in 10% Invert Sugar in Normal Saline (4-h stability).
- Administer IM by deep intragluteal injection to avoid irritation.
- Administer IV slowly to avoid irritation to the vein.

Adverse effects in *Italics* are most common; those in **Bold** are life-threatening.

- Arrange to continue treatment for 48–72 h after patient is asymptomatic.
- Do not give IM injections repeatedly in the same site; atrophy can occur. Monitor injection sites.

Drug-specific teaching points
- Be aware that this drug can only be given by injection.
- Know that upset stomach, nausea, diarrhea, mouth sores, pain or discomfort at injection sites may occur. Report difficulty breathing, rashes, severe diarrhea, severe pain at injection site, mouth sores.

methimazole

(meth *im' a zole*)
Tapazole

Pregnancy Category D

Drug classes
Antithyroid drug

Therapeutic actions
Inhibits the synthesis of thyroid hormones.

Indications
- Hyperthyroidism

Contraindications/cautions
- Allergy to antithyroid products, pregnancy (use only if absolutely necessary and when mother has been informed about potential harm to the fetus; if an antithyroid agent is required, propylthiouracil is the drug of choice), lactation.

Dosage
Administer only PO, usually in three equal doses q8h.
Adult: Initial dose: 15 mg/d PO up to 30–60 mg/d in severe cases. *Maintenance dose:* 5–15 mg/d PO.
Pediatric: Initial dose: 0.4 mg/kg per day PO. *Maintenance:* approximately half the initial dose; actual dose is determined by the patient's response, or initial dose 0.5–0.7 mg/kg per day or 15–20 mg/m^2 per day PO in three divided doses. *Maximum dose:* 30 mg/24 h.

Pharmacokinetics

Route	Onset	Peak	Duration
Oral	30–40 min	60 min	2–4 h

Metabolism: $T_{1/2}$: 6–13 h
Distribution: Crosses placenta; enters breast milk
Excretion: Urine

Adverse effects
- **CNS:** *Paresthesias, neuritis,* vertigo, drowsiness, neuropathies, depression, headache
- **GI:** *Nausea,* vomiting, epigastric distress, loss of taste, sialadenopathy, jaundice, hepatitis
- **Hematologic:** *Agranulocytosis, granulocytopenia, thrombocytopenia, hypoprothrombinemia, bleeding,* vasculitis, periarteritis
- **GU:** Nephritis
- **Dermatologic:** *Skin rash,* urticaria, pruritus, skin pigmentation, exfoliative dermatitis, lupuslike syndrome, loss of hair
- **Other:** Arthralgia, myalgia, edema, lymphadenopathy, drug fever

Clinically important drug-drug interactions
- Increased theophylline clearance and decreased effectiveness if given to hyperthyroid patients; clearance will change as patient approaches euthyroid state • Altered effects of oral anticoagulants if given concurrently with methimazole • Increased therapeutic effects and toxicity of digitalis glycosides, metroprolol, propranolol when hyperthyroid patients become euthyroid

Nursing Considerations

Assessment
- *History:* Allergy to antithyroid poroducts, pregnancy, lactation
- *Physical:* Skin—color, lesions, pigmentation; orientation, reflexes, affect; liver evaluation; CBC, differential, prothrombin time, liver and renal function tests

Implementation
- Administer drug in three equally divided doses at 8-h intervals; try to schedule to

- allow patient to sleep at his or her regular time.
- Arrange for regular, periodic blood tests to monitor bone marrow depression and bleeding tendencies.
- Advise medical personnel who may be doing surgical procedures with this patient that he or she is on this drug and therefore at greater risk for bleeding problems.

Drug-specific teaching points
- Take this drug around the clock at 8-h intervals. Work with your nurse or physician to establish a schedule that best fits into your routine.
- Be aware that this drug will need to be taken for a prolonged period to achieve the desired effects.
- Know that the following side effects may occur: dizziness, weakness, vertigo, drowsiness (use caution if operating a car or dangerous machinery if these effects occur); nausea, vomiting, loss of appetite (small, frequent meals may help); rash, itching.
- Report fever, sore throat, unusual bleeding or bruising, headache, general malaise.

methocarbamol

*(meth ob **kar'** ba mole)*
Robaxin

Pregnancy Category C

Drug classes
Centrally acting skeletal muscle relaxant

Therapeutic actions
Precise mechanism of action not known but may be due to general CNS depression; does not directly relax tense skeletal muscles or directly affect the motor end plate or motor nerves.

Indications
- Relief of discomfort associated with acute, painful musculoskeletal conditions, as an adjunct to rest, physical therapy, and other measures
- May have a beneficial role in the control of neuromuscular manifestations of tetanus

Contraindications/cautions
- Contraindicated in the presence of hypersensitivity to methocarbamol; known or suspected renal pathology (parenteral methocarbamol is contraindicated because of presence of polyethylene glycol 300 in vehicle).
- Use caution in the presence of epilepsy, pregnancy, lactation.

Dosage
Adult
- ***Parenteral:*** IV and IM use only. Do not use SC. Do not exceed total dosage of 3 g/d for more than 3 consecutive d, except in the treatment of tetanus. Repeat course of treatment after a lapse of 48 h if condition persists. Ordinarily, injection need not be repeated, because tablets will sustain the relief.
- *IV:* Administer undiluted at a maximum rate of 3 ml/min.
- ***Tetanus:*** Give 1–2 g directly IV and add 1–2 g to IV infusion bottle so that initial dose is 3 g. Repeat q6h until conditions allow for insertion of nasogastric tube and administration of crushed tablets suspended in water or saline. Total daily oral doses up to 24 g may be required.
- *IM:* Do not administer more than 5 ml at any one gluteal injection site. Repeat q8h if needed.
- *Oral:* Initially, 1.5 g qid PO. For the first 48–72 h, 6 g/d or up to 8 g/d is recommended. Maintenance: 1 g qid or 750 mg q4h IV or 1.5 g bid–tid for total dosage of 4 g/d.

Pediatric
- ***Tetanus:*** A minimum initial dose of 15 mg/kg IV by direct IV injection or IV infusion. Repeat q6h as needed.

Pharmacokinetics

Route	Onset	Peak
Oral	30 min	2 h
IM/IV	Rapid	Unknown

Metabolism: Hepatic, $T_{1/2}$: 1–2 h
Distribution: Crosses placenta; may enter breast milk
Excretion: Urine and feces

IV facts
Preparation: Administer undiluted. May be added to IV drip of Sodium Chloride Injection or 5% Dextrose Injection; do not dilute one vial given as a single dose to more than 250 ml for IV infusion.
Infusion: Inject directly 1 or 2 g into IV tubing at maximum rate of 3 ml/min; may add 1–2 g to infusion for a total of 3 g.

Adverse effects
Parenteral
- **CNS:** *Syncope, dizziness, lightheadedness, vertigo, headache, mild muscular incoordination,* convulsions during IV administration, blurred vision
- **GI:** GI upset, metallic taste
- **CV:** *Hypotension*
- **Dermatologic:** *Urticaria,* pruritus, rash, flushing
- **Local:** Sloughing or pain at injection site
- **Other:** Nasal congestion

Oral
- **CNS:** *Lightheadedness, dizziness, drowsiness,* headache, fever, blurred vision
- **GI:** *Nausea*
- **Dermatologic:** *Urticaria,* pruritus, rash
- **Other:** Conjuctivitis with nasal congestion

Drug-lab test interferences
- May cause interference with color reactions in tests for 5-HIAA and vanilylmandelic acid

■ Nursing Considerations

Assessment
- *History:* Hypersensitivity to methocarbamol; known or suspected renal pathology, epilepsy (use caution with parenteral administration)
- *Physical:* Body temperature; skin—color, lesions; nasal mucous membranes, conjunctival exam; orientation, affect, vision exam, reflexes; P, BP; bowel sounds, normal output; urinalysis, renal function tests

Implementation
- Ensure that patient is recumbent during IV injection and for at least 15 min thereafter.
- Administer IV slowly to minimize risk of CVS reactions, seizures.
- Monitor IV injection sites carefully to prevent extravasation; solution is hypertonic; can cause sloughing of tissue.
- Ensure that patients receiving methocarbamol for tetanus receive other appropriate care—débridement of wound, penicillin, tetanus antitoxin, tracheotomy, attention to fluid/electrolyte balance.
- Provide epinephrine, injectable steroids, or injectable antihistamines on standby in case syncope, hypotension occur with IV administration.
- Be aware that patient's urine may darken on standing.

Drug-specific teaching points
- Take this drug exactly as prescribed. Do not take a higher dosage than that prescribed for you, and do not take drug longer than prescribed.
- Avoid alcohol, sleep-inducing, or OTC drugs while you are on this drug. These could cause dangerous effects.
- Be aware that your urine may darken to a brown, black, or green color on standing. This is expected while you are taking this drug and should not worry you.
- Know that the following side effects may occur: drowsiness, dizziness, blurred vision (avoid driving a car or engaging in activities that require alertness if these occur); nausea (taking drug with food and eating frequent, small meals may help).
- Report skin rash, itching, fever, or nasal congestion.

Adverse effects in *Italics* are most common; those in **Bold** are life-threatening.

methotrexate

*(meth oh **trex' ate**)*

amethopterin, MTX
Folex PFS, Rheumatrex Dose Pak (treatment of psoriasis or rheumatoid arthritis)

Pregnancy Category X

Drug classes
Antimetabolite
Antineoplastic drug

Therapeutic actions
Inhibits folic acid reductase, leading to inhibition of DNA synthesis and inhibition of cellular replication; selectively affects the most rapidly dividing cells (neoplastic and psoriatic cells).

Indications
- Treatment of gestational choriocarcinoma, chorioadenoma destruens, hydatidiform mole
- Treatment and prophylaxis of meningeal leukemia
- Symptomatic control of severe, recalcitrant, disabling psoriasis
- Management of severe, active, classical, or definite rheumatoid arthritis
- Unlabeled uses: high-dose regimen followed by leucovorin rescue for adjuvant therapy of nonmetastatic osteosarcoma (orphan drug designation); to reduce corticosteriod requirements in patients with severe corticosteroid-dependent asthma

Contraindications/cautions
- Contraindicated in the presence of allergy to methotrexate, lactation, proriasis with renal or hepatic disorders, pregnancy or childbearing age.
- Use caution in the presence of hematopoietic depression; leukopenia, thrombocytopenia, anemia, severe hepatic or renal disease, infection, peptic ulcer, ulcerative colitis, debility.

Dosage
Adult
- **Choriocarcinoma and other trophoblastic diseases:** 15–30 mg PO or IM daily for a 5-d course. Repeat courses three to five times as required, with rest periods of 1 wk or more between courses until toxic symptoms subside. Continue 1–2 courses of methotrexate after chorionic gonadotropin hormone levels are normal.
- **Leukemia:** Induction: 3.3 mg/m^2 of methorexate PO or IM with 60 mg/m^2 of prednisone daily for 4–6 wk. Maintenance: 30 mg/m^2 methotrexate PO or IM twice weekly or 2.5 mg/m^2 IV every 14 d. If relapse occurs, return to induction doses.
- **Meningeal leukemia:** Administer methotrexate intrathecally in cases of lymphocytic leukemia as prophylaxis. 12 mg/m^2 intrathecally at intervals of 2–5 d and repeat until cell count of CSF is normal.
- **Lymphomas:** Burkitt's tumor, Stages I and II: 10–25 mg/d PO for 4–8 d. In stage III, combine with other neoplastic drugs. All usually require several courses of therapy with 7- to 10-d rest periods between doses.
- **Mycosis fungoides:** 2.5–10 mg/d PO for weeks or months or 50 mg IM once weekly or 25 mg IM twice weekly.
- **Osteosarcoma:** Starting dose is 12 g/m^2 or up to 15 g/m^2 PO, IM or IV to give a peak serum concentration of 1,000 μmol. Must be used as part of a cytotoxic regimen with leucovorin rescue.
- **Severe psoriasis:** 10–25 mg/wk PO, IM, or IV as a single weekly dose. Do not exceed 50 mg/wk or 2.5 mg PO at 12-h intervals for three doses or at 8-h intervals for four doses each week. Do not exceed 30 mg/wk. Alternatively, 2.5 mg/d PO for 5 d followed by at least 2 d rest. Do not exceed 6.25 mg/d. After optimal clinical response is achieved, reduce dosage to lowest possible with longest rest periods and consider return to conventional, topical therapy.
- **Severe rheumatoid arthritis:** Starting dose: single doses of 7.5 mg/wk PO or divided dosage of 2.5 mg PO at 12-h intervals for three doses given as a course once weekly. Dosage may be gradually increased, based on patient re-

sponse. Do not exceed 20 mg/wk. Therapeutic response usually begins within 3–6 wk, and improvement may continue for another 12 wk. Improvement may be maintained for up to 2 y with continued therapy.

Pharmacokinetics

Route	Onset	Peak
Oral	Varies	1–4 h
IM/IV	Rapid	½–2 h

Metabolism: $T_{1/2}$: 2–4 h
Distribution: Crosses placenta; enters breast milk
Excretion: Urine

IV facts

Preparation: Reconstitute 20- and 50-mg vials with an appropriate sterile preservative free medium, 5% Dextrose Solution or Sodium Chloride Injection to a concentration no greater than 25 mg/ml; reconstitute 1-g vial with 19.4 ml to a concentration of 50 mg/ml.

Infusion: Administer diluted drug by direct IV injection at a rate of not more than 10 mg/min.

Adverse effects

- CNS: Headache, drowsiness, blurred vision, aphasia, hemiparesis, paresis, seizures, *fatigue, malaise, dizziness*
- GI: *Ulcerative stomatitis*, gingivitis, pharyngitis, anorexia, *nausea,* vomiting, diarrhea, hematemesis, melena, GI ulceration and bleeding, enteritis, **hepatic toxicity**
- Respiratory: Interstitial pneumonitis, chronic interstitial obstructive pulmonary disease
- Hematologic: **Bone marrow depression, increased susceptibility to infection**
- GU: Renal failure, *effects on fertility* (defective oogenesis, defective spermatogenesis, transient oligospermia, menstrual dysfunction, infertility, abortion, fetal defects)
- Dermatologic: *Erythematous rashes*, pruritus, urticaria, photosensitivity, depigmentation, *alopecia*, ecchymosis, telangiectasia, acne, furunculosi
- Hypersensitivity: Anaphylaxis, sudden death
- Other: *Chills and fever*, metabolic changes (diabetes, osteoporosis), cancer

Clinically important drug-drug interactions

- Increased risk of methotrexate toxicity if taken concurrently with salicylates, phenytoin, probenecid, sulfonamides • Decreased serum levels and therapeutic effects of digoxin if taken concurrently with methotrexate

■ Nursing Considerations

Assessment

- *History:* Allergy to methotrexate, hematopoietic depression, severe hepatic or renal disease, infection, peptic ulcer, ulcerative colitis, debility, psorosis, pregnancy, lactation
- *Physical:* Weight; temperature; skin—lesions, color; hair; vision, speech, orientation, reflexes, sensation; R, adventitious sounds; mucous membranes, liver evaluation, abdominal exam; CBC, differential; renal and liver function tests; urinalysis, blood and urine glucose, glucose tolerance test, chest x-ray

Implementation

- Arrange for tests to evaluate CBC, urinalysis, renal and liver function tests, chest x-ray before beginning therapy, at appropriate intervals during therapy, and for several weeks after drug therapy.
- Arrange for reduced dosage or discontinuation of drug therapy if renal failure occurs.
- Reconstitute powder for intrathecal use with preservative free sterile Sodium Chloride Injection; intended for one dose only; discard remainder. The solution for injection contains benzyl alcohol and should *not* be given intrathecally.
- Arrange to have leucovorin readily available as antidote for methotrexate over-

Adverse effects in *Italics* are most common; those in **Bold** are life-threatening.

dose or when large doses are used. In general, the dose of leucovorin (calcium leucovorin) should equal or be higher than the dose of methotrexate and should be administered within the first hour. Up to 75 mg IV within 12 h, followed by 12 mg IM q6h for four doses. For average doses of methotrexate that cause adverse effects, give 6–12 mg leucovorin IM, q6h for four doses or 10 mg/m^2 PO followed by 10 mg/m^2 q6h for 72 h.
- Arrange for an antiemetic if nausea and vomiting are severe.
- Arrange for adequate hydration during the course of therapy to reduce the risk of hyperuricemia.
- Do not administer any other medications containing alcohol.

Drug-specific teaching points
- Prepare a calendar of treatment days to follow.
- Know that the following side effects may occur: nausea, vomiting (medication may be ordered to help; small, frequent meals may also help); numbness, tingling, dizziness, drowsiness, blurred vision, difficulty speaking (these are all effects of the drug; dosage adjustment may be needed; it is advisable to avoid driving or operating dangerous machinery if these occur): mouth sores (frequent mouth care will be needed); infertility; loss of hair (you may wish to obtain a wig or other suitable head covering; it is important to keep the head covered at extremes of temperature); skin rash, sensitivity to sunlight and ultraviolet light (avoid exposure to the sun; use a sunscreen and protective clothing if exposed to sun).
- Be aware that this drug may cause birth defects or miscarriages. It is advisable to use birth control while on this drug and for 8 wk thereafter.
- Avoid alcohol while on this drug; serious side effects may occur.
- Arrange for frequent, regular medical follow-up, including frequent blood tests to follow the effects of the drug on your body.
- Report black, tarry stools; fever; chills; sore throat; unusual bleeding or bruising; cough or shortness of breath; darkened or bloody urine; abdominal, flank, or joint pain; yellow color to the skin or eyes; mouth sores.

☐ methotrimeprazine hydrochloride

*(meth oh trye **mep'** ra zeen)*
Levoprome, Nozinan (CAN)

Pregnancy Category C

Drug classes
Analgesic
Phenothiazine

Therapeutic actions
CNS depressant; suppresses sensory impulses; reduces motor activity; produces sedation and tranquilization; raises pain threshold; produces amnesia. Also has antihistaminic, anticholinergic, antiadrenergic activity.

Indications
- Relief of moderate to marked pain in nonambulatory patients
- Obstetric analgesia and sedation where respiratory depression is to be avoided
- Preanesthetic for producing sedation, somnolence, relief of apprehension and anxiety

Contraindications/cautions
- Contraindicated in the presence of hypersensitivity to phenothiazines, sulfites; coma; severe myocardial, hepatic or renal disease; hypotension.
- Use caution in the presence of heart disease, pregnancy prior to labor, lactation.

Dosage
For IM use only. Do *not* give SC or IV. Do *not* administer for longer than 30 d, unless narcotic analgesics are contraindicated or patient has terminal illness.
Adult
- ***Analgesia:*** 10–20 mg IM q4–6h as required (range, 5–40 mg q1–24h)

- **Obstetric analgesia:** During labor, an initial dose of 15–20 mg PO. May be repeated or adjusted as needed.
- **Preanesthetic medication:** 2–20 mg IM 45 min–3 h before surgery; 10 mg is often satisfactory. 15–20 mg IM may be given for more sedation. Atropine sulfate or scopolamine HBr may be used concurrently in lower than usual doses.
- **Postoperative analgesia:** 2.5–7.5 mg IM in the immediate postoperative period. Supplement q4–6h as needed.

Pediatric younger than 12 y: Not recommended.
Geriatric: Initial dose of 5–10 mg IM; gradually increase subsequent doses if needed and tolerated.

Pharmacokinetics

Route	Onset	Peak	Duration
IM	20 min	30–90 min	4 h

Metabolism: Hepatic, $T_{1/2}$: 15–30 h
Distribution: Crosses placenta; enters breast milk
Excretion: Urine

Adverse effects
- CNS: *Weakness,* disorientation, dizziness, excessive sedation, slurring of speech
- GI: Abdominal discomfort, nausea, vomiting, *dry mouth,* jaundice
- CV: *Orthostatic hypotension, fainting, syncope*
- GU: Difficult urination, uterine inertia
- Local: Local inflammation, swelling, pain at injection site
- Other: Nasal congestion, agranulocytosis, chills

Clinically important drug-drug interactions
• Additive anticholinergic effects and possibly decreased antipsychotic efficacy with anticholinergic drugs • Increased likelihood of seizures with metrizamide (contrast agent used in myelography)

Drug-lab test interferences
• False-positive pregnancy tests (less likely if serum test is used) • Increase in protein-bound iodine, not attributable to an increase in thyroxine

■ Nursing Considerations
Assessment
- *History:* Hypersensitivity to phenothiazines, sulfites; coma; severe myocardial, hepatic, renal or heart disease; hypotension; lactation
- *Physical:* Body weight, temperature; reflexes, orientation, intraocular pressure; P, BP, orthostatic BP; R, adventitious sounds; bowel sounds and normal output, liver evaluation; urinary output, prostate size; CBC, urinalysis, thyroid, liver and kidney function tests

Implementation
- Do not mix drugs other than atropine or scopolamine in the same syringe with methotrimeprazine.
- Rotate IM injection sites.
- Keep patient supine for about 6–12 h after injection to prevent severe hypotension, syncope; tolerance to hypotensive effects usually occurs with repeated administration but may be lost if dosage is interrupted for several days.
- Provide methoxamine, phenylephrine on standby in case severe hypotension occurs. Do not give epinephrine; paradoxical hypotension may occur.

Drug-specific teaching points
- Know that the following side effects may occur: dizziness, sedation, drowsiness (it is important for you to remain supine for 12 h after the injection; request assistance if you feel you need to sit or stand for any reason); nausea, vomiting (frequent, small meals may minimize these effects).
- Report severe nausea, vomiting, urinary difficulty, yellowing of the skin or eyes, pain at injection site.

❒ methoxsalen

(meth ox' a len)
8-MOP

Pregnancy Category C

methoxsalen

Drug classes
Psoralen

Therapeutic actions
Strong photosensitizing effect on epidermal cells, combined with ultraviolet light (UVA) produces an inflammatory reaction that produces an increased synthesis of melanin, increased number of melanocytes.

Indications
- Repigmentation of vitiliginous skin
- Symptomatic treatment of severe disabling psoriasis that is refractory to other forms of therapy
- Unlabeled use: with UVA for the treatment of mycosis fungoides

Contraindications/cautions
- Contraindicated in the presence of allergies to psoralens, sensitivity to sun, diseases associated with photosensitivity, squamous cell carcinoma, cataracts, pregnancy.
- Use caution in the presence of hepatic dysfunction, chronic infection, GI diseases, immunosuppression, cardiovascular disease, lactation.

Dosage
Adult
- **Oral:** < 30 kg, 10 mg; 30–50 kg, 20 mg; 51–65 kg, 30 mg; 66–80 kg, 40 mg; 81–90 kg, 50 mg; 91–115 kg, 60 mg; > 115 kg, 70 mg. Administer 90–120 min before exposure to UV light, two to three times per week.
- **Topical:** Apply lotion to skin 1–2 h before exposure to UV light.

Pharmacokinetics

Route	Peak	Duration
PO	2 h	8–10 h
Topical	Slow	8–10 h

Metabolism: Hepatic, $T_{1/2}$: 45–125 min
Distribution: Crosses placenta; may enter breast milk
Excretion: Urine

Adverse effects
- CNS: Nervousness, depression, headache, dizziness, malaise
- GI: *Nausea*
- Dermatologic: *Burns,* hypopigmentation, vesicultion and bullae formation, rash, urticaria, skin carcinoma

■ Nursing Considerations

Assessment
- *History:* Allergies to psoralens, sensitivity to sun, diseases associated with photosensitivity, squamous cell carcinoma, cataracts, use of drugs known to cause photosensitivity, pregnancy, hepatic dysfunction, chronic infection, GI diseases, immunosuppression, cardiovascular disease, lactation
- *Physical:* Culture infected area; skin—color, lesion; orientation, reflexes

Implementation
- Store in light-resistant containers.
- Administer oral drug with food or meals to reduce GI upset.
- Apply topical drug to only a small area; protect borders of lesion with petrolatum and sunscreen lotion to prevent hypopigmentation.
- Use finger cot or rubber glove to apply lotion.
- Know that drug is administered in combination with ultraviolet light; should only be used by physician experienced with these procedures.
- Do not give patients methoxsalen topical to self-administer.

Drug-specific teaching points
- Be aware that drug is given in conjunction with ultraviolet light treatments; timing of drug use is important.
- Take oral drug with food or meals and consistently each time.
- Do not expose yourself to additional ultraviolet light during treatments (use sunscreen if outdoors).
- Know that upset stomach, skin rash, and burning may occur.
- Report new psoratic lesions, burning, dizziness.

Adverse effects in *Italics* are most common; those in **Bold** are life-threatening.

methscopolamine bromide

*(meth skoe **pol'** a meen)*
Pamine

Pregnancy Category C

Drug classes
Anticholinergic (quaternary)
Antimuscarinic
Parasympatholytic drug
Antispasmodic

Therapeutic actions
Competitively blocks the effects of acetylcholine at muscarinic cholinergic receptors that mediate the effects of parasympathetic postganglionic impulses, relaxing the GI tract and inhibiting gastric acid secretion.

Indications
- Adjunctive therapy in the treatment of peptic ulcer

Contraindications/cautions
- Contraindicated in the presence of glaucoma; adhesions between iris and lens, stenosing peptic ulcer, pyloroduodenal obstruction, paralytic ileus, intestinal atony, severe ulcerative colitis, toxic megacolon, symptomatic prostatic hypertrophy, bladder neck obstruction, bronchial asthma, COPD, cardiac arrhythmias, myocardial ischemia; sensitivity to anticholinergic drugs; bromides, tartrazine (tartrazine sensitivity is rare but is more common in patients allergic to aspirin), impaired metabolic, liver or kidney function, myasthenia gravis.
- Use caution in the presence of Down's syndrome, brain damage, spasticity, hypertension, hyperthyroidism, pregnancy, lactation.

Dosage
Adult: 2.5 mg PO 30 min before meals and 2.5–5 mg at bedtime.
Pediatric: Safety and efficacy not established.

Pharmacokinetics

Route	Onset	Duration
Oral	1 h	4–6 h

Metabolism: Hepatic, $T_{1/2}$: 2–3 h
Distribution: Crosses placenta; may enter breast milk
Excretion: Urine and bile

Adverse effects
- **CNS:** *Blurred vision*, mydriasis, cycloplegia, photophobia, increased intraocular pressure
- **GI:** *Dry mouth, altered taste perception, nausea, vomiting, dysphagia,* heartburn, constipation, bloated feeling, paralytic ileus, gastroesophageal reflux
- **CV:** Palpitations, tachycardia
- **GU:** *Urinary hesitancy and retention;* impotence
- **Local:** *Irritation at site of IM injection*
- **Other:** Decreased sweating and predisposition to heat prostration, suppression of lactation, nasal congestion

Clinically important drug-drug interactions
- Decreased antipsychotic effectiveness of haloperidol when given with anticholinergic drugs

■ Nursing Considerations
Assessment
- *History:* Glaucoma, adhesions between iris and lens, stenosing peptic ulcer, pyloroduodenal obstruction, paralytic ileus, intestinal atony, severe ulcerative colitis, toxic megacolon, symptomatic prostatic hypertrophy, bladder neck obstruction, bronchial asthma, COPD, cardiac arrhythmias, myocardial ischemia; sensitivity to anticholinergic drugs; bromides, tartrazine, impaired metabolic, liver or kidney function, myasthenia gravis, Down's syndrome, brain damage, spasticity, hypertension, hyperthyroidism, pregnancy, lactation
- *Physical:* Bowel sounds, normal output; urinary output, prostate palpation; R adventitious sounds; P, B; intraocular pressure, vision; bilateral grip strength, re-

Adverse effects in *Italics* are most common; those in **Bold** are life-threatening.

flexes; liver palpation, liver and renal function tests; skin color, lesions, texture

Implementation
- Ensure adequate hydration; provide environmental control (temperature) to prevent hyperpyrexia.
- Encourage patient to void before each dose of medication if urinary retention becomes a problem.

Drug-specific teaching points
- Take drug exactly as prescribed.
- Avoid hot environments while taking this drug (you will be heat intolerant, and dangerous reactions may occur).
- Know that the following side effects may occur: constipation (ensure adequate fluid intake, proper diet); dry mouth (sugarless lozenges, frequent mouth care may help; this effect sometimes lessens with time); blurred vision, sensitivity to light (avoid tasks that require acute vision; wear sunglasses when in bright light if these occur); impotence (this is a drug effect that will go away when you discontinue the drug); difficulty in urination (it may help to empty the bladder immediately before taking each dose of drug).
- Report skin rash, flushing, eye pain, difficulty breathing, tremors, loss of coordination, irregular heartbeat, palpitations, headache, abdominal distention, hallucinations, severe or persistent dry mouth, difficulty swallowing, difficulty in urination, severe constipation, sensitivity to light.

☐ methsuximide

*(meth **sux**' i mide)*
Celontin Kapseals

Pregnancy Category C

Drug classes
Antiepileptic
Succinimide

Therapeutic actions
Suppresses the paroxysmal three-cycle-per-second spike and wave EEG pattern associated with lapses of consciousness in absence (petit mal) seizures; reduces frequency of attacks; mechanism of action not understood.

Indications
- Control of absence (petit mal) seizures when refractory to other drugs

Contraindications/cautions
- Contraindicated in the presence of hypersensitivity to succinimides.
- Use caution in the presence of hepatic, renal abnormalities; pregnancy (data suggest an association between use of antiepileptic drugs by women with epilepsy and an elevated incidence of birth defects in children born to these women; however, antiepileptic therapy should not be discontinued in pregnant women who are receiving such therapy to prevent major seizures; the effect of even minor seizures on the developing fetus is unknown, and this should be considered when deciding whether to continue antiepileptic therapy in pregnant women); lactation.

Dosage
Determine optimal dosage by trial.
Adult: Suggested schedule is 300 mg/d PO for the first week. If required, increase at weekly intervals by increments of 300 mg/d for 3 wk, up to a dosage of 1.2 g/d. Individualize therapy according to response. May be administered with other antiepileptic drugs when other forms of epilepsy coexist with absence (petit mal) seizures.
Pediatric: 150 mg half-strength capsules aid pediatric administration; determine dosage by trial.

Pharmacokinetics

Route	Onset	Peak
Oral	Rapid	1–4 h

Metabolism: Hepatic, $T_{1/2}$: 2.6–4 h
Distribution: Crosses placenta; may enter breast milk
Excretion: Urine

Adverse effects
Succinimides
- CNS: *Drowsiness, ataxia, dizziness,* irritability, nervousness, headache, blurred

methyclothiazide ■ 721

vision, myopia, photophobia, hiccups, euphoria, dreamlike state, lethargy, hyperactivity, fatigue, insomnia, confusion, instability, mental slowness, depression, hypochondriacal behavior, sleep disturbances
- **GI:** *Nausea, vomiting, vague gastric upset, epigastric and abdominal pain,* cramps, anorexia, diarrhea, contipation, weight loss, swelling of tongue, gum hypertrophy
- **Hematologic:** Eosinophilia, granulocytopenia, leukopenia, agranulocytosis, aplastic anemia, monocytosis, **pancytopenia**
- **Dermatologic:** Pruritus, urticaria, Stevens-Johnson syndrome, pruritic erythematous rashes, skin eruptions, erythema multiforme, systemic lupus erythematosus, alopecia, hirsutism
- **Other:** Periorbital edema, hyperemia, muscle weakness, abnormal liver and kidney function tests, vaginal bleeding

Clinically important drug-drug interactions
- Decreased serum levels and therapeutic effects of primidone if taken concurrently with methsoxumide

■ Nursing Considerations

Assessment
- *History:* Hypersensitivity to succinimides; hepatic, renal abnormalities; pregnancy; lactation
- *Physical:* Skin—color, lesions; orientation, affect, reflexes, bilateral grip strength, vision exam; bowel sounds, normal output, liver evaluation; liver and kidney function tests, urinalysis, CBC with differential, EEG

Implementation
- Arrange to reduce dosage, discontinue methsuximide, or substitute other antiepileptic medication gradually; abrupt discontinuation may precipitate absence (petit mal) seizures.
- Monitor CBC and differential before therapy is instituted and frequently during therapy.
- Arrange to discontinue drug if skin rash, depression of blood count, or unusual depression, aggressiveness, or behavioral alterations occur.

Drug-specific teaching points
- Take this drug exactly as prescribed; do not discontinue this drug abruptly or change dosage, except on the advice of your physician.
- Avoid alcohol, sleep-inducing, or OTC drugs while you are on this drug. These could cause dangerous effects. If you feel that you need one of these preparations, consult your nurse or physician.
- Arrange for frequent check-ups to monitor your response to this drug.
- Know that the following side effects may occur: drowsiness, dizziness, confusion, blurred vision (avoid driving a car or performing other tasks requiring alertness or visual acuity if these occur); GI upset (taking the drug with food or milk and eating frequent, small meals may help).
- Wear a medical alert tag at all times so that any emergency medical personnel taking care of you will know that you are an epileptic taking antiepileptic medication.
- Report skin rash, joint pain, unexplained fever, sore throat, unusual bleeding or bruising, drowsiness, dizziness, blurred vision, pregnancy.

❒ methyclothiazide

*(meth i kloe **thye**' a zide)*
Aquatensen, Duretic (CAN), Enduron, Ethon

Pregnancy Category C

Drug classes
Thiazide diuretic

Therapeutic actions
Inhibits reabsorption of sodium and chloride in distal renal tubule, thereby increasing excretion of sodium, chloride, and water by the kidney.

Adverse effects in *Italics* are most common; those in **Bold** are life-threatening.

methyclothiazide

Indications
- Adjunctive therapy in edema associated with CHF, cirrhosis, corticosteroid and estrogen therapy, renal dysfunction
- Hypertension, as sole therapy or in combination with other antihypertensives
- Unlabeled use: diabetes insipidus, especially nephrogenic diabetes insipidus

Contraindications/cautions
- Contraindicated in the presence of hypersensitivity to thiazides, pregnancy.
- Use caution in the presence of fluid or electrolyte imbalances, renal or liver disease, gout, SLE, glucose tolerance abnormalities, hyperparathyroidism, manic-depressive disorders, lactation.

Dosage
Adult
- ***Edema:*** 2.5–10 mg qd PO. Maximum single dose is 10 mg.
- ***Hypertension:*** 2.5–5 mg qd PO. If BP is not controlled by 5 mg qd within 8–12 wk, another antihypertensive may be needed.

Pharmacokinetics

Route	Onset	Peak	Duration
Oral	2 h	6 h	24 h

Metabolism: $T_{1/2}$: unknown
Distribution: Crosses placenta; enters breast milk
Excretion: Urine

Adverse effects
- **CNS:** *Dizziness, vertigo,* paresthesias, weakness, headache, drowsiness, fatigue, leukopenia, thrombocytopenia, **agranulocytosis, aplastic anemia,** neutropenia
- **GI:** *Nausea, anorexia, vomiting, dry mouth,* diarrhea, constipation, jaundice, hepatitis
- **CV:** Orthostatic hypotension, venous thrombosis, volume depletion, cardiac arrhythmias, chest pain
- **GU:** *polyuria, nocturia,* impotence, loss of libido
- **Dermatologic:** Photosensitivity, rash, purpura, exfoliative dermatitis, hives
- **Other:** Muscle cramp

Clinically important drug-drug interactions
- Risk of hyperglycemia if taken with diazoxide • Decreased absorption of methyclothiazide if taken with cholestyramine, colestipol • Increased risk of digitalis glycoside toxicity if hypokalemia occurs • Increased risk of lithium toxicity when taken with thiazides • Increased fasting blood glucose leading to need to adjust dosage of antidiabetic agents

Drug-lab test interferences
- Decreased PBI levels without clinical signs of thyroid disturbances

■ Nursing Considerations

Assessment
- *History:* Fluid or electrolyte imbalances, renal or liver disease, gout, SLE, glucose tolerance abnormalities, hyperparathyroidism, manic-depressive disorders, pregnancy, lactation
- *Physical:* Skin—color and lesions; orientation, reflexes, muscle strength; pulses, BP, orthostatic BP, perfusion, edema, baseline ECG; R, adventitious sounds; liver evaluation, bowel sounds; CBC, serum electrolytes, blood glucose, liver and renal function tests, serum uric acid, urinalysis

Implementation
- Administer with food or milk if GI upset occurs.
- Administer early in the day so increased urination will not disturb sleep.
- Measure and record regular body weights to monitor fluid changes.

Drug-specific teaching points
- Take drug early in the day so sleep will not be disturbed by increased urination.
- Weigh yourself daily, and record weights on a calendar.
- Protect skin from exposure to sun or bright lights (sensitivity to the sun may occur).
- Know that increased urination will occur (stay close to bathroom facilities).
- Use caution if dizziness, drowsiness, feeling faint occur.

Adverse effects in *Italics* are most common; those in **Bold** are life-threatening.

methyldopa ■ 723

- Report rapid weight gain or loss, swelling in ankles or fingers, unusual bleeding or bruising, muscle cramps.

☐ methyldopa

(meth ill doe' pa)

methyldopate hydrochloride
Aldomet, Dopamet (CAN), Medimet (CAN), Novomedopa (CAN)

Pregnancy Category C

Drug classes
Antihypertensive drug
Centrally acting sympatholytic drug

Therapeutic actions
Mechanism of action not conclusively demonstrated; probably due to drug's metabolism to alpha-methyl norepinephrine, which lowers arterial blood pressure by stimulating central (CNS) alpha$_2$-adrenergic receptors, which in turn decreases sympathetic outflow from the CNS.

Indications
- Hypertension
- Acute hypertensive crises (IV methyldopate); not drug of choice because of slow onset of action

Contraindications/cautions
- Contraindicated in the presence of hypersensitivity to methyldopa, active hepatic disease, previous methyldopa therapy associated with liver disorders.
- Use caution in the presence of previous liver disease, renal failure, dialysis, bilateral cerebrovascular disease, pregnancy, lactation.

Dosage
Adult
- ***Oral therapy (methyldopa):*** Initial therapy: 250 mg bid—tid in the first 48 h. Adjust dosage at intervals of no less than 2 d until an adequate response is achieved. Increase dosage in the evening to minimize sedation. Maintenance: 500 mg–3 g/d in two to four doses. Usually given in two doses; some patients may be controlled with a single bedtime dose.
- ***Concomitant therapy:*** When given with antihypertensives other than thiazides, limit initial dosage to 500 mg/d in divided doses. When added to a thiazide, dosage of thiazide need not be changed.
- ***IV therapy (methyldopate):*** 250–500 mg q6h as required (maximum 1 g q6h). Switch to oral therapy as soon as control is attained, using the same dosage schedule as used for parenteral therapy.

Pediatric
- ***Oral therapy (methyldopa):*** Individualize dosage; initial dosage is based on 10 mg/kg per day in two to four doses. Maximum dosage is 65 mg/kg per day or 3 g/d, whichever is less.
- ***IV therapy (methyldopate):*** 20–40 mg/kg per day in divided doses q6h. Maximum dosage is 65 mg/kg or 3 g/d, whichever is less.

Geriatric or impaired renal function: Reduce dosage. Drug is largely excreted by the kidneys.

Pharmacokinetics

Route	Onset	Peak	Duration
Oral	Varies	2–4 h	24–48 h
IV	4–6 h	Unknown	10–16 h

Metabolism: Hepatic, T$_{1/2}$: 1.7 h
Distribution: Crosses placenta; enters breast milk
Excretion: Urine

IV facts
Preparation: Add the dose to 100 ml of 5% Dextrose, or give in 5% Dextrose in Water in a concentration of 10 mg/ml.
Infusion: Administer over 30–60 min.

Adverse effects
- CNS: *Sedation, headache, asthenia, weakness* (usually early and transient), dizziness, lightheadedness, symptoms of cerebrovascular insufficiency, paresthe-

Adverse effects in *Italics* are most common; those in **Bold** are life-threatening.

sias, parkinsonism, Bell's palsy, decreased mental acuity, involuntary choreoathetotic movements, psychic disturbances
- GI: *Nausea, vomiting, distention, constipation*, flatus, diarrhea, colitis, dry mouth, sore or "black" tongue, pancreatitis, sialadenitis, abnormal liver function tests, jaundice, hepatitis, **fatal hepatic necrosis**
- CV: *Bradycardia*, prolonged carotid sinus hypersensitivity, aggravation of angina pectoris, paradoxical pressor response, pericarditis, **myocarditis** (fatal), orthostatic hypotension, edema
- Hematologic: Positive Coombs' test, hemolytic anemia, bone marrow depression, leukopenia, granulocytopenia, thrombocytopenia, positive tests for antinuclear antibody, LE cells, and rheumatoid factor
- Dermatologic: Rash as in eczema or lichenoid eruption, toxic epidermal necrolysis fever, lupuslike syndrome
- Endocrine: Breast enlargement, gynecomastia, lactation, hyperprolactinemia, amenorrhea, galactorrhea, impotence, failure to ejaculate, decreased libido
- Other: Nasal stuffiness, mild arthralgia, myalgia, septic shocklike syndrome

Clinically important drug-drug interactions
- Potentiation of the pressor effects of sympathomimetic amines

Drug-lab test interferences
- Methyldopa may interfere with tests for urinary uric acid, serum creatinine, SGOT, urinary catecholamines

■ Nursing Considerations

Assessment
- *History:* Hypersensitivity to methyldopa; hepatic disease; previous methyldopa therapy associated with liver disorders; renal failure; dialysis; bilateral cerebrovascular disease; lactation
- *Physical:* Body weight; body temperature; skin—color, lesions; mucous membranes—color, lesions; orientation, affect, reflexes; P, BP, orthostatic BP, perfusion, edema, auscultation; bowel sounds, normal output, liver evaluation; breast exam; liver and kidney function tests, urinalysis, CBC and differential, direct Coombs' test

Implementation
- Administer IV slowly; monitor injection site.
- Arrange to monitor hepatic function periodically, especially during the first 6–12 wk of therapy or when unexplained fever appears. Discontinue drug if fever, abnormalities in liver function tests, or jaundice occur. Ensure that methyldopa is not reinstituted in such patients.
- Arrange to monitor blood counts periodically to detect hemolytic anemia; a direct Coombs' test before therapy and 6 and 12 mo later may be helpful. Arrange to discontinue drug if Coombs' positive hemolytic anemia occurs. If hemolytic anemia is related to methyldopa, ensure that methyldopa is not reinstituted.
- Arrange to discontinue methyldopa therapy if involuntary choreoathetotic movements occur.
- Arrange to discontinue methyldopa if edema progresses or signs of heart failure occur.
- Arrange to add a thiazide to drug regimen or increase dosage of methyldopa if methyldopa tolerance occurs (usually between the second and third mo of therapy).
- Monitor blood pressure carefully when discontinuing methyldopa; drug has short duration of action, and hypertension usually returns within 48 h.

Drug-specific teaching points
- Take this drug exactly as prescribed; it is important that you not miss doses.
- Know that the following side effects may occur: drowsiness, dizziness, lightheadedness, headache, weakness (these are often transient symptoms that occur when you begin treatment or when the dosage is increased; avoid driving a car or engaging in tasks that require alertness while you are experiencing these symptoms); GI upset (frequent, small meals may help); dreams, nightmares, memory impairment (it may help to know that

these are drug effects that will go away when the drug is discontinued; dizziness, lightheadedness when you get up (get up slowly; use caution when climbing stairs); urine that darkens on standing (this is an expected effect due to the presence of drug metabolites in your urine); impotence, failure of ejaculation, decreased libido; breast enlargement, sore breasts.
- Report unexplained, prolonged general tiredness; yellowing of the skin or eyes; fever; bruising; skin rash.

☐ methylene blue

(meth' i leen)
Urolene Blue

Pregnancy Category C

Drug classes
Urinary Anti-infective
Antidote

Therapeutic actions
Oxidation-reduction agent that converts the ferrous iron of reduced hemoglobin to the ferric form, producing methemoglobin; weak germicide in lower doses; tissue staining.

Indications
- Treatment of cyanide poisoning and drug-induced methemoglobinemia
- GU antiseptic for cystitis and urethritis
- Unlabeled uses: delineation of body structures and fistulas through dye effect; diagnosis/confirmation of rupture of amniotic membranes

Contraindications/cautions
- Contraindicated in the presence of allergy to methylene blue, renal insufficiency, intraspinal injections.
- Use caution in the presence of G6PD deficiency; anemias; cardiovascular deficiencies.

Dosage
Adult
- **Oral:** 65–130 mg tid with a full glass of water.
- **IV:** 1–2 mg/kg (0.1–0.2 ml/kg) injected over several minutes.

Pharmacokinetics

Route	Onset	Peak
Oral	Varies	Unknown
IV	Immediate	End of infusion

Metabolism: Tissue, $T_{1/2}$: unknown
Excretion: Urine, bile, and feces

IV facts
Preparation: No preparation required.
Infusion: Inject directly IV or into tubing of actively running IV; inject slowly over several minutes.

Adverse effects
- **CNS:** Dizziness, headache, mental confusion, sweating
- **GI:** *Nausea*, vomiting, diarrhea, abdominal pain, *blue-green stool*
- **CV:** Precordial pain
- **GU:** *Discolored urine* (blue-green); bladder irritation
- **Other:** Necrotic absess (SC injection); fetal anemia and distress (amniotic injection); neural damage, paralysis (intrathecal injection); *skin stained blue*

■ Nursing Considerations

Assessment
- *History:* Allergy to methylene blue, renal insufficiency, presence of G6PD deficiency; anemias; cardiovascular deficiencies
- *Physical:* Skin—color, lesions; urinary output, bladder palpation; abdominal exam, normal output; CBC with differential

Implementation
- Administer oral drug after meals with a full glass of water.
- Administer IV slowly over several minutes; avoid exceeding recommended dosage.
- Use care to avoid SC injection; monitor any intrathecal site used for diagnostic injection for signs of necrosis and damage.

Adverse effects in *Italics* are most common; those in **Bold** are life-threatening.

- Contact with skin will dye the skin blue; stain may be removed by hypochlorite solution.
- Monitor CBC for signs of marked anemia.

Drug-specific teaching points
- Take drug after meals with a full glass of water.
- Avoid bubble baths, excessive ingestion of citrus juice, and sexual contacts if bladder infection or urethritis is being treated.
- Know that the following side effects may occur: urine or stool discolored blue-green; abdominal pain, nausea, vomiting (small frequent meals may help).
- Report difficulty breathing, severe nausea or vomiting, fatigue.

☐ methylergonovine maleate

*(meth ill er goe **noe'** veen)*
Methergine
Pregnancy Category C

Drug classes
Oxytocic

Therapeutic actions
A partial agonist or antagonist at alpha receptors; as a result, it increases the strength, duration, and frequency of uterine contractions.

Indications
- Routine management after delivery of the placenta
- Treatment of postpartum atony and hemorrhage; subinvolution of the uterus
- Uterine stimulation during the second stage of labor following the delivery of the anterior shoulder, under strict medical supervision

Contraindications/cautions
- Contraindicated in the presence of allergy to methylergonovine, hypertension, toxemia, lactation.
- Use caution in the presence of sepsis, obliterative vascular disease, hepatic or renal impairment, pregnancy.

Dosage
Adult
- ***IM:*** 0.2 mg after delivery of the placenta, after delivery of the anterior shoulder, during puerperium. May be repeated q2–4h.
- ***IV:*** Same dosage as IM; infuse slowly over at least 60 sec. Monitor BP very carefully as severe hypertensive reaction can occur.
- ***Oral:*** 0.2 mg tid or qid daily in the puerperium for up to 1 wk.

Pharmacokinetics

Route	Onset	Peak	Duration
Oral	5–10 min	30–60 min	3 h
IM	2–5 min	30 min	3 h
IV	Immediate	2–3 min	1–3 h

Metabolism: Hepatic, $T_{1/2}$: 30 min
Distribution: Crosses placenta; enters breast milk
Excretion: Urine

IV facts
Preparation: No additional preparation required.
Infusion: Inject directly IV or into tubing of running IV; inject very slowly, over no less than 60 sec; rapid infusion can result in sudden hypertension or cerebral events.

Adverse effects
- CNS: *Dizziness, headache,* tinnitus, diaphoresis
- GI: *Nausea,* vomiting
- CV: *Transient hypertension,* palpitations, chest pain, dyspnea

■ Nursing Considerations

Assessment
- *History:* Allergy to methylergonovine, hypertension, toxemia, sepsis, obliterative vascular disease, hepatic or renal impairment, lactation
- *Physical:* Uterine tone, vaginal bleeding; orientation, reflexes, affect; P, BP, edema; CBC, renal and liver function tests

Adverse effects in *Italics* are most common; those in **Bold** are life-threatening.

Implementation
- Administer by IM injection or orally unless emergency requires IV use. Complications are more frequent with IV use.
- Monitor postpartum women for BP changes and amount and character of vaginal bleeding.
- Arrange for discontinuation of drug if signs of toxicity occur.
- Avoid prolonged use of the drug.

Drug-specific teaching points
- The patient receiving a parenteral oxytocic is usually receiving it as part of an immediate medical situation, and the drug teaching should be incorporated into the teaching about delivery. The patient needs to know the name of the drug and what she can expect once it is administered.
- Be aware that the drug should not be needed for longer than 1 wk.
- Know that the following side effects may occur: nausea, vomiting, dizziness, headache, ringing in the ears (as the drug is only given for a short time, these may be tolerable).
- Report difficulty breathing, headache, numb or cold extremities, severe abdominal cramping.

methylphenidate hydrochloride

(meth ill fen'i date)
Ritalin

Pregnancy Category C
C-II controlled substance

Drug classes
CNS stimulant

Therapeutic actions
Mild cortical stimulant with CNS actions similar to those of the amphetamines; efficacy in hyperkinetic syndrome, attention-deficit disorders in children appears paradoxical and is not understood.

Indications
- Narcolepsy
- Attention-deficit disorders, hyperkinetic syndrome, minimal brain dysfunction in children with a behavioral syndrome characterized by the following symptoms: moderate to severe distractibility, short attention span, hyperactivity, emotional lability and impulsivity, not secondary to environmental factors or psychiatric disorders
- Unlabeled use: treatment of depression in the elderly, cancer and stroke patients

Contraindications/cautions
- Contraindicated in the presence of hypersensitivity to methylphenidate; marked anxiety, tension, and agitation; glaucoma; motor tics, family history or diagnosis of Gilles de la Tourette's syndrome; severe depression of endogenous or exogenous origin; normal fatigue states.
- Use caution in the presence of seizure disorders; hypertension; drug dependence, alcoholism; emotional instability; lactation.

Dosage
Adult: Individualize dosage. Administer orally in divided doses bid–tid, preferably 30–45 min before meals. dosage ranges from 10–60 mg/d PO. If insomnia is a problem, drug should be taken before 6 PM. Timed-release tablets have a duration of 8 h and may be used when timing and dosage are titrated to the 8-h regimen.
Pediatric: Start with small oral doses (eg, 5 mg PO before breakfast and lunch with gradual increments of 5–10 mg weekly. Daily dosage > 60 mg not recommended. Discontinue use after 1 mo if no improvement. Discontinue periodically to assess condition; usually discontinued after puberty.

Pharmacokinetics

Route	Onset	Peak	Duration
Oral	Varies	1–3 h	4–6 h

Metabolism: Hepatic, $T_{1/2}$: 1–3 h
Distribution: Crosses placenta; enters breast milk
Excretion: Urine

Adverse effects
- CNS: *Nervousness, insomnia,* dizziness, headache, dyskinesia, chorea, drowsiness, Gilles de la Tourette's syndrome, toxic

psychosis, blurred vision, accommodation difficulties
- GI: *Anorexia, nausea, abdominal pain*, weight loss
- CV: *Increased or decreased pulse and blood pressure; tachycardia*, angina, cardiac arrhythmias, palpitations
- Hematologic: Leukopenia, anemia
- Dermatologic: Skin rash, urticaria, fever, arthralgia, exfoliative dermatitis, erythema multiforme with necrotizing vasculitis and thrombocytopenic purpura, loss of scalp hair
- Other: Tolerance, psychological dependence, abnormal behavior with abuse

Drug-lab test interferences
- Methylphenidate may increase the urinary excretion of epinephrine

■ Nursing Considerations

Assessment
- *History:* Hypersensitivity to methylphenidate; marked anxiety, tension and agitation; glaucoma; motor tics, Gilles de la Tourette's syndrome; severe depression; normal fatigue state; seizure disorders; hypertension; drug dependence, alcoholism, emotional instability
- *Physical:* Body weight; body temperature; skin—color, lesions; orientation, affect, ophthalmic exam (tonometry); P, BP, auscultation; R, adventitious sounds; bowel sounds, normal output; CBC with differential, platelet count, baseline ECG

Implementation
- Ensure proper diagnosis before administering to children for behavioral syndromes; drug should not be used until other causes/concomitants of abnormal behavior (learning disability, EEG abnormalities, neurologic deficits) are ruled out.
- Arrange to interrupt drug dosage periodically in children being treated for behavioral disorders to determine if symptoms recur at an intensity that warrants continued drug therapy.
- Monitor growth of children on long-term methylphenidate therapy.
- Ensure that timed-release tablets are swallowed whole, not chewed or crushed.
- Arrange to dispense the least feasible amount of drug at any one time to minimize risk of overdosage.
- Administer drug before 6 PM to prevent insomnia.
- Arrange to monitor CBC, platelet counts periodically in patients on long-term therapy.
- Monitor blood pressure frequently early in treatment.

Drug-specific teaching points
- Take this drug exactly as prescribed. Timed-release tablets must be swallowed whole, not chewed or crushed.
- Take drug before 6 PM to avoid nighttime sleep disturbance.
- Avoid alcohol and OTC drugs, including nose drops, cold remedies, while taking this drug; some OTC drugs could cause dangerous effects.
- Know that the following side effects may occur: nervousness, restlessness, dizziness, insomnia, impaired thinking (these effects may become less pronounced after a few days; avoid driving a car or engaging in activities that require alertness if these occur; headache, loss of appetite, dry mouth.
- Report nervousness, insomnia, palpitations, vomiting, skin rash, fever.

☐ methylprednisolone

*(meth ill pred **niss**' oh lone)*
Oral: Medrol

methylprednisolone acetate
IM, intra-articular, soft-tissue injection, retention enema, topical dermatologic ointment:: dep Medalone, Depoject, Depo-Medrol, Depopred, Duralone, Medralone, Medrol Acetate, M-Prednisol

methylprednisolone sodium succinate
IV, IM injection: Solu-Medrol

Pregnancy Category C

methylprednisolone ■ 729

Drug classes
Corticosteroid (intermediate acting)
Glucocorticoid
Hormonal agent

Therapeutic actions
Enters target cells and binds to intracellular corticosteroid receptors, initiating many complex reactions that are responsible for its anti-inflammatory and immunosuppressive effects.

Indications
Systemic Administration
- Hypercalcemia associated with cancer
- Short-term management of various inflammatory and allergic disorders, such as rheumatoid arthritis, collagen diseases (eg, SLE), dermatologic diseases (eg, pemphigus), status asthmaticus, and auroimmune disorders
- Hematologic disorders: thrombocytopenia purpura, erythroblastopenia
- Ulcerative colitis, acute exacerbations of mutiple sclerosis and palliation in some leukemias and lymphomas
- Trichinosis with neurologic or myocardial involvement
- Unlabeled use: septic shock

Intra-articular or Soft-Tissue Administration
- Arthritis, psoriatic plaques, and so forth

Dermatologic Preparations
- Relief of inflammatory and pruritic manifestations of dermatoses that are steroid responsive

Contraindications/cautions
- Contraindicated in the presence of infections, especially tuberculosis, fungal infections, amebiasis, vaccinia and varicella, and antibiotic-resistant infections; lactation; allergy to tartrazine or aspirin in products labeled *Medrol*.
- Use caution in the presence of kidney or liver disease, hypothyroidism, ulcerative colitis with impending perforation, diverticulitis, active or latent peptic ulcer, inflammatory bowel disease, CHF, hypertension, thromboembolic disorders, osteoporosis, convulsive disorders, diabetes mellitus.

Dosage
Adult
- **Systemic Administration:** Individualize dosage, depending on the severity of the condition and the patient's response. Give daily dose before 9 AM to minimize adrenal suppression. For maintenance, reduce initial dose in small increments at intervals until the lowest dose that maintains satisfactory clinical response is reached. If long-term therapy is needed, alternate-day therapy with a short-acting corticosteroid should be considered. After long-term therapy, withdraw drug slowly to prevent adrenal insufficiency.
  – *Oral (methylprednisolone, oral):* 4–48 mg/d. Alternate-day therapy: twice the usual dose every other morning.
  – *IM (methylprednisolone acetate):* As temporary substitute for oral therapy, give total daily dose as a single IM injection.
  – *Adrenogenital syndrome:* 40 mg every 2 wk PO or IM.
  – *Rheumatoid arthritis:* 40–120 mg once a week PO or IM.
  – *Dermatologic lesions:* 40–120 mg weekly for 1–4 wk PO or IM; in severe dermatitis, 80–120 mg as a single dose.
  – *Seborrheic dermatitis:* 80 mg once a week PO or IM.
  – *Asthma, allergic rhinitis:* 80–120 mg PO or IM.
  – *IV, IM (methylprednisolone sodium succinate):* 10–40 mg IV administered over 1 to several min. Give subsequent doses IV or IM. *Caution:* Rapid IV administration of large doses (more than 0.5–1.0 g in less than 10–120 min) has caused serious cardiac complications.

Pediatric: Individualize dosage on the basis of the severity of the condition and the patient's response rather than by strict adherence to formulae that correct adult doses for age or body weight. Carefully observe growth and development in infants and children on prolonged therapy. Not less than 0.5 mg/kg per 24 h. High-dose therapy: 30 mg/kg IV infused over 10–20 min; may repeat q4–6h, but not beyond 48–72 h.

Intra-articular, intralesional (methylprednisolone acetate): 4–80 mg intra-articular, soft tissue; 20–60 mg intralesional (depending on joint or soft-tissue injection site).

Topical dermatologic ointment (methylprednisolone acetate): Apply sparingly to affected area bid–qid.

Pharmacokinetics

Route	Onset	Peak	Duration
Oral	Varies	1–2 h	1.2–1.5 d
IV	Rapid	Rapid	Unknown
IM	Rapid	4–8 d	1–5 wk

Metabolism: Hepatic, $T_{1/2}$: 78–188 min
Distribution: Crosses placenta; enters breast milk
Excretion: Urine

IV facts

Preparation: No additional preparation in required.
Infusion: Inject directly into vein or into tubing of running IV; administer slowly, over 1–20 min to reduce cardiac effects.

Adverse effects

Effects depend on dose, route, and duration of therapy. The following are primarily associated with systemic absorption and are more likely to occur with systemically administered steroids than with locally administered preparations.

- **CNS:** *Vertigo, headache,* paresthesias, insomnia, convulsions, psychosis, cataracts, increased intraocular pressure, glaucoma
- **GI:** Peptic or esophageal ulcer, pancreatitis, abdominal distention, nausea, vomiting, *increased appetite, weight gain*
- **CV:** Hypotension, shock, hypertension and CHF secondary to fluid retention, thromboembolism, thrombophlebitis, fat embolism, cardiac arrhythmias
- **MS:** Muscle weakness, steroid myopathy, loss of muscle mass, osteoporosis, spontaneous fractures
- **Endocrine:** Amenorrhea, irregular menses, growth retardation, decreased carbohydrate tolerance, diabetes mellitus, cushingoid state (long-term effect), increased blood sugar, increased serum cholesterol, decreased T_3 and T_4 levels, hypothalamic-pituitary-adrenal (HPA) suppression with systemic therapy longer than 5 d
- **Electrolyte imbalance:** *Na^+ and fluid retention,* hypokalemia, hypocalcemia
- **Hypersensitivity or anaphylactoid reactions:**
- **Other:** *Immunosuppression, aggravation, or masking of infections; impaired wound healing;* thin, fragile skin; petechiae, ecchymoses, purpura, striae; subcutaneous fat atrophy
- The following effects are related to various local routes of steroid administration:
- **Intra-articular:** Osteonecrosis, tendon rupture, infection
- **Intralesional therapy:** Blindness—face and head
- **Topical dermatologic ointments, creams, sprays:** *Local burning, irritation,* acneiform lesions, striae, skin atrophy

Systemic absorption can lead to HPA suppression, growth retardation in children, and other systemic adverse effects. Children may be at special risk of systemic absorption because of their larger skin surface area to body weight ratio.

Clinically important drug-drug interactions

- Increased therapeutic and toxic effects of methylprednisolone if taken concurrently with erythromycin, ketoconazole, troleandomycin • Risk of severe deterioration of muscle strength when given to myasthenia gravis patients who are receiving ambenonium, edrophonium, neostigmine, pyridostigmine • Decreased steroid blood levels when taken with barbiturates, phenytoin, rifampin • Decreased effectiveness of salicylates when taken with methylprednisolone

Drug-lab test interferences

- False-negative nitroblue-tetrazolium test for bacterial infection • Suppression of skin test reactions

Adverse effects in *Italics* are most common; those in **Bold** are life-threatening.

methyprylon ■ 731

■ Nursing Considerations

Assessment
- *History:* Infections; kidney or liver disease, hypothyroidism, ulcerative colitis, diverticulitis, active or latent peptic ulcer, inflammatory bowel disease, CHF, hypertension, thromboembolic disorders, osteoporosis, convulsive disorders, diabetes mellitus; pregnancy; lactation
- *Physical:* Body weight, temperature, reflexes and grip strength, affect and orientation, P, BP, peripheral perfusion, peripheral perfusion, prominence of superficial veins, R and adventitious sounds, serum electrolytes, blood glucose

Implementation

Systemic (Oral and Parenteral) Administration
- Use caution with the 24-mg tablets marketed under the brand name *Medrol*; these contain tartrazine, which may cause allergic reactions, especially in people who are allergic to aspirin.
- Administer once-a-day doses before 9 AM to mimic normal peak corticosteroid blood levels.
- Arrange for increased dosage when patient is subject to stress.
- Taper doses when discontinuing high-dose or long-term therapy.
- Do not give live virus vaccines with immunosuppressive doses of corticosteroids.

Topical Dermatologic Preparations
- Assess affected area for infections, skin integrity.
- Administer cautiously to pregnant patients; topical corticosteroids have caused teratogenic effects in preclinical studies.
- Use caution when occlusive dressings, tight diapers cover affect area; these can increase systemic absorption of the drug.
- Avoid prolonged use near the eyes, in genital and rectal areas, and in skin creases.

Drug-specific teaching points

Systemic (Oral and Parenteral) Administration
- Do not stop taking the drug (oral) without consulting your health-care provider.
- Avoid exposure to infections.
- Report unusual weight gain, swelling of the extremities, muscle weakness, black or tarry stools, fever, prolonged sore throat, colds or other infections, worsening of the disorder for which the drug is being taken.

Intra-articular Therapy
- Do not overuse the joint after therapy, even if the pain is gone.

Topical Dermatologic Preparations
- Apply sparingly.
- Avoid contact with the eyes.
- Report irritation or infection at the site of application.

❒ methyprylon

(meth i prye' lon)

Pregnancy Category B
C-III controlled substance

Drug classes
Sedative/hypnotic (nonbarbiturate)

Therapeutic actions
Increases the threshold of the arousal centers of the brain stem and produces CNS depression similar to that of barbiturates.

Indications
- Hypnotic: effective for at least 7 consecutive nights; prolonged administration is not generally recommended

Contraindications/cautions
- Contraindicated in the presence of hypersensitivity to methyprylon.
- Use caution in the presence of acute intermittent porphyria, impaired hepatic or renal function, addiction-prone patients, lactation.

Dosage
Adult: Usual dosage is 200–400 mg PO at bedtime. Dosage should not exceed 400 mg/d.
Pediatric: Older than 12 y: Dosage varies greatly. Initiate treatment with 50 mg PO at bedtime, increase to 200 mg if required. Younger than 12 y: Safety and efficacy not established.

Geriatric: Increased chance of confusion, acute brain syndrome; monitor dosage and use with caution.

Pharmacokinetics

Route	Onset	Peak	Duration
Oral	45 min	1–2 h	5–8 h

Metabolism: Hepatic, $T_{1/2}$: 4 h
Distribution: Crosses placenta; may enter breast milk
Excretion: Urine

Adverse effects

- CNS: Convulsions, hallucinations, ataxia, EEG changes, pyrexia, *morning drowsiness, hangover, headache, dizziness,* vertigo, acute brain syndrome and confusion; paradoxical excitation, anxiety, depression, nightmares, dreaming, diplopia, blurred vision, *suppression of REM sleep; REM rebound when drug is discontinued*
- GI: *Esophagitis,* vomiting, nausea, diarrhea, constipation
- CV: Hypotension, syncope
- Hematologic: Aplastic anemia, thrombocytopenic purpura, neutropenia
- Hypersensitivity: Generalized allergic reactions; pruritus, rash
- Other: Physical, psychological dependence; tolerance; withdrawal reaction

■ Nursing Considerations

Assessment

- *History:* Hypersensitivity to methyprylon, acute intermittent porphyria, impaired hepatic or renal function, addiction-prone patients, lactation
- *Physical:* Body temperature; skin—color, lesions; orientation, affect, reflexes, vision exam; P, BP; bowel sounds, normal output, liver evaluation; CBC with differential, hepatic and renal function tests

Implementation

- Supervise carefully dose and amount of drug prescribed in patients who are addiction prone or likely to increase dosage on their own initiative.
- Dispense least amount of drug feasible to patients who are depressed or suicidal.
- Withdraw drug gradually if patient has used drug long term or if patient has developed tolerance. Supportive therapy similar to that for withdrawal from barbiturates may be necessary to prevent dangerous withdrawal symptoms.
- Arrange for re-evaluation of patients with prolonged insomnia; therapy of the underlying cause of insomnia (eg, pain, depression) is preferable to prolonged therapy with sedative/hypnotic drugs.

Drug-specific teaching points

- Take this drug exactly as prescribed. Do not exceed prescribed dosage. Long-term use is not recommended.
- Know that the following side effects may occur: drowsiness, dizziness, blurred vision (avoid driving a car or performing other tasks requiring alertness or visual acuity if these occur); GI upset (frequent, small meals may help).
- Report skin rash, sore throat, fever, bruising.

☐ methysergide maleate

(meth i ser' jide)
Sansert

Pregnancy Category X

Drug classes
Antimigraine drug
Semisynthetic ergot derivative

Therapeutic actions
Mechanism of action unknown; inhibits the effects of serotonin; serotonin may be involved in vascular headaches and may be a "headache substance," lowering pain threshold during headaches; methysergide also inhibits histamine release from mast cells and stabilizes platelets against serotonin release.

Indications
- Prevention or reduction in intensity and frequency of vascular headaches in spe-

Adverse effects in *Italics* are most common; those in **Bold** are life-threatening.

cific patients: patients suffering from one or more severe vascular headaches per week, from vascular headaches that are so severe that preventive measures are necessary
- Prophylaxis of vascular headache; not for management of acute attacks

Contraindications/cautions
- Allergy to ergot preparations, tartrazine (more likely in patients with aspirin sensitivity) contained in 2-mg tablets marketed as *Sansert;* peripheral vascular disease, severe arteriosclerosis, severe hypertension, coronary artery disease, phlebitis or cellulitis of the lower limbs, pulmonary disease, collagen disease, fibrotic processes, impaired liver or renal function, valvular heart disease, debilitated states, serious infection, pregnancy, lactation.

Dosage
Adult: 4–8 mg/d PO, taken with meal. There must be a 3- to 4-wk drug free interval after every 6-mo course of treatment. If efficacy has not been demonstrated after a 3-wk trial period, benefit is unlikely to occur.
Pediatric: Not recommended for children.

Pharmacokinetics

Route	Onset	Peak
Oral	Varies	1–2 d

Metabolism: Hepatic, $T_{1/2}$: 10 h
Distribution: Crosses placenta; enters breast milk
Excretion: Urine

Adverse effects
- CNS: *Insomnia, drowsiness, mild euphoria, dizziness,* ataxia, weakness, lightheadedness, hyperesthesia, hallucinatory experiences
- GI: *Nausea, vomiting, diarrhea, heartburn,* abdominal pain
- CV: *Vascular insufficiency of lower limbs, intense vasoconstriction* (chest pain; abdominal pain; cold, numb, painful extremities), postural hypotension
- Hematologic: Neutropenia, eosinophilia
- Dermatologic: *Facial flushing,* telangiectasia, rashes, hair loss, peripheral edema, dependent edema
- Other: Arthralgia, myalgia, weight gain; retroperitoneal fibrosis, pleuropulmonary fibrosis and fibrotic thickening of cardiac valves with long-term therapy

Clinically important drug-drug interactions
- Increased risk of peripheral ischemia if taken concurrently with beta-blockers

■ Nursing Considerations
Assessment
- *History:* Allergy to ergot preparations, tartrazine; peripheral vascular disease, severe arteriosclerosis, severe hypertension, coronary artery disease, phlebitis or cellulitis of the lower limbs, pulmonary disease, collagen disease, fibrotic processes, impaired liver or renal function, valvular heart disease, debilitated states, serious infection; pregnancy; lactation
- *Physical:* Skin—color, edema, lesions; weight; body temperature; orientation, gait, reflexes, affect; P, BP, peripheral perfusion, auscultation; R, adventitious sounds; liver evaluation, bowel sounds; CBC, liver and renal function tests

Implementation
- Do not administer continuously for longer than 6 mo; ensure a drug free interval for 3–4 wk after each 6-mo course.
- Arrange to reduce dosage gradually during the last 2–3 wk of each treatment course to avoid "headache rebound."
- Administer drug with food to prevent GI upset.

Drug-specific teaching points
- Take drug with meals to prevent GI upset. Drug is meant to prevent migraines, not as treatment of acute attacks. Drug is given in treatment courses of 6 mo; a 3- to 4-wk drug-free interval is necessary between treatment courses.
- Know that the following side effects may occur: weight gain (monitor caloric in-

Adverse effects in *Italics* are most common; those in **Bold** are life-threatening.

take if this occurs); drowsiness, dizziness, weakness, lightheadedness (use caution if driving or operating dangerous machinery if this occurs); diarrhea; nausea, vomiting, heartburn (these may gradually subside).
- Be aware that this drug should not be taken during pregnancy. If you become pregnant or desire to become pregnant, consult with your physician. Contraception is recommnended while you are using this drug.
- Report cold, numb, painful extremities, leg cramps when walking, girdle, flank or chest pain, painful urination, shortness of breath.

metoclopramide

*(met oh kloe **pra'** mide)*

Maxeran (CAN), Maxolon, Octamide PFS, Reglan

Pregnancy Category B

Drug classes
GI stimulant
Antiemetic
Dopaminergic-blocking drug

Therapeutic actions
Stimulates motility of upper GI tract without stimulating gastric, biliary, or pancreatic secretions; appears to sensitize tissues to action of acetylcholine; relaxes pyloric sphincter, which, when combined with effects on motility, accelerates gastric emptying and intestinal transit; little effect on gallbladder or colon motility; increases lower esophageal sphincter pressure; has sedative properties; induces release of prolactin.

Indications
- Relief of symptoms of acute and recurrent diabetic gastroparesis
- Short-term therapy (4–12 wk) for adults with documented symptomatic gastroesophageal reflux who fail to respond to conventional therapy
- Prevention of nausea and vomiting associated with emetogenic cancer chemotherapy (parenteral)
- Prophylaxis of postoperative nausea and vomiting when nasogastric suction is undesirable
- Facilitation of small bowel intubation when tube does not pass the pylorus with conventional maneuvers (single-dose parenteral use)
- Stimulation of gastric emptying and intestinal transit of barium when delayed emptying interferes with radiologic exam of the stomach or small intestine (single dose parenteral use)
- Unlabeled uses: improvement of lactation (doses of 30–45 mg/d); treatment of nausea and vomiting of a variety of etiologies: emesis during pregnancy and labor, gastric ulcer, anorexia nervosa

Contraindications/cautions
- Contraindicated in the presence of allergy to metoclopramide; GI hemorrhage, mechanical obstruction or perforation; pheochromocytoma (may cause hypertensive crisis); epilepsy.
- Use caution in the presence of previously detected breast cancer (one-third of such tumors are prolactin-dependent); lactation.

Dosage
Adult
- ***Relief of symptoms of gastroparesis:*** 10 mg PO 30 min before each meal and at bedtime for 2–8 wk. If symptoms are severe, initiate therapy with IM or IV administration for up to 10 d until symptoms subside.
- ***Symptomatic gastroesophageal reflux:*** 10–15 mg PO up to four times a day 30 min before meals and at bedtime. If symptoms occur only at certain times or in relation to specific stimuli, single doses of 20 mg may be preferable; guide therapy by endoscopic results. Do not use longer than 12 wk.
- ***Prevention of postoperative nausea and vomiting:*** 10–20 mg IM at the end of surgery.
- ***Prevention of chemotherapy-induced emesis:*** Dilute and give by IV infusion over not less than 15 min. Give first dose $\frac{1}{2}$ h before chemotherapy; repeat q2h for two doses, then q3h for

three doses. The initial two doses should be 2 mg/kg for highly emetogenic drugs (cisplatin, dacarbazine); 1 mg/kg may suffice for other chemotherapeutic agents.
- **_Facilitation of small bowel intubation, gastric emptying:_** 10 mg (2 ml) by direct IV injection over 1–2 min.

Pediatric
- **_Facilitation of intubation, gastric emptying:_** *6–14 y:* 2.5–5 mg by direct IV injection over 1–2 min. *< 6 y:* 0.1 mg/kg by direct IV injection over 1–2 min.

Pharmacokinetics

Route	Onset	Peak	Duration
Oral	30–60 min	60–90 min	1–2 h
IM	10–15 min	60–90 min	1–2 h
IV	1–3 min	60–90 min	1–2 h

Metabolism: Hepatic, $T_{1/2}$: 5–6 h
Distribution: Crosses placenta; enters breast milk
Excretion: Urine

IV facts
Preparation: Dilute dose in 50 ml of a parenteral solution (Dextrose 5% in Water, Sodium Chloride Injection, Dextrose 5% in 0.45% Sodium Chloride, Ringer's Injection, or Lactated Ringer's Injection). May be stored for up to 48 h if protected from light or up to 24 h under normal light.
Infusion: Give direct IV doses slowly (over 1–2 min); give infusions over at least 15 min.
Incompatabilities: Do not mix with solutions containing cephalothin, chloramphenicol, sodium bicarbonate.

Adverse effects
- **CNS:** *Restlessness, drowsiness, fatigue, lassitude,* insomnia, *extrapyramidal reactions, parkinsonism-like reactions,* akathisia, dystonia, myoclonus, dizziness, anxiety
- **GI:** *Nausea, diarrhea*
- **CV:** Transient hypertension

Clinically important drug-drug interactions
- Decreased absorption of digoxin from the stomach when taken with metoclopramide • Increased toxic and immunosuppressive effects of cyclosporine if taken concurrently

■ Nursing Considerations
Assessment
- *History:* Allergy to metoclopramide, GI hemorrhage, mechanical obstruction or perforation, pheochromocytoma, epilepsy, lactation, previously detected breast cancer
- *Physical:* Orientation, reflexes, affect; P, BP; bowel sounds, normal output; EEG

Implementation
- Monitor BP carefully during IV administration.
- Monitor for extrapyramidal reactions, and consult physician if they occur.
- Monitor diabetic patients, and arrange for alteration in insulin dose or timing, as appropriate, if diabetic control is compromised by alterations in timing of food absorption.
- Provide diphenhydramine injection on standby in case extrapyramidal reactions occur (50 mg IM).
- Provide phentolamine on standby in case of hypertensive crisis (most likely to occur in patients with undiagnosed pheochromocytoma).

Drug-specific teaching points
- Take this drug exactly as prescribed.
- Do not use alcohol, sleep remedies, sedatives while you are taking this drug; serious sedation could occur.
- Know that the following side effects may occur: drowsiness, dizziness (do not drive a car or perform other tasks that require alertness if these occur); restlessness, anxiety, depression, headache, insomnia (it may help to know that these are drug effects that will not persist after you discontinue the drug); nausea, diarrhea.

Adverse effects in *Italics* are most common; those in **Bold** are life-threatening.

- Report involuntary movement of the face, eyes, or limbs, severe depression, severe diarrhea.

metolazone

(me tole' a zone)
Mykrox, Zaroxolyn

Pregnancy Category B

Drug classes
Thiazide-like diuretic

Therapeutic actions
Inhibits reabsorption of sodium and chloride in distal renal tubule, increasing excretion of sodium, chloride, and water by the kidney.

Indications
- Adjunctive therapy in edema associated with CHF, cirrhosis, corticosteroid and estrogen therapy, renal dysfunction
- Hypertension, as sole therapy or in combination with other antihypertensives
- Unlabeled uses: calcium nephrolithiasis alone or with amiloride or allopurinol to prevent recurrences in hypercalciuric or normal calciuric patients; diabetes insipidus, especially nephrogenic diabetes insipidus

Contraindications/cautions
- Contraindicated in the presence of hypersensitivity to thiazides, hepatic coma, fluid or electrolyte imbalances, renal or liver disease.
- Use caution in the presence of gout, SLE, glucose tolerance abnormalities, hyperparathyroidism, manic-depressive disorders, lactation.

Dosage
Adult
- **Zaroxolyn**
– *Hypertension:* 2.5–5 mg qd PO.
– *Edema of renal disease:* 5–20 mg qd PO.
– *Edema of CHF:* 5–10 mg qd PO.
– *Calcium nephrolithiasis:* 2.5–10 mg/d PO.
- **Mykrox**
– *Mild to moderate hypertension:* 0.5 mg qd PO taken as a single dose early in the morning. May be increased to 1 mg qd; do not exceed 1 mg/d. If switching from Zaroxolyn to Mykrox, determine the dose by titration starting at 0.5 mg qd and increasing to 1 mg qd.

Pediatric: Not recommended.

Pharmacokinetics

Brand	Onset	Peak	Duration
Mykrox	20–30 min	2–4 h	12–24 h
Zaroxolyn	1 h	2 h	12–24 h

Metabolism: Hepatic, $T_{1/2}$: 14 h (*Mykrox*), unknown (*Zaroxolyn*)
Distribution: Crosses placenta; enters breast milk
Excretion: Urine

Adverse effects
- **CNS:** *Dizziness, vertigo,* paresthesias, weakness, *headache,* drowsiness, *fatigue*
- **GI:** *Nausea, anorexia, vomiting, dry mouth, diarrhea, constipation,* jaundice, hepatitis, pancreatitis
- **CV:** Orthostatic hypotension, venous thrombosis, volume depletion, cardiac arrhythmias, chest pain
- **Hematologic:** Leukopenia, thrombocytopenia, agranulocytosis, aplastic anemia, neutropenia, fluid and electrolyte imbalances
- **GU:** *Polyuria, nocturia, impotence,* loss of libido
- **Dermatologic:** Photosensitivity, rash, purpura, exfoliative dermatitis
- **Other:** Muscle cramps and muscle spasms, fever, hives, gouty attacks, flushing

Clinically important drug-drug interactions
- Increased thiazide effects and chance of acute hyperglycemia if taken with diazoxide • Decreased absorption with cholestyramine, colestipol • Increased risk of cardiac glycoside toxicity if hypokalemia occurs • Increased risk of lithium toxicity • Increased dosage of antidiabetic

agents may be needed • Increased risk of hyperglycemia if taken concurrently with diazoxide

Drug-lab test interferences
• Decreased PBI levels without clinical signs of thyroid disturbances

■ Nursing Considerations
Assessment
- *History:* Fluid or electrolyte imbalances, renal or liver disease, gout, SLE, glucose tolerance abnormalities, hyperparathyroidism, manic-depressive disorders, hepatic coma or precoma, lactation
- *Physical:* Skin—color and lesions; orientation, reflexes, muscle strength; pulses, BP, orthostatic BP, perfusion, edema, baseline ECG; R, adventitious sounds; liver evaluation, bowel sounds; CBC, serum electrolytes, blood glucose, liver and renal function tests, serum uric acid, urinalysis

Implementation
- Withdraw drug 2–3 d before elective surgery; if emergency surgery is indicated, reduce dosage of preanesthetic or anesthetic agents.
- Administer with food or milk if GI upset occurs.
- Measure and record regular body weights to monitor fluid changes.

Drug-specific teaching points
- Take drug early in the day so sleep will not be disturbed by increased urination.
- Weigh yourself daily, and record weights.
- Protect skin from exposure to the sun or bright lights.
- Know that the following side effects may occur: increased urination; dizziness, drowsiness, feeling faint (use caution; avoid driving or operating dangerous machinery if this occurs); headache.
- Report rapid weight gain or loss, swelling in ankles or fingers, unusual bleeding or bruising, muscle cramps.

❏ metoprolol tartrate

(me toe' proe lole)
Betaloc (CAN), Lopresor (CAN), Lopressor, Toprxol XL

Pregnancy Category B

Drug classes
Beta-adrenergic blocking agent (β_1-selective)
Antihypertensive agent

Therapeutic actions
Competitively blocks beta-adrenergic receptors in the heart and juxtaglomerular apparatus, decreasing the influence of the sympathetic nervous system on these tissues and the excitability of the heart, decreasing cardiac output and the release of renin, and lowering blood pressure; acts in the CNS to reduce sympathetic outflow and vasoconstrictor tone.

Indications
- Hypertension, alone or with other drugs, especially diuretics
- Prevention of reinfarction in MI patients who are hemodynamically stable or within 3–10 d of the acute MI
- Treatment of angina pectoris

Contraindications/cautions
- Contraindicated in the presence of sinus bradycardia (HR < 45 beats/min), second- or third-degree heart block (PR interval > 0.24 sec), cardiogenic shock, CHF, systolic BP < 100 mm Hg; lactation.
- Use caution in the presence of diabetes or thyrotoxicosis; asthma or COPD; pregnancy.

Dosage
Adult
- ***Hypertension:*** Initially 100 mg/d PO in single or divided doses; gradually increase dosage at weekly intervals. Usual maintenance dose is 100–450 mg/d.
- ***Angina pectoris:*** Initially 100 mg/d PO in two divided doses; may be increased gradually, effective range 100–400 mg/d.
- ***MI, early treatment:*** Three IV bolus doses of 5 mg each at 2-min intervals with careful monitoring. If these are tolerated, give 50 mg PO 15 min after the last IV dose and q6h for 48 h. Thereafter, give a maintenance dosage of 100 mg PO bid. Reduce initial PO doses to 25 mg, or discontinue the drug in patients who do not tolerate the IV doses.

- **MI, late treatment:** 100 mg PO bid as soon as possible after infarct, continuing for at least 3 mo and possibly for 1–3 y.
- **Extended-release tablets:** *Hypertension:* 50–100 mg/d PO as one dose. *Angina:* 100 mg/d PO as a single dose.

Pediatric: Safety and efficacy not established.

Pharmacokinetics

Route	Onset	Peak	Duration
Oral	15 min	90 min	15–19 h
IV	Immediate	60–90 min	15–19 h

Metabolism: Hepatic, $T_{1/2}$: 3–4 h
Distribution: Crosses placenta; enters breast milk
Excretion: Urine

IV facts

Preparation: No additional preparation is required.
Infusion: Inject directly into vein or into tubing of running IV. Inject as a bolus; monitor carefully; wait 2 min between doses.

Adverse effects

- **CNS:** Dizziness, vertigo, tinnitus, fatigue, emotional depression, paresthesias, sleep disturbances, hallucinations, disorientation, memory loss, slurred speech
- **GI:** *Gastric pain, flatulence, constipation, diarrhea, nausea, vomiting,* anorexia, ischemic colitis, renal and mesenteric arterial thrombosis, retroperitoneal fibrosis, hepatomegaly, acute pancreatitis
- **CV:** *CHF, cardiac arrhythmias,* peripheral vascular insufficiency, claudication, CVA, pulmonary edema, hypotension
- **Respiratory:** Bronchospasm, dyspnea, cough, bronchial obstruction, nasal stuffiness, rhinitis, pharyngitis
- **GU:** *Impotence, decreased libido,* Peyronie's disease, dysuria, nocturia, frequent urination
- **MS:** Joint pain, arthralgia, muscle cramp
- **EENT:** Eye irritation, dry eyes, conjunctivitis, blurred vision
- **Dermatologic:** Rash, pruritus, sweating, dry skin
- **Allergic:** Pharyngitis, erythematous rash, fever, sore throat, laryngospasm
- **Other:** *Decreased exercise tolerance, development of antinuclear antibodies (ANA),* hyperglycemia or hypoglycemia, elevated serum transaminase, alkaline

Clinically important drug-drug interactions

- Increased effects of metoprolol if taken with verapamil, cimetidine, methimazole, propylthiouracil • Increased effects of both drugs if metoprolol is taken concurrently with hydralazine • Increased serum levels and toxicity of IV lidocaine, if given concurrently • Increased risk of postural hypotension if taken concurrently with prazosin • Decreased antihypertensive effects if taken with NSAIDs, clonidine, rifampinDecreased therapeutic effects if taken concurrently with barbiturates • Hypertension followed by severe bradycardia if given concurrently with epinephrine

Drug-lab test interferences

- Possible false results with glucose or insulin tolerance tests (oral)

■ Nursing Considerations

Assessment

- *History:* Sinus bradycardia (HR < 45 beats/min), second- or third-degree heart block (PR interval > 0.24 sec), cardiogenic shock, CHF, systolic BP < 100 mg Hg; diabetes or thyrotoxicosis; asthma or COPD; lactation
- *Physical:* Body weight, skin condition, neurologic status, P, BP, ECG, respiratory status, kidney and thyroid function, blood and urine glucose

Implementation

- Do not discontinue drug abruptly after chronic therapy (hypersensitivity to catecholamines may have developed, causing exacerbation of angina, MI, and ventricular dysrhythmias). Taper drug gradually over 2 wk with monitoring.

Adverse effects in *Italics* are most common; those in **Bold** are life-threatening.

- Consult with physician about withdrawing drug if patient is to undergo surgery (controversial).
- Give oral drug with food to facilitate absorption.
- Provide continual cardiac monitoring for patients receiving IV metoprolol.

Drug-specific teaching points
- Do not to stop taking this drug unless instructed to do so by a health care provider.
- Know that the following side effects may occur: dizziness, drowsiness, lightheadedness, blurred vision (avoid driving or dangerous activities if these effects occur); nausea, loss of appetite (small, frequent meals may help); nightmares, depression (notify your health care provider who may be able to change the medication); sexual impotence.
- Report difficulty breathing, night cough, swelling of extremities, slow pulse, confusion, depression, rash, fever, sore throat

▢ metronidazole

*(me troe **ni'** da zole)*

Apo-Metronidazole (CAN), Femazole, Flagyl, MetroGel, Metro I.V., Metronidazole Redi-Infusion, Neo-Tric (CAN), Novonidazol (CAN), PMS-Metronidazole (CAN), Protostat, Trikacide (CAN)

Pregnancy Category B

Drug classes
Antibiotic
Antibacterial
Amebicide
Antiprotozoal agent

Therapeutic actions
Bactericidal: inhibits DNA synthesis in specific (obligate) anaerobes, causing cell death; antiprotozoal-trichomonacidal, amebicidal: biochemical mechanism of action is not known.

Indications
- Acute infection with susceptible anaerobic bacteria
- Acute intestinal amebiasis
- Amebic liver abscess
- Trichomoniasis (acute and partners of patients with acute infection)
- Preoperative, intraoperative, postoperative prophylaxis for patients undergoing colorectal surgery
- Topical application in the treatment of inflammatory papules, pustules, and erythema of rosacea
- Unlabeled uses: prophylaxis for patients undergoing gynecologic, abdominal surgery; hepatic encephalopathy; Crohn's disease; antibiotic-associated pseudomembranous colitis; treatment of *Gardnerella vaginalis*, giardiasis (use recommended by the CDC)

Contraindications/cautions
- Contraindicated in the presence of hypersensitivity to metronidazole; pregnancy (do not use for trichomoniasis in first trimester).
- Use caution in the presence of CNS diseases, hepatic disease, candidiasis (moniliasis), blood dyscrasias, lactation.

Dosage
Adult
- ***Anaerobic bacterial infection:*** 15 mg/kg IV infused over 1 h; then 7.5 mg/kg infused over 1 h q6h for 7–10 d, not to exceed 4 g/d.
- ***Amebiasis:*** 750 mg/tid PO for 5–10 d. (In amebic dysentary, combine with iodoquinol 650 mg PO tid for 20 d).
- ***Trichomoniasis:*** 2 g PO in one day (1-d treatment) *or* 250 mg tid PO for 7 d.
- ***Prophylaxis:*** 15 mg/kg infused IV over 30–60 min and completed about 1 h before surgery. Then 7.5 mg/kg infused over 30–60 min at 6- to 12-h intervals after initial dose during the day of surgery only.
- ***Gardnerella Vaginalis:*** 500 mg bid PO for 7 d.
- ***Giardiasis:*** 250 mg tid PO for 7 d.
- ***Antibiotic-associated pseudomembranous colitis:*** 1–2 g/d PO for 7–10 d.
- ***Treatment of inflammatory papules, pustules, and erythema of rosacea (MetroGel):*** Apply and

rub in a thin film twice daily, morning and evening, to entire affected areas after washing; results should be seen within 3 wk; treatment through 9 wk has been effective.

Pediatric
- **Anaerobic bacterial infection:** Not recommended.
- **Amebiasis:** 35–50 mg/kg per day PO in three doses for 10 d.

Pharmacokinetics

Route	Onset	Peak
Oral	Varies	1–2 h
IV	Rapid	1–2 h
Topical	Not generally absorbed systemically	

Metabolism: Hepatic, $T_{1/2}$: 6–8 h
Distribution: Crosses placenta; enters breast milk
Excretion: Urine and feces

IV facts

Preparation: Reconstitute by adding 4.4 ml of Sterile Water for Injection, Bacteriostatic Water for Injection, 0.9% Sodium Chloride Injection, Bacteriostatic 0.9% Sodium Chloride Injection to the vial and mix thoroughly. Resultant volume is 5 ml with a concentration of 100 mg/ml. Solution should be clear to pale yellow to yellow-green; do not use if cloudy or if containing precipitates; use within 24 h; protect from light. Add reconstituted solution to glass or plastic container containing 0.9% Sodium Chloride Injection, 5% Dextrose Injection or Lactated Ringer's; discontinue other solutions while running metronidazole.

Infusion: Prior to administration, add 5 mEq Sodium Bicarbonate Injection for each 500 mg used, mix thoroughly. Do not refrigerate neutralized solution. Do not administer solution that has not been neutralized. Infuse over 1 h.

Adverse effects

- CNS: *Headache, dizziness, ataxia,* vertigo, incoordination, insomnia, seizures, peripheral neuropathy, fatigue
- GI: *Unpleasant metallic taste, anorexia, nausea, vomiting, diarrhea,* GI upset, cramps
- GU: Dysuria, incontinence, *darkening of the urine*
- Local: Thrombophlebitis (IV); *redness, burning, dryness, and skin irritation* (topical)
- Other: Severe disulfiramlike interaction with alcohol, candidiasis (superinfection)

Clinically important drug-drug interactions

- Decreased effectiveness of drug if taken with barbiturates • Disulfiram-like reaction (flushing, tachycardia, nausea, vomiting) if taken concurrently with alcohol • Psychosis if taken concurrently with disulfiram • Increased bleeding tendencies if taken with oral anticoagulants

Drug-lab test interferences

- Falsely low (or zero) values in SGOT (AST), SGPT (ALT), LDH, triglycerides, hexokinase glucose tests

■ Nursing Considerations

Assessment

- *History:* CNS or hepatic disease; candidiasis (moniliasis); blood dyscrasias; pregnancy; lactation
- *Physical:* Reflexes, affect; skin—lesions, color (with topical application); abdominal exam, liver palpation; urinalysis, CBC, liver function tests

Implementation

- Avoid use unless necessary. Metronidazole is carcinogenic in some rodents.
- Administer oral doses with food.
- Apply topically (*MetroGel*) after cleansing the area. Advise patient that cosmetics may be used over the area after application.
- Reduce dosage in hepatic disease.

Drug-specific teaching points

- Take full course of drug therapy; take the drug with food if GI upset occurs.
- Know that the following side effects may occur: dry mouth with strange metallic

Adverse effects in *Italics* are most common; those in **Bold** are life-threatening.

taste (frequent mouth care, sucking sugarless candies may help, and the sensation will go away when the drug is stopped); nausea, vomiting, diarrhea (small, frequent meals may help).
- Do not drink alcohol (ie, beverages or preparations containing alcohol, cough syrups) while taking this drug; severe reactions may occur.
- Be aware that your urine may appear dark while taking this drug; this is expected and should not be a cause for alarm.
- Refrain from sexual intercourse unless partner wears a condom during treatment for trichomoniasis.
- Report severe GI upset, dizziness, unusual fatigue or weakness, fever, chills.

Topical Application
- Apply the topical preparation by cleansing the area and then rubbing a thin film into the affected area. Avoid contact with the eyes. Cosmetics may be applied to the area after application.

☐ metyrosine

(me tye' roe seen)
Demser

Pregnancy Category C

Drug classes
Enzyme inhibitor

Therapeutic actions
Blocks the enzyme tyrosine hydroxylase; inhibits the conversion of tyrosine to DOPA, which is the first step in the synthesis of catecholamines. In patients with pheochromocytoma, this reduces catecholamine synthesis, substantially reducing hypertensive attacks and associated symptoms.

Indications
- Preoperative preparation of patients for surgery for pheochromocytoma
- Management of pheochromocytoma when surgery is contraindicated
- Chronic treatment for malignant pheochromocytoma

Contraindications/cautions
- Contraindicated in the presence of hypersensitivity to metyrosine.
- Use caution in the presence of pregnancy, lactation.

Dosage
Adult and children older than 12 y: Initial dose of 250 mg PO qid; may be increased by 250–500 mg qd to a maximum of 4 g/d.
- ***Preoperative:*** 2–3 g/d PO for 5–7 d.

Pediatric: Not recommended.

Pharmacokinetics

Route	Onset	Peak	Duration
Oral	Slow	2–3 d	3–4 d

Metabolism: Hepatic, $T_{1/2}$: 3.4–3.7 h
Distribution: Crosses placenta; may enter breast milk
Excretion: Urine and feces

Adverse effects
- CNS: *Sedation,* drooling, tremor, speech difficulty, depression, hallucinations
- GI: *Diarrhea,* dry mouth, nausea, vomiting, abdominal pain
- GU: Impotence, failure of ejaculation, dysuria, hematuria, crystalluria
- Other: Nasal congestion, breast swelling

■ Nursing Considerations

Assessment
- *History:* Hypersensitivity to metyrsoine, pregnancy, lactation
- *Physical:* Orientation, affect, reflexes; bowel sounds, normal output; urinalysis

Implementation
- Ensure a very liberal intake of fluids while on drug therapy.
- Arrange for use of antidiarrheals if diarrhea is severe and metryosine needs to be used.
- Monitor urine for changes associated with drug use; less likely when fluids are encouraged.

Adverse effects in *Italics* are most common; those in **Bold** are life-threatening.

Drug-specific teaching points
- Drink plenty of fluids while you are on this drug.
- Avoid alcohol, sleep-inducing, or OTC drugs while you are on this drug. These could cause dangerous effects.
- Know that the following side effects may occur: drowsiness, dizziness, blurred vision (avoid driving a car or engaging in activities that require alertness if these occur); nausea, dry mouth (good mouth care, taking drug with food, and eating frequent, small meals may help); diarrhea (medication may be ordered if this is severe).
- Report drooling, speech difficulty, tremors, disorientation, severe diarrhea, painful urination.

☐ mexiletine HCl

*(mex **ill**' i teen)*
Mexitil

Pregnancy Category C

Drug classes
Antiarrhythmic

Therapeutic actions
Type 1 antiarrhythmic: decreases automaticity of ventricular cells by membrane stabilization.

Indications
- Treatment of documented life-threatening ventricular arrhythmias (use with lesser arrhythmias is not recommended)
- Unlabeled uses: prophylactic use to decrease arrhythmias in acute phase of acute MI (mortality may not be affected); reduction of pain, dysesthesia, and paresthesia associated with diabetic neuropathy

Contraindications/cautions
- Contraindicated in the presence of allergy to mexiletine, CHF, cardiogenic shock, hypotension, second- or third-degree heart block (without artificial pacemaker), lactation.
- Use caution in the presence of hepatic disease, seizure disorders, pregnancy.

Dosage
Adult: 200 mg q8h PO. Increase in 50- to 100-mg increments every 2–3 d until desired antiarrhythmic effect is obtained. Maximum dose: 1,200 mg/d PO. Rapid control: 400 mg loading dose, then 200 mg q8h PO.
- ***Transferring from other antiarrhythmics:*** *Lidocaine:* Stop the lidocaine with the first dose of mexiletine; leave IV line open until adequate arrhythmia suppression is assured. *Quinidine sulfate:* Initial dose of 200 mg 6–12 h PO after the last dose of quinidine. *Procainamide:* Initial dose of 200 mg 3–6 h PO after the last dose of procainamide. *Disopyramide:* 200 mg 6–12 h PO after the last dose of disopyramide. *Tocainide:* 200 mg 8–12 h PO after the last dose of tocainide.

Pediatric: Safety and efficacy not established.

Pharmacokinetics

Route	Onset	Peak
Oral	Varies	2–3 h

Metabolism: Hepatic, $T_{1/2}$: 10–12 h
Distribution: Crosses placenta; enters breast milk
Excretion: Urine

Adverse effects
- **CNS:** *Dizziness/lightheadedness, headache,* fatigue, drowsiness, *tremors, coordination difficulties, visual disturbances,* numbness, nervousness, *sleep difficulties*
- **GI:** *Nausea, vomiting, heart burn,* abdominal pain, diarrhea, liver injury
- **CV:** *Cardiac arrhythmias, chest pain*
- **Respiratory:** *Dyspnea*
- **Hematologic:** Positive ANA, thrombocytopenia, leukopenia
- **Other:** *Rash*

Clinically important drug-drug interactions
- Decreased mexiletine levels if given with phenytoins • Increased theophylline levels

Adverse effects in *Italics* are most common; those in **Bold** are life-threatening.

and toxicity if theophyllines are given with mexiletine

Nursing Considerations

Assessment
- *History:* Allergy to mexiletine, CHF, cardiogenic shock, hypotension, second- or third-degree heart block, hepatic disease, seizure disorders, lactation
- *Physical:* Weight; orientation, reflexes; P, BP, auscultation, ECG, edema; R, adventitious sounds; bowel sounds, liver evaluation; urinalysis, urine pH, CBC, electrolytes, liver and renal function tests

Implementation
- Monitor patient response carefully, especially when beginning therapy.
- Reduce dosage in patients with hepatic failure.
- Monitor for safe and effective serum levels (0.5–2 μg/ml).

Drug-specific teaching points
- Take with food to reduce GI problems.
- Be aware that frequent monitoring of cardiac rhythm will be necessary.
- Know that the following side effects may occur: drowsiness, dizziness, numbness, visual disturbances (avoid driving or working with dangerous machinery until you know your response to the drug); nausea, vomiting, heartburn (small, frequent meals may help); diarrhea; headache; sleep disturbances.
- Do not stop taking this drug for any reason without checking with your health care provider.
- Return for regular follow-up visits to check your heart rhythm; you also may have a blood test.
- Do not make any changes in your diet that could change the acidity of your urine; should you change your diet to include a large amount of any particular type of food (such as fruit or vegetables), check with your health care provider.
- Report fever, chills, sore throat, excessive GI discomfort, chest pain, excessive tremors, numbness, lack of coordination, headache, sleep disturbances.

☐ mezlocillin sodium

*(mez loe **sill'** in)*
Mezlin

Pregnancy Category B

Drug classes
Antibiotic
Penicillin with extended spectrum

Therapeutic actions
Bactericidal: inhibits synthesis of cell wall in sensitive organisms, causing cell death.

Indications
- Lower respiratory tract infections caused by *Haemophilus influenzae; Klebsiella*, including *Klebsiella pneumoniae; Proteus mirabilis; Pseudomonas* species, including *Pseudomonas aeruginosa; Escherichia coli; Bacteroides* species, including *Bacteroides fragilis*
- Intra-abdominal infections caused by *E. coli, P. mirabilis, Klebsiella, Pseudomonas, Streptococcus faecalis, Bacteroides, Peptococcus, Peptostreptococcus*
- UTIs caused by *E. coli, Proteus mirabilis, Proteus, Morganella morganii, Klebsiella, Enterobacter, Serratia, Pseudomonas, S. faecalis*
- Gynecologic infections caused by *Neisseria gonorrhoeae, Peptococcus, Peptostreptococcus, Bacteroides, E. coli, P. mirabilis, Klebsiella, Enterobacter*
- Skin and skin-structure infections caused by *S. faecalis, E. coli, P. mirabilis, Proteus, Proteus vulgaris, Providencia rettgeri, Klebsiella, Enterobacter, Pseudomonas, Peptococcus, Bacteroides*
- Septicemia caused by *E. coli, Klebsiella, Enterobacter, Pseudomonas, Bacteroides, Peptococcus*
- Infections caused by *Streptococcus*
- Severe life threatening infections caused by *P. aeruginosa*, in combination with an aminoglycoside antibiotic
- Prophylaxis to decrease the incidence of infections in patients undergoing "dirty" surgical procedures

Contraindications/cautions
- Contraindicated in the presence of allergies to penicillins, cephalosporins, or other allergens.
- Use caution in the presence of renal disorders; lactation (may cause diarrhea or candidiasis in the infant).

Dosage
Do not exceed 24 g/d.
Adult: 200–300 mg/kg per day IV or IM, given in four to six divided doses, up to 350 mg/kg per day in severe cases.
- ***Gonococcal urethritis:*** 1–2 g IV or IM with 1 g probenecid PO.

Pediatric: Older than 1 mo, up to 12 y: 50 mg/kg q4h, IM or by IV infusion over 30 min. *< 2,000 g body weight:* younger than 7 d, 75 mg/kg q12h; 7 d, 75 mg/kg q8h. *> 2,000 g body weight:* younger than 7 d, 75 mg/kg q12h; older than 7 d, 75 mg/kg q6h.
Geriatric or renal insufficiency:

Creatinine Clearance (ml/min)	Dosage— UTIs	Systemic Infection
>30	Usual dosage	Usual dosage
10–30	1.5 g q6–8h	3 g q8h
<10	1.5 g q8h	2 g q8h

Pharmacokinetics

Route	Onset	Peak
IM	Rapid	45 min
IV	Immediate	5 min

Metabolism: Hepatic, $T_{1/2}$: 50–55 min
Distribution: Crosses placenta; enters breast milk
Excretion: Urine and bile

IV facts
Preparation: Reconstitute each gram of mezlocillin for IV use by vigorous shaking with 10 ml of Sterile Water for Injection, 5% Dextrose Injection, 0.9% Sodium Chloride Injection. Date reconstituted solution; reconstituted solution is stable for 24–48 h at room temperature, up to 7 d if refrigerated, depending on concentration and diluent—see manufacturer's instructions. Product may darken during storage. If precipitation occurs while refrigerated, warm solution to 37°C, and shake well.
Infusion: Direct injection—administer as slowly as possible (3–5 min) to avoid vein irritation. Infusion should be run over a 30-min period. Discontinue any other IV solution running in the same line while mezlocillin is being administered.
Compatibilities: Compatible diluents include Sterile Water for Injection, 0.9% Sodium Chloride Injection, 5% Dextrose Injection, 5% Dextrose in 0.225% or 0.45% Sodium Chloride, Lactated Ringer's Injection, 5% Dextrose in Electrolyte #75 Injection, Ringer's Injection, 10% Dextrose Injection, 5% Fructose Injection.

Adverse effects
- **CNS:** Lethargy, hallucinations, seizures
- **GI:** *Glossitis, stomatitis, gastritis, sore mouth,* furry tongue, black "hairy" tongue, *nausea, vomiting, diarrhea,* abdominal pain, bloody diarrhea, enterocolitis, pseudomembranous colitis, nonspecific hepatitis
- **Hematologic:** Anemia, thrombocytopenia, leukopenia, neutropenia, prolonged bleeding time
- **GU:** Nephritis—oliguria, proteinuria, hematuria, casts, azotemia, pyuria
- **Hypersensitivity reactions:** *Rash, fever, wheezing,* anaphylaxis
- **Local:** *Pain, phlebitis,* thrombosis at injection site
- **Other:** *Superinfections,* vaginitis, sodium overload leading to CHF

Clinically important drug-drug interactions
- Decreased effectiveness of mezlocillin if taken concurrently with tetracyclines
- Inactivation of parenteral aminoglycosides (amikacin, gentamicin, kanamycin, neomycin, metilmicin, streptomycin, tobramycin) if taken concurrently

Drug-lab test interferences
- False-positive Coombs' test with IV use; false-positive urine protein tests if using sulfosalicylic acid and boiling test, acetic acid test, biuret reaction, nitric acid test

miconazole ■ 745

■ Nursing Considerations
Assessment
- *History:* Allergies to penicillins, cephalosporins, or other allergens; renal disorders, lactation
- *Physical:* Culture infected area; skin—color, lesion; R, adventitious sounds; bowel sounds; CBC, liver and renal function tests, serum electrolytes, Hct, urinalysis

Implementation
- Culture infected area before beginning treatment; reculture area if response is not as expected.
- Administer by IV and IM routes only.
- Reconstitute each gram of mezlocillin for IM use by vigorous shaking with 3–4 ml Sterile Water for Injection, 0.5% or 1.0% Lidocaine HCl without epinephrine. Do not exceed 2 g per injection. Inject deep into a large muscle, such as upper outer quadrant of the buttock; slow injection (12–15 sec) will minimize the pain of injection.
- Carefully check IV site for signs of thrombosis or local drug reaction.
- Do not give IM injections repeatedly in the same site; atrophy can occur. Monitor injection sites.

Drug-specific teaching points
- Be aware that this drug can only be given IV or IM.
- Know that upset stomach, nausea, diarrhea, mouth sores, pain, or discomfort at injection sites may occur.
- Report difficulty breathing, rashes, severe diarrhea, severe pain at injection site, mouth sores.

☐ miconazole

*(mi **kon**' a zole)*
Parenteral: Monistat I.V.

miconazole nitrate

Vaginal suppositories, topical: Micatin, Monistat 3, Monistat 7, Monistat-Derm, Monistat Dual Pak

Pregnancy Category B

Drug classes
Antifungal

Therapeutic actions
Fungicidal: alters fungal cell membrane permeability, causing cell death; also may alter fungal cell DNA and RNA metabolism or cause accumulation of toxic peroxides intracellularly.

Indications
- Treatment of severe systemic fungal infections: coccidioidomycosis, candidiasis, cryptococcosis, petriellidiosis, paracoccidioidomycosis, chronic mucocutaneous candidiasis (parenteral)
- Fungal meningitis or fungal urinary bladder infections (intrathecal, bladder instillation)
- Local treatment of vulvovaginal candidiasis (moniliasis; vaginal suppositories)
- Tinea pedis, tinea cruris, tinea corporis caused by *Trichophyton rubrum, Trichophyton mentagrophytes, Epidermophyton floccosum;* cutaneous candidiasis (moniliasis), tinea versicolor (topical administration)

Contraindications/cautions
- Contraindicated in the presence of allergy to miconazole or components used in preparation.
- Use caution in the presence of pregnancy, lactation.

Dosage
Adult: Daily dosage for parenteral administration may be divided into three infusions. Recommended dosage varies with organism involved:

Organism	Total Daily Dosage Range	Duration (weeks)
Coccidioidomycosis	1,800–3,600 mg	3 to >20
Cryptococcosis	1,200–2,400 mg	3 to >12
Petriellidiosis	600–3,000 mg	5 to >20
Candidiasis	600–1,800 mg	1 to >20
Paracoccidioidomycosis	200–1,200 mg	2 to >16

miconazole

- **Intrathecal administration:** 20 mg/dose administered undiluted as an adjunct to IV treatment. Alternate injections between lumbar, cervical, and cisternal punctures q3–7 d.
- **Bladder instillation:** 200 mg diluted solution for urinary bladder mycoses.
- **Vaginal suppositories:** Monistat 3: Insert 1 suppository intravaginally once daily at bedtime for 3 d. Monistat 7: one applicator cream or 1 suppository in the vagina daily at bedtime for 7 d. Repeat course if necessary.
- **Topical:** Cream and lotion: Cover affected areas bid, morning and evening. Powder: Spray or sprinkle powder liberally over affected area in the morning and evening.

Pediatric
- **Parenteral:** 20–40 mg/kg IV as a total dose. Do not exceed 15 mg/kg per dose.
- **Topical:** Not recommended for children younger than 2 y.

Pharmacokinetics

Route	Onset	Peak
IV	Rapid	Unknown

Metabolism: Hepatic, $T_{1/2}$: 21–24 h
Distribution: Crosses placenta; may enter breast milk
Excretion: Urine and feces

IV facts
Preparation: Dilute in at least 200 ml of fluid, preferably 0.9% Sodium Chloride or 5% Dextrose Solution.
Infusion: Administer initial IV dose of 200 mg with physician in attendance, monitoring patient response. Infuse IV over 30–60 min; avoid rapid infusion; transient tachycardia or arrhythmias may occur.

Adverse effects
Systemic Administration
- GI: *Nausea, vomiting,* diarrhea, anorexia
- Dermatologic: *Phlebitis, pruritus, rash,* flushes
- Hematologic: Decreased hematocrit, thrombocytopenia, aggregation of erythrocytes or rouleau formation, hyperlipemia (associated with vehicle used), Cremophor EL (PEG 40, castor oil)
- Other: *Febrile reactions,* drowsiness, anaphylactoid reactions

Vaginal Suppositories
- Local: *Irritation,* sensitization or vulvovaginal burning, pelvic cramps
- Other: Skin rash, headache

Topical Application
- Local: *Irritation, burning, maceration,* allergic contact dermatitis

■ Nursing Considerations

Assessment
- *History:* Allergy to miconazole or components used in preparation, lactation
- *Physical:* Skin—color, lesions, area around lesions; body temperature; orientation, affect; CBC and differential, serum sodium; serum hemoglobin and lipids (IV administration); culture of area involved

Implementation
- Arrange for culture of fungus involved before beginning therapy.
- Arrange to continue IV treatments until clinical and laboratory tests no longer indicate presence of active fungal infection; suggested length of treatment varies with the causative organism.
- Alternate intrathecal injections between lumbar, cervical, and cisternal sites every 3–7 d.
- Insert vaginal suppositories high into the vagina; have patient remain recumbent for 10–15 min after insertion; provide sanitary napkin to protect clothing from stains.
- Monitor response to drug therapy; if no response is noted, arrange for further cultures to determine causative organism.
- Apply lotion to intertriginous areas if topical application is required; if cream is used, apply sparingly to avoid maceration of the area.

Adverse effects in *Italics* are most common; those in **Bold** are life-threatening.

- Ensure that patient receives the full course of therapy to eradicate the fungus and to prevent recurrence.
- Discontinue topical or vaginal administration if rash or sensitivity occurs.

Drug-specific teaching points

- Take the full course of drug therapy even if symptoms improve. Continue during menstrual period if vaginal route is being used. Long-term use of the drug will be needed; beneficial effects may not be seen for several weeks. Vaginal suppositories should be inserted high into the vagina.
- Use hygiene measures to prevent reinfection or spread of infection.
- Be aware that this drug is specific for the fungus being treated; do not self-medicate other problems with this drug.
- Refrain from sexual intercourse, or advise partner to use a condom to avoid reinfection; use a sanitary napkin to prevent staining of clothing (vaginal use)
- Know that the following side effects may occur: nausea, vomiting, diarrhea (medications may be provided to help this problem); local use: irritation, burning, stinging.
- Report local irritation, burning (topical application); rash, irritation, pelvic pain (vaginal use); drowsiness, difficulty breathing, rash, nausea (parenteral administration).

▯ milrinone lactate

(mill' ri none)
Primacor
Pregnancy Category C

Drug classes
Cardiotonic drug

Therapeutic actions
Increases force of contraction of ventricles (positive inotropic effect); causes vasodilation by a direct relaxant effect on vascular smooth muscle.

Indications
- CHF: short-term IV management of those patients who are receiving digitalis and diuretics

Contraindications/cautions
- Contraindicated in the presence of allergy to milrinone or bisulfites; severe aortic or pulmonic valvular disease.
- Use caution in the elderly, pregnancy.

Dosage
Adult: Loading dose: 50 µg/kg IV bolus, given over 10 min. Maintenance infusion: 0.375–0.75 µg/kg per minute. Do not exceed a total of 1.13 mg/kg per day.
Pediatric: Not recommended.
Geriatric or renal impairment: Creatinine clearance: 5 (0.2 µg/kg per min IV), 10 (0.23 µg/kg per min IV), 20 (0.28 µg/kg per min IV); 30 (0.3 µg/kg per min IV); 40 (0.38 µg/kg per min IV); 50 (0.43 µg/kg per min IV). Do not exceed 1.13 mg/kg per day.

Pharmacokinetics

Route	Onset	Peak	Duration
IV	Immediate	5–15 min	8 h

Metabolism: Hepatic, $T_{1/2}$: 2.3–2.5 h
Distribution: Crosses placenta; may enter breast milk
Excretion: Urine

IV facts
Preparation: Add diluent of 0.45% or 0.9% Sodium Chloride Injection, USP or 5% Dextrose Injection, USP. Add 180 ml per 20-mg vial to prepare solution of 100 µg/ml²; 113 ml per 20-mg vial to prepare a solution of 150 µg/ml²; add 80 ml diluent to 20-mg vial to prepare solution of 200 µg/ml².
Infusion: Administer while carefully monitoring patient's hemodynamic and clinical response.
Incompatibilities: Do not mix directly with furosemide.

Adverse effects
- **CV:** *Ventricular arrhythmias*, hypotension, supraventricular arrhythmias, chest pain, angina, death

Adverse effects in *Italics* are most common; those in **Bold** are life-threatening.

- Hematologic: Thrombocytopenia, hypokalemia

Clinically important drug-drug interactions
- Precipitate formation in solution if given in the same IV line with furosemide

■ Nursing Considerations
Assessment
- *History:* Allergy to milrinone or bisulfites, severe aortic or pulmonic valvular disease, lactation
- *Physical:* Weight, orientation, P, BP, cardiac auscultation, peripheral pulses and perfusion, R, adventitious sounds, serum electrolyte levels, platelet count, ECG

Implementation
- Monitor cardiac rhythm continually during treatment.
- Monitor BP and P and reduce dose if marked decreases occur.
- Monitor intake and output and electrolyte levels.

Drug-specific teaching points
- Know that, because of the effects of this drug, you will need frequent BP and P and heart activity monitoring during drug therapy.
- Be aware that you may experience increased voiding while on this drug; appropriate bathroom arrangements will be made.
- Report pain at IV injection site, numbness or tingling, shortness of breath, chest pain.

☐ minocycline hydrochloride

(mi noe sye' kleen)
Minocin

Pregnancy Category D

Drug classes
Antibiotic
Tetracycline

Therapeutic actions
Bacteriostatic: inhibits protein synthesis of susceptible bacteria, causing cell death.

Indications
- Infections caused by rickettsiae; *Mycoplasma pneumoniae;* agents of psittacosis, ornithosis, lymphogranuloma venereum and granuloma inguinale; *Borrelia recurrentis; Hemophilus ducreyi; Pasteurella pestis; Pasteurella tularensis; Bartonella bacilliformis; Bacteroides; Vibrio comma; Vibrio fetus; Brucella; E. coli; Enterobacter aerogenes; Shigella; Acinetobacter calcoaceticus; H. influenzae; Klebsiella; Diplococcus pneumoniae; S. aureus*
- When penicillin is contraindicated, infections caused by *N. gonorrhoeae, Treponema pallidum, Treponema pertenue, Listeria monocytogenes, Clostridium, Bacillus anthracis.* As an adjunct to amebicides in acute intestinal amebiasis
- *Oral* tetracyclines are indicated for treatment of acne, uncomplicated urethral, endocervical, or rectal infections in adults caused by *Chlamydia trachomatis*
- *Oral* minocycline is indicated in treatment of asymptomatic carriers of *Neisseria meningitidis* (not useful for treating the infection); infections caused by *Mycobacterium marinum;* uncomplicated urethral, endocervical, or rectal infections caused by *Ureaplasma urealyticum;* uncomplicated gonococcal urethritis in men due to *N. gonorrhoeae*
- Unlabeled use: alternative to sulfonamides in the treatment of nocardiosis

Contraindications/cautions
- Contraindicated in the presence of allergy to tetracylines.
- Use caution in the presence of renal or hepatic dysfunction, pregnancy, lactation.

Dosage
Adult: 200 mg followed by 100 mg q12h IV. Do not exceed 400 mg/d. Or 200 mg initially, followed by 100 mg q12h PO. May be given as 100–200 mg initially and then 50 mg qid PO.
- ***Syphilis:*** Usual PO dose for 10–15 d.
- ***Urethral, endocervical, rectal infections:*** 100 mg bid PO for 7 d.

minocycline hydrochloride ■ 749

- ***Gonococcal urethritis in men:*** 100 mg bid PO for 5 d.
- ***Gonorrhea:*** 200 mg PO followed by 100 mg q12h for 4 d.
- ***Meningococcal carrier state:*** 100 mg q12h PO for 5 d.

Pediatric: Older than 8 y: 4 mg/kg IV followed by 2 mg/kg q12h IV or PO.
Geriatric or renal failure patients: IV doses of minocycline are not as toxic as other tetracyclines in these patients.

Pharmacokinetics

Route	Onset	Peak
Oral	Rapid	2–3 h
IV	Immediate	End of infusion

Metabolism: Hepatic, $T_{1/2}$: 11–26 h
Distribution: Crosses placenta; enters breast milk
Excretion: Urine and feces

IV facts
Preparation: Dissolve powder and then further dilute to 500–1,000 ml with Sodium Chloride Injection, Dextrose Injection, Dextrose and Sodium Chloride Injection, Ringer's Injection, or Lactated Ringer's Injection; administer immediately.
Infusion: Infuse slowly; discard any diluted solution not used within 24 h.
Incompatibilities: Avoid solutions with calcium; a precipitate may form.

Adverse effects
- GI: Fatty liver, **liver failure**, *anorexia, nausea, vomiting, diarrhea, glossitis,* dysphagia, enterocolitis, esophageal ulcer
- Hematologic: Hemolytic anemia, thrombocytopenia, neutropenia, eosinophilia, leukocytosis, leukopenia
- Dermatologic: *Phototoxic reactions, rash,* exfoliative dermatitis (more frequent and more severe with this tetracycline than with any others)
- Dental: *Discoloring and inadequate calcification of primary teeth of fetus if used by pregnant women; discoloring and inadequate calcification of permanent teeth if used during period of dental development*
- Local: Local irritation at injection site
- Other: Superinfections, nephrogenic diabetes insipidus syndrome

Clinically important drug-drug interactions
- Decreased absorption of minocycline if taken with antacids, iron, alkali • Increased digoxin toxicity if taken with minocycline • Increased nephrotoxicity if taken with methoxyflurane • Decreased activity of penicillin if taken with minocycline

Clinically important drug-food interactions
- Decreased absorption of minocycline if taken with food, dairy products

■ Nursing Considerations

Assessment
- *History:* Allergy to tetracylines, renal or hepatic dysfunction, pregnancy, lactation
- *Physical:* Skin—status, orientation and reflexes, R and sounds, GI function and liver evaluation, urinalysis and BUN, liver and renal function tests; culture infected area

Implementation
- Administer oral medication without regard to food or meals; if GI upset occurs, give with meals.

Drug-specific teaching points
- Take this drug throughout the day for best results.
- Take the drug with meals if GI upset occurs.
- Know that the following side effects may occur: sensitivity to sunlight (wear protective clothing, and use a sunscreen if in the sun); diarrhea, nausea (taking the drug with meals, small, frequent meals may help).
- Report rash, itching; difficulty breathing; dark urine or light-colored stools; severe cramps, watery diarrhea.

Adverse effects in *Italics* are most common; those in **Bold** are life-threatening.

minoxidil

*(mi **nox**' i dill)*
Oral: Loniten
Topical: Rogaine
Pregnancy Category C

Drug classes
Antihypertensive drug
Vasodilator

Therapeutic actions
Acts directly on vascular smooth muscle to cause vasodilation, reducing elevated systolic and diastolic blood pressure; does not interfere with cardiovascular reflexes; does not usually cause orthostatic hypotension but does cause reflex tachycardia and renin release, leading to sodium and water retention; mechanism of action in stimulating hair growth is not known, possibly related to arterial dilation.

Indications
- Severe hypertension that is symptomatic or associated with target organ damage and is not manageable with maximum therapeutic doses of a diuretic plus two other antihypertensive drugs; use in milder hypertension not recommended
- Alopecia areata and male pattern alopecia—topical use when compounded as a 1%–5% lotion or 1% ointment

Contraindications/cautions
- Contraindicated in the presence of hypersensitivity to minoxidil or any component of the topical preparation (topical); pheochromocytoma (may stimulate release of catecholamines from tumor); acute MI; dissecting aortic aneurysm; lactation.
- Use caution in the presence of malignant hypertension; CHF (use with diuretic); angina pectoris (use with a beta-blocker); pregnancy.

Dosage
Adult: Initial dosage is 5 mg/d PO as a single dose. Daily dosage can be increased to 10, 20, then 40 mg in single or divided doses if required. Effective range is usally 10–40 mg/d PO. Maximum dosage is 100 mg/d. Magnitude of within-day fluctuation in BP is directly proportional to extent of BP reduction. If supine diastolic BP has been reduced less than 30 mm Hg, administer the drug only once a day. If reduced more than 30 mm Hg, divide the daily dosage into two equal parts. Dosage adjustment should normally be at least 3 d (q6h with careful monitoring).
- ***Concomitant therapy:*** *Diuretics:* Use minoxidil with a diuretic in patients relying on renal function for maintaining salt and water balance; the following diuretic dosages have been used when starting minoxidil therapy: hydrochlorothiazide, 50 mg bid; chlorthalidone, 50–100 mg qd; furosemide, 40 mg bid. If excessive salt and water retention result in weight gain > 5 lb, change diuretic therapy to furosemide; if patient already takes furosemide, increase dosage. *Beta-adrenergic blockers or other sympatholytics:* The following dosages are recommended when starting minoxidil therapy: propranolol, 80–160 mg/d; other beta-blockers, dosage equivalent to the above, methyldopa 250–750 mg bid (start methyldopa at least 24 h before minoxidil); clonidine, 0.1–0.2 mg bid.
- ***Topical:*** Apply 1 ml to the total affected areas of the scalp twice daily. The total daily dosage should not exceed 2 ml. Twice daily appliation for > 4 mo may be required before evidence of hair regrowth is observed. Once hair growth is realized, twice daily application is necessary for continued and additional hair regrowth. Balding process reported to return to untreated state 3–4 mo after cessation of the drug.

Pediatric: Experience is limited, particularly in infants; the following recommendations are only a guide; careful titration is necessary. *12 y or older:* As adult. *Younger than 12 y:* Initial dosage is 0.2 mg/kg per day PO as a single dose. May increase 50%–100% increments until optimum BP control is achieved. Effective range is usually 0.25–1 mg/kg per day; maximum dosage is 50 mg daily. Experience in children is limited; monitor carefully.

Geriatric or impaired renal function: Smaller doses may be required; closely supervise to prevent cardiac failure or exacerbation of renal failure.

Pharmacokinetics

Route	Onset	Peak	Duration
Oral	30 min	2–3 h	75 h
Topical	Not generally absorbed systemically.		

Metabolism: Hepatic, $T_{1/2}$: 4.2 h
Distribution: Crosses placenta; enters breast milk
Excretion: Urine

Adverse effects

- **CNS:** Fatigue, headache
- **GI:** Nausea, vomiting
- **CV:** Tachycardia (unless given with beta-adrenergic blocker or other sympatholytic drug), pericardial effusion and tamponade; *changes in direction and magnitude of T-waves*; cardiac necrotic lesions in preclinical studies, reported in humans who had taken minoxidil only in patients with known ischemic heart disease, but possibility of minoxidil-associated cardiac damage cannot be excluded
- **Respiratory:** *bronchitis, upper respiratory infection, sinusitis* (topical use)
- **Hematologic:** Initial decrease in hematocrit, hemoglobin, RBC count
- **Dermatologic:** *Temporary edema, hypertrichosis* (elongation, thickening, and enhanced pigmentation of fine body hair occurring within 3–6 wk of starting therapy; usually first noticed on temples, between eyebrows and extending to other parts of face, back, arms, legs, scalp); rashes including bullous eruptions; Stevens-Johnson syndrome; darkening of the skin
- **Local:** *Irritant dermatitis, allergic contact dermatitis, eczema, pruritus, dry skin/scalp, flaking, alopecia* (topical use)

■ Nursing Considerations
Assessment

- *History:* Hypersensitivity to minoxidil or any component of the topical preparation; pheochromocytoma; acute MI, dissecting aortic aneurysm; malignant hypertension; CHF; angina pectoris; lactation
- *Physical:* Skin—color, lesions, hair, scalp; P, BP, orthostatic BP, supine BP, perfusion, edema, auscultation; bowel sounds, normal output; CBC with differential, kidney function tests, urinalysis, ECG

Implementation

- Apply topical preparation to total affected area; if fingertips are used to facilitate drug application, wash hands thoroughly afterward.
- Do not apply other topical agents, including topical corticosteroids, retinoids, and petrolatum or agents known to enhance cutaneous drug absorption.
- Do not apply topical preparation to open lesions or breaks in the skin, which could increase risk of systemic absorption.
- Arrange to withdraw drug gradually, especially from children; rapid withdrawal may cause a possible sudden increase in BP (rebound hypertension has been reported in children, even with gradual withdrawal of minoxidil; use caution and monitor BP closely when withdrawing drug from children).
- Arrange for echocardiographic evaluation of possible pericardial effusion; more vigorous diuretic therapy, dialysis, other treatment (including withdrawal of minoxidil) may be required.

Drug-specific teaching points

- Take this drug exactly as prescribed. Take all other medications that have been prescribed for you. Do not discontinue any drug prescribed for you or reduce the dosage without consulting your nurse or physician.
- Know that the following side effects may occur: enhanced growth and darkening of fine body and face hair (this may be bothersome, but do not discontinue the medication without consulting your nurse or physician); GI upset (frequent small meals may help).

Adverse effects in *Italics* are most common; those in **Bold** are life-threatening.

- Report increased heart rate of ≥ 20 beats per minute over normal (your normal heart rate is ___ beats per minute); rapid weight gain of greater than 5 lb; unusual swelling of the extremities, face, or abdomen; difficulty breathing, especially when lying down; new or aggravated symptoms of angina (chest, arm, or shoulder pain); severe indigestion; dizziness, lightheadedness, or fainting.

Topical
- Apply the prescribed amount to the total affected area twice a day. If using the fingers to facilitate application, wash hands thoroughly after application. It may take 4 mo or longer for any noticeable hair regrowth to appear. Response to this drug is very individual. If no response is seen within 4 mo, consult with your nurse or physician about the efficacy of continued use.
- Do not apply more frequent or larger applications. This will not speed up or increase hair growth but may increase side effects.
- Be aware that if one or two daily applications are missed, restart twice-daily applications, and return to usual schedule. Do not attempt to make up missed applications.
- Do not apply any other topical medication to the area while you are using this drug.
- Do not apply to any sunburned, broken skin or open lesions; this increases the risk of systemic effects. Do not apply to any part of the body other than the scalp.
- Be aware that continued use of the drug twice a day will be necessary to retain or continue the hair regrowth.

☐ misoprostol

*(mye soe **prost'** ole)*
Cytotec
Pregnancy Category X

Drug classes
Prostaglandin

Therapeutic actions
A synthetic prostaglandin E_1 analog; inhibits gastric acid secretion and increases bicarbonate and mucus production, protecting the lining of the stomach.

Indications
- Prevention of NSAID (including aspirin)-induced gastric ulcers in patients at high risk of complications from a gastric ulcer (elderly, patients with concomitant debilitating disease, patients with a history of ulcers)
- Unlabeled use: appears effective in treating duodenal ulcers in those patients unresponsive to H_2 antagonists

Contraindications/cautions
- History of allergy to prostaglandins; pregnancy (abortifacient property; women of childbearing age need to receive written and oral warnings of such drug use, have a negative serum pregnancy test within 2 wk prior to the beginning of therapy, have contraceptive measures available for use, and begin therapy on the second or third day of the next normal menstrual period); lactation.

Dosage
Adult: 200 μg four times daily PO with food. If this dose cannot be tolerated, 100 μg can be used. Take misoprostol for the duration of the NSAID therapy. Take the last dose of the day at bedtime.
Pediatric: Safety and efficacy in children younger than 18 y not established.
Geriatric or renal impaired: Adjustment in dosage is usually not necessary, but dosage can be reduced if 200-μg PO dose cannot be tolerated.

Pharmacokinetics

Route	Onset	Peak
Oral	Rapid	12–15 min

Metabolism: Hepatic, $T_{1/2}$: 20–40 min
Distribution: Crosses placenta; enters breast milk
Excretion: Urine

Adverse effects
- GI: *Nausea, diarrhea, abdominal pain, flatulence,* vomiting, dyspepsia, constipation

- GU: *Miscarriage,* excessive bleeding, death; *spotting, cramping,* hypermenorrhea, menstrual disorders, dysmenorrhea
- Other: Headache

■ Nursing Considerations
Assessment
- *History:* Allergy to prostaglandins, pregnancy, lactation
- *Physical:* Abdominal exam, normal output; urinary output

Implementation
- Administer only to patients at high risk for developing NSAID-induced gastric ulcers; administer for the full term of the NSAID use.
- Arrange for serum pregnancy test for any woman of childbearing age who is to receive this drug; must have a negative test within 2 wk of beginning therapy.
- Arrange for oral and written explanation of the risks to pregnancy; appropriate contraceptive measures must be taken; begin therapy on the second or third day of a normal menstrual period.

Drug-specific teaching points
- Take this drug four times a day, with meals and at bedtime. Continue to take your NSAID while on this drug. Take the drug exactly as prescribed. Do not give this drug to anyone else to take.
- Know that the following side effects may occur: abdominal pain, nausea, diarrhea, flatulence (take drug with meals); menstrual cramping, abnormal menstrual periods, spotting, even in postmenopausal women (this is a direct effect of the drug; consult with your nurse or physician for appropriate analgesics); headache.
- Be aware that this drug can cause miscarriage, often associated with dangerous bleeding. Do not take misoprostol if pregnant; do not become pregnant while taking this medication. If pregnancy occurs, discontinue drug, and consult physician immediately.
- Report severe diarrhea, spotting or menstrual pain, severe menstrual bleeding, pregnancy.

mitomycin ■ 753

☐ mitomycin

*(mye toe **mye'** sin)*

mitomycin-C, MTC
Mutamycin

Pregnancy Category D

Drug classes
Antibiotic
Antineoplastic agent

Therapeutic actions
Cytotoxic: inhibits DNA synthesis and cellular RNA and protein synthesis in susceptible cells, causing cell death.

Indications
- Disseminated adenocarcinoma of the stomach or pancreas; part of combination therapy or as palliative measure when other modalities fail
- Unlabeled use: superficial bladder cancer (intravesical route)

Contraindications/cautions
- Allergy to mitomycin; thrombocytopenia, coagulation disorders, or increase in bleeding tendencies, impaired renal function (creatinine > 17 mg%); myelosuppression; pregnancy; lactation.

Dosage
Adult: After hematologic recovery from previous chemotherapy, use either of the following schedules at 6- to 8-wk intervals: 20 mg/m^2 IV as a single dose or 2 mg/m^2 per day IV for 5 d followed by a drug-free interval of 2 d, and then by 2 mg/m^2 per day for 5 d (total of 20 mg/m^2 for 10 d). Reevaluate patient for hematologic response between courses of therapy; adjust dose accordingly:

Nadir After Prior Dose (count/mm^3)		% of Prior Dose to Be Given
Leukocytes	Platelets	
>4,000	>100,000	100
3,000–3,999	75,000–99,999	100
2,000–2,999	25,000–74,999	70
<2,000	<25,000	50

Adverse effects in *Italics* are most common; those in **Bold** are life-threatening.

754 ■ mitotane

- Do not repeat dosage until leukocyte count has returned to 3,000/mm³ and platelet count to 75,000/mm³.

Pharmacokinetics

Route	Onset	Peak
IV	Slow	Unknown

Metabolism: Hepatic, T_{1/2}: 17 min
Distribution: Crosses placenta; enters breast milk
Excretion: Urine

IV facts

Preparation: Reconstitute 5- to 20-mg vial with 10 or 40 ml of Sterile Water for Injection, respectively; if product does not dissolve immediately, allow to stand at room temperature until solution is obtained. This solution is stable for 14 d if refrigerated, 7 d at room temperature; further dilution in various IV fluids reduces stability—check manufacturer's insert.
Infusion: Infuse slowly; monitor injection site to avoid local reaction.

Adverse effects

- CNS: Headache, blurred vision, confusion, drowsiness, syncope, fatigue
- GI: *Anorexia, nausea, vomiting,* diarrhea, hematemesis, stomatitis
- Respiratory: **Pulmonary toxicity**
- Hematologic: *Bone marrow toxicity,* microangiopathic hemolytic anemia (a syndrome of anemia, thrombocytopenia, renal failure, hypertension)
- GU: Renal toxicity
- Other: *Fever,* cancer in preclinical studies, *cellulitis at injection site, alopecia*

■ Nursing Considerations

Assessment

- *History:* Allergy to mitomycin; thrombocytopenia, coagulation disorders or increase in bleeding tendencies, impaired renal function; myelosuppression; pregnancy; lactation
- *Physical:* Temperature; skin—color, lesions; weight; hair; local injection site; orientation, reflexes; R, adventitious sounds; mucus membranes; CBC, clotting tests, renal function tests

Implementation

- Do not administer IM or SC because severe local reaction and tissue necrosis occur.
- Monitor injection site for extravasation: reports of burning or stinging; discontinue infusion immediately and restart in another vein.
- Monitor patient's response to therapy frequently at beginning of therapy (CBC, renal function tests, pulmonary exam); adverse effects may require a decrease in drug dose or discontinuing of the drug; consult with physician.

Drug-specific teaching points

- Prepare a calendar of dates you will need to return for drug therapy; this drug can only be given IV.
- Know that the following side effects may occur: rash, skin lesions, loss of hair (you may want to invest in a wig before hair loss occurs; skin care may help somewhat); loss of appetite, nausea, mouth sores (frequent mouth care, small frequent meals may help; you will need to try to maintain good nutrition if at all possible; a dietician may be able to help; an antiemetic also may be ordered); drowsiness, dizziness, syncope, headache (use caution if driving or operating dangerous machinery; take special precautions to prevent injuries).
- Arrange for regular medical follow-up, which will include blood tests to monitor the drug's effects.
- Report difficulty breathing, sudden weight gain, swelling, burning or pain at injection site, unusual bleeding or bruising.

❒ mitotane

(mye' toe tane)
o, p' - DDD
Lysodren

Pregnancy Category C

Adverse effects in *Italics* are most common; those in **Bold** are life-threatening.

Drug classes
Antineoplastic drug
Adrenal cytotoxic drug

Therapeutic actions
Acts by unknown mechanism to reduce plasma and urinary levels of adrenocorticosteroids; selectively cytotoxic to normal and neoplastic adrenal cortical cells.

Indications
- Treatment of inoperable adrenal cortical carcinoma, functional (hormone-secreting) and nonfunctional

Contraindications/cautions
- Contraindicated in the presence of allergy to mitotane, lactation.
- Use caution in the presence of impaired liver function, pregnancy.

Dosage
Adult: Institute therapy in a hospital. Start at 2–6 g/d PO in divided doses tid or qid. Increase dose incrementally to 9–10 g/d. If severe side effects occur, reduce to maximum tolerated dose (2–16 g/d), usually 9–10 g/d. Continue therapy as long as benefits are observed. If no clinical benefits are seen after 3 mo, consider the case a clinical failure.

Pharmacokinetics

Route	Onset	Peak	Duration
Oral	Slow	Varies	10 wk

Metabolism: Hepatic, $T_{1/2}$: 18–159 d
Distribution: Crosses placenta; may enter breast milk
Excretion: Urine and bile

Adverse effects
- CNS: *Depression, sedation, lethargy, vertigo, dizziness,* visual blurring, diplopia, lens opacity, toxic retinopathy, brain damage and possible behavioral and neurologic changes (therapy longer than 2 y)
- GI: *Nausea, vomiting, diarrhea, anorexia*
- CV: Hypertension, orthostatic hypotension, flushing
- GU: Hematuria, hemorrhagic cystitis, proteinuria
- **Endocrine:** *Adrenal insufficiency*
- Other: *Rash*, fever, generalized aching

Drug-lab test interferences
- Decreased levels of protein-bound iodine, urinary 17-hydroxycorticsteroids

■ Nursing Considerations

Assessment
- *History:* Allergy to mitotane; impaired liver function; lactation
- *Physical:* Body weight, skin integrity; orientation, affect, vestibular nerve function, ophthalmologic exam; BP, P, orthostatic BP; bowel sounds, output; liver and renal function tests, urinalysis, plasma cortisol, serum electrolytes

Implementation
- Be aware that large metastatic tumor masses are usually removed surgically before therapy to minimize risk of tumor infarction and hemorrhage due to rapid therapeutic effect.
- Administer cautiously to patients with impaired liver function; drug metabolism may be impaired, and drug may accumulate to toxic levels if usual dosage is continued.
- Monitor for adrenal insufficiency; adrenal steroid replacement therapy may be necessary.

Drug-specific teaching points
- Arrange for frequent follow-up visits and monitoring.
- Be aware that you should use contraceptive measures during therapy; this drug can cause birth defects or fetal death.
- Know that the following side effects may occur: dizziness, drowsiness, tiredness (avoid driving a car or performing hazardous tasks); nausea, vomiting, diarrhea (small, frequent meals may help, proper nutrition is important); aching muscles, fever (medication may be available to help).
- Report severe nausea, vomiting, loss of appetite, diarrhea, aching muscles, mus-

Adverse effects in *Italics* are most common; those in **Bold** are life-threatening.

cle twitching, fever, flushing, emotional depression, rash or darkening of skin.

☐ mitoxantrone hydrochloride

*(mye toe **zan'** trone)*
Novantrone

Pregnancy Category D

Drug classes
Antibiotic
Antineoplastic

Therapeutic actions
Mechanism of action is not fully understood; a DNA-reactive agent causes cell death in proliferating and nonproliferating cells; cell cycle nonspecific.

Indications
- In combination with other drugs in the initial therapy of acute nonlymphocytic leukemia in adults (includes myelogenous, promyelocytic, monocytic, and erythroid acute leukemias)
- Unlabeled uses: alone or in combination with other agents in the treatment of breast cancer, refractory lymphomas
- Orphan drug use: treatment of acute myelogenous leukemia

Contraindications/cautions
- Contraindicated in the presence of hypersensitivity to mitoxantrone; pregnancy; lactation.
- Use caution in the presence of preexisting cardiac disease; prior mediastinal radiotherapy; prior treatment with anthracycline.

Dosage
Adult
- ***Combination therapy:*** For induction, 12 mg/m^2 per day on days 1–3 given as an IV infusion, and 100 mg/m^2 of cytosine arabinoside for 7 d given as a continuous 24-h infusion on days 1–7. In the event of an incomplete remission, a second induction course may be given: mitoxantrone for 2 d and cytosine arabinoside for 5 d.
- ***Consolidation therapy:*** Mitoxantrone 12 mg/m^2 given by IV infusion daily for days 1 and 2, and cytosine arabinoside 100 mg/m^2 for 5 d given as a continuous 24-h infusion on days 1–5. The first course generally given about 6 wk after the final induction course; the second was generally administered 4 wk after the first.

Pediatric: Safety and efficacy not established.

Pharmacokinetics

Route	Onset	Peak	Duration
IV	Varies	10–14 d	28 d

Metabolism: Hepatic, T$_{1/2}$: 5.8 d
Distribution: Crosses placenta; may enter breast milk
Excretion: Feces and urine

IV facts
Preparation: Dilute solution to at least 50 ml with either 0.9% Sodium Chloride Injection or 5% Dextrose Injection. Discard unused infusion solutions in appropriate manner.

Infusion: Introduce solution slowly into tubing of a freely running IV solution of 0.9% Sodium Chloride or 5% Dextrose Injection over no less than 3 min.

Adverse effects
- CNS: *Headache,* seizures, *conjunctivitis*
- GI: *Nausea, vomiting, diarrhea, abdominal pain, stomatitis, GI bleeding*
- CV: *CHF, arrhythmias,* chest pain, tachycardia, ECG changes
- Respiratory: *Dyspnea, cough*
- Dermatologic: *Bluish discoloration of the sclera,* rash
- Other: *Infections, fever, alopecia,* blue-green color to the urine

■ Nursing Considerations
Assessment
- *History:* Hypersensitivity to mitoxantrone, preexisting cardiac disease, prior

mediastinal radiotherapy, prior treatment with anthracycline, pregnancy, lactation
- *Physical:* Temperature, hair, skin—lesions, rashes; reflexes, affect, eye exam; BP, P, ECG, peripheral pulses, auscultation; R, auscultation; abdominal exam, mucous membrane evaluation; CBC, Hct, liver function tests, serum uric acid

Implementation
- Administer by IV route only.
- Arrange for careful monitoring of hematologic and chemical laboratory parameters before beginning therapy and frequently during therapy.
- Monitor injection site for extravastation. If extravasation occurs, stop administration immediately, and restart in another vein.
- Use goggles, gloves, and protective gown when preparing and administering drug. Avoid exposure of the skin and eyes to the mitoxantrone solution. If exposure does occur, rinse copiously with warm water.
- Do not mix in the same infusion with any other drug.
- Monitor patient for infections, which commonly occur during the use of this drug; arrange to treat them concurrently as appropriate.
- Monitor cardiac rhythm, ECG, and cardiac output during course of therapy.
- Monitor serum uric acid levels periodically during therapy. Institute hypouricemic therapy prior to antileukemic therapy as appropriate.

Drug-specific teaching points
- Prepare a calendar of treatment days; this drug can only be given IV.
- Arrange for frequent blood tests to determine the effects of the drug on your blood count and to determine the appropriate dosage needed. It is important that you keep appointments for these tests.
- Be aware that this drug cannot be taken during pregnancy. It is important to use contraceptive measures while you are on this drug. If you become pregnant, notify your physician immediately.
- Know that the following side effects may occur: nausea, vomiting, diarrhea (proper nutrition is important; ensure ready access to bathroom facilities); cough, difficulty breathing (notify your nurse or physician for appropriate treatment if needed); loss of hair (you may want to obtain a wig before hair loss occurs; it is important to keep the head covered in extremes of temperature); blue-green color of the urine (this is a normal effect of the drug and should not cause concern; the whites of the eyes also may be tinted blue-green).
- Report difficulty breathing, chest pain, palpitations, unusual bleeding, fever, sore throat, swollen or tender joints, pain or redness at IV injection site.

molindone hydrochloride

(moe lin' done)
Moban

Pregnancy Cateogry C

Drug classes
Dopaminergic blocking drug
Antispychotic drug

Therapeutic actions
Mechanism of action not fully understood: antipsychotic drugs block postsynaptic dopamine receptors in the brain, but this may not be necessary and sufficient for antipsychotic activity; clinically resembles the piperazine phenothiazines (eg, fluphenazine).

Indications
- Management of manifestations of psychotic disorders

Contraindications/cautions
- Contraindicated in the presence of coma or severe CNS depression, bone marrow depression, blood dyscrasia, circulatory collapse, subcortical brain damage, Parkinson's disease, liver damage, cerebral arteriosclerosis, coronary disease, severe hypotension or hypertension.

molindone hydrochloride

- Use caution in the presence of respiratory disorders ("silent pneumonia" may develop); glaucoma, prostatic hypertrophy; epilepsy or history of epilepsy (drug lowers seizure threshold); breast cancer (elevations in prolactin may stimulatea prolactin-dependent tumor); thyrotoxicosis; peptic ulcer, decreased renal function; exposure to heat or phosphorous insecticides; pregnancy; lactation; children younger than 12 y, especially those with chickenpox, CNS infections (children are especially susceptible to dystonias that may confound the diagnosis of Reye's syndrome).

Dosage
Adult: Initially 50–75 mg/d PO increased to 100 mg/d in 3–4 d. Individualize dosage; patients with severe symptoms may require up to 225 mg/d. *Maintenance therapy:* mild symptoms, 5–15 mg PO tid–qid; moderate symptoms, 10–25 mg PO tid–qid; severe symptoms, 225 mg/d.
Pediatric: Not recommended for children younger than 12 y.
Geriatric: Use lower doses and increase dosage more gradually than in younger patients.

Pharmacokinetics

Route	Onset	Peak	Duration
Oral	Varies	1½ h	24–36 h

Metabolism: Hepatic, $T_{1/2}$: 1.5 h
Distribution: Crosses placenta; enters breast milk
Excretion: Urine and feces

Adverse effects
Antipsychotic Drugs
- CNS: *Drowsiness*, insomnia, vertigo, headache, weakness, tremor, ataxia, slurring, cerebral edema, seizures, exacerbation of psychotic symptoms, extrapyramidal syndromes—*pseudoparkinsonism; dystonias; akathisia*, tardive dyskinesias, potentially irreversible (no known treatment), **NMS**—extrapyramidal symptoms, hyperthermia, autonomic disturbances (rare, but 20% fatal)
- CV: Hypotension, orthostatic hypotension, hypertension, tachycardia, bradycardia, cardiac arrest, CHF, cardiomegaly, **refractory arrhythmias** (some fatal), pulmonary edema
- Respiratory: Bronchospasm, laryngospasm, dyspnea; suppression of cough reflex and potential for aspiration (sudden death related to asphyxia or cardiac arrest has been reported)
- Hematologic: Eosinophilia, leukopenia, leukocytosis, anemia; aplastic anemia; hemolytic anemia; thrombocytopenic or nonthrombocytopenic purpura
- Hypersensitivity: Jaundice, urticaria, angioneurotic edema, laryngeal edema, eczema, asthma, anaphylactoid reactions, exfoliative dermatitis
- Endocrine: Lactation, breast engorgement in females, galactorrhea; SIADH; amenorrhea, menstrual irregularities; gynecomastia in males; changes in libido; hyperglycemia or hypoglycemia; glycosuria; hyponatremia; pituitary tumor with hyperprolactinemia; inhibition of ovulation, infertility, pseudopregnancy; reduced urinary levels of gonadotropins, estrogens, progestins
- Autonomic: Dry mouth, salivation, nasal congestion, nausea, vomiting, anorexia, fever, pallor, flushed facies, sweating, constipation, paralytic ileus, urinary retention, incontinence, polyuria, enuresis, priapism, ejaculation inhibition, male impotence

Clinically important drug-drug interactions
- Decreased absorption of oral phenytoin, tetracycline if given concurrently

Drug-lab test interferences
- False-positive pregnancy tests (less likely if serum test is used) • Increase in protein-bound iodine, not attributable to an increase in thyroxine

■ Nursing Considerations
Assessment
- *History:* Coma or severe CNS depression; bone marrow depression; circulatory collapse; subcortical brain damage; Parkin-

Adverse effects in *Italics* are most common; those in **Bold** are life-threatening.

son's disease; liver damage; cerebral arteriosclerosis; coronary disease; severe hypotension or hypertension; respiratory disorders; glaucoma, prostatic hypertrophy; epilepsy; breast cancer; thyrotoxicosis; peptic ulcer, decreased renal function; exposure to heat or phosphorous insecticides; pregnancy; lactation; children younger than 12 y
- *Physical:* Body weight, temperature; reflexes, orientation, intraocular pressure; P, BP, orthostatic BP; R, adventitious sounds; bowel sounds and normal output, liver evaluation; urinary output, prostate size; CBC, urinalysis, thyroid, liver and kidney function tests

Implementation
- Arrange for discontinuation of drug is serum creatinine, BUN become abnormal or if WBC count is depressed.
- Monitor elderly patients for dehydration, and institute remedial measures promptly; sedation and decreased sensation of thirst related to CNS effects of drug can lead to severe dehydration.
- Consult physician regarding appropriate warning of patient or patient's guardian about tardive dyskinesias.
- Consult physician about dosage reduction, use of anticholinergic antiparkinsonian drugs (controversial) if extrapyramidal effects occur.

Drug-specific teaching points
- Take drug exactly as prescribed.
- Avoid driving a car or engaging in other dangerous activities if CNS, vision changes occur.
- Maintain fluid intake, and use precautions against heatstroke in hot weather.
- Report sore throat, fever, unusual bleeding or bruising, rash, weakness, tremors, impaired vision, dark urine (pink or reddish brown urine is to be expected), pale stools, yellowing of the skin or eyes.

❑ monoctanoin

*(mon ok ta **no'** in)*
Moctanin
Pregnancy Category C

Drug classes
Gallstone-solubilizing agent

Therapeutic actions
An esterified glycerol that solubilizes cholesterol gallstones in the biliary tract.

Indications
- Dissolution of cholesterol gallstones retained in the biliary tract following cholecystectomy when other means of stone removal have failed or are contraindicated

Contraindications/cautions
- Allergy to monoctanoin; hepatic dysfunction, clinical jaundice, biliary tract infection; recent duodenal ulcer; recent jejunitis; pregnancy; lactation.

Dosage
Adult: 3–5 ml/h on a 24-h basis at a pressure of 10 cm H_2O as a continuous perfusion through a catheter inserted directly into the common bile duct. Therapy is continued for 7–21 d.
Pediatric: Safety and efficacy not established.

Pharmacokinetics
Metabolized to fatty acids and glycerol, which are absorbed into the portal vein. Not absorbed systemically.

Adverse effects
- **GI:** *GI pain/discomfort, nausea, vomiting, diarrhea,* anorexia, indigestion, burning, gastric, duodenal and bile duct irritation
- **Hematologic:** Leukopenia, metabolic acidosis
- **Other:** *Fever,* pruritus, fatigue/lethargy

■ Nursing Considerations

Assessment
- *History:* Allergy to monoctanoin; hepatic dysfunction, clinical jaundice, biliary tract infection; recent duodenal ulcer; recent jejunitis; pregnancy; lactation
- *Physical:* Body temperature; liver evaluation, abdominal exam; liver function tests, CBC

Adverse effects in *Italics* are most common; those in **Bold** are life-threatening.

Implementation
- Do not administer IV or IM.
- Administer drug as a continuous perfusion through a catheter inserted directly into the common bile duct using a perfusion pump that does not exceed perfusion pressure of 15 cm H_2O. Administration may be interrupted during meals.
- Warm monoctanoin to 60–80°F before perfusion.
- Continue administration for 7–21 d if periodic x-rays show response to therapy.
- Discontinue drug and consult with physician if fever, chills, leukocytosis, upper right quadrant pain, or jaundice occurs.
- Arrange for periodic, regular monitoring of liver function tests.
- Arrange for patient to be scheduled for periodic oral cholecystograms or ultrasonograms to evaluate drug effectiveness.
- Arrange for outpatients to have the use of battery-operated infusion pumps and home follow-up.

Drug-specific teaching points
- Be aware that this drug should be continually perfused through the infusion pump as ordered. Infusion can be interrupted during meals.
- Be aware that this drug may dissolve the gallstones that you have now. It does not "cure" the problem that caused the stones in the first place, and in many cases the stones can recur; medical follow-up is important.
- Arrange for periodic x-rays or ultrasound tests of your gallbladder. You also will need periodic blood tests to evaluate your response to this drug.
- Know that abdominal pain/discomfort and GI upset may occur; small, frequent meals may help a little.
- Report fever, chills, upper right quadrant pain, yellowing of skin or eyes, rapid, difficult breathing.

☐ moricizine hydrochloride

(mor i' siz een)
Ethmozine

Pregnancy Category B

Drug classes
Antiarrhythmic

Therapeutic actions
Type I antiarrhythmic with potent local anesthetic acitivity; decreases diastolic depolarization, decreasing automaticity of ventricular cells; increases ventricular fibrillation threshold.

Indications
- Treatment of documented ventricular arrhythmias, such as sustained ventricular tachycardias, that are deemed to be life threatening; because of proarrhythmic effects, reserve use for patients in whom the benefit outweighs the risk

Contraindications/cautions
- Contraindicated in the presence of hypersensitivity to moricizine; preexisiting second- or third-degree AV block; right bundle branch block when associated with left hemiblock (unless a pacemaker is present), cardiogenic shock, CHF; pregnancy; lactation.
- Use caution in the presence of sick sinus syndrome, hepatic or renal impairment.

Dosage
Adult: 600–900 mg/d PO, given q8h in three equally divided doses. Adjust dosage within this range in increments of 150 mg/d at 3-d intervals until the desired effect is seen. Patients with good response may be retained on the same dosage at q12h intervals instead of q8h if this is more convenient. Patients with malignant arrhythmias who respond well may be maintained on long-term therapy.
- ***Transfer from another antiarrhythmic:*** Withdraw previous antiarrhythmic for 1–2 half-lives before starting moricizine therapy. Hospitalize patients in whom withdrawal may precipitate serious arrhythmias. Transferring from quinidine, disopyramide, start moricizine 6–12 h after last dose; procainamide, start moricizine 3–6 h after last dose; encainide, propafenone, tocainide, mexiletine, start moricizine 8–12 h after last dose.

moricizine hydrochloride ■ 761

Pediatric: Safety and efficacy not established for children younger than 18 y.
Geriatric or hepatic impaired: Start < 600 mg/d, and monitor closely, including measurement of ECG intervals, before adjusting dosage.

Pharmacokinetics

Route	Onset	Peak	Duration
Oral	2 h	½–2 h	10–24 h

Metabolism: Hepatic, $T_{1/2}$: 1.5–3.5 h
Distribution: Crosses placenta; enters breast milk
Excretion: Urine

Adverse effects

- CNS: *Headache, dizziness, fatigue, hypoesthesias, asthenia, nervousness, sleep disorders,* tremor, anxiety, depression, euphoria, confusion, seizure, nystagmus, ataxia, loss of memory
- GI: *Nausea, vomiting, diarrhea, abdominal pain, dyspepsia,* flatulence, anorexia, bitter taste, ileus
- CV: *Arrhythmias, palpitations, ventricular tachycardia, CHF,* **death** (up to 5% occurence), conduction defects, heart block, hypotension, **cardiac arrest**, MI
- GU: Urinary retention, dysuria, urinary incontinence, kidney pain, impotence
- Respiratory: *Dyspnea,* hyperventilation, apnea, asthma, pharyngitis, cough, sinusitis
- Other: Sweating, muscle pain, dry mouth, blurred vision, fever

Clinically important drug-drug interactions

• Increased serum levels of moricizine if taken concurrently with cimetidine • Increased risk of heart block if taken concurrently with digoxin, propranolol • Decreased serum levels and therapeutic effects of theophylline if taken concurrently

■ Nursing Considerations

Assessment

- *History:* Hypersensitivity to moricizine; preexisiting second- or third-degree AV block; right bundle branch block associated with left hemiblock; cardiogenic shock, CHF; sick sinus syndrome; hepatic or renal impairment; lactation
- *Physical:* Temperature; reflexes, affect; BP, P, ECG including interval monitoring, exercise testing; R, auscultation; abdominal exam, normal output; urinary output; liver and renal function tests, serum electrolytes

Implementation

- Administer only to patients with life threatening arrhythmias who do not respond to conventional therapy and in whom the benefits outweigh the risks of therapy.
- Correct electrolyte disturbances (hypokalemia, hyperkalemia, hypomagnesemia), which may alter the effects of class I antiarrhythmics, before beginning therapy.
- Know that patient should be hospitalized and monitored continually during initiation of therapy.
- Arrange for reduced dosage for patients with hepatic failure.
- Maintain life support equipment and vasopressor agents on standby in case of severe reactions or generation of arrhythmias.
- Administer with food if severe GI upset occurs; food delays but does not change peak serum levels.
- Arrange for frequent monitoring of heart rhythm, including ECG intervals during long-term therapy.

Drug-specific teaching points

- Take drug exactly as prescribed. Arrange most convenient schedule to decrease interruptions in your day.
- Know that frequent monitoring will be necessary to determine the effects of the drug on your heart and to determine the appropriate dosage needed. It is important that you keep appointments for these tests, which may include Holter monitoring, stress tests.
- Know that the following side effects may occur: arrhythmias or abnormal heart rhythm (because of this, hospitalization

Adverse effects in *Italics* are most common; those in **Bold** are life-threatening.

is required to start drug therapy and to monitor your response to the drug until your dosage is determined and stabilized); dizziness, headache, fatigue, nervousness (avoid driving a car or performing hazardous tasks if these occur); nausea, vomiting, diarrhea (small, frequent meals may help; proper nutrition is important; cough, difficulty breathing, sweating.
- Report palpitations, lethargy, vomiting, difficulty breathing, edema of the extremities, chest pain.

☐ morphine sulfate

(mor' feen)

Immediate-release tablets: MSIR

Timed-release tablets: MS Contin, Roxanol SR

Oral solution: Roxanol

Rectal suppositories: RMS

Injection: Astramorph PF, Duramorph, Epimorph (CAN)

Concentrate for microifusion devices for intraspinal use: Infumorph

Pregnancy Category C
C-II controlled substance

Drug classes
Narcotic agonist analgesic

Therapeutic actions
Principal opium alkaloid; acts as agonist at specific opioid receptors in the CNS to produce analgesia, euphoria, sedation; the receptors mediating these effects are thought to be the same as those mediating the effects of endogenous opioids (enkephalins, endorphins).

Indications
- Relief of moderate to severe acute and chronic pain
- Preoperative medication to sedate and allay apprehension, facilitate induction of anesthesia, and reduce anesthetic dosage
- Analgesic adjunct during anesthesia
- Component of most preparations that are referred to as Brompton's Cocktail or Mixture, an oral alcoholic solution that is used for chronic severe pain, especially in terminal cancer patients
- Intraspinal use with microinfusion devices for the relief of intractable pain
- Unlabeled use: dyspnea associated with acute left ventricular failure and pulmonary edema

Contraindications/cautions
- Contraindicated in the presence of hypersensitivity to narcotics; diarrhea caused by poisoning until toxins are eliminated; during labor or delivery of a premature infant (may cross immature blood–brain barrier more readily); after biliary tract surgery or following surgical anastomosis; pregnancy; labor (can cause respiratory depression of neonate, may prolong labor).
- Use caution in the presence of head injury and increased intracranial pressure; acute asthma, COPD, cor pulmonale, preexisting respiratory depression, hypoxia, hypercapnia (may decrease respiratory drive and increase airway resistance); lactation (may be safer to wait 4–6 h after administration to nurse the baby); acute abdominal conditions, cardiovascular disease, supraventricular tachycardias, myxedema, convulsive disorders, acute alcoholism, delirium tremens, cerebral arteriosclerosis, ulcerative colitis, fever, kyphoscoliosis, Addison's disease, prostatic hypertrophy, urethral stricture, recent GI or GU surgery, toxic psychosis, renal or hepatic dysfunction.

Dosage
Adult
- ***Oral:*** $1/3$ to $1/6$ as effective as parenteral administration because of first-pass metabolism; 10–30 mg q4h PO. *Controlled-release:* 30 mg q8–12h PO or as directed by physician.
- ***SC/IM:*** 10 mg (5–20 mg)/70 kg q4h or as directed by physician.
- ***IV:*** 2.5–15 mg/70 kg in 4–5 ml Water for Injection administered over 4–5 min, or as directed by physician. *Continuous*

morphine sulfate ■ 763

IV infusion: 0.1–1 mg/ml in 5% Dextrose in Water by controlled infusion device.
- ***Rectal:*** 10–20 mg q4h or as directed by physician.
- ***Epidural:*** Initial injection of 5 mg in the lumbar region may provide pain relief for up to 24 h. If adequate pain relief is not achieved within 1 h, incremental doses of 1–2 mg may be given at intervals sufficient to assess effectiveness, up to 10 mg/24 h. For continuous infusion, initial dose of 2–4 mg/24 h is recommended. Further doses of 1–2 mg may be given if pain relief is not achieved intitially.
- ***Intrathecal:*** Dosage is usually $\frac{1}{10}$ that of epidural dosage; a single injection of 0.2–1 mg may provide satisfactory pain relief for up to 24 h. Do not inject more than 2 ml of the 5 mg/10 ml ampule or more than 1 ml of the 10 mg/10 ml ampule. Use only in the lumbar area. Repeated intrathecal injections are not recommended; use other routes if pain recurs.

Pediatric: Do not use in premature infants.
- ***SC/IM:*** 0.1–0.2 mg/kg (up to 15 mg) q4h or as directed by physician.

Geriatric or impaired adult: Use caution. Respiratory depression may occur in elderly, the very ill, those with respiratory problems. Reduced dosage may be necessary.
- ***Epidural:*** Use extreme caution; injection of < 5 mg in the lumbar region may provide adequate pain relief for up to 24 h.
- ***Intrathecal:*** Use lower dosages than recommended for adults above.

Pharmacokinetics

Route	Onset	Peak	Duration
Oral	Varies	60 min	5–7 h
PR	Rapid	20–60 min	5–7 h
SC	Rapid	50–90 min	5–7 h
IM	Rapid	30–60 min	5–6 h
IV	Immediate	20 min	5–6 h

Metabolism: Hepatic, $T_{1/2}$: 1.5–2 h

Distribution: Crosses placenta; enters breast milk
Excretion: Urine and bile

IV facts
Preparation: No further preparation needed for direct injection; prepare infusion by adding 0.1–1 mg/ml to 5% Dextrose in Water.
Infusion: Inject slowly directly IV or into tubing of running IV; monitor by controlled infusion device to maintain pain control.

Adverse effects
- CNS: *Lightheadedness, dizziness, sedation,* euphoria, dysphoria, delirium, insomnia, agitation, anxiety, fear, hallucinations, disorientation, drowsiness, lethargy, impaired mental and physical performance, coma, mood changes, weakness, headache, tremor, convulsions, miosis, visual disturbances, suppression of cough reflex
- GI: *Nausea, vomiting,* dry mouth, anorexia, constipation, biliary tract spasm; increased colonic motility in patients with chronic ulcerative colitis
- CV: Facial flushing, peripheral circulatory collapse, tachycardia, bradycardia, arrhythmia, palpitations, chest wall rigidity, hypertension, hypotension, orthostatic hypotension, syncope
- GU: Ureteral spasm, spasm of vesical sphincters, urinary retention or hesitancy, oliguria, antidiuretic effect, reduced libido or potency
- Dermatologic: Pruritus, urticaria, laryngospasm, bronchospasm, edema
- Local: Tissue irritation and induration (SC injection)
- Major hazards: **Respiratory depression, apnea, circulatory depression, respiratory arrest, shock, cardiac arrest**
- Other: *Sweating,* physical tolerance and dependence, psychological dependence

Clinically important drug-drug interactions
- Increased likelihood of respiratory depression, hypotension, profound sedation or

Adverse effects in *Italics* are most common; those in **Bold** are life-threatening.

coma in patients receiving barbiturate general anesthetics

Drug-lab test interferences
- Elevated biliary tract pressure (an effect of narcotics) may cause increases in plasma amylase, lipase; determinations of these levels may be unreliable for 24 h

■ Nursing Considerations

Assessment
- *History:* Hypersensitivity to narcotics; diarrhea caused by poisoning; labor or delivery of a premature infant; biliary tract surgery or surgical anastomosis; head injury and increased intracranial pressure; acute asthma, COPD, cor pulmonale, preexisting respiratory depression; acute abdominal conditions, cardiovascular disease, supraventricular tachycardias, myxedema, convulsive disorders, acute alcoholism, delirium tremens, cerebral arteriosclerosis, ulcerative colitis, fever, kyphoscoliosis, Addison's disease, prostatic hypertrophy, urethral stricture, recent GI or GU surgery, toxic psychosis, renal or hepatic dysfunction; pregnancy; lactation
- *Physical:* Body temperature; skin—color, texture, lesions; orientation, reflexes, bilateral grip strength, affect; P, auscultation, BP, orthostatic BP, perfusion; R, adventious sounds; bowel sounds, normal output; urinary frequency, voiding pattern, normal output; ECG; EEG; thyroid, liver, kidney function tests

Implementation
- Caution patient not to chew or crush controlled-release preparations.
- Dilute and administer slowly IV to minimize likelihood of adverse effects.
- Direct patient to lie down during IV administration.
- Provide narcotic antagonist, facilities for assisted or controlled respiration on standby during IV administration.
- Use caution when injecting SC or IM into chilled areas or in patients with hypotension or in shock; impaired perfusion may delay absorption; with repeated doses, an excessive amount may be absorbed when circulation is restored.
- Reassure patient about addiction liability; most patients who receive opiates for medical reasons do not develop dependence syndromes.

Drug-specific teaching points
- Take this drug exactly as prescribed. Avoid alcohol, antihistamines, sedatives, tranquilizers, OTC drugs while you are taking this drug.
- Know that the following side effects may occur: nausea, loss of appetite (taking the drug with food and lying quietly should minimize these effects); constipation (a laxative may help); dizziness, sedation, drowsiness, impaired visual acuity (avoid driving a car or performing other tasks that require alertness, visual acuity).
- Do not take any leftover medication for other disorders, and do not let anyone else take your prescription.
- Report severe nausea, vomiting, constipation, shortness of breath or difficulty breathing, skin rash.

▢ muromonab-CD3

(mew ro' mon ab)
Orthoclone OKT3

Pregnancy Category C

Drug classes
Immunosuppressive

Therapeutic actions
A murine monoclonal antibody to the antigen of human T cells; functions as an immunosuppressant by enabling T cells.

Indications
- Acute allograft rejection in renal transplant patients

Contraindications/cautions
- Contraindicated in the presence of allergy to muromonab or any murine product, fluid overload as evidenced by chest x-ray, or > 3% weight gain in 1 wk.

- Use caution in the presence of fever (antipyretics should be used to decrease fever before beginning therapy); previous administration of muromonab-CD3 (antibodies frequently develop, causing a risk of serious reactions on repeat administration); pregnancy.

Dosage
Administer only as an IV bolus in < 1 min. Do not infuse or give by any other route.
Adult: 5 mg/d for 10–14 d. Begin treatment once acute renal rejection is diagnosed. It is strongly recommended that methylprednisolone sodium succinate 1 mg/kg IV be given prior to muromonab-CD3 and IV hydrocortisone sodium succinate 100 mg be given 30 min after muromonab-CD3 administration.
Pediatric: Safety and efficacy not established.

Pharmacokinetics

Route	Onset	Peak	Duration
IV	Minutes	2–7 d	7 d

Metabolism: Tissue, $T_{1/2}$: 47–100 h
Distribution: Crosses placenta

IV facts
Preparation: Draw solution into a syringe through a low protein-binding 0.2- or 0.22-μm filter. Discard filter and attach needle for IV bolus injection. Solution may develop fine translucent particles that do not affect its potency. Refrigerate solution; do not freeze or shake.
Infusion: Administer as an IV bolus over < 1 min. Do not give as an IV infusion or with other drug solutions.
Incompatabilities: Do not mix with any other drug solution.

Adverse effects
- CNS: Malaise, *tremors*
- GI: *Vomiting, nausea, diarrhea*
- General: *Fever, chills*
- Respiratory: Acute pulmonary edema, *dyspnea, chest pain*, wheezing
- Other: Lymphomas, *increased susceptibility to infection*

Clinically important drug-drug interactions
- Reduce dosage of other immunosuppressive agents; severe immunosuppression can lead to increased susceptibility to infection and increased risk of lymphomas; other immunosuppressives can be restarted about 3 d prior to cessation of muromonab

■ Nursing Considerations
Assessment
- *History:* Allergy to muromonab or any murine product; fluid overload; fever; previous administration of muromonab-CD3; pregnancy; lactation
- *Physical:* Body temperature, body weight; P, BP; R, adventitious sounds; chest x-ray, CBC

Implementation
- Arrange for chest x-ray within 24 h of beginning therapy to ensure that chest is clear.
- Arrange for the use of antipyretics (acetaminophen) if patient is febrile before beginning therapy.
- Monitor WBC levels and circulating T cells periodically during therapy.
- Monitor patient very closely after first dose; acetaminophen prn should be ordered to cover febrile reactions; cooling blanket may be needed in severe cases. Equipment for intubation and respiratory support should be on standby for severe pulmonary reactions.

Drug-specific teaching points
- Know that there is often a severe reaction to the first dose, including high fever and chills, difficulty breathing, and chest congestion (you will be closely watched, and comfort measures will be taken to make you as comfortable as possible).
- Avoid infection while you are on this drug; people may wear masks and rubber gloves when caring for you; visitors may have to be limited.
- Report chest pain, difficulty breathing, nausea, chills.

Adverse effects in *Italics* are most common; those in **Bold** are life-threatening.

nabumetone

(nab byew' meh tone)
Relafen
Pregnancy Category B

Drug classes
NSAID
Analgesic (non-narcotic)

Therapeutic actions
Analgesic, anti-inflammatory, and antipyretic activities largely related to inhibition of prostaglandin synthesis; exact mechanisms of action are not known.

Indications
- Acute and chronic treatment of signs and symptoms of rheumatoid arthritis and osteoarthritis

Contraindications/cautions
- Contraindicated in the presence of significant renal impairment, pregnancy, lactation.
- Use caution in the presence of impaired hearing; allergies; hepatic, cardiovascular, and GI conditions

Dosage
Adult: 1,000 mg as a single dose with or without food. 1,500–2,000 mg/d have been used. May be given in divided doses.
Pediatric: Safety and efficacy have not been established.

Pharmacokinetics

Route	Onset	Peak
Oral	30–60 min	2.5–4 h

Metabolism: Hepatic, $T_{1/2}$: 22.5–30 h
Distribution: Crosses placenta; enters breast milk
Excretion: Urine.

Adverse effects
NSAIDs
- CNS: *Headache, dizziness, somnolence, insomnia,* fatigue, tiredness, dizziness, tinnitus, ophthamological effects
- GI: *Nausea, dyspepsia, GI pain,* diarrhea, vomiting, *constipation,* flatulence
- Respiratory: Dyspnea, hemoptysis, pharyngitis, bronchospasm, rhinitis
- Hematologic: Bleeding, platelet inhibition with higher doses, neutropenia, eosinophilia, leukopenia, pancytopenia, thrombocytopenia, agranulocytosis, granulocytopenia, aplastic anemia, decreased hemoglobin or hematocrit, bone marrow depression, mennorhagia
- GU: Dysuria, **renal impairment**
- Dermatologic: *Rash*, pruritus, sweating, dry mucous membranes, stomatitis
- Other: Peripheral edema, **anaphylactoid reactions to fatal anaphylactic shock**

■ Nursing Considerations

Assessment
- *History:* Renal impairment; impaired hearing; allergies; hepatic, cardiovascular, and GI conditions; lactation
- *Physical:* Skin—color and lesions; orientation, reflexes, ophthalmological and audiometric evaluation, peripheral sensation; P, edema; R, adventitious sounds; liver evaluation; CBC, clotting times, renal and liver function tests; serum electrolytes, stool guaiac

Implementation
- Administer drug with food or after meals if GI upset occurs.
- Arrange for periodic ophthalmologic examination during long-term therapy.
- Institute emergency procedures if overdose occurs: gastric lavage, induction of emesis, supportive therapy.

Drug-specific teaching points
- Take drug with food or meals if GI upset occurs; take only the prescribed dosage.
- Know that dizziness, drowsiness can occur (avoid driving or the use of dangerous machinery while on this drug).
- Report sore throat, fever, rash, itching, weight gain, swelling in ankles or fingers; changes in vision; black, tarry stools.

☐ nadolol

*(nay **doe'** lol)*
Corgard

Pregnancy Category C

Drug classes
Beta-blocking agent (nonselective beta-blocker)
Antianginal drug
Antihypertensive drug

Therapeutic actions
Competitively blocks beta-adrenergic receptors in the heart and juxtaglomerular apparatus, decreasing the influence of the sympathetic nervous system on these tissues and decreasing the excitability of the heart, cardiac output, oxygen consumption, and the release of renin, and lowering blood pressure.

Indications
- Hypertension alone or with other drugs, especially diuretics
- Long-term management of angina pectoris caused by atherosclerosis
- Unlabeled uses: treatment of ventricular arrhythmias, migraines, lithium induced tremors, aggressive behavior, essential tremors, rebleeding from esophageal varices, reduction of intraocular pressure, situational anxiety

Contraindications/cautions
- Contraindicated in the presence of sinus bradycardia (HR < 45 beats/min), second- or third-degree heart block (PR interval > 0.24 sec), cardiogenic shock, CHF, asthma, COPD, pregnancy, lactation.
- Use caution in the presence of diabetes or thyrotoxicosis.

Dosage
Adult
- ***Hypertension:*** Initially 40 mg PO qd; gradually increase dosage in 40- to 80-mg increments until optimum response is achieved. Usual maintenance dose is 40–80 mg/d; up to 320 mg qd may be needed.
- ***Angina:*** Initially 40 mg PO qd; gradually increase dosage in 40- to 80-mg increments at 3- to 7-d intervals until optimum response is achieved or heart rate markedly decreases. Usual maintenance dose is 40–80 mg qd; up to 240 mg/d may be needed. Safety and efficacy of larger doses not established. To discontinue, reduce dosage gradually over 1- to 2-wk period.

Pediatric: Safety and efficacy not established.

Geriatric or renal failure:

Creatinine Clearance (ml/min)	Dosage Intervals (h)
>50	24
31–50	24–36
10–30	24–48
<10	40–60

Pharmacokinetics

Route	Onset	Peak	Duration
Oral	Varies	2–4 h	17–24 h

Metabolism: $T_{1/2}$: 20–24 h
Distribution: Crosses placenta; enters breast milk
Excretion: Urine

Adverse effects
- CNS: Dizziness, vertigo, tinnitus, fatigue, emotional depression, paresthesias, sleep disturbances, hallucinations, disorientation, memory loss, slurred speech
- GI: *Gastric pain, flatulence, constipation, diarrhea, nausea, vomiting,* anorexia, ischemic colitis, renal and mesenteric arterial thrombosis, retroperitoneal fibrosis, hepatomegaly, acute pancreatitis
- CV: **CHF, cardiac arrhythmias,** peripheral vascular insufficiency, claudication, CVA, pulmonary edema, hypotension
- Respiratory: Bronchospasm, dyspnea, cough, bronchial obstruction, nasal stuffiness, rhinitis, pharyngitis (less likely than with propranolol)
- GU: *Impotence, decreased libido,* Peyronie's disease, dysuria, nocturia, frequency

Adverse effects in *Italics* are most common; those in **Bold** are life-threatening.

- **MS:** Joint pain, arthralgia, muscle cramp
- **EENT:** Eye irritation, dry eyes, conjunctivitis, blurred vision
- **Dermatologic:** Rash, pruritus, sweating, dry skin
- **Allergic reactions:** Pharyngitis, erythematous rash, fever, sore throat, laryngospasm, respiratory distress
- **Other:** *Decreased exercise tolerance, development of antinuclear antibodies,* hyperglycemia or hypoglycemia, elevated serum transaminase, alkaline phosphatase

Clinically important drug-drug interactions
- Increased effects of metoprolol if taken with verapamil • Increased serum levels and toxicity of IV lidocaine, aminophylline if given concurrently • Increased risk of postural hypotension if taken concurrently with prazosin • Increased risk of peripheral ischemia if taken concurrently with ergotamine, methysergide, dihydroergotamine • Decreased antihypertensive effects if taken with NSAIDs, clonidine • Hypertension followed by severe bradycardia if given concurrently with epinephrine

Drug-lab test interferences
- Possible false results with glucose or insulin tolerance tests

■ Nursing Considerations

Assessment
- *History:* Sinus bradycardia, second- or third-degree heart block, cardiogenic shock, CHF, asthma, COPD; diabetes or thyrotoxicosis; pregnancy; lactation
- *Physical:* Body weight, skin condition, neurologic status, P, BP, ECG, respiratory status, kidney and thyroid function, blood and urine glucose

Implementation
- Do not discontinue drug abruptly after chronic therapy (hypersensitivity to catecholamines may have developed, causing exacerbation of angina, MI, and ventricular dysrhythmias). Taper drug gradually over 2 wk with monitoring.
- Consult with physician about withdrawing drug if patient is to undergo surgery (controversial).

Drug-specific teaching points
- Do not to stop taking this drug unless instructed to do so by a health care provider.
- Avoid driving or dangerous activities if CNS effects occur.
- Report difficulty breathing, night cough, swelling of extremities, slow pulse, confusion, depression, rash, fever, sore throat.

☐ nafarelin acetate

(naf a re lin)
Synarel

Pregnancy Category X

Drug classes
Gonadotropin releasing hormone
Hormone

Therapeutic actions
A potent agonistic analog of gonadotropic-releasing hormone (GnRH) which is released from the hypothalamus to stimulate LH and FSH release from the pituitary; these hormones are responsible for regulating reproductive status. Repeated dosing abolishes the stimulatory effect on the pituitary gland, leading to decreased secretion of gonadal steroids by about 4 wk; consequently, tissues and functions that depend on gonadal steroids for their maintenance become quiescent.

Indications
- Treatment of endometriosis, including pain relief and reduction of endometriotic lesions
- Treatment of central precocious puberty in children of both sexes

Contraindications/cautions
- Known sensitivity to GnRH, GnRH-agonist analogs, excipients in the product; undiagnosed abnormal genital bleeding;

nafarelin acetate

pregnancy; lactation (potential androgenic effects on the fetus).

Dosage
Adult
- **Endometriosis:** 400 μg/d. One spray (200 μg) into one nostril in the morning and one spray into the other nostril in the evening. Start treatment between days 2 and 4 of the menstrual cycle. 800-μg dose may administered as one spray into each nostril in the morning (a total of two sprays) and again in the evening for patients with persistent regular menstruation after months of treatment. Treatment for 6 mo is recommended. Retreatment is not recommended because safety has not been established.

Pediatric
- **Central precocious puberty:** 1,600 μg/d. Two sprays (400 μg) in each nostril in the morning and two sprays in each nostril in the evening; may be increased to 1,800 μg/d. Continue until resumption of puberty is desired.

Pharmacokinetics

Route	Onset	Peak
Nasal	Rapid	4 wk

Metabolism: $T_{1/2}$: 85.5 h
Distribution: Crosses placenta; enters breast milk
Excretion: Urine

Adverse effects
- **CNS:** Dizziness, headache, sleep disorders, fatigue, tremor
- **GI:** Hepatic dysfunction
- **GU:** Fluid retention
- **Endocrine:** *Androgenic effects* (acne, edema, mild hirsutism, decrease in breast size, deepening of the voice, oily skin or hair, weight gain, clitoral hypertrophy or testicular atrophy), *hypoestrogenic effects* (flushing, sweating, vaginitis, nervousness, emotional lability)
- **Local:** *Nasal irritation*
- **Other:** With prolonged therapy, bone density loss has been noted

■ Nursing Considerations
Assessment
- *History:* Sensitivity to GnRH, GnRH-agonist analogs, excipients in the product; undiagnosed abnormal genital bleeding; pregnancy; lactation
- *Physical:* Body weight; hair distribution pattern; skin—color, texture, lesions; breast exam; nasal mucosa; orientation, affect, reflexes; P, auscultation, BP, peripheral edema; liver evaluation; bone density studies in long-term therapy

Implementation
- Ensure that patient is not pregnant before beginning therapy; begin therapy for endometriosis during menstrual period, days 2–4.
- Store drug upright; protect from exposure to light.
- Arrange for bone density studies before beginning therapy if retreatment is suggested because of return of endometriosis.
- Ensure that patient has enough of the drug on hand to prevent interruption of therapy during the duration of treatment.
- Caution patient that androgenic effects may not be reversible when the drug is withdrawn.
- Monitor nasal mucosa for signs of erosion during course of therapy.
- Arrange for use of topical decongestant if needed during therapy at least 30 min after dosing with nafarelin.

Drug-specific teaching points
- Use this drug without interruption; make sure that you have enough on hand to prevent interruption. Store the drug upright. Protect the bottle from exposure to light.
- Be aware that regular menstruation should cease within 4–6 wk of beginning therapy. Breakthrough bleeding or ovulation may still occur.
- Know that the following side effects may occur: masculinizing effects (acne, hair growth, deepening of voice, oily skin or hair; these effects may not be reversible when the drug is withdrawn); low estrogen effects (flushing, sweating,

Adverse effects in *Italics* are most common; those in **Bold** are life-threatening.

vaginal irritation, nervousness); nasal irritation.
- Consult with your nurse or physician if you need a topical nasal decongestant during the course of this drug therapy; a decongestant should be used at least 30 min after nafarelin use.
- Be aware that this drug is contraindicated during pregnancy; use a nonhormonal form of birth control during drug therapy. If you become pregnant, discontinue the drug and consult with your physician immediately.
- Report abnormal growth of facial hair, deepening of the voice, unusual bleeding or bruising, fever, chills, sore throat, vaginal itching or irritation; nasal irritation, burning.

▢ nafcillin sodium

(naf sill'in)
Nafcil, Nallpen, Unipen

Pregnancy Category B

Drug classes
Antibiotic
Penicillinase-resistant pencillin

Therapeutic actions
Bactericidal: inhibits cell wall synthesis of sensitive organisms, causing cell death

Indications
- Infections due to penicillinase-producing staphylococci
- Infections caused by group A beta-hemolytic streptococci, *Streptococcus viridans*

Contraindications/cautions
- Contraindicated in the presence of allergies to penicillins, cephalosporins, or other allergens.
- Use caution in the presence of renal disorders, pregnancy, lactation (may cause diarrhea or candidiasis in the infant).

Dosage
Adult
- *IV:* 500–1,000 mg q4h for short-term (24–48 h) therapy only, especially in the elderly
- *IM:* 500 mg q6h (q4h in severe infections).
- *PO:* 250–500 mg q4–6h, up to 1 g q4–6h in severe infections.

Pediatric
- *IM:* 25 mg/kg bid; newborns, 10 mg/kg bid.
- *PO*
  - *Staphylococcal infections:* 50 mg/kg per day in four divided doses; newborns, 10 mg/kg tid–qid.
  - *Scarlet fever, pneumonia:* 25 mg/kg per day in four divided doses.
  - *Streptococcal pharyngitis:* 250 mg tid (penicillin G is preferred).

Pharmacokinetics

Route	Onset	Peak	Duration
Oral	Varies	60 min	4 h
IM	Rapid	3–90 min	4–6 h
IV	Immediate	15 min	4 h

Metabolism: Hepatic, $T_{1/2}$: 1 h
Distribution: Crosses placenta; enters breast milk
Excretion: Urine and bile

IV facts
Preparation: Dilute solution for IV use in 15–30 ml Sodium Chloride Injection or Sterile Water for Injection; dilute reconstituted solution with compatible IV solution: 0.9% Sodium Chloride Injection, Sterile Water for Injection, 5% Dextrose in Water or in 0.4% Sodium Chloride Solution, M/6 Sodium Lactate Solution, or Ringer's Solution. Solutions at concentrations of 2–40 mg/ml are stable for 24 h at room temperature or 4 d refrigerated; discard solution after this time.
Infusion: Infuse slowly.
Incompatibilities: Do not mix in the same IV solution as other antibiotics.

Adverse effects
- CNS: Lethargy, hallucinations, seizures
- GI: *Glossitis, stomatitis, gastritis, sore mouth,* furry tongue, black "hairy" tongue, *nausea, vomiting, diarrhea,* abdominal pain, bloody diarrhea, enterocolitis, pseudomembranous colitis, nonspecific hepatitis
- Hematologic: Anemia, thrombocytopenia, leukopenia, neutropenia, prolonged bleeding time (more common with this drug than with other penicillinase-resistant penicillins)
- GU: Nephritis—oliguria, proteinuria, hematuria, casts, azotemia, pyuria
- Hypersensitivity reactions: *Rash, fever, wheezing,* anaphylaxis
- Local: *Pain, phlebitis,* thrombosis at injection site
- Other: *Superinfections*—oral and rectal moniliasis, vaginitis

Clinically important drug-drug interactions
- Decreased effectiveness of nafcillin if taken concurrently with tetracyclines
- Inactivation of parenteral aminoglycosides (amikacin, gentamicin, kanamycin, neomycin, metilmicin, streptomycin, tobramycin) if taken concurrently with nafcillin

Drug-lab test interferences
- False-positive Coombs' test with IV use.

■ Nursing Considerations

Assessment
- *History:* Allergies to penicillins, cephalosporins, or other allergens; renal disorders; pregnancy; lactation
- *Physical:* Culture infected area; skin—color, lesions; R, adventitious sounds; bowel sounds: CBC, liver and renal function tests, serum electrolytes, Hct, urinalysis

Implementation
- Culture infected area before beginning treatment; reculture area if response is not as expected.
- Arrange to continue therapy for at least 2 d after signs of infection have disappeared, usually 7–10 d.
- Reconstitute powder for IM use with Sterile or Bacteriostatic Water for Injection or Sodium Chloride Injection. Administer by deep intragluteal injection. Reconstituted solution is stable for 7 d if refrigerated or 3 d at room temperature.
- Do not give IM injections repeatedly in the same site; atrophy can occur; monitor injection sites.
- Administer oral drug on an empty stomach, 1 h before or 2 h after meals, with a full glass of water. Do not administer with fruit juices or soft drinks.

Drug-specific teaching points
- Take oral drug on an empty stomach with a full glass of water; take the full course of drug therapy.
- Avoid self-treating other infections with this antibiotic because it is specific for the infection being treated. Know that nausea, vomiting, diarrhea, mouth sores, pain at injection sites may occur.
- Report difficulty breathing, rashes, severe diarrhea, severe pain at injection site, mouth sores, unusual bleeding or bruising.

❒ nalbuphine hydrochloride

(nal' byoo feen)
Nubain

Pregnancy Category C

Drug classes
Narcotic agonist-antagonist analgesic

Therapeutic actions
Nalbuphine acts as an agonist at specific opioid receptors in the CNS to produce analgesia, sedation but also acts to cause hallucinations and is an antagonist at μ receptors.

Indications
- Relief of moderate to severe pain
- Preoperative analgesia, as a supplement to surgical anesthesia, and for obstetric analgesia during labor and delivery

Adverse effects in *Italics* are most common; those in **Bold** are life-threatening.

772 ■ nalbuphine hydrochloride

Contraindications/cautions
- Contraindicated in the presence of hypersensitivity to nalbuphine, sulfites; lactation.
- Use caution in the presence of emotionally unstable patients or those with a history of narcotic abuse; pregnancy prior to labor (neonatal withdrawal may occur in infants born to mothers who used this drug during pregnancy), labor or delivery (use with caution in women delivering premature infants who are especially sensitive to the respiratory depressant effects of narcotics), bronchial asthma, COPD, respiratory depression, anoxia, increased intracranial pressure, acute MI when nausea and vomiting are present, biliary tract surgery (may cause spasm of the sphincter of Oddi).

Dosage
Adult: Usual dose is 10 mg/70 kg, SC, IM, or IV q 3–6 h as necessary. Individualize dosage. In nontolerant patients, the recommended single maximum dose is 20 mg, with a maximum total daily dose of 160 mg. Patients dependent on narcotics may experience withdrawal symptoms with administration of nalbuphine; control by small increments of morphine by slow IV administration until relief occurs. If the previous narcotic was morphine, meperidine, codeine, or another narcotic with similar duration of activity, administer ¼ the anticipated nalbuphine dose initially, and observe for signs of withdrawal. If no untoward symptoms occur, progressively increase doses until analgesia is obtained.
Pediatric: Younger than 18 y: Not recommended.
Geriatric or renal or hepatic impairment: Reduce dosage.

Pharmacokinetics

Route	Onset	Peak	Duration
IV	2–3 min	15–20 min	3–6 h
SC/IM	< 15 min	30–60 min	3–6 h

Metabolism: Hepatic, $T_{1/2}$: 5 h

Distribution: Crosses placenta; enters breast milk
Excretion: Urine

IV facts
Preparation: No additional preparation is required.
Infusion: Administer by direct injection or into the tubing of a running IV.

Adverse effects
- CNS: *Sedation, clamminess, sweating, headache,* nervousness, restlessness, depression, crying, confusion, faintness, hostility, unusual dreams, hallucinations, euphoria, dysphoria, unreality, *dizziness, vertigo,* floating feeling, feeling of heaviness, numbness, tingling, flushing, warmth, blurred vision
- GI: Nausea, vomiting, cramps, dyspepsia, bitter taste, *dry mouth*
- CV: Hypotension, hypertension, bradycardia, tachycardia
- Respiratory: Respiratory depression, dyspnea, asthma
- GU: Urinary urgency
- Dermatologic: Itching, burning, urticaria

Clinically important drug-drug interactions
- Potentiation of effects of nalbuphine when given with other barbiturate anesthetics.

■ Nursing Considerations

Assessment
- *History:* Hypersensitivity to nalbuphine, sulfites; lactation; emotionally unstable patients or those with a history of narcotic abuse; pregnancy; bronchial asthma, COPD, respiratory depression, anoxia, increased intracranial pressure, MI, biliary tract surgery
- *Physical:* Orientation, reflexes, bilateral grip strength, affect; pupil size, vision; pulse, auscultation, BP; R, adventitious sounds; bowel sounds, normal output; urine output; liver, kidney function tests

Adverse effects in *Italics* are most common; those in **Bold** are life-threatening.

Implementation
- Arrange to taper dosage when discontinuing drug after prolonged use to avoid withdrawal symptoms.
- Provide narcotic antagonist, facilities for assisted or controlled respiration on standby in case respiratory depression occurs.
- Reassure patient about addiction liability; most patients who receive opiates for medical reasons do not develop dependence syndromes.

Drug-specific teaching points
- Know that the following side effects may occur: dizziness, sedation, drowsiness, impaired visual acuity (avoid driving a car, performing other tasks that require alertness); nausea, loss of appetite (lying quietly, eating frequent, small meals should minimize these effects).
- Report severe nausea, vomiting, palpitations, shortness of breath, or difficulty breathing.

▢ nalidixic acid

(nal i dix' ik)
NegGram

Pregnancy Category C

Drug classes
Urinary tract anti-infective
Antibacterial drug

Therapeutic actions
Bactericidal; interferes with DNA and RNA synthesis in susceptible gram-negative bacteria, causing cell death.

Indications
- Urinary tract infections caused by susceptible gram-negative bacteria, including *Proteus* strains, *Klebsiella* species, *Enterobacter* species, *Escherichia coli*

Contraindications/cautions
- Contraindicated in the presence of allergy to nalidixic acid, seizures, epilepsy, pregnancy, lactation.
- Use caution in the presence of G-6-PD deficiency, renal or liver dysfunction, cerebral arteriosclerosis.

Dosage
Adult: Initial therapy, 1 g PO qid for 1–2 wk. For prolonged therapy, total dose may be reduced to 2 g/d.
Pediatric: < 12 y: Exact dosage is based on weight; total daily dose for initial therapy, 55 mg/kg per day PO divided into four equal doses. For prolonged therapy, may be reduced to 33 mg/kg per day. Not recommended under 3 mo.

Pharmacokinetics

Route	Onset	Peak
Oral	Varies	1–2 h

Metabolism: Hepatic, $T_{1/2}$: 1–2.5 h
Distribution: Crosses placenta; enters breast milk
Excretion: Urine

Adverse effects
- **CNS:** *Drowsiness, weakness, headache, dizziness, vertigo,* visual disturbances
- **GI:** *Abdominal pain, nausea, vomiting, diarrhea*
- **Hematologic:** Thrombocytopenia, leukopenia, hemolytic anemia
- **Dermatologic:** Photosensitivity reactions
- **Hypersensitivity:** Rash, pruritus, urticaria, angioedema, eosinophilia, arthralgia

Clinically important drug-drug interactions
- Increased risk of bleeding if given with oral anticoagulants

Drug-lab test interferences
- False-positive urinary glucose results when using Benedict's reagent, Fehling's reagent, Clinitest tablets • False elevations of urinary 17-keto and ketogenic steroids when assay uses m-dinitrobenzene

■ Nursing Considerations
Assessment
- *History:* Allergy to nalidixic acid, seizures, epilepsy, G-6-PD deficiency, renal

Adverse effects in *Italics* are most common; those in **Bold** are life-threatening.

774 ■ naloxone hydrochloride

or liver dysfunction, cerebral arteriosclerosis, pregnancy, lactation
- *Physical:* Skin—color, lesions; joints; orientation, reflexes; CBC, liver and renal function tests

Implementation
- Arrange for culture and sensitivity tests.
- Administer drug with food if GI upset occurs.
- Arrange for periodic blood counts, renal and liver function tests during prolonged therapy.
- Monitor clinical response; if no improvement is seen or a relapse occurs, send urine for repeat culture and sensitivity.

Drug-specific teaching points
- Take drug with food. Complete the full course of drug therapy to ensure resolution of the infection.
- Know that the following side effects may occur: nausea, vomiting, abdominal pain (small, frequent meals may help); diarrhea; sensitivity to sunlight (wear protective clothing, and use sunscreen if exposed to sunlight); drowsiness, blurring of vision, dizziness (observe caution if driving or using dangerous equipment).
- Report severe rash, visual changes, weakness, tremors.

▢ naloxone hydrochloride

(nal ox' one)
Narcan

Pregnancy Category B

Drug classes
Narcotic antagonist
Diagnostic agent

Therapeutic actions
Pure narcotic antagonist; reverses the effects of opioids, including respiratory depression, sedation, hypotension; can reverse the psychotomimetic and dysphoric effects of narcotic agonist-antagonists, such as pentazocine.

Indications
- Complete or partial reversal of narcotic depression, including respiratory depression induced by opioids, including natural and synthetic narcotics, propoxyphene, methadone, nalbuphine, butorphanol, pentazocine
- Diagnosis of suspected acute opioid overdosage
- Unlabeled uses: improvement of circulation in refractory shock, reversal of alcoholic coma

Contraindications/cautions
- Contraindicated in the presence of allergy to narcotic antagonists.
- Use caution in the presence of narcotic addiction, cardiovascular disorders, pregnancy, lactation.

Dosage
IV administration is recommended in emergency situations when rapid onset of action is required.
Adult
- ***Narcotic overdose:*** Initial dose of 0.4–2 mg, IV. Additional doses may be repeated at 2- to 3-min intervals. If no response after 10 mg, question the diagnosis. IM or SC routes may be used if IV route is unavailable.
- ***Postoperative narcotic depression:*** Titrate dose to patient's response. Initial dose of 0.1–0.2 mg IV at 2–3 min intervals until desired degree of reversible. Repeat doses may be needed within 1- to 2-h intervals, depending on the amount and type of narcotic. Supplemental IM doses produce a longer lasting effect.

Pediatric
- ***Narcotic overdose:*** Initial dose is 0.01 mg/kg IV. Subsequent dose of 0.1 mg/kg may be administered if needed. May be given IM or SC in divided doses.
- ***Postoperative narcotic depression:*** For the initial reversal of respiratory depression, inject in increments of 0.005–0.01 mg IV at 2- to 3-min intervals to the desired degree of reversal.

Neonates
- ***Narcotic-induced depression:*** Initial dose if 0.01 mg/kg IV, SC, IM.

May be repeated as indicated in the adult guidelines.

Pharmacokinetics

Route	Onset	Duration
IV	2 min	4–6 h
IM/SC	3–5 min	4–6 h

Metabolism: Hepatic, $T_{1/2}$: 30–81 min
Distribution: Crosses placenta; enters breast milk
Excretion: Urine

IV facts

Preparation: Dilute in Normal Saline or 5% Dextrose Solutions for IV infusions. The addition of 2 mg in 500 ml of solution provides a concentration of 0.004 mg/ml; titrate rate by patient's response. Use diluted mixture within 24 h. After that time, discard any remaining solution.

Infusion: Inject directly or titrate rate of infusion based on patient's response.

Incompatibilities: Do not mix naloxone with preparations containing bisulfite, metabisulfite, high molecular weight anions, alkaline pH solutions.

Adverse effects

- CNS: Reversal of analgesia and excitement (postoperative use)
- CV: *Hypotension, hypertension*, ventricular tachycardia and fibrillation, pulmonary edema (postoperative use)
- Acute narcotic abstinence syndrome: *nausea, vomiting, sweating, tachycardia, increased blood pressure, tremulousness*

■ Nursing Considerations

Assessment
- *History:* Allergy to narcotic antagonists; narcotic addiction; cardiovascular disorders; lactation
- *Physical:* Sweating; reflexes; pupil size; P, BP; R, adventitious sounds

Implementation
- Monitor patient continuously after use of naloxone; repeat doses may be necessary, depending on duration of narcotic and time of last dose.
- Maintain open airway, and provide artificial ventilation, cardiac massage, vasopressor agents if needed to counteract acute narcotic overdosage.

Drug-specific teaching points
- Report sweating, feelings of tremulousness.

☐ naltrexone hydrochloride

*(nal **trex'** one)*
ReVia

Pregnancy Category C

Drug classes
Narcotic antagonist

Therapeutic actions
Pure opiate antagonist; markedly attenuates or completely, reversibly blocks the subjective effects of IV opioids, including those with mixed narcotic agonist-antagonist properties.

Indications
- Adjunct to treatment of alcohol or narcotic dependence as part of a comprhensive treatment program
- Unlabeled uses: treatment of postconcussional syndrome unresponsive to other treatments; eating disorders

Contraindications/cautions
- Contraindicated in the presence of allergy to narcotic antagonists, pregnancy.
- Use caution in the presence of narcotic addiction (may produce withdrawal symptoms; do not administer unless patient has been opioid free for 7–10 d); opioid withdrawal; acute hepatitis, liver failure; lactation; depression, suicidal tendencies.

Dosage
Adult: Administer naloxone challenge before use.
- **IV:** Draw 2 ampules of naloxone, 2 ml into a syringe. Inject 0.5 ml. Leave needle

in vein, and observe for 30 sec. If no signs of withdrawal occur, inject remaining 1.5 ml, and observe for 20 min for signs and symptoms of withdrawal (eg, stuffiness or running nose, tearing, yawning, sweating, tremor, vomiting, piloerection, feeling of temperature change, joint or bone and muscle pain, abdominal cramps, skin crawling).
- **SC:** Administer 2 ml, and observe for signs and symptoms of withdrawal for 45 min. If any of the signs and symptoms of withdrawal occur or if there is any doubt that the patient is opioid free, do not administer naltrexone. Confirmatory rechallenge can be done within 24 h. Inject 4 ml IV, and observe for signs and symptoms of withdrawal. Repeat until no signs and symptoms are seen and patient is no longer at risk.
- *Naltrexone maintenance:* Alcoholism: 50 mg PO per day. *Narcotic dependence:* Initial dose of 25 mg PO. Observe for 1 h; if no signs or symptoms are seen, complete dose with 25 mg. Usual maintenance dose is 50 mg/24 h PO. Flexible dosing schedule can be used with 100 mg every other day or 150 mg every third day, and so forth.

Pediatric: Safety has not been established in children younger than 18 y.

Pharmacokinetics

Route	Onset	Peak	Duration
Oral	15–30 min	60 min	24–72 h

Metabolism: Hepatic, T$_{1/2}$: 3.9–12.9 h
Distribution: Crosses placenta; enters breast milk
Excretion: Urine

Adverse effects

- **CNS:** *Difficulty sleeping, anxiety, nervousness, headache, low energy,* increased energy, irritability, dizziness, blurred vision, burning, light sensitivity
- **GI:** Hepatocellular injury, *abdominal pain/cramps, nausea, vomiting,*, loss of appetite, diarrhea, constipation
- **CV:** Phlebitis, edema, increased blood pressure, nonspecific ECG changes
- **Respiratory:** Nasal congestion, rhinorrhea, sneezing, sore throat, excess mucus or phlegm, sinus trouble, epistaxis
- **GU:** *Delayed ejaculation, decreased potency,* increased frequency/discomfort voiding
- **Dermatologic:** Skin rash, itching, oily skin, pruritus, acne
- **Other:** *Chills, increased thirst,* increased appetite, weight loss or gain, yawning, swollen glands, *joint and muscle pain*

■ Nursing Considerations

Assessment
- *History:* Allergy to narcotic antagonists; narcotic addiction; opioid withdrawal; acute hepatitis, liver failure; lactation; depression, suicidal tendencies
- *Physical:* Sweating; skin—lesions, color; reflexes, affect, orientation, muscle strength; P, BP, edema, baseline ECG; R, adventitious sounds; liver evaluation; urine screen for opioids, liver function tests

Implementation
- Do not use until patient has been opioid free for 7–10 d; check urine opioid levels.
- Do not administer until patient has passed a naloxone challenge.
- Initiate treatment slowly, and monitor patient continuously until patient has been given naltrexone in the full daily dose with no signs and symptoms of withdrawal.
- Arrange for periodic monitoring of liver function tests during therapy; discontinue therapy at any signs of increasing liver dysfunction.
- Do not use opioid drugs for analgesia, cough, and cold; do not use opioid antidiarrheal preparations; patient will not have a response to these drugs; use a nonopioid preparation if possible.
- Assure that patient is actively participating in a comprehensive treatment program.

Drug-specific teaching points
- Be aware that this drug will help facilitate abstinence from alcohol.

Adverse effects in *Italics* are most common; those in **Bold** are life-threatening.

- Be aware that this drug blocks the effects of narcotics and other opiates.
- Wear a medical alert tag indicating that you are on this drug so that medical personnel will know how to treat any emergency situation.
- Be aware that small doses of heroin or other opiate drugs will not have an effect. Self-administration of large doses of heroin or other narcotics can overcome the blockade effect of this drug and may cause death or serious injury or coma.
- Know that the following side effects may occur: drowsiness, dizziness, blurred vision, anxiety (avoid driving or operating dangerous machinery if these occur); diarrhea, nausea, vomiting; decreased sexual function.
- Report unusual bleeding or bruising; dark, tarry stools; yellowing of eyes or skin; running nose; tearing; sweating; chills; joint or muscle pain.

☐ nandrolone decanoate

(nan' droe lone)

Andralone-D, Deca-Durabolin, Hybolin Decanoate, Nandrobolic, Neo-Durabolic

nandrolone phenpropionate

Durabolin, Hybolin Improved, Nandrobolic

Pregnancy Category X
C-III controlled substance

Drug classes
Anabolic steroid
Hormonal agent

Therapeutic actions
Testosterone analogue; promotes body tissue-building processes and reverses catabolic or tissue-depleting processes; increases hemoglobin and red cell mass.

Indications
- Nandrolone decanoate: Management of anemia related to renal insufficiency
- Nandrolone phenpropionate: Control of metastatic breast cancer

Contraindications/cautions
- Known sensitivity to nandrolone or anabolic steroids; prostate or breast cancer in males; benign prostatic hypertrophy; breast cancer (females); pituitary insufficiency; MI (contraindicated because of effects on cholesterol); nephrosis; liver disease; hypercalcemia; pregnancy; lactation.

Dosage
Administer by deep IM injection; therapy should be intermittent.
Anemia of renal insufficiency (nandrolone decanoate): Women: 50–100 mg/wk IM; *men:* 100–200 mg/wk IM; *children (2–13 y):* 25–50 mg IM every 3–4 wk.
Control of metastatic breast cancer (nandrolone phenpropionate): 50–100 mg/wk IM based on therapeutic response.
Infants: Contraindicated because of possibility of serious disruption of growth and development.

Pharmacokinetics

Route	Onset	Peak
IM	Slow	Unknown

Metabolism: Hepatic, $T_{1/2}$: unknown
Distribution: Crosses placenta; enters breast milk
Excretion: Unknown

Adverse effects
- **CNS:** *Excitation, insomnia,* chills, toxic confusion
- **GI:** Hepatotoxicity, peliosis, hepatitis with life threatening liver failure or intra-abdominal hemorrhage; liver cell tumors, sometimes malignant and fatal, *nausea, vomiting, diarrhea, abdominal fullness, loss of appetite, burning of tongue*
- **Hematologic:** *Blood lipid changes* (increased risk of atherosclerosis); iron-deficiency anemia, hypercalcemia, altered serum cholesterol levels; *retention of so-*

Adverse effects in *Italics* are most common; those in **Bold** are life-threatening.

778 ■ naproxen

dium, chloride, water, potassium, phosphates and calcium
- GU: Possible increased risk of prostatic hypertrophy, carcinoma in geriatric patients
- **Endocrine:** *Virilization, prepubertal males,* phallic enlargement, hirsutism, increased skin pigmentation; *postpubertal males,* inhibition of testicular function, gynecomastia, testicular atrophy, priapism, baldness, epidiymitis, change in libido; *females,* hirsutism, hoarseness, deepening of the voice, clitoral enlargement, menstrual irregularities, baldness; decreased glucose tolerance
- **Other:** *Acne,* premature closure of the epiphyses

Clinically important drug-drug interactions
- Potentiation of oral anticoagulants if taken with anabolic steroids • Decreased need for insulin, oral hypoglycemica agents if anabolic steroids are used

Drug-lab test interferences
- Altered glucose tolerance tests • Decrease in thyroid function tests, which may persist for 2–3 wk after stopping therapy • Increased creatinine, creatinine clearance, which may last for 2 wk after therapy

■ Nursing Considerations

Assessment
- *History:* Sensitivity to nandrolone or anabolic steroids; prostate or breast cancer in males; benign prostatic hypertrophy; breast cancer in females; pituitary insufficiency; MI; nephrosis; liver disease; hypercalcemia; pregnancy; lactation
- *Physical:* Skin—color, texture; hair distribution pattern; affect, orientation; abdominal exam, liver evaluation; serum electrolytes, serum cholesterol levels, glucose tolerance tests, thyroid function tests, long-bone x-ray (in children)

Implementation
- Inject nandrolone deeply into gluteal muscle.
- Administer nandrolone intermittently to decrease adverse effects.
- Monitor effect on children with long-bone x-rays every 3–6 mo during therapy; discontinue drug well before the bone age reaches the norm for the patient's chronologic age.
- Monitor patient for occurrence of edema; arrange for appropriate diuretic therapy as needed.
- Arrange to monitor liver function, serum electrolytes periodically during therapy, and consult with physician for appropriate corrective measures as needed.
- Arrange to measure cholesterol levels periodically in patients who are at high risk for coronary artery disease.
- Monitor diabetic patients closely as glucose tolerance may change; adjustments may be needed in insulin, oral hypoglycemic dosage, and diet.

Drug-specific teaching points
- Be aware that this drug can only be given IM; mark calendar indicating days to return for injection.
- Know that the following side effects may occur: nausea, vomiting, diarrhea, burning of the tongue (small, frequent meals may help; body hair growth, baldness, deepening of the voice, loss of libido, impotence; most of these effects will be reversible when the drug is stopped); excitation, confusion, insomnia (avoid driving, performing tasks that require alertness if these effects occur); swelling of the ankles, fingers (medication may be ordered to help).
- Diabetic patients—monitor urine sugar closely because glucose tolerance may change. Report any abnormalities to physician, so corrective action can be taken.
- Report ankle swelling, skin color changes, severe nausea, vomiting, hoarseness, body hair growth, deepening of the voice, acne, menstrual irregularities (women).

❒ naproxen

*(na **prox**' en)*

Apo-Naproxen (CAN),
Naprosyn, Naxen (CAN),
Novonaprox (CAN)

Adverse effects in *Italics* are most common; those in **Bold** are life-threatening.

naproxen sodium
Aleve, Anaprox, Anaprox DS

Pregnancy Category B

Drug classes
NSAID
Non-narcotic analgesic

Therapeutic actions
Analgesic, anti-inflammatory, and antipyretic activities largely related to inhibition of prostaglandin synthesis; exact mechanisms of action are not known.

Indications
- Mild to moderate pain
- Treatment of primary dysmenorrhea, rheumatoid arthritis, osteoarthritis, ankylosing spondylitis, tendinitis, bursitis, acute gout
- OTC use: temporary relief of minor aches and pains associated with the common cold, headache, toothache, muscular aches, backache, minor pain of arthritis, pain of menstrual cramps, reduction of fever
- Treatment of juvenile arthritis (naproxen only)

Contraindications/cautions
- Contraindicated in the presence of allergy to naproxen, salicylates, other NSAIDs; pregnancy; lactation.
- Use caution in the presence of asthma, chronic urticaria, cardiovascular dysfunction; hypertension; GI bleeding; peptic ulcer; impaired hepatic or renal function.

Dosage
Do not exceed 1,250 mg/d (1,375 mg/d naproxen sodium).

Adult
- **Rheumatoid arthritis/osteoarthritis, ankylosing spondylitis:** *Naproxen:* 250–500 mg bid, PO. May increase to 1.5 g/d for a limited period. *Naproxen sodium:* 275–550 mg bid PO. May increase to 1.65 g/d for a limited period.
- **Acute gout:** *Naproxen:* 750 mg PO followed by 250 mg q8h until the attack subsides. *Naproxen sodium:* 825 mg, PO followed by 275 mg q8h until the attack subsides.
- **Mild to moderate pain:** Naproxen sodium is used more often than naproxen as an analgesic because it is absorbed more quickly. *Naproxen:* 500 mg PO followed by 250 mg q6–8h. *Naproxen sodium:* 550 mg PO followed by 275 mg q6–8h.
- **OTC:** 200 mg PO q8–12h with a full glass of liquid while symptoms persist. Do not exceed 600 mg in 24 h.

Pediatric
- **Juvenile arthritis:** Naproxen: total daily dose of 10 mg/kg PO in two divided doses. Suspension, 13 kg, 2.5 ml bid; 25 kg, 5 ml bid; 38 kg, 7.5 ml bid. Naproxen sodium: safety and efficacy not established.
- **OTC:** Do not give to children younger than 12 y unless under advise of physician.

Geriatric: Do not take > 200 mg q12h PO.

Pharmacokinetics

Drug	Onset	Peak	Duration
Naproxen	1 h	2–4 h	up to 7 h
Naproxen sodium	1 h	1–2 h	up to 7 h

Metabolism: Hepatic, $T_{1/2}$: 12–15 h
Distribution: Crosses placenta; enters breast milk
Excretion: Urine

Adverse effects
NSAIDs
- CNS: *Headache, dizziness, somnolence, insomnia,* fatigue, tiredness, dizziness, tinnitus, ophthalmologic effects
- GI: *Nausea, dyspepsia, GI pain,* diarrhea, vomiting, *constipation,* flatulence
- Respiratory: Dyspnea, hemoptysis, pharyngitis, bronchospasm, rhinitis
- Hematologic: Bleeding, platelet inhibition with higher doses, neutropenia, eosinophilia, leukopenia, pancytopenia, thrombocytopenia, agranulocytosis, gra-

Adverse effects in *Italics* are most common; those in **Bold** are life-threatening.

nulocytopenia, aplastic anemia, decreased hemoglobin or hematocrit, bone marrow depression, mennorhagia
- GU: Dysuria, renal impairment, including renal failure, interstitial nephritis, hematuria
- Dermatologic: *Rash*, pruritus, sweating, dry mucous membranes, stomatitis
- Other: Peripheral edema, **anaphylactoid reactions to fatal anaphylactic shock**

Clinically important drug-drug interactions
- Increased serum lithium levels and risk of toxicity if taken concurrently with naproxen.

Drug-lab test interferences
- Falsely increased values for urinary 17-ketogenic steroids; discontinue naproxen therapy for 72 h before adrenal function tests • Inaccurate measurement of urinary 5-hydroxy indoleacetic acid

■ Nursing Considerations
Assessment
- *History:* Allergy to naproxen, salicylates, other NSAIDs; asthma, chronic urticaria, cardiovascular dysfunction; hypertension; GI bleeding; peptic ulcer; impaired hepatic or renal function; pregnancy; lactation
- *Physical:* Skin—color and lesions; orientation, reflexes, ophthalmologic and audiometric evaluation, peripheral sensation; P, edema; R, adventitious sounds; liver evaluation; CBC, clotting times, renal and liver function tests; serum electrolytes, stool guaiac

Implementation
- Administer drug with food or after meals if GI upset occurs.
- Arrange for periodic ophthalmologic examination during long-term therapy.
- Institute emergency procedures if overdose occurs: gastric lavage, induction of emesis, supportive therapy.

Drug-specific teaching points
- Take drug with food or meals if GI upset occurs; take only the prescribed dosage.
- Know that dizziness, drowsiness can occur (avoid driving or the use of dangerous machinery while on this drug).
- Report sore throat; fever; rash; itching; weight gain; swelling in ankles or fingers; changes in vision; black, tarry stools.

▢ nedocromil sodium

(nee doc' ro mill)
Tilade

Pregnancy Category B

Drug classes
Antiasthmatic drug (prophylactic)
Antiallergic drug

Therapeutic actions
Inhibits the mediators of a variety of inflammatory cells, including eosinophils, neutrophils, macrophages, mast cells; decreases the release of histamine and blocks the overall inflammatory reaction.

Indications
- Maintenance therapy in the management of patients with mild to moderate bronchial asthma

Contraindications/cautions
- Allergy to nedocromil or any other ingredients in the preparation, pregnancy, lactation.

Dosage
Adults, children older than 12 y: 2 inhalations qid at regular intervals to provide 14 mg/d; to lower dose, first reduce to tid inhalations (10.5 mg/d), then after several weeks to bid (7 mg/d).

Pharmacokinetics

Route	Onset	Peak	Duration
Inhal.	Rapid	28 min	10–12 h

Metabolism: Hepatic, $T_{1/2}$: 3.3 h
Distribution: Crosses placenta; may enter breast milk
Excretion: Urine

Adverse effects
- CNS: Dizziness, *headache*, fatigue, lacrimation
- GI: *Nausea,* vomiting, dyspepsia, diarrhea, *unpleasant taste*
- Respiratory: *Cough, pharyngitis, rhinitis, URI,* increased sputum, dyspnea, bronchitis

■ Nursing Considerations

Assessment
- *History:* Allergy to nedocromil, lactation
- *Physical:* Skin—color, lesions; orientation; R, auscultation, patency of nasal passages; abdominal exam, normal output; kidney and liver function tests, urinalysis

Implementation
- Do not use during acute bronchospasm; begin therapy when acute episode has been controlled and patient can inhale adequately.
- Arrange for continuation of treatment as appropriate; to be successful, nedocromil therapy must be continuous, even during periods with no asthmatic attacks.
- Use caution if cough or bronchospasm occurs after inhalation; this may (rarely) preclude continuation of treatment.
- Administer corticosteroids concomitantly if indicated.

Drug-specific teaching points
- Take drug at regular intervals, even during periods with no asthmatic attacks. Do not use during acute bronchospasm.
- Administer the drug according to guidelines in manufacturer's insert; the therapeutic effect of the drug depends on contact with the lungs; it is very important that you follow the manufacturer's directions.
- Do not discontinue drug abruptly except on advice of your health care provider
- Know that you may experience dizziness, drowsiness, fatigue while you are taking this drug (avoid driving or operating dangerous machinery); headache (if severe, proper analgesics may help); coughing, running nose.
- Report coughing, wheezing, dizziness.

◻ nefazodone hydrochloride

(ne faz' oh don)
Serzone

Pregnancy Category C

Drug classes
Antidepressant

Therapeutic actions
Acts as an antidepressant by inhibiting CNS neuronal uptake of serotonin and norepinephrine; also thought to antagonize α_1-adrenergic receptors.

Indications
- Treatment of depression

Contraindications/cautions
- Contraindicated in the presence of pregnancy.
- Use caution in the presence of cardiovascular or cerebrovascular disorders, dehydration, hypovolemia, mania, hypomania, suicidal patients, hepatic cirrhosis, electroshock therapy, debilitation, lactation.

Dosage
Adult: 200 mg PO in 2 divided doses; increase at 1 wk intervals in increments of 100–200 mg/d; usual range is 300–600 mg/d.
Pediatric: Not recommended in children <18 yr.
Geriatric or debilitated: Initially 100 mg/d in 2 divided doses.

Pharmacokinetics

Route	Onset	Peak
Oral	Slow	2d

Metabolism: Hepatic metabolism; $T_{1/2}$: 2–3 days
Distribution: Crosses placenta; passes into breast milk
Excretion: Urine and feces

Adverse effects in *Italics* are most common; those in **Bold** are life-threatening.

Adverse effects
- CNS: *headache, nervousness, insomnia, drowsiness, anxiety, tremor, dizziness, lightheadedness,* agitation, sedation, abnormal gait, confusion
- GI: *nausea, vomiting, diarrhea, dry mouth, anorexia, dyspepsia, constipation, taste changes,* flatulence, gastroenteritis, dysphagia, gingivitis
- CV: *postural hypotension*
- Dermatologic: *sweating, rash, pruritus,* acne, alopecia, contact dermatitis

Clinically important drug-drug interactions
- Increased risk of severe toxic effects if taken with MAOIs, astemizole, terfenadine; avoid these combinations • Risk of increased depression with general anesthetics

■ Nursing Considerations
Assessment
- *History*: Pregnancy, cardiovascular or cerebrovascular disorders, dehydration, hypovolemia, mania, hypomania, suicidal patients, hepatic cirrhosis, electroshock therapy, debilitation, lactation.
- *Physical*: Weight, temperature, skin—rash, lesions; reflexes, affect; bowel sounds, liver evaluation; P, BP, peripheral perfusion; urinary output, renal function; renal and liver function tests

Implementation
- Arrange for lower dose or less frequent administration in elderly or debilitated patients.
- Establish suicide precautions for severely depressed patients. Dispense only a small number of capsules at a time to these patients.
- Ensure that patient is well hydrated while on this therapy; monitor for postural hypotension.

Drug-specific teaching points
- Take this drug exactly as prescribed; do not increase dosage or combine with any other drugs without first consulting prescriber.
- Know that the following side effects may occur : dizziness, drowsiness, nervousness, insomnia (avoid driving a car or performing hazardous tasks, change positions slowly, take care in conditions of extremes of temperature); nausea, vomiting, weight loss (small, frequent meals may help; monitor your weight loss; if it becomes marked, consult with your heath care provider.
- Report changes in stool or urine; chest pain, dizziness, vision changes

☐ neomycin sulfate

*(nee o **mye**' sin)*
Systemic: *Mycifradin Sulfate*
Topical dermatologic preparations: *Mycifradin (CAN), Myciguent, Neocin (CAN)*

Pregnancy Category C

Drug classes
Aminoglycoside antibiotic

Therapeutic actions
Bactericidal: inhibits protein synthesis in susceptible strains of gram-negative bacteria; functional integrity of bacterial cell membrane appears to be disrupted, causing cell death

Indications
- Preoperative suppression of GI bacterial flora (oral)
- Hepatic coma to reduce ammonia-forming bacteria in the GI tract (oral)
- Infection prophylaxis in minor skin wounds and treatment of superficial skin infections due to susceptible organisms (topical dermatologic preparations)
- Unlabeled oral use: lowering of plasma lipids (LDL cholesterol)

Contraindications/cautions
- Contraindicated in the presence of allergy to aminoglycosides, intestinal obstruction, pregnancy, lactation.
- Use caution in the presence of the elderly or to any patient with diminished hearing, decreased renal function, dehydra-

neomycin sulfate ■ 783

tion, neuromuscular disorders (myasthenia gravis, parkinsonism, infant botulism).

Dosage
Adult
- **IM:** 15 mg/kg per day in divided doses q6h. 300 mg q6h for four doses, then 300 mg q12h yields blood concentrations of 12–30 μg/ml in 48–72 h. Do not exceed 1 g/d. Do not continue therapy for more than 10 d.
- **Oral:** Preoperative preparation for elective colorectal surgery: see manufacturer's recommendations for a complex 3-d regimen that includes oral erythromycin, magnesium sulfate, enemas, and dietary restrictions.
- *Hepatic coma:* 4–12 g/d in divided doses for 5–6 d, as adjunct to protein-free diet and supportive therapy, including transfusions, as needed.
- **Topical dermatologic:** Apply to affected area one to five times daily, except burns affecting more than 20% of the body surface should be treated once daily.

Pediatric
- **IM:** Do not use in infants and children.
- **Oral**
- *Hepatic coma:* 50–100 mg/kg per day in divided doses for 5–6 d, as adjunct to protein-free diet and supportive therapy including transfusions, as needed.

Geriatric or renal failure patients: Reduce dosage and carefully monitor serum drug levels and renal function tests throughout treatment. If this is not possible, reduce frequency of administration.

Pharmacokinetics

Route	Onset	Peak
Oral	Varies	1–4 h
IM	Rapid	½–1 h
Topical	Not generally absorbed systemically.	

Metabolism: $T_{1/2}$: 3 h
Distribution: Crosses placenta; enters breast milk
Excretion: Feces and urine (IM)

Adverse effects
Although oral neomycin is absorbed only negligibly across the intact GI mucosa, the risk of absorption from ulcerated area dictates that all of the listed side effects should be considered with oral and parenteral therapy. These side effects also should be considered with applications of the dermatologic preparations to ulcerated or burned skin or to large areas of skin, where absorption is possible.

- **CNS:** Ototoxicity—*tinnitus, dizziness, ringing in the ears,* vertigo, deafness (partially reversible to irreversible), vestibular paralysis, confusion, disorientation, depression, lethargy, nystagmus, visual disturbances, headache, *numbness, tingling,* tremor, paresthesias, muscle twitching, convulsions
- **GI:** Hepatic toxicity, *nausea, vomiting, anorexia,* weight loss, stomatitis, increased salivation
- **CV:** Palpitations, hypotension, hypertension
- **Hematologic:** *Leukemoid reaction,* agranulocytosis, granulocytosis, leukopenia, leukocytosis, thrombocytopenia, eosinophilia, pancytopenia, anemia, hemolytic anemia, increased or decreased reticulocyte count, electrolyte disturbances
- **GU:** *Nephrotoxicity*
- **Hypersensitivity:** Hypersensitivity reactions: *purpura, rash,* urticaria, exfoliative dermatitis, itching
- **Local:** *Pain, irritation, arachnoiditis at IM injection sites*
- **Other:** Fever, apnea, splenomegaly, joint pain, *superinfections*

Clinically important drug-drug interactions
- Increased ototoxic, nephrotoxic, neurotoxic effects if taken with other aminoglycosides, cephalothin, potent diuretics • Increased neuromuscular blockade and muscular paralysis when given with anesthetics, nondepolarizing neuromuscular blocking drugs, succinylcholine, citrate-anticoagulated blood • Potential inactivation

Adverse effects in *Italics* are most common; those in **Bold** are life-threatening.

of both drugs if mixed with beta-lactam-type antibiotics • Increased bactericidal effect if combined with penicillins, cephalosporins, carbenicillin, ticarcillin • Decreased absorption and therapeutic effects of digoxin if taken concurrently

Drug-lab test interferences
• Falsely low serum aminoglycoside levels in patients receiving concomitant penicillin or cephalosporin therapy; these antibiotics can inactivate aminoglycosides after the blood sample is drawn.

■ Nursing Considerations

Assessment
- *History:* Allergy to aminoglycosides; intestinal obstruction, diminished hearing, decreased renal function, dehydration, neuromuscular disorders; pregnancy, lactation
- *Physical:* Renal function, eighth cranial nerve function, state of hydration, CBC, skin color and lesions, orientation and affect, reflexes, bilateral grip strength, body weight, bowel sounds

Implementation
- Arrange culture and sensitivity tests of infection before beginning therapy.
- Administer parenteral preparation only by deep IM injection. Prepare solution by adding 2 ml Sodium Chloride Injection to 500-mg vial. Store unreconstituted solution at room temperature; refrigerate reconstituted solution; protect from light and use within 1 wk.
- Ensure that the patient is well hydrated.

Drug-specific teaching points
- Report hearing changes, dizziness, severe diarrhea.

❐ neostigmine bromide, oral

(nee oh stig' meen)
Prostigmin

neostigmine methylsulfate, parenteral
Prostigmin

Pregnancy Category C

Drug classes
Cholinesterase inhibitor
Parasympathomimetic drug (indirectly acting)
Urinary tract stimulant
Antimyasthenic drug
Antidote

Therapeutic actions
Increases the concentration of acetylcholine at the sites of cholinergic transmission, and prolongs and exaggerates the effects of acetylcholine by reversibly inhibiting the enzyme acetylcholinesterase, causing parasympathomimetic effects and facilitating transmission at the skeletal neuromuscular junction; also has direct cholinomimetic activity on skeletal muscle; may have direct cholinomimetic activity on neurons in autonomic ganglia and the CNS.

Indications
- Prevention and treatment of postoperative distention and urinary retention (neostigmine methylsulfate)
- Symptomatic control of myasthenia gravis
- Diagnosis of myasthenia gravis (edrophonium preferred)
- Antidote for nondepolarizing neuromuscular junction blockers (eg, tubocurarine) after surgery

Contraindications/cautions
- Contraindicated in the presence of hypersensitivity to anticholinesterases; adverse reactions to bromides (neostigmine bromide); intestinal or urogenital tract obstruction, peritonitis; pregnancy (may stimulate uterus and induce premature labor); lactation.
- Use caution in the presence of asthma, peptic ulcer, bradycardia, cardiac arrhythmias, recent coronary occlusion, vagotonia, hyperthyroidism, epilepsy.

Dosage
Adult
- ***Prevention of postoperative distention and urinary retention:*** 1 ml of the 1:4,000 solution (0.25 mg) neostigmine methylsulfate SC or IM as

- Use caution in the presence of the elderly or any patient with diminished hearing, decreased renal function, dehydration, neuromuscular disorders (myasthenia gravis, parkinsonism, infant botulism).

Dosage
IM or IV (dosage is the same).
Adult
- ***Complicated UTIs:*** 1.5–2 mg/kg q12h.
- ***Systemic infections:*** 1.3–2.2 mg/kg q8h or 2–3.25 mg/kg q12h.

Pediatric (6 wk–12 y): 1.8–2.7 mg/kg q8h or 2.7–4 mg/kg q12h.
Neonates: 2–3.25 mg/kg q12h.
Geriatric or renal failure patients: Reduce dosage, and carefully monitor serum drug levels and renal function tests throughout treatment. Manufacturer suggests three ways to adjust dosage based on serum creatinine or creatinine clearance; see package insert.

Pharmacokinetics

Route	Onset	Peak
IM	Rapid	30–60 min
IV	Immediate	End of infusion

Metabolism: Hepatic, $T_{1/2}$: 2–2.5 h
Distribution: Crosses placenta; enters breast milk
Excretion: Urine

IV facts
Preparation: Dilute with 50–200 ml of solution. Stable when stored in glass in concentrations of 2.1–3 mg/ml for up to 72 h at room temperature or refrigerated. Discard after that time.
Infusion: Infuse over ½–2 h.
Compatibilities: Compatible with Sterile Water for Injection; 0.9% Sodium Chloride Injection alone or with 5% Dextrose; 5% or 10% Dextrose Injection in Water; 5% Dextrose with Electrolyte #48 or #75; Ringer's and Lactated Ringer's; Lactated Ringer's and 5% Dextrose Injecton; Plasma-Lyte 56 or 148 Injection with 5% Dextrose; 10% Travert with Electrolyte #2 or #3 Injection; Isolyte E, M, or P with 5% Dextrose Injection; 10% Dextran 40 or 6% Dextran 75 in 5% Dextrose Injection; Plasma-Lyte M Injection with 5% Dextrose; Ionosol B in D5W; Normosol-R; Plasma-Lyte 148 Injection; 10% Fructose Injection; Electrolyte #3 with 10% Invert Sugar Injection; Normosol-M or R in D5W, Isolyte H or S with 5% Dextrose; Isolyte S; Plasma-Lyte 148 Injection in Water; Normosol-R pH 7.4.

Adverse effects
- CNS: Ototoxicity—*tinnitus, dizziness, ringing in the ears*, vertigo, deafness (partially reversible to irreversible), vestibular paralysis, confusion, disorientation, depression, lethargy, nystagmus, visual disturbances, headache, *numbness, tingling*, tremor, paresthesias, muscle twitching, convulsions, muscular weakness, neuromuscular blockade
- GI: Hepatic toxicity, *nausea, vomiting, anorexia*, weight loss, stomatitis
- CV: Palpitations, hypotension, hypertension
- Hematologic: **Leukemoid reaction,** agranulocytosis, granulocytosis, leukopenia, leukocytosis, thrombocytopenia, eosinophilia, pancytopenia, anemia, hemolytic anemia, increased or decreased reticulocyte count, electrolyte disturbances
- GU: *Nephrotoxicity*
- Hypersensitivity: *Purpura, rash*, urticaria, exfoliative dermatitis, itching
- Local: *Pain, irritation, arachnoiditis at IM injection sites*
- Other: Fever, apnea, splenomegaly, joint pain, *superinfections*

Clinically important drug-drug interactions
- Increased ototoxic, nephrotoxic, neurotoxic effects if taken with other aminoglycosides, cephalothin, potent diuretics • Increased neuromuscular blockade and muscular paralysis when given with anesthetics, nondepolarizing neuromuscular blocking drugs, succinylcholine, citrate-anticoagulated blood • Potential inactivation

788 ■ nicardipine hydrochloride

of both drugs if mixed with beta-lactam-type antibiotics Increased bactericidal effect if combined with penicillins, cephalopsorins, carbenicillin, ticarcillin

■ Nursing Considerations

Assessment
- *History:* Allergy to aminoglycosides; intestinal obstruction (oral); pregnancy; lactation; diminished hearing; decreased renal function, dehydration, neuromuscular disorders
- *Physical:* Body weight, renal function, eighth cranial nerve function, state of hydration, hepatic function, CBC, skin—color and lesions, orientation and affect, reflexes, bilateral grip strength, bowel sounds

Implementation
- Arrange culture and sensitivity tests of infection before beginning therapy.
- Limit duration of treatment to short term to reduce the risk of toxicity; usual duration of treatment is 7–14 d.
- Administer IM dose by deep intramuscular injection.
- Ensure that patient is well hydrated before and during therapy.

Drug-specific teaching points
- Know that the following side effects may occur: nausea, loss of appetite (small, frequent meals may help); diarrhea; superinfections in mouth, vagina (report for appropriate treatment).
- Report any hearing changes, dizziness, lesions in mouth, vaginal itching.

☐ nicardipine hydrochloride

(nye kar' de peen)
Cardene, Cardene SR, Cardene IV

Pregnancy Category C

Drug classes
Calcium channel-blocker
Antianginal drug
Antihypertensive

Therapeutic actions
Inhibits the movement of calcium ions across the membranes of cardiac and arterial muscle cells; calcium is involved in the generation of the action potential in specialized automatic and conducting cells in the heart, in arterial smooth muscle, and in excitation-contraction coupling in cardiac muscle cells. Inhibition of calcium flow results in the depression of impulse formation in specialized cardiac pacemaker cells, in slowing of the velocity of conduction of the cardiac impulse, in the depression of myocardial contractility, and in the dilation of coronary arteries and arterioles and peripheral arterioles; these effects lead to decreased cardiac work, decreased cardiac energy consumption, and increased delivery of oxygen to myocardial cells.

Indications
- Chronic stable (effort-associated) angina. Use alone or with beta-blockers.
- Management of essential hypertension alone or with other antihypertensives (immediate release and sustained release)
- Short-term treatment of hypertension when oral use is not feasible (IV)

Contraindications/cautions
- Contraindicated in the presence of allergy to nicardipine, pregnancy, lactation.
- Use caution in the presence of impaired hepatic or renal function, sick sinus syndrome, heart block (second or third degree).

Dosage
Adult
- *Angina:* Immediate release only. Individualize dosage. Usual initial dose is 20 mg tid PO. Range 20–40 mg tid PO. Allow at least 3 d before increasing dosage to ensure steady-state plasma levels.
- *Hypertension:* Immediate release. *Initial dose:* 20 mg tid PO. Range 20–40 mg tid. The maximum blood pressure-lowering effect occurs in 1–2 h. Adjust dosage based on BP response, allow at least 3 d before increasing dosage. *Sustained release:* Initial dose is 30 mg bid PO. *Range:* 30–60 mg bid.

niclosamide ■ 789

Pediatric: Safety and efficacy not established.

Geriatric or renal or hepatic impairment
- **Renal impairment:** Titrate dose beginning with 20 mg tid PO (immediate release).
- **Hepatic impairment:** Starting dose 20 mg bid PO (immediate release) with individual titration.

Pharmacokinetics

Route	Onset	Peak
Oral	20 min	0.5–2 h

Metabolism: Hepatic, $T_{1/2}$: 2–4 h
Distribution: Crosses placenta; enters breast milk
Excretion: Urine

IV facts
Preparation: Dilute each amp with 240 ml of solution; store at room temperature; protect from light; stable for 24 h.
Infusion: Slow IV infusion.
Compatibilities: Dextrose 5% Injection, Dextrose 5% and Sodium Chloride 0.45% or 0.9% Injection; Dextrose 5% with Potassium; 0.45% or 0.9% Sodium Chloride. Do not mix with 5% Sodium Bicarbonate or Lactated Ringer's.

Adverse effects
- CNS: *Dizziness, lightheadedness, headache, asthenia,* fatigue
- GI: *Nausea,* hepatic injury
- CV: *Peripheral edema, angina,* hypotension, arrhythmias, *bradycardia, AV block,* **asystole**
- Dermatologic: *Flushing,* rash

Clinically important drug-drug interactions
- Increased serum levels and toxicity of cyclosporine if taken concurrently

■ Nursing Considerations

Assessment
- *History:* Allergy to nicardipine, impaired hepatic or renal function, sick sinus syndrome, heart block (second or third degree), pregnancy, lactation
- *Physical:* Skin—lesions, color, edema; P, BP, baseline ECG, peripheral perfusion, auscultation; R, adventitious sounds; liver evaluation, normal GI output; liver and renal function tests, urinalysis

Implementation
- Monitor patient carefully (BP, cardiac rhythm, and output) while drug is being titrated to therapeutic dose; dosage may be increased more rapidly in hospitalized patients under close supervision.
- Monitor BP very carefully if patient is on concurrent doses of nitrates.
- Monitor cardiac rhythm regularly during stabilization of dosage and periodically during long-term therapy.
- Provide small, frequent meals if GI upset occurs.

Drug-specific teaching points
- Know that the following side effects may occur: nausea, vomiting (small, frequent meals may help); headache (monitor the lighting, noise, and temperature; medication may be ordered if this becomes severe).
- Report irregular heart beat, shortness of breath, swelling of the hands or feet, pronounced dizziness, constipation.

❒ niclosamide

*(ni **kloe**' sa mide)*
Niclocide

Pregnancy Category B

Drug classes
Anthelmintic

Therapeutic actions
Inhibits oxidative phosphorylation in the mitochondria of cestodes. The scolex and proximal segments of the cestode are killed on contact with the drug.

Adverse effects in *Italics* are most common; those in **Bold** are life-threatening.

Indications
- Treatment of *Taenia saginata* (beef tapeworm), *Diphyllobothrium latum* (fish tapeworm), *Hymenolepis nana* (dwarf tapeworm)

Contraindications/cautions
- Allergy to niclosamide, pregnancy, lactation.

Dosage
Adult
- ***T. saginata, D. latum (beef tapeworm):*** 4 tablets (2 g) PO as a single dose. Repeat dose if stool culture is positive after seventh day after therapy.
- ***H. nana (dwarf tapeworm):*** 4 tablets (2 g) PO as a single dose for 7 d.

Pediatric: Safety for use in children younger than 2 y not established.
- ***T. saginata, D. latum:*** > 34 kg, 3 tablets (1.5 g) PO as a single dose. 11–34 kg, 2 tablets (1 g) PO as a single dose. Repeat dose if stool culture is positive after seventh day after therapy.
- ***H. nana:*** > 34 kg, 3 tablets (1.5 g) PO on the first day, then 2 tablets (1 g) for next 6 d. 11–34 kg, 2 tablets (1 g) PO on the first day, then 1 tablet (0.5 g) for the next 6 d.

Pharmacokinetics
Not generally absorbed systemically.
Excretion: Feces

Adverse effects
- **CNS:** Drowsiness, dizziness, headache
- **GI:** *Nausea, vomiting, abdominal discomfort, loss of appetite,* diarrhea, constipation, rectal bleeding, oral irritation, bad taste in mouth
- **Dermatologic:** Skin rash, pruritus ani, alopecia
- **Other:** Fever, sweating, palpitations, irritability, backache

■ Nursing Considerations
Assessment
- *History:* Allergy to niclosamide, pregnancy, lactation
- *Physical:* Skin—color, lesions; temperature; orientation, reflexes; bowel sounds, output

Implementation
- Culture for ova and parasites. Reculture at least 4 d after therapy is finished and periodically for 3 mo.
- Administer drug with food, preferably after a light meal; have patient chew tablets and swallow with a little water; tablet may be crushed and mixed to a paste with food or water.

Drug-specific teaching points
- Be aware that this drug should be chewed and swallowed with a small amount of water. Children may have the tablet crushed and mixed with food. Take after a light meal.
- Know that the following side effects may occur: nausea, abdominal pain, GI upset (small, frequent meals may help); constipation (a mild laxative may be needed); drowsiness, dizziness (use caution if driving a car or operating dangerous equipment if these occur).
- Report fever, rash, severe abdominal pain, marked weakness, dizziness.

▢ nicotine polacrilex

(nik' oh teen)

nicotine resin complex
Nicorette, Nicorette DS

Pregnancy Category X

Drug classes
Smoking deterrent

Therapeutic actions
Acts as an agonist at nicotinic receptors in the peripheral and CNS; produces behavioral stimulation and depression, cardiac acceleration, peripheral vasoconstriction, and elevated blood pressure.

Indications
- Temporary aid to the cigarette smoker seeking to give up smoking while in a behavioral modification program under medical supervision

---

Adverse effects in *Italics* are most common; those in **Bold** are life-threatening.

Contraindications/cautions
- Contraindicated in the presence of allergy to nicotine or resin used; nonsmoker; post-MI period; arrhythmias; angina pectoris; active TMJ disease; pregnancy; lactation.
- Use caution in the presence of hyperthyroidism, pheochromocytoma, type II diabetes (releases catecholamines from the adrenal medulla); hypertension, peptic ulcer disease.

Dosage
Adult: Have patient chew one piece of gum whenever the urge to smoke occurs. Chew each piece slowly and intermittently for about 30 min to promote even, slow, buccal absorption of nicotine. Patients often require 10 pieces/d during the first month. Do not exceed 30 pieces/d (2 mg) or 20 pieces/d (4 mg). Therapy may be effective for up to 3 mo; 4–6 mo for complete cessation has been used. Should not be used for longer than 6 mo.

Pediatric: Safety and efficacy in children and adolescents who smoke have not been established.

Pharmacokinetics

Route	Onset	Peak
Oral	Slow	15–30 min

Metabolism: Hepatic, $T_{1/2}$: 30–120 min
Distribution: Crosses placenta; enters breast milk
Excretion: Urine

Adverse effects
- **CNS:** Dizziness, lightheadedness
- **GI:** *Mouth or throat soreness; hiccoughs, nausea, vomiting,* nonspecific GI distress, excessive salivation
- **Local:** Mechanical effects of chewing gum—traumatic injury to oral mucosa or teeth, *jaw ache,* eructation secondary to air swallowing

Clinically important drug-drug interactions
- Increased circulating levels of cortisol, catecholamines with nicotine use, smoking—dosage of adrenergic agonists, adrenergic blockers may need to adjusted according to nicotine, smoking status of patient. Smoking increases metabolism and lowers blood levels of caffeine, theophylline, imipramine, pentazocine; decreases effects of furosemide, propranolol • Cessation of smoking may decrease absorption of glutethimide, decrease metabolism of propoxyphene

■ Nursing Considerations

Assessment
- *History:* Allergy to nicotine or resin used; nonsmoker; post-MI period; arrhythmias; angina pectoris; active TMJ disease; hyperthyroidism, pheochromocytoma, type II diabetes; hypertension, peptic ulcer disease; pregnancy; lactation
- *Physical:* Jaw strength, symmetry; orientation, affect; P, auscultation, BP; oral mucous membranes, abdominal exam; thyroid function tests

Implementation
- Review mechanics of chewing gum with patient; patient must chew the gum slowly and intermittently to promote even, slow absorption of nicotine; discard chewed gum in wrapper to prevent access by children or pets.
- Arrange to withdraw or taper use of gum in abstainers at 3 mo; effectiveness after that time has not been established, and patients may be using gum as substitute source for nicotine dependence.

Drug-specific teaching points
- Chew one piece of gum every time you have the desire to smoke. Chew slowly and intermittently for about 30 min; do not chew more than 30 pieces of gum each day. Discard chewed gum in wrapper to prevent access by children or pets.
- Abstain from smoking while you are using this drug.
- Know that the following side effects may occur: dizziness, headache, lightheadedness (use caution if driving or performing tasks that require alertness if this occurs); nausea, vomiting, increased

Adverse effects in *Italics* are most common; those in **Bold** are life-threatening.

nicotine transdermal

burping; jaw muscle ache (modifying your chewing technique may help).
- Report nausea and vomiting, increased salivation, diarrhea, cold sweat, headache, disturbances in hearing or vision, chest pain, palpitations.
- Do not offer to nonsmokers; serious reactions can occur if used by nonsmokers.

▢ nicotine transdermal

(nik' oh teen)
Habitrol, Nicoderm, Nicotrol, ProStep

Pregnancy Category X

Drug classes
Smoking deterrent

Therapeutic actions
Nicotine acts at nicotinic receptors in the peripheral and CNS; produces behavioral stimulation and depression, cardiac acceleration, peripheral vasoconstriction, and elevated blood pressure.

Indications
- Temporary aid to the cigarette smoker seeking to give up smoking while in a behavioral modification program under medical supervision
- Unlabeled use: improvement of symptoms of Gilles de la Tourette's syndrome

Contraindications/cautions
- Contraindicated in the presence of allergy to nicotine; nonsmokers; post-MI period; arrhythmias; angina pectoris; pregnancy; lactation
- Use caution in the presence of hyperthyroidism, pheochromocytoma, type II diabetes (releases catecholamines from the adrenal medulla); hypertension, peptic ulcer disease.

Dosage
Adult: Apply system, 5–22 mg, once every 24 h. Dosage is based on individual response and stage of withdrawal *Habitrol, Nicoderm*: 21 mg/d for first 6 wk; 14 mg/d for next 2 wk; 7 mg/d for next 2 wk. *Nicotrol*: 15 mg/d for first 6 wk; 10 mg/d for next 2 wk; 5 mg/d for last 2 wk. *ProStep*: 22 mg/d for 4–6 wk; 11 mg/d for 2–4 wk.
Pediatric: Safety and efficacy in children and adolescents who smoke have not been established.

Pharmacokinetics

Route	Onset	Peak	Duration
Derma	1–2 h	4–6 min	4–24 h

Metabolism: Hepatic, $T_{1/2}$: 3–4 h
Distribution: Crosses placenta; enters breast milk
Excretion: Urine

Adverse effects
- **CNS:** *Headache, insomnia,* abnormal dreams, dizziness, lightheadedness, sweating
- **GI:** Diarrhea, constipation, nausea, dyspepsia, abdominal pain, dry mouth
- **Respiratory:** Cough, pharyngitis, sinusitis
- **Local:** *Erythema, burning, pruritus* at site of patch, local edema
- **Other:** Back ache, chest pain, asthenia, dysmenorrhea

Clinically important drug-drug interactions
- Increased circulating levels of cortisol, catecholamines with nicotine use; smoking—dosage of adrenergic agonists, adrenergic blockers may need to be adjusted according to nicotine, smoking status of patient • Smoking increases metabolism and lowers blood levels of caffeine, theophylline, imipramine, pentazocine; decreases effects of furosemide, propranolol • Cessation of smoking may decrease absorption of glutethimide, decrease metabolism of propoxyphene

■ Nursing Considerations

Assessment
- *History:* Allergy to nicotine; nonsmoker; post-MI period; arrhythmias; angina pectoris; hyperthyroidism, pheochromocy-

Adverse effects in *Italics* are most common; those in **Bold** are life-threatening.

toma, type II diabetes; hypertension, peptic ulcer disease; pregnancy; lactation
- *Physical:* Jaw strength, symmetry; orientation, affect; P, auscultation, BP; oral mucous membranes, abdominal exam; thyroid function tests

Implementation
- Protect systems from heat; slight discoloration of system is not significant.
- Apply system to nonhairy, clean, dry skin site on upper body or upper outer arm; use only when the pouch is intact; use immediately after removal from pouch; use each system only once.
- Wash hands thoroughly after application; do not touch eyes.
- Wrap used system in foil pouch of newly applied system; fold over and dispose of immediately to prevent access by pets or children.
- Apply new system after 24 h; do not reuse same site for at least 1 wk. *Nicotrol:* apply a new system each day after waking, and remove at bedtime.
- Ensure that patient has stopped smoking; if the patient is unable to stop smoking within the first 4 wk of therapy, drug therapy should be stopped.
- Encourage patients who have been unsuccessful at any dose to take a "therapy holiday" before trying again; counseling should explore factors contributing to their failure and other means of success.

Drug-specific teaching points
- Protect systems from heat; slight discoloration of system is not significant.
- Apply system to nonhairy, clean, dry skin site on upper body or upper outer arm; use only when the pouch is intact; use immediately after removal from pouch; use each system only once.
- Wash hands thoroughly after application; do not touch eyes. Wrap used system in foil pouch of newly applied system; fold over and dispose of immediately to prevent access by pets or children.
- Apply new system after 24 h; do not reuse same site for at least 1 wk. *Nicotrol:* apply a new system each day after waking, and remove at bedtime.
- Abstain from smoking while you are using this drug.
- Know that the following side effects may occur: dizziness, headache, lightheadedness (use caution if driving or performing tasks that require alertness if this occurs); nausea, vomiting, constipation or diarrhea (small, frequent meals, regular mouth care may help); skin redness, swelling at application site (good skin care, switching sites daily may help).
- Report nausea and vomiting, diarrhea, cold sweat, chest pain, palpitations, burning or swelling at application site.

▢ nifedipine

(nye fed' i peen)
Adalat, Procardia, Procardia XL

Pregnancy Category C

Drug classes
Calcium channel-blocker
Antianginal drug
Antihypertensive

Therapeutic actions
Inhibits the movement of calcium ions across the membranes of cardiac and arterial muscle cells; inhibition of transmembrane calcium flow results in the depression of impulse formation in specialized cardiac pacemaker cells, in slowing of the velocity of conduction of the cardiac impulse, in the depression of myocardial contractility, and in the dilation of coronary arteries and arterioles and peripheral arterioles; these effects lead to decreased cardiac work, decreased cardiac energy consumption, and increased delivery of oxygen to myocardial cells.

Indications
- Angina pectoris due to coronary artery spasm (Prinzmetal's variant angina)
- Chronic stable angina (effort-associated angina)
- Treatment of hypertension (sustained-release preparation only)

- Orphan drug use: treatment of interstitial cystitis

Contraindications/cautions
- Contraindicated in the presence of allergy to nifedipine, pregnancy. Use caution in the presence of lactation.

Dosage
Adult: 10 mg tid PO initial dose. Maintenance range: 10–20 mg tid. Higher doses (20–30 mg tid–qid) may be required, depending on patient response. Titrate over 7–14 d. More than 180 mg/d is not recommended.
- ***Sustained release:*** 30–60 mg once daily. Titrate over 7–14 d.

Pharmacokinetics

Route	Onset	Peak
Oral	20 min	30 min
SR	20 min	6 h

Metabolism: Hepatic, $T_{1/2}$: 2–5 h
Distribution: Crosses placenta; enters breast milk
Excretion: Urine and feces

Adverse effects
- CNS: *Dizziness, lightheadedness, headache, asthenia,* fatigue, *nervousness,* sleep disturbances, blurred vision
- GI: *Nausea, diarrhea, constipation,* cramps, flatulence, hepatic injury
- CV: *Peripheral edema, angina,* hypotension, arrhythmias, *bradycardia, AV block,* asystole
- Dermatologic: *Flushing, rash,* dermatitis, pruritus, urticaria
- Other: *Nasal congestion, cough,* fever, chills, shortness of breath, muscle cramps, joint stiffnes, sexual difficulties

Clinically important drug-drug interactions
- Increased effects of nifedipine if taken concurrently with cimetidine, ranitidine

■ Nursing Considerations

Assessment
- *History:* Allergy to nifedipine; pregnancy; lactation
- *Physical:* Skin—lesions, color, edema; orientation, reflexes; P, BP, baseline ECG, peripheral perfusion, auscultation; R, adventitious sounds; liver evaluation, normal GI output; liver function tests

Implementation
- Monitor patient carefully (BP, cardiac rhythm, and output) while drug is being titrated to therapeutic dose; the dosage may be increased more rapidly in hospitalized patients under close supervision. *Do not exceed 30 mg/dose.*
- Ensure that patients do not chew or divide sustained-release tablets.
- Arrange to taper dosage of beta-blockers before beginning nifedipine therapy.
- Protect drug from light and moisture.

Drug-specific teaching points
- Do not chew or divide sustained-release tablets. Swallow whole.
- Know that the following side effects may occur: nausea, vomiting (small, frequent meals may help); dizziness, lightheadedness, vertigo (avoid driving, operating dangerous machinery while on this drug; take special precautions to avoid falling); muscle cramps, joint stiffness, sweating, sexual difficulties (these are all uncomfortable and should disappear when the drug therapy is stopped).
- Report irregular heart beat, shortness of breath, swelling of the hands or feet, pronounced dizziness, constipation.

▢ nimodipine

(nye moe' di peen)
Nimotop

Pregnancy Category C

Drug classes
Calcium channel-blocker

Therapeutic actions
Inhibits the movement of calcium ions across the membranes of cardiac and arterial muscle cells; inhibition of transmembrane calcium flow results in the

Adverse effects in *Italics* are most common; those in **Bold** are life-threatening.

depression of impulse formation in specialized cardiac pacemaker cells, in slowing of the velocity of conduction of the cardiac impulse, in the depression of myocardial contractility, and in the dilation of coronary arteries and arterioles and peripheral arterioles.

Indications
- Improvement of neurologic deficits due to spasm following subarachnoid hemorrhage (SAH) from ruptured congenital intracranial aneurysms in patients who are in good neurologic condition postictus (eg, Hunt and Hess Grades I–III)
- Unlabeled uses: treatment of common and classic migraines and chronic cluster headaches

Contraindications/cautions
- Allergy to nimodipine, impaired hepatic function, pregnancy (teratogenic), lactation.

Dosage
Adult: Begin therapy within 96 h of the SAH. 60 mg q4h PO for 21 consecutive d.
Pediatric: Safety and efficacy not established.

Pharmacokinetics

Route	Onset	Peak
Oral	Unknown	> 60 min

Metabolism: Hepatic, $T_{1/2}$: 1–2 h
Distribution: Crosses placenta; enters breast milk
Excretion: Urine

Adverse effects
- CNS: Dizziness, lightheadedness, *headache*, asthenia, fatigue
- GI: *Diarrhea,* nausea, hepatic injury
- CV: Peripheral edema, angina, *hypotension*, **arrhythmias**, bradycardia, AV block, asystole
- Dermatologic: Flushing, *rash*

■ Nursing Considerations

Assessment
- *History:* Allergy to nimodipine, impaired hepatic function, pregnancy, lactation
- *Physical:* Skin—lesions, color, edema; reflexes, affect, complete neurologic exam; P, BP, baseline ECG, peripheral perfusion, auscultation; R, adventitious sounds; liver evaluation, normal output; liver function tests, urinalysis

Implementation
- Begin therapy within 96 h of subarachnoid hemorrhage.
- Administer PO. If patient is unable to swallow capsule, make a hole in both ends of the capsule with an 18-gauge needle, and extract the contents into a syringe. Empty the contents into the patient's in-situ nasogastric tube, and wash down the tube with 30 ml of normal saline.
- Monitor neurologic effects closely to determine progress and patient response.

Drug-specific teaching points
- Take drug for 21 consecutive d.
- Know that the following side effects may occur: nausea, diarrhea (small, frequent meals may help); headache (monitor the lighting, noise, and temperature; medication may be ordered if this becomes severe).
- Report irregular heart beat, shortness of breath, swelling of the hands or feet, pronounced dizziness, constipation.

◻ nitrofurantoin

*(nye troe fyoor **an'** toyn)*

Furadantin, Furanite,
Nephronex (CAN), Nitrofan,
Novofuran (CAN)

nitrofurantoin macrocrystals
Macrodantin

Pregnancy Category B

Drug classes
Urinary tract anti-infective
Antibacterial drug

Therapeutic actions
Bacteriostatic in low concentrations, possibly by interfering with bacterial carbohy-

Adverse effects in *Italics* are most common; those in **Bold** are life-threatening.

drate metabolism; bactericidal in high concentrations, possibly by disrupting bacterial cell wall formation, causing cell death.

Indications
- Treatment of urinary tract infections caused by susceptible strains of *E. coli, S. aureus, Klebsiella, Enterobacter, Proteus*

Contraindications/cautions
- Contraindicated in the presence of allergy to nitrofurantoin, renal dysfunction, pregnancy, lactation.
- Use caution in the presence of G-6-PD deficiency, anemia, diabetes.

Dosage
Adult: 50–100 mg PO qid for 10–14 d. Do not exceed 400 mg/d.
- ***Chronic suppressive therapy:*** 25–50 mg PO qid.

Pediatric: Not recommended in children younger than 1 mo. 5–7 mg/kg per day in four divided doses PO.
- ***Chronic suppressive therapy:*** As low as 1 mg/kg per day in one to two doses.

Pharmacokinetics

Route	Onset	Peak
Oral	Rapid	30 min

Metabolism: Hepatic, $T_{1/2}$: 20–60 min
Distribution: Crosses placenta; enters breast milk
Excretion: Urine

Adverse effects
- **CNS:** Peripheral neuropathy, headache, dizziness, nystagmus, drowsiness, vertigo
- **GI:** *Nausea, abdominal cramps, vomiting, diarrhea, anorexia*, parotitis, pancreatitis, **hepatotoxicity**, sometimes fatal
- **Respiratory:** Pulmonary hypersensitivity, sometimes fatal
- **Hematologic:** Hemolytic anemia in G-6-PD deficiency; granulocytopenia, agranulocytosis, leukopenia, thrombocytopenia, eosinophilia, megaloblastic anemia
- **Dermatologic:** Exfoliative dermatitis, Stevens-Johnson syndrome, alopecia, pruritus, urticartia, angioedema
- **Other:** Superinfections of the GU tract, hypotension, muscular aches; *brown-rust urine*

Clinically important drug-drug interactions
- Delayed or decreased absorption of nitrofurantoin if taken with magnesium trisilicate, magaldrate

Drug-lab test interferences
- False elevations of serum glucose, bilirubin, alkaline phosphatase, BUN, urinary creatinine • False-positive urine glucose when using Benedict's reagent.

■ Nursing Considerations

Assessment
- *History:* Allergy to nitrofurantoin, renal dysfunction, G-6-PD deficiency, anemia, diabetes, pregnancy, lactation
- *Physical:* Skin—color, lesions; orientation, reflexes; R, adventitious sounds; liver evaluation; CBC; liver and kidney function tests; serum electrolytes; blood, urine glucose

Implementation
- Arrange for culture and sensitivity tests before and during therapy.
- Administer drug with food or milk to prevent GI upset.
- Arrange to continue drug for at least 3 d after a sterile urine specimen is obtained.
- Monitor clinical response; if no improvement is seen or a relapse occurs, send urine for repeat culture and sensitivity.
- Monitor pulmonary function carefully; reactions can occur within hours or weeks of nitrofurantoin therapy.
- Arrange for periodic CBC and liver function tests during long-term therapy.

Drug-specific teaching points
- Take drug with food or milk. Complete the full course of drug therapy to ensure

Adverse effects in *Italics* are most common; those in **Bold** are life-threatening.

a resolution of the infection. Take this drug at regular intervals around the clock; consult your nurse or pharmacist for help in setting up a schedule that does not interfere with your usual activities.
- Know that the following side effects may occur: nausea, vomiting, abdominal pain (small, frequent meals may help); diarrhea; drowsiness, blurring of vision, dizziness (observe caution if driving or using dangerous equipment); brown or yellow-rust urine (do not be concerned; this is an expected effect of the drug therapy).
- Report fever, chills, cough, chest pain, difficulty breathing, rash, numbness or tingling of the fingers or toes.

nitroglycerin, intravenous

(nye troe gli' ser in)
Nitro-Bid IV, Nitrostat IV, Tridil

nitroglycerin, sublingual
Nitrostat

nitroglycerin, sustained release
Nitroglyn, Nitrong

nitroglycerin, topical
Nitrobid, Nitrol, Nitrong, Nitrostat

nitroglycerin, transdermal
Nitro-Dur, Nitrodisc, Transderm-Nitro

nitroglycerin, translingual
Nitrolingual

nitroglycerin, transmucosal
Nitrogard

Pregnancy Category C

Drug classes
Antianginal drug
Nitrate

Therapeutic actions
Relaxes vascular smooth muscle with a resultant decrease in venous return and decrease in arterial blood pressure, which reduces left ventricular workload and decreases myocardial oxygen consumption.

Indications
- Acute angina: sublingual, translingual preparations
- Prophylaxis of angina: oral sustained release, sublingual, topical, transdermal, translingual, transmucosal preparations
- Angina unresponsive to recommended doses of organic nitrates or β-blockers (IV preparations)
- Perioperative hypertension (IV preparations)
- CHF associated with acute MI (IV preparations)
- To produce controlled hypertension during surgery (IV preparations)
- Unlabeled uses: reduction of cardiac workload in acute MI and in CHF (sublingual, topical); adjunctive treatment of Raynaud's disease (topical)

Contraindications/cautions
- Contraindicated in the presence of allergy to nitrates, severe anemia, early MI, head trauma, cerebral hemorrhage, hypertrophic cardiomyopathy, pregnancy, lactation.
- Use caution in the presence of hepatic or renal disease, hypotension or hypovolemia, increased intracranial pressure, constrictive pericarditis, pericardial tamponade, low ventricular filling pressure or low PCWP.

Dosage
Adult
- **Intravenous:** *Initial:* 5 μg/min delivered through an infusion pump. Increase by 5-μg increments every 3–5 min as needed. If no response at 20 μg, increase increments to 10–20 μg. Once a partial blood pressure response is obtained, reduce dose and lengthen dosage intervals; continually monitor patient response and titrate carefully.
- **Sublingual**
 – *Acute attack:* Dissolve 1 tablet under

tongue or in buccal pouch at first sign of anginal attack; repeat every 5 min until relief is obtained. Do not take more than 3 tablets/15 min. If pain continues or increases, patient should call physician or go to hospital.
- *Prophylaxis:* Use 5–10 min before activities that might precipitate an attack.
- **Sustained release (oral):** *Initial:* 2.5–2.6 mg tid or qid. Titrate upward by 2.5- or 2.6-mg increments until side effects limit the dose. Doses as high as 26 mg given four times daily have been used.
- **Topical:** *Initial dose:* ½ in q8h. Increase by ½ in to achieve desired results. Usual dose is 1–2 in q8h; up to 4–5 in q4h have been used. 1 inch = 15 mg nitroglycerin.
- **Transdermal:** Apply one pad each day. Titrate to higher doses by using pads that deliver more drug or by applying more than one pad.
- **Translingual:** Spray preparation delivers 0.4 mg/metered dose. At onset of attack, 1–2 metered doses into oral mucosa; no more than 3 doses/15 min should be used. If pain persists, seek medical attention. May be used prophylactically 5–10 min prior to activity that might precipitate an attack.
- **Transmucosal:** 1 mg q3–5h during waking hours. Place tablet between lip and gum above incisors, or between cheek and gum.

Pediatric: Safety and efficacy not established.

Pharmacokinetics

Route	Onset	Duration
IV	1–2 min	3–5 min
Sublingual	1–3 min	30–60 min
TL spray	2 min	30–60 min
Trans/tablet	1–2 min	3–5 h
Oral, SR	20–45 min	3–8 h
Topical ointment	30–60 min	2–12 h
Transdermal	30–60 min	24 h

Metabolism: Hepatic, $T_{1/2}$: 47–100 h

Distribution: Crosses placenta; enters breast milk
Excretion: Urine

IV facts

Preparations: Dilute in 5% Dextrose Injection or 0.9% Sodium Chloride Injection. Do not mix with other drugs; check the manufacturer's instructions carefully because products vary considerably in concentration and volume per vial. Use only with glass IV bottles and the administration sets provided. Protect from light and extremes of temperature.

Infusion: Do not give by IV push; regulate rate based on patient response.

Adverse effects

- CNS: Headache, apprehension, restlessness, weakness, vertigo, dizziness, faintness
- GI: Nausea, vomiting, incontinence of urine and feces, abdominal pain
- CV: Tachycardia, retrosternal discomfort, palpitations, **hypotension**, syncope, collapse, postural hypotension, angina
- Dermatologic: Rash, exfoliative dermatitis, cutaneous vasodilation with flushing, pallor, perspiration, cold sweat, contact dermatitis—transdermal preparations, topical allergic reactions—topical nitroglycerin ointment
- Local: Local burning sensation at the point of dissolution (sublingual)
- Other: Ethanol intoxication with high dose IV use (alcohol in diluent)

Clinically important drug-drug interactions

• Increased risk of hypertension and decreased antianginal effect if taken concurrently with ergot alkaloids • Decreased pharmacologic effects of heparin if taken concurrently

Drug-lab test interferences

• False report of decreased serum cholesterol if done by the Zlatkis-Zak color reaction

Adverse effects in *Italics* are most common; those in **Bold** are life-threatening.

nitroglycerin, intravenous ■ 799

■ Nursing Considerations

Assessment

- *History:* Allergy to nitrates, severe anemia, early MI, head trauma, cerebral hemorrhage, hypertrophic cardiomyopathy, hepatic or renal disease, hypotension or hypovolemia, increased intracranial pressure, constrictive pericarditis, pericardial tamponade, low ventricular filling pressure or low PCWP, pregnancy, lactation
- *Physical:* Skin—color, temperature, lesions; orientation, reflexes, affect; P, BP, orthostatic BP, baseline ECG, peripheral perfusion; R, adventitious sounds; liver evaluation, normal output; liver and renal function tests (IV); CBC, Hgb

Implementation

- Administer sublingual preparations under the tongue or in the buccal pouch. Encourage patient not to swallow. Ask patient if the tablet "fizzles" or burns. Always check the expiration date on the bottle; store at room temperature, protected from light. Discard unused drug 6 mo after bottle is opened (conventional tablets); stabilized tablets (*Nitrostat*) are less subject to loss of potency.
- Administer sustained-release preparations with water; tell the patient not to chew the tablets or capsules; do not crush these preparations.
- Administer topical ointment by applying the ointment over a 6 × 6 inch area in a thin, uniform layer using the applicator. Cover area with plastic wrap held in place by adhesive tape. Rotate sites of application to decrease the chance of inflammation and sensitization; close tube tightly when finished.
- Administer transdermal systems to skin site free of hair and not subject to much movement. Shave areas that have a lot of hair. Do not apply to distal extremities. Change sites slightly to decrease the chance of local irritation and sensitization. Remove transdermal system before attempting defibrillation or cardioversion.
- Administer transmucosal tablets by placing them between the lip and gum above the incisors or between the cheek and gum. Encourage patient not to swallow and not to chew the tablet.
- Administer the translingual spray directly onto the oral mucosa; preparation is not to be inhaled.
- Arrange to withdraw drug gradually. 4–6 wk is the recommended withdrawal period for the transdermal preparations.

Drug-specific teaching points

- Place sublingual tablets under your tongue or in your cheek; do not chew or swallow the tablet; the tablet should burn or "fizzle" under the tongue. Take the nitroglycerin before chest pain begins, when you anticipate that your activities or situation may precipitate an attack. Do not buy large quantities; this drug does not store well. Keep the drug in a dark, dry place, in a dark-colored glass bottle with a tight lid; do not combine with other drugs. You may repeat your dose every 5 min for a total of ___ tablets. If the pain is still not relieved, go to an emergency room.
- Do not chew or crush the timed-release preparations; take on an empty stomach.
- Spread a thin layer of topical ointment on the skin using the applicator. Do not rub or massage the area. Cover with plastic wrap held in place with adhesive tape. Wash your hands after application. Keep the tube tightly closed. Rotate the sites frequently to prevent local irritation.
- Use transdermal systems, you may need to shave an area for application. Apply to a slightly different area each day. Use care if changing brands; each system has a different concentration.
- Place transmucosal tablets these between the lip and gum or between the gum and cheek. Do not chew; try not to swallow.
- Spray translingual spray directly onto oral mucous membranes; do not inhale. Use 5–10 min before activities that you anticipate will precipitate an attack.
- Know that the following side effects may occur: dizziness, lightheadedness (this may pass as you adjust to the drug; use care to change positions slowly); headache (lying down in a cool environment

and resting may help; OTC preparations may not help); flushing of the neck or face (this usually passes as the drug's effects pass).
- Report blurred vision, persistent or severe headache, skin rash, more frequent or more severe angina attacks, fainting.

☐ nitroprusside, sodium

*(nye troe **pruss**' ide)*

Nitropress

Pregnancy Category C

Drug classes
Antihypertensive drug (hypertensive emergencies)
Vasodilator

Therapeutic actions
Acts directly on vascular smooth muscle to cause vasodilation (arterial and venous) and reduce blood pressure. Mechanism involves interference with calcium influx and intracellular activation of calcium. Cardiovascular reflexes are not inhibited and reflex tachycardia, increased renin release occur.

Indications
- Hypertensive crises for immediate reduction of BP
- Controlled hypotension during anesthesia to reduce bleeding in surgical procedures in which this is appropriate
- Unlabeled use: severe refractory CHF and acute MI, alone or with dopamine

Contraindications/cautions
- Contraindicated in the treatment of compensatory hypertension; to produce controlled hypotension during surgery in patients with known inadequate cerebral circulation; emergency use in moribund patients.
- Use caution in the presence of hepatic, renal insufficiency (drug decomposes by cyanide, which is metabolized by the liver and kidneys to thiocyanate ion); hypothyroidism (thiocyanate inhibits the uptake and binding of iodine); pregnancy; lactation.

Dosage
Administer only by continuous IV infusion with Sterile 5% Dextrose in Water.

Adult and Pediatric: In patients not receiving antihypertensive medication, the average dose is 3 μg/kg per minute (range 0.5–10.0 μg/kg per minute). At this rate, diastolic BP is usually lowered by 30%–40% below pretreatment diastolic levels. Use smaller doses in patients on antihypertensive medication. Do not exceed infusion rate of 10 μg/kg per minute. If this rate of infusion does not reduce BP within 10 min, discontinue administration.

Geriatric or renal impaired: Use with caution and in initial low dosage. The elderly may be more sensitive to the hypotensive effects.

Pharmacokinetics

Route	Onset	Duration
IV	1–2 min	1–10 min

Metabolism: Hepatic, $T_{1/2}$: 2 min
Distribution: Crosses placenta; may enter breast milk
Excretion: Urine

IV facts
Preparation: Dissolve the contents of the 50-mg vial in 2–3 ml of 5% Dextrose in Water. Dilute the prepared stock solution in 250–1,000 ml of 5% Dextrose in Water, and promptly wrap container in aluminum foil or other opaque material to protect from light; the administration set tubing does not need to be covered. Observe solution for color changes. The freshly prepared solution has a faint brown tint; discard it if it is highly colored (blue, green, or dark red). If properly protected from light, reconstituted solution is stable for 24 h. Do not use the infusion fluid for administration of any other drugs.

Infusion: Infuse slowly to reduce likelihood of adverse effects; use an infusion pump, micro-drip regulator, or similar device to allow precise control of flow rate.
Incompatibilities: Do not mix in solution with any other drugs.

Adverse effects
- **CNS:** *Apprehension, headache, restlessness, muscle twitching*, dizziness
- **GI:** *Nausea, vomiting, abdominal pain*
- **CV:** *Restrosternal pressure, palpitations*, bradycardia, tachycardia, ECG changes
- **Hematologic:** Methemoglobinemia, antiplatelet effects
- **Dermatologic:** *Diaphoresis*, flushing
- **Endocrine:** Hypothyroidism
- **Local:** Irritation at injection site
- **Cyanide toxicity:** Increasing tolerance to drug and metabolic acidosis are early signs, followed by dyspnea, headache, vomiting, dizziness, ataxia, loss of consciousness, imperceptible pulse, absent reflexes, widely dilated pupils, pink color, distant heart sounds, shallow breathing (seen in overdose)

■ Nursing Considerations
Assessment
- **History:** Hepatic, renal insufficiency, hypothyroidism, pregnancy, lactation
- **Physical:** Reflexes, affect, orientation, pupil size; BP, P, orthostatic BP, supine BP, perfusion, edema, auscultation; R, adventitious sounds; renal, liver and thyroid function tests, blood acid–base balance

Implementation
- Monitor injection site carefully to prevent extravasation.
- Do not allow BP to drop too rapidly; do not lower systolic BP below 60 mm Hg.
- Provide amyl nitrate inhalation, materials to make 3% sodium nitrite solution, sodium thiosulfate on standby in case overdose of nitroprusside; depletion of patient's body stores of sulfur occur, leading to cyanide toxicity.
- Monitor blood acid–base balance (metabolic acidosis is early sign of cyanide toxicity), serum thiocyanate levels daily during prolonged therapy, especially in patients with renal impairment.

Drug-specific teaching points
- Anticipate frequent monitoring of BP, blood tests, checks of IV dosage, rate.

- Report pain at injection site, chest pain.

❒ nizatidine

(ni za' ti deen)
Axid Pulvules

Pregnancy Category C

Drug classes
Histamine H_2 antagonist

Therapeutic actions
Inhibits the action of histamine at the histamine H_2 receptors of the parietal cells of the stomach, inhibiting basal gastric acid secretion and gastric acid secretion that is stimulated by food, caffeine, insulin, histamine, cholinergic agonists, gastrin and pentagastrin. Total pepsin output also is reduced.

Indications
- Short-term and maintenance treatment of duodenal ulcer
- Short-term treatment of benign gastric ulcer
- Gastroesophageal reflux disease

Contraindications/cautions
- Contraindicated in the presence of allergy to nizatidine, lactation.
- Use caution in the presence of impaired renal or hepatic function, pregnancy.

Dosage
Adult
- ***Active duodenal ulcer:*** 300 mg PO qd at bedtime. 150 mg PO bid may be used.
- ***Maintenance of healed duodenal ulcer:*** 150 mg PO qd at bedtime.
- ***GERD:*** 150 mg PO bid.
- ***Benign gastric ulcer:*** 150 mg PO bid or 300 mg qd.

Pediatric: Safety and efficacy not established.

Geriatric or renal impaired: Creatinine clearance 20–50 ml/min: 150 mg/d PO for active ulcer; 150 mg every other day for maintenance. *Creatinine*

Adverse effects in *Italics* are most common; those in **Bold** are life-threatening.

802 ■ norepinephrine bitartrate

clearance < 20 ml/min: 150 mg PO every other day for active ulcer; 150 mg PO every 3 d for maintenance.

Pharmacokinetics

Route	Onset	Peak
Oral	Varies	$\frac{1}{2}$–3 h

Metabolism: Hepatic, $T_{1/2}$: 1–2 h
Distribution: Crosses placenta; enters breast milk
Excretion: Urine

Adverse effects

- **CNS:** *Dizziness, somnolence, headache, confusion, hallucinations,* peripheral neuropathy; symptoms of brainstem dysfunction (dysarthria, ataxia, diplopia)
- **GI:** *Diarrhea,* hepatitis, pancreatitis, hepatic fibrosis
- **CV:** Cardiac arrhythmias, **arrest**
- **Hematologic:** Neutropenia, agranulocytosis, increases in plasma creatinine, serum transaminase
- **Other:** *Impotence,* gynecomastia, rash, arthralgia, myalgia

Clinically important drug-drug interactions

- Increased serum salicylate levels if taken concurrently with aspirin

Drug-lab test interferences

- False-positive tests for urobilinogen

■ Nursing Considerations

Assessment

- *History:* Allergy to nizatidine, impaired renal or hepatic function, pregnancy, lactation
- *Physical:* Skin—lesions; orientation, affect; P, baseline ECG; liver evaluation, abdominal exam, normal output; CBC, liver and renal function tests

Implementation

- Administer drug at bedtime.
- Arrange for decreased doses in renal dysfunction and liver dysfunction.
- Prepare liquid by mixing 150 or 300 mg in apple juice, Gatorade, Ocean Spray; stable for 48 h refrigerated or at room temperature.
- Arrange for regular follow-up, including blood tests to evaluate effects.

Drug-specific teaching points

- Take drug at bedtime. Therapy may continue for 4–6 wk or longer.
- Take antacids exactly as prescribed, being careful of the times of administration. Do not take any OTC drugs, and avoid alcohol while you are on this medication. Many of these drugs contain ingredients that might interfere with this drug's effectiveness.
- Tell any physician, nurse, or dentist who is taking care of you that you are taking this drug. If you are on other medications, the dosage and timing of all of these drugs must be coordinated. If anything changes the drugs that you are taking, consult with your nurse or physician.
- Arrange to have regular medical follow-up while you are on this drug to evaluate your response to it.
- Report sore throat, fever, unusual bruising or bleeding, tarry stools, confusion, hallucinations, dizziness, muscle or joint pain.

☐ norepinephrine bitartrate

*(nor ep i **nef** rin)*
levarterenol

Pregnancy Category D

Drug classes

Sympathomimetic drug
Alpha-adrenergic agonist
Beta-1 adrenergic agonist
Cardiac stimulant
Vasopressor

Therapeutic actions

Vasopressor and cardiac stimulant; effects are mediated by alpha or beta-1 adrenergic receptors in target organs; potent norepinephrine bitartrate ■ 803

vasoconstrictor (alpha effect) acting in arterial and venous beds; potent positive inotropic agent (beta-1 effect), increasing the force of myocardial contraction and increasing coronary blood flow.

Indications
- Restoration of blood pressure in controlling certain acute hypotensive states (pheochromocytomectomy, sympathectomy, poliomyelitis, spinal anesthesia, MI, septicemia, blood transfusion, and drug reactions)
- Adjunct in the treatment of cardiac arrest and profound hypotension

Contraindications/cautions
- Hypovolemia (not a substitute for restoration of fluids, plasma, electrolytes, and should not be used in the presence of blood volume deficits except as an emergency measure to maintain coronary and cerebral perfusion until blood volume replacement can be effected; if administered continuously to maintain BP in the presence of hypovolemia, perfusion of vital organs may be severely compromised and tissue hypoxia may result); general anesthesia with halogenated hydrocarbons or cyclopropane, profound hypoxia or hypercarbia, mesenteric or peripheral vascular thrombosis (risk of extending the infarct); pregnancy.

Dosage
Individualize infusion rate on the basis of the patient's response.
Adult
- ***Restoration of BP in acute hypotensive states:*** Add 4 ml of the solution (1 mg/ml) to 1,000 ml of 5% Dextrose Solution for a concentration of 4 μg base/ml. Initially give 2–3 ml (8–12 μg base) per minute, IV. Adjust flow to establish and maintain a low normal blood pressure (usually 80–100 mm Hg systolic) sufficient to maintain circulation to vital organs; average maintenance rate of infusion is 2–4 μg/min. Occasionally enormous daily doses are necessary (68 mg base/d). Continue the infusion until adequate BP and tissue perfusion are maintained without therapy. Treatment may be required up to 6 d (vascular collapse due to acute MI). Reduce infusion gradually.
- ***Adjunct in cardiac arrest:*** Administer IV during cardiac resuscitation to restore and maintain BP after effective heartbeat and ventilation established.

Pharmacokinetics

Route	Onset	Duration
IV	Rapid	1–2 min

Metabolism: Neural, $T_{1/2}$: unknown
Distribution: Crosses placenta
Excretion: Urine

IV facts
Preparation: Dilute drug in 5% Dextrose Solution in Distilled Water or 5% Dextrose in Saline Solution; these dextrose solutions protect against oxidation. Do not administer in saline solution alone.
Infusion: Infusion rate is determined by patient response with constant BP monitoring.

Adverse effects
- CNS: *Headache*
- CV: *Bradycardia*, hypertension

Clinically important drug-drug interactions
- Increased hypertensive effects when given to patients receiving tricyclic antidepressants (eg, imipramine), guanethidine or reserpine, furazolidone, methyldopa • Decreased vasopressor effects when given with phenothiazines

■ Nursing Considerations
Assessment
- *History:* Hypovolemia, general anesthesia with halogenated hydrocarbons or cyclopropane, profound hypoxia or hypercarbia, mesenteric or peripheral vascular thrombosis, lactation
- *Physical:* Body weight, skin—color, temperature, turgor; P, BP; R, adventitious sounds; urine output; serum electrolytes, ECG

Adverse effects in *Italics* are most common; those in **Bold** are life-threatening.

Implementation
- Administer whole blood or plasma separately, if indicated.
- Administer IV infusions into a large vein, preferably of the antecubital fossa, to prevent extravasation.
- Do not infuse into femoral vein in elderly patients or those suffering from occlusive vascular disease (atherosclerosis, arteriosclerosis, diabetic endarteritis, Buerger's disease); occlusive vascular disease is more likely to occur in lower extremity.
- Avoid catheter tie-in technique, if possible, because stasis around tubing may lead to high local concentrations of drug.
- Monitor blood pressure every 2 min from the start of infusion until desired blood pressure is achieved, then monitor every 5 min if infusion is continued.
- Monitor infusion site for extravasation.
- Provide phentolamine on standby in case extravasation occurs (5–10 mg phentolamine in 10–15 ml saline should be used to infiltrate the affected area).
- Do not use drug solutions that are pink or brown; drug solutions should be clear and colorless.

Drug-specific teaching points
- Because norepinephrine is used only in acute emergency situations, patient teaching will depend on patient's awareness and will relate mainly to patient's status, monitors, and so forth rather than specifically to therapy with norepinephrine.

❏ norethindrone

(nor eth in' drone)
Norlutin

norethindrone acetate
Aygestin, Norlutate

Pregnancy Category X

Drug classes
Hormonal agent
Progestin

Therapeutic actions
Progesterone derivative. Progesterone transforms proliferative endometrium into secretory endometrium; inhibits the secretion of pituitary gonadotropins, which prevents follicular maturation and ovulation; and inhibits spontaneous uterine contraction. Progestins have varying profiles of estrogenic, antiestrogenic, anabolic, and androgenic activity.

Indications
- Treatment of amenorrhea; abnormal uterine bleeding due to hormonal imbalance
- Treatment of endometriosis
- Component of some oral contraceptive preparations

Contraindications/cautions
- Contraindicated in the presence of allergy to progestins; thrombophlebitis, thromboembolic disorders, cerebral hemorrhage or history of these conditions; hepatic disease, carcinoma of the breast or genital organs, undiagnosed vaginal bleeding, missed abortion; pregnancy; lactation.
- Use caution in the presence of epilepsy, migraine, asthma, cardiac or renal dysfunction.

Dosage
Administer PO only
Adult
- ***Amenorrhea; abnormal uterine bleeding:*** *Norethindrone*: 5–20 mg starting on day 5 and ending on day 25 of the menstrual cycle. *Norethindrone acetate*: 2.5–10 mg starting with day 5 of the menstrual cycle and ending on day 25.
- ***Endometriosis:*** *Norethindrone*: 10 mg/d for 2 wk. Increase in increments of 5 mg/d every 2 wk until 30 mg/d is reached. May be maintained for 6–9 mo or until breakthrough bleeding demands temporary termination. *Norethindrone acetate*: 5 mg/d for 2 wk. Increase in increments of 2.5 mg/d every 2 wk until 15 mg/d is reached. May be maintained for 6–9 mo or until breakthrough bleeding demands temporary termination.

Pharmacokinetics

Route	Onset
Oral	Varies

Metabolism: Hepatic, $T_{1/2}$: unknown
Distribution: Crosses placenta; enters breast milk
Excretion: Urine and feces

Adverse effects

- **CNS:** Sudden, partial or complete loss of vision, proptosis, diplopia, migraine, precipitation of acute intermittent porphyria, mental depression, pyrexia, insomnia, somnolence
- **GI:** Cholestatic jaundice, nausea
- **CV:** Thrombophlebitis, cerebrovascular disorders, retinal thrombosis, pulmonary embolism, thromboembolic and thrombotic disease, increased blood pressure
- **GU:** *Breakthrough bleeding, spotting, change in menstrual flow, amenorrhea,* changes in cervical erosion and cervical secretions, breast tenderness and secretion
- **Dermatologic:** *Rash with or without pruritus, acne,* melasma or chloasma, alopecia, hirsutism, photosensitivity
- **General:** *Fluid retention, edema, increase in weight*
- **Other:** Decreased glucose tolerance

Clinically important drug-drug interactions

- Inaccurate tests of hepatic and endocrine function.

■ Nursing Considerations

Assessment

- *History:* Allergy to progestins; thrombophlebitis, thromboembolic disorders, cerebral hemorrhage; hepatic disease, carcinoma of the breast or genital organs, undiagnosed vaginal bleeding, missed abortion; pregnancy; lactation; epilepsy, migraine, asthma, cardiac or renal dysfunction
- *Physical:* Skin—color, lesions, turgor; hair; breasts; pelvic exam; orientation, affect; ophthalmologic exam; P, auscultation, peripheral perfusion, edema; R, adventitious sounds; liver evaluation; liver and renal function tests, glucose tolerance, Pap smear

Implementation

- Arrange for pretreatment and periodic (at least annual) history and physical, which should include BP, breasts, abdomen, pelvic organs, and a Pap smear.
- Caution patient before beginning therapy of the need to prevent pregnancy during treatment, the need for frequent medical follow-up.
- Use caution when administering drug to ensure which preparation has been ordered and which one is being used; norethindrone acetate is approximately twice as potent as norethindrone.
- Arrange to discontinue medication and consult physician if sudden partial or complete loss of vision occurs; if papilledema or retinal vascular lesions are present on exam, the drug should be discontinued.
- Arrange to discontinue medication and consult physician at the first sign of thromboembolic disease: leg pain, swelling, peripheral perfusion changes, shortness of breath.

Drug-specific teaching points

- Follow a calendar with drug days marked.
- Know that the following side effects may occur: sensitivity to light (avoid exposure to the sun; use sunscreen and protective clothing if exposure is necessary); dizziness, sleeplessness, depression (use caution if driving or performing tasks that require alertness if these occur); skin rash, color changes, loss of hair; fever; nausea.
- Avoid pregnancy while taking this drug; serious fetal abnormalities or fetal death could occur.
- Report pain or swelling and warmth in the calves, acute chest pain or shortness of breath, sudden severe headache or vomiting, dizziness or fainting, numbness or tingling in the arm or leg.

Adverse effects in *Italics* are most common; those in **Bold** are life-threatening.

☐ norfloxacin

(nor *flox'* a sin)
Noroxin

Pregnancy Category C

Drug classes
Urinary tract anti-infective
Antibacterial drug

Therapeutic actions
Bactericidal; interferes with DNA replication in susceptible gram-negative bacteria, leading to cell death.

Indications
- For the treatment of adults with urinary tract infections caused by susceptible gram-negative bacteria, including *E. coli, Proteus mirabilis, K. pneumoniae, Enterobacter cloacae, Proteus vulgaris, Providencia rettgeri, Morganella morganii, Proteus aeruginosa, Citrobacter freundii, S. aureus, Staphylococcus epidermidis,* group D streptococci
- Uncomplicated urethral and cervical gonorrhea caused by *Neisseria gonorrhoeae*

Contraindications/cautions
- Contraindicated in the presence of allergy to norfloxacin, nalidixic acid or cinoxacin; pregnancy; lactation.
- Use caution in the presence of renal dysfunction, seizures.

Dosage
Adult
- **Uncomplicated urinary tract infections:** 400 mg q12h PO for 7–10 d. Maximum dose of 800 mg/d.
- **Complicated urinary tract infections:** 400 mg q12h PO for 10–21 d. Maximum dose of 800 mg/d.
- **Uncomplicated sexually transmitted disease:** 800 mg PO as a single dose.

Pediatric: Not recommended; produced lesions of joint cartilage in immature experimental animals.

Geriatric or impaired renal function: Creatinine clearance < 30 ml/min/1.73 m^2: 400 mg/d, PO for 7–10 d.

Pharmacokinetics

Route	Onset	Peak
Oral	Varies	2–3 h

Metabolism: Hepatic, $T_{1/2}$: 3–4.5 h
Distribution: Crosses placenta; enters breast milk
Excretion: Urine

Adverse effects
- **CNS:** *Headache*, dizziness, insomnia, fatigue, somnolence, depression, blurred vision
- **GI:** *Nausea*, vomiting, dry mouth, diarrhea, abdominal pain, dyspepsia, flatulence, constipation, heartburn
- **Hematologic:** Elevated BUN, SGOT, SGPT, serum creatinine and alkaline phosphatase; decreased WBC, neutrophil count, hematocrit
- **Other:** Fever, rash

Clinically important drug-drug interactions
- Decreased therapeutic effect of nofloxacin if taken concurrently with iron salts, sulcrafate • Decreased absorption of norfloxacin if taken with antacids • Increased serum levels and toxic effects of theophyllines if taken concurrently

■ Nursing Considerations
Assessment
- *History:* Allergy to norfloxacin, nalidixic acid or cinoxacin; renal dysfunction; seizures; pregnancy; lactation
- *Physical:* Skin—color, lesions; body temperature; orientation, reflexes, affect; mucous membranes, bowel sounds; renal and liver function tests

Implementation
- Arrange for culture and sensitivity tests before beginning therapy.
- Administer drug 1 h before or 2 h after meals with a glass of water.
- Ensure that patient is well hydrated during course of drug therapy.

Adverse effects in *Italics* are most common; those in **Bold** are life-threatening.

- Administer antacids if needed at least 2 h after dosing.
- Monitor clinical response; if no improvement is seen or a relapse occurs, send urine for repeat culture and sensitivity.

Drug-specific teaching points
- Take drug on an empty stomach, 1 h before or 2 h after meals. If an antacid is needed, do not take it within 2 h of norfloxacin dose.
- Drink plenty of fluids while you are on this drug.
- Know that the following side effects may occur: nausea, vomiting, abdominal pain (small, frequent meals may help); diarrhea or constipation; drowsiness, blurring of vision, dizziness (observe caution if driving or using dangerous equipment).
- Report rash, visual changes, severe GI problems, weakness, tremors.

❏ norgestrel

*(nor **jess'** trel)*
Ovrette
Pregnancy Category X

Drug classes
Hormonal agent
Progestin
Oral contraceptive

Therapeutic actions
Progestational agent; the endogenous female progestin, progesterone, transforms proliferative endometrium into secretory endometrium; inhibits the secretion of pituitary gonadotropins, which prevents follicular maturation and ovulation; and inhibits spontaneous uterine contractions. The primary mechanism by which norgestrel prevents conception is not known, but progestin-only oral contraceptives alter the cervical mucus, exert a progestional effect on the endometrium that interferes with implantation, and in some patients, suppress ovulation.

Indications
- Prevention of pregnancy in women who elect to use oral contraceptives; somewhat less efficacious (3 pregnancies per 100 woman years) than the combined estrogen/progestin oral contraceptives (about 1 pregnancy per 100 woman years, depending on the specific formulation)

Contraindications/cautions
- Contraindicated in the presence of allergy to progestins, tartrazine; thrombophlebitis, thromboembolic disorders, cerebral hemorrhage or history of these conditions; coronary artery disease; hepatic disease, carcinoma of the breast or genital organs, undiagnosed vaginal bleeding, missed abortion; as a diagnostic test for pregnancy; pregnancy (fetal abnormalities, including masculinization of the female fetus, congenital heart defects, and limb reduction defects have occurred); lactation.
- Use caution in the presence of epilepsy, migraine, asthma, cardiac or renal dysfunction.

Dosage
Adult: Administer daily, starting on the first day of menstruation. Take one tablet, PO, at the same time each day, every day of the year. *Missed dose:* 1 tablet—take as soon as remembered, then take the next tablet at regular time; 2 consecutive tablets—take 1 of the missed tablets, discard the other, and take daily tablet at usual time; 3 consecutive tablets—discontinue immediately.

Pharmacokinetics

Route	Onset
Oral	Varies

Metabolism: Hepatic, $T_{1/2}$: unknown
Distribution: Crosses placenta; enters breast milk
Excretion: Urine

Adverse effects
- CNS: Neuro-ocular lesions, mental depression, migraine, *changes in corneal curvature,* contact lens intolerance

Adverse effects in *Italics* are most common; those in **Bold** are life-threatening.

- **GI:** Gallbladder disease, liver tumors, hepatic lesions, *nausea, vomiting*, abdominal cramps, bloating, cholestatic jaundice MDNMO
- **CV:** *Thrombophlebitis, thrombosis*, pulmonary embolism, coronary thrombosis, MI, cerebral thrombosis, Raynaud's disease, arterial thromboembolism, renal artery thrombosis, cerebral hemorrhage, hypertension
- **GU:** *Breakthrough bleeding, spotting, change in menstrual flow, amenorrhea,* changes in cervical erosion and cervical secretions, endocervical hyperplasia, vaginal candidiasis
- **Dermatologic:** Rash with or without pruritus, acne, melasma
- **Other:** *Breast tenderness and secretion, enlargement*; fluid retention, edema, increase or decrease in weight

■ Nursing Considerations
Assessment
- *History:* Allergy to progestins, tartrazine; thrombophlebitis, thromboembolic disorders, cerebral hemorrhage; CAD; hepatic disease, carcinoma of the breast or genital organs, undiagnosed vaginal bleeding, missed abortion; epilepsy, migraine, asthma, cardiac or renal dysfunction; pregnancy; lactation
- *Physical:* Skin—color, lesions, turgor; hair; breasts; pelvic exam; orientation, affect; ophthalmologic exam; P, auscultation, peripheral perfusion, edema; R, adventitious sounds; liver evaluation; liver and renal function tests, glucose tolerance, Pap smear, pregnancy test if appropriate

Implementation
- Arrange for pretreatment and periodic (at least annual) history and physical, which should include BP, breasts, abdomen, pelvic organs and a Pap smear.
- Arrange to discontinue medication and consult physician if sudden partial or complete loss of vision occur; if papilledema or retinal vascular lesions are present on exam, the drug should be discontinued.
- Arrange to discontinue medication and consult physician at the first sign of thromboembolic disease: leg pain, swelling, peripheral perfusion changes, shortness of breath.

Drug-specific teaching points
- Take exactly as prescribed at intervals not exceeding 24 h. Take at bedtime or with a meal to establish a routine; medication must be taken daily for desired prevention of pregnancy; if you miss one tablet, take as soon as remembered, then take the next tablet at regular time. If you miss two consecutive tablets, take 1 of the missed tablets, discard the other, and take daily tablet at usual time. If you miss three consecutive tablets, discontinue immediately, and use another method of birth control until your cycle starts again. It is a good idea to use an additional method of birth control if any tablets are missed.
- Discontinue drug and consult your nurse or physician if you decide to become pregnant. It may be suggested that you use a nonhormonal form of birth control for a few months after stopping this drug and before becoming pregnant.
- Know that the following side effects may occur: sensitivity to light (avoid exposure to the sun; use sunscreen and protective clothing if exposure is necessary); dizziness, sleeplessness, depression (use caution if driving or performing tasks that require alertness if these occur); skin rash, skin color changes, loss of hair; fever; nausea; breakthrough bleeding or spotting (this may occur during the first month of therapy); intolerance to contact lenses due to corneal changes.
- Do not take this drug during pregnancy; serious fetal abnormalities have been reported. If you think that you are pregnant consult physician immediately.
- Tell any nurse, physician, or dentist who takes care of you that you are on this drug. This is important if another medication is prescribed, because some drugs are known to decrease the effectiveness

Adverse effects in *Italics* are most common; those in **Bold** are life-threatening.

of oral contraceptives and an additional method of birth control may be needed.
- Report pain or swelling and warmth in the calves, acute chest pain or shortness of breath, sudden severe headache or vomiting, dizziness or fainting, visual disturbances, numbness or tingling in the arm or leg, breakthrough bleeding or spotting that lasts into the second month of therapy.

◻ nortriptyline hydrochloride

*(nor **trip'** ti leen)*
Aventyl, Pamelor

Pregnancy Category C

Drug classes
Tricyclic antidepressant (TCA; secondary amine)

Therapeutic actions
Mechanism of action unknown; the TCAs are structurally related to the phenothiazine antipsychotic drugs (eg, chlorpromazine), but inhibit the presynaptic reuptake of the neurotransmitters norepinephrine and serotonin; anticholinergic at CNS and peripheral receptors; sedating; the relationship of these effects to clinical efficacy is unknown.

Indications
- Relief of symptoms of depression (endogenous depression most responsive)
- Unlabeled uses: treatment of panic disorders (25–75 mg/d), premenstrual depression (50–125 mg/d), dermatologic disorders (75 mg/d)

Contraindications/cautions
- Contraindicated in the presence of hypersensitivity to any tricyclic drug; concomitant therapy with an MAO inhibitor; recent MI; myelography within previous 24 h or scheduled within 48 h; pregnancy (limb reduction abnormalities reported); lactation.
- Use caution in the presence of electroshock therapy (increased hazard with TCAs); preexisting cardiovascular disorders (possibly increased risk of serious CVS toxicity with TCAs); angle-closure glaucoma, increased intraocular pressure, urinary retention, ureteral or urethral spasm (anticholinergic effects of TCAs may exacerbate these conditions); seizure disorders; hyperthyroidism (predisposes to CVS toxicity, including cardiac arrhythmias); impaired hepatic, renal function; psychiatric patients (schizophrenic or paranoid patients may exhibit a worsening of psychosis with TCA therapy); manic-depressive patients (may shift to hypomanic or manic phase); elective surgery (TCAs should be discontinued as long as possible before surgery).

Dosage
Adult: 25 mg tid–qid PO. Begin with low dosage and gradually increase as required and tolerated. Doses > 150 mg/d are not recommended.
Pediatric, adolescents: 30–50 mg/d PO in divided doses. Not recommended for use in children younger than 12 y.
Geriatric: 30–50 mg/d PO in divided doses.

Pharmacokinetics

Route	Onset	Peak	Duration
Oral	Varies	2–4 h	2–4 wk

Metabolism: Hepatic, $T_{1/2}$: 18–28 h
Distribution: Crosses placenta; enters breast milk
Excretion: Urine

Adverse effects
- CNS: *Sedation and anticholinergic (atropine-like) effects* (dry mouth, blurred vision, disturbance of accommodation for near vision, mydriasis, increased intraocular pressure), *confusion* (especially in elderly), *disturbed concentration*, hallucinations, disorientation, decreased memory, feelings of unreality, delusions, anxiety, nervousness, restless-

Adverse effects in *Italics* are most common; those in **Bold** are life-threatening.

ness, agitation, panic, insomnia, nightmares, hypomania, mania, exacerbation of psychosis, drowsiness, weakness, fatigue, headache, numbness, tingling, paresthesias of extremities, incoordination, motor hyperactivity, akathisia, ataxia, tremors, peripheral neuropathy, extrapyramidal symptoms, *seizures*, speech blockage, dysarthria
- **GI:** *Dry mouth, constipation*, paralytic ileus, *nausea*, vomiting, anorexia, epigastric distress, diarrhea, flatulence, dysphagia, peculiar taste, increased salivation, stomatitis, glossitis, parotid swelling, abdominal cramps, black tongue, hepatitis; elevated transaminase, altered alkaline phosphatase
- **CV:** *Orthostatic hypotension*, hypertension, syncope, tachycardia, palpitations, MI, arrhythmias, heart block, precipitation of CHF, stroke
- **Hematologic:** Bone marrow depression, including agranulocytosis; eosinophila; purpura; thrombocytopenia; leukopenia
- **GU:** Urinary retention, delayed micturition, dilation of the urinary tract, gynecomastia, testicular swelling in men; breast enlargement, menstrual irregularity and galactorrhea in women; increased or decreased libido; impotence
- **Hypersensitivity:** Skin rash, pruritus, vasculitis, petechiae, photosensitization, edema (generalized or of face and tongue), drug fever
- **Endocrine:** Elevated or depressed blood sugar; elevated prolactin levels; inappropriate ADH secretion
- **Withdrawal:** Symptoms with abrupt discontinuation of prolonged therapy: nausea, headache, vertigo, nightmares, malaise
- **Other:** Nasal congestion, excessive appetite, weight gain or loss; sweating, alopecia, lacrimation, hyperthermia, flushing, chills

Clinically important drug-drug interactions

- Increased TCA levels and pharmacologic (especially anticholinergic) effects when given with cimetidine, fluoxetine, ranitidine • Increased half-life and therefore increased bleeding if taken concurrently with dicumarol • Altered response, including dysrhythmias and hypertension if taken with sympathomimetics • Risk of severe hypertension when taken concurrently with clonidine • Hyperpyretic crises, severe convulsions, hypertensive episodes and deaths when MAO inhibitors are given with TCAs • Decreased hypotensive activity of guanethidine if taken concurrently • *Note:* MAOIs and tricyclic antidepressants have been used successfully in some patients resistant to therapy with single agents; however, case reports indicate that the combination can cause serious and potentially fatal adverse effects.

■ Nursing Considerations

Assessment

- *History:* Hypersensitivity to any tricyclic drug; concomitant therapy with an MAO inhibitor; recent MI; myelography within previous 24 h or scheduled within 48 h; pregnancy; lactation; electroshock therapy; preexisting cardiovascular disorders; angle-closure glaucoma, increased intraocular pressure, urinary retention, ureteral or urethral spasm; seizure disorders; hyperthyroidism; impaired hepatic, renal function; psychiatric patients; manic-depressive patients; elective surgery
- *Physical:* Body weight; temperature; skin—color, lesions; orientation, affect, reflexes, vision and hearing; P, BP, orthostatic BP, perfusion; bowel sounds, normal output, liver evaluation; urine flow, normal output; usual sexual function, frequency of menses, breast and scrotal examination; liver function tests, urinalysis, CBC, ECG

Implementation

- Ensure that depressed and potentially suicidal patients have access to only limited quantities of the drug.

Adverse effects in *Italics* are most common; those in **Bold** are life-threatening.

- Administer major portion of dose at bedtime if drowsiness, severe anticholinergic effects occur.
- Arrange to reduce dosage if minor side effects develop; arrange to discontinue the drug if serious side effects occur.
- Arrange for CBC if patient develops fever, sore throat, or other sign of infection during therapy.

Drug-specific teaching points
- Take drug exactly as prescribed; do not stop taking this drug abruptly or without consulting the physician or nurse.
- Avoid alcohol, other sleep-inducing, OTC drugs while on this drug.
- Avoid prolonged exposure to sunlight or sunlamps; use a sunscreen or protective garments if long exposure to sunlight is unavoidable.
- Know that the following side effects may occur: headache, dizziness, drowsiness, weakness, blurred vision (these effects are reversible; safety measures may need to be taken if these become severe, and you should avoid driving an automobile or performing tasks that require alertness while these persist); nausea, vomiting, loss of appetite, dry mouth (small, frequent meals, frequent mouth care and sucking sugarless candies may help); nightmares, inability to concentrate, confusion; changes in sexual function.
- Report dry mouth, difficulty in urination, excessive sedation.

☐ nystatin

(nye stat' in)
Oral, oral suspensions, oral troche: Mycostatin, Nadostine (CAN), Nilstat, Nystex
Vaginal preparations: Mycostatin
Topical application: Mycostatin, Nadostine (CAN), Nilstat, Nystex
Pregnancy Category A

Drug classes
Antifungal antibiotic

Therapeutic actions
Fungicidal and fungistatic: binds to sterols in the cell membrane of the fungus with a resultant change in membrane permeability, allowing leakage of intracellular components and causing cell death.

Indications
- Treatment of intestinal candidiasis (oral)
- Treatment of oral candidiasis (oral suspension, troche)
- Local treatment of vaginal candidiasis (moniliasis; vaginal)
- Treatment of cutaneous or mucocutaneous mycotic infections caused by *Candida albicans* and other *Candida* species (topical applications)

Contraindications/cautions
- Allergy to nystatin or components used in preparation.

Dosage
Oral: 500,000–1,000,000 U tid. Continue for at least 48 h after clinical cure.
Oral suspension: 400,000–600,000 U qid ($\frac{1}{2}$ of dose in each side of mouth, retaining the drug as long as possible before swallowing). *Troche:* Dissolve 1–2 tablets in mouth 4–5 times/day for up to 14 days.
- **Infants:** 200,000 U qid (100,000 in each side of mouth).
- **Premature and low–birth-weight infants:** 100,000 U qid.

Vaginal preparations: 1 tablet (100,000 U) intravaginally qd for 2 wk.
Topical: Apply to affected area two to three times per day until healing is complete. For fungal infections of the feet, dust powder on feet and in shoes and socks.

Pharmacokinetics
Not generally absorbed systemically. Excreted unchanged in the feces after oral use.

Adverse effects
Oral Doses
- GI: *Diarrhea, GI distress, nausea,* vomiting

Oral Suspension
- GI: *Nausea, vomiting, diarrhea*, GI distress

Vaginal
- Local: *Irritation, vulvovaginal burning*

Topical
- Local: *Local irritation*

■ Nursing Considerations

Assessment
- *History:* Allergy to nystatin or components used in preparation
- *Physical:* Skin—color, lesions, area around lesions; bowel sounds; culture of area involved

Implementation
- Arrange for appropriate culture of fungus involved before beginning therapy.
- Have patient retain oral suspension in mouth as long as possible before swallowing. Paint suspension on each side of the mouth. Continue local treatment for at least 48 h after clinical improvement is noted.
- Prepare nystatin in the form of frozen flavored popsicles to improve oral retention of the drug for local application.
- Administer nystatin troche orally for the treatment of oral candidiasis; have patient dissolve 1–2 tablets in mouth.
- Insert vaginal suppositories high into the vagina. Have patient remain recumbent for 10–15 min after insertion. Provide sanitary napkin to protect clothing from stains.
- Cleanse affected area before topical application, unless otherwise indicated.
- Monitor response to drug therapy. If no response is noted, arrange for further cultures to determine causative organism.
- Ensure that patient receives the full course of therapy to eradicate the fungus and to prevent recurrence.
- Discontinue topical or vaginal administration if rash or sensitivity occurs.

Drug-specific teaching points
- Take the full course of drug therapy even if symptoms improve. Continue during menstrual period if vaginal route is being used. Long-term use of the drug may be needed; beneficial effects may not be seen for several weeks. Vaginal suppositories should be inserted high into the vagina.
- Use appropriate hygiene measures to prevent reinfection or spread of infection.
- Be aware that this drug is specific for the fungus being treated; do not self-medicate other problems.
- Refrain from sexual intercourse or advise partner to use a condom to avoid reinfection; use a sanitary napkin to prevent staining of clothing with vaginal use.
- Know that the following side effects may occur: nausea, vomiting, diarrhea (oral use); irritation, burning, stinging (local use).
- Report worsening of the condition being treated; local irritation, burning (topical application); rash, irritation, pelvic pain (vaginal use); nausea, GI distress (oral administration).

☐ octreotide acetate

*(ok **trye'** oh tide)*
Sandostatin

Pregnancy Category B

Drug classes
Hormonal agent

Therapeutic actions
Mimics the natural hormone somatostatin; suppresses secretion of serotonin, gastrin, vasoactive intestinal peptide, insulin, glucagon, secretin, motilin, and pancreatic polypeptide; also suppresses growth hormone and decreases sphlanchnic blood flow.

Indications
- Symptomatic treatment of patients with metastatic carcinoid tumors to suppress or inhibit the associated severe diarrhea and flushing episodes
- Treatment of the profuse watery diarrhea associated with vasoactive intestinal polypeptide tumors (VIPomas)

Adverse effects in *Italics* are most common; those in **Bold** are life-threatening.

Contraindications/cautions
- Contraindicated in the presence of hypersensitivity to octreotide or any of its components.
- Use caution in the presence of renal impairment, thyroid disease, diabetes mellitus, pregnancy, lactation.

Dosage
Adult: SC injection is the route of choice. Initial dose is 50 μg SC qd or bid; the number of injections is increased based on patient response, usually two to three times per day. IV bolus injections have been used in emergency situations—not recommended.
- *Carcinoid tumors:* First 2 wk of therapy: 100–600 μg/d SC in two to four divided doses (mean daily dosage 300 μg).
- *VIPomas:* 200–300 μg SC in two to four divided doses during initial 2 wk of therapy to control symptoms. Range: 150–750 μg SC; doses above 450 μg are usually not required.

Pediatric: Safety and efficacy not established.
Geriatric or renal impaired: Half-life may be prolonged; adjustment of dosage may be necessary.

Pharmacokinetics

Route	Onset	Peak
SC	Rapid	15 min

Metabolism: Hepatic, $T_{1/2}$: 1.5 h
Distribution: Crosses placenta; may enter breast milk
Excretion: Urine

Adverse effects
- CNS: *Headache, dizziness, lightheadedness,* fatigue, anxiety, convulsions, depression, drowsiness, vertigo, hyperesthesia, irritability, forgetfulness, malaise, nervousness, visual disturbances
- GI: *Nausea, vomiting, diarrhea, abdominal pain, loose stools,* fat malabsorption, constipation, flatulence, hepatitis, rectal spasm, GI bleeding, heartburn, cholelithiasis, dry mouth, burning mouth
- CV: Shortness of breath, hypertension, thrombophlebitis, ischemia, CHF, palpitations
- **Respiratory:** Rhinorrhea
- **MS:** Asthenia/weakness, leg cramps, muscle pain
- **Dermatologic:** *Flushing,* edema, hair loss, thinning of skin, skin flaking, bruising, pruritus, rash
- **Endocrine:** *Hyperglycemia, hypoglycemia,* galactorrhea, clinical hypothyroidism
- **Local:** *Injection site pain*

■ Nursing Considerations

Assessment
- *History:* Hypersensitivity to octreotide or any of its components; renal impairment; thyroid disease, diabetes mellitus; lactation
- *Physical:* Skin—lesions, hair; reflexes, affect; BP, P, orthostatic BP; abdominal exam, liver evaluation, mucous membranes; renal and thyroid function tests, blood glucose, electrolytes

Implementation
- Administer by SC injection; avoid multiple injections in the same site within short periods of time.
- Monitor patients with renal function impairment closely; reduced dosage may be necessary.
- Store ampules in the refrigerator; may be at room temperature on day of use. Do not use if particulates or discoloration are observed.
- Monitor patient closely for endocrine reactions: blood glucose alterations, thyroid hormone changes.
- Arrange for baseline and periodic gall bladder ultrasound to pick up cholelithiasis.
- Monitor blood glucose, especially in the beginning of therapy, to detect hypoglycemia or hyperglycemia. Diabetic patients will require close monitoring.

Adverse effects in *Italics* are most common; those in **Bold** are life-threatening.

Drug-specific teaching points
- Be aware that this drug must be injected. You and a significant other can be instructed in the procedure of SC injections. Review technique and process periodically. Do not use the same site for repeated injections; rotate injection sites. Dosage will be adjusted based on your response to the drug.
- Know that the following side effects may occur: headache, dizziness, lightheadedness, fatigue (avoid driving or performing tasks that require alertness if these effects occur); nausea, diarrhea, abdominal pain (small, frequent meals may help; it is important to maintain your nutrition); flushing, dry skin, flaking of skin (appropriate skin care will help prevent breakdown); pain at the injection site.
- Arrange for periodic medical exams, including blood tests and gall bladder tests.
- Report sweating, dizziness, severe abdominal pain, fatigue, fever, chills, infection, or severe pain at injection sites.

ofloxacin

(oe flox' a sin)
Floxin, Ocuflox

Pregnancy Category C

Drug classes
Antibacterial drug

Therapeutic actions
Bactericidal; interferes with DNA replication in susceptible gram-negative bacteria, preventing cell reproduction.

Indications
- Lower respiratory tract infections caused by *Haemophilus influenzae, Streptococcus pneumoniae*
- Acute, uncomplicated urethral and cervical gonorrhea due to *Neisseria gonorrhoeae*, nongonococcal urethritis, and cervicitis due to *Chlamydia trachomatis*, mixed infections due to both
- Skin and skin-structure infections due to *Staphylococcus aureus, Staphylococcus pyogenes, Proteus mirabilis*
- Urinary tract infections due to *Citrobacter diversus, Enterobacter aerogenes, Escherichia coli, Klebsiella pneumoniae, Pseudomonas aeruginosa*
- Prostatitis due to *E. coli*
- Treatment of ocular infections caused by susceptible organisms
- Orphan drug use: treatment of bacterial corneal ulcers

Contraindications/cautions
- Contraindicated in the presence of allergy to fluoroquinolones, pregnancy, lactation.
- Use caution in the presence of renal dysfunction, seizures.

Dosage
Adult
- ***Uncomplicated urinary tract infections:*** 200 mg q12h PO or IV for 3 d.
- ***Complicated urinary tract infections:*** 200 mg bid PO or IV for 10 d.
- ***Lower respiratory tract infections:*** 400 mg q12h PO or IV for 10 d.
- ***Mild to moderate skin infections:*** 400 mg q12h PO or IV for 10 d.
- ***Prostatitis:*** 300 mg q12h PO or IV for 6 weeks.
- ***Acute, uncomplicated gonorrhea:*** 400 mg PO or IV as a single dose.
- ***Cervicitis, urethritis:*** 300 mg q12h PO or IV for 7 d.

Pediatric: Not recommended; produced lesions of joint cartilage in immature experimental animals.

Geriatric or impaired renal function: Ccr 10–50 ml/min, use a 24-h interval and adjust dosage; Ccr < 10 ml/min, use a 2-h interval and half the recommended dose.

Pharmacokinetics

Route	Onset	Peak	Duration
Oral	Varies	1–2 h	9 h
IV	10 min	30 min	9 h

Metabolism: Hepatic, $T_{1/2}$: 5–10 h

olsalazine sodium ■ 815

Distribution: Crosses placenta; enters breast milk
Excretion: Urine and bile

IV facts
Preparation: Dilute the single-dose vial to a final concentration of 4 mg/ml 0.9% NaCl Injection, 5% Dextrose Injection, 5% Dextrose/0.9% Sodium Chloride; 5% Dextrose in Lactated Ringer's; 5% Sodium Bicarbonate; Plasma-Lyte 56 in 5% Dextrose; 5% Dextrose, 0.45% Sodium Chloride and 0.15% Potassium Chloride; Sodium Lactate (M/6); Water for Injection. Premixed bottles require no further dilution. Discard any unused portion.

Infusion: Administer slowly over 60 min.

Adverse effects
- CNS: *Headache*, dizziness, *insomnia*, fatigue, somnolence, depression, blurred vision
- GI: *Nausea*, vomiting, dry mouth, *diarrhea*, abdominal pain
- Hematologic: Elevated BUN, SGOT, SGPT, serum creatinine and alkaline phosphatase; decreased WBC, neutrophil count, hematocrit
- Other: Fever, rash

Clinically important drug-drug interactions
- Decreased therapeutic effect of ofloxacin if taken concurrently with iron salts, sulcrafate • Decreased absorption of ofloxacin if taken with antacids

■ Nursing Considerations

Assessment
- *History:* Allergy to fluoroquinolones, renal dysfunction, seizures, lactation
- *Physical:* Skin—color, lesions; body temperature; orientation, reflexes, affect; mucous membranes, bowel sounds; renal and liver function tests

Implementation
- Arrange for culture and sensitivity tests before beginning therapy.
- Continue therapy for 2 d after the signs and symptoms of infection have disappeared.
- Administer oral drug 1 h before or 2 h after meals with a glass of water.
- Ensure that patient is well hydrated during course of drug therapy.
- Administer antacids, if needed, at least 2 h after dosing.
- Monitor clinical response; if no improvement is seen or a relapse occurs, repeat culture and sensitivity.

Drug-specific teaching points
- Take oral drug on an empty stomach, 1 h before or 2 h after meals. If an antacid is needed, do not take it within 2 h of ofloxacin dose.
- Drink plenty of fluids while you are on this drug.
- Know that the following side effects may occur: nausea, vomiting, abdominal pain (small, frequent meals may help); diarrhea or constipation; drowsiness, blurring of vision, dizziness (observe caution if driving or using dangerous equipment).
- Report rash, visual changes, severe GI problems, weakness, tremors.

❒ olsalazine sodium

*(ole **sal'** a zeen)*
Dipentum

Pregnancy Category C

Drug classes
Anti-inflammatory

Therapeutic actions
Mechanism of action is unknown; thought to be a direct, local anti-inflammatory effect in the colon where olsalazine is converted to mesalamine (5-ASA), which blocks cyclooxygenase and inhibits prostaglandin production in the colon.

Indications
- Maintenance of remission of ulcerative colitis in patients intolerant of sulfasalazine

Contraindications/cautions
- Contraindicated in the presence of hypersensitivity to salicylates, pregnancy

Adverse effects in *Italics* are most common; those in **Bold** are life-threatening.

(caused fetal abnormalities in preclinical studies).
- Use caution in the presence of lactation.

Dosage
Adult: 1 g/d PO in two divided doses.
Pediatric: Safety and efficacy not established.

Pharmacokinetics

Route	Onset	Peak
Oral	Varies	60 min

Metabolism: Hepatic, $T_{1/2}$: 0.9 h
Distribution: Crosses placenta; may enter breast milk
Excretion: Feces and urine

Adverse effects
- CNS: *Headache, fatigue, malaise, depression,* dizziness, asthenia, insomnia
- GI: *Abdominal pain, cramps, discomfort; gas; flatulence; nausea; diarrhea, dyspepsia,* bloating, hemmorhoids, rectal pain, constipation
- Other: *Flulike symptoms, rash,* fever, cold, rash, back pain, hair loss, peripheral edema, *arthralgia*

■ Nursing Considerations

Assessment
- *History:* Hypersensitivity to salicylates, pregnancy, lactation
- *Physical:* Temperature, hair status; reflexes, affect; abdominal and rectal exam; urinary output, renal function tests

Implementation
- Administer with meals in evenly divided doses.
- Monitor patients with renal impairment for possible adverse effects.

Drug-specific teaching points
- Take the drug with meals in evenly divided doses.
- Know that the following side effects may occur: abdominal cramping, discomfort, pain, diarrhea (taking the drug with meals may help); headache, fatigue, fever, flulike symptoms (medications may be available to help); skin rash, itching (skin care may help).
- Report severe diarrhea, malaise, fatigue, fever, blood in the stool.

☐ omeprazole

*(oh **me'** pray zol)*
Prilosec

Pregnancy Category C

Drug classes
Antisecretory agent

Therapeutic actions
Gastric acid-pump inhibitor: suppresses gastric acid secretion by specific inhibition of the hydrogen/potassium ATPase enzyme system at the secretory surface of the gastric parietal cells; blocks the final step of acid production.

Indications
- Short-term treatment of active duodenal ulcer
- Gastroesophageal reflux disease (GERD), severe erosive esophagitis, poorly responsive symptomatic GERD
- Treatment of pathologic hypersecretory conditions (eg, Zollinger-Ellison syndrome, multiple adenomas, systemic mastocytosis) (long-term therapy)
- Unlabeled use: treatment of duodenal ulcers at a dose of 20–40 mg/d

Contraindications/cautions
- Contraindicated in the presence of hypersensitivity to omeprazole or any of its components.
- Use caution in the presence of pregnancy, lactation.

Dosage
Adult
- ***Active duodenal ulcer:*** 20 mg PO qd for 4–8 wk.
- ***Severe erosive esophagitis or poorly responsive GERD:*** 20 mg PO daily for 4–8 wk. Do not use as maintenance therapy.

Adverse effects in *Italics* are most common; those in **Bold** are life-threatening.

- **Pathologic hypersecretory conditions:** Individualize dosage. Initial dose is 60 mg PO qd. Doses up to 120 mg tid have been used. Administer daily doses of > 80 mg in divided doses.

Pediatric: Safety and efficacy not established.

Pharmacokinetics

Route	Onset	Peak
Oral	Varies	0.5–3.5 h

Metabolism: Hepatic, $T_{1/2}$: 0.5–1 h
Distribution: Crosses placenta; may enter breast milk
Excretion: Urine and bile

Adverse effects
- CNS: *Headache, dizziness,* asthenia, vertigo, insomnia, apathy, anxiety, paresthesias, dream abnormalities
- GI: *Diarrhea, abdominal pain, nausea, vomiting,* constipation, dry mouth, tongue atrophy
- Respiratory: *URI symptoms,* cough, epistaxis
- Dermatologic: Rash, inflammation, urticaria, pruritus, alopecia, dry skin
- Other: Cancer in preclinical studies, back pain, fever

Clinically important drug-drug interactions
- Increased serum levels and potential increase in toxicity of benzodiazepines when taken concurrently

Nursing Considerations

Assessment
- *History:* Hypersensitivity to omeprazole or any of its components, pregnancy, lactation
- *Physical:* Skin—lesions; body temperature; reflexes, affect; urinary output, abdominal exam; respiratory auscultation

Implementation
- Administer before meals. Caution patient to swallow capsules whole, not to open, chew, or crush.
- Arrange for further evaluation of patient after 8 wk of therapy for gastroreflux disorders; not intended for maintenance therapy. Symptomatic improvement does not rule out gastric cancer, which did occur in preclinical studies.
- Administer antacids concomitantly with omeprazole, if needed.

Drug-specific teaching points
- Take the drug before meals. Swallow the capsules whole; do not chew, open, or crush. This drug will need to be taken for up to 8 wk (short-term therapy) or for a prolonged period (> 5 y in some cases), depending on the condition being treated.
- Arrange to have regular medical follow-up while you are on this drug.
- Know that the following side effects may occur: dizziness (avoid driving a car or performing hazardous tasks); headache (medications may be available to help); nausea, vomiting, diarrhea (proper nutrition is important); symptoms of upper respiratory tract infection, cough (it may help to know that this is a drug effect; do not self-medicate; consult with your nurse or physician if this becomes uncomfortable).
- Report severe headache, worsening of symptoms, fever, chills.

ondansetron hydrochloride

*(on **dan'** sah tron)*
Zofran

Pregnancy Category B

Drug classes
Antiemetic

Therapeutic actions
Blocks specific receptor sites (5-HT$_3$), which are associated with nausea and vomiting in the CTZ (chemoreceptor trigger zone) centrally and at specific sites peripherally. It is not known whether its antiemetic actions are from actions at the central, peripheral, or combined sites.

Adverse effects in *Italics* are most common; those in **Bold** are life-threatening.

ondansetron hydrochloride

Indications
- Treatment of nausea and vomiting associated with emetogenic cancer chemotherapy (parenteral and oral)
- Treatment of postoperative nausea and vomiting—to prevent further episodes or, when postoperative nausea and vomiting must be avoided, prophylactically (parenteral)

Contraindications/cautions
- Contraindicated in the presence of allergy to ondansetron.
- Use caution in the presence of pregnancy, lactation.

Dosage
Adult
- ***Antiemetic***
  - *Parenteral: Three 0.15 mg/kg doses IV:* first dose is given over 15 min, beginning 20 min before the chemotherapy; subsequent doses are given at 4 and 8 h, or a single 32-mg dose infused over 30 min beginning 30 min before the start of the chemotherapy.
  - *Oral:* 8 mg PO tid; administer the first dose 30 min before beginning the chemotherapy at 4 and 8 h; continue q8h for 1–2 d after the chemotherapy treatment.
- ***Prevention of postoperative nausea and vomiting:*** 4 mg undiluted IV over 2–5 min.

Pediatric
- ***Antiemetic:*** 4–18 y, IV dose same as adult; younger than 3 y, safety and efficacy not established; 4–12 y, 4 mg PO tid, using same schedule as adults.
- ***Prevention of postoperative nausea and vomiting:*** Safety and efficacy not established.
- ***Hepatic impairment:*** Do not exceed 8 mg PO; maximum daily dose of 8 mg IV.

Pharmacokinetics

Route	Onset	Peak
Oral	30–60 min	1.7–2.2 h
IV	Immediate	Immediate

Metabolism: Hepatic, $T_{1/2}$: 3.5–6 h

Distribution: Crosses placenta; may enter breast milk
Excretion: Urine

IV facts
Preparation: Dilute in 50 ml of 5% Dextrose Injection or 0.9% Sodium Chloride Injection; stable for 48 h at room temperature after dilution.
Infusion: Infuse slowly over 15 min diluted or 2–5 min undiluted.
Compatibilities: May be diluted with 0.9% Sodium Chloride Injection, 5% Dextrose Injection, 5% Dextrose and 0.9% Sodium Chloride injection; 5% Dextrose and 0.45% Sodium Chloride Injection; 3% Sodium Chloride Injection; do not mix with alkaline solutions.

Adverse effects
- **CNS:** *Headache, dizziness,* drowsiness, shivers, malaise, fatigue, weakness, *myalgia*
- **GI:** Abdominal pain, constipation
- **CV:** Chest pain, hypotension
- **GU:** Urinary retention
- **Dermatologic:** Pruritis
- **Local:** Pain at injection site

Clinically important drug-food interactions
- Increased extent of absorption of ondansetron if taken orally with food

■ Nursing Considerations

Assessment
- *History:* Allergy to ondansetron, pregnancy, lactation, nausea and vomiting
- *Physical:* Skin color and texture; orientation, reflexes, bilateral grip strength, affect; P, BP; abdominal exam; urinary output

Implementation
- Ensure that doses of drug are administered in the correct timing to the chemotherapy being given.
- Administer oral drug for 1–2 d following completion of chemotherapy.

Adverse effects in *Italics* are most common; those in **Bold** are life-threatening.

Drug-specific teaching points
- Take oral drug for 1–2 d following chemotherapy to maximize prevention of nausea and vomiting. Take the drug every 8 h around the clock for best results.
- Know that the following side effects may occur: weakness, dizziness (change position slowly to avoid injury); drowsiness (do not drive a car or perform tasks that require alertness if you experience these effects).
- Report continued nausea and vomiting, pain at injection site, chest pain, palpitations.

❐ opium preparations

(oh' pee um)
Paregoric, Camphorated Tincture of Opium

Pregnancy Category C
C-III controlled substance

Drug classes
Narcotic agonist analgesic
Antidiarrheal drug

Therapeutic actions
Activity is primarily due to morphine content; acts as agonist at specific opioid receptors in the CNS to produce analgesia, euphoria, sedation; the receptors mediating these effects are thought to be the same as those mediating the effects of endogenous opioids (enkephalins, endorphins); inhibits peristalsis and diarrhea by producing spasm of GI tract smooth muscle.

Indications
- Antidiarrheal
- Disorders in which the analgesic, sedative/hypnotic narcotic, or effect of an opiate is needed (no longer a drug of choice)
- For relief of severe pain in place of morphine (no longer a drug of choice)

Contraindications/cautions
- Contraindicated in the presence of hypersensitivity to narcotics, diarrhea caused by poisoning (before toxins are eliminated), pregnancy, labor or delivery (administration of narcotics to the mother can cause respiratory depression of neonate; premature infants are at special risk; may prolong labor), bronchial asthma, COPD, cor pulmonale, respiratory depression, anoxia, kyphoscoliosis, acute alcoholism, increased intracranial pressure.
- Use caution in the presence of acute abdominal conditions, cardiovascular disease, supraventricular tachycardias, myxedema, convulsive disorders, delirium tremens, cerebral arteriosclerosis, ulcerative colitis, fever, Addison's disease, prostatic hypertrophy, urethral stricture, recent GI or GU surgery, toxic psychosis, renal or hepatic dysfunction.

Dosage
Adult
- **Paregoric:** 5–10 ml PO qd–qid (5 ml is equivalent to 2 mg morphine).

Pediatric: Contraindicated in premature infants.
- **Paregoric:** 0.25–0.5 ml/kg PO qd–qid.

Geriatric or impaired adult: Use caution; respiratory depression may occur in elderly, the very ill, those with respiratory problems: reduced dosage may be necessary.

Pharmacokinetics

Route	Onset	Peak	Duration
Oral	Varies	0.5–1	3–7 h

Metabolism: Hepatic, $T_{1/2}$: 1.5–2 h
Distribution: Crosses placenta; enters breast milk
Excretion: Urine

Adverse effects
- CNS: *Lightheadedness, dizziness, sedation,* euphoria, dysphoria, delirium, insomnia, agitation, anxiety, fear, hallucinations, disorientation, drowsiness, lethargy, impaired mental and physical performance, **coma**, mood changes, weakness, headache, tremor, **convulsions**, miosis, visual disturbances

Adverse effects in *Italics* are most common; those in **Bold** are life-threatening.

- **GI:** *Nausea, vomiting, sweating,* dry mouth, anorexia, constipation, biliary tract spasm; increased colonic motility in patients with chronic ulcerative colitis
- **CV:** Facial flushing, peripheral circulatory collapse, tachycardia, bradycardia, arrhythmia, palpitations, chest wall rigidity, hypertension, hypotension, orthostatic hypotension, syncope, circulatory depression, shock, cardiac arrest
- **Respiratory:** Suppression of cough reflex, respiratory depression, apnea, respiratory arrest, laryngospasm, bronchospasm
- **GU:** Ureteral spasm, spasm of vesical sphincters, urinary retention or hesitancy, oliguria, antidiuretic effect, reduced libido or potency
- **Dermatologic:** Pruritus, urticaria, edema, hemorrhagic urticaria (rare)
- **Other:** Physical tolerance and dependence, psychological dependence

Clinically important drug-drug interactions
- Increased likelihood of respiratory depression, hypotension, profound sedation or coma in patients receiving barbiturate general anesthetics.

Drug-lab test interferences
- Elevated biliary tract pressure may cause increases in plasma amylase, lipase; determinations 24 h after administration

■ Nursing Considerations

Assessment
- *History:* Hypersensitivity to narcotics, diarrhea caused by poisoning, bronchial asthma, COPD, cor pulmonale, respiratory depression, kyphoscoliosis, acute alcoholism, increased intracranial pressure, acute abdominal conditions, cardiovascular disease, supraventricular tachycardias, myxedema, convulsive disorders, delirium tremens, cerebral arteriosclerosis, ulcerative colitis, fever, Addison's disease, prostatic hypertrophy, urethral stricture, recent GI or GU surgery, toxic psychosis, renal or hepatic dysfunction
- *Physical:* Body temperature; skin—color, texture, lesions; orientation, reflexes, bilateral grip strength, affect, pupil size; P, auscultation, BP, orthostatic BP, perfusion; R, adventious sounds; bowel sounds, normal output; frequency and pattern of voiding, normal output; thyroid, liver, kidney function tests

Implementation
- Administer to women who are lactating 4–6 h before the next scheduled feeding to minimize the amount in milk.
- Reassure patient about addiction liability; most patients who receive opiates for medical reasons do not develop dependence syndromes.

Drug-specific teaching points
- Take this drug exactly as prescribed.
- Know that the following side effects may occur: nausea, loss of appetite (taking the drug with food and lying quietly, eating frequent, small meals should minimize these effects); constipation (a laxative may help); dizziness, sedation, drowsiness, impaired visual acuity (avoid driving a car, performing other tasks that require alertness, visual acuity)
- Do not to take any leftover medication for other disorders, and do not to let anyone else take the prescription.
- Report severe nausea, vomiting, constipation, shortness of breath, or difficulty breathing.

❒ orphenadrine citrate

*(or **fen' a dreen**)*
Banflex, Flexoject, Norflex

Pregnancy Category C

Drug classes
Centrally acting skeletal muscle relaxant

Therapeutic actions
Precise mechanisms of action not known; acts in the CNS; does not directly relax tense skeletal muscles; does not directly

Adverse effects in *Italics* are most common; those in **Bold** are life-threatening.

affect the motor endplate or motor nerves.

Indications
- Relief of discomfort associated with acute, painful musculoskeletal conditions, as an adjunct to rest, physical therapy and other measures
- Unlabeled use: 100 mg at bedtime for the treatment of quinidine-resistant leg cramps

Contraindications/cautions
- Contraindicated in the presence of hypersensitivity to orphenadrine; glaucoma, pyloric, or duodenal obstruction; stenosing peptic ulcers; achalasia; cardiospasm (megaesophagus); prostatic hypertrophy; obstruction of bladder neck; myasthenia gravis; lactation.
- Use caution in the presence of cardiac decompensation, coronary insufficiency, cardiac arrhythmias, hepatic or renal dysfunction, pregnancy.

Dosage
Adult: 60 mg IV or IM. May repeat q12h. Inject IV over 5 min.
Pediatric: Safety and efficacy not established; not recommended.
Geriatric: Use caution and regulate dosage carefully; patients older than 60 y frequently develop increased sensitivity to adverse CNS effects of anticholinergic drugs.

Pharmacokinetics

Route	Onset	Peak	Duration
IM/IV	Rapid	2 h	4–6 h

Metabolism: Hepatic, $T_{1/2}$: 14 h
Distribution: Crosses placenta; enters breast milk
Excretion: Urine and feces

IV facts
Preparation: No further preparation is required.
Infusion: Administer slowly IV.

Adverse effects
- CNS: *Weakness, headache, dizziness, confusion* (especially in elderly), hallucinations, drowsiness, memory loss, psychosis, agitation, nervousness, delusions, delirium, paranoia, euphoria, depression, paresthesia, blurred vision, pupil dilation, increased intraocular tension
- **GI:** *Dry mouth, gastric irritation, vomiting, nausea, constipation*, dilation of the colon, paralytic ileus
- **CV:** *Tachycardia*, palpitation, transient syncope, hypotension, orthostatic hypotension
- **GU:** *Urinary hesitancy and retention*, dysuria, difficulty achieving or maintaining an erection
- **Dermatologic:** Urticaria, other dermatoses
- **General:** *Flushing, decreased sweating*, elevated temperature, muscle weakness, cramping

Clinically important drug-drug interactions
- Additive anticholinergic effects when given with other anticholinergic drugs
- Additive adverse CNS effects when given with phenothiazines • Possible masking of the development of persistent extrapyramidal symptoms, tardive dyskinesia in patients on long-term therapy with phenothiazines, halperidol • Decreased antipsychotic efficacy of phenothiazines, halperidol given concurrently

■ Nursing Considerations

Assessment
- *History:* Hypersensitivity to orphenadrine; glaucoma, pyloric, or duodenal obstruction; stenosing peptic ulcers; achalasia; cardiospasm; prostatic hypertrophy; obstruction of bladder neck; myasthenia gravis; cardiac, hepatic or renal dysfunction; lactation
- *Physical:* Body weight; body temperature; skin—color, lesions; orientation, affect, reflexes, bilateral grip strength, vision exam with tonometry; P, BP, orthostatic BP, auscultation; bowel sounds, normal output, liver evaluation; prostate palpation, normal output, voiding pattern; urinalysis, CBC with differential, liver and renal function tests, ECG

Adverse effects in *Italics* are most common; those in **Bold** are life-threatening.

Implementation
- Ensure that patient is recumbent during IV injection and for at least 15 min thereafter; assist patient from the recumbent position after parenteral treatment.
- Arrange to decrease dosage or discontinue drug temporarily if dry mouth is so severe that swallowing or speaking becomes difficult.
- Give with caution and arrange dosage reduction in hot weather, as appropriate to patient's lifestyle; drug interferes with sweating and body's ability to thermoregulate in hot environments.
- Arrange for analgesics if headache occurs (and possibly as adjunct to orphenadrine for relief of discomfort of muscle spasm).

Drug-specific teaching points
- Know that the following side effects may occur: drowsiness, dizziness, blurred vision (avoid driving a car or engaging in activities that require alertness and visual acuity if these occur); dry mouth (sucking on sugarless lozenges or ice chips may help); nausea (frequent, small meals may help); difficulty urinating (be sure that you empty the bladder just before taking the medication); constipation (increasing your fluid and fiber intake and exercising regularly as appropriate may help); headache (it may be possible for you to use an analgesic).
- Report dry mouth, difficult urination, constipation, headache, or GI upset that persists; skin rash or itching; rapid heart rate or palpitations; mental confusion; eye pain; fever; sore throat; bruising.

❐ oxacillin sodium

(ox a sill'in)
Bactocill, Prostaphilin

Pregnancy Category B

Drug classes
Antibiotic
Penicillinase-resistant pencillin

Therapeutic actions
Bactericidal: inhibits cell wall synthesis of sensitive organisms, causing cell death.

Indications
- Infections due to penicillinase-producing staphylococci
- Infections caused by streptococci

Contraindications/cautions
- Contraindicated in the presence of allergies to penicillins, cephalosporins, or other allergens.
- Use caution in the presence of renal disorders, pregnancy, lactation (may cause diarrhea or candidiasis in the infant).

Dosage
Maximum recommended dosage is 6 g/d.
Adult
- **PO:** 500 mg q4–6h PO for at least 5 d. *Follow-up therapy after parenteral oxacillin in severe infections:* 1 g q4–6h PO for up to 1–2 wk.
- **Parenteral:** 250–500 mg q4–6h IM or IV. Up to 1 g q4–6h in severe infections.

Pediatric
- **PO:** < 40 kg: 50 mg/kg per day in equally divided doses q6h for at least 5 d. Follow-up therapy after parenteral oxacillin for severe infections: 100 mg/kg per day in equally divided doses q4–6h for 1–2 wk.
- **Parenteral:** < 40 kg: 50 mg/kg per day IM or IV in equally divided doses q6h. Up to 100 mg/kg per day in equally divided doses q4–6h in severe infections.

Prematures and neonates: 25 mg/kg per day IM or IV.

Pharmacokinetics

Route	Onset	Peak	Duration
Oral	Varies	30–60 min	4 h
IM	Rapid	30–120 min	4–6 h
IV	Rapid	15 min	Length of infusion

Metabolism: Hepatic, $T_{1/2}$: 0.5–1 h
Distribution: Crosses placenta; enters breast milk
Excretion: Urine and bile

IV facts
Preparation: Dilute for direct IV administration to a maximum concentration of 1

g/10 ml using Sodium Chloride Injection or Sterile Water for Injection. For IV infusion: reconstituted solution may be diluted with compatible IV solution: 0.9% Sodium Chloride Injection, 5% Dextrose in Water or in Normal Saline, 10% D-Fructose in Water or in Normal Saline, Lactated Ringer's Solution, Lactated Potassic Saline Injections, 10% Invert Sugar in Water or in Normal Saline, 10% Invert Sugar plus 0.3% Potassium Chloride in Water, Travert 10% Electrolyte #1, #2, or #3. 0.5–40 mg/ml solutions are stable for up to 6h at room temperature. Discard after that time.
Infusion: Give by direct administration slowly to avoid vein irritation.
Incompatibilities: *Do not* mix in the same IV solution as other antibiotics.

Adverse effects
- CNS: Lethargy, hallucinations, seizures
- GI: *Glossitis, stomatitis, gastritis, sore mouth,* furry tongue, black "hairy" tongue, *nausea, vomiting, diarrhea,* abdominal pain, bloody diarrhea, enterocolitis, pseudomembranous colitis, nonspecific hepatitis
- Hematologic: Anemia, thrombocytopenia, leukopenia, neutropenia, prolonged bleeding time (more common with this drug than with other penicillinase-resistant penicillins)
- GU: Nephritis—oliguria, proteinuria, hematuria, casts, azotemia, pyuria
- Hypersensitivity reactions: *Rash, fever, wheezing,* anaphylaxis
- Local: *Pain, phlebitis,* thrombosis at injection site
- Other: *Superinfections,* sodium overload leading to CHF

Clinically important drug-drug interactions
- Decreased effectiveness of oxacillin if taken concurrently with tetracyclines
- Inactivation of aminoglycosides if combined in parenteral solutions with oxacillin.

Drug-lab test interferences
- False-positive Coombs' test with IV oxacillin

■ Nursing Considerations
Assessment
- *History:* Allergies to penicillins, cephalosporins, or other allergens; renal disorders; pregnancy; lactation
- *Physical:* Culture infected area; skin—color, lesions; R, adventitious sounds; bowel sounds: CBC, liver and renal function tests, serum electrolytes, Hct, urinalysis

Implementation
- Culture infected area before beginning treatment; reculture area if response is not as expected.
- Arrange to continue therapy for at least 2 d after signs of infection have disappeared, usually 7–10 d.
- Reconstitute for IM use to a dilution of 250 mg/1.5 ml using Sterile Water for Injection or Sodium Chloride Injection. Discard after 3 d at room temperature or after 7 d if refrigerated.
- Maintain epinephrine, IV fluids, vasopressors, bronchodilators, oxygen, and emergency equipment on standby in case of serious hypersensitivity reaction.

Drug-specific teaching points
- Know that the following side effects may occur: upset stomach, nausea, diarrhea (small, frequent meals may help), mouth sores (frequent mouth care may help), pain or discomfort at the injections site may occur.
- Report difficulty breathing, rashes, severe diarrhea, severe pain at injection site, mouth sores.

❑ oxamniquine

(ox **am'** ni kwin)
Vansil

Pregnancy Category C

Drug classes
Anthelmintic

Therapeutic actions
Antischistosomal versus *Schistosoma mansoni*; causes worms to move from mesen-

Adverse effects in *Italics* are most common; those in **Bold** are life-threatening.

tery to liver where tissue reactions trap male worms; female worms move back, but cease to lay eggs; mechanism of action not fully understood.

Indications
- Treatment of all stages of *S. mansoni* infection
- Unlabeled use: concurrent low-dose administration with praziquantel as a single-dose treatment of neurocysticercosis

Contraindications/cautions
- Allergy to oxamniquine, seizures, pregnancy, lactation.

Dosage
Adult: 12–15 mg/kg PO as a single dose.
Pediatric (< 30 kg): 20 mg/kg PO, in two divided doses of 10 mg/kg PO with 2–8 h between doses.

Pharmacokinetics

Route	Onset	Peak
Oral	Varies	1–1½ h

Metabolism: Hepatic, $T_{1/2}$: 1–2.5 h
Distribution: Crosses placenta; may enter breast milk
Excretion: Urine

Adverse effects
- **CNS:** *Drowsiness, dizziness, headache,* **epileptiform convulsions**
- **GI:** *Nausea,* vomiting, abdominal discomfort, loss of appetite
- **Dermatologic:** Urticaria

■ Nursing Considerations

Assessment
- *History:* Allergy to oxamniquine, seizures, pregnancy, lactation
- *Physical:* Skin—color, lesions; orientation, reflexes

Implementation
- Culture for ova.
- Administer drug with food to improve tolerance.

Drug-specific teaching points
- Take drug with meals to avoid GI upset.
- Know that the following side effects may occur: nausea, abdominal pain, GI upset (small, frequent meals may help); drowsiness, dizziness (if these occur, use caution if driving a car or operating dangerous equipment).
- Report rash, severe abdominal pain, marked weakness, dizziness.

❐ oxandrolone

(ox an' droh lone)
Oxandrin

Pregnancy Category X

Drug classes
Anabolic steroid
Hormonal agent

Therapeutic actions
Testosterone analog with androgenic and anabolic activity; promotes body tissue-building processes and reverses catabolic or tissue-depleting processes; increases hemoglobin and red cell mass.

Indications
- Adjunctive therapy to promote weight gain after weight loss following extensive surgery, chronic infections, trauma
- Offset the protein catabolism associated with prolonged administration of corticosteroids
- Relief of bone pain accompanying osteoporosis
- Unlabeled use: alcoholic hepatitis
- Orphan drug uses: short stature associated with Turner syndrome, HIV wasting syndrome, and HIV-associated muscle weakness

Contraindications/cautions
- Known sensitivity to anabolic steroids; prostate or breast cancer in males; benign prostatic hypertrophy; breast cancer in females; pituitary insufficiency; MI (contraindicated because of effects on cholesterol); nephrosis; liver disease; hypercalcemia; pregnancy, lactation.

Adverse effects in *Italics* are most common; those in **Bold** are life-threatening.

Dosage
Adult: 2.5 mg PO bid–qid; up to 20 mg has been used to achieve the desired effect; 2–4 wk of therapy is needed to evaluate response.
Pediatric: Total daily dose of < 0.1 mg/kg or < 0.045 mg/lb PO, which may be repeated intermittently.

Pharmacokinetics

Route	Onset
Oral	Slow

Metabolism: Hepatic, $T_{1/2}$: 9 h
Distribution: Crosses placenta; enters breast milk
Excretion: Urine

Adverse effects
- CNS: *Excitation, insomnia,* chills, toxic confusion
- GI: Hepatotoxicity, peliosis, **hepatitis** with life threatening liver failure or intraabdominal hemorrhage; liver cell tumors, sometimes malignant and fatal, *nausea, vomiting, diarrhea, abdominal fullness, loss of appetite, burning of tongue*
- Hematologic: *Blood lipid changes;* iron deficiency anemia, hypercalcemia, alterred serum cholesterol levels; *retention of sodium, chloride, water,* potassium, phosphates and calcium
- GU: Possible increased risk of prostatic hypertrophy, carcinoma in geriatric patients
- Endocrine: *Virilization: prepubertal males*—phallic enlargement, hirsutism, increased skin pigmentation; *postpubertal males*—inhibition of testicular function, gynecomastia, testicular atrophy, priapism, baldness, epidiymitis, change in libido; *females* — hirsutism, hoarseness, deepening of the voice, clitoral enlargement, menstrual irregularities, baldness; decreased glucose tolerance
- Other: *Acne,* premature closure of the epiphyses

Clinically important drug-drug interactions
- Potentiation of oral anticoagulants if taken with anabolic steroids • Decreased need for insulin, oral hypoglycemica agents if anabolic steroids are used

Drug-lab test interferences
- Altered glucose tolerance tests • Decrease in thyroid function tests (may persist for 2–3 wk after stopping therapy) • Increased creatinine, creatinine clearance, which may last for 2 wk after therapy

■ Nursing Considerations

Assessment
- *History:* Sensitivity to anabolic steroids; prostate or breast cancer; benign prostatic hypertrophy; pituitary insufficiency; MI; nephrosis; liver disease; hypercalcemia; pregnancy; lactation
- *Physical:* Skin—color, texture; hair distribution pattern; affect, orientation; abdominal exam, liver evaluation; serum electrolytes and cholesterol levels, glucose tolerance tests, thyroid function tests, long bone x-ray (in children)

Implementation
- Administer with food if GI upset or nausea occurs.
- Monitor effect on children with longbone x-rays every 3–6 mo during therapy; discontinue drug well before the bone age reaches the norm for the patient's chronologic age because effects may continue for 6 mo after therapy.
- Monitor patient for occurrence of edema; arrange for appropriate diuretic therapy as needed.
- Arrange to monitor liver function, serum electrolytes periodically during therapy, and consult with physician for appropriate corrective measures as needed.
- Arrange to measure cholesterol levels periodically in patients who are at high risk for coronary artery disease.
- Monitor diabetic patients closely because glucose tolerance may change. Adjustments may be needed in insulin, oral hypoglycemic dosage, and diet.

Adverse effects in *Italics* are most common; those in **Bold** are life-threatening.

Drug-specific teaching points

- Take drug with food if nausea or GI upset occur.
- Know that the following side effects may occur: nausea, vomiting, diarrhea, burning of the tongue (small, frequent meals may help); body hair growth, baldness, deepening of the voice, loss of libido, impotence (most of these effects will be reversible when the drug is stopped); excitation, confusion, insomnia (avoid driving, performing tasks that require alertness if these effects occur); swelling of the ankles, fingers (medication may be ordered to help).
- Be aware that diabetic patients need to monitor urine sugar closely because glucose tolerance may change; report any abnormalities to physician, so corrective action can be taken.
- Be aware that these drugs do not enhance athletic ability but do have serious effects and should not be used for increasing muscle strength.
- Report ankle swelling, skin color changes, severe nausea, vomiting, hoarseness, body hair growth, deepening of the voice, acne, menstrual irregularities.

oxaprozin

(oks a pro' zin)
Daypro

Pregnancy Category C

Drug classes
Analgesic (non-narcotic)
Antipyretic
NSAID

Therapeutic actions
Inhibits prostaglandin synthetase to cause antipyretic and anti-inflammatory effects; the exact mechnanism of action is not known.

Indications
- Acute or long-term use in the management of signs and symptoms of osteoarthritis and rheumatoid arthritis

Contraindications/cautions
- Contraindicated in the presence of significant renal impairment, pregnancy, lactation.
- Use caution in the presence of impaired hearing, allergies, hepatic, cardiovascular, and GI conditions.

Dosage
Titrate to the lowest effective dose to minimize side effects. Maximum daily dose: 1,800 mg or 26 mg/kg, whichever is lower.
Adult
- ***Osteoarthritis:*** 1,200 mg PO qd; use initial dose of 600 mg in patients with known low body weight or milder disease.
- ***Rheumatoid arthritis:*** 1,200 mg PO qd.

Pediatric: Safety and efficacy not established.

Pharmacokinetics

Route	Onset	Peak	Duration
Oral	Varies	3–5 h	24–36 h

Metabolism: Hepatic, $T_{1/2}$: 42–50 h
Distribution: Crosses placenta; enters breast milk
Excretion: Urine and feces

Adverse effects
- CNS: Dizziness, somnolence, insomnia, fatigue, tiredness, dizziness, tinnitus, ophthalmologic effects
- GI: *Nausea, dyspepsia,* GI pain, *diarrhea,* vomiting, *constipation,* flatulence
- Hematologic: Bleeding, platelet inhibition with higher doses
- GU: Dysuria, renal impairment
- Dermatologic: Rash, pruritus, sweating, dry mucous membranes, stomatitis
- Other: Peripheral edema, **anaphylactoid reactions** to fatal anaphylactic shock

■ Nursing Considerations

Assessment
- *History:* Renal impairment, impaired hearing, allergies, hepatic, cardiovascular, and GI conditions, lactation

Adverse effects in *Italics* are most common; those in **Bold** are life-threatening.

- *Physical:* Skin—color and lesions; orientation, reflexes, ophthalmologic and audiometric evaluation, peripheral sensation; P, edema; R, adventitious sounds; liver evaluation; CBC, clotting times, renal and liver function tests; serum electrolytes, stool guaiac

Implementation
- Administer drug with food or after meals if GI upset occurs.
- Arrange for periodic ophthalmologic examination during long-term therapy.
- Institute emergency procedures if overdose occurs (gastric lavage, induction of emesis, supportive therapy).

Drug-specific teaching points
- Take drug with food or meals if GI upset occurs.
- Know that dizziness, drowsiness can occur (avoid driving or the use of dangerous machinery while on this drug).
- Report sore throat, fever, rash, itching, weight gain, swelling in ankles or fingers, changes in vision, black, tarry stools.

▢ oxazepam

(ox a' ze pam)
Apo-Oxazepam (CAN), Novoxapam (CAN), Ox-Pam(CAN), Serax, Zapex (CAN)

Pregnancy Category D
C-IV controlled drug

Drug classes
Benzodiazepine
Antianxiety drug

Therapeutic actions
Exact mechanisms of action not understood; acts mainly at subcortical levels of the CNS, leaving the cortex relatively unaffected; main sites of action may be the limbic system and reticular formation; benzodiazepines potentiate the effects of GABA, an inhibitory neurotransmitter; anxiolytic effects occur at doses well below those necessary to cause sedation, ataxia.

Indications
- Management of anxiety disorders or for short-term relief of symptoms of anxiety; anxiety associated with depression also is responsive
- Management of anxiety, tension, agitation, and irritability in older patients
- Alcoholics with acute tremulousness, inebriation, or anxiety associated with alcohol withdrawal

Contraindications/cautions
- Contraindicated in the presence of hypersensitivity to benzodiazepines, tartrazine (in the tablets); psychoses; acute narrow-angle glaucoma; shock; coma; acute alcoholic intoxication with depression of vital signs; pregnancy (increased risk of congenital malformations, neonatal withdrawal syndrome); labor and delivery ("floppy infant" syndrome reported when mothers were given benzodiazepines during labor); lactation (may cause infants to become lethargic and lose weight).
- Use caution in the presence of impaired liver or kidney function, debilitation.

Dosage
Increase dosage gradually to avoid adverse effects.
Adult: 10–15 mg PO or up to 30 mg, PO tid–qid, depending on severity of symptoms of anxiety. The higher dosage range is recommended in alcoholics.
Pediatric: 6–12 y: Dosage not established.
Geriatric patients or those with debilitating disease: Initially 10 mg PO tid. Gradually increase to 15 mg PO tid–qid if needed and tolerated.

Pharmacokinetics

Route	Onset	Peak
Oral	Slow	2–4 h

Metabolism: Hepatic, $T_{1/2}$: 5–20 h
Distribution: Crosses placenta; enters breast milk
Excretion: Urine

Adverse effects

- **CNS:** *Transient, mild drowsiness* (initially), *sedation, depression, lethargy, apathy, fatigue, lightheadedness, disorientation*, restlessness, confusion, crying, delirium, headache, slurred speech, dysarthria, stupor, rigidity, tremor, dystonia, vertigo, euphoria, nervousness, difficulty in concentration, vivid dreams, psychomotor retardation, extrapyramidal symptoms, mild paradoxical excitatory reactions during first 2 wk of treatment, visual and auditory disturbances, diplopia, nystagmus, depressed hearing
- **GI:** *Constipation, diarrhea, dry mouth*, salivation, nausea, anorexia, vomiting, difficulty in swallowing, gastric disorders
- **CV:** Bradycardia, tachycardia, cardiovascular collapse, hypertension and hypotension, palpitations, edema
- **Hematologic:** Elevations of blood enzymes, hepatic dysfunction, blood dyscrasias: agranulocytosis, leukopenia
- **GU:** *Incontinence, urinary retention*, changes in libido, menstrual irregularities
- **Dermatologic:** Urticaria, pruritus, skin rash, dermatitis
- **Other:** *Nasal congestion, hiccups, fever, diaphoresis*, paresthesias, muscular disturbances, gynecomastia, drug dependence with withdrawal syndrome when drug is discontinued: more common with abrupt discontinuation of higher dosage used for longer than 4 mo

Clinically important drug-drug interactions

- Increased CNS depression when taken with alcohol • Decreased sedation when given to heavy smokers of cigarettes or if taken concurrently with theophyllines

■ Nursing Considerations

Assessment

- *History:* Hypersensitivity to benzodiazepines, tartrazine; psychoses; acute narrow-angle glaucoma; shock; coma; acute alcoholic intoxication; pregnancy; labor and delivery; lactation; impaired liver or kidney function, debilitation
- *Physical:* Skin—color, lesions; body temperature; orientation, reflexes, affect, ophthalmologic exam; P, BP; R, adventitious sounds; liver evaluation, abdominal exam, bowel sounds, normal output; CBC, liver and renal function tests.

Implementation

- Arrange to taper dosage gradually after long-term therapy, especially in epileptic patients.

Drug-specific teaching points

- Take this drug exactly as prescribed; do not stop taking drug (long-term therapy) without consulting health care provider.
- Know that the following side effects may occur: drowsiness, dizziness (these may become less pronounced after a few days; avoid driving a car or engaging in other dangerous activities if these occur); GI upset (taking the drug with food may help); depression, dreams, emotional upset, crying.
- Report severe dizziness, weakness, drowsiness that persists, palpitations, swelling of the extremities, visual changes, difficulty voiding, rash or skin lesion.

▢ oxtriphylline

*(ox **trye**' fi lin)*

choline theophyllinate
Choledyl, Choledyl SA

Pregnancy Category C

Drug classes
Bronchodilator
Xanthine

Therapeutic actions
Oxtriphylline, the choline salt of theophylline, is 64% theophylline; it relaxes bronchial smooth muscle, causing bronchodilation and increasing vital capacity, which has been impaired by bronchospasm and air trapping; actions may be mediated by inhibition of phosphodiesterase, which increases the concentration

Adverse effects in *Italics* are most common; those in **Bold** are life-threatening.

of cyclic adenosine monophosphate (cAMP).

Indications

- Symptomatic relief or prevention of bronchial asthma and reversible bronchospasm associated with chronic bronchitis and emphysema

Contraindications/cautions

- Contraindicated in the presence of hypersensitivity to any xanthine, peptic ulcer, active gastritis.
- Use caution in the presence of cardiac arrhythmias, acute myocardial injury, CHF, cor pulmonale, severe hypertension, severe hypoxemia, renal or hepatic disease, hyperthyroidism, alcoholism, labor, pregnancy (tachycardia, jitteriness, and withdrawal apnea have been observed in neonates), lactation.

Dosage

Individualize dosage, basing adjustments on clinical responses with monitoring of serum theophylline levels, if possible, to maintain levels in the therapeutic range of 10–20 µg/ml. Base dosage on lean body mass.
Adult: 4.7 mg/kg PO q8h. Sustained release, 400–600 mg PO q12h.
Pediatric: Use in children younger than 6 mo not recommended. Use of timed-release products in children younger than 6 y not recommended. Children are very sensitive to CNS stimulant action of theophylline. Use caution in younger children who cannot complain of minor side effects. 9–16 y, 4.7 mg/kg PO q6h; 1–9 y, 6.2 mg/kg PO q6h.

Pharmacokinetics

Route	Onset	Peak
Oral	Rapid	2 h

Metabolism: Hepatic, $T_{1/2}$: 3–15 h
Distribution: Crosses placenta; enters breast milk
Excretion: Urine

Adverse effects

- CNS: *Irritability (especially children); restlessness,* dizziness, muscle twitching, convulsions, severe depression, stammering speech; abnormal behavior characterized by withdrawal, mutism and unresponsiveness alternating with hyperactive periods
- GI: *Loss of appetite,* hematemesis, epigastric pain, gastroesophageal reflux
- CV: Palpitations, sinus tachycardia, ventricular tachycardia, **life threatening ventricular arrhythmias**, circulatory failure
- **Respiratory:** Tachypnea, respiratory arrest
- GU: Proteinuria, increased excretion of renal tubular cells and RBCs; diuresis, urinary retention in men with prostate enlargement
- Other: Fever, flushing, hyperglycemia, SIADH, rash, increased SGOT
- Serum theophylline levels < 20 µg/ml: Adverse effects uncommon.
- Serum theophylline levels > 20–25 µg/ml: Nausea, vomiting, diarrhea, headache, insomnia, irritability (75% of patients)
- Serum theophylline levels > 30–35 µg/ml: Hyperglycemia, hypotension, cardiac arrhythmias, tachycardia (> 10 µg/ml in premature newborns); **seizures, brain damage, death**

Clinically important drug-drug interactions

- Increased effects and toxicity when given with cimetidine, erythromycin, troleandomycin, ciprofloxacin, norfloxacin, enoxacin, pefloxacin, oral contraceptives, ticlopidine, rifampin • Increased serum levels and risk of toxicity in hypothyroid patients; decreased drug levels in patients who are hyperthyroid; monitor patients on thioamines, thyroid hormones for changes in serum levels as patients become euthyroid • Increased cardiac toxicity when given with halothane • Decreased effects in patients who are cigarette smokers (1–2 packs/d) • Decreased effects when given with barbiturates • Decreased effects of phenytoins, benzodiazepines, nondepolarizing neuromuscular blockers, and theophylline preparations when given concomitantly • Mutually antagonistic effects of beta-blockers and theophylline preparations

Clinically important drug-food interactions

- Elimination of theophylline preparations is increased by a low-carbohydrate, high-protein diet and by charcoal broiled beef • Elimination of theophylline preparations is decreased by a high-carbohydrate, low-protein diet • Food may alter bioavailability, absorption of timed-release theophylline preparations; these may rapidly release their contents in the presence of food and cause toxicity; timed-release forms should be taken on an empty stomach

Drug-lab test interferences

- Interference with spectrophotometric determinations of serum theophylline levels by furosemide, phenylbutazone, probenecid, theobromine; coffee, tea, cola beverages, chocolate, acetaminophen, which cause falsely high values • Alteration in assays of uric acid, urinary catecholamines, plasma free fatty acids by theophylline preparations

■ Nursing Considerations

Assessment

- *History:* Hypersensitivity to any xanthine, peptic ulcer, active gastritis, cardiac disorders, cor pulmonale, severe hypertension, severe hypoxemia, renal or hepatic disease, hyperthyroidism, alcoholism, pregnancy, lactation
- *Physical:* Bowel sounds, normal output; P, auscultation, BP, perfusion, ECG; R, adventitious sounds; urinary frequency, voiding, normal output pattern, urinalysis; liver palpation; liver, renal, thyroid function tests; skin—color, texture, lesions; reflexes, bilateral grip strength, affect, EEG

Implementation

- Caution patient not to chew or crush enteric-coated timed-release preparations.
- Give immediate-release, liquid dosage forms with food if GI effects occur.
- Do not give timed-release preparations with food; these should be given on an empty stomach, 1 h before or 2 h after meals.
- Monitor results of serum theophylline level determinations carefully, and arrange for reduced dosage if serum levels exceed therapeutic range of 10–20 µg/ml.
- Monitor patient carefully for clinical signs of adverse effects, particularly if serum theophylline levels are not available.
- Maintain diazepam on standby to treat seizures.

Drug-specific teaching points

- Take this drug exactly as prescribed; if a timed-release product is prescribed, take this drug on an empty stomach, 1 h before or 2 h after meals; it may be necessary to take this drug around the clock for adequate control of asthma attacks.
- Do not chew or crush timed-release preparations.
- Avoid excessive intake of coffee, tea, cocoa, cola beverages, chocolate.
- Be aware that smoking cigarettes or other tobacco products may markedly influence the effects of theophylline; it is preferable not to smoke while taking this drug. Notify the nurse or physician if smoking habits change while taking this drug.
- Be aware that frequent blood tests may be necessary to monitor the effect of this drug and ensure safe and effective dosage.
- Know that the following side effects may occur: nausea, loss of appetite (taking this drug with food may help—applies only to immediate-release or liquid dosage forms); difficulty sleeping, depression, emotional lability (it may be reassuring to know that these are drug effects).
- Report nausea, vomiting, severe GI pain, restlessness, convulsions, irregular heartbeat.

☐ oxybutynin chloride

*(ox i **byoo'** ti nin)*
Ditropan

Pregnancy Category C

oxybutynin chloride ■ 831

Drug classes
Urinary antispasmodic

Therapeutic actions
Acts directly to relax smooth muscle and inhibits the effects of acetylcholine at muscarinic receptors; reported to be less potent an anticholinergic than atropine but more potent as antispasmodic and devoid of antinicotinic activity at skeletal neuromuscular junctions or autonomic ganglia.

Indications
- Relief of symptoms of bladder instability associated with voiding in patients with uninhibited neurogenic and reflex neurogenic bladder

Contraindications/cautions
- Contraindicated in the presence of allergy to oxybutynin, pyloric or duodenal obstruction, obstructive intestinal lesions or ileus, intestinal atony, megacolon, colitis, obstructive uropathies, glaucoma, myasthenia gravis, cardiovascular instability in acute hemorrhage.
- Use caution in the presence of hepatic, renal impairment; pregnancy; lactation.

Dosage
Adult: 5 mg PO bid or tid. Maximum dose is 5 mg qid.
Pediatric (older than 5 y): 5 mg PO bid. Maximum dose is 5 mg tid.

Pharmacokinetics

Route	Onset	Peak	Duration
Oral	30–60 min	3–6 h	6–10 h

Metabolism: Hepatic, $T_{1/2}$: unknown
Distribution: Crosses placenta; may enter breast milk
Excretion: Urine

Adverse effects
- **CNS:** *Drowsiness, dizziness, blurred vision,* dilatation of the pupil, cycloplegia, increased ocular tension, weakness
- **GI:** *Dry mouth, nausea,* vomiting, constipation, bloated feeling
- **CV:** Tachycardia, palpitations
- **GU:** *Urinary hesitancy,* retention, impotence
- **Hypersensitivity:** Allergic reactions including urticaria, dermal effect
- **Other:** *Decreased sweating,* heat prostration in high environmental temperatures secondary to loss of sweating

Clinically important drug-drug interactions
- Decreased effectiveness of phenothiazines if taken concurrently with oxybutynin
- Decreased effectiveness of haloperidol and development of tardive dyskinesia if taken concurrently with oxybutynin

■ Nursing Considerations
Assessment
- *History:* Allergy to oxybutynin, intestinal obstructions or lesions, intestinal atony, obstructive uropathies, glaucoma, myasthenia gravis, cardiovascular instability in acute hemorrhage, hepatic or renal impairment, pregnancy
- *Physical:* Skin—color, lesions; body temperature; orientation, affect, reflexes, ophthalmic exam, ocular pressure measurement; P, rhythm, BP; bowel sounds, liver evaluation; renal and liver function tests, cystometry

Implementation
- Arrange for cystometry and other appropriate diagnostic tests before beginning treatment and periodically during treatment to evaluate response to treatment.
- Arrange for ophthalmic exam before beginning therapy and periodically during therapy.

Drug-specific teaching points
- Take this drug as prescribed.
- Be aware that periodic bladder exams will be needed during the course of treatment to evaluate your response to therapy.
- Know that the following side effects may occur: dry mouth, GI upset (sucking on sugarless lozenges and frequent mouth care may help); drowsiness, blurred vision (avoid driving or performing tasks that require alertness while on this drug);

Adverse effects in *Italics* are most common; those in **Bold** are life-threatening.

decreased sweating (avoid high temperatures; serious complications can occur because your body will not be able to cool itself efficiently).
- Report blurred vision, fever, skin rash, nausea, vomiting.

☐ oxycodone hydrochloride

(ox i koe' done)
Roxicodone, Supeudol (CAN)

Pregnancy Category C
C-II controlled substance

Drug classes
Narcotic agonist analgesic

Therapeutic actions
Acts as agonist at specific opioid receptors in the CNS to produce analgesia, euphoria, sedation; the receptors mediating these effects are thought to be the same as those mediating the effects of endogenous opioids (enkephalins, endorphins).

Indications
- Relief of moderate to moderately severe pain

Contraindications/cautions
- Contraindicated in the presence of hypersensitivity to narcotics, diarrhea caused by poisoning (before toxins are eliminated); pregnancy (readily crosses placenta; neonatal withdrawal has occurred in infants born to mothers who used narcotics during pregnancy); labor or delivery (administration of narcotics to the mother can cause respiratory depression of neonate; premature infants are at special risk; may prolong labor); bronchial asthma, COPD, cor pulmonale, respiratory depression, anoxia, kyphoscoliosis, acute alcoholism, increased intracranial pressure, lactation.
- Use caution in the presence of acute abdominal conditions, cardiovascular disease, supraventricular tachycardias, myxedema, convulsive disorders, delirium tremens, cerebral arteriosclerosis, ulcerative colitis, fever, Addison's disease, prostatic hypertrophy, urethral stricture, recent GI or GU surgery, toxic psychosis, renal or hepatic dysfunction.

Dosage
Individualize dosage.
Adult: 5 mg or 5 ml PO q6h as needed.
Pediatric: Not recommended.
Geriatric or impaired adult: Use caution. Respiratory depression may occur in elderly, the very ill, those with respiratory problems.

Pharmacokinetics

Route	Onset	Peak	Duration
Oral	15–30 min	1 h	4–6 h

Metabolism: Hepatic, $T_{1/2}$: unknown
Distribution: Crosses placenta; enters breast milk
Excretion: Urine

Adverse effects
- CNS: *Lightheadedness, dizziness, sedation,* euphoria, dysphoria, delirium, insomnia, agitation, anxiety, fear, hallucinations, disorientation, drowsiness, lethargy, impaired mental and physical performance, coma, mood changes, weakness, headache, tremor, convulsions, miosis, visual disturbances
- GI: *Nausea, vomiting, sweating* (more common in ambulatory patients and those without severe pain), dry mouth, anorexia, constipation, biliary tract spasm; increased colonic motility in patients with chronic ulcerative colitis
- CV: Facial flushing, peripheral circulatory collapse, tachycardia, bradycardia, arrhythmia, palpitations, chest wall rigidity, hypertension, hypotension, orthostatic hypotension, syncope, circulatory depression, shock, cardiac arrest
- **Respiratory**: Suppression of cough reflex, respiratory depression, apnea, respiratory arrest, laryngospasm, bronchospasm
- GU: Ureteral spasm, spasm of vesical sphincters, urinary retention or hesi-

Adverse effects in *Italics* are most common; those in **Bold** are life-threatening.

tancy, oliguria, antidiuretic effect, reduced libido or potency
- **Dermatologic:** Pruritus, urticaria, edema, hemorrhagic urticaria (rare)
- **Other:** Physical tolerance and dependence, psychological dependence

Clinically important drug-drug interactions
- Increased likelihood of respiratory depression, hypotension, profound sedation or coma in patients receiving barbiturate general anesthetics

Drug-lab test interferences
- Elevated biliary tract pressure may cause increases in plasma amylase, lipase; determinations for 24 h after administration

■ Nursing Considerations

Assessment
- *History:* Hypersensitivity to narcotics, diarrhea caused by poisoning, pregnancy, labor or delivery, bronchial asthma, COPD, cor pulmonale, respiratory depression, kyphoscoliosis, acute alcoholism, increased intracranial pressure, acute abdominal conditions, cardiovascular disease, myxedema, convulsive disorders, cerebral arteriosclerosis, ulcerative colitis, fever, Addison's disease, prostatic hypertrophy, urethral stricture, recent GI or GU surgery, toxic psychosis, renal or hepatic dysfunction
- *Physical:* Body temperature; skin—color, texture, lesions; orientation, reflexes, bilateral grip strength, affect, pupil size; pulse, auscultation, BP, orthostatic BP, perfusion; R, adventious sounds; bowel sounds, normal output; frequency and pattern of voiding, normal output; ECG; EEG; thyroid, liver, kidney function tests

Implementation
- Administer to women who are lactating 4–6 h before the next scheduled feeding to minimize the amount in milk.
- Provide narcotic antagonist, facilities for assisted or controlled respiration on standby during parenteral administration.
- Reassure patient about addiction liability; most patients who receive opiates for medical reasons do not develop dependence syndromes.

Drug-specific teaching points
- Take drug exactly as prescribed.
- Know that the following side effects may occur: nausea, loss of appetite (taking the drug with food and lying quietly, eating frequent, small meals should minimize these effects); constipation (a laxative may help); dizziness, sedation, drowsiness, impaired visual acuity (avoid driving a car, performing other tasks that require alertness, visual acuity).
- Do not take any leftover medication for other disorders, and do not to let anyone else take the prescription.
- Report severe nausea, vomiting, constipation, shortness of breath, or difficulty breathing.

▢ oxymetazoline

(ox i met az' oh leen)
Afrin, Allerest 12-hour Nasal, Dristan Long Lasting, Duramist Plus, Genasal, Neo-Synephrine, Nostrilla, Sinex Long Lasting, Twice-A-Day
Pregnancy Category C

Drug classes
Nasal decongestant

Therapeutic actions
Acts directly on alpha receptors to produce vasoconstriction of arterioles in nasal passages, which produces a decongestant response; no effect on beta receptors.

Indications
- Symptomatic relief of nasal and nasopharyngeal mucosal congestion due to colds, hay fever, or other respiratory allergies (topical)

Contraindications/cautions
- Contraindicated in the presence of allergy to oxymetalozine, angle-closure glau-

coma, anesthesia with cyclopropane or halothane; thyrotoxicosis, diabetes, hypertension, cardiovascular disorders, women in labor whose BP > 130/80.
- Use caution in the presence of angina, arrhythmias, prostatic hypertrophy, unstable vasomotor syndrome, lactation.

Dosage
Adult: 2–3 sprays or 2–3 drops of 0.05% solution in each nostril bid, morning and evening or q10–12h.
Pediatric: Older than 6 y, adult dosage; 2–5 y, 2–3 drops of 0.0025% solution in each nostril twice daily, morning and evening.

Pharmacokinetics

Route	Onset	Duration
Nasal	5–10 min	6–10 h

Metabolism: Hepatic, $T_{1/2}$: unknown
Distribution: Crosses placenta; may enter breast milk
Excretion: Urine

Adverse effects
Systemic effects are less likely with topical administration than with systemic administration, but because systemic absorption can take place, the systemic effects should be considered:
- CNS: *Fear, anxiety, tenseness, restlessness, headache, lightheadedness, dizziness*, drowsiness, tremor, insomnia, hallucinations, psychological disturbances, convulsions, CNS depression, weakness, blurred vision, ocular irritation, tearing, photophobia, symptoms of paranoid schizophrenia
- GI: *Nausea*, vomiting, anorexia
- CV: Arrhythmias, hypertension resulting in intracranial hemorrhage, cardiovascular collapse with hypotension, palpitations, tachycardia, precordial pain in patients with ischemic heart disease
- GU: Constriction of renal blood vessels, *dysuria, vesical sphincter spasm* resulting in difficult and painful urination, urinary retention in males with prostatism
- Local: *Rebound congestion* with topical nasal application
- Other: *Pallor*, respiratory difficulty, orofacial dystonia, sweating

Clinically important drug-drug interactions
- Severe hypertension when taken with MAO-inhibitors, tricyclic antidepressants, furazolidone • Additive effects and increased risk of toxicity if taken with urinary alkalinizers • Decreased vasopressor response if taken with reserpine, methyldopa, urinary acidifiers • Decreased hypotensive action of guanethidine if taken concurrently

■ Nursing Considerations

Assessment
- *History:* Allergy to oxymetazoline; angle-closure glaucoma; anesthesia with cyclopropane or halothane; thyrotoxicosis, diabetes, hypertension, cardiovascular disorders; prostatic hypertrophy, unstable vasomotor syndrome; lactation
- *Physical:* Skin—color, temperature; orientation, reflexes, peripheral sensation, vision; P, BP, auscultation, peripheral perfusion; R, adventitious sounds; urinary output pattern, bladder percussion, prostate palpation; nasal mucous membrane evaluation

Implementation
- Monitor cardiovascular effects carefully; patients with hypertension who take this drug may experience changes in blood pressure because of the additional vasoconstriction. If a nasal decongestant is needed, pseudoephedrine is the drug of choice.

Drug-specific teaching points
- Do not exceed recommended dose. Demonstrate proper administration technique for topical nasal application. Avoid prolonged use because underlying medical problems can be disguised.
- Know that the following side effects may occur: dizziness, weakness, restlessness, lightheadedness, tremor (avoid driving or operating dangerous equipment when these effects occur); urinary retention

Adverse effects in *Italics* are most common; those in **Bold** are life-threatening.

(emptying the bladder before taking the drug may help).
- Be aware that a rebound congestion may occur when this drug is stopped; drink plenty of fluids, use a humidifier, and avoid smoke-filled areas to help decrease problems.
- Report nervousness, palpitations, sleeplessness, sweating.

☐ oxymetholone

(ox i meth' oh lone)
Anadrol-50, Anapolon 50 (CAN)

Pregnancy Category X
C-III Controlled Substance

Drug classes
Anabolic steroid
Hormonal agent

Therapeutic actions
Testosterone analog with androgenic and anabolic activity; promotes body tissue-building processes and reverses catabolic or tissue-depleting processes; increases hemoglobin and red cell mass.

Indications
- Anemias caused by deficient red cell production
- Acquired or congenital aplastic anemia
- Myelofibrosis and hypoplastic anemias due to administration of myelotoxic drugs

Contraindications/cautions
- Known sensitivity to oxymetholone or anabolic steroids, prostate or breast cancer; benign prostatic hypertrophy, pituitary insufficiency, MI, nephrosis, liver disease, hypercalcemia, pregnancy, lactation.

Dosage
Adults: 1–5 mg/kg per day PO. Usual effective dose is 1–2 mg/kg per day. Give for a minimum trial of 3–6 mo. Following remission, patients may be maintained without the drug or on a lower daily dose. Continuous therapy is usually needed in cases of congenital aplastic anemia.

Pediatric: Long-term therapy is contraindicated because of possibility of serious disruption of growth and development; weigh benefits and risks.

Pharmacokinetics

Route	Onset
Oral	Rapid

Metabolism: Hepatic, $T_{1/2}$: 9 h
Distribution: Crosses placenta; enters breast milk
Excretion: Urine

Adverse effects
- **CNS:** *Excitation, insomnia,* chills, toxic confusion
- **GI:** Hepatotoxicity, peliosis, **hepatitis** with life-threatening liver failure or intra-abdominal hemorrhage; liver cell tumors, sometimes malignant and fatal, *nausea, vomiting, diarrhea, abdominal fullness, loss of appetite, burning of tongue*
- **Hematologic:** *Blood lipid changes:* decreased HDL and sometimes increased LDL; iron deficiency anemia, hypercalcemia, altered serum cholesterol levels; *retention of sodium, chloride, water,* potassium, phosphates and calcium
- **GU:** Possible increased risk of prostatic hypertrophy, carcinoma in geriatric patients
- **Endocrine:** *Virilization: prepubertal males*—phallic enlargement, hirsutism, increased skin pigmentation; *postpubertal males*—inhibition of testicular function, gynecomastia, testicular atrophy, priapism, baldness, epidiymitis, change in libido; *females* — hirsutism, hoarseness, deepening of the voice, clitoral enlargement, menstrual irregularities, baldness; decreased glucose tolerance
- **Other:** *Acne,* premature closure of the epiphyses

Adverse effects in *Italics* are most common; those in **Bold** are life-threatening.

oxymorphone hydrochloride

Clinically important drug-drug interactions
- Potentiation of oral anticoagulants if taken with anabolic steroids • Decreased need for insulin, oral hypoglycemica agents if anabolic steroids are used

Drug-lab test interferences
- Altered glucose tolerance tests • Decrease in thyroid function tests, which may persist for 2–3 wk after therapy • Increased creatinine, creatinine clearance, which may last for 2 wk after therapy

■ Nursing Considerations

Assessment
- *History:* Known sensitivity to oxymetholone or anabolic steroids; prostate or breast cancer; benign prostatic hypertrophy; pituitary insufficiency; MI; nephrosis; liver disease; hypercalcemia; pregnancy; lactation
- *Physical:* Skin—color, texture; hair distribution pattern; affect, orientation; abdominal exam, liver evaluation; serum electrolytes and cholesterol levels, glucose tolerance tests, thyroid function tests, long bone x-ray (in children)

Implementation
- Administer with food if GI upset or nausea occurs.
- Monitor effect on children with long-bone x-rays every 3–6 mo during therapy; discontinue drug well before the bone age reaches the norm for the patient's chronologic age because effects may continue for 6 mo after therapy.
- Monitor patient for occurrence of edema; arrange for appropriate diuretic therapy as needed.
- Arrange to monitor liver function, serum electrolytes periodically during therapy, and consult with physician for appropriate corrective measures as needed.
- Arrange to measure cholesterol levels periodically in patients who are at high risk for coronary artery disease.
- Monitor diabetic patients closely because glucose tolerance may change. Adjustments may be needed in insulin, oral hypoglycemic dosage, and diet.

Drug-specific teaching points
- Take drug with food if nausea or GI upset occurs.
- Know that the following side effects may occur: nausea, vomiting, diarrhea, burning of the tongue (small, frequent meals may help); body hair growth, baldness, deepening of the voice, loss of libido, impotence (most of these effects will be reversible when the drug is stopped); excitation, confusion, insomnia (avoid driving, performing tasks that require alertness if these effects occur); swelling of the ankles, fingers (medication may be ordered to help).
- Be aware that diabetic patients need to monitor urine sugar closely as glucose tolerance may change; report any abnormalities to physician, so corrective action can be taken.
- Be aware that these drugs do not enhance athletic ability but do have serious effects and should not be used for increasing muscle strength.
- Report ankle swelling, skin color changes, severe nausea, vomiting, hoarseness, body hair growth, deepening of the voice, acne, menstrual irregularities in women.

▢ oxymorphone hydrochloride

(ox i mor' fone)
Numorphan

Pregnancy Category C
C-II controlled substance

Drug classes
Narcotic agonist analgesic

Therapeutic actions
Acts as agonist at specific opioid receptors in the CNS to produce analgesia, euphoria, sedation; the receptors mediating these effects are thought to be the same as those mediating the effects of endogenous opioids (enkephalins, endorphins).

Indications
- Relief of moderate to moderately severe pain

oxymorphone hydrochloride ■ 837

- Parenterally for preoperative medication, support of anesthesia, obstetric analgesia
- For relief of anxiety in patients with dyspnea associated with acute left ventricular failure and pulmonary edema

Contraindications/cautions
- Contraindicated in the presence of hypersensitivity to narcotics, diarrhea caused by poisoning (before toxins are eliminated), pregnancy (readily crosses placenta; neonatal withdrawal has occurred in infants born to mothers who used narcotics during pregnancy), labor or delivery (administration of narcotics to the mother can cause respiratory depression of neonate; premature infants are at special risk; may prolong labor), bronchial asthma, COPD, cor pulmonale, respiratory depression, anoxia, kyphoscoliosis, acute alcoholism, increased intracranial pressure, lactation.
- Use caution in the presence of acute abdominal conditions, cardiovascular disease, supraventricular tachycardias, myxedema, convulsive disorders, delirium tremens, cerebral arteriosclerosis, ulcerative colitis, fever, Addison's disease, prostatic hypertrophy, urethral stricture, recent GI or GU surgery, toxic psychosis, renal or hepatic dysfunction

Dosage
Adult
- ***IV:*** Initially 0.5 mg.
- ***SC or IM:*** Initially 1–1.5 mg q4–6h as needed. For analgesia during labor, 0.5–1 mg IM.
- ***Rectal suppositories:*** 5 mg q4–6h. After initial dosage, cautiously increase dose in nondebilitated patients until pain relief is obtained.

Pediatric: Safety and efficacy not established for children younger than 12 y.

Geriatric or impaired adult: Use caution; respiratory depression may occur in elderly, the very ill, those with respiratory problems.

Pharmacokinetics
Metabolism: Hepatic, $T_{1/2}$: 2.6–4 h

Route	Onset	Peak	Duration
IV	5–10 min	½–1 h	3–6 h
IM/SC	10–15 min	½–1 h	3–6 h
PR	15–30 min	1–1½ h	3–6 h

Distribution: Crosses placenta; enters breast milk
Excretion: Urine

IV facts
Preparation: No further preparation needed.
Infusion: Inject slowly directly into vein or into tubing of running IV.

Adverse effects
- **CNS:** *Lightheadedness, dizziness, sedation,* euphoria, dysphoria, delirium, insomnia, agitation, anxiety, fear, hallucinations, disorientation, drowsiness, lethargy, impaired mental and physical performance, coma, mood changes, weakness, headache, tremor, convulsions, miosis, visual disturbances
- **GI:** *Nausea, vomiting, sweating* (more common in ambulatory patients and those without severe pain), dry mouth, anorexia, constipation, biliary tract spasm; increased colonic motility in patients with chronic ulcerative colitis
- **CV:** Facial flushing, peripheral circulatory collapse, tachycardia, bradycardia, arrhythmia, palpitations, chest wall rigidity, hypertension, hypotension, orthostatic hypotension, syncope, circulatory depression, shock, cardiac arrest
- **Respiratory:** Suppression of cough reflex, respiratory depression, apnea, respiratory arrest, laryngospasm, bronchospasm
- **GU:** Ureteral spasm, spasm of vesical sphincters, urinary retention or hesitancy, oliguria, antidiuretic effect, reduced libido or potency
- **Dermatologic:** Pruritus, urticaria, edema, hemorrhagic urticaria (rare)
- **Local:** Pain at injection site, tissue irritation and induration (SC injection)
- **Other:** Physical tolerance and dependence, psychological dependence

Adverse effects in *Italics* are most common; those in **Bold** are life-threatening.

Clinically important drug-drug interactions
- Increased likelihood of respiratory depression, hypotension, profound sedation or coma in patients receiving barbiturate general anesthetics

Drug-lab test interferences
- Elevated biliary tract pressure may cause increases in plasma amylase, lipase; determinations for 24 h after administration of narcotics

■ Nursing Considerations

Assessment
- *History:* Hypersensitivity to narcotics, diarrhea caused by poisoning, pregnancy; labor or delivery; bronchial asthma, COPD, cor pulmonale, respiratory depression, kyphoscoliosis, acute alcoholism, increased intracranial pressure, acute abdominal conditions, cardiovascular disease, myxedema, convulsive disorders, delirium tremens, cerebral arteriosclerosis, ulcerative colitis, fever, Addison's disease, prostatic hypertrophy, urethral stricture, recent GI or GU surgery, toxic psychosis, renal or hepatic dysfunction
- *Physical:* Body temperature; skin—color, texture, lesions; orientation, reflexes, bilateral grip strength, affect, pupil size; P, auscultation, BP, orthostatic BP, perfusion; R, adventitious sounds; bowel sounds, normal output; frequency and pattern of voiding, normal output; ECG; EEG; thyroid, liver, kidney function tests

Implementation
- Administer to women who are lactating 4–6 h before the next scheduled feeding to minimize the amount in milk.
- Refrigerate rectal suppositories.
- Provide narcotic antagonist, facilities for assisted or controlled respiration on standby during parenteral administration.
- Use caution when injecting SC into chilled areas or in patients with hypotension or in shock; impaired perfusion may delay absorption; with repeated doses, an excessive amount may be absorbed when circulation is restored.
- Reassure patient about addiction liability; most patients who receive opiates for medical reasons do not develop dependence syndromes.

Drug-specific teaching points
- Take drug exactly as prescribed.
- Know that the following side effects may occur: nausea, loss of appetite (taking the drug with food and lying quietly, eating frequent small meals should minimize these effects); constipation (a laxative may help); dizziness, sedation, drowsiness, impaired visual acuity (avoid driving a car, performing other tasks that require alertness, visual acuity).
- Do not to take any leftover medication for other disorders, and do not to let anyone else take the prescription.
- Report severe nausea, vomiting, constipation, shortness of breath or difficulty breathing.

▢ oxyphencyclimine hydrochloride

(oks' ee fen cy' kli meen)
Daricon

Pregnancy Category C

Drug classes
Antispasmodic
Anticholinergic
Antimuscarinic
Parasympatholytic

Therapeutic actions
Direct GI smooth muscle relaxant; competitively blocks the effects of acetylcholine at muscarinic cholinergic receptors that mediate the effects of parasympathetic postganglionic impulses, thus relaxing the GI tract.

Indications
- Treatment of functional bowel/irritable bowel syndrome (irritable colon, spastic colon, mucous colitis)
- Adjunctive treatment of peptic ulcer

Contraindications/cautions
- Contraindicated in the presence of glaucoma; adhesions between iris and lens;

stenosing peptic ulcer, pyloroduodenal obstruction, paralytic ileus, intestinal atony, severe ulcerative colitis, toxic megacolon; symptomatic prostatic hypertrophy, bladder neck obstruction; bronchial asthma, COPD; cardiac arrhythmias, tachycardia, myocardial ischemia; impaired metabolic, liver or kidney function; myasthenia gravis; lactation
- Use caution in the presence of Down's syndrome, brain damage, spasticity, hypertension, hyperthyroidism.

Dosage
Adult: 5–10 mg PO bid–tid, in the morning and at bedtime.
Pediatric: Not recommended for children younger than 12 y.

Pharmacokinetics

Route	Onset	Duration
Oral	1–2 h	> 12 h

Metabolism: Hepatic, $T_{1/2}$: 9–10 h
Distribution: Crosses placenta; enters breast milk
Excretion: Urine and feces

Adverse effects
- **CNS:** *Blurred vision*, mydriasis, cycloplegia, photophobia, increased intraocular pressure
- **GI:** *Dry mouth, altered taste perception, nausea, vomiting, dysphagia*, heartburn, constipation, bloated feeling, paralytic ileus, gastroesophageal reflux
- **CV:** Palpitations, tachycardia
- **GU:** *Urinary hesitancy and retention*, impotence
- **Other:** Decreased sweating and predisposition to heat prostration, suppression of lactation

Clinically important drug-drug interactions
- Decreased antipsychotic effectiveness of haloperidol when given with anticholinergic drugs • Decreased effectiveness of phenothiazines given with anticholinergic drugs but increased incidence of paralytic ileus

■ Nursing Considerations
Assessment
- *History:* Glaucoma; adhesions between iris and lens; stenosing peptic ulcer; pyloroduodenal obstruction; intestinal atony; severe ulcerative colitis; symptomatic prostatic hypertrophy; bladder neck obstruction; bronchial asthma; COPD; cardiac arrhythmias; myocardial ischemia; impaired metabolic, liver, or kidney function; myasthenia gravis; Down syndrome; brain damage; spasticity; hypertension; hyperthyroidism; lactation
- *Physical:* Bowel sounds, normal output; normal urinary output, prostate palpation; R, adventitious sounds; P, BP; intraocular pressure, vision; bilateral grip strength, reflexes; liver palpation, liver and renal function tests; skin color, lesions, texture

Implementation
- Encourage patient to void before each dose of medication if urinary retention becomes a problem.

Drug-specific teaching points
- Take drug exactly as prescribed.
- Avoid hot environments while taking this drug (you will be heat intolerant, and dangerous reactions may occur).
- Know that the following side effects may occur: constipation (ensure adequate fluid intake, proper diet); dry mouth (sugarless lozenges, frequent mouth care may help; this effect sometimes lessens with time); blurred vision, sensitivity to light (avoid tasks that require acute vision; wear sunglasses when in bright light if these occur); impotence (this is a drug effect that will go away when you discontinue the drug); difficulty in urination (it may help to empty the bladder immediately before taking each dose of drug).
- Report skin rash, flushing, eye pain, difficulty breathing, tremors, loss of coordination, irregular heartbeat, palpitations, headache, abdominal distention, hallucinations, severe or persistent dry mouth, difficulty swallowing, difficulty in urina-

Adverse effects in *Italics* are most common; those in **Bold** are life-threatening.

tion, severe constipation, sensitivity to light.

☐ oxytetracycline

(ox i tet ra sye' kleen)
Terramycin, Uri-Tet

Pregnancy Category D

Drug classes
Antibiotic
Tetracycline

Therapeutic actions
Bacteriostatic: inhibits protein synthesis of susceptible bacteria, causing cell death.

Indications
- Infections caused by rickettsiae; *Mycoplasma pneumoniae;* agents of psittacosis, ornithosis, lymphogranuloma venereum and granuloma inguinale; *Borrelia recurrentis; Hemophilus ducreyi; Pasteurella pestis; Pasteurella tularensis; Bartonella bacilliformis; Bacteroides; Vibrio comma; Vibrio fetus; Brucella; E. coli; E. aerogenes; Shigella; Acinetobacter calcoaceticus; H. influenzae; Klebsiella; Streptococcus pneumoniae; S. aureus*
- When penicillin is contraindicated, infections caused by *N. gonorrhoeae, Treponema pallidum, Treponema pertenue, Listeria monocytogenes, Clostridium, Bacillus anthracis, Fusobacterium fusiforme, Actinomyces, Neisseria meningitidis*
- As an adjunct to amebicides in acute intestinal amebiasis

Contraindications/cautions
- Allergy to tetracylines, renal or hepatic dysfunction, pregnancy, lactation.

Dosage
Adult: 250 mg qd or 300 mg in divided doses q8–12h IM. 250–500 mg q12h IV. *Do not exceed 500 mg q6h.* 1–2 g/d PO in two to four equal doses up to 500 mg qid PO.

Pediatric: Older than 8 y, 15–25 mg/kg per day IM. May be given in single dose of up to 250 mg, or divided into equal doses q8–12h. 12 mg/kg per day divided into two doses IV. Up to 10–20 mg/kg per day IV in severe cases. 25–50 mg/kg per day in 2–4 equal doses PO.

Geriatric or renal failure patients: IV and IM doses of tetracyclines have been associated with severe hepatic failure and death when used in patients with renal dysfunction. Lower than normal doses are required, and serum levels should be checked regularly.

Pharmacokinetics

Route	Onset	Peak
Oral	Varies	2–4 h
IM	Rapid	2–4 h
IV	Immediate	Minutes

Metabolism: Hepatic, $T_{1/2}$: 6–12 h
Distribution: Crosses placenta; enters breast milk
Excretion: Urine

IV facts
Preparation: Dissolve powder in 10 ml of Sterile Water for Injection or 5% Dextrose Injection. Dilute further with at least 100 ml of Ringer's Solution, Isotonic Sodium Chloride Solution, or 5% Dextrose in Water.
Infusion: Administer slowly.

Adverse effects
- **GI:** Fatty liver, **liver failure**, *anorexia, nausea, vomiting, diarrhea, glossitis,* dysphagia, enterocolitis, esophageal ulcer
- **Hematologic:** Hemolytic anemia, thrombocytopenia, neutropenia, eosinophilia, leukocytosis, leukopenia
- **Dermatologic:** *Phototoxic reactions, rash,* exfoliative dermatitis (more frequent and more severe with this tetracycline than with any others)
- **Dental:** *Discoloring and inadequate calcification of primary teeth of fetus if used by pregnant women; discoloring and inadequate calcification of perma-*

nent teeth if used during period of dental development
- **Local:** Local irritation at injection site
- **Other:** Superinfections, nephrogenic diabetes insipidus syndrome

Clinically important drug-drug interactions
- Decreased absorption of oxytetracycline if taken with antacids, iron, alkali, food, dairy products, urine alkalinizers • Increased digoxin toxicity if taken with oxytetracycline • Increased nephrotoxicity if taken with methoxyflurane • Decreased activity of penicillins if taken with oxytetracycline

■ Nursing Considerations

Assessment
- *History:* Allergy to tetracylines, renal or hepatic dysfunction, pregnancy, lactation
- *Physical:* Skin status, orientation and reflexes, R, sounds, GI function and liver evaluation, urinalysis and BUN, liver and renal function tests; culture infected area before beginning therapy

Implementation
- Administer oral medication without regard to food or meals; if GI upset occurs, give with meals.

Drug-specific teaching points
- Take the drug throughout the day for best results.
- Take the drug with meals if GI upset occurs.
- Know that sensitivity to sunlight may occur (wear protective clothing, and use a sunscreen if out in the sun).
- Report rash, itching; difficulty breathing; dark urine or light-colored stools; severe cramps, watery diarrhea.

☐ oxytocin

(ox i toe' sin)
Parenteral: Pitocin, Syntocinon
Nasal spray: Syntocinon
Pregnancy Category C

Drug classes
Oxytocic
Hormonal agent

Therapeutic actions
Synthetic form of an endogenous hormone produced in the hypothalamus and stored in the posterior pituitary; stimulates the uterus, especially the gravid uterus just before parturition, and causes myoepithelium of the lacteal glands to contract, which results in milk ejection in lactating women.

Indications
- Antepartum: to initate or improve uterine contractions to achieve early vaginal delivery when the delivery is in the best interest of the mother and baby; stimulation or reinforcement of labor in selected cases of uterine inertia; management of inevitable or incomplete abortion; second trimester abortion (parenteral)
- Postpartum: to produce uterine contractions during the third stage of labor and to control postpartum bleeding or hemorrhage (parenteral)
- To stimulate initial milk let-down (nasal)
- Unlabeled use: antepartum fetal heart rate testing (oxytocin challenge test), treatment of breast engorgement

Contraindications/cautions
- Significant cephalopelvic disproportion, unfavorable fetal positions or presentations, obstetric emergencies that favor surgical intervention, prolonged use in severe toxemia, uterine inertia, hypertonic uterine patterns, induction or augmentation of labor when vaginal delivery is contraindicated, previous cesarean section, pregnancy (nasal).

Dosage
Dosage must be adjusted based on uterine response.
Adult
- ***Induction or stimulation of labor:*** Initial dose of no more than 1–2 mU/min (0.001–0.002 U/min) by IV infusion through an infusion pump. In-

crease the dose in increments of no more than 1–2 mU/min at 15- to 30-min intervals until a contraction pattern similar to normal labor is established. Do not exceed 20 mU/min. Discontinue in event of uterine hyperactivity, fetal distress.
- ***Control of postpartum uterine bleeding***
- *IV drip:* Add 10–40 U to 1,000 ml of a nonhydrating diluent, run at a rate to control uterine atony.
- *IM:* Administer 10 U after delivery of the placenta.
- ***Treatment of incomplete or inevitable abortion:*** IV infusion of 10 U of oxytocin with 500 ml physiologic saline solution or 5% dextrose in physiologic saline infused at a rate of 10–20 mU (20–40 drops)/min.
- ***Initial milk let-down:*** One spray into one or both nostrils 2–3 min before nursing or pumping of breasts.

Pharmacokinetics

Route	Onset	Duration
IV	Immediate	60 min
IM	3–5 min	2–3 h
Nasal	Varies	20 min

Metabolism: Hepatic, $T_{1/2}$: 1–6 min
Distribution: Crosses placenta; enters breast milk
Excretion: Urine

IV facts

Preparation: Add 1 ml (10 U) to 1,000 ml of 0.9% Aqueous Sodium Chloride or other IV fluid; the resulting solution will contain 10 mU/ml (0.01 U/ml).

Infusion: Infuse constant infusion pump to ensure accurate control of rate; rate determined by uterine response.

Compatibilities: Compatible at a concentration of 5 U/L in dextrose–Ringer's combinations; Dextrose–Lactated Ringer's combinations; Dextrose–Saline combinations; Dextrose 2%, 5%, and 10% in Water; Fructose 10% in Water; Ringer's Injection; Lactated Ringer's Injection; Sodium Chloride 0.45% and 0.9% Injection; and $\frac{1}{6}$ M Sodium Lactate.

Adverse effects

- **GI:** *Nausea, vomiting*
- **CV:** *Cardiac arrhythmias*, PVCs, hypertension, subarachnoid hemorrhage
- **GU:** Postpartum hemorrhage, uterine rupture, pelvic hematoma, *uterine hypertonicity*, spasm, tetanic contraction, rupture of the uterus with excessive dosage or hypersensitivity
- **Hypersensitivity:** Anaphylactic reaction
- **Fetal effects:** *Fetal bradycardia,* neonatal jaundice, low Apgar scores
- **Other:** Maternal and fetal deaths when used to induce labor or in first or second stages of labor; fatal afibrinogenemia; **severe water intoxication** with convulsions and coma, **maternal death** (associated with slow oxytocin infusion over 24 h; oxytocin has antidiuretic effects)

■ Nursing Considerations
Assessment
- *History:* Significant cephalopelvic disproportion, unfavorable fetal positions or presentations, severe toxemia, uterine inertia, hypertonic uterine patterns, previous cesarean section
- *Physical:* Fetal heart rate (continuous monitoring is recommended); fetal positions; fetal-pelvic proportions; uterine tone; timing and rate of contractions; breast exam; orientation, reflexes; P, BP, edema; R, adventitious sounds; CBC, bleeding studies, urinary output

Implementation
- Ensure fetal position and size and absence of complications that are contraindications to the use of oxytocin before beginning administration.
- Administer nasal preparation by having patient hold the squeeze bottle upright; patient should be sitting, not lying down. If preferred, the solution can be instilled in drop form by inverting the squeeze bottle and exerting gentle pressure to allow drop formation.

paclitaxel ■ 843

- Ensure continuous observation of patient receiving IV oxytocin for induction or stimulation of labor; fetal monitoring is preferred. A physician should be immediately available to deal with complications if they arise.
- Regulate rate of oxytocin delivery to establish uterine contractions that are similar to normal labor; monitor rate and strength of contractions; discontinue drug and notify physician at any sign of uterine hyperactivity or spasm.
- Monitor maternal BP during oxytocin administration, discontinue drug and notify physician with any sign of hypertensive emergency.
- Monitor neonate for the occurrence of jaundice.

Drug-specific teaching points
- The patient receiving parenteral oxytocin is usually receiving it as part of an immediate medical situation, and the drug teaching should be incorporated into the teaching about the procedure, labor, or complication of delivery that is involved. The patient needs to know the name of the drug and what she can expect once it is administered.
- Administer one spray into one or both nostrils 2–3 min before nursing or pumping breasts to initate milk let-down. Proper administration is important; hold the bottle upright and squeeze into nostril while sitting up, not lying down.
- Report sores in the nostrils, palpitations, unusual bleeding or bruising.

❐ paclitaxel

*(pass leh **tax' **ell)*
Taxol
Pregnancy Category D

Drug classes
Antineoplastic

Therapeutic actions
Inhibits the normal dynamic reorganization of the microtubule network that is essential for dividing cells; leads to cell death in rapidly dividing cells.

Indications
- Treatment of metastatic carcinoma of the ovary after failure of first-line or subsequent therapy
- Unlabeled uses: treatment of advanced head and neck cancer, previously untreated extensive-stage small-cell lung cancer, adenocarcinoma of the upper GI tract, hormone-refractory prostate cancer, advanced non–small-cell lung cancer, metastatic breast cancer, leukemias

Contraindications/cautions
- Contraindicated in the presence of hypersensitivity to paclitaxel or drug formulated with polyoxethylated castor oil, bone marrow depression, severe neurologic toxicity, lactation, pregnancy.
- Use caution in the presence of cardiac conduction defects, severe hepatic impairment.

Dosage
Adult: 135 mg/m^2 IV over 24 h every 3 wk. Do not repeat until neutrophil count is at least 1,500 cells/mm^2 and platelet count is at least 100,000 cells/mm^2.
Pediatric: Safety and efficacy not established.

Pharmacokinetics

Route	Onset	Duration
IV	Rapid	6–12 h

Metabolism: Hepatic, T$_{1/2}$: 5.3–17.4 h
Distribution: Crosses placenta; enters breast milk
Excretion: Bile

IV facts
Preparation: Use extreme caution when handling drug; dilute prior to infusion in 0.9% Sodium Chloride, 5% Dextrose Injection, 5% Dextrose and 0.9% Sodium Chloride Injection, 5% Dextrose in Ringer's Injection to a concentration of 0.3–1.2 mg/ml; stable at room temperature for 24 h. Refrigerate unopened vials; avoid use of PVC infusion bags and tubing.
Infusion: Administer over 24 h through an in-line filter not greater than 0.22 μm.

Adverse effects
- CNS: Peripheral sensory neuropathy, mild to severe
- GI: *Nausea, vomiting*, mucositis, anorexia, elevated liver enzymes
- CV: Bradycardia, hypotension, severe cardiovascular events
- Hematologic: **Bone marrow depression,** *infection*
- Other: *Hypersensitivity reactions, myalgia, arthralgia, alopecia*

Clinically important drug-drug interactions
- Increased myelosuppression if taken concurrently with cisplatin • Decreased paclitaxel effects if taken concurrently with ketoconazole

■ Nursing Considerations

Assessment
- *History:* Hypersensitivity to paclitaxel, castor oil; bone marrow depression; cardiac conduction defects; severe hepatic impairment; pregnancy; lactation
- *Physical:* Neurologic status, body temperature; P, BP, peripheral perfusion; skin—color, texture, hair distribution; abdominal exam, mucous membranes; kidney and liver function tests, CBC

Implementation
- Do not administer drug unless blood counts are within acceptable parameters.
- Handle drug with great care; gloves are recommended. If drug comes in contact with skin, wash immediately with soap and water.
- Premedicate patient before administration to prevent severe hypersensitivity reactions: oral dexamethasone 20 mg, 12 h and 6 h before paclitaxel; diphenhydramine 50 mg IV 30–60 min before paclitaxel; or cimetidine 300 mg IV 30–60 min before paclitaxel.
- Monitor blood pressure and pulse during administration.
- Arrange for blood counts before beginning therapy and at least monthly during treatment.
- Monitor patient's neurologic status frequently during treatment.

Drug-specific teaching points
- Be aware that drug will need to be given over a 24-h period once every 3 wk. Mark a calendar noting drug days.
- Arrange to have regular blood tests and neurologic exams while receiving this drug.
- Know that the following side effects may occur: nausea and vomiting (this may be severe; antiemetics may be helpful and can be ordered for you; small frequent meals also may help); weakness, lethargy (frequent rest periods will help); increased susceptibility to infection (avoid crowds and situations that might expose you to many people or diseases); numbness and tingling in the fingers or toes (use care to avoid injury to these areas; use care if trying to perform tasks that require precision); loss of hair (you may want to arrange for a wig or other head covering; it is important to keep the head covered at extremes of temperature).
- Report severe nausea and vomiting; fever, chills, sore throat; unusual bleeding or bruising; numbness or tingling in your fingers or toes; chest pain.

☐ pamidronate disodium

(pah mih' dro nate)

Aredia

Pregnancy Category C

Drug classes
Calcium regulator

Therapeutic actions
Slows normal and abnormal bone resorption without inhibiting bone formation and mineralization.

Indications
- Treatment of hypercalcemia of malignancy

pancreatic enzymes ■ 845

- Unlabeled uses: Paget's disease, postmenopausal osteoporosis, bone metastases from breast cancer, hyperparathyroidism, prostatic carcinoma, mutiple myeloma, immobilization-related hypercalcemia to prevent fractures and bone pain

Contraindications/cautions
- Contraindicated in the presence of allergy to pamidronate disodium or biphosphates.
- Use caution in the presence of renal failure, enterocolitis, pregnancy, lactation.

Dosage
Adult: 60–90 mg IV given over 24 h.
Pediatric: Safety and efficacy not established.

Pharmacokinetics

Route	Onset	Duration
IV	Rapid	72 h

Metabolism: Hepatic, $T_{1/2}$: 1.6 h, then 27.3 h
Distribution: Crosses placenta; may enter breast milk
Excretion: Urine

IV facts
Preparation: Reconstitute by adding 10 ml Sterile Water for Injection to each vial; resulting solution contains 30 mg/10 ml; allow drug to dissolve. May be further diluted in 1,000 ml sterile 0.45% or 0.9% Sodium Chloride or 5% Dextrose Injection; stable for 24 h at room temperature.
Infusion: Infuse over 24 h.
Incompatibilities: Do not mix with calcium-containing infusions, such as Ringer's.

Adverse effects
- GI: *Nausea, diarrhea*
- MS: *Increased or recurrent bone pain* at pagetic sites, focal osteomalacia

■ Nursing Considerations
Assessment
- *History:* Allergy to pamidronate disodium or any biphosphates, renal failure, enterocolitis, lactation
- *Physical:* Skin—lesions, color, temperature; muscle tone, bone pain; bowel sounds; urinalysis, serum calcium

Implementation
- Provide saline hydration before administration.
- Monitor serum calcium levels before, during, and after therapy. Consider retreatment if hypercalcemia recurs, but allow a minimum of 7 wk between treatments.
- Do not give foods high in calcium, vitamins with mineral supplements, or antacids high in metals within 2 h of dosing.
- Maintain adequate nutrition, particularly intake of calcium and vitamin D.
- Monitor patients with renal impairment carefully; arrange for reduction of dosage if glomerular filtration rate is reduced.
- Maintain calcium on standby in case hypocalcemic tetany develops.

Drug-specific teaching points
- Do not take foods high in calcium, antacids, or vitamins with minerals within 2 h of taking this drug.
- Know that the following side effects may occur: nausea, diarrhea; recurrent bone pain.
- Report twitching, muscle spasms, dark urine, severe diarrhea.

☐ pancreatic enzymes

(pan kre li' pase)

pancrelipase
Prescription products:
Cotazym, Ilozyme, Ku-Zyme HP Capsules, Pancrease Capsules, Protilase, Ultrase MT 8, 12, 20, 24;, Viokase

pancreatin
Creon Capsules, Donnazyme, Entozyme

Adverse effects in *Italics* are most common; those in **Bold** are life-threatening.

OTC products: Dizymes Capsules, Pancreatin Enseals, Pancrezyme, 4X and 8X Pancreatin

Pregnancy Category C

Drug classes
Digestive enzyme

Therapeutic actions
Replacement of pancreatic enzymes: helps to digest and absorb fat, proteins, and carbohydrates.

Indications
- Replacement therapy in patients with deficient exocrine pancreatic secretions, cystic fibrosis, chronic pancreatitis, postpancreatectomy, ductal obstructions, pancreatic insufficiency, steatorrhea or malabsorption syndrome, and postgastrectomy
- Presumptive test for pancreatic function

Contraindications/cautions
- Contraindicated in the presence of allergy to any component, pork products.
- Use caution in the presence of pregnancy, lactation.

Dosage
Adult
- **Pancrelipase:** *Capsules and tablets:* 4,000–48,000 U PO with each meal and with snacks, usually 1–3 capsules or tablets before or with meals and snacks. May be increased to 8 tablets in severe cases. Patients with pancreatectomy or obstruction, 8,000–16,000 U PO lipase at 2-h intervals, may be increased to 64,000–88,000 U.
- **Powder:** 0.7 g PO with meals.
- **Pancreatin:** Capsules and tablets: 1–2 PO with meals or snacks.

Pediatric
- *6 mo–1 y:* 2,000 U lipase PO per meal.
- *1–6 y:* 4,000–8,000 U PO lipase with each meal and 4,000 U with snacks.
- *7–12 y:* 4,000–12,000 U PO lipase with each meal and with snacks.

Pharmacokinetics
Not known.

Adverse effects
- **GI:** *Nausea, abdominal cramps, diarrhea*
- **GU:** Hyperuricosuria, hyperuricemia with extremely high doses
- **Hypersensitivity:** Asthma with inhalation of fine-powder concentrates in sensitized individuals

■ Nursing Considerations

Assessment
- *History:* Allergy to any component, pork products; pregnancy; lactation
- *Physical:* R, adventitious sounds; abdominal exam, bowel sounds; pancreatic function tests

Implementation
- Administer before or with meals and snacks.
- Avoid inhaling or spilling powder on hands because it may irritate skin or mucous membranes.
- Do not crush or let patient chew the enteric-coated capsules; drug will not survive acid environment of the stomach.

Drug-specific teaching points
- Take drug before or with meals and snacks.
- Do not crush or chew the enteric-coated capsules; swallow whole.
- Do not inhale powder dosage forms; severe reaction can occur.
- Know that the following side effects may occur: abdominal discomfort, diarrhea.
- Report joint pain, swelling, soreness; difficulty breathing; GI upset.

❑ paraldehyde

(par al' de hyde)
Paral

Pregnancy Category C
C-IV controlled substance

Adverse effects in *Italics* are most common; those in **Bold** are life-threatening.

Drug classes
Sedative/hypnotic (nonbarbiturate)

Therapeutic actions
Hypnotic that produces nonspecific, reversible depression of the CNS.

Indications
- Oral, rectal: sedative and hypnotic; quiets the patient and produces sleep in delirium tremens and other psychiatric states characterized by excitement
- Emergency treatment of tetanus, eclampsia, status epilepticus, and poisoning by convulsive drugs

Contraindications/cautions
- Contraindicated in the presence of hypersensitivity to paraldehyde, gastroenteritis.
- Use caution in the presence of bronchopulmonary disease, hepatic insufficiency, pregnancy, lactation.

Dosage
All doses expressed in volume refer to the 1 g/ml solution of paraldehyde that is commercially available.
Adult
- **Oral:** 4–8 ml in milk or iced fruit juice to mask the taste and odor. *For hypnosis:* 10–30 ml. *For sedation:* 5–10 ml. *For delirium tremens:* 10–35 ml.
- **Rectal:** Dissolve in oil as a retention enema; mix 10–20 ml, as appropriate, with 1 or 2 parts of olive oil or isotonic sodium chloride solution. *For hypnosis:* 10–30 ml of the 1 g/ml solution diluted as described above. *For sedation:* 5–10 ml of the 1 g/ml solution.

Pediatric
- *Hypnosis:* Give 0.3 ml/kg or 12 ml/m^2 of the 1 g/ml solution PO or rectally.
- *Sedation:* Give 0.15 ml/kg or 6 ml/m^2 PO, rectally, or IM.
- *Control of convulsions, tetanus, and so forth: Rectally:* 0.3 ml/kg diluted in 1–2 parts olive or cottonseed oil, q4–6h (this route is not generally recommended).

Pharmacokinetics

Route	Onset	Peak	Duration
Oral	10–15 min	30–60 min	8–12 h
PR	Slow	2½ h	8–12 h

Metabolism: Hepatic, $T_{1/2}$: 3.4–9.8 h
Distribution: Crosses placenta; may enter breast milk
Excretion: Lungs and bile

Adverse effects
- **GI:** GI upset, *irritation of the mucous membranes,* esophagitis, gastritis, proctitis, hepatitis, *strong, unpleasant breath for up to 24 h after ingestion*
- **CV:** Unusually slow heart beat, right heart edema, dilation, and failure
- **Respiratory:** Shortness of breath, troubled breathing, coughing
- **Hematologic:** *Metabolic acidosis,* particularly with high dosage or addiction
- **Dermatologic:** Skin rash, redness
- **Local:** Swelling or pain at injection site (thrombophlebitis), severe and permanent nerve damage, including paralysis, particularly of the sciatic nerve, when injected too close to a nerve trunk
- **Other:** *Addiction resembling alcoholism,* with withdrawal syndrome characterized by delirium tremens, hallucinations (prolonged use)

■ Nursing Considerations
Assessment
- *History:* Hypersensitivity to paraldehyde, bronchopulmonary disease, hepatic insufficiency, gastroenteritis, lactation
- *Physical:* Skin—injection site; orientation, reflexes; P, BP, perfusion; R, depth, adventitious sounds; bowel sounds, liver evaluation; liver function tests

Implementation
- Dilute before oral or rectal use, as described in dosage section.
- Give with food or mix with milk or iced fruit juice to improve taste and reduce GI upset when administering drug orally.
- Do not let paraldehyde contact plastic surfaces (eg, syringes, glasses, spoons); paraldehyde reacts with plastic.

Adverse effects in *Italics* are most common; those in **Bold** are life-threatening.

- Discard any unused paraldehyde after opening bottle; paraldehyde decomposes to acetaldehyde when exposed to light and air.
- Do not use drug solutions that are brownish or have a sharp odor of acetic acid (vinegar).
- Keep away from heat, open flame, or sparks.
- Liquefy drug solution that has solidified due to exposure to temperatures less than 12°C or 54°F.
- Do not store in direct sunlight or expose to temperatures > 25°C (77°F).
- Arrange to withdraw drug slowly after chronic use.

Drug-specific teaching points
- Take this drug exactly as directed, diluted in iced fruit juice or milk.
- Do not let this drug contact plastic; avoid plastic glasses, spoons, and so forth.
- Do not use if liquid is brownish or has a strong odor of vinegar.
- Discard any unused paraldehyde after opening bottle.
- Know that the following side effects may occur: drowsiness (use caution and avoid driving a car or performing other tasks that require alertness if you experience daytime drowsiness); GI upset (taking this drug with food or with milk or iced juices should help); strong unpleasant smelling breath for up to 24 h after you have taken a dose of this drug (you may be unaware of this).
- Report yellowing of the skin or eyes, pale stools, bloody stools.

☐ paramethadione

*(par a meth a **dye**' one)*
Paradione

Pregnancy Category D

Drug classes
Anticonvulsant

Therapeutic actions
Increases seizure threshold; sedative effects may progress to ataxia.

Indications
- Control of absence (petit mal) seizures refractory to treatment with other drugs

Contraindications/cautions
- Contraindicated in the presence of hypersensitivity to oxazolidinediones, tartrazine (300-mg tablets); pregnancy; lactation.
- Use caution in the presence of hepatic, renal abnormalities; pregnancy.

Dosage
Adult: 300 mg PO tid; may increase by 300 mg/d at weekly intervals; maximum dose, 2.4 g/d.
Pediatric
- ***Older than 6 y:*** 300 mg PO tid or qid.
- ***2–6 y:*** 200 mg PO tid.
- ***Younger than 2 y:*** 100 mg PO tid.

Pharmacokinetics

Route	Onset	Peak	Duration
Oral	15–30 min	1–2 h	4–6 h

Metabolism: Hepatic, $T_{1/2}$: 1–4 h
Distribution: Crosses placenta; enters breast milk
Excretion: Urine

Adverse effects
- **CNS:** *Drowsiness, ataxia, dizziness,* sedation, headache, paresthesias
- **GI:** GI distress, abnormal liver function tests, hepatitis
- **Hematologic:** Aplastic anemia
- **Dermatologic:** *Pruritus,* **exfoliative dermatitis**
- **Other:** Vaginal bleeding, **lupus-like syndrome**, fetal malformations, *photosensitivity*

■ Nursing Considerations

Assessment
- *History:* Hypersensitivity to oxazolidinediones; hepatic, renal abnormalities; lactation, pregnancy
- *Physical:* Skin—color, lesions; orientation, affect, reflexes, bilateral grip strength, vision exam; bowel sounds, normal output, liver evaluation; liver and

Adverse effects in *Italics* are most common; those in **Bold** are life-threatening.

850 ■ paroxetine

Adverse effects
- CNS: Vertigo, headache, change in hearing, ringing in the ears
- GI: *Nausea, abdominal cramps, diarrhea,* heartburn, vomiting
- GU: BUN increase, decrease in urinary output, hematuria
- Other: *Superinfections*

Clinically important drug-drug interactions
- Increased or decreased bioavailability of digoxin if taken concurrently • Increased neuromuscular blockade if given concurrently with succinylcholine; delay administration of paromomycin as long as possible after recovery of spontaneous respirations after use of succinylcholine

■ Nursing Considerations

Assessment
- *History:* Allergy to paromomycin, renal failure, intestinal obstruction, lactation
- *Physical:* Reflexes, eighth cranial nerve function; bowel sounds; BUN, urinalysis

Implementation
- Administer drug with meals.

Drug-specific teaching points
- Take drug three times a day with meals; small, frequent meals will help if stomach upset occurs.
- Be aware that nausea, vomiting, diarrhea may occur.
- Report ringing in the ears, dizziness, skin rash, fever, severe GI upset.

☐ paroxetine

*(pah **rox'** a teen)*
Paxil

Pregnancy Category B

Drug classes
Antidepressant

Therapeutic actions
Potentiates serotonergic activity in the CNS, resulting in antidepressant effect.

Indications
- Treatment of depression

Contraindications/cautions
- Contraindicated in the presence of MAO inhibitor use.
- Use caution in the presence of renal or hepatic impairment, the elderly, pregnancy, lactation, suicidal patients.

Dosage
Adult: 20 mg/d PO as a single daily dose.
Range: 20–50 mg/d.
- ***Switching to or from an MAO inhibitor:*** At least 14 d should elapse between discontinuation of MAO inhibitor and initiation of paroxetine therapy; similarly, allow 14 d between discontinuing paroxetine and beginning MAO inhibitor.

Pediatric: Safety and efficacy not established.
Geriatric, renal, or hepatic impairment: 10 mg/d PO. Do not exceed 40 mg/d.

Pharmacokinetics

Route	Onset
Oral	Slow

Metabolism: Hepatic, $T_{1/2}$: 1 h
Distribution: Crosses placenta; enters breast milk
Excretion: Urine

Adverse effects
- CNS: *Somnolence, dizziness, insomnia, tremor, nervousness, headache,* anxiety, paresthesia, blurred vision
- GI: *Nausea, dry mouth, constipation, diarrhea,* anorexia, flatulence, vomiting
- CV: Palpitations, vasodilation, postural hypotension, hypertension
- Respiratory: Yawns, pharyngitis, cough
- GU: *Ejaculatory disorders, male genital disorders,* urinary frequency
- Dermatologic: *Sweating,* skin rash, redness
- General: *Headache, asthenia*

Adverse effects in *Italics* are most common; those in **Bold** are life-threatening.

Clinically important drug-drug interactions

- Increased paroxetine levels and toxicity if taken with cimetidine, MAOIs • Decreased therapeutic effects of phenytoin, digoxin if taken with paroxetine • Decreased effectiveness of paroxetine if taken with phenobarbital, phenytoin • Increased serum levels of procyclidine, tryptophane, warfarin if taken with paroxetine

■ Nursing Considerations

Assessment

- *History:* Hypersensitivity to paroxetine, lactation, renal or hepatic impairment, seizure disorder
- *Physical:* Orientation, reflexes; P, BP, perfusion; R, adventitious sounds; bowel sounds, normal output; urinary output; liver evaluation; liver and renal function tests

Implementation

- Administer once a day in the morning.
- Encourage patient to continue use for 1–4 wk, as directed, to ensure adequate levels to affect depression.
- Limit amount of drug given in prescription to potentially suicidal patients.
- Advise patient to avoid use if pregnant or lactating.

Drug-specific teaching points

- Take this drug exactly as directed and as long as directed.
- Know that the following side effects may occur: drowsiness, dizziness, tremor (use caution and avoid driving a car or performing other tasks that require alertness if you experience daytime drowsiness); GI upset (small, frequent meals, frequent mouth care may help); alterations in sexual function (it may help to know that this is a drug effect and will pass when drug therapy is ended).
- Be aware that this drug should not be taken during pregnancy or when lactating.
- Report severe nausea, vomiting; palpitations; blurred vision; excessive sweating.

☐ pegasparagase

(peg ass par' a gase)
PEG-L, Oncaspar

Pregnancy Category C

Drug classes
Antineoplastic agent

Therapeutic actions
Formulation of L-asparaginase, an enzyme that hydrolyzes the amino acid asparagine, which is needed by some malignant cells (but not normal cells) for protein synthesis; thus, it inhibits malignant cell proliferation by interrupting protein synthesis; maximal effect in G_1 phase of the cell cycle; causes less frequent and less severe hypersensitivity reactions than asparaginase.

Indications
- Acute lymphocytic leukemia (ALL) in patients hypersensitive to native forms of L-asparaginase

Contraindications/cautions
- Allergy to asparaginase, severe response to asparaginase, pancreatitis or history of pancreatitis, immunosuppression, pregnancy, lactation

Dosage
Adults and children older than 1 y: 2500 IU/m^2 IM (preferred) or IV every 14 d.
Pediatric (BSA < 0.6 m^2): 82.5 IU/kg IM or IV every 14 d.

Pharmacokinetics

Route	Onset
IM	Varies
IV	30–40 min

Metabolism: T$_{1/2}$: 5 d
Distribution: Crosses placenta; enters breast milk
Excretion: Small amount in urine

IV facts
Preparation: No further preparation necessary. Single-use vial; discard any extra.

Infusion: Infuse over not less than 30 min into an already running IV infusion of Sodium Chloride Injection or 5% Dextrose Injection.

Adverse effects
- CNS: CNS depression
- GI: Hepatotoxicity, **pancreatitis** (sometimes fatal), *nausea, vomiting, anorexia*, abdominal cramps, pancreatitis
- Hematologic: Bleeding problems, hyperurecemia, **bone marrow depression**
- GU: Uric acid nephropathy; **renal toxicity**
- Hypersensitivity: *Skin rashes, urticaria, arthralgia*, respiratory distress to anaphylaxis
- Endocrine: Hyperglycemia—glucosuria, polyuria, hypoglycemia
- Other: Chills, fever, weight loss, **fatal hyperthermia**

Clinically important drug-drug interactions
- Diminished or decreased effect of methotrexate on malignant cells if given with or immediately following asparaginase • Increased toxicity of anticoagulants, immunosuppressives if given concurrently

Drug-lab test interferences
- Inaccurate interpretation of thyroid-function tests in patients taking asparaginase because of decreased serum levels of thyroxine-binding globulin; levels usually return to pretreatment levels within 4 wk of the last dose of asparaginase

■ Nursing Considerations

Assessment
- *History:* Allergy to asparaginase, pancreatitis, impaired hepatic function, bone marrow depression, lactation
- *Physical:* Weight; temperature; skin—color, lesions; orientation, reflexes; liver evaluation, abdominal exam; CBC, blood sugar, liver, andrenal function tests, serum amylase, clotting time, urinalysis, serum uric acid levels

Implementation
- Arrange for laboratory tests (CBC, serum amylase, blood glucose, liver function tests, uric acid) before beginning therapy and frequently during therapy.
- Administer IM if at all possible; reserve IV use for extreme situations.
- Monitor for any sign of hypersensitivity (eg, rash, difficulty breathing). If any of these occur, discontinue drug and consult with physician.
- Maintain life support equipment for dealing with anaphylaxis on standby anytime the drug is used.
- Monitor for pancreatitis; if serum amylase levels rise, discontinue drug and consult with physician.
- Monitor for hyperglycemia; reaction may resemble hyperosmolar, nonketotic hyperglycemia. If present, discontinue drug, and be prepared for use of IV fluids and insulin if required.

Drug-specific teaching points
- Prepare a calendar for patients who will need to return for specific treatment days and additional courses of drug therapy. Drug can be given only in the hospital under the direct supervision of physician.
- Know that the following side effects may occur: loss of appetite, nausea, vomiting (frequent mouth care, small, frequent meals may help; you will need to try to maintain good nutrition if at all possible; an antiemetic also may be ordered); fatigue, confusion, agitation, hallucinations, depression (it may help to know that these are drug effects; use special precautions to avoid injury if these occur).
- Arrange to have regular blood tests to monitor the drug's effects.
- Report fever, chills, sore throat; unusual bleeding or bruising; yellow skin or eyes; light-colored stools, dark urine; thirst, frequent urination.

◻ pemoline

(pem' oh leen)
Cylert

Pregnancy Category B
C-IV controlled substance

Adverse effects in *Italics* are most common; those in **Bold** are life-threatening.

Drug classes
CNS stimulant

Therapeutic actions
CNS actions similar to those of the amphetamines and methylphenidate but has minimal sympathomimetic effects; may act through dopaminergic mechanisms; efficacy in hyperkinetic syndrome, attention-deficit disorders in children appears paradoxical and is not understood.

Indications
- Attention-deficit disorders, hyperkinetic syndrome, minimal brain dysfunction in children with a behavioral syndrome characterized by the following symptoms: moderate to severe distractibility, short attention span, hyperactivity, emotional lability and impulsivity, not secondary to environmental factors or psychiatric disorders (as part of a total treatment program)
- Unlabeled use: narcolepsy and excessive daytime sleepiness

Contraindications/cautions
- Contraindicated in the presence of hypersensitivity to pemoline, impaired hepatic function.
- Use caution in the presence of impaired renal function, psychosis in children, epilepsy, drug dependence, alcoholism, emotional instability, lactation.

Dosage
Administer as a single oral dose each morning. Recommended starting dose is 37.5 mg/d PO. Gradually increase at 1-wk intervals using increments of 18.75 mg until desired response is obtained. Mean effective dose range is 56.25–75 mg/d. Do not exceed 112.5 mg/d. Not recommended in children younger than 6 y.
Narcolepsy: 50–200 mg PO in two divided doses daily.

Pharmacokinetics

Route	Onset	Peak
Oral	Gradual	2–4 h

Metabolism: Hepatic, $T_{1/2}$: 12 h

Distribution: Crosses placenta; may enter breast milk
Excretion: Urine

Adverse effects
- **CNS**: *Insomnia, anorexia with weight loss* (most common), dyskinetic movements of tongue, lips, face, and extremities; Gilles de la Tourette's syndrome; nystagmus; oculogyric crisis; convulsive seizures; increased irritability; mild depression; dizziness; headache; drowsiness; hallucinations
- **GI**: *Stomach ache*, nausea, hepatitis; elevations of SGOT, SGPT, LDH; jaundice
- **Dermatologic**: Skin rashes
- **Other**: Aplastic anemia; tolerance, psychological or physical dependence

■ Nursing Considerations

Assessment
- *History:* Hypersensitivity to pemoline; impaired hepatic or renal function, psychosis in children, epilepsy; drug dependence, alcoholism, emotional instability; lactation
- *Physical:* Body weight; body temperature; skin—color, lesions; orientation, affect, reflexes; P, BP, auscultation; R, adventitious sounds; bowel sounds, normal output; CBC with differential, liver and kidney function tests, baseline ECG

Implementation
- Ensure proper diagnosis before administering to children for behavioral syndromes: drug should not be used until other causes/concomitants of abnormal behavior (learning disability, EEG abnormalities, neurologic deficits) are ruled out.
- Arrange to interrupt drug dosage periodically in children being treated for behavioral disorders to determine if symptoms recur at an intensity that warrants continued drug therapy.
- Monitor growth of children on long-term pemoline therapy.
- Arrange to dispense the least feasible amount of drug at any time to minimize risk of overdosage.

Adverse effects in *Italics* are most common; those in **Bold** are life-threatening.

- Administer drug in the morning to prevent insomnia.
- Arrange to monitor liver function tests periodically in patients on long-term therapy.

Drug-specific teaching points
- Take this drug exactly as prescribed.
- Know that the following side effects may occur: insomnia, nervousness, restlessness, dizziness, impaired thinking (these effects may become less pronounced after a few days; avoid driving a car or engaging in activities that require alertness if these occur); diarrhea; headache, loss of appetite, weight loss.
- Report insomnia, abnormal body movements, skin rash, severe diarrhea, pale stools, yellowing of the skin or eyes.

❏ penbutolol sulfate

*(pen **byoo'** toe lole)*
Levatol

Pregnancy Category C

Drug classes
Beta-adrenergic blocking agent
Antihypertensive drug

Therapeutic actions
Competitively blocks beta-adrenergic receptors in the heart and juxtaglomerular apparatus, reducing the influence of the sympathetic nervous system on these tissues; decreasing the excitability of the heart, cardiac output, and release of renin; and lowering blood pressure.

Indications
- Treatment of mild to moderate hypertension

Contraindications/cautions
- Contraindicated in the presence of sinus bradycardia, second- or third-degree heart block, cardiogenic shock, CHF, pregnancy, lactation.
- Use caution in the presence of renal failure, diabetes or thyrotoxicosis, asthma, COPD, impaired hepatic function.

Dosage
Adult: Usual starting dose, maintenance dose, and dose used in combination with other antihypertensives: 20 mg PO qd. Doses of 40–80 mg qd have been used but with no additional antihypertensive effect.
Pediatric: Safety and efficacy not established.

Pharmacokinetics

Route	Onset	Peak	Duration
Oral	Varies	2–3 h	20 h

Metabolism: Hepatic, $T_{1/2}$: 5 h
Distribution: Crosses placenta; enters breast milk
Excretion: Urine

Adverse effects
- **CNS:** Dizziness, vertigo, tinnitus, fatigue, emotional depression, paresthesias, sleep disturbances, hallucinations, disorientation, memory loss, slurred speech
- **GI:** *Gastric pain, flatulence, constipation, diarrhea, nausea, vomiting,* anorexia, ischemic colitis, renal and mesenteric arterial thrombosis, retroperitoneal fibrosis, hepatomegaly, acute pancreatitis
- **CV:** **Bradycardia, CHF,** *cardiac arrhythmias, sinoartial or AV nodal block, tachycardia,* peripheral vascular insufficiency, claudication, CVA, pulmonary edema, hypotension
- **Respiratory:** Bronchospasm, dyspnea, cough, bronchial obstruction, nasal stuffiness, rhinitis, pharyngitis (less likely than with propranolol)
- **GU:** *Impotence, decreased libido,* Peyronie's disease, dysuria, nocturia, frequent urination
- **MS:** Joint pain, arthralgia, muscle cramp
- **EENT:** Eye irritation, dry eyes, conjunctivitis, blurred vision
- **Dermatologic:** Rash, pruritus, sweating, dry skin
- **Allergic reactions:** Pharyngitis, erythematous rash, fever, sore throat, laryngospasm, respiratory distress

Adverse effects in *Italics* are most common; those in **Bold** are life-threatening.

- **Other:** *Decreased exercise tolerance, development of antinuclear antibodies (ANA)*, hyperglycemia or hypoglycemia, elevated serum transaminase, alkaline phosphatase, and LDH

Clinically important drug-drug interactions

- Increased effects of penbutolol with verapamil • Decreased effects of penbutolol with epinephrine • Increased risk of peripheral ischemia, even gangrene, when given concurrently with ergot alkaloids (dihydroergotamine, methysergide, ergotamine) • Prolonged hypoglycemic effects of insulin • Increased "first-dose response" to prazosin • Paradoxical hypertension when clonidine is given with beta-blockers; increased rebound hypertension when clonidine is discontinued in patients on beta-blockers • Decreased hypertensive effect if given with NSAIDs (piroxicam, indomethacin, ibuprofen) • Decreased bronchodilator effects of theophylline and decreased bronchial and cardiac effects of sympathomimetics with penbutolol

Drug-lab test interferences

- Possible false results with glucose or insulin tolerance tests

■ Nursing Considerations

Assessment

- *History:* Sinus bradycardia, heart block, cardiogenic shock, CHF, renal failure, diabetes or thyrotoxicosis, asthma or COPD, impaired hepatic function, lactation
- *Physical:* Body weight, skin condition, neurologic status, P, BP, ECG, respiratory status, kidney and thyroid function, blood and urine glucose

Implementation

- Administer penbutolol once a day. Monitor response and maintain at lowest possible dose.
- Do not discontinue drug abruptly after chronic therapy (hypersensitivity to catecholamines may have developed, causing exacerbation of angina, MI, and ventricular dysrhythmias; taper drug gradually over 2 wk with monitoring).
- Consult with physician about withdrawing drug if patient is to undergo surgery (withdrawal is controversial).

Drug-specific teaching points

- Do not stop taking this drug unless instructed to do so by a health care provider.
- Avoid driving or dangerous activities if dizziness, drowsiness occur.
- Report difficulty breathing, night cough, swelling of extremities, slow pulse, confusion, depression, rash, fever, sore throat.

☐ penicillamine

(pen i sill' a meen)
Cuprimine, Depen

Pregnancy Category C

Drug classes

Chelating agent
Antirheumatic agent

Therapeutic actions

Chelating agent that removes excessive copper in Wilson's disease; exact mechanism of action as antirheumatoid agent is not known, but penicillamine lowers IgM rheumatoid factor; reduces excessive cystine excretion by disulfide interchange with cystine, resulting in a substance more soluble than cystine that is readily excreted.

Indications

- Rheumatoid arthritis: severe active disease in patients in whom other therapies have failed
- Wilson's disease
- Cystinuria when conventional measures are inadequate to control stone formation
- Unlabeled uses: primary biliary cirrhosis, scleroderma

Contraindications/cautions

- Contraindicated in the presence of allergy to penicillamine, penicillin; history of

penicillamine-related aplastic anemia or agranulocytosis; renal insufficiency; pregnancy (teratogenic).
- Use caution in the presence of lactation.

Dosage
Warning: interruptions of daily therapy of Wilson's disease or cystinuria for even a few days have been followed by sensitivity reactions when the drug is reinstituted.

Adult
- **Wilson's disease:** Base dosage on urinary copper excretion. Suggested initial dosage is 1 g/d PO given in divided doses qid. Up to 2 g/d may be needed.
- **Rheumatoid arthritis (2–3 mo may be required for a clinical response):** *Initial therapy:* a single daily dose of 125–250 mg PO. Thereafter increase dose at 1- to 3-mo intervals by 125 or 250 mg/d based on patient response, tolerance, and toxicity. Continue increases at 2- to 3-mo intervals. Doses of 1,000–1,500 mg/d for 3–4 mo with no improvement probably indicates that patient will not respond. *Maintenance:* many patients respond to 500–750 mg/d PO. Dosage above 1 g/d is unusual. *Exacerbations:* some patients experience exacerbation of disease activity that can subside in 12 wk. Treatment with NSAIDs is usually sufficient for control. Increase maintenance dose only if flare fails to subside within the 12-wk time period. *Duration of therapy:* after 6 mo of remission, attempt a gradual, stepwise dosage reduction in decrements of 125–250 mg/d at 3-mo intervals.
- **Cystinuria:** Usual dosage is 2 g/d (range 1–4 g/d) PO in divided doses qid, with the last dose at bedtime. Initiate dosage with 250 mg/d and increase gradually. Individualize dosage to limit cystine excretion to 100–200 mg/d in those with no history of stones, and to <100 mg/d in those with a history of stones.

Pediatric
- **Wilson's disease:** Base dosage on urinary copper excretion. Suggested initial dosage is 1 g/d PO given in divided doses qid. Up to 2 g/d may be needed.
- **Rheumatoid arthritis:** Efficacy in juvenile rheumatoid arthritis has not been established.
- **Cystinuria:** 30 mg/kg per day PO in divided doses qid with the last dose at bedtime. Consider patient's age, size, and rate of growth in determining dosage.

Pharmacokinetics

Route	Onset	Peak
Oral	Varies	1–3 h

Metabolism: Hepatic, $T_{1/2}$: 1.7–3.2 h
Distribution: Crosses placenta; enters breast milk
Excretion: Urine

Adverse effects
- CNS: Tinnitus, reversible optic neuritis, **myasthenic syndrome**, sometimes fatal
- GI: *Anorexia, epigastric pain, nausea, vomiting, diarrhea, altered taste perception,* intrahepatic cholestasis and toxic hepatitis, *oral ulcerations,* cheilosis, glossitis, colitis
- Hematologic: *Bone marrow depression*—leukopenia, thrombocytopenia, thrombocytic thrombocytopenic purpura, hemolytic anemia, red cell aplasia, monocytosis, leukocytosis, eosinophilia—fatalities from thrombocytopenia, agranulocytosis, and aplastic anemia
- GU: *Proteinuria,* hematuria, which may progress to nephrotic syndrome
- Hypersensitivity: Allergic reactions: *generalized pruritus,* lupus erythematosus-like syndrome, pemphigoid-type reactions, drug eruptions, uritcaria and exfoliative dermatitis, migratory polyarthralgia, **polymyositis**, Goodpasture's syndrome, alveolitis, obliterative bronchiolitis

Clinically important drug-drug interactions
- Decreased absorption of penicillamine if taken with iron salts, antacids, food • De-

creased serum levels of digoxin if taken with penicillamine

■ Nursing Considerations
Assessment
- *History:* Allergy to penicillamine, penicillin; history of penicillamine related aplastic anemia or agranulocytosis; renal insufficiency; pregnancy; lactation
- *Physical:* Skin—color, lesions; temperature; orientation, reflexes, ophthalmologic evaluation, audiometric evaluation, peripheral sensation; R, adventitious sounds; liver evaluation, bowel sounds, mucous membranes; CBC, clotting times, urinalysis, renal and liver function tests, x-ray for renal stones

Implementation
- Use caution when administering this drug because of the potential serious side effects.
- Arrange for monitoring of urinalysis, CBC before beginning therapy and every 2 wk during the first 6 mo of therapy and monthly thereafter; also monitor liver function tests and x-ray for renal stones before beginning therapy and periodically during therapy.
- Discontinue drug therapy if drug fever occurs—for a short period of time in Wilson's disease and cystinuria, permanently in rheumatoid arthritis—and switch to another therapy.
- Consult physician about the advisability of decreasing dosage to 250 mg/d when surgery is contemplated; wound healing may be delayed by the effects on collagen and elastin.
- Administer drug on an empty stomach, 1 h before or 2 h after meals and at least 1 h apart from any other drug, food, or milk.
- Administer drug for Wilson's disease on an empty stomach, 30–60 min before meals and at bedtime, at least 2 h after the evening meal.
- Administer drug for cystinuria in four equal doses; if this is not possible, give the larger dose at bedtime; the bedtime dose is of utmost importance.
- Ensure that patient with cystinuria drinks 1 pint of fluid at bedtime and another pint once during night; the greater the fluid intake, the lower the dose of penicillamine required.
- Arrange for nutritional consultation; pyridoxine supplements may be needed; ensure that multivitamin preparations do not contain copper for patients with Wilson's disease; iron deficiency also may occur; if iron supplements are used, ensure that they are given with at least a 2-h interval between iron and penicillamine; hypogeusia (loss of taste) may lead to anorexia or inappropriate eating habits.

Drug-specific teaching points
- Take drug on an empty stomach 1 h before or 2 h after meals and at least 1 h apart from any other drug, food, or milk. Wilson's disease: take 30–60 min before meals and at bedtimes. Cystinuria: be sure to take the bedtime dose; drink one pint of fluid at bedtime and one pint of fluid during the night; drink copious amounts of fluid during the day.
- Know that the following side effects may occur: nausea, GI upset, vomiting (taking the drug with food may help); diarrhea; rash, delays in healing (use good skin care; try to avoid injury); mouth sores, loss of taste perception (frequent mouth care will help; taste perception usually returns within 2–3 mo after therapy).
- Be aware that this drug is not to be used during pregnancy; if you become pregnant or want to become pregnant, consult your physician.
- Report skin rash, unusual bruising or bleeding, sore throat, difficulty breathing, cough or wheezing, fever, chills.
- Keep this drug and all medications out of the reach of children; this drug can be very dangerous for children.

☐ penicillin G benzathine

(pen i sill' in)
Bicillin L-A, Permapen

Pregnancy Category B

penicillin G benzathine

Drug classes
Antibiotic
Penicillin

Therapeutic actions
Bactericidal: inhibits synthesis of cell wall of sensitive organisms, causing cell death.

Indications
- Severe infections caused by sensitive organisms (streptococci)
- Treatment of syphilis, neurosyphilis, congenital syphilis, yaws, uncomplicated erysipeloid infection

Contraindications/cautions
- Contraindicated in the presence of allergies to penicillins, cephalosporins, or other allergens.
- Use caution in the presence of renal disorders, pregnancy, lactation (may cause diarrhea or candidiasis in the infant).

Dosage
Adult
- ***Streptococcal infections (including otitis media, URIs of mild to moderate severity):*** A single injection of 1.2 million U IM.
- ***Early syphilis:*** 2.4 million U IM in a single dose.
- ***Congenital syphilis:*** 50,000 U/kg IM in a single dose.
- ***Syphilis lasting more than 1 y:*** 7.2 million U given as 2.4 million U IM weekly for 3 wk.
- ***Yaws:*** 1.2 million U IM as a single dose.
- ***Erysipeloid:*** 1.2 million U IM as a single dose.

Pediatric
- ***Streptococcal infections (including otitis media, URIs of mild to moderate severity):*** A single injection of 900,000–1.2 million U in older children. A single injection of 300,000–600,000 U for children under 60 lb.
- ***Neonates:*** 50,000 U/kg

Pharmacokinetics

Route	Onset	Peak	Duration
IM	Slow	12–24 h	Days

Metabolism: Hepatic, $T_{1/2}$: 30–60 min
Distribution: Crosses placenta; enters breast milk
Excretion: Urine

Adverse effects
- **CNS:** Lethargy, hallucinations, seizures
- **GI:** *Glossitis, stomatitis, gastritis, sore mouth,* furry tongue, black "hairy" tongue, *nausea, vomiting, diarrhea,* abdominal pain, bloody diarrhea, enterocolitis, pseudomembranous colitis, nonspecific hepatitis
- **Hematologic:** Anemia, thrombocytopenia, leukopenia, neutropenia, prolonged bleeding time (more common with this drug than with other penicillinase-resistant penicillins)
- **GU:** Nephritis
- **Hypersensitivity reactions:** *Rash, fever, wheezing,* anaphylaxis
- **Local:** *Pain, phlebitis,* thrombosis at injection site, Jarisch-Herxheimer reaction when used to treat syphilis
- **Other:** *Superinfection,* sodium overload, leading to CHF

Clinically important drug-drug interactions
- Decreased effectiveness of penicillin G benzathine if taken concurrently with tetracyclines • Inactivation of parenteral aminoglycosides (amikacin, gentamicin, kanamycin, neomycin, metilmicin, streptomycin, tobramycin) if taken concurrently

■ Nursing Considerations

Assessment
- *History:* Allergies to penicillins, cephalosporins, other allergens, renal disorders, pregnancy, lactation
- *Physical:* Culture infected area; skin—color, lesions; R, adventitious sounds; bowel sounds: CBC, liver and renal function tests, serum electrolytes, Hct, urinalysis

Adverse effects in *Italics* are most common; those in **Bold** are life-threatening.

penicillin G potassium ■ 859

Implementation
- Culture infected area before beginning treatment; reculture area if response is not as expected.
- Administer by IM route only.
- Arrange to continue therapy for at least 2 d after signs of infection have disappeared, usually 7–10 d.
- Administer IM injection in upper outer quadrant of the buttock. In infants and small children, the midlateral aspect of the thigh may be preferred.

Drug-specific teaching points
- Be aware that you will need to receive a full course of drug therapy.
- Know that nausea, vomiting, diarrhea, mouth sores, pain at injection sites may occur.
- Report difficulty breathing, rashes, severe diarrhea, severe pain at injection site, mouth sores, unusual bleeding or bruising.

☐ penicillin G potassium

(pen i sill' in)

penicillin G (aqueous)
Falapen (CAN), Megacillin (CAN), Pfizerpen

penicillin G sodium
Crystapen (CAN)

Drug classes
Antibiotic
Penicillin

Therapeutic actions
Bactericidal: inhibits synthesis of cell wall of sensitive organisms, causing cell death.

Indications
- Treatment of severe infections caused by sensitive organisms—streptococci, pneumococci, staphylococci, *Neisseria gonorrhoeae*, *Treponema pallidum*, meningococci, *Actinomyces israelii*, *Clostridium perfringens* and *tetani*, *Leptotrichia buccalis* (Vincent's disease), *Spirillum minus* or *Streptobacillus moniliformis*, *Listeria monocytogenes*, *Pasteurella multocida*, *Erysipelothrix insidiosa*, *Escherichia coli*, *Enterobacter aerogenes*, *Alcaligenes faecalis*, *Salmonella*, *Shigella*, *Proteus mirabilis*, *Corynebacterium diphtheriae*, *Bacillus anthracis*
- Treatment of syphilis, gonococcal infections
- Unlabeled uses: treatment of Lyme disease

Contraindications/cautions
- Contraindicated in the presence of allergy to penicillins, cephalosporins, other allergens.
- Use caution in the presence of renal disease, pregnancy, lactation (may cause diarrhea or candidiasis in the infant).

Dosage
Adult
- ***Meningococcal meningitis:*** 1–2 million U q2h IM or by continuous IV infusion of 20–30 million U/d.
- ***Actinomycosis:*** 1–6 million U/d IM or IV for cervicofacial cases. 10–20 million U/d IM or IV for thoracic and abdominal diseases.
- ***Clostridial infections:*** 20 million U/d IM or IV with antitoxin therapy.
- ***Fusospirochetal infections (Vincent's disease):*** 5–10 million U/d IM or IV *or* 200,000–500,000 U q6–8h PO for milder infections.
- ***Rat-bite fever:*** 12–15 million U/d IM or IV for 3–4 wk.
- ***Listeria infections:*** 15–20 million U/d IM or IV for 2 or 4 wk (meningitis or endocarditis, respectively).
- ***Pasteurella infections:*** 4–6 million U/d IM or IV for 2 wk.
- ***Erysipeloid endocarditis:*** 12–20 million U/d IM or IV for 4–6 wk.
- ***Gram-negative bacillary bacteremia:*** 20–30 million U/d IM or IV.
- ***Diphtheria (adjunctive therapy with antitoxin to prevent carrier state):*** 2–3 million U/d IM or IV in divided doses for 10–12 d.
- ***Anthrax:*** Minimum of 5 million U/d IM or IV in divided doses.

- **Pneumococcal infections:** 5–24 million U/d in divided doses.
- **Syphilis:** 12–24 million U/d IV for 10 d followed by benzathine penicillin G 2.4 million U IM weekly for 3 wk.
- **Gonorrhea:** 10 million U/d IV until improvement occurs, followed by amoxicillin or ampicillin 500 mg qid PO for 7 d.

Pediatric
- **Meningitis:** 100,000–250,000 U/kg per day IM or IV in divided doses q4h.
- **Listeria infections:** *Neonates:* 500,000–1 million U/d IM or IV.
- **Infants born to mothers with gonococcal infections:** 50,000 U in a single IM or IV injection to full-term infants. 20,000 U to low–birth-weight infants.

Pharmacokinetics

Route	Onset	Peak
IM/IV	Rapid	¼–½ h

Metabolism: Hepatic, $T_{1/2}$: 30–60 min
Distribution: Crosses placenta; enters breast milk
Excretion: Urine

IV facts
Preparation: Prepare solution using Sterile Water for Injection, Isotonic Sodium Chloride Injection, or Dextrose Injection. Do not use with carbohydrate solutions at alkaline pH; do not refrigerate powder; sterile solution is stable for 1 wk refrigerated. IV solutions are stable at 24 h at room temperature. Discard solution after 24 h.
Infusion: Administer doses of 10–20 million U by slow infusion.

Adverse effects
- CNS: Lethargy, hallucinations, **seizures**
- GI: *Glossitis, stomatitis, gastritis, sore mouth,* furry tongue, black "hairy" tongue, *nausea, vomiting, diarrhea,* abdominal pain, bloody diarrhea, enterocolitis, pseudomembranous colitis, nonspecific hepatitis
- Hematologic: Anemia, thrombocytopenia, leukopenia, neutropenia, prolonged bleeding time
- GU: Nephritis—oliguria, proteinuria, hematuria, casts, azotemia, pyuria
- Hypersensitivity reactions: *Rash, fever, wheezing,* **anaphylaxis**
- Local: *Pain, phlebitis,* thrombosis at injection site, Jarisch-Herxheimer reaction when used to treat syphilis
- Other: *Superinfections,* sodium overload, leading to CHF

Clinically important drug-drug interactions
- Decreased effectiveness of penicillin G if taken concurrently with tetracyclines
- Inactivation of parenteral aminoglycosides (amikacin, gentamicin, kanamycin, neomycin, metilmicin, streptomycin, tobramycin) if taken concurrently

Drug-lab test interferences
- False-positive Coombs' test (IV)

■ Nursing Considerations
Assessment
- *History:* Allergy to penicillins, cephalosporins, other allergens, renal disease, lactation
- *Physical:* Culture infected area; skin—rashes, lesions; R, adventitious sounds; bowel sounds, normal output; CBC, liver and renal function tests, serum electrolytes, Hct, urinalysis; skin test with benzylpenicylloyl-polylysine if hypersensitivity reactions to penicillin have occurred

Implementation
- Culture infected area before beginning treatment; reculture area if response is not as expected.
- Use the smallest dose possible for IM injection to avoid pain and discomfort.
- Arrange to continue treatment for 48–72 h beyond the time that the patient becomes asymptomatic.
- Monitor serum electrolytes and cardiac status if penicillin G is given by IV infusion. Sodium or potassium preparations have been associated with severe electrolyte imbalances.

Adverse effects in *Italics* are most common; those in **Bold** are life-threatening.

- Explain the reason for parenteral routes of administration; offer support and encouragement to deal with therapy.
- Maintain epinephrine, IV fluids, vasopressors, bronchodilators, oxygen, and emergency equipment on standby in case of serious hypersensitivity reaction.
- Arrange for the use of corticosteroids, antihistamines for skin reactions.

Drug-specific teaching points
- Be aware that this drug must be given by injection.
- Know that the following side effects may occur: upset stomach, nausea, vomiting (small, frequent meals may help); sore mouth (frequent mouth care may help); diarrhea; pain or discomfort at the injection site.
- Report unusual bleeding, sore throat, rash, hives, fever, severe diarrhea, difficulty breathing.

☐ penicillin G procaine

(pen i sill' in)

penicillin G procaine, aqueous, APPG

Ayercillin (CAN), Crysticillin, Pfizerpen-AS, Wycillin

Pregnancy Category B

Drug classes
Antibiotic
Penicillin, long-acting, parenteral

Therapeutic actions
Bactericidal: inhibits cell wall synthesis of sensitive organisms, causing cell death.

Indications
- Treatment of moderately severe infections caused by sensitive organisms—streptococci, pneumococci, staphylococci, meningococci, *A. israelii, C. perfringens* and *tetani, L. buccalis* (Vincent's disease), *S. minus* or *S. moniliformis, L. monocytogenes, P. multocida, E. insidiosa, E. coli, E. aerogenes, A. faecalis, Salmonella, Shigella, P. mirabilis, C. diphtheriae, B. anthracis*
- Treatment of specific sexually transmitted diseases

Contraindications/cautions
- Contraindicated in the presence of allergies to penicillins, cephalosporins, procaine, or other allergens.
- Use caution in the presence of renal disorders, pregnancy, lactation (may cause diarrhea or candidiasis in the infant).

Dosage
Adult
- ***Moderately severe infections caused by sensitive strains of streptococci, pneumococci, staphylococci:*** Minimum of 600,000–1.2 million U/d IM.
- ***Bacterial endocarditis (group A streptococci):*** 600,000–1.2 million U/d IM.
- ***Fusospirochetal infections:*** 600,000–1.2 million U/d IM.
- ***Rat-bite fever:*** 600,000–1.2 million U/d IM.
- ***Erysipeloid:*** 600,000–1.2 million U/d IM.
- ***Diphtheria:*** 300,000–600,000 U/d IM with antitoxin.
- ***Diphtheria carrier state:*** 300,000 U/d IM for 10 d.
- ***Anthrax:*** 600,000–1.2 million U/d IM.
- ***Syphilis (negative spinal fluid):*** 600,000 U/d IM for 8 d.
- ***Late syphilis:*** 600,000 U/d for 10–15 d.
- ***Neurosyphilis:*** 2–4 million U/d IM with 500 mg probenecid PO qid for 10 d, followed by 2.4 million U IM benzathine penicillin G weekly for three doses.
- ***Uncomplicated gonococcal infections:*** 4.8 million U IM in divided doses at two sites together with 1 g probenecid.

Pediatric
- ***Congenital syphilis:*** Patients weighing < 70 lb: 50,000 U/kg per day IM for 10–14 d.
- ***Neurosyphilis:*** *Infants:* 50,000 U/kg per day IM for at least 10 d.

Pharmacokinetics

Route	Onset	Peak	Duration
IM	Varies	4 h	15–20 h

Metabolism: Hepatic, $T_{1/2}$: 30–60 min
Distribution: Crosses placenta; enters breast milk
Excretion: Urine

Adverse effects

- **CNS:** Lethargy, hallucinations, **seizures**
- **GI:** *Glossitis, stomatitis, gastritis, sore mouth,* furry tongue, black "hairy" tongue, *nausea, vomiting, diarrhea,* abdominal pain, bloody diarrhea, enterocolitis, pseudomembranous colitis, nonspecific hepatitis
- **Hematologic:** Anemia, thrombocytopenia, leukopenia, neutropenia, prolonged bleeding time
- **GU:** Nephritis—oliguria, proteinuria, hematuria, casts, azotemia, pyuria
- **Hypersensitivity reactions:** *Rash, fever, wheezing,* **anaphylaxis**
- **Local:** *Pain, phlebitis,* thrombosis at injection site, Jarisch-Herxheimer reaction when used to treat syphilis
- **Other:** *Superinfections,* sodium overload, leading to CHF

Clinically important drug-drug interactions

- Decreased effectiveness of penicillin G procaine if taken concurrently with tetracyclines • Inactivation of parenteral aminoglycosides (amikacin, gentamicin, kanamycin, neomycin, metilmicin, streptomycin, tobramycin) if taken concurrently

■ Nursing Considerations

Assessment

- *History:* Allergies to penicillins, cephalosporins, procaine, other allergens, renal disorders, pregnancy, lactation
- *Physical:* Culture infected area; skin—color, lesions; R, adventitious sounds; bowel sounds; CBC, liver and renal function tests, serum electrolytes, Hct, urinalysis

Implementation

- Culture infected area before beginning treatment; reculture area if response is not as expected.
- Administer by IM route only.
- Arrange to continue therapy for at least 2 d after signs of infection have disappeared, usually 7–10 d.
- Administer IM injection in upper outer quadrant of the buttock. In infants and small children, the midlateral aspect of the thigh may be preferred.

Drug-specific teaching points

- Be aware that this drug can be given only by IM injection.
- Know that nausea, vomiting, diarrhea, mouth sores, pain at injection sites may occur.
- Report difficulty breathing, rashes, severe diarrhea, severe pain at injection site, mouth sores, unusual bleeding or bruising.

☐ penicillin V

(pen i sill' in)

pencillin V potassium

Beepen VK, Betapen VK, Ledercillin VK, Nadopen-V (CAN), Novopen VK (CAN), Penbec-V (CAN), Pen-Vee-K, Robicillin VK, V-Cillin K, Veetids

Pregnancy Category B

Drug classes

Antibiotic
Penicillin (acid stable)

Therapeutic actions

Bactericidal: inhibits cell wall synthesis of sensitive organisms, causing cell death.

Indications

- Mild to moderately severe infections caused by sensitive organisms—streptococci, pneumococci, staphylococci, fusospirochetes

Adverse effects in *Italics* are most common; those in **Bold** are life-threatening.

penicillin V ■ 863

- Prophylaxis against bacterial endocarditis in patients with valvular heart disease undergoing dental or upper respiratory tract surgery
- Unlabeled uses: prophylactic treatment of children with sickle cell anemia, mild to moderate anaerobic infections, Lyme disease

Contraindications/cautions
- Contraindicated in the presence of allergies to penicillins, cephalosporins, or other allergens.
- Use caution in the presence of renal disorders, pregnancy, lactation (may cause diarrhea or candidiasis in the infant).

Dosage
125 mg = 200,000 U.
Adult
- ***Fusospirochetal infections:*** 250–500 mg q6–8h PO.
- ***Streptococcal infections (including otitis media, URIs of mild to moderate severity, scarlet fever, erysipelas):*** 125–250 mg q6–8h PO for 10 d.
- ***Pneumococcal infections:*** 250–500 mg q6h PO until afebrile for 48h.
- ***Staphylococcal infections of skin and soft tissues:*** 250–500 mg q6–8h PO.
- ***Prophylaxis against bacterial endocarditis, dental or upper respiratory procedures:*** 2 g PO ½–1 h before the procedure, then 500 mg q6h for eight doses.
- ***Alternate prophylaxis:*** 1 million U penicillin G IM mixed with 600,000 U procaine penicillin G ½–1 h before the procedure, then 500 mg penicillin V PO q6h for 8-h doses.
- ***Lyme disease:*** 250–500 mg PO qid for 10–20 d.

Pediatric
- ***< 12 y:*** 25–50 mg/kg per day PO given q6–8h. Calculate specific doses according to body weight.
- ***Prophylaxis against bacterial endocarditis, dental or upper respiratory procedures:*** *Children > 60 lb:* 2 g PO ½–1 h before the procedure, then 500 mg q6h for eight doses. *Children < 60 lb:* 1 g PO ½–1 h before the procedure, then 250 mg q6h for eight doses.
- ***Alternate prophylaxis:*** *< 30kg:* 30,000 U penicillin G/kg IM mixed with 600,000 U procaine penicillin G ½–1 h before the procedure and then 250 mg penicillin V PO q6h for eight doses.
- ***Sickle cell anemia:*** 125 mg PO bid.
- ***Lyme disease:*** 50 mg/kg per day PO in four divided doses for 10–20 d

Pharmacokinetics

Route	Onset	Peak
Oral	Varies	60 min

Metabolism: Hepatic, $T_{1/2}$: 30–60 min
Distribution: Crosses placenta; enters breast milk
Excretion: Urine

Adverse effects
- CNS: Lethargy, hallucinations, **seizures**
- GI: *Glossitis, stomatitis, gastritis, sore mouth,* furry tongue, black "hairy" tongue, *nausea, vomiting, diarrhea,* abdominal pain, bloody diarrhea, enterocolitis, pseudomembranous colitis, nonspecific hepatitis
- Hematologic: Anemia, thrombocytopenia, leukopenia, neutropenia, prolonged bleeding time
- GU: Nephritis—oliguria, proteinuria, hematuria, casts, azotemia, pyuria
- Hypersensitivity reactions: *Rash, fever, wheezing,* **anaphylaxis** (sometimes fatal)
- Other: *Superinfections,* sodium overload leading to CHF; potassium poisoning—hyperreflexia, coma, cardiac arrhythmias, cardiac arrest (potassium preparations)

Clinically important drug-drug interactions
- Decreased effectiveness of penicillin V if taken concurrently with tetracyclines

Adverse effects in *Italics* are most common; those in **Bold** are life-threatening.

Nursing Considerations

Assessment
- *History:* Allergies to penicillins, cephalosporins, or other allergens; renal disorders; pregnancy; lactation
- *Physical:* Culture infected area; skin—color, lesions; R, adventitious sounds; bowel sounds: CBC, liver and renal function tests, serum electrolytes, Hct, urinalysis

Implementation
- Culture infected area before beginning treatment; reculture area if response is not as expected.
- Arrange to continue therapy for at least 2 d after signs of infection have disappeared, usually 7–10 d.
- Administer drug on an empty stomach, 1 h before or 2 h after meals, with a full glass of water.
- Do not administer oral drug with milk, fruit juices, or soft drinks; a full glass of water is preferred; this oral penicillin is less affected by food than other penicillins.

Drug-specific teaching points
- Take drug on an empty stomach with a full glass of water.
- Avoid self-treating other infections with this antibiotic because it is specific for the infection being treated.
- Know that nausea, vomiting, diarrhea, mouth sores may occur.
- Report difficulty breathing, rashes, severe diarrhea, mouth sores, unusual bleeding or bruising.

☐ pentamidine isethionate

(pen ta' ma deen)
Parenteral: Pentam 300
Inhalation: NebuPent
Pregnancy Category C

Drug classes
Antiprotozoal drug

Therapeutic actions
Antiprotozoal acitivity in susceptible *Pneumocystis carinii* infections; mechanism of action is not fully understood, but the drug interferes with nuclear metabolism and inhibits the synthesis of DNA, RNA, phospholipids, and proteins, which leads to cell death.

Indications
- Treatment of *P. carinii* pneumonia, especially in patients who do not respond to therapy with the less toxic trimethoprim/sulfamethoxazole combination (injection)
- Prevention of *P. carinii* pneumonia in high-risk, HIV-infected patients (inhalation)
- Unlabeled use (injection): treatment of trypanosomiasis, visceral leishmaniasis

Contraindications/cautions
- If the diagnosis of *P.carinii* pneumonia has been confirmed, there are no absolute contraindications to the use of this drug.
- Contraindicated in the presence of history of anaphylactic reaction to inhaled or parenteral pentamidine isethionate (inhalation therapy); pregnancy; lactation.
- Use caution in the presence of hypotension, hypertension, hypoglycemia, hyperglycemia, hypocalcemia, leukopenia, thrombocytopenia, anemia, hepatic or renal dysfunction.

Dosage
Adult and Pediatric
- ***Parenteral:*** 4 mg/kg once a day for 14 d by deep IM injection or IV infusion over 60 min.
- ***Inhalation:*** 300 mg once every 4 wk administered through the Respirgard II nebulizer.

Pharmacokinetics

Route	Onset
IM	Slow
Inhalation	Rapid

Metabolism: $T_{1/2}$: 6.4–9.4 h
Distribution: Crosses placenta; enters breast milk
Excretion: Urine

IV facts
Preparation: Prepare solution by dissolving contents of 1 vial in 3–5 ml of Sterile

pentamidine isethionate ■ 865

Water for Injection or 5% Dextrose Injection. Dilute the calculated dose further in 50–250 ml of 5% Dextrose solution; solutions of 1 and 2.5 mg/ml in 5% Dextrose are stable at room temperature for up to 24 h. Protect from light.
Infusion: Infuse the diluted solution over 60 min.

Adverse effects
Parenteral
- GI: *Nausea, anorexia*
- CV: *Hypotension,* tachycardia
- **Hematologic:** *Leukopenia, hypoglycemia,* thrombocytopenia, hypocalcemia, elevated liver function tests
- GU: *Elevated serum creatinine,* acute renal failure
- Local: *Pain, abscess at injection site*
- Other: Stevens-Johnson syndrome, *fever, rash,* **deaths due to severe hypotension, hypoglycemia and cardiac arrhythmias**

Inhalation
- CNS: *Fatigue, dizziness,* headache, tremors, confusion, anxiety, memory loss, seizure, insomnia, drowsiness
- GI: *Metallic taste to mouth, anorexia, nausea, vomiting,* gingivitis, dyspepsia, oral ulcer, gastritis, hypersalivation, dry mouth, melena, colitis, abdominal pain
- CV: Tachycardia, hypotension, hypertension, palpitations, syncope, vasodilatation
- Respiratory: *Shortness of breath, cough, pharyngitis, congestion, bronchospasm,* rhinitis, laryngitis, laryngospasm, hyperventilation, pneumothorax
- Other: *Rash, night sweats, chill*

■ Nursing Considerations
Assessment
- *History:* History of anaphylactic reaction to inhaled or parenteral pentamidine isethionate, hypotension, hypertension, hypoglycemia, hyperglycemia, hypocalcemia, leukopenia, thrombocytopenia, anemia, hepatic or renal dysfunction, pregnancy, lactation
- *Physical:* Skin—lesions, color; temperature; reflexes, affect (inhalation); BP, P, baseline ECG; BUN, serum creatinine, blood glucose, CBC, platelet count, liver function tests, serum calcium

Implementation
- Monitor patient closely during administration; fatalities have been reported.
- Arrange for the following tests to be performed before, during, and after therapy: daily BUN, daily serum creatinine, daily blood glucose; regular CBC, platelet counts, liver function tests, serum calcium; periodic ECG.
- Position patient in supine position before parenteral administration to protect patient if blood pressure changes occur.
- Reconstitute for inhalation: Dissolve contents of 1 vial in 6 ml of Sterile Water for Injection. Use only sterile water. Saline cannot be used, precipitates will form. Place entire solution in nebulizer reservoir. Solution is stable for 48 h in original vial at room temperature if protected from light. Do not mix with other drugs.
- Administer inhalation using the *Respirgard II* nebulizer. Deliver the dose until the chamber is empty (30–45 min).
- For IM use: Prepare IM solution by dissolving contents of 1-g vial in 3 ml of Sterile Water for Injection; protect from light. Discard any unused portions. Inject deeply into large muscle group. Inspect injection site regularly; rotate injection sites.
- Arrange to instruct patient and significant other in the reconstitution of inhalation solutions and appropriate administration for outpatient use.

Drug-specific teaching points
- Be aware that parenteral drug can be given only IV or IM and must be given every day. Inhalation drug must be given using the *Respirgard II* nebulizer. Prepare the solution as instructed by your nurse, using only Sterile Water for Injection. Protect the medication from exposure to light. Use freshly reconstituted solution. The drug must be used once every 4 wk. Prepare a calendar with drug

Adverse effects in *Italics* are most common; those in **Bold** are life-threatening.

days marked as a reminder. Do not mix any other drugs in the nebulizer.
- Arrange for frequent blood tests and blood pressure checks while you are on this drug because this drug may cause many changes in your body.
- Be aware that you may feel weak and dizzy with sudden position changes; take care to change position slowly.
- Know that if using the inhalation, metallic taste and GI upsets may occur. Small, frequent meals and mouth care may help.
- Report pain at injection site, confusion, hallucinations, unusual bleeding or bruising, weakness, fatigue.

☐ pentazocine lactate

*(pen **taz**' oh seen)*
Parenteral: Talwin

pentazocine hydrochloride with naloxone hydrochloride, 0.5 mg
Oral: Talwin NX

Pregnancy Category C
C-IV controlled substance

Drug classes
Narcotic agonist-antagonist analgesic

Therapeutic actions
Pentazocine acts as an agonist at specific (kappa) opioid receptors in the CNS to produce analgesia, sedation; acts as an agonist at *sigma* opioid receptors to cause dysphoria, hallucinations; acts at *mu* opioid receptors to antagonize the analgesic and euphoric activities of some other narcotic analgesics. Has lower abuse potential than morphine, other pure narcotic agonists; the oral preparation contains the opioid antagonist, naloxone, which has poor bioavailability when given orally and does not interfere with the analgesic effects of pentazocine but serves as a deterrent to the unintended IV injection of solutions made from the oral tablets.

Indications
- Relief of moderate to severe pain (oral)
- Preanesthetic medication and as supplement to surgical anesthesia (parenteral)

Contraindications/cautions
- Contraindicated in the presence of hypersensitivity to narcotics, to naloxone (oral form); pregnancy (neonatal withdrawal has occurred in infants born to mothers who used narcotics during pregnancy); labor or delivery (administration of narcotics to the mother can cause respiratory depression of neonate; premature infants are especially at risk; may prolong labor); lactation.
- Use caution in the presence of physical dependence on a narcotic analgesic (can precipitate a withdrawal syndrome); bronchial asthma, COPD, cor pulmonale, respiratory depression, anoxia, increased intracranial pressure; acute MI with hypertension, left ventricular failure or nausea and vomiting; renal or hepatic dysfunction.

Dosage
Adult
- **Oral:** Initially, 50 mg q3–4h. Increase to 100 mg if necessary. Do not exceed a total dose of 600 mg/24 h.
- **Parenteral:** 30 mg IM, SC, or IV. May repeat q3–4h. Doses > 30 mg IV or 60 mg IM or SC are not recommended. Do not exceed 360 mg/24 h. Give SC only when necessary; repeat injections should be given IM.

Patients in labor: A single 30-mg IM dose is most common. A 20-mg IV dose given two to three times at 2- to 3-h intervals relieves pain when contractions become regular.
Pediatric (> 12 y): Not recommended.
Geriatric or impaired adult: Use caution; respiratory depression may occur in elderly, very ill, those with respiratory problems. Reduced dosage may be necessary.

Pharmacokinetics

Route	Onset	Peak	Duration
Oral, IM, SC	15–30 min	1–3 h	3 h
IV	2–3 min	15 min	1 h

pentazocine lactate

Metabolism: Hepatic, T$_{1/2}$: 2–3 h
Distribution: Crosses placenta; enters breast milk
Excretion: Urine and feces

IV facts
Preparation: No further preparation is required.
Infusion: Inject directly into vein or into tubing of actively running IV; infuse slowly.
Incompatibilities: Do not mix in same syringe as barbiturates; precipitate will form.

Adverse effects
- CNS: *Lightheadedness, dizziness, sedation, euphoria,* dysphoria, delirium, insomnia, agitation, anxiety, fear, hallucinations, disorientation, drowsiness, lethargy, impaired mental and physical performance, coma, mood changes, weakness, headache, tremor, convulsions, miosis, visual disturbances
- GI: *Nausea, vomiting, sweating* (more common in ambulatory patients and those without severe pain), dry mouth, anorexia, constipation, biliary tract spasm; increased colonic motility in patients with chronic ulcerative colitis
- CV: Facial flushing, peripheral circulatory collapse, tachycardia, bradycardia, arrhythmia, palpitations, chest wall rigidity, hypertension, hypotension, orthostatic hypotension, syncope, circulatory depression, shock, cardiac arrest
- Respiratory: Suppression of cough reflex, **respiratory depression, apnea, respiratory arrest, laryngospasm, bronchospasm**
- GU: Ureteral spasm, spasm of vesical sphincters, urinary retention or hesitancy, oliguria, antidiuretic effect, reduced libido or potency
- Dermatologic: Pruritus, urticaria, edema
- Local: Pain at injection site, tissue irritation and induration (SC injection)
- Other: Physical tolerance and dependence, psychological dependence (the oral form of the drug has especially been abused in combination with tripelennamine—"Ts and Blues"—with serious and fatal consequences; the addition of naloxone to the oral formulation may decrease this abuse)

Clinically important drug-drug interactions
- Increased likelihood of respiratory depression, hypotension, profound sedation, or coma in patients receiving barbiturate general anesthetics • Precipitation of withdrawal syndrome in patients previously given other narcotic analgesics, including morphine, methadone (note that this applies to the parenteral preparation without naloxone and to the oral preparation that includes naloxone).

■ Nursing Considerations

Assessment
- *History:* Hypersensitivity to narcotics, to naloxone (oral form); physical dependence on a narcotic analgesic; pregnancy; labor or delivery; lactation; respiratory disease; anoxia; increased intracranial pressure; acute MI; renal or hepatic dysfunction.
- *Physical:* Body temperature; skin—color, texture, lesions; orientation, reflexes, bilateral grip strength, affect, pupil size; P, auscultation, BP, orthostatic BP, perfusion; R, adventitious sounds; bowel sounds, normal output; frequency and pattern of voiding, normal output; liver, kidney function tests, CBC with differential.

Implementation
- Do not mix parenteral pentazocine in same syringe as barbiturates; precipitate will form.
- Provide narcotic antagonist, facilities for assisted or controlled respiration on standby during parenteral administration.
- Use caution when injecting SC into chilled areas or in patients with hypotension or in shock; impaired perfusion may delay absorption; with repeated doses, an

Adverse effects in *Italics* are most common; those in **Bold** are life-threatening

excessive amount may be absorbed when circulation is restored.
- Arrange to withdraw drug gradually if it has been given for 4–5 d, especially to emotionally unstable patients or those with a history of drug abuse; a withdrawal syndrome sometimes occurs in these circumstances.
- Reassure patient about addiction liability; most patients who receive opiates for medical reasons do not develop dependence syndromes.

Drug-specific teaching points
- Take drug exactly as prescribed.
- Avoid alcohol, antihistamines, sedatives, tranquilizers, OTC drugs while taking this drug.
- Know that the following may be experienced while taking this drug: nausea, loss of appetite (taking the drug with food and lying quietly, eating frequent small meals should minimize these effects); constipation (a laxative may help); dizziness, sedation, drowsiness, impaired visual acuity (avoid driving a car, performing other tasks that require alertness, visual acuity).
- Do not take any leftover medication for other disorders, and do not let anyone else take the prescription.
- Report severe nausea, vomiting, constipation, shortness of breath or difficulty breathing.

pentobarbital

*(pen toe **bar'** bi tal)*

pentobarbital sodium

Nembutal, Nembutal Sodium, Novopentobarb (CAN)

Pregnancy Category D
C-II controlled substance

Drug classes
Barbiturate (short acting)
Sedative
Hypnotic
Anticonvulsant

Therapeutic actions
General CNS depressant; barbiturates inhibit impulse conduction in the ascending reticular activating system, depress the cerebral cortex, alter cerebellar function, depress motor output, and can produce excitation, sedation, hypnosis, anesthesia, and deep coma; at anesthetic doses, has anticonvulsant activity.

Indications
- Sedative or hypnotic for short-term treatment of insomnia (appears to lose effectiveness for sleep induction and maintenance after 2 wk; oral)
- Preanesthetic medication (oral)
- Sedation when oral or parenteral administration may be undesirable (rectal)
- Hypnotic for short-term treatment of insomnia (rectal)
- Sedative (parenteral)
- Anticonvulsant, in anesthetic doses, for emergency control of certain acute convulsive episodes (eg, status epilepticus, eclampsia, meningitis, tetanus, toxic reactions to strychnine or local anesthetics; parenteral)

Contraindications/cautions
- Contraindicated in the presence of hypersensitivity to barbiturates, manifest or latent porphyria, marked liver impairment, nephritis, severe respiratory distress, previous addiction to sedative-hypnotic drugs, pregnancy (has caused fetal damage, neonatal withdrawal syndrome), lactation.
- Use caution in the presence of acute or chronic pain (paradoxical excitement or masking of important symptoms could result); seizure disorders (abrupt discontinuation of daily doses of drug can result in status epilepticus); fever, hyperthyroidism, diabetes mellitus, severe anemia, pulmonary or cardiac disease, status asthmaticus, shock, uremia.

Dosage
Adult
- ***Oral***
  - *Daytime sedation:* 20 mg tid–qid.
  - *Hypnotic:* 100 mg at bedtime.
- ***Rectal:*** 120–200 mg.

pentobarbital ■ 869

- **Parenteral**
  - *IV:* Restrict IV use to conditions in which other routes are not feasible or prompt action is imperative. Give by slow IV injection, 50 mg/min. Initial dose is 100 mg in a 70-kg adult. Wait at least 1 min for full effect. Base dosage on patient response. Additional small increments may be given up to a total of 200–500 mg. Minimize dosage in convulsive states to avoid compounding the depression that may follow convulsions.
  - *IM:* Inject deeply into a muscle mass. Usual adult dose is 150–200 mg. Do not exceed a volume of 5 ml at any one site because of possibility of tissue irritation.

Pediatric: Use caution: barbiturates may produce irritability, aggression, inappropriate tearfulness.

- **Oral**
  - *Preoperative sedation:* 2–6 mg/kg per day (maximum: 100 mg), depending on age, weight, degree of sedation desired.
  - *Hypnotic:* Base dosage on age and weight.
- **Rectal:** Do not divide suppositories.
  - *12–14 y (80–110 lb):* 60 or 120 mg.
  - *5–12 y (40–80 lb):* 60 mg.
  - *1–4 y (20–40 lb):* 30 or 60 mg.
  - *2 mo–1 y (10–20 lb):* 30 mg.
- **Parenteral**
  - *IV:* Reduce initial adult dosage on basis of age, weight, and patient's condition.
  - *IM:* Dosage frequently ranges from 25 to 80 mg or 2–6 mg/kg.

Geriatric patients or those with debilitating disease: Reduce dosage and monitor closely. May produce excitement, depression, confusion.

Pharmacokinetics

Route	Onset	Duration
Oral	10–15 min	3–4 h
IM/IV	rapid	2–3 h

Metabolism: Hepatic, $T_{1/2}$: 15–20 h
Distribution: Crosses placenta; enters breast milk
Excretion: Urine

IV facts
Preparation: No further preparation is required.
Infusion: Infuse slowly, monitor patient response to dosage.

Adverse effects

- CNS: *Somnolence, agitation, confusion, hyperkinesia, ataxia, vertigo, CNS depression, nightmares, lethargy, residual sedation (hangover), paradoxical excitement, nervousness, psychiatric disturbance, hallucinations, insomnia, anxiety, dizziness, thinking abnormality*
- GI: *Nausea, vomiting, constipation, diarrhea, epigastric pain*
- CV: *Bradycardia, hypotension, syncope*
- Respiratory: *Hypoventilation, apnea, respiratory depression,* laryngospasm, bronchospasm, circulatory collapse
- Hypersensitivity: Skin rashes, angioneurotic edema, serum sickness, morbiliform rash, urticaria; rarely, exfoliative dermatitis, **Stevens-Johnson syndrome** (sometimes fatal)
- Local: *Pain, tissue necrosis at injection site,* gangrene; arterial spasm with inadvertent intra-arterial injection; thrombophlebitis; permanent neurologic deficit if injected near a nerve
- Other: Tolerance, psychological and physical dependence; **withdrawal syndrome** (sometimes fatal)

Clinically important drug-drug interactions

• Increased CNS depression when taken with alcohol • Increased nephrotoxicity if given concurrently with methoxyflurane • Decreased effects of the following drugs given with barbiturates: oral anticoagulants, corticosteroids, oral contraceptives and estrogens, beta-adrenergic blockers (especially propranolol, metoprolol), theophylline, metronidazole, doxycycline, griseofulvin, phenylbutazones, quinidine

Adverse effects in *Italics* are most common; those in **Bold** are life-threatening.

Nursing Considerations

Assessment
- *History:* Hypersensitivity to barbiturates, manifest or latent porphyria, marked liver impairment, nephritis, severe respiratory distress, previous addiction to sedative-hypnotic drugs, acute or chronic pain, seizure disorders, pregnancy, lactation, fever, hyperthyroidism, diabetes mellitus, severe anemia, pulmonary or cardiac disease, shock, uremia
- *Physical:* Body weight; body temperature; skin—color, lesions, injection site; orientation, affect, reflexes; P, BP, orthostatic BP; R, adventitious sounds; bowel sounds, normal output, liver evaluation; liver and kidney function tests, blood and urine glucose, BUN

Implementation
- Do not administer intra-arterially; may produce arteriospasm, thrombosis, gangrene.
- Administer IV doses slowly.
- Administer IM doses deep in a muscle mass.
- Do not use parenteral dosage forms if solution is discolored or contains a precipitate.
- Monitor injection sites carefully for irritation, extravasation (IV use); solutions are alkaline and very irritating to the tissues.
- Monitor P, BP, respiration carefully during IV administration.
- Arrange to taper dosage gradually after repeated use, especially in epileptic patients.

Drug-specific teaching points
- Be aware that this drug will make you drowsy and less anxious.
- Do not try to get up after you have received this drug (request assistance if you feel you must sit up or move about for any reason).
  #### Outpatients
- Take this drug exactly as prescribed. This drug is habit-forming; its effectiveness in facilitating sleep disappears after a short time. Do not take this drug longer than 2 wk (for insomnia) and do not increase the dosage without consulting your physician. If the drug appears to be ineffective, consult your nurse or physician.
- Avoid alcohol, sleep-inducing, or OTC drugs while you are on this drug. These could cause dangerous effects.
- Avoid becoming pregnant while you are taking this drug. The use of contraception other than oral contraceptive preparations is recommended; these may lose their effectiveness while you are taking this drug.
- Know that the following side effects may occur: drowsiness, dizziness, "hangover," impaired thinking (these effects may become less pronounced after a few days; avoid driving a car or engaging in activities that require alertness if these occur); GI upset (taking the drug with food may help); dreams, nightmares, difficulty concentrating, fatigue, nervousness (it may help to know that these are effects of the drug that will go away when the drug is discontinued).
- Report severe dizziness, weakness, drowsiness that persists, rash or skin lesions, pregnancy.

pentostatin

(pen' toe stah tin)
2'-doxycoformycin

DCF, Nipent

Pregnancy Category D

Drug classes
Antineoplastic agent
Antibiotic

Therapeutic actions
Potent inhibitor of the enzyme ADA, which has its greatest activity in the T cells and B cells of the immune system; presence of pentostatin leads to cell toxicity and death; exact mechanism of action in hairy cell leukemia is not understood.

Indications
- Single agent for the treatment of adult patients with alpha-interferon-refractory hairy cell leukemia

Contraindications/cautions
- Contraindicated in the presence of hypersensitivity to pentostatin, pregnancy, lactation.
- Use caution in the presence of myelosuppression, renal failure.

Dosage
Adult: 4 mg/m^2 IV every other week. Hydrate with 500–1,000 ml 5% Dextrose in 0.5% Normal Saline before administration, and administer an additional 500 ml 5% Dextrose after pentostatin.
Pediatric: Safety and efficacy not established.
Geriatric or renal impaired: Decrease dose and monitor patient carefully. 2 mg/m^2 IV may be sufficient.

Pharmacokinetics

Route	Onset	Peak
IV	Rapid	11 min

Metabolism: Hepatic, T$_{1/2}$: 5.7 h
Distribution: Crosses placenta; enters breast milk
Excretion: Urine

IV facts
Preparation: Transfer 5 ml Sterile Water for Injection to the vial containing pentostatin; mix thoroughly to obtain a solution of 2 mg/ml; dilute further, if desired, in 25 or 50 ml of 5% Dextrose Injection or 0.9% Sodium Chloride Injection; results in a solution of 0.33 or 0.18 mg/ml respectively. Stable at room temperature for up to 8 h; discard after that time.
Infusion: Administer by bolus injection, or slowly infuse more dilute solution.

Adverse effects
- CNS: *Headache,* tremor, anxiety, confusion, depression, insomnia, nervousness
- GI: *Nausea, vomiting, anorexia, diarrhea,* constipation, flatulence, stomatitis
- CV: Angina, chest pain, arrhythmia
- Respiratory: *Cough, URI, lung disorders,* dyspnea, epistaxis, pneumonia, **fatal pulmonary toxicity**
- Hematologic: *Leukopenia, anemia, thrombocytopenia,* petechiae, ecchymosis
- Dermatologic: *Rash,* urticaria, eczema, pruritus, seborrhea, sweating
- General: *Fever, infection, fatigue, pain, allergic reaction, fever,* **death**, sepsis

Clinically important drug-drug interactions
- Increased incidence of severe skin rashes if taken with allopurinol • Fatal pulmonary toxicity if taken with fludarabine • Increased risk of toxicity and side effects of pentostatin and vidarabine if taken concurrently

■ Nursing Considerations
Assessment
- *History:* Hypersensitivity to pentostatin, pregnancy, lactation, myelosuppression, renal failure
- *Physical:* Body temperature; skin—color, temperature; orientation, reflexes; P, BP; liver evalution, bowel sounds; R, adventitious sounds; urinary output; liver and renal function tests; CBC with differential

Implementation
- Monitor laboratory tests for renal function, myelosuppression before and frequently during therapy.
- Hold drug and notify physician in cases of active infection, neutrophil count < 200 cells/mm^3, severe CNS toxicity, severe rash, signs of pulmonary toxicity, elevated creatinine.
- Wear protective clothing and gloves while preparing drug; arrange for proper disposal of chemotherapeutic agent.
- Hydrate patient with 500–1,000 ml of 5% Dextrose in 0.5 Normal Saline prior to drug administration; infuse an additional 500 ml of 5% Dextrose after administration.

Drug-specific teaching points
- Be aware that this drug can only be given IV and only every other week. Mark calendar with days to return for drug therapy.

Adverse effects in *Italics* are most common; those in **Bold** are life-threatening.

- Arrange for frequent blood tests and monitoring to determine your body's response to this drug. Frequent monitoring will be needed and will determine the timing of the next dose if adverse effects occur.
- Know that the following side effects may occur: nausea, vomiting (medication may be ordered to help; frequent mouth care may also help); dizziness, nervousness, confusion (avoid driving a car or operating dangerous machinery if this occurs); increased susceptibility to infection (avoid crowded areas and people known to have infections while on this drug); headache, muscle aches and pains (medication may be ordered that will help).
- Report bleeding, bruising, fatigue, abcesses, severe nausea or vomiting, difficulty breathing, hallucinations, severe headache, swelling.

☐ pentoxifylline

(pen tox i' fi leen)
Trental

Pregnancy Category C

Drug classes
Hemorheologic agent
Xanthine

Therapeutic actions
Reduces RBC aggregation and local hyperviscosity, decreases platelet aggregation, decreases fibrinogen concentration in the blood; precise mechanism of action is not known.

Indications
- Intermittent claudication
- Unlabeled use: cerebrovascular insufficiency, to improve psychopathologic symptoms

Contraindications/cautions
- Contraindicated in the presence of allergy to pentoxifylline or methylxanthines (eg, caffeine, theophylline; drug is a dimethylxanthine derivative), lactation.
- Use caution in the presence of pregnancy.

Dosage
Adult: 400 mg tid PO with meals. Decrease to 400 mg bid if adverse side effects occur. Continue for at least 8 wk.
Pediatric: Safety and efficacy not established.

Pharmacokinetics

Route	Onset	Peak
Oral	Varies	60 min

Metabolism: Hepatic, $T_{1/2}$: 0.4–1.6 h
Distribution: Crosses placenta; enters breast milk
Excretion: Urine

Adverse effects
- **CNS:** *Dizziness, headache*, tremor, anxiety, confusion
- **GI:** *Dyspepsia, nausea*, vomiting
- **CV:** Angina, chest pain, arrhythmia, hypotension, dyspnea
- **Hematologic:** Pancytopenia, purpura, thrombocytopenia
- **Dermatologic:** Brittle fingernails, pruritus, rash, urticaria

Clinically important drug-drug interactions
- Increased therapeutic and toxic effects of pentoxifylline if taken with cimetidine

■ Nursing Considerations

Assessment
- *History:* Allergy to pentoxifylline or methylxanthines, pregnancy, lactation
- *Physical:* Skin—color, temperature; orientation, reflexes; P, BP, peripheral perfusion; CBC

Implementation
- Monitor patient for angina, arrhythmias.
- Administer drug with meals.

Drug-specific teaching points
- Take drug with meals.
- Be aware that this drug helps the signs and symptoms of claudication, but additional definitive therapy is still needed.
- Know that dizziness may occur as a result of drug therapy; if this happens, avoid driving and operating dangerous ma-

Adverse effects in *Italics* are most common; those in **Bold** are life-threatening.

chinery; take precautions to prevent injury.
- Report chest pain, flushing, loss of consciousness, twitching, numbness and tingling.

☐ pergolide mesylate

(per' go lide)
Permax

Pregnancy Category B

Drug classes
Antiparkinsonian drug

Therapeutic actions
Potent dopamine receptor agonist; inhibits the secretion of prolactin, causes a transient rise in growth hormone and decrease in luteinizing hormone; directly stimulates postsynaptic dopamine receptors in the nigrostriatal system.

Indications
- Adjunctive treatment to levodopa-carbidopa in the management of the signs and symptoms of Parkinson's disease

Contraindications/cautions
- Contraindicated in the presence of hypersensitivity to pergolide or ergot derivatives, lactation (suppression of prolactin may inhibit nursing).
- Use caution in the presence of cardiac dysrhythmias, hallucinations, confusion, dyskinesias, pregnancy.

Dosage
Adult: Initiate with a daily dose of 0.05 mg PO for the first 2 d. Gradually increase dosage by 0.1 or 0.15 mg/d every third day over the next 12 d of therapy. May then be increased by 0.25 mg/d every third day until an optimal therapeutic dosage is achieved. *Usual dose:* 3 mg given in three equally divided doses per day.
Pediatric: Safety and efficacy not established.

Pharmacokinetics

Route	Onset	Peak
Oral	Varies	Unknown

Metabolism: Hepatic, $T_{1/2}$: unknown
Distribution: May cross placenta; may enter breast milk
Excretion: Urine and lungs

Adverse effects
- **CNS:** *Dyskinesias, dizziness, hallucinations, dystonias, confusion, somnolence, insomnia, anxiety, tremor,* fatigue, anxiety, convulsions, depression, drowsiness, vertigo, hyperesthesia, irritability, nervousness, visual disturbances
- **GI:** *Nausea, constipation, diarrhea, dyspepsia,* anorexia, dry mouth, vomiting
- **CV:** *Postural hypotension, vasodilation,* palpitation, hypotension, syncope, hypertension, arrhythmia
- **Respiratory:** *Rhinitis, dyspnea,* epistaxis, hiccups
- **GU:** Urinary frequency, urinary tract infection, hematuria
- **Dermatologic:** Rash, sweating
- **General:** *Pain, abdominal pain, headache, asthenia,* chest pain, neck pain, chills, *peripheral edema,* edema, weight gain, anemia

■ Nursing Considerations

Assessment
- *History:* Hypersensitivity to pergolide or ergot derivatives, cardiac dysrhythmias, hallucinations, confusion, dyskinesias, lactation
- *Physical:* Reflexes, affect; BP, P, peripheral perfusion; abdominal exam, normal output; auscultation, R; urinary output

Implementation
- Administer with extreme caution to patients with a history of cardiac arrhythmias, hallucinations, confusion, or dyskinesias.
- Monitor patient while titrating drug to establish therapeutic dosage. Dosage of levodopa/carbidopa may need to be ad-

Adverse effects in *Italics* are most common; those in **Bold** are life-threatening.

justed accordingly to balance therapeutic effects.

Drug-specific teaching points
- Take this drug with your levodopa/carbidopa. The drug dosage will need to be adjusted carefully over the next few weeks to determine the correct dosage to get the best effect for you. It is important that you keep appointments to have this dosage evaluated. It is important to instruct a family member or significant other about this medication, because confusion and hallucinations are common effects; you may not be able to remember or follow instructions.
- Know that the following side effects may occur: dizziness, confusion, shaking (avoid driving a car or performing hazardous tasks; change position slowly; use caution when climbing stairs); nausea, diarrhea, constipation (proper nutrition is important); pain, swelling (generalized pain and discomfort may occur; running nose (this is a common problem; do not self-medicate).
- Report hallucinations, palpitations, tingling in the arms or legs, chest pain.

perindopril erbumine

*(per **in'** doh pril)*
Aceon

Pregnancy Category D

Drug classes
Antihypertensive
Angiotensin-converting enzyme (ACE) inhibitor

Therapeutic actions
Renin, synthesized by the kidneys, is released into the circulation where it acts on a plasma precursor to produce angiotensin I, which is converted by ACE to angiotensin II, a potent vasoconstrictor that also causes release of aldosterone from the adrenals; perindopril blocks the conversion of angiotensin I to angiotensin II, leading to decreased blood pressure, decreased aldosterone secretion, a small increase in serum potassium levels, and sodium and fluid loss; increased prostaglandin synthesis also may be involved in the antihypertensive action.

Indications
- Treatment of hypertension, alone or in combination with thiazide-type diuretics

Contraindications/cautions
- Contraindicated in the presence of allergy to perindopril or other ACE inhibitors, pregnancy, angioedema related to previous ACE inhibitor therapy.
- Use caution in the presence of impaired renal function, CHF, salt/volume depletion, lactation.

Dosage
Adult: Initial dose 4 mg PO qd, given as a single dose. Usual range 4–8 mg/d.
Maximum: 16 mg/d.
Pediatric: Safety and efficacy not established.

Pharmacokinetics

Route	Onset	Peak	Duration
Oral	1 h	3 h	24 h

Metabolism: Hepatic, $T_{1/2}$: 12 h
Distribution: Crosses placenta; enters breast milk
Excretion: Urine and feces

Adverse effects
- **GI:** *Nausea*, abdominal pain, vomiting, dairrhea
- **CV:** Angina pectoris, orthostatic hypotension in salt/volume depleted patients, palpitations
- **Respiratory:** *Cough,* asthma, bronchitis, dyspnea, sinusitis
- **Dermatologic:** Rash, pruritus, diaphoresis, flushing
- **Other:** Angioedema, asthenia, myalgia, arthralgia

■ Nursing Considerations
Assessment
- *History:* Allergy to perindopril and other ACE inhibitors, impaired renal function,

CHF, salt/volume depletion, lactation, angioedema
- *Physical:* Skin—color, lesions, turgor; body temperature; P, BP, peripheral perfusion; mucous membranes, bowel sounds, liver evaluation; urinalysis, renal and liver function tests, CBC and differential

Implementation
- Alert surgeon and mark patient's chart with notice that perindopril is being taken; the angiotensin II formation subsequent to compensatory renin release during surgery will be blocked; hypotension may be reversed with volume expansion.
- Monitor patient closely in any situation that may lead to a fall in blood pressure secondary to reduction in fluid volume—excessive perspiration and dehydration, vomiting, diarrhea—because excessive hypotension may occur.

Drug-specific teaching points
- Do not stop taking the medication without consulting your physician.
- Know that the following side effects may occur: GI upset, loss of appetite (these may be limited effects that will pass with time); lightheadedness (this usually passes after the first few days of therapy; if it occurs, change position slowly, and limit your activities to those that do not require alertness and precision); dry cough (this is irritating but not harmful).
- Be careful in any situation that may lead to a drop in blood pressure (diarrhea, sweating, vomiting, dehydration); if lightheadedness or dizziness should occur, consult your nurse or physician.
- Report mouth sores; sore throat, fever, chills; swelling of the hands, feet; irregular heartbeat, chest pains; swelling of the face, eyes, lips, tongue; difficulty in breathing, persistent cough.

▢ perphenazine

(per fen' a zeen)
Apo-Perphenazine (CAN),
Phenazine (CAN), Trilafon

Pregnancy Category C

Drug classes
Phenothiazine (piperazine)
Dopaminergic-blocking drug
Antipsychotic drug
Antiemetic drug

Therapeutic actions
Mechanism of action not fully understood: antipsychotic drugs block postsynaptic dopamine receptors in the brain, but this may not be necessary and sufficient for antipsychotic activity; depresses the reticular activating system, including the parts of the brain involved with wakefulness and emesis; anticholinergic, antihistaminic (H_1), and alpha-adrenergic blocking activity also may contribute to some of its therapeutic (and adverse) actions.

Indications
- Management of manifestations of psychotic disorders
- Control of severe nausea and vomiting, intractable hiccups

Contraindications/cautions
- Contraindicated in the presence of coma or severe CNS depression, bone marrow depression, blood dyscrasia, circulatory collapse, subcortical brain damage, Parkinson's disease, liver damage, cerebral arteriosclerosis, coronary disease, severe hypotension or hypertension.
- Use caution in the presence of respiratory disorders ("silent pneumonia" may develop); glaucoma, prostatic hypertrophy; epilepsy or history of epilepsy; breast cancer; thyrotoxicosis; peptic ulcer, decreased renal function; myelography within previous 24 h or scheduled within 48 h; exposure to heat or phosphorous insecticides; pregnancy; lactation; children younger than 12 y, especially those with chickenpox, CNS infections (children are especially susceptible to dystonias that may confound the diagnosis of Reye's syndrome).

Dosage
Full clinical antipsychotic effects may require 6 wk–6 mo of therapy.
Adult
- ***Moderately disturbed nonhospitalized patients:*** 4–8 mg PO tid;

reduce as soon as possible to minimum effective dosage.
- **Hospitalized patients:** 8–16 mg PO bid–qid. Avoid dosages > 64 mg/d.
- **IM:** Initial dose 5–10 mg q6h. Total dosage should not exceed 15 mg/d in ambulatory, 30 mg/d in hospitalized patients. Switch to oral dosage as soon as possible.
- **Antiemetic:** 8–16 mg/d PO in divided doses (occasionally 24 mg may be needed); 5–10 mg IM for rapid control of vomiting; 5 mg IV in divided doses by slow infusion of dilute solutions. Give IV only when necessary to control severe vomiting.

Pediatric: Not recommended for children < 12 y; children > 12 y may receive lowest adult dosage.

Geriatric or debilitated: Use lower doses (one-third to one-half adult dose), and increase dosage more gradually than in younger patients.

Pharmacokinetics

Route	Onset	Peak	Duration
Oral	Varies	Unknown	
IM/IV	5–10 min	1–2 h	6 h

Metabolism: Hepatic, $T_{1/2}$: unknown
Distribution: Crosses placenta; enters breast milk
Excretion: Urine

IV facts
Preparation: Dilute drug to 0.5 mg/ml.
Infusion: Give by either fractional injection or slow drip infusion. When giving as divided doses, give no more than 1 mg/injection at not less than 1- to 2-min intervals. Do not exceed 5 mg total dose; hypotensive and extrapyramidal effects may occur.

Adverse effects
- CNS: *Drowsiness,* insomnia, vertigo, headache, weakness, tremor, ataxia, slurring, cerebral edema, seizures, exacerbation of psychotic symptoms, extrapyramidal syndromes—*pseudoparkinsonism; dystonias; akathisia,* tardive dyskinesias, potentially irreversible (no known treatment), **neuroleptic malignant syndrome**
- CV: Hypotension, orthostatic hypotension, hypertension, tachycardia, bradycardia, cardiac arrest, CHF, cardiomegaly, **refractory arrhythmias** (some fatal), pulmonary edema
- Respiratory: Bronchospasm, laryngospasm, dyspnea; suppression of cough reflex and potential for aspiration (**sudden death related to asphyxia** or cardiac arrest has been reported)
- Hematologic: Eosinophilia, leukopenia, leukocytosis, anemia; aplastic anemia; hemolytic anemia; thrombocytopenic or nonthrombocytopenic purpura; pancytopenia
- EENT: Glaucoma, *photophobia, blurred vision,* miosis, mydriasis, deposits in the cornea and lens (opacities), pigmentary retinopathy
- Hypersensitivity: Jaundice, urticaria, angioneurotic edema, laryngeal edema, photosensitivity, eczema, asthma, anaphylactoid reactions, exfoliative dermatitis
- Endocrine: Lactation, breast engorgement in females, galactorrhea; syndrome of inappropriate ADH secretion (SIADH); amenorrhea, menstrual irregularities; gynecomastia in males; changes in libido; hyperglycemia or hypoglycemia; glycosuria; hyponatremia; pituitary tumor with hyperprolactinemia; inhibition of ovulation, infertility, pseudopregnancy; reduced urinary levels of gonadotropins, estrogens, progestins
- Autonomic: Dry mouth, salivation, nasal congestion, nausea, vomiting, anorexia, fever, pallor, flushed facies, sweating, constipation, paralytic ileus, urinary retention, incontinence, polyuria, enuresis, priapism, ejaculation inhibition, male impotence
- Other: *urine discolored pink to red-brown*

Adverse effects in *Italics* are most common; those in **Bold** are life-threatening.

Clinically important drug-drug interactions

- Additive CNS depression with alcohol
- Additive anticholinergic effects and possibly decreased antipsychotic efficacy with anticholinergic drugs
- Increased likelihood of seizures with metrizamide (contrast agent used in myelography)
- Increased chance of severe neuromuscular excitation and hypotension if given to patients receiving barbiturate anesthetics (methohexital, thiamylal, phenobarbital, thiopental)
- Decreased antihypertensive effect of guanethidine when taken with antipsychotics

Drug-lab test interferences

- False-positive pregnancy tests (less likely if serum test is used) • Increase in protein-bound iodine, not attributable to an increase in thyroxine

■ Nursing Considerations

Assessment

- *History:* Coma or severe CNS depression; bone marrow depression; circulatory collapse; subcortical brain damage; Parkinson's disease; liver damage; cerebral arteriosclerosis; coronary disease; severe hypotension or hypertension; respiratory disorders; glaucoma, prostatic hypertrophy; epilepsy; breast cancer; thyrotoxicosis; peptic ulcer, decreased renal function; myelography within previous 24 h or myelography scheduled within 48 h; exposure to heat or phosphorus insecticides; pregnancy; children younger than 12 y
- *Physical:* Body weight, temperature; reflexes, orientation, intraocular pressure; P, BP, orthostatic BP; R, adventitious sounds; bowel sounds and normal output, liver evaluation; urinary output, prostate size; CBC, urinalysis, thyroid, liver, and kidney function tests

Implementation

- Dilute oral concentrate *only* with water, saline, 7-Up, homogenized milk, carbonated orange drink, and pineapple, apricot, prune, orange, V-8, tomato, and grapefruit juices; use 60 ml of diluent for each 16 mg (5 ml) of concentrate.
- Do *not* mix with beverages that contain caffeine (coffee, cola), tannics (tea), or pectinates (apple juice); physical incompatibility may result.
- Give IM injections only to seated or recumbent patients, and observe for adverse effects for a brief period afterward.
- Monitor pulse and BP continuously during IV administration.
- Do not change dosage in chronic therapy more often than weekly; drug requires 4–7 d to achieve steady-state plasma levels.
- Avoid skin contact with oral solution; contact dermatitis has occurred.
- Arrange for discontinuation of drug if serum creatinine, BUN become abnormal or if WBC count is depressed.
- Monitor elderly patients for dehydration, and institute remedial measures promptly; sedation and decreased sensation of thirst related to CNS effects of drug can lead to severe dehydration.
- Consult physician regarding appropriate warning of patient or patient's guardian about tardive dyskinesias.
- Consult physician about dosage reduction, use of anticholinergic antiparkinsonian drugs (controversial) if extrapyramidal effects occur.

Drug-specific teaching points

- Take drug exactly as prescribed.
- Avoid skin contact with drug solutions.
- Avoid driving a car or engaging in other dangerous activities if CNS, vision changes occur.
- Avoid prolonged exposure to sun, or use a sunscreen or covering garments if this is necessary.
- Maintain fluid intake, and use precautions against heatstroke in hot weather.
- Report sore throat, fever, unusual bleeding or bruising, rash, weakness, tremors, impaired vision, dark urine (pink or reddish brown urine is to be expected), pale stools, yellowing of the skin or eyes.

☐ phenacemide

(fen ace' a myde)
Phenurone

Pregnancy Category D

Drug classes
Anticonvulsant

Therapeutic actions
Mechanism of action not understood; elevates the threshold for minimal electroshock convulsions and abolishes the tonic phase of maximal electroshock seizures.

Indications
- Severe epilepsy, particularly mixed forms of complex partial seizures refractory to other drugs

Contraindications/cautions
- Contraindicated in the presence of pregnancy, lactation.
- Use caution in the presence of hepatic failure, hypersensitivity to other convulsants.

Dosage
Adult: Starting dose of 1.5 g/d PO in three divided doses of 500 mg each; up to 5 g/d has been used to cover seizures. Because of the serious nature of side effects, use smallest dose possible to prevent seizures.
Pediatric: Safety and efficacy not established.

Pharmacokinetics

Route	Onset
Oral	Rapid

Metabolism: Hepatic, $T_{1/2}$: unknown
Distribution: Crosses placenta; may enter breast milk
Excretion: Urine

Adverse effects
- **CNS:** Dizziness, insomnia, headache, *drowsiness*
- **GI:** Dyspepsia, anorexia, weight loss
- **Renal: Nephritis**

Clinically important drug-drug interactions
- Increased serum levels of hydantoins if taken concurrently

■ Nursing Considerations
Assessment
- *History:* Hypersensitivity to anticonvulsants, lactation, pregnancy, hepatic failure
- *Physical:* Body weight; body temperature; skin—color, lesions; orientation, affect, reflexes; P; R, adventitious sounds; bowel sounds, normal output; liver and renal function tests, CBC

Implementation
- Monitor renal and hepatic function, CBC before and periodically during therapy; abnormal findings are an indication to discontinue therapy.
- Caution patient to avoid pregnancy; serious fetal harm could result.

Drug-specific teaching points
- Take this drug exactly as prescribed.
- Do not discontinue this drug abruptly or change dosage, except on the advice of your prescriber.
- Know that the following side effects may occur: dizziness, drowsiness (avoid driving a car or performing other tasks requiring alertness or visual acuity if this occurs); GI upset (taking the drug with food or milk and eating frequent, small meals may help); headache (medication can be ordered).
- Wear a medical alert tag at all times so that any emergency medical personnel taking care of you will know that you are an epileptic taking antiepileptic medication.
- Report yellowing of skin, abdominal pain, changes in color of urine or stools, fever, sore throat, mouth sores, unusual bleeding or bruising, skin rash.

☐ phenazopyridine hydrochloride

*(fen az oh **peer'** i deen)*
phenylazo-diaminopyridine hydrochloride

Azo-Standard, Baridium, Geridium, Phenazo (CAN), Phenazodine, Pyridate,

Adverse effects in *Italics* are most common; those in **Bold** are life-threatening.

phenelzine sulfate ■ 879

Pyridium, Pyronium (CAN), Urodine

Pregnancy Category B

Drug classes
Urinary analgesic

Therapeutic actions
An azo dye that is excreted in the urine and exerts a direct topical analgesic effect on urinary tract mucosa; exact mechanism of action is not understood.

Indications
- Symptomatic relief of pain, urgency, burning, frequency, and discomfort related to irritation of the lower urinary tract mucosa caused by infection, trauma, surgery, endoscopic procedures, passage of sounds or catheters

Contraindications/cautions
- Contraindicated in the presence of allergy to phenazopyridine, renal insufficiency.
- Use caution in the presence of pregnancy, lactation.

Dosage
Adult: 200 mg PO tid after meals. Do not exceed 2 d of use if used concomitantly with antibacterial agent.
Pediatric
- *6–12 y:* 12 mg/kg per day or 350 mg/m² per day divided into three doses PO.

Pharmacokinetics

Route	Onset
Oral	Rapid

Metabolism: Hepatic, $T_{1/2}$: unknown
Distribution: Crosses placenta; may enter breast milk
Excretion: Urine

Adverse effects
- CNS: *Headache*
- GI: *GI disturbances*
- Hematologic: Methemoglobinemia, hemolytic anemia
- Dermatologic: *Rash*, yellowish tinge to skin or sclera
- Other: Renal and hepatic toxicity, cancer, *yellow-orange discoloration of urine*

Drug-lab test interferences
- Interference with colorimetric laboratory test procedures

■ Nursing Considerations
Assessment
- *History:* Allergy to phenazopyridine, renal insufficiency, pregnancy
- *Physical:* Skin—color, lesions; urinary output; normal GI output, bowel sounds, liver palpation; urinalysis, renal and liver function tests, CBC

Implementation
- Administer after meals to avoid GI upset.
- Do not administer longer than 2 d if being given with antibacterial agent for treatment of UTI.
- Alert patient to the fact that urine may be reddish-orange and that it may stain fabric.
- Arrange to discontinue drug if skin or sclera become yellowish, a sign of drug accumulation.

Drug-specific teaching points
- Take drug after meals to avoid GI upset.
- Know that there may be a reddish-orange discoloration of the urine (do not be alarmed; this is a normal effect of this drug; this urine may stain fabric).
- Report yellowish stain to skin or eyes, headache, unusual bleeding or bruising, fever, sore throat.

▢ phenelzine sulfate

(fen' el zeen)
Nardil

Pregnancy Category C

Drug classes
Antidepressant
Monoamine oxidase inhibitor (MAOI; hydrazine derivative)

Adverse effects in *Italics* are most common; those in **Bold** are life-threatening.

Therapeutic actions
Irreversibly inhibits MAO, an enzyme that breaks down biogenic amines, such as epinephrine, norepinephrine, and serotonin, thus allowing these biogenic amines to accumulate in neuronal storage sites. According to the "biogenic amine hypothesis," this accumulation of amines is responsible for the clinical efficacy of MAOIs as antidepressants.

Indications
- Treatment of patients with depression characterized as "atypical," "nonendogenous," or "neurotic"; patients who are unresponsive to other antidepressive therapy; and patients in whom other antidepressive therapy is contraindicated

Contraindications/cautions
- Contraindicated in the presence of hypersensitivity to any MAOI, pheochromocytoma, CHF, history of liver disease or abnormal liver function tests, severe renal impairment, confirmed or suspected cerebrovascular defect, cardiovascular disease, hypertension, history of headache, myelography within previous 24 h or scheduled within 48 h.
- Use caution in the presence of seizure disorders; hyperthyroidism; impaired hepatic, renal function; psychiatric patients (agitated or schizophrenic patients may show excessive stimulation; manic-depressive patients may shift to hypomanic or manic phase); patients scheduled for elective surgery; pregnancy; lactation.

Dosage
Adult: Initially, 15 mg PO tid. Increase dosage to at least 60 mg/d at a fairly rapid pace consistent with patient tolerance. Many patients require therapy at 60 mg/d for at least 4 wk before response. Some patients may require 90 mg/d. After maximum benefit is achieved, reduce dosage slowly over several weeks. Maintenance may be 15 mg/d or every other day.

Pediatric: Not recommended for children younger than 16 y.
Geriatric: Patients older than 60 y are more prone to develop adverse effects; adjust dosage accordingly.

Pharmacokinetics

Route	Onset	Duration
Oral	Slow	48–96 h

Metabolism: Hepatic, $T_{1/2}$: unknown
Distribution: Crosses placenta; enters breast milk
Excretion: Urine

Adverse effects
- **CNS:** *Dizziness, vertigo, headache, overactivity, hyperreflexia, tremors, muscle twitching, mania, hypomania, jitteriness, confusion, memory impairment, insomnia, weakness, fatigue, drowsiness, restlessness, overstimulation, increased anxiety, agitation, blurred vision, sweating,* akathisia, ataxia, coma, euphoria, neuritis, repetitious babbling, chills, glaucoma, nystagmus
- **GI:** *Constipation, diarrhea, nausea, abdominal pain, edema, dry mouth, anorexia, weight changes*
- **CV: Hypertensive crises** (sometimes fatal, sometimes with intracranial bleeding, usually attributable to ingestion of contraindicated food or drink containing tyramine; see "Drug-Food Interactions" below; symptoms include some or all of the following: occipital headache, which may radiate frontally; palpitations; neck stiffness or soreness; nausea; vomiting; sweating; dilated pupils; photophobia; tachycardia or bradycardia; chest pain); *orthostatic hypotension, sometimes associated with falling; disturbed cardiac rate and rhythm,* palpitations, tachycardia
- **GU:** Dysuria, incontinence, urinary retention, sexual disturbances
- **Dermatologic:** Minor skin reactions, spider telangiectases, photosensitivity
- **Other:** Hematologic changes, black tongue, hypernatremia

Adverse effects in *Italics* are most common; those in **Bold** are life-threatening.

Clinically important drug-drug interactions

- Increased sympathomimetic effects (hypertensive crisis) when given with sympathomimetic drugs (norepinephrine, epinephrine, dopamine, dobutamine, levodopa, ephedrine), amphetamines, other anorexiants, local anesthetic solutions containing sympathomimetics • Hypertensive crisis, coma, severe convulsions when given with tricyclic antidepressants (eg, imipramine, desipramine). Note: MAOIs and tricyclic antidepressants have been used successfully in some patients resistant to therapy with single agents; however, case reports indicate that the combination can cause serious and potentially fatal adverse effects.
- Additive hypoglycemic effect when given with insulin, oral sulfonylureas • Increased risk of adverse interactive actions if taken concurrently with meperidine

Clinically important drug-food interactions

- Tyramine (and other pressor amines) contained in foods are normally broken down by MAO enzymes in the GI tract; in the presence of MAOIs, these vasopressors may be absorbed in high concentrations; in addition, tyramine releases accumulated norepinephrine from nerve terminals; thus, hypertensive crisis may occur when the following foods that contain tyramine or other vasopressors are ingested by a patient on an MAOI:

Dairy products (blue, camembert, cheddar, mozzarella, parmesan, romano, roquefort, Stilton cheeses; sour cream; yogurt); meats, fish (liver, pickled herring, fermented sausages—bologna, pepperoni, salami; caviar; dried fish; other fermented or spoiled meat or fish); undistilled beverages (imported beer, ale; red wine, especially Chianti; sherry; coffee, tea, colas containing caffeine; chocolate drinks); fruit/vegetables (avocado, fava beans, figs, raisins, bananas, yeast extracts, soy sauce, chocolate)

■ Nursing Considerations

Assessment

- *History:* Hypersensitivity to any MAOI; pheochromocytoma, CHF; abnormal liver function tests; severe renal impairment; cerebrovascular defect; cardiovascular disease, hypertension; history of headache; myelography within previous 24 h or scheduled within 48 h; seizure disorders; hyperthyroidism; impaired hepatic, renal function; psychiatric patients; elective surgery; lactation
- *Physical:* Body weight; temperature; skin—color, lesions; orientation, affect, reflexes, vision; P, BP, orthostatic BP, auscultation, perfusion; bowel sounds, normal output, liver evaluation; urine flow, normal output; thyroid palpation; liver, kidney and thyroid function tests, urinalysis, CBC, ECG, EEG

Implementation

- Limit amount of drug that is available to suicidal patients.
- Monitor BP and orthostatic BP carefully; arrange for more gradual increase in dosage initially in patients who show tendency for hypotension.
- Arrange for periodic liver function tests during therapy; arrange for discontinuation of drug at first sign of hepatic dysfunction or jaundice.
- Arrange to discontinue drug and monitor BP carefully if patient reports unusual or severe headache.
- Provide phentolamine or another α-adrenergic blocking drug on standby in case hypertensive crisis occurs.
- Provide diet that is low in tyramine-containing foods

Drug-specific teaching points

- Take drug exactly as prescribed. Do not stop taking this drug abruptly or without consulting your physician or nurse.
- Avoid ingestion of tyramine-containing foods while you are taking this drug and for 2 wk afterward (patient and significant other should receive a list of such foods).
- Avoid alcohol; other sleep-inducing drugs; all OTC drugs, including nose drops, cold, and hay fever remedies; and appetite suppressants while you are on this drug. Many of these contain substances that could cause serious or even life-threatening problems.

- Know that the following side effects may occur: dizziness, weakness or fainting when arising from a horizontal or sitting position (you should change position slowly; these effects usually disappear after a few days of therapy); drowsiness, blurred vision (these effects are reversible; safety measures may need to be taken if these become severe; you should avoid driving an automobile or performing tasks that require alertness while these persist); nausea, vomiting, loss of appetite (small, frequent meals, frequent mouth care may help); memory changes, irritability, emotional changes, nervousness (it may help to know that these are drug effects).
- Report headache, skin rash, darkening of the urine, pale stools, yellowing of the eyes or skin, fever, chills, sore throat, any other unusual symptoms.

phenobarbital

*(fee noe **bar'** bi tal)*

Oral preparations: Gardenal (CAN), Solfoton

phenobarbital sodium
Parenteral: Luminal Sodium

Pregnancy Category D
C-IV controlled substance

Drug classes
Barbiturate (long acting)
Sedative
Hypnotic
Anticonvulsant
Antiepileptic

Therapeutic actions
General CNS depressant; barbiturates inhibit impulse conduction in the ascending reticular activating system, depress the cerebral cortex, alter cerebellar function, depress motor output, and can produce excitation, sedation, hypnosis, anesthesia and deep coma; at subhypnotic doses, has anticonvulsant activity, making it suitable for long-term use as an antiepileptic.

Indications
- Sedative (oral)
- Hypnotic, short-term (up to 2 wk) treatment of insomnia (oral)
- Long-term treatment of generalized tonic-clonic and cortical focal seizures (oral)
- Emergency control of certain acute convulsive episodes (e.g., those associated with status epilepticus, eclampsia, meningitis, tetanus and toxic reactions to strychnine or local anesthetics; oral)
- Sedative (parenteral)
- Hypnotic, short-term (up to 2 wk) treatment of insomnia (parenteral)
- Preanesthetic (parenteral)
- Anticonvulsant treatment of generalized tonic-clonic and cortical focal seizures (parenteral)
- Emergency control of acute convulsions (tetanus, eclampsia, epilepticus; parenteral)

Contraindications/cautions
- Contraindicated in the presence of hypersensitivity to barbiturates, manifest or latent porphyria; marked liver impairment; nephritis; severe respiratory distress; previous addiction to sedative-hypnotic drugs (drug may be ineffective, and use may contribute to further addiction); pregnancy (has caused fetal damage, neonatal withdrawal syndrome).
- Use caution in the presence of acute or chronic pain (drug may cause paradoxical excitement or mask important symptoms); seizure disorders (abrupt discontinuation of daily doses of drug can result in status epilepticus); lactation (secreted in breast milk; has caused drowsiness in nursing infants); fever, hyperthyroidism, diabetes mellitus, severe anemia, pulmonary or cardiac disease, status asthmaticus, shock, uremia; impaired liver or kidney function, debilitation.

Dosage
Adult
- **Oral**
- *Sedation:* 30–120 mg/d in two to three divided doses.
- *Hypnotic:* 100–200 mg.
- *Anticonvulsant:* 60–100 mg/d.

phenobarbital

- **Parenteral (IM or IV)**
- *Sedation:* 30–120 mg/d IM or IV in two to three divided doses.
- *Preoperative sedation:* 100–200 mg IM, 60–90 min before surgery.
- *Hypnotic:* 100–320 mg IM or IV.
- *Acute convulsions:* 200–320 mg IM or IV repeated in 6 h if necessary.

Pediatric
- **Oral**
- *Sedation:* 8–32 mg/d.
- *Hypnotic:* Determine dosage using age and weight charts.
- *Anticonvulsant:* 3–6 mg/kg per day.
- **Parenteral**
- *Preoperative sedation:* 1–3 mg/kg IM or IV.
- *Anticonvulsant:* 4–6 mg/kg per day for 7–10 d to a blood level of 10–15 μg/ml *or* 10–15 mg/kg per day IV or IM.
- *Status epilepticus:* 15–20 mg/kg IV over 10–15 min.

Geriatric patients or those with debilitating disease, renal or hepatic impairment: Reduce dosage and monitor closely—may produce excitement, depression, confusion.

Pharmacokinetics

Route	Onset	Duration
Oral	30–60 min	10–16 h
IM, SC	10–30 min	4–6 h
IV	5 min	4–6 h

Metabolism: Hepatic, $T_{1/2}$: 79 h
Distribution: Crosses placenta; enters breast milk
Excretion: Urine

IV facts
Preparation: No further preparation is needed.
Infusion: Infuse very slowly directly IV or into tubing or running IV; inject partial dose and observe for response before continuing.

Adverse effects
- CNS: *Somnolence, agitation, confusion, hyperkinesia, ataxia, vertigo, CNS depression, nightmares, lethargy, residual sedation (hangover), paradoxical excitement, nervousness, psychiatric disturbance, hallucinations, insomnia, anxiety, dizziness, thinking abnormality*
- GI: *Nausea, vomiting, constipation, diarrhea, epigastric pain*
- CV: *Bradycardia, hypotension, syncope*
- Respiratory: *Hypoventilation, apnea, respiratory depression,* laryngospasm, bronchospasm, circulatory collapse
- Hypersensitivity: Skin rashes, angioneurotic edema, serum sickness, morbiliform rash, urticaria; rarely, exfoliative dermatitis, **Stevens-Johnson syndrome**
- Local: *Pain, tissue necrosis at injection site,* gangrene; arterial spasm with inadvertent intra-arterial injection; thrombophlebitis; permanent neurologic deficit if injected near a nerve
- Other: Tolerance, psychological and physical dependence, **withdrawal syndrome**

Clinically important drug-drug interactions
- Increased serum levels and therapeutic and toxic effects of phenobarbital when taken concurrently with valproic acid • Increased CNS depression when taken with alcohol • Increased risk of nephrotoxicity if taken with methoxyflurane • Increased risk of neuromuscular excitation and hypotension if taken concurrently with barbiturate anesthetics • Decreased effects of the following drugs given with barbiturates: theophyllines, oral anticoagulants, beta-blockers, doxycycline, griseofulvin corticosteroids, oral contraceptives and estrogens, metronidazole, phenylbutazones, quinidine

■ Nursing Considerations
Assessment
- *History:* Hypersensitivity to barbiturates, manifest or latent porphyria; marked liver impairment; nephritis; severe respiratory distress; previous addiction to sedative-hypnotic drugs; pregnancy; acute or chronic pain; seizure disorders; lactation, fever; hyperthyroidism; diabetes mellitus;

Adverse effects in *Italics* are most common; those in **Bold** are life-threatening.

severe anemia; cardiac disease; shock; uremia; impaired liver or kidney function; debilitation
- *Physical:* Body weight; body temperature; skin—color, lesions; orientation, affect, reflexes; P, BP, orthostatic BP; R, adventitious sounds; bowel sounds, normal output, liver evaluation; liver and kidney function tests, blood and urine glucose, BUN

Implementation

- Monitor patient responses, blood levels (as appropriate) if any of the above interacting drugs are given with phenobarbital; suggest alternate means of contraception to women on oral contraceptives for whom phenobarbital is prescribed.
- Do not administer intra-arterially; may produce arteriospasm, thrombosis, gangrene.
- Administer IV doses slowly.
- Administer IM doses deep in a large muscle mass (gluteus maximus, vastus lateralis) or other areas where there is little risk of encountering a nerve trunk or major artery.
- Monitor injection sites carefully for irritation, extravasation (IV use). Solutions are alkaline and very irritating to the tissues.
- Monitor P, BP, respiration carefully during IV administration.
- Arrange for periodic laboratory tests of hematopoietic, renal, and hepatic systems during long-term therapy.
- Arrange to taper dosage gradually after repeated use, especially in epileptic patients. When changing from one antiepileptic medication to another, arrange to taper dosage of the drug being discontinued as the dosage of the replacement drug is increased.

Drug-specific teaching points

- Be aware that this drug will make you drowsy and less anxious; do not try to get up after you have received this drug (request assistance if you feel you must sit up or move around for any reason).
- Take this drug exactly as prescribed; this drug is habit forming; its effectiveness in facilitating sleep disappears after a short time.
- Do not take this drug longer than 2 wk (for insomnia), and do not increase the dosage without consulting the prescriber.
- Do not reduce the dosage or discontinue this drug (when used for epilepsy); abrupt discontinuation of the drug could result in a serious increase in seizures.
- Know that the following side effects may occur: drowsiness, dizziness, "hangover," impaired thinking (these effects may become less pronounced after a few days; avoid driving a car or engaging in dangerous activities if these occur); GI upset (taking the drug with food may help); dreams, nightmares, difficulty concentrating, fatigue, nervousness (it may help to know that these are effects of the drug that will go away when the drug is discontinued). Wear a medical alert tag so that emergency medical personnel would immediately know that you are an epileptic taking this medication.
- Be aware that you should not become pregnant while taking this drug; use a means of contraception other than oral contraceptives while on this drug.
- Report severe dizziness, weakness, drowsiness that persists, rash or skin lesions, fever, sore throat, mouth sores, easy bruising or bleeding, nosebleed, petechiae, pregnancy.

phenoxybenzamine hydrochloride

*(fen ox ee **ben'** za meen)*
Dibenzyline
Pregnancy Category C

Drug classes
Alpha-adrenergic blocking drug

Therapeutic actions
Irreversibly blocks postsynaptic alpha$_1$-adrenergic receptors, decreasing sympathetic tone on the vasculature, dilating blood vessels, and lowering arterial blood pressure (no longer used to treat essential hypertension because it also blocks

presynaptic alpha$_2$-adrenergic receptors that are believed to mediate a feedback inhibition of further norepinephrine release; this accentuates the reflex tachycardia caused by the lowering of blood pressure); produces a "chemical sympathectomy."

Indications
- Pheochromocytoma to control episodes of hypertension and sweating (concomitant treatment with a beta-adrenergic blocker may be necessary to control excessive tachycardia)
- Unlabeled use: micturition disorders resulting from neurogenic bladder, functional outlet obstruction, partial prostatic obstruction

Contraindications/cautions
- Contraindicated in the presence of hypersensitivity to phenoxybenzamine or related drugs, MI, evidence of coronary artery disease.
- Use caution in the presence of pregnancy, lactation.

Dosage
Adult: Give small initial doses and increase dosage gradually until desired effects are obtained or side effects become troublesome. Initially, give 10 mg PO bid. Increase dosage every other day until an optimal dosage is obtained. Usual dosage range is 20–40 mg PO bid–tid.
Pediatric: 1–2 mg/kg per day divided every 6–8 h PO.

Pharmacokinetics

Route	Onset	Peak	Duration
Oral	2 h	4–6 h	3–4 d

Metabolism: Hepatic, T$_{1/2}$: 24 h
Distribution: Crosses placenta; may enter breast milk
Excretion: Urine and bile

Adverse effects
- **CNS:** *Miosis*, drowsiness, fatigue
- **GI:** GI upset
- **CV:** *Postural hypotension, tachycardia*
- **Respiratory:** *Nasal congestion*
- **GU:** *Inhibition of ejaculation*

■ Nursing Considerations
Assessment
- *History:* Hypersensitivity to phenoxybenzamine or related drugs, evidence of coronary artery disease, lactation
- *Physical:* Orientation, affect, reflexes; ophthalmologic exam; P, BP, orthostatic BP, supine BP, perfusion, edema, auscultation; bowel sounds, normal output

Implementation
- Monitor blood pressure response, heart rate carefully.

Drug-specific teaching points
- Take this drug exactly as prescribed. Do not stop taking this drug without consulting your nurse or physician.
- Do not ingest alcohol while you are taking this drug.
- Know that the following side effects may occur: dizziness when you change position (change position slowly; use caution when exercising, climbing stairs); drowsiness, fatigue (avoid driving a car or performing tasks that require alertness if these occur); GI upset (frequent, small meals may help); nasal stuffiness (do not use nose drops or cold remedies); constricted pupils and difficulty with far vision (avoid tasks that require visual acuity); inhibition of ejaculation (these effects generally diminish with time as therapy continues).
- Report increased heart rate; rapid weight gain; unusual swelling of the extremities; difficulty in breathing, especially when lying down; new or aggravated symptoms of angina (chest, arm, or shoulder pain); severe indigestion; dizziness, lightheadedness, or fainting.

☐ phensuximide

*(fen **sux**' i mide)*
Milontin Kapseals

Pregnancy Category C

Adverse effects in *Italics* are most common; those in **Bold** are life-threatening.

phensuximide

Drug classes
Antiepileptic
Succinimide

Therapeutic actions
Suppresses the paroxysmal three cycle per second spike and wave EEG pattern associated with lapses of consciousness in absence (petit mal) seizures; reduces frequency of attacks; mechanism of action not understood, but may act in inhibitory neuronal systems that are important in the generation of the three per second rhythm.

Indications
- Control of absence (petit mal) seizures when refractory to other drugs

Contraindications/cautions
- Contraindicated in the presence of hypersensitivity to succinimides.
- Use caution in the presence of hepatic, renal abnormalities, acute intermittent porphyria, pregnancy (association between use of antiepileptic drugs by women with epilepsy and an elevated incidence of birth defects in children born to these women; however, antiepileptic therapy should not be discontinued in pregnant women who are receiving such therapy to prevent major seizures; the effect of even minor seizures on the developing fetus is unknown, and this should be considered when deciding whether to continue antiepileptic therapy in pregnant women), lactation.

Dosage
Adult and Pediatric: Administer 500–1,000 mg PO bid–tid. The total dosage, irrespective of age, may vary between 1 and 3 g/d (average, 1.5 g/d). May be administered with other antiepileptic drugs when other forms of epilepsy coexist with absence (petit mal) seizures.

Pharmacokinetics

Route	Onset	Peak
Oral	Varies	1–4 h

Metabolism: Hepatic, $T_{1/2}$: 4 h

Distribution: Crosses placenta; enters breast milk
Excretion: Urine and bile

Adverse effects
Succinimides
- CNS: *Drowsiness, ataxia, dizziness*, irritability, nervousness, headache, blurred vision, myopia, photophobia, hiccups, euphoria, dreamlike state, lethargy, hyperactivity, fatigue, insomnia, increased frequency of grand mal seizures may occur when used alone in some patients with mixed types of epilepsy, confusion, instability, mental slowness, depression, hypochondriacal behavior, sleep disturbances, night terrors, aggressiveness, inability to concentrate
- GI: *Nausea, vomiting, vague gastric upset, epigastric and abdominal pain,* cramps, anorexia, diarrhea, constipation, weight loss, swelling of tongue, gum hypertrophy
- Hematologic: Eosinophilia, granulocytopenia, leukopenia, agranulocytosis, aplastic anemia, monocytosis, **pancytopenia**
- Dermatologic: Pruritus, urticaria, Stevens-Johnson syndrome, pruritic erythematous rashes, skin eruptions, erythema multiforme, systemic lupus erythematosus, alopecia, hirsutism
- Other: Periorbital edema, hyperemia, muscle weakness, abnormal liver and kidney function tests, vaginal bleeding, *discoloration of urine* (pink, red, or brown; not harmful)

Clinically important drug-drug interactions
- Decreased serum levels and therapeutic effects of primidone if taken concurrently

■ Nursing Considerations
Assessment
- *History:* Hypersensitivity to succinimides; hepatic, renal abnormalities; acute intermittent porphyria; pregnancy; lactation
- *Physical:* Skin—color, lesions; orientation, affect, reflexes, bilateral grip

Adverse effects in *Italics* are most common; those in **Bold** are life-threatening.

strength, vision exam; bowel sounds, normal output, liver evaluation; liver and kidney function tests, urinalysis, CBC with differential, EEG

Implementation
- Arrange to reduce dosage, discontinue phensuximide, or substitute other antiepileptic medication gradually; abrupt discontinuation may precipitate absence (petit mal) status.
- Monitor CBC and differential before therapy is instituted and frequently during therapy.
- Arrange to discontinue drug if skin rash, depression of blood count, or unusual depression, aggressiveness, or behavioral alterations occur.

Drug-specific teaching points
- Take this drug exactly as prescribed; do not discontinue this drug abruptly or change dosage, except on the advice of your prescriber.
- Arrange for frequent checkups to monitor your response to this drug.
- Know that the following side effects may occur: drowsiness, dizziness, confusion, blurred vision (avoid driving a car or performing other tasks requiring alertness or visual acuity if these occur); GI upset (taking the drug with food or milk and eating frequent, small meals may help).
- Wear a medical alert tag at all times so that any emergency medical personnel taking care of you will know that you are an epileptic taking antiepileptic medication.
- Report skin rash, joint pain, unexplained fever, sore throat, unusual bleeding or bruising, drowsiness, dizziness, blurred vision, pregnancy.

☐ phentolamine mesylate

*(fen **tole'** a meen)*
Regitine, Rogitine (CAN)
Pregnancy Category C

Drug classes
Alpha-adrenergic blocking drug
Diagnostic agent

Therapeutic actions
Competitively blocks postsynaptic alpha$_1$-adrenergic receptors, decreasing sympathetic tone on the vasculature, dilating blood vessels, and lowering arterial blood pressure (no longer used to treat essential hypertension because it also blocks presynaptic alpha$_2$-adrenergic receptors that are believed to mediate a feedback inhibition of further norepinephrine release; this accentuates the reflex tachycardia caused by the lowering of blood pressure); use of phentolamine injection as a test for pheochromocytoma depends on the premise that a greater blood pressure reduction will occur with pheochromocytoma than with other etiologies of hypertension.

Indications
- Pheochromocytoma—prevention or control of hypertensive episodes that may occur as a result of stress or manipulation during preoperative preparation and surgical excision
- Pharmacologic test for pheochromocytoma (not the method of choice; urinary assays of catecholamines, other biochemical tests have largely supplanted the phentolamine test)
- Prevention and treatment of dermal necrosis and sloughing following IV administration or extravasation of norepinephrine or dopamine
- Unlabeled use: treatment of hypertensive crises secondary to MAOI/sympathomimetic amine interactions, or secondary to rebound hypertension on withdrawal of clonidine, propranolol, or other antihypertensive drugs

Contraindications/cautions
- Contraindicated in the presence of hypersensitivity to phentolamine or related drugs, evidence of coronary artery disease.
- Use caution in the presence of pregnancy.

Dosage

Adult

- **Prevention or control of hypertensive episodes in pheochromocytoma:** For use in preoperative reduction of elevated BP, inject 5 mg IV or IM 1–2 h before surgery. Repeat if necessary. Administer 5 mg IV during surgery as indicated to control paroxysms of hypertension, tachycardia, respiratory depression, convulsions.
- **Prevention and treatment of dermal necrosis following IV administration or extravasation of norepinephrine, and so forth:** For prevention, add 10 mg to each liter of solution containing norepinephrine. The pressor effect of norepinephrine is not affected. For treatment, inject 5–10 mg in 10 ml saline into the area of extravasation within 12 h.
- **Diagnosis of pheochromocytoma:** See manufacturer's recommendations. This test should be used only for additional confirmatory evidence and after the risks have been carefully considered.

Pediatric

- **Prevention or control of hypertensive episodes in pheochromocytoma:** For use in preoperative reduction of elevated BP, inject 1 mg IV or IM 1–2 h before surgery. Repeat if necessary. Administer 1 mg IV during surgery as indicated to control paroxysms of hypertension, tachycardia, respiratory depression, convulsions.

Pharmacokinetics

Route	Onset	Peak	Duration
IM	rapid	20 min	30–45 min
IV	immediate	2 min	15–30 min

Metabolism: Unknown
Distribution: Unknown
Excretion: Kidneys

IV facts

Preparation: No further preparation is required.

Infusion: Inject slowly directly into vein or into tubing of actively running IV.

Adverse effects

- CNS: *Weakness, dizziness*
- GI: *Nausea*, vomiting, diarrhea
- CV: *Acute and prolonged hypotensive episodes*, orthostatic hypotension, MI, cerebrovascular spasm, cerebrovascular occlusion, *tachycardia, arrhythmias*
- Other: Flushing, nasal stuffiness

Clinically important drug-drug interactions

- Decreased vasoconstrictor and hypertensive effects of epinephrine, ephedrine if given with phentolamine

■ Nursing Considerations

Assessment

- *History:* Hypersensitivity to phentolamine or related drugs, evidence of coronary artery disease
- *Physical:* Orientation, affect, reflexes; ophthalmologic exam; P, BP, orthostatic BP, supine BP, perfusion, edema, auscultation; bowel sounds, normal output

Implementation

- Monitor blood pressure response, heart rate carefully.

Drug-specific teaching points

- Report dizziness, palpitations.

☐ phenylephrine hydrochloride

(fen ill ef rin)

Parenteral: Neo-Synephrine

Topical OTC Nasal Decongestants: Alcon-Efrin, Allerest Nasal, Coricidin, Doktors, Duration Mild, Neo-Synephrine, Nostril, Rhinall, Sinarest Nasal

Ophthalmic preparations (0.12% solutions are OTC): AK-Dilate, AK-Nefrin, Isopto Frin, Mydfrin, Neo-Synephrine

Pregnancy Category C

Adverse effects in *Italics* are most common; those in **Bold** are life-threatening.

phenylephrine hydrochloride ■ 889

Drug classes
Sympathomimetic amine
Alpha-adrenergic agonist
Vasopressor
Nasal decongestant
Ophthalmic vasoconstrictor/mydriatic

Therapeutic actions
Powerful postsynaptic alpha-adrenergic receptor stimulant that causes vasoconstriction and increased systolic and diastolic blood pressure with little effect on the beta receptors of the heart. Topical application causes vasoconstriction of the mucous membranes, which in turn relieves pressure and promotes drainage of the nasal passages. Topical ophthalmic application causes contraction of the dilator muscles of the pupil (mydriasis), vasoconstriction, and increased outflow of aqueous humor.

Indications
- Treatment of vascular failure in shock, shocklike states, drug-induced hypotension, or hypersensitivity (parenteral)
- To overcome paroxysmal supraventricular tachycardia (parenteral)
- To prolong spinal anesthesia (parenteral)
- Vasoconstrictor in regional anesthesia (parenteral)
- To maintain an adequate level of BP during spinal and inhalation anesthesia (parenteral)
- Symptomatic relief of nasal and nasopharyngeal mucosal congestion due to the common cold, hay fever, or other respiratory allergies (topical)
- Adjunctive therapy of middle ear infections by decreasing congestion around the eustachian ostia (topical)
- 10% solution: decongestant and vasoconstrictor and for pupil dilation in uveitis, wide-angle glaucoma and surgery (ophthalmic solution)
- 2.5% solution: decongestant and vasoconstrictor and for pupil dilation in uveitis, open-angle glaucoma in conjunction with miotics, refraction, ophthalmoscopic examination, diagnostic procedures, and before intraocular surgery (ophthalmic solution)
- 0.12% solution: decongestant to provide temporary relief of minor eye irritations caused by hay fever, colds, dust, wind, smog, or hard contact lenses (ophthalmic solution)

Contraindications/cautions
- Contraindicated in the presence of hypersensitivity to phenylephrine; severe hypertension, ventricular tachycardia; narrow-angle glaucoma; pregnancy.
- Use caution in the presence of thyrotoxicosis, diabetes, hypertension, cardiovascular disorders; prostatic hypertrophy, unstable vasomotor syndrome; lactation.

Dosage
Parenteral preparations may be given IM, SC, by slow IV injection, or as a continuous IV infusion of dilute solutions; for supraventricular tachycardia and emergency use, give by direct IV injection.

Adult
- ***Mild to moderate hypotension (adjust dosage on basis of BP response):*** 1–10 mg SC or IM; do not exceed an initial dose of 5 mg. A 5-mg IM dose should raise BP for 1–2 h.
  - *IV:* 0.1–0.5 mg. Do not exceed initial dose of 5 mg. Do not repeat more often than q10–15 min. 5 mg IV should raise the pressure for 15 min.
- ***Severe hypotension and shock:*** Continuous infusion: add 10 mg to 500 ml of Dextrose Injection or Sodium Chloride Injection. Start infusion at 100–180 μg/min (based on a drop factor of 20 drops/ml; this would be 100–180 drops/min). When BP is stabilized, maintain at 40–60 μg/min. If prompt vasopressor response is not obtained, add 10-mg increments to infusion bottle.
- ***Spinal anesthesia:*** 2–3 mg SC or IM 3–4 min before injection of spinal anesthetic.
- ***Hypotensive emergencies during anesthesia:*** Give 0.2 mg IV. Do not exceed 0.5 mg/dose.
- ***Prolongation of spinal anesthesia:*** Addition of 2–5 mg to the anesthetic solution increases the duration of motor block by as much as 50%.

phenylephrine hydrochloride

- ***Vasoconstrictor for regional anesthesia:*** 1:20,000 concentration (add 1 mg of phenylephrine to every 20 ml of local anesthetic solution).
- ***Paroxysmal supraventricular tachycardia:*** Rapid IV injection (within 20–30 sec) is recommended. Do not exceed an initial dose of 0.5 mg. Subsequent doses should not exceed the preceding dose by more than 0.1–0.2 mg and should never exceed 1 mg.
- ***Nasal decongestant:*** 1–2 sprays of the 0.25% solution in each nostril q3–4h. In severe cases, the 0.5% or 1% solutions may be needed.
- ***Vasoconstriction and pupil dilation:*** 1 drop of 2.5% or 10% solution on the upper limbus. May be repeated in 1 h. Precede instillation with a local anesthetic to prevent tearing and dilution of the drug solution.
- ***Uveitis to prevent posterior synechiae:*** 1 drop of the 2.5% or 10% solution on the surface of the cornea with atropine.
- ***Glaucoma:*** 1 drop of 10% solution on the upper surface of the cornea repeated as often as necessary and in conjunction with miotics in patients with wide-angle glaucoma.
- ***Intraocular surgery:*** 2.5% or 10% solution may be instilled in the eye 30–60 min before the operation.
- ***Refraction:*** 1 drop of a cycloplegic drug followed in 5 min by 1 drop of phenylephrine 2.5% solution and in 10 min by another drop of the cycloplegic.
- ***Ophthalmoscopic exam:*** 1 drop of 2.5% phenylephrine solution in each eye. Mydriasis is produced in 15–30 min and lasts for 1–3 h.
- ***Minor eye irritation:*** 1–2 drops of the 0.12% solution in eye bid to qid as needed.

Pediatric
- ***Hypotension during spinal anesthesia:*** 0.5–1 mg/25 lb SC or IM.
- ***Nasal decongestion:*** > 6 y: 1–2 sprays of the 0.25% solution in each nostril q3–4h. *Infants*: 1 drop of the 0.125%–0.2% solution in each nostril q2–4h.
- ***Refraction:*** 1 drop of atropine sulfate 1% in each eye. Follow in 10–15 min with 1 drop of phenylephrine 2.5% solution and in 5–10 min with a second drop of atropine. Eyes will be ready for refraction in 1–2 h.

Geriatric: These patients are more likely to experience adverse reactions; use with caution.

Pharmacokinetics

Route	Onset	Duration
IV	Immediate	15–20 min
IM/SC	10–15 min	30–120 min

Topical routes are generally not absorbed systemically.

Metabolism: Hepatic and tissue, $T_{1/2}$: 47–100 h
Distribution: Crosses placenta; enters breast milk

IV facts

Preparation: Inject directly for emergency use; dilute phenylephrine 1 mg/L is compatible with Dextrose-Ringer's combinations; Dextrose-Lactated Ringer's combinations; Dextrose-Saline combinations; Dextrose 2½%, 5%, and 10% in Water; Ringer's Injection; Lactated Ringer's Injection; 0.45% and 0.9% Sodium Chloride Injection; ⅙ M Sodium Lactate Injection.

Infusion: Determine actual rate of infusion by patient response.

Adverse effects

Less likely with topical administration.
Systemic Administration
- CNS: *Fear, anxiety, tenseness, restlessness, headache, lightheadedness, dizziness,* drowsiness, tremor, insomnia, hallucinations, psychological disturbances, convulsions, CNS depression, weakness, blurred vision, ocular irritation, tearing, photophobia, symptoms of paranoid schizophrenia
- CV: Cardiac arrhythmias
- GI: *Nausea,* vomiting, anorexia

phenylephrine hydrochloride ■ 891

- GU: Constriction of renal blood vessels and *decreased urine formation* (initial parenteral administration), *dysuria, vesical sphincter spasm* resulting in difficult and painful urination, urinary retention in males with prostatism
- Local: Necrosis and sloughing if extravasation occurs with IV use
- Other: *Pallor*, respiratory difficulty, orofacial dystonia, sweating

Nasal Solution
- EENT: *Blurred vision*, ocular irritation, tearing, photophobia
- Local: *Rebound congestion, local burning and stinging,* sneezing, dryness, contact dermatitis

Ophthalmic Solutions
- CNS: *Headache, browache, blurred vision,* photophobia, difficulty with night vision, photophobia, *pigmentary (adrenochrome) deposits in the cornea,* conjunctiva, or lids if applied to damaged cornea
- Local: *Transitory stinging on initial instillation*
- Other: Rebound miosis, decreased mydriatic response in older patients; significant BP elevation in compromised elderly patients with cardiac problems

Clinically important drug-drug interactions

- Severe headache, hypertension, hyperpyrexia, possibly resulting in hypertensive crisis if given concurrently with MAO inhibitors (isocarboxazid, pargyline, phenelzine, tranylcypromine. *Do not* administer sympathomimetic amines to patients on MAOIs • Increased sympathomimetic effects when given with tricyclic antidepressants (eg, imipramine), rauwolfia alkaloids • Excessive hypertension when phenylephrine is given with furazolidone • Decreased antihypertensive effect of guanethidine, methyldopa, when given with phenylephrine

■ Nursing Considerations

Assessment
- *History:* Hypersensitivity to phenylephrine; severe hypertension, ventricular tachycardia; narrow-angle glaucoma; thyrotoxicosis; diabetes, cardiovascular disorders; prostatic hypertrophy; unstable vasomotor syndrome; pregnancy; lactation
- *Physical:* Skin—color, temperature; orientation, reflexes, affect, peripheral sensation, vision, pupils; BP, P, auscultation, peripheral perfusion; R, adventitious sounds; urinary output, bladder percussion, prostate palpation; ECG

Implementation
- Protect parenteral solution from light; do not administer unless solution is clear; discard unused portion.
- Maintain an alpha-adrenergic blocking agent on standby in case of severe reaction or overdose.
- Infiltrate area of extravasation with phentolamine (5–10 mg in 10–15 ml of saline), using a fine hypodermic needle; usually effective if area is infiltrated within 12 h of extravasation.
- Monitor P, BP continuously during parenteral administration.
- Do not administer ophthalmic solution that has turned brown or contains precipitates; prevent prolonged exposure to air and light.
- Administer ophthalmic solution as follows: have patient lie down or tilt head backward and look at ceiling. Hold dropper above eye; drop medicine inside lower lid while patient is looking up. Do not touch dropper to eye, fingers, or any surface. Have patient keep eye open and avoid blinking for at least 30 sec. Apply gentle pressure with fingers to inside corner of the eye for about 1 min. Caution patient not to close eyes tightly and not to blink more often than usual.
- Do not administer other eye drops for at least 5 min after phenylephrine.
- Do not administer nasal decongestant for longer than 3–5 d.
- Do not administer ophthalmic solution for longer than 72 h.
- Monitor BP and cardiac response regularly in patients with any cardiovascular disorders.

Adverse effects in *Italics* are most common; those in **Bold** are life-threatening.

- Arrange for use of topical anesthetics if ophthalmic preparations are painful and burning.
- Monitor cardiovascular effects carefully; patients with hypertension who take this drug may experience changes in BP because of the additional vasoconstriction. If a nasal decongestant is needed, pseudoephedrine is the drug of choice.

Drug-specific teaching points
- Do not exceed recommended dose. Demonstrate proper administration technique for topical nasal and ophthalmic preparations.
- Avoid prolonged use, because underlying medical problems can be disguised. Limit is 3–5 d for nasal decongestant, 72 h for ophthalmic preparations.
- Know that the following side effects may occur: dizziness, drowsiness, fatigue, apprehension (use caution if driving or performing tasks that require alertness if these effects occur); *nasal solution*, burning or stinging when first used (these effects are transient and usually cease to be a problem after several treatments); *ophthalmic solution*, slight stinging when first used (this is usually transient and usually ceases to be a problem after several uses); blurring of vision.
- Report nervousness, palpitations, sleeplessness, sweating; *ophthalmic solution*, severe eye pain, vision changes, floating spots, eye redness or sensitivity to light, headache.

☐ phenytoin

(fen' i toe in)
phenytoin sodium,
diphenylhydantoin
Dilantin

Pregnancy Category D

Drug classes
Antiepileptic
Hydantoin

Therapeutic actions
Has antiepileptic activity without causing general CNS depression; stabilizes neuronal membranes and prevents hyperexcitability caused by excessive stimulation; limits the spread of seizure activity from an active focus; also effective in treating cardiac arrhythmias, especially those induced by digitalis; antiarrhythmic properties are very similar to those of lidocaine; both are Class IB antiarrhythmics.

Indications
- Control of grand mal (tonic-clonic) and psychomotor seizures
- Prevention and treatment of seizures occurring during or following neurosurgery
- Control of status epilepticus of the grand mal type (parenteral administration)
- Unlabeled uses: antiarrhythmic, particularly in digitalis-induced arrhythmias (IV preparations); treatment of trigeminal neuralgia (tic douloureux)

Contraindications/cautions
- Contraindicated in the presence of hypersensitivity to hydantoins, sinus bradycardia, sinoatrial block, Stokes-Adams syndrome, pregnancy (data suggest an association between use of antiepileptic drugs by women with epilepsy and an elevated incidence of birth defects in children born to these women; however, do not discontinue antiepileptic therapy in pregnant women who are receiving such therapy to prevent major seizures; discontinuing medication is likely to precipitate status epilepticus, with attendant hypoxia and risk to both mother and unborn child), lactation.
- Use caution in the presence of acute intermittent porphyria, hypotension, severe myocardial insufficiency, diabetes mellitus, hyperglycemia.

Dosage
Adult

- ***Phenytoin sodium, parenteral***
  – *Status epilepticus:* 10–15 mg/kg by slow IV. Maintenance: 100 mg PO or IV q6–8h. Higher doses may be required. Dosage also may be calculated on the basis of 10–15 mg/kg administered in divided doses of 5–10 mg/kg. Do not exceed an infusion rate of 50 mg/min.

phenytoin ■ 893

Follow each IV injection with an injection of sterile saline through the same needle or IV catheter to avoid local venous irritation by the alkaline solution. Continuous IV infusion is not recommended.
- *Neurosurgery (prophylaxis):* 100–200 mg IM q4h during surgery and the postoperative period (in general, the IM route is not recommended because of erratic absorption of phenytoin, pain and muscle damage at the injection site).
- *IM therapy in a patient previously stabilized on oral dosage:* Increase dosage by 50% over oral dosage. When returning to oral dosage, decrease dose by 50% of the original oral dose for 1 wk to prevent excessive plasma levels due to continued absorption from IM tissue sites.
- *Phenytoin and phenytoin sodium, oral:* Individualize dosage. Determine serum levels for optimal dosage adjustments. The clinically effective serum level is usually between 10 and 20 μg/ml.
- *Loading dose (hospitalized patients without renal or liver disease):* Initially, 1 g of phenytoin capsules (phenytoin sodium, prompt) is divided into three doses (400 mg, 300 mg, 300 mg) and administered q2h. Normal maintenance dosage is then instituted 24 h after the loading dose with frequent serum determinations.
- *No previous treatment:* Start with 100 mg tid PO. Satisfactory maintenance dosage is usually 300–400 mg/d. An increase to 600 mg/d may be necessary.
- *Single daily dosage (phenytoin sodium, extended):* If seizure control is established with divided doses of three 100-mg extended phenytoin sodium capsules per day, once-a-day dosage with 300 mg PO may be considered.

Pediatric
- **Phenytoin sodium, parenteral**
- *Status epilepticus:* Administer phenytoin IV. Determine dosage according to weight in proportion to dose for a 150 lb (70 kg) adult (see adult dosage above; see Appendix C for calculation of pediatric doses). Pediatric dosage may be calculated on the basis of 250 mg/m^2. Dosage for infants and children also may be calculated on the basis of 10–15 mg/kg, given in divided doses of 5–10 mg/kg. For neonates, 15–20 mg/kg in divided doses of 5–10 mg/kg is recommended.
- **Phenytoin and phenytoin sodium, oral**
- *Children not previously treated:* Initially, 5 mg/kg per day in two to three equally divided doses. Subsequent dosage should be individualized to a maximum of 300 mg/d. Daily maintenance dosage is 4–8 mg/kg. Children older than 6 y may require the minimum adult dose of 300 mg/d.

Geriatric and hepatic impairment: Use caution and monitor for early signs of toxicity; phenytoin is metabolized in the liver.

Pharmacokinetics

Route	Onset	Peak	Duration
Oral	Slow	2–12 h	6–12 h
IV	1–2 h	Rapid	12–24 h

Metabolism: Hepatic, $T_{1/2}$: 6–24 h
Distribution: Crosses placenta; enters breast milk
Excretion: Urine

IV facts
Preparation: Administration by IV infusion is not recommended because of low solubility of drug and likelihood of precipitation; however, this may be feasible if proper precautions are observed. Use suitable vehicle of 0.9% Sodium Chloride or Lactated Ringer's Injection, appropriate concentration; prepare immediately before administration, and use an inline filter.

Infusion: Infuse slowly in small increments; infuse flush immediately after drug to reduce the risk of damage to vein and tissues.

Adverse effects
Some adverse effects are related to plasma concentrations, as follows:

Adverse effects in *Italics* are most common; those in **Bold** are life-threatening.

phenytoin

5–10 μg/ml	may be therapeutic for some patients
10–20 μg/ml	usual therapeutic range
>20 μg/ml	far-lateral nystagmus may occur
>30 μg/ml	ataxia is usually seen
>40 μg/ml	significantly diminished mental capacity

- CNS: *Nystagmus, ataxia, dysarthria, slurred speech, mental confusion, dizziness, drowsiness, insomnia, transient nervousness, motor twitchings, fatigue, irritability, depression, numbness, tremor, headache*, photophobia, diplopia, conjunctivitis
- GI: *Nausea*, vomiting, diarrhea, constipation, *gingival hyperplasia*, toxic hepatitis, **liver damage,** sometimes fatal; hypersensitivity reactions with hepatic involvement, including hepatocellular degeneration and fatal hepatocellular necrosis
- Respiratory: Pulmonary fibrosis, acute pneumonitis
- Hematologic: **Hematopoietic complications,** sometimes fatal: thrombocytopenia, leukopenia, granulocytopenia, agranulocytosis, pancytopenia; macrocytosis and megaloblastic anemia that usually respond to folic acid therapy; eosinophilia, monocytosis, leukocytosis, simple anemia, hemolytic anemia, aplastic anemia, hyperglycemia
- GU: Nephrosis
- Dermatologic: Dermatologic reactions, scarlatiniform, morbilliform, maculopapular, urticarial and nonspecific rashes; serious and sometimes fatal dermatologic reactions—**bullous, exfoliative, or purpuric dermatitis, lupus erythematosus, and Stevens-Johnson syndrome;** toxic epidermal necrolysis, hirsutism, alopecia, coarsening of the facial features, enlargement of the lips, Peyronie's disease
- Other: Lymph node hyperplasia, sometimes progressing to frank malignant lymphoma, monoclonal gammopathy and multiple myeloma (prolonged therapy), polyarthropathy, osteomalacia, weight gain, chest pain, periarteritis nodosa
- IV use complications: Hypotension, transient hyperkinesia, drowsiness, nystagmus, circumoral tingling, vertigo, nausea, cardiovascular collapse, CNS depression

Clinically important drug-drug interactions

- Increased pharmacologic effects of hydantoins when given with chloramphenicol, cimetidine, disulfiram, isoniazid, phenacemide, phenylbutazone, sulfonamides, trimethoprim • Complex interactions and effects when phenytoin and valproic acid are given together; phenytoin toxicity with apparently normal serum phenytoin levels; decreased plasma levels of valproic acid given with phenytoin; breakthrough seizures when the two drugs are given together • Decreased pharmacologic effects of hydantoins when given with antineoplastics, diazoxide, folic acid, sucralfate, rifampin, theophylline (applies only to oral hydantoins, absorption of which is decreased) • Increased pharmacological effects and toxicity when primidone, oxyphenbutazone, amiodarone, chloramphenicol, fluconazole, isoniazid are given concurrently with hydantoins • Increased hepatotoxicity if given concurrently with acetaminophen • Decreased pharmacologic effects of the following drugs when given with hydantoins: corticosteroids, cyclosporine, dicumarol, disopyramide, doxycycline, estrogens, furosemide, levodopa, methadone, metyrapone, mexiletine, oral contraceptives, quinidine, atracurium, gallamine triethiodide, metocurine, pancuronium, tubocurarine, vecuronium, carbamazepine, diazoxide • Severe hypotension and bradycardia when IV phenytoin given with dopamine

Drug-lab test interferences

- Interference with the metyrapone and the 1 mg dexamethasone tests for at least 7 d

Adverse effects in *Italics* are most common; those in **Bold** are life-threatening.

Nursing Considerations

Assessment
- *History:* Hypersensitivity to hydantoins; sinus bradycardia, AV heart block, Stokes-Adams syndrome, acute intermittent porphyria, hypotension, severe myocardial insufficiency, diabetes mellitus, hyperglycemia, pregnancy, lactation
- *Physical:* Body temperature; skin—color, lesions; lymph node palpation; orientation, affect, reflexes, vision exam; P, BP; R, adventitious sounds; bowel sounds, normal output, liver evaluation; periodontal exam; liver function tests, urinalysis, CBC and differential, blood proteins, blood and urine glucose, EEG and ECG

Implementation
- Use only clear parenteral solutions; a faint yellow color may develop, but this has no effect on potency. If the solution is refrigerated or frozen, a precipitate might form, but this will dissolve if the solution is allowed to stand at room temperature. Do not use solutions that have haziness or a precipitate.
- Administer IV slowly to prevent severe hypotension; the margin of safety betwen full therapeutic and toxic doses is small. Continually monitor patient's cardiac rhythm and check blood pressure frequently and regularly during IV infusion.
- Monitor injection sites carefully; drug solutions are very alkaline and irritating.
- Monitor for therapeutic serum levels of 10–20 μg/ml.
- Give oral drug with food to enhance absorption and to reduce GI upset.
- Recommend that a patient's prescription for oral phenytoin be filled with the same brand each time; differences in bioavailability have been documented.
- Suggest that adult patients who are controlled with 300-mg extended phenytoin capsules try once-a-day dosage to increase compliance and convenience.
- Arrange to reduce dosage, discontinue phenytoin, or substitute other antiepileptic medication gradually; abrupt discontinuation may precipitate status epilepticus.
- Be aware that phenytoin is ineffective in controlling absence (petit mal) seizures. Patients with combined seizures will need other medication for their absence seizures.
- Arrange to discontinue drug if skin rash, depression of blood count, enlarged lymph nodes, hypersensitivity reaction, signs of liver damage, or Peyronie's disease (induration of the corpora cavernosa of the penis) occurs. Arrange to institute another antiepileptic drug promptly.
- Monitor hepatic function periodically during chronic therapy; monitor blood counts, urinalysis monthly.
- Monitor blood or urine sugar of patients with diabetes mellitus regularly. Adjustment of dosage of hypoglycemic drug may be necessary because antiepileptic drug may inhibit insulin release and induce hyperglycemia.
- Arrange to have lymph node enlargement occurring during therapy evaluated carefully. Lymphadenopathy that simulates Hodgkin's disease has occurred. Lymph node hyperplasia may progress to lymphoma.
- Monitor blood proteins, as appropriate, to detect early malfunction of the immune system (eg, multiple myeloma).
- Arrange dental consultation to instruct patients on long-term hydantoin therapy in proper oral hygiene technique to prevent development of gum hyperplasia.

Drug-specific teaching points
- Take this drug exactly as prescribed, with food to enhance absorption and reduce GI upset; be especially careful not to miss a dose if you are on once-a-day therapy.
- Do not discontinue this drug abruptly or change dosage, except on the advice of your prescriber.
- Maintain good oral hygiene (regular brushing and flossing) while you are taking this drug to prevent gum disease; arrange frequent dental checkups to prevent serious gum disease.
- Arrange for frequent checkups to monitor your response to this drug.

- Monitor your blood or urine sugar regularly, and report any abnormality to your nurse or physician if you are a diabetic.
- Be aware that this drug is not recommended for use during pregnancy. It is advisable to use some form of contraception other than birth control pills while you are on this drug.
- Know that the following side effects may occur: drowsiness, dizziness, confusion, blurred vision (avoid driving a car or performing other tasks requiring alertness or visual acuity if these occur); GI upset (taking the drug with food and eating frequent, small meals may help).
- Wear a medical alert tag at all times so that any emergency medical personnel taking care of you will know that you are an epileptic taking antiepileptic medication.
- Report skin rash, severe nausea or vomiting, drowsiness, slurred speech, impaired coordination (ataxia), swollen glands, bleeding, swollen or tender gums, yellowish discoloration of the skin or eyes, joint pain, unexplained fever, sore throat, unusual bleeding or bruising, persistent headache, malaise, any indication of an infection or bleeding tendency, abnormal erection, pregnancy.

pimozide

(pi' moe zyde)
Orap

Pregnancy Category C

Drug classes
Diphenylbutylpiperdine
Antipsychotic

Therapeutic actions
Blocks CNS dopaminergic receptors with no effect on the norephinephrine receptors.

Indications
- Suppression of severely compromising motor and phonic tics in patients with Gilles de la Tourette's syndrome who have failed to respond adequately to standard treatment

Contraindications/cautions
- Contraindicated in the presence of simple tics or tics not associated with Gilles de la Tourette's syndrome, drug-induced motor tics, congential long Q-T intervals, history of cardiac arrhythmias, severe toxic CNS depression, comatose states, hypersensitivity to pimozide, lactation.
- Use caution in the presence of pregnancy, hepatic or renal impairment, hypokalemia.

Dosage
Adult: 1–2 mg/d PO in divided doses; increase every other day to maintenance of not more than 10 mg/d.
Pediatric (younger than 12 y): Not recommended.

Pharmacokinetics

Route	Onset	Peak
Oral	Varies	6–8 h

Metabolism: Hepatic, $T_{1/2}$: 55 h
Distribution: Crosses placenta; may enter breast milk
Excretion: Urine

Adverse effects
- **CNS:** *Lightheadedness, dizziness, sedation,* extrapyramidal effects, persistent tardive dyskinesia, neuroleptic malignant syndrome, *headache, visual disturbances*
- **GI:** Nausea, vomiting, dry mouth, anorexia, constipation, diarrhea, belching
- **CV:** Prolonged Q-T intervals, cardiac arrhythmias, hypotension, postural hypotension
- **GU:** Impotence, nocturia, urinary frequency
- **Dermatologic:** Rash, sweating, skin irritation
- **Other:** Weight gain, weight loss, periorbital edema

Adverse effects in *Italics* are most common; those in **Bold** are life-threatening.

Nursing Considerations

Assessment
- *History:* Simple tics or tics not associated with Gilles de la Tourette's syndrome, congenital long Q-T intervals, history of cardiac arrhythmias, severe toxic CNS depression, hypersensitivity to pimozide, lactation, hepatic or renal impairment, hypokalemia
- *Physical:* Body temperature; skin—color, texture, lesions; orientation, reflexes, affect, orientation; pulse, auscultation, BP, orthostatic BP, perfusion; bowel sounds, normal output; frequency and pattern of voiding, normal output; liver, kidney function tests, electrolytes, ECG

Implementation
- Monitor serum potassium; correct any deficiencies before administration.
- Obtain baseline ECG and Q-T interval measurement before and periodically during treatment.
- Increase dosage very slowly every other day; monitor ECG during treatment.
- Caution patient about the development of tardive dyskinesia, extrapyramidal effects; support patient if these occur; consider the use of antiparkinsonian drugs if needed.
- Do not stop drug suddenly, withdraw gradually to decrease adverse effects.

Drug-specific teaching points
- Take drug exactly as prescribed; do not stop drug suddenly; take only the prescribed dose; sudden deaths have occurred with overdose.
- Know that the following may be experienced while taking this drug: nausea, loss of appetite (taking the drug with food and lying quietly, eating frequent, small meals should minimize these effects); dizziness, sedation, drowsiness, impaired visual acuity (avoid driving a car, performing other tasks that require alertness, visual acuity); restlessness, drooling, lack of coordination (medication may be ordered to help; in some cases the drug may need to be stopped); headache (medication may be ordered to help).
- Report shortness of breath or difficulty breathing, drooling, inability to walk, palpitation, feeling faint, "blacking out."

pindolol

(pin' doe lole)
Visken

Pregnancy Category B

Drug classes
Beta-adrenergic blocking agent (nonselective beta-blocker)
Antihypertensive drug

Therapeutic actions
Competitively blocks beta-adrenergic receptors, but also has some intrinsic sympathomimetic activity; however, the mechanism by which it lowers BP is unclear, because it only slightly decreases resting cardiac output and inconsistently affects plasma renin levels.

Indications
- Management of hypertension, alone or with other drugs, especially diuretics
- Unlabeled uses: treatment of ventricular arrhythmias, antipsychotic-induced akathisia, situational anxiety

Contraindications/cautions
- Contraindicated in the presence of sinus bradycardia, second- or third-degree heart block, cardiogenic shock, CHF, pregnancy (embryotoxic in preclinical studies), lactation.
- Use caution in the presence of diabetes or thyrotoxicosis.

Dosage
Adult: Initially 5 mg PO bid. Ajdust dose as necessary in increments of 10 mg/d at 3- to 4-wk intervals to a maximum of 60 mg/d. Usual maintenance dose is 5 mg tid.
Pediatric: Safety and efficacy not established.

Pharmacokinetics

Route	Onset
Oral	Varies

898 ■ piperacillin sodium

Metabolism: Hepatic, $T_{1/2}$: 3–4 h
Distribution: Crosses placenta; enters breast milk
Excretion: Urine

Adverse effects

- **CNS:** Dizziness, vertigo, tinnitus, fatigue, emotional depression, paresthesias, sleep disturbances, hallucinations, disorientation, memory loss, slurred speech
- **GI:** *Gastric pain, flatulence, constipation, diarrhea, nausea, vomiting,* anorexia, ischemic colitis, renal and mesenteric arterial thrombosis, retroperitoneal fibrosis, hepatomegaly, acute pancreatitis
- **CV:** **Bradycardia, CHF, cardiac arrhythmias, sinoatrial or AV nodal block, tachycardia,** peripheral vascular insufficiency, claudication, CVA, pulmonary edema, hypotension
- **Respiratory:** Bronchospasm, dyspnea, cough, bronchial obstruction, nasal stuffiness, rhinitis, pharyngitis (less likely than with propranolol)
- **GU:** *Impotence, decreased libido,* Peyronie's disease, dysuria, nocturia, frequency
- **MS:** Joint pain, arthralgia, muscle cramp
- **EENT:** Eye irritation, dry eyes, conjunctivitis, blurred vision
- **Dermatologic:** Rash, pruritus, sweating, dry skin
- **Allergic reactions:** Pharyngitis, erythematous rash, fever, sore throat, laryngospasm, respiratory distress
- **Other:** *Decreased exercise tolerance, development of ANAs,* hyperglycemia or hypoglycemia, elevated serum transaminase, alkaline phosphatase, and LDH

Clinically important drug-drug interactions

- Increased effects of pindolol with verapamil • Decreased effects of pindolol with indomethacin, ibuprofen, piroxicam, sulindac • Prolonged hypoglycemic effects of insulin if taken concurrently with pindolol • Peripheral ischemia possible if pindolol combined with ergot alkaloids • Initial hypertensive episode followed by bradycardia if taken concurrently with epinephrine • Increased "first-dose response" to prazosin when taken concurrently with pindolol • Increased serum levels and toxic effects if taken concurrently with lidocaine • Paradoxical hypertension when clonidine is given with beta-blockers; increased rebound hypertension when clonidine is discontinued in patients on beta-blockers • Decreased bronchodilator effects of theophyllines taken with pindolol

Drug-lab test interferences

- Possible false results with glucose or insulin tolerance tests.

■ Nursing Considerations

Assessment

- *History:* Sinus bradycardia, second- or third-degree heart block, cardiogenic shock, CHF, pregnancy, lactation, diabetes, thyrotoxicosis
- *Physical:* Body weight, skin condition, neurologic status, P, BP, ECG, respiratory status, kidney and thyroid function, blood and urine glucose

Implementation

- Do not discontinue drug abruptly after chronic therapy (hypersensitivity to catecholamines may have developed, causing exacerbation of angina, MI, and ventricular dysrhythmias). Taper drug gradually over 2 wk with monitoring.
- Consult with physician about withdrawing drug if patient is to undergo surgery (withdrawal is controversial).

Drug-specific teaching points

- Do not to stop taking this drug unless instructed to do so by a health care provider.
- Avoid driving or dangerous activities if CNS effects occur.
- Report difficulty breathing, night cough, swelling of extremities, slow pulse, confusion, depression, rash, fever, sore throat.

🗀 piperacillin sodium

*(pi **per'** a sill in)*
Pipracil

Pregnancy Category B

Adverse effects in *Italics* are most common; those in **Bold** are life-threatening.

Drug classes
Antibiotic
Penicillin with extended spectrum

Therapeutic actions
Bactericidal: inhibits synthesis of cell wall of sensitive organisms, causing cell death.

Indications
- Treatment of mixed infections and presumptive therapy prior to identification of organisms
- Lower respiratory tract infections caused by *Haemophilus influenzae, Klebsiella, Pseudomonas aeruginosa, Serratia, E. coli, Bacteroides, Enterobacter*
- Intra-abdominal infections caused by *E. coli, P. aeruginosa, Clostridium, Bacteroides* species, including *Bacteroides fragilis*
- UTIs caused by *E. coli, Proteus* species, including *Proteus mirabilis, Klebsiella, P. aeruginosa,* enterococci
- Gynecologic infections caused by *Neisseria gonorrhoeae, Bacteroides,* enterococci, anaerobic cocci
- Skin and skin-structure infections caused by *E. coli, P. mirabilis,* indole-positive *Proteus, P. aeruginosa, Klebsiella, Enterobacter, Bacteroides, Serratia, Acinetobacter*
- Bone and joint infections caused by *P. aeruginosa, Bacteroides,* enterococci, anaerobic cocci
- Septicemia caused by *E. coli, Klebsiella, Enterobacter, Serratia, P. mirabilis, Streptococcus pneumoniae, P. aeruginosa, Bacteroides,* enterococci, anaerobic cocci
- Infections caused by *Streptococcus* (narrower spectrum antibiotic usually used)
- Prophylaxis in abdominal surgery

Contraindications/cautions
- Contraindicated in the presence of allergies to penicillins, cephalosporins, procaine, or other allergens.
- Use caution in the presence of pregnancy, lactation (may cause diarrhea or candidiasis in the infant).

Dosage
Adult: 3–4 g q4–6h IV or IM. Do not exceed 24 g/d.

Surgery	First Dose	Second Dose	Third Dose
Intra-abdominal	2 g IV just before surgery	2 g during surgery	2 g q6h, no longer than 24 h
Vaginal hysterectomy	2 g IV just before surgery	2 g at 6 h	2 g at 12 h
Caesarian section	2 g IV after cord is clamped	2 g at 4 h	2 g at 8 h
Abdominal hysterectomy	2 g IV just before surgery	2 g in recovery room	2 g after 6 h

Pediatric: Dosage not established for children younger than 12 y.
Geriatric or renal insufficiency:

Creatinine Clearance (ml/min)	Dosage, UTIs	Systemic Infection
>40	Usual dosage	Usual dosage
20–40	3 g q8h	4 g q8h
<20	3 g q12h	4 g q12h

Pharmacokinetics

Route	Onset	Peak
IV	Rapid	End of infusion
IM	Rapid	30–60 min

Metabolism: Hepatic, $T_{1/2}$: 0.7–1.3 h
Distribution: Crosses placenta; enters breast milk
Excretion: Urine

IV facts
Preparation: Reconstitute each gram for IV use with 5 ml of Bacteriostatic Water for Injection, Bacteriostatic Sodium Chloride Injection, Bacteriostatic or Sterile Water for Injection, Dextrose 5% in Water, 0.9% Sodium Chloride, Dextrose 5% and 0.9% Sodium Chloride, Lactated Ringer's Injection, Dextran 6% in 0.9% Sodium Chloride, Ringer's Injection; stable for 24 h at room temperature, up to 7 d if refrigerated.
Infusion: Direct injection: Administer as slowly as possible (3–5 min) to avoid vein

irritation. Infusion should be run over 20–30 min.

Incompatibilities: Do not mix in solution with aminoglycoside solution; **do not mix** in the same IV solution as other antibiotics.

Adverse effects
- CNS: Lethargy, hallucinations, **seizures**
- GI: *Glossitis, stomatitis, gastritis, sore mouth,* furry tongue, black "hairy" tongue, *nausea, vomiting, diarrhea,* abdominal pain, bloody diarrhea, enterocolitis, pseudomembranous colitis, nonspecific hepatitis
- Hematologic: Anemia, thrombocytopenia, leukopenia, neutropenia, prolonged bleeding time
- GU: Nephritis
- Hypersensitivity reactions: *Rash, fever, wheezing,* **anaphylaxis**
- Other: *Superinfections,* sodium overload—**CHF**
- Local: *Pain, phlebitis,* thrombosis at injection site

Clinically important drug-drug interactions
- Decreased effectiveness of piperacillin if taken concurrently with tetracyclines
- Inactivation of parenteral aminoglycosides (amikacin, gentamicin, kanamycin, neomycin, metilmicin, streptomycin, tobramycin) if taken concurrently

Drug-lab test interferences
- False-positive Coombs' test with IV piperacillin.

■ Nursing Considerations

Assessment
- *History:* Allergies to penicillins, cephalosporins, procaine, or other allergens; pregnancy; lactation
- *Physical:* Culture infected area; skin—color, lesions; R, adventitious sounds; bowel sounds: CBC, liver and renal function tests, serum electrolytes, Hct, urinalysis

Implementation
- Culture infected area before beginning treatment; reculture area if response is not as expected.
- Arrange to continue therapy for at least 2 d after signs of infection have disappeared, usually 7–10 d.
- Administer by IM or IV routes only.
- Reconstitute each gram for IM use with 2 ml Sterile or Bacteriostatic Water for Injection, 0.5% or 1.0% lidocaine HCl without epinephrine, Bacteriostatic Sodium Chloride Injection, Sodium Chloride Injection. Do not exceed 2 g per injection. Inject deep into a large muscle, such as upper outer quadrant of the buttock. Do not inject into lower or mid-third of upper arm.
- Carefully check IV site for signs of thrombosis or drug reaction.
- Do not give IM injections repeatedly in the same site, atrophy can occur; monitor injection sites.
- Maintain epinephrine, IV fluids, vasopressors, bronchodilators, oxygen, and emergency equipment on standby in case of serious hypersensitivity reaction.

Drug-specific teaching points
- Be aware that this drug must be given by injection.
- Know that the following side effects may occur: upset stomach, nausea, diarrhea (small, frequent meals may help), mouth sores (frequent mouth care may help), pain or discomfort at the injection site.
- Report difficulty breathing, rashes, severe diarrhea, severe pain at injection site, mouth sores.

☐ piperazine citrate

(pi' per a zeen)
Entacyl (CAN)

Pregnancy Category B

Adverse effects in *Italics* are most common; those in **Bold** are life-threatening.

Drug classes
Anthelmintic

Therapeutic actions
Paralyzes ascarids by hyperpolarizing ascarid muscles; the ascarids are then dislodged and expelled from the intestine through peristalsis. Mechanism of action against *Enterobius* is not understood.

Indications
- Treatment of enterobiasis (pinworm infection)
- Treatment of ascariasis (roundworm infection)

Contraindications/cautions
- Contraindicated in the presence of allergy to piperazine, renal or hepatic dysfunction, convulsive disorders, pregnancy, lactation.
- Use caution in the presence of anemia, malnutrition.

Dosage
Adult
- ***Ascariasis:*** 3.5 g PO as single daily dose for 2 consecutive d. Severe infections, repeat treatment after 1 wk interval.
- ***Enterobiasis:*** 65 mg/kg PO in a single daily dose for 7 consecutive days (maximum daily dose of 2.5 g). Severe infections, repeat treatment course after 1 wk.

Pediatric
- ***Ascariasis:*** 75 mg/kg PO as a single daily dose for 2 consecutive d. Maximum daily dose of 3.5 g. Severe infections, repeat treatment after 1 wk.
- ***Enterobiasis:*** 65 mg/kg PO in a single daily dose for 7 consecutive d (maximum daily dose of 2.5 g). Severe infections, repeat treatment course after 1 wk.

Pharmacokinetics

Route	Onset
Oral	Slow

Metabolism: Hepatic, $T_{1/2}$: unknown
Distribution: May cross placenta or enter breast milk
Excretion: Urine

Adverse effects
- **CNS:** *Headache, vertigo*, ataxia, tremors, chorea, muscular weakness, hyporeflexia, paresthesia, seizures, EEG abnormalities, memory defect, cataracts, blurred vision, nystagmus, paralytic strabismus
- **GI:** *Nausea, vomiting, abdominal cramps, diarrhea*
- **Hypersensitivity reactions:** Urticaria, erythema multiforme, purpura, fever, arthralgia, eczematous skin reactions, lacrimation, rhinorrhea, cough, bronchospasm

■ Nursing Considerations

Assessment
- *History:* Allergy to piperazine, hepatic or renal dysfunction, convulsive disorders, anemia, malnutrition, pregnancy, lactation
- *Physical:* Skin—color, lesions, turgor; orientation, reflexes, affect, ocular exam; bowel sounds; renal and liver function tests, CBC

Implementation
- Culture for ova and parasites.
- Administer drug on an empty stomach; surface contact between drug and parasite is diminished by presence of food.
- Discontinue drug, and consult with physician if severe CNS, GI, or hypersensitivity reactions occur.
- Avoid prolonged, repeated, or excessive treatment to avoid neurotoxicity.
- Arrange for treatment of all family members (pinworm infestations).
- Arrange for disinfection of toilet facilities after patient use (pinworms).

Drug-specific teaching points
- Take on an empty stomach, 1 h before or 2 h after meals.
- Be aware that pinworms are easily transmitted; all family members should be treated for complete eradication.
- Observe strict handwashing and hygiene measures; launder undergarments, bedlinens, nightclothes daily; disinfect toilet

Adverse effects in *Italics* are most common; those in **Bold** are life-threatening.

facilities daily and bathroom floors periodically.
- Know that the following side effects may occur: dizziness, tremors, weakness (avoid driving a car or operating dangerous equipment if any of these occur); nausea, abdominal pain, diarrhea (small, frequent meals may help).
- Report skin rash, joint pain, headache, weakness, tremors, vision changes, severe GI upset.

☐ pirbuterol acetate

(peer byoo' ter ole)
Maxair

Pregnancy Category C

Drug classes
Sympathomimetic drug
Beta-2 selective adrenergic agonist
Bronchodilator
Antiasthmatic drug

Therapeutic actions
Relatively selective beta-adrenergic stimulator; acts at beta$_2$-adrenergic receptors to cause bronchodilation (and vasodilation); at higher doses, beta$_2$-selectivity is lost, and the drug also acts at beta$_1$ receptors to cause typical sympathomimetic cardiac effects.

Indications
- Prophylaxis and treatment of reversible bronchospasm, including asthma

Contraindications/cautions
- Contraindicated in the presence of hypersensitivity to pirbuterol, tachyarrhythmias, general anesthesia with halogenated hydrocarbons or cyclopropane, unstable vasomotor system disorders, hypertension.
- Use caution in the presence of coronary insufficiency, history of stroke, COPD patients who have developed degenerative heart disease, hyperthyroidism, history of seizure disorders, psychoneurotic individuals, pregnancy, lactation.

Dosage
Each actuation of aerosol dispenser delivers 0.2 mg pirbuterol.
Adult: 2 inhalations (0.4 mg) repeated q4–6h. One inhalation (0.2 mg) may be sufficient for some patients. Do not exceed a total daily dose of 12 inhalations.
Pediatric
- ***Older than 12 y:*** Same as adult; safety and efficacy in children younger than 12 y not established.

Pharmacokinetics

Route	Onset	Duration
Inhalation	5 min	5 h

Metabolism: Hepatic and tissue, T$_{1/2}$: unknown
Distribution: Crosses placenta; may enter breast milk
Excretion: Urine

Adverse effects
- **CNS:** *Restlessness, apprehension,* anxiety, fear, CNS stimulation, hyperkinesia, *insomnia,* tremor, drowsiness, *irritability,* weakness, vertigo, headache
- **GI:** *Nausea,* vomiting, heartburn, unusual or bad taste
- **CV:** Cardiac arrhythmias, tachycardia, palpitations, PVCs (rare), anginal pain (less likely with bronchodilator doses of this drug than with bronchodilator doses of a nonselective beta-agonist; ie, isoproterenol), changes in BP, sweating, pallor, flushing
- **Respiratory:** Respiratory difficulties, pulmonary edema, coughing, bronchospasm, paradoxical airway resistance with repeated, excessive use of inhalation preparations
- **Hypersensitivity:** Immediate hypersensitivity (allergic) reactions

Clinically important drug-drug interactions
- Increased sympathomimetic effects when given with other sympathomimetic drugs

---

Adverse effects in *Italics* are most common; those in **Bold** are life-threatening.

piroxicam ■ 903

■ Nursing Considerations

Assessment
- *History:* Hypersensitivity to pirbuterol, tachyarrhythmias, general anesthesia with halogenated hydrocarbons or cyclopropane, unstable vasomotor system disorders, hypertension, coronary insufficiency, history of stroke, COPD, hyperthyroidism, seizure disorders, psychoneurotic individuals, pregnancy, lactation
- *Physical:* Body weight, skin—color, temperature, turgor; orientation, reflexes, affect; P, BP; R, adventitious sounds; blood and urine glucose, serum electrolytes, thyroid and liver function tests, ECG, CBC

Implementation
- Use minimal doses for minimal periods of time; drug tolerance can occur with prolonged use.
- Maintain a beta-adrenergic blocker (a cardioselective beta-blocker, such as atenolol should be used in patients with respiratory distress) on standby in case cardiac arrhythmias occur.
- Do not exceed recommended dosage; administer during second half of inspiration, as the airways are open wider and the aerosol distribution is more extensive.

Drug-specific teaching points
- Do not exceed recommended dosage; adverse effects or loss of effectiveness may result. Read the instructions that come with the product, and ask your health care provider or pharmacist if you have any questions.
- Know that the following side effects may occur: drowsiness, dizziness, fatigue, apprehension (use caution if driving or performing tasks that require alertness if these occur); nausea, heartburn, change in taste (small, frequent meals may help); sweating, flushing, rapid heart rate.
- Report chest pain, dizziness, insomnia, weakness, tremor or irregular heart beat, difficulty breathing, productive cough, failure to respond to usual dosage.

▢ piroxicam

(peer ox' i kam)
Apo-Piroxicam (CAN), Feldene, Novo-Pirocam (CAN)

Pregnancy Category B

Drug classes
NSAID (oxicam derivative)

Therapeutic actions
Anti-inflammatory, analgesic, and antipyretic activities related to inhibition of prostaglandin synthesis; exact mechanisms of action are not known.

Indications
- Relief of the signs and symptoms of acute and chronic rheumatoid arthritis and osteoarthritis

Contraindications/cautions
- Contraindicated in the presence of pregnancy, lactation.
- Use caution in the presence of allergies, renal, hepatic, cardiovascular, GI conditions.

Dosage
Adult: Single daily dose of 20 mg PO. Dose may be divided if desired. Steady-state blood levels are not achieved for 7–12 d. Therapeutic response occurs early but progresses over several weeks; do not evaluate for 2 wk.
Pediatric: Safety and efficacy not established.

Pharmacokinetics

Route	Onset	Peak
Oral	1 h	3–5 h

Metabolism: Hepatic, $T_{1/2}$: 30–86 h
Distribution: Crosses placenta; enters breast milk
Excretion: Urine

Adverse effects
NSAIDs
- CNS: *Headache, dizziness, somnolence, insomnia,* fatigue, tiredness, dizziness, tinnitus, ophthalmologic effects

Adverse effects in *Italics* are most common; those in **Bold** are life-threatening.

- **GI:** *Nausea, dyspepsia, GI pain,* diarrhea, vomiting, *constipation,* flatulence
- **Respiratory:** Dyspnea, hemoptysis, pharyngitis, bronchospasm, rhinitis
- **Hematologic:** Bleeding, platelet inhibition with higher doses, neutropenia, eosinophilia, leukopenia, pancytopenia, thrombocytopenia, agranulocytosis, granulocytopenia, aplastic anemia, decreased hemoglobin or hematocrit, bone marrow depression, mennorhagia
- **GU:** Dysuria, renal impairment
- **Dermatologic:** *Rash,* pruritus, sweating, dry mucous membranes, stomatitis
- **Other:** Peripheral edema, anaphylactoid reactions to fatal anaphylactic shock

Clinically important drug-drug interactions

- Increased serum lithium levels and risk of toxicity if taken concurrently • Decreased antihypertensive effects of beta-blockers if taken concurrently • Decreased therapeutic effects of piroxicam if taken concurrently with cholestyramine

■ Nursing Considerations

Assessment

- *History:* Allergies; renal, hepatic, cardiovascular, and GI conditions; history of ulcers; pregnancy; lactation
- *Physical:* Skin—color and lesions; orientation, reflexes, ophthalmologic and audiometric evaluation, peripheral sensation; P, edema; R, adventitious sounds; liver evaluation; CBC, clotting times, renal and liver function tests; serum electrolytes, stool guaiac

Implementation

- Administer drug with food or milk if GI upset occurs.
- Arrange for periodic ophthalmologic examination during long-term therapy.
- Institute emergency procedures if overdose occurs (gastric lavage, induction of emesis, supportive therapy).

Drug-specific teaching points

- Take drug with food or meals if GI upset occurs.
- Know that dizziness, drowsiness can occur (avoid driving or the use of dangerous machinery while on this drug).
- Report sore throat, fever, rash, itching, weight gain, swelling in ankles or fingers, changes in vision, black, tarry stools.

☐ plasma protein fraction

Plasmanate, Plasma-Plex, Plasmatein, Protenate

Pregnancy Category C

Drug classes
Blood product
Plasma protein

Therapeutic actions
Maintains plasma colloid osmotic pressure and carries intermediate metabolites in the transport and exchange of tissue products; important in the maintenance of normal blood volume.

Indications

- Supportive treatment of shock due to burns, trauma, surgery, and infections
- Hypoproteinemia—nephrotic syndrome, hepatic cirrhosis, toxemia of pregnancy, postoperative patients, tuberculous patients, premature infants
- Acute liver failure
- Sequestration of protein-rich fluids
- Hyperbilirubinemia and erythroblastosis fetalis as an adjunct to exchange transfusions

Contraindications/cautions

- Contraindicated in the presence of allergy to albumin, severe anemia, cardiac failure, normal or increased intravascular volume, current use of cardiopulmonary bypass.
- Use caution in the presence of hepatic or renal failure, pregnancy.

Dosage
Administer by IV infusion only. Contains 130–160 mEq sodium/L. Do not give more

than 250 g in 48 h; if it seems that more is required, patient probably needs whole blood or plasma.

Adult
- *Hypovolemic shock:* 250–500 ml as an initial dose. Do not exceed 10 ml/min. Regulate dose based on patient response.
- *Hypoproteinemia:* Daily doses of 1,000–1,500 ml are appropriate. Do not exceed 5–8 ml/min. Adjust the rate of infusion based on patient response.

Pediatric
- *Hypovolemic shock:* Infuse a dose of 20–30 ml/kg at a rate not to exceed 10 ml/min. Dose may be repeated depending on patient's response.

Pharmacokinetics

Route

IV
Stays in the intravascular space

Metabolism: $T_{1/2}$: unknown
Excretion: Unknown

IV facts

Preparation: No further preparation required; store at room temperature; discard within 4 h of entering a bottle; store at room temperature; do not use if there is sediment in the bottle.

Infusion: Regulate base on patient response. Do not exceed 10 ml/min.

Incompatibilities: Administer in combination with or through the same administration set as the usual IV solutions of saline or carbohydrates. Do not use with alcohol or protein hydrolysates; precipitates may form.

Adverse effects

- CV: *Hypotension,* CHF, pulmonary edema following rapid infusion
- **Hypersensitivity reactions:** Fever, chills, changes in blood pressure, flushing, nausea, vomiting, changes in respiration, rashes

■ Nursing Considerations

Assessment
- *History:* Allergy to albumin, severe anemia, cardiac failure, normal or increased intravascular volume, current use of cardiopulmonary bypass, renal or hepatic failure
- *Physical:* Skin—color, lesions; body temperature; P, BP, peripheral perfusion; R, adventitious sounds; liver and renal function tests, Hct, serum electrolytes

Implementation
- Administer by IV infusion only.
- Administer without regard to blood group or type.
- Consider the need for whole blood based on the patient's clinical condition; this infusion only provides symptomatic relief of the patient's hypoproteinemia.
- Monitor blood pressure during infusion; discontinue if hypotension occurs.
- Stop infusion if headache, flushing, fever, changes in blood pressure occur. Arrange to treat reaction with antihistamines. If a plasma protein is still needed, try material from a different lot number.
- Monitor patient's clinical response and adjust infusion rate accordingly.

Drug-specific teaching points
- Be aware that rate will be adjusted based on your response, so constant monitoring will be necessary.
- Report headache, nausea, vomiting, difficulty breathing, back pain.

❏ plicamycin

*(plye kay **mye'** sin)*

mithramycin
Mithracin

Pregnancy Category X

Drug classes
Antibiotic
Antineoplastic agent

Therapeutic actions
Tumoricidal: binds to DNA and inhibits DNA-dependent and DNA-directed RNA synthesis. Exhibits a calcium-lowering effect, acts on osteoclasts, and blocks the action of parathyroid hormone.

Adverse effects in *Italics* are most common; those in **Bold** are life-threatening.

plicamycin

Indications
- Malignant testicular tumors not amenable to successful treatment by surgery or radiation
- Hypercalcemia and hypercalciuria not responsive to other treatments in symptomatic patients with advanced neoplasms

Contraindications/cautions
- Contraindicated in the presence of allergy to plicamycin, bone marrow suppression, thrombocytopenia, thrombocytopathy, coagulation disorders or increased susceptibility to bleeding, electrolyte imbalance, pregnancy, lactation.
- Use caution in the presence of hepatic or renal impairment.

Dosage
Adult

- ***Testicular tumors:*** 25–30 μg/kg per day IV for 8–10 d unless limited by toxicity. Do not exceed 30 μg/d. Do not use course of therapy longer than 10 d. If tumor masses remain unchanged after 3–4 wk, additional courses of therapy at monthly intervals may be prescribed.
- ***Hypercalcemia, hypercalciuria:*** 25 μg/kg per day IV for 3–4 d. May be repeated at 1-wk intervals until the desired effect is reached. Serum calcium may be maintained with single, weekly doses or 2–3 doses/wk.

Pharmacokinetics

Route	Onset	Peak
IV	Rapid	4 h

Metabolism: Hepatic, $T_{1/2}$: unknown
Distribution: Crosses placenta; enters breast milk
Excretion: Urine

IV facts
Preparation: Reconstitute with 4.9 ml Sterile Water for Injection to prepare a solution of 500 mg plicamycin/ml. Prepare fresh solutions each day of therapy; dilute daily dose in 1 L of 5% Dextrose Injection or Sodium Chloride Injection.

Infusion: Administer by slow infusion over 4–6 h.

Adverse effects
- CNS: Drowsiness, weakness, lethargy, malaise, headache, depression
- GI: *Anorexia, nausea, vomiting, diarrhea, stomatitis,* hepatic impairment
- Hematologic: Hemorrhagic syndrome—epistaxis to severe bleeding and death; depression of platelet count, WBC count, hemoglobin, and prothrombin content; elevated clotting time and bleeding time, abnormal clot retraction; *electrolyte abnormalities—decreased serum calcium, phosphorus, and potassium*
- GU: Renal impairment
- Local: *Cellulitis, local reaction at injection site*
- Other: Fever, phlebitis, facial flushing, skin rash

■ Nursing Considerations

Assessment
- *History:* Allergy to plicamycin, bone marrow suppression, thrombocytopenia, thrombocytopathy, coagulation disorders, electrolyte imbalance, hepatic or renal impairment, pregnancy, lactation
- *Physical:* Temperature; skin—color, lesions; weight; orientation, reflexes, affect; mucous membranes, abdominal exam; CBC, platelet count, coagulation studies, renal and liver function tests, serum electrolytes, urinalysis

Implementation
- Do not administer IM or SC as severe local reaction and tissue necrosis occurs.
- Base daily dose on body weight, using ideal weight if patient has abnormal fluid retention.
- Monitor injection site for extravasation: reports of burning or stinging. Discontinue infusion immediately, and restart in another vein. Apply moderate heat to the extravasation area.
- Monitor patient's response to therapy frequently at beginning of therapy and for

several days following the last dose: monitor platelet count, prothrombin, and bleeding time; discontinue drug, and consult with physician if significant prolongation of prothrombin or bleeding times or thrombocytopenia occurs.
- Advise patients to avoid pregnancy while on this drug; serious fetal defects could occur; suggest contraceptive use.

Drug-specific teaching points
- Be aware that this drug must be given by injection. Prepare a calendar for dates to return for additional courses of drug therapy.
- Know that the following side effects may occur: loss of appetite, nausea, vomiting, mouth sores (frequent mouth care, small, frequent meals may help; you will need to try to maintain good nutrition if at all possible; an antiemetic also may be ordered); drowsiness, fatigue, lethargy, weakness (use caution if driving or operating dangerous machinery if these changes occur; use caution to avoid injury); serious fetal deformities if used during pregnancy (use contraceptive measures while on this drug).
- Arrange to have regular blood tests to monitor the drug's effects.
- Report severe GI upset, diarrhea, vomiting, burning or pain at injection site, unusual bleeding or bruising, fever, chills, sore throat, pregnancy.

▢ polymyxin B sulfate

(pol i mix' in)
Parenteral: Aerosporin
Ophthalmic: Polymyxin B Sulfate Sterile Ophthalmic
Pregnancy Category B

Drug classes
Antibiotic

Therapeutic actions
Bactericidal: has surfactant (detergent) activity that allows it to penetrate and disrupt the cell membranes of susceptible gram-negative bacteria, causing cell death; not effective against *Proteus* species.

Indications
- Acute infections caused by susceptible strains of *P. aeruginosa, H. influenzae, E. coli, E. aerogenes, Klebsiella pneumoniae* when less toxic drugs are ineffective or contraindicated
- Infections of the eye caused by susceptible strains of *P. aeruginosa* (ophthalmic preparations)
- Meningeal infections caused by *P. aeruginosa* (intrathecal)

Contraindications/cautions
- Contraindicated in the presence of allergy to polymyxins (polymyxin B, colistin, colistimethate).
- Use caution in the presence of renal disease, pregnancy, lactation.

Dosage
Adults and Pediatric
- ***IV:*** 15,000–25,000 U/kg per day may be given q12h. Do not exceed 25,000 U/d.
- ***IM:*** 25,000–30,000 U/kg per day divided and given at 4- to 6-h intervals.
- ***Intrathecal:*** 50,000 U once daily for 3–4 d; then 50,000 U every other day for at least 2 wk after cultures of CSF are negative, and glucose content is normal.
- ***Ophthalmic:*** 1–2 drops in infected eye bid–q4h or as often as needed.

Infants
- ***IV:*** Up to 40,000 U/kg per day.
- ***IM:*** Up to 40,000 U/kg per day; doses as high as 45,000 U/kg per day have been used in cases of sepsis caused by *P. aeruginosa*.
- ***Intrathecal (younger than 2 y):*** 20,000 U once daily for 3–4 d or 25,000 U once every other day. Continue with 25,000 U once every other day for at least 2 wk after cultures of CSF are negative and glucose content is normal.

Geriatric or renal failure: Reduce dosage downward from the recommended dose, and follow renal function tests during therapy.

Pharmacokinetics
Metabolism: $T_{1/2}$: 4.3–6 h

908 ■ polythiazide

Route	Onset	Peak
IV	Rapid	Unknown
IM	Gradual	2 h

Distribution: Does not cross placenta
Excretion: Urine

IV facts
Preparation: Dissolve 500,000 U in 300–500 ml of 5% Dextrose in Water. Dissolve 500,000 U in 2 ml sterile distilled water or Sodium Chloride Injection, or 1% procaine hydrochloride solution; refrigerate and discard any unused portion after 72 h.
Infusion: Administer by continuous IV drip.

Adverse effects
- CNS: Neurotoxicity—*facial flushing, dizziness, ataxia, drowsiness*, paresthesias
- Respiratory: Apnea (high dosage)
- GU: *Nephrotoxicity*
- Dermatologic: Rash, urticaria
- Local: *Pain at IM injection site; thrombophlebitis at IV injection sites; irritation, burning, stinging, itching, blurring of vision* (ophthalmic preparations)
- Other: Drug fever, superinfections

Clinically important drug-drug interactions
- Increased neuromuscular blockade, apnea, and muscular paralysis when given with nondepolarizing neuromuscular blocking drugs

■ Nursing Considerations

Assessment
- *History:* Allergy to polymyxins, renal disease, lactation
- *Physical:* Site of infection, skin—color, lesions; orientation, reflexes, speech; R; urinary output; urinalysis, serum creatinine, renal function tests

Implementation
- Store drug solutions in refrigerator, and discard any unused portion after 72 h.
- For intrathecal use: Dissolve 500,000 U in 10 ml sterile physiologic saline for a concentration of 50,000 U/ml.
- For ophthalmic use: Reconstitute powder with 20–50 ml of diluent.
- Culture infected area before beginning therapy.
- Monitor renal function tests during therapy.

Drug-specific teaching points
- Administer ophthalmic preparation as follows: tilt head back; place medication into eyelid and close eyes; gently hold the inner corner of the eye for 1 min. Do not touch dropper to the eye.
- Know that the following side effects may occur: vertigo, dizziness, drowsiness, slurring of speech (avoid driving or using hazardous equipment while on this drug); numbness, tingling of the tongue, extremities (decreasing the dosage may help to alleviate this problem); superinfections (frequent hygiene measures will help; at times medications may be required); burning, stinging, blurring of vision (ophthalmic; this sensation usually passes within a few minutes).
- Report difficulty breathing, rash or skin lesions, pain at injection site or IV site, change in urinary voiding patterns, fever, flulike symptoms, changes in vision, severe stinging or itching (ophthalmic).

☐ polythiazide

(pol i thye' a zide)
Renese

Pregnancy Category C

Drug classes
Thiazide diuretic

Therapeutic actions
Inhibits reabsorption of sodium and chloride in distal renal tubule, thereby increasing excretion of sodium, chloride, and water by the kidney.

Adverse effects in *Italics* are most common; those in **Bold** are life-threatening.

Indications
- Adjunctive therapy in edema associated with CHF, cirrhosis, corticosteroid and estrogen therapy, renal dysfunction
- Hypertension, as sole therapy or in combination with other antihypertensives
- Unlabeled use: diabetes insipidus, especially nephrogenic diabetes insipidus

Contraindications/cautions
- Contraindicated in the presence of fluid or electrolyte imbalances, pregnancy, lactation.
- Use caution in the presence of renal or liver disease, gout, SLE, glucose tolerance abnormalities, hyperparathyroidism, manic-depressive disorders.

Dosage
Adult
- **Edema:** 1–4 mg qd PO.
- **Hypertension:** 2–4 mg qd PO.

Pediatric: Safety and efficacy not established.

Pharmacokinetics

Route	Onset	Peak	Duration
Oral	2 h	6 h	24–48 h

Metabolism: $T_{1/2}$: 25.7 h
Distribution: Crosses placenta; enters breast milk
Excretion: Urine

Adverse effects
- **CNS:** *Dizziness, vertigo,* paresthesias, weakness, headache, drowsiness, fatigue, leukopenia, thrombocytopenia, agranulocytosis, aplastic anemia, neutropenia
- **GI:** *Nausea, anorexia, vomiting, dry mouth,* diarrhea, constipation, jaundice, hepatitis, pancreatitis
- **CV:** Orthostatic hypotension, venous thrombosis, volume depletion, cardiac arrhythmias, chest pain
- **GU:** *Polyuria, nocturia,* impotence, loss of libido
- **Dermatologic:** Photosensitivity, rash, purpura, exfoliative dermatitis, hives
- **Other:** Muscle cramps and muscle spasms, fever, gouty attacks, flushing, weight loss, rhinorrhea

Clinically important drug-drug interactions
- Risk of hyperglycemia if taken with diazoxide • Decreased absorption of polythiazide if taken with cholestyramine, colestipol • Increased risk of digitalis glycoside toxicity if hypokalemia occurs • Increased risk of lithium toxicity when taken with thiazides • Increased fasting blood glucose leading to need to adjust dosage of antidiabetic agents.

Drug-lab test interferences
- Monitor for decreased PBI levels without clinical signs of thyroid disturbances.

■ Nursing Considerations

Assessment
- *History:* Electrolyte imbalances, renal or liver disease, gout, SLE, glucose tolerance abnormalities, hyperparathyroidism, manic-depressive disorders, pregnancy, lactation
- *Physical:* Skin—color, lesions; orientation, reflexes, muscle strength; pulses, BP, orthostatic BP, perfusion, edema, baseline ECG; R, adventitious sounds; liver evaluation, bowel sounds; CBC, serum electrolytes, blood glucose, liver and renal function tests, serum uric acid, urinalysis

Implementation
- Administer with food or milk if GI upset occurs.
- Administer early in the day so increased urination will not disturb sleep.
- Measure and record regular body weights to monitor fluid changes.

Drug-specific teaching points
- Take drug early in the day so sleep will not be disturbed by increased urination.
- Weigh yourself daily and record weights.
- Protect skin from exposure to sun or bright lights
- Be aware that increased urination will occur.
- Use caution if dizziness, drowsiness, feeling faint occur.

Adverse effects in *Italics* are most common; those in **Bold** are life-threatening.

- Report rapid weight gain or loss, swelling in ankles or fingers, unusual bleeding or bruising, muscle cramps.

☐ potassium acetate

*(po **tass'** ee um)*

potassium chloride
Oral: Cena-K, Gen-K, Kaochlor, Kaon-C1, Kato, Kay Ciel, K-Lor, Klor-Con, Klorvess, Klotrix, K-Lyte/C1, Kolyum, Potachlor, Potasalan, Rum-K, Slow-K, Ten K

Injection: Potassium Chloride

potassium gluconate
Duo-K, Kaon, Kaylixir, K-G Elixir, Kolyum, Tri-K, Trikates, Twin-K

Pregnancy Category C

Drug classes
Electrolyte

Therapeutic actions
Principal intracellular cation of most body tissues, participates in a number of physiologic processes—maintaining intracellular tonicity, transmission of nerve impulses, contraction of cardiac, skeletal and smooth muscle, maintenance of normal renal function; also plays a role in carbohydrate metabolism and various enzymatic reactions.

Indications
- Prevention and correction of potassium deficiency; when associated with alkalosis, use potassium chloride; when associated with acidosis, use potassium acetate, bicarbonate, citrate, or gluconate
- Treatment of cardiac arrhythmias due to cardiac glycosides (IV)

Contraindications/cautions
- Contraindicated in the presence of allergy to tartrazine, aspirin (tartrazine is found in some preparations marketed as *Kaon-Cl, Klor-Con*); severe renal impairment with oliguria, anuria, azotemia; untreated Addison's disease; hyperkalemia; adynamia episodica hereditaria; acute dehydration; heat cramps; GI disorders that cause delay in passage in the GI tract.
- Use caution in the presence of cardiac disorders, especially if treated with digitalis, pregnancy, lactation.

Dosage
Individualize dosage based on patient response using serial ECG and electrolyte determinations in severe cases.
Adult
- ***Prevention of hypokalemia:*** 16–24 mEq/d PO.
- ***Treatment of potassium depletion:*** 40–100 mEq/d PO.
- ***IV infusion:*** Do not administer undiluted. Dilute in dextrose solution to 40–80 mEq/L. Use the following as a guide to administration:

Serum K+ in mEq/L	Maximum infusion rate	Maximum concentration	Maximum 24-h dose
> 2.6	10 mEq/h	40 mEq/L	200 mEq
< 2.0	40 mEq/h	80 mEq/L	400 mEq

Pediatric: Replacement: 3 mEq/Kg/d or 40 mg/m^2/d PO or IV.
Geriatric and renal impaired: Carefully monitor serum potassium concentration and reduce dosage appropriately.

Pharmacokinetics

Route	Onset	Peak
Oral	Slow	1–2 h
IV	Rapid	

Metabolism: Cellular, T$_{1/2}$: unknown
Distribution: Crosses placenta; enters breast milk
Excretion: Urine

IV facts
Preparation: Do not administer undiluted potassium IV; dilute in dextrose solution to 40–80 mEq/L; in critical states, potassium chloride can be administered in saline.

Infusion: Adjust dosage based on patient response.

Adverse effects
- **GI:** *Nausea, vomiting, diarrhea, abdominal discomfort,* GI obstruction, GI bleeding, GI ulceration or perforation
- **Hematologic:** Hyperkalemia—increased serum K+, ECG changes (peaking of T waves, loss of P waves, depression of ST segment, prolongation of QT interval)
- **Dermatologic:** Skin rash
- **Local:** Tissue sloughing, local necrosis, local phlebitis, and venospasm with injection

Clinically important drug-drug interactions
- Increased risk of hyperkalemia if taken with potassium-sparing diuretics, salt substitutes using potassium

■ Nursing Considerations

Assessment
- *History:* Allergy to tartrazine, aspirin; severe renal impairment; untreated Addison's disease; hyperkalemia; adynamia episodica hereditaria; acute dehydration; heat cramps, GI disorders that cause delay in passage in the GI tract, cardiac disorders, lactation
- *Physical:* Skin—color, lesions, turgor; injection sites; P, baseline ECG; bowel sounds, abdominal exam; urinary output; serum electrolytes, serum bicarbonate

Implementation
- Arrange for serial serum potassium levels before and during therapy.
- Administer liquid preparations to any patient with delayed GI emptying.
- Administer oral drug after meals or with food and a full glass of water to decrease GI upset.
- Caution patient not to chew or crush tablets; have patient swallow tablet whole.
- Mix or dissolve oral liquids, soluble powders, and effervescent tablets completely in 3–8 oz of cold water, juice, or other suitable beverage, and have patient drink it slowly.
- Arrange for further dilution or dose reduction if GI effects are severe.
- Agitate prepared IV solution to prevent "layering" of potassium; do not add potassium to an IV bottle in the hanging position.
- Monitor IV injection sites regularly for necrosis, tissue sloughing, phlebitis.
- Monitor cardiac rhythm carefully during IV administration.
- Caution patient that expended wax matrix capsules will be found in the stool.
- Caution patient not to use salt substitutes while taking this drug.

Drug-specific teaching points
- Take drug after meals or with food and a full glass of water to decrease GI upset. Do not chew or crush tablets, swallow tablets whole. Mix or dissolve oral liquids, soluble powders, and effervescent tablets completely in 3–8 oz of cold water, juice, or other suitable beverage, and drink it slowly. Take the drug as prescribed; do not take more than prescribed.
- Know that nausea, vomiting, diarrhea may occur (taking the drugs with meals, diluting them further may help).
- Do not use salt substitutes while taking this drug.
- Be aware that you may find wax matrix capsules in the stool if you are taking this form of drug. The wax matrix is not absorbed in the GI tract.
- Arrange to have periodic blood tests and medical evaluation while you are on this drug.
- Report tingling of the hands or feet, unusual tiredness or weakness, feeling of heaviness in the legs, severe nausea, vomiting, abdominal pain, black or tarry stools, pain at IV injection site

❏ pralidoxime chloride

*(pra li **dox'** eem)*

PAM

Protopam Chloride

Pregnancy Category C

Adverse effects in *Italics* are most common; those in **Bold** are life-threatening.

Drug classes
Antidote

Therapeutic actions
Reactivates cholinesterase (mainly outside the CNS) inactivated by phosphorylation due to organophosphate pesticide or related compound.

Indications
- Antidote in poisoning due to organophosphate pesticides and chemicals with anticholinesterase activity
- IM use as an adjunct to atropine in poisoning by nerve agents having anticholinesterase activity (autoinjector)
- Control of overdosage by anticholinesterase drugs used to treat myasthenia gravis

Contraindications/cautions
- Contraindicated in the presence of allergy to any component of drug.
- Use caution in the presence of impaired renal function, myasthenia gravis, pregnancy, lactation.

Dosage
Adult
- ***Organophosphate poisoning:*** In absence of cyanosis, give atropine 2–4 mg IV. If cyanosis is present, give 2–4 mg atropine IM while improving ventilation; repeat every 5–10 min until signs of atropine toxicity appear. Maintain atropinization for at least 48 h. *Give pralidoxime concomitantly:* inject an initial dose of 1–2 g pralidoxime IV, preferably as a 15- to 30-min infusion in 100 ml of saline. After 1 h, give a second dose of 1–2 g IV if muscle weakness is not relieved. Give additional doses cautiously. If IV administration is not feasible or if pulmonary edema is present, give IM or SC.
- ***Anticholinesterase overdosage (eg, neostigmine, pyridostigmine, ambenonium):*** 1–2 g IV followed by increments of 250 mg q5 min.
- ***Exposure to nerve agents:*** Administer atropine and pralidoxime as soon as possible after exposure. Use the autoinjectors, giving the atropine first; repeat after 15 min. If symptoms exist after an additional 15 min, repeat injections. If symptoms persist after third set of injections, seek medical help.

Pediatric
- ***Organophosphate poisoning:*** 20–40 mg/kg IV per dose given as above.

Pharmacokinetics

Route	Onset	Peak
IV	Rapid	5–15 min
IM	Rapid	10–20 min

Metabolism: Hepatic, $T_{1/2}$: 0.8–2.7 h
Distribution: May cross placenta or enter breast milk
Excretion: Urine

IV facts
Preparation: Dilute 1–2 g pralidoxime in 100 ml saline.
Infusion: Administer over 15–30 min.

Adverse effects
- **CNS:** *Dizziness, blurred vision, diplopia,* impaired accommodation, *headache,* drowsiness, nausea
- **CV:** Tachycardia
- **Respiratory:** Hyperventilation
- **Hematologic:** *Transient SGOT, SGPT, CPK elevations*
- **Local:** *Mild to moderate pain at the injection site* 40–60 min after IM injection
- **Other:** Muscular weakness

■ Nursing Considerations

Assessment
- *History:* Allergy to any component of drug; impaired renal function; myasthenia gravis; lactation
- *Physical:* Reflexes, orientation, vision exam, muscle strength; P, auscultation, baseline ECG; liver evaluation; renal and liver function tests

Implementation
- Remove secretions, maintain patent airway, and provide artificial ventilation as needed for acute organophosphate poisoning; then begin drug therapy.

- Institute treatment as soon as possible after exposure to the poison.
- Remove clothing; thoroughly wash hair and skin with sodium bicarbonate or alcohol as soon as possible after dermal exposure to organophosphate poisoning.
- Arrange for use of IV sodium thiopental or diazepam if convulsions interfere with respiration after organophosphate poisoning.
- Administer by slow IV infusion; tachycardia, laryngospasm, muscle rigidity have occurred with rapid injection.

Drug-specific teaching points
- Be aware that discomfort may be experienced at IM injection site. If you receive the autoinjector, you need to understand the indications and proper use of the mechanism, review the signs, and symptoms of poisoning.
- Report blurred or double vision, dizziness, nausea.

☐ pravastatin

(prah va sta' tin)
Pravachol

Pregnancy Category X

Drug classes
Antihyperlipidemic agent
HMG CoA inhibitor

Therapeutic actions
A fungal metabolite that inhibits the enzyme HMG CoA that catalyzes the first step in the cholesterol synthesis pathway, resulting in a decrease in serum cholesterol, serum LDLs (associated with increased risk of coronary artery disease), and either an increase or no change in serum HDLs (associated with decreased risk of coronary artery disease).

Indications
- As an adjunct to diet in the treatment of elevated total cholesterol and LDL cholesterol in patients with primary hypercholesterolemia (types IIa and IIb) whose response to dietary restriction of saturated fat and cholesterol and other nonpharmacologic measures has not been adequate.

Contraindications/cautions
- Contraindicated in the presence of allergy to pravastatin, fungal byproducts, pregnancy, lactation.
- Use caution in the presence of impaired hepatic function, cataracts.

Dosage
Adult: Initially, 10–20 mg/d PO administered at bedtime. Maintenance doses range from 10–40 mg/d PO, as a single bedtime use.
Pediatric: Safety and efficacy not established.
Geriatric: 10 mg PO once daily at bedtime.

Pharmacokinetics

Route	Onset	Peak
Oral	Slow	1–1½ h

Metabolism: Hepatic, $T_{1/2}$: 77 h
Distribution: Crosses placenta; enters breast milk
Excretion: Bile and feces

Adverse effects
- CNS: *Headache, blurred vision*, dizziness, insomnia, fatigue, muscle cramps, cataracts
- GI: *Flatulence, abdominal pain, cramps, constipation, nausea, vomiting*, heartburn
- Hematologic: Elevations of CPK, alkaline phosphatase, and transaminases

Clinically important drug-drug interactions
- Possible severe myopathy or rhabdomyolysis if taken with cyclosporine, erythromycin, gemfibrozil, niacin

■ Nursing Considerations

Assessment
- *History:* Allergy to pravastatin, fungal byproducts; impaired hepatic function; cataracts; pregnancy; lactation

Adverse effects in *Italics* are most common; those in **Bold** are life-threatening.

- *Physical:* Orientation, affect, ophthalmologic exam; liver evaluation; lipid studies, liver function tests

Implementation
- Administer drug at bedtime; highest rates of cholesterol synthesis are between midnight and 5 AM.
- Arrange for periodic ophthalmologic exam to check for cataract development.

Drug-specific teaching points
- Take drug at bedtime.
- Know that the following side effects may occur: nausea (small, frequent meals may help); headache, muscle and joint aches and pains (these may lessen with time).
- Arrange to have periodic ophthalmic exams while you are on this drug.
- Report severe GI upset, changes in vision, unusual bleeding or bruising, dark urine or light colored stools.

▯ prazepam

(pra' ze pam)
Centrax

Pregnancy Category D
C-IV controlled substance

Drug classes
Benzodiazepine
Antianxiety drug

Therapeutic actions
Exact mechanisms of action not understood; acts mainly at subcortical levels of the CNS, leaving the cortex relatively unaffected; main sites of action may be the limbic system and reticular formation; benzodiazepines potentiate the effects of gamma-aminobutyrate, an inhibitory neurotransmitter; anxiolytic effects occur at doses well below those necessary to cause sedation, ataxia.

Indications
- Management of anxiety disorders or for short-term relief of symptoms of anxiety

Contraindications/cautions
- Contraindicated in the presence of hypersensitivity to benzodiazepines, tartrazine (in the tablets); psychoses; acute narrow-angle glaucoma; shock; coma; acute alcoholic intoxication with depression of vital signs; pregnancy (increased risk of congenital malformations, neonatal withdrawal syndrome); labor and delivery ("floppy infant" syndrome reported when mothers were given benzodiazepines during labor); lactation (has caused infants to become lethargic and lose weight).
- Use caution in the presence of impaired liver or kidney function, debilitation.

Dosage
Adult: Usual dose is 30 mg/d PO in divided doses. Optimal dosage usually ranges from 20–60 mg/d. Also may be given as single daily dose at bedtime; starting dose is 20 mg/night. Adjust dosage to maximize antianxiety effect with minimum daytime drowsiness.
Pediatric: Safety and efficacy not established for children younger than 18 y.
Geriatric patients or those with debilitating disease: Initially, 10–15 mg/d PO in divided doses. Adjust as needed and tolerated.

Pharmacokinetics

Route	Onset	Peak
Oral	Slow	6 h

Metabolism: Hepatic, $T_{1/2}$: 30–100 h
Distribution: Crosses placenta; enters breast milk
Excretion: Urine

Adverse effects
- CNS: *Transient, mild drowsiness* (initially), *sedation, depression, lethargy, apathy, fatigue, lightheadedness, disorientation*, restlessness, confusion, crying, delirium, headache, slurred speech, dysarthria, stupor, rigidity, tremor, dystonia, vertigo, euphoria, nervousness, difficulty in concentration, vivid dreams, psychomotor retardation, extrapyramidal symp-

Adverse effects in *Italics* are most common; those in **Bold** are life-threatening.

toms, mild paradoxical excitatory reactions, during first two weeks of treatment, visual and auditory disturbances, diplopia, nystagmus, depressed hearing
- **GI:** *Constipation, diarrhea, dry mouth*, salivation, nausea, anorexia, vomiting, difficulty in swallowing, gastric disorders
- **CV:** Bradycardia, tachycardia, cardiovascular collapse, hypertension and hypotension, palpitations, edema
- **Hematologic:** Elevations of blood enzymes (LDH, alkaline phosphatase, SGOT, SGPT); hepatic dysfunction, blood dyscrasias: agranulocytosis, leukopenia
- **GU:** *Incontinence, urinary retention*, changes in libido, menstrual irregularities
- **Dermatologic:** Urticaria, pruritus, skin rash, dermatitis
- **Other:** *Nasal congestion, hiccups, fever, diaphoresis*, paresthesias, muscular disturbances, gynecomastia, drug dependence with withdrawal syndrome

Clinically important drug-drug interactions
- Increased CNS depression when taken with alcohol • Increased effect when given with cimetidine, disulfiram, oral contraceptives, omeprazole • Decreased sedation when given to heavy smokers of cigarettes or if taken concurrently with theophyllines

■ Nursing Considerations
Assessment
- *History:* Hypersensitivity to benzodiazepines, tartrazine; psychoses; acute narrow-angle glaucoma; shock; coma; acute alcoholic intoxication; pregnancy; lactation; impaired liver or kidney function, debilitation
- *Physical:* Skin—color, lesions; body temperature; orientation, reflexes, affect, ophthalmologic exam; P, BP; R, adventitious sounds; liver evaluation, abdominal exam, bowel sounds, normal output; CBC, liver and renal function tests

Implementation
- Arrange to taper dosage gradually after long-term therapy, especially in epileptic patients.

Drug-specific teaching points
- Take drug exactly as prescribed; do not stop taking drug (long-term therapy) without consulting health care provider.
- Know that the following side effects may occur: drowsiness, dizziness (these may become less pronounced after a few days; avoid driving a car or engaging in other dangerous activities if these occur); GI upset (taking the drug with food may help); depression, dreams, emotional upset, crying.
- Report severe dizziness, weakness, drowsiness that persists, palpitations, swelling of the extremities, visual changes, difficulty voiding, rash or skin lesions.

❏ praziquantel

*(pray zi **kwon'** tel)*
Biltricide

Pregnancy Category B

Drug classes
Anthelmintic

Therapeutic actions
Increases cell membrane permeability in susceptible worms, resulting in a loss of intracellular calcium, massive contractions, and paralysis of the worm's musculature; also causes a disintegration of the schistosome's tegument.

Indications
- Infections caused by *Schistosoma mekongi, Schistosoma japonicum, Schistosoma mansoni, Schistosoma haematobium,* liver flukes
- Orphan drug use: treatment of neurocysticercosis

Contraindications/cautions
- Allergy to praziquantel; pregnancy (abortifacient in some high-dose preclinical studies); lactation (secreted in breast milk; should not nurse on the day of treatment or for 72 h thereafter).

Adverse effects in *Italics* are most common; those in **Bold** are life-threatening.

Dosage
Adult and Pediatric (older than 4 y)
- **Schistosomiasis:** Three doses of 20 mg/kg PO as a 1-d treatment, with intervals of 4–6 h between doses.
- **Clonorchiasis and opisthorchiasis:** Three doses of 25 mg/kg PO as a 1-d treatment.

Pediatric (younger than 4 y): Safety not established.

Pharmacokinetics

Route	Onset	Peak
Oral	Varies	1–3 h

Metabolism: Hepatic, $T_{1/2}$: 0.8–1.5 h
Distribution: Crosses placenta; enters breast milk
Excretion: Urine

Adverse effects
- CNS: Malaise, headache, dizziness
- GI: Abdominal discomfort, slight increase in liver enzymes
- Other: Fever, urticaria

■ Nursing Considerations

Assessment
- *History:* Allergy to praziquantel, pregnancy, lactation
- *Physical:* Skin—color, lesions; orientation, reflexes; liver function tests

Implementation
- Culture urine or feces, as appropriate, for ova.
- Do not administer if the patient has ocular cysticercosis.
- Do not administer on an outpatient basis to patients with cerebral cysticercosis; consult with physician regarding hospital admission.
- Administer drug with food; have patient swallow the tablets unchewed with some liquid. If the patient keeps the tablets in the mouth, a bitter taste may result that could cause gagging or vomiting.

Drug-specific teaching points
- Be aware that tablets should be swallowed unchewed during meals, with a small amount of liquid. Do not hold the tablet in your mouth; it gives a bitter taste that could cause gagging or vomiting.
- Know that the following side effects may occur: nausea, abdominal pain, GI upset (small, frequent meals may help); drowsiness, dizziness (if these occur, use caution when driving a car or operating dangerous equipment).
- Report rash, severe abdominal pain, marked weakness, dizziness.

▢ prazosin hydrochloride

(pra' zoe sin)
Apo-Prazo (CAN), Minipress, Novo-Prazin (CAN), Nu-Prazo (CAN)

Pregnancy Category C

Drug classes
Antihypertensive drug
Alpha-adrenergic blocking drug

Therapeutic actions
Selectively blocks postsynaptic alpha$_1$-adrenergic receptors, decreasing sympathetic tone on the vasculature, dilating arterioles and veins, and lowering supine and standing blood pressure; unlike conventional alpha-adrenergic blocking agents (eg, phentolamine), it does not also block alpha$_2$ presynaptic receptors, so it does not cause reflex tachycardia.

Indications
- Treatment of hypertension, alone or in combination with other agents
- Unlabeled uses: refractory CHF, management of Raynaud's vasospasm, treatment of prostatic outflow obstruction

Contraindications/cautions
- Contraindicated in the presence of hypersensitivity to prazosin, lactation.
- Use caution in the presence of CHF, renal failure, pregnancy.

Adverse effects in *Italics* are most common; those in **Bold** are life-threatening.

prazosin hydrochloride ■ 917

Dosage

Adult: First dose may cause syncope with sudden loss of consciousness. First dose should be limited to 1 mg PO and given at bedtime. Initial dosage is 1 mg PO bid–tid. Increase dosage to a total of 20 mg/d given in divided doses. When increasing dosage, give the first dose of each increment at bedtime. Maintenance dosages most commonly range from 6–15 mg/d given in divided doses.

- ***Concomitant therapy:*** When adding a diuretic or other antihypertensive drug, reduce dosage to 1–2 mg PO tid and then retitrate.

Pediatric: Safety and efficacy not established.

Pharmacokinetics

Route	Onset	Peak
Oral	Varies	1–3 h

Metabolism: Hepatic, $T_{1/2}$: 2–3 h
Distribution: Crosses placenta; may enter breast milk
Excretion: Bile/feces, urine

Adverse effects

- CNS: *Dizziness, headache, drowsiness, lack of energy, weakness,* nervousness, vertigo, depression, paresthesia
- GI: *Nausea,* vomiting, diarrhea, constipation, abdominal discomfort or pain
- CV: *Palpitations,* sodium and water retention, increased plasma volume, edema, dyspnea, syncope, tachycardia, orthostatic hypotension
- GU: Urinary frequency, incontinence, impotence, priapism
- EENT: Blurred vision, reddened sclera, epistaxis, tinnitus, dry mouth, nasal congestion
- **Dermatologic:** Rash, pruritus, alopecia, lichen planus
- Other: Diaphoresis, lupus erythematosus

Clinically important drug-drug interactions

- Severity and duration of hypotension following first dose of prazosin may be greater in patients receiving beta-adrenergic blocking drugs (eg, propranolol), verapamil; first dose of prazosin should be only 0.5 mg or less

■ Nursing Considerations

Assessment

- *History:* Hypersensitivity to prazosin, CHF, renal failure, lactation
- *Physical:* Body weight; skin—color, lesions; orientation, affect, reflexes; ophthalmologic exam; P, BP, orthostatic BP, supine BP, perfusion, edema, auscultation; R, adventitious sounds; status of nasal mucous membranes; bowel sounds, normal output; voiding pattern, normal output; kidney function tests, urinalysis

Implementation

- Arrange to administer, or have patient take, first dose just before bedtime to lessen likelihood of first dose effect (syncope)—believed due to excessive postural hypotension.
- Place patient in recumbent position and treat supportively if syncope occurs; condition is self-limiting.
- Monitor patient for orthostatic hypotension, which is most marked in the morning and is accentuated by hot weather, alcohol, exercise.
- Monitor edema, body weight in patients with incipient cardiac decompensation, and arrange to add a thiazide diuretic to the drug regimen if sodium and fluid retention, signs of impending CHF occur.

Drug-specific teaching points

- Take this drug exactly as prescribed. Take the first dose just before bedtime. Do not drive a car or operate machinery for 4 h after the first dose.
- Know that the following side effects may occur: dizziness, weakness (these are more likely to occur when you change position, in the early morning, after exercise, in hot weather, and when you have consumed alcohol; some tolerance may occur after you have taken the drug for a while, but you should avoid driving a car or engaging in tasks that require alertness while you are experiencing

Adverse effects in *Italics* are most common; those in **Bold** are life-threatening.

these symptoms; change position slowly, and use caution when climbing stairs; lie down for a while if dizziness persists); GI upset (frequent, small meals may help); impotence; dry mouth (sucking on sugarless lozenges, ice chips may help); stuffy nose. Most of these effects will gradually disappear with continued therapy.
- Report frequent dizziness or faintness.

prednisolone

*(pred **niss'** oh lone)*
Oral: Delta-Cortef, Novoprednisolone (CAN), Prelone

prednisolone acetate

IM, ophthalmic solution: AK-Tate, Articulose, Econopred, Key-Pred, Predaject, Predcor, Pred-Forte, Pred Mild, and others

prednisolone acetate and sodium phosphate IM, intra-articular, prednisolone sodium phosphate

IV, IM, intra-articular injection, ophthalmic solution: AK-Pred, Hydeltrasol, Hydrocortone, Inflamase, Key-Pred, Metreton

prednisolone tebutate

Intra-articular, intralesional injection: Hydeltra, Hydeltrasol, Nor-Pred, Predcor-TBA, Prednisol TBA

Pregnancy Category C

Drug classes
Corticosteroid (intermediate acting)
Glucocorticoid
Hormonal agent

Therapeutic actions
Enters target cells and binds to intracellular corticosteroid receptors, thereby initiating many complex reactions that are responsible for its anti-inflammatory and immunosuppressive effects.

Indications
- Hypercalcemia associated with cancer (systemic)
- Short-term management of various inflammatory and allergic disorders, such as rheumatoid arthritis, collagen diseases (eg, SLE), dermatologic diseases (eg, pemphigus), status asthmaticus, and autoimmune disorders (systemic)
- Hematologic disorders: thrombocytopenia purpura, erythroblastopenia (systemic)
- Ulcerative colitis, acute exacerbations of mutiple sclerosis and palliation in some leukemias and lymphomas (systemic)
- Trichinosis with neurologic or myocardial involvement (systemic)
- Arthritis, psoriatic plaques (intra-articular, soft tissue administration)
- Inflammation of the lid, conjunctiva, cornea, and globe (ophthalmic)
- Prednisolone has weaker mineralocorticoid activity than hydrocortisone and is not used as physiologic replacement therapy (ophthalmic)

Contraindications/cautions
- Contraindicated in the presence of infections, especially tuberculosis, fungal infectons, amebiasis, vaccinia and varicella, and antibiotic-resistant infections; lactation.
- Use caution in the presence of kidney or liver disease, hypothyroidism, ulcerative colitis with impending perforation, diverticulitis, active or latent peptic ulcer, inflammatory bowel disease, CHF, hypertension, thromboembolic disorders, osteoporosis, convulsive disorders, diabetes mellitus, pregnancy.

Ophthalmic Preparations
- Contraindicated in the presence of acute superficial herpes simplex keratitis; fungal infections of ocular structures; vaccinia, varicella, and other viral diseases of the cornea and conjunctiva; ocular tuberculosis.

Dosage
Adult: Individualize dosage, depending on the severity of the condition and the patient's response. Administer daily dose before 9 AM to minimize adrenal suppression.

If long-term therapy is needed, alternate-day therapy should be considered. After long-term therapy, withdraw drug slowly to avoid adrenal insufficiency. For maintenance therapy, reduce initial dose in small increments at intervals until the lowest dose that maintains satisfactory clinical response is reached.

Pediatric: Individualize dosage, depending on the severity of the condition and the patient's response rather than by strict adherence to formulae that correct adult doses for age or body weight. Carefully observe growth and development in infants and children on prolonged therapy.

- ***Oral (prednisolone):*** 5–60 mg/d. Acute exacerbations of multiple sclerosis: 200 mg/d for 1 wk, followed by 80 mg every other day for 1 mo.
- ***IM (prednisolone acetate):*** 4–60 mg/d. Acute exacerbations of multiple sclerosis: 200 mg/d for 1 wk followed by 80 mg every other day for 1 mo.
- ***IM, IV (prednisolone sodium phosphate):*** Initial dosage, 4–60 mg/day. Acute exacerbations of multiple sclerosis: 200 mg/d for 1 wk followed by 80 mg every other day for 1 mo.
- ***IM (prednisolone acetate and sodium phosphate):*** Initial dose 0.25–1.0 ml. Repeat within several days, up to 3–4 wk or more often as necessary.
- ***Intra-articular, intralesional (dose will vary with joint or soft tissue site to be injected)***
- *Prednisolone acetate:* 5–100 mg.
- *Predisolone acetate and sodium phosphate:* 0.25–0.5 ml.
- *Prednisolone sodium phosphate:* 2–30 mg.
- *Prednisolone tebutate:* 4–30 mg.
- ***Ophthalmic (prednisolone acetate suspension; prednisolone sodium phosphate solution):*** 1–2 drops into the conjunctival sac every hour during the day and every 2 h during the night. After a favorable response, reduce dose to 1 drop q4h and then 1 drop tid or qid.

Pharmacokinetics

Route	Onset	Peak	Duration
Oral	Varies	1–2 h	1–1½ d

Metabolism: Hepatic, $T_{1/2}$: 3.5 h
Distribution: Crosses placenta; enters breast milk
Excretion: Urine

Adverse effects

Effects depend on dose, route, and duration of therapy. The following are primarily associated with systemic absorption.

- **CNS:** *Vertigo, headache,* paresthesias, insomnia, convulsions, psychosis, cataracts, increased intraocular pressure, glaucoma (long-term therapy)
- **GI:** Peptic or esophageal ulcer, pancreatitis, abdominal distention, nausea, vomiting, *increased appetite, weight gain* (long-term therapy)
- **CV:** Hypotension, shock, hypertension and CHF secondary to fluid retention, thromboembolism, thrombophlebitis, fat embolism, cardiac arrhythmias
- **MS:** Muscle weakness, steroid myopathy, loss of muscle mass, osteoporosis, spontaneous fractures (long-term therapy)
- **Hypersensitivity:** Hypersensitivity or anaphylactoid reactions
- **Endocrine:** Amenorrhea, irregular menses, growth retardation, decreased carbohydrate tolerance, diabetes mellitus, cushingoid state (long-term effect), increased blood sugar, increased serum cholesterol, decreased T_3 and T_4 levels, hypothalamic-pituitary-adrenal (HPA) suppression with systemic therapy longer than 5 d
- **Electrolyte imbalance:** *Na$^+$ and fluid retention,* hypokalemia, hypocalcemia
- **Other:** *Immunosuppression, aggravation, or masking of infections; impaired wound healing;* thin, fragile skin; petechiae, ecchymoses, purpura, striae; subcutaneous fat atrophy
- The following effects are related to various local routes of steroid administration:

Adverse effects in *Italics* are most common; those in **Bold** are life-threatening.

Intra-articular
- Local: Osteonecrosis, tendon, rupture, infection

Intralesional (Face and Head)
- Local: Blindness (rare)

Ophthalmic Solutions, Ointments
- Local: Infections, especially fungal; glaucoma, cataracts with long-term therapy
- Other: Systemic absorption and adverse effects (see above) with prolonged use

Clinically important drug-drug interactions
- Increased therapeutic and toxic effects of prednisolone if taken concurrently with troleandomycin, ketoconazole • Increased therapeutic and toxic effects of estrogens, including oral contraceptives, if taken concurrently with prednisolone • Risk of severe deterioration of muscle strength when given to myasthenia gravis patients who also are receiving ambenonium, edrophonium, neostigmine, pyridostigmine • Decreased steroid blood levels when taken with barbiturates, phenytoin, rifampin • Decreased effectiveness of salicylates when taken with prednisolone

Drug-lab test interferences
- False-negative nitroblue-tetrazolium test for bacterial infection • Suppression of skin test reactions

■ Nursing Considerations

Assessment
- *History:* Infections; kidney or liver disease; hypothyroidism; ulcerative colitis with impending perforation; diverticulitis; active or latent peptic ulcer; inflammatory bowel disease; CHF; hypertension; thromboembolic disorders; osteoporosis; convulsive disorders; diabetes mellitus; pregnancy; lactation. Ophthalmic: acute superficial herpes simplex keratitis; fungal infections of ocular structures; vaccinia, varicella, and other viral diseases of the cornea and conjunctiva; ocular tuberculosis
- *Physical:* Body weight, temperature, reflexes and grip strength, affect and orientation, P, BP, peripheral perfusion, prominence of superficial veins, R, adventitious sounds, serum electrolytes, blood glucose

Implementation
- Administer once-a-day doses before 9 AM to mimic normal peak corticosteroid blood levels.
- Arrange for increased dosage when patient is subject to stress.
- Arrange to taper doses when discontinuing high-dose or long-term therapy.
- Do not give live virus vaccines with immunosuppressive doses of corticosteroids.

Drug-specific teaching points

Systemic
- Do not stop taking the drug without consulting your health care provider.
- Avoid exposure to infections.
- Report unusual weight gain, swelling of the extremities, muscle weakness, black or tarry stools, fever, prolonged sore throat, colds or other infections, worsening of the disorder for which the drug is being taken.

Intra-articular Administration
- Do not overuse joint after therapy, even if pain is gone.

Ophthalmic Preparations
- Learn the proper administration technique: Lie down or tilt head backward, and look at ceiling. Drop suspension inside lower eyelid while looking up. After instilling eye drops, release lower lid, but do not blink for at least 30 sec; apply gentle pressure to the inside corner of the eye for 1 min. Do not close eyes tightly, and try not to blink more often than usual. Do not touch dropper to eye, fingers, or any surface. Wait at least 5 min before using any other eye preparations.
- Be aware that the eyes may be sensitive to bright light; sunglasses may help.
- Report worsening of the condition, pain, itching, swelling of the eye, failure of the condition to improve after 1 wk.

prednisone

(pred' ni sone)
Apo-Prednisone (CAN), Deltasone, Liquid Pred, Meticorten, Novoprednisone (CAN), Orasone, Panasol, Prednicen-M, Prednisone-Intensol, Winpred (CAN)

Pregnancy Category C

Drug classes
Corticosteroid (intermediate acting)
Glucocorticoid
Hormonal agent

Therapeutic actions
Enters target cells and binds to intracellular corticosteroid receptors, thereby initiating many complex reactions that are responsible for its anti-inflammatory and immunosuppressive effects.

Indications
- Replacement therapy in adrenal cortical insufficiency
- Hypercalcemia associated with cancer
- Short-term management of various inflammatory and allergic disorders, such as rheumatoid arthritis, collagen diseases (eg, SLE), dermatologic diseases (eg, pemphigus), status asthmaticus, and autoimmune disorders
- Hematologic disorders: thrombocytopenia purpura, erythroblastopenia
- Ulcerative colitis, acute exacerbations of multiple sclerosis and palliation in some leukemias and lymphomas
- Trichinosis with neurologic or myocardial involvement

Contraindications/cautions
- Contraindicated in the presence of infections, especially tuberculosis, fungal infections, amebiasis, vaccinia and varicella, and antibiotic-resistant infections; lactation.
- Use caution in the presence of kidney or liver disease, hypothyroidism, ulcerative colitis with impending perforation, diverticulitis, active or latent peptic ulcer, inflammatory bowel disease, CHF, hypertension, thromboembolic disorders, osteoporosis, convulsive disorders, diabetes mellitus; hepatic disease; pregnancy (monitor infants born to mothers who have received substantial corticosteroid doses during pregnancy for adrenal insufficiency).

Dosage
Adult: Individualize dosage, depending on the severity of the condition and the patient's response. Administer daily dose before 9 AM to minimize adrenal suppression. If long-term therapy is needed, alternate-day therapy should be considered. After long-term therapy, withdraw drug slowly to avoid adrenal insufficiency. Initial dose, 5–60 mg/d PO. For maintenance therapy, reduce initial dose in small increments at intervals until the lowest dose that maintains satisfactory clinical response is reached.

Pediatric
- ***Physiologic replacement:*** 0.1–0.15 mg/kg per day PO or 4–5 mg/m^2 per day PO in equal divided doses q12h.
- ***Other indications:*** Individualize dosage, depending on the severity of the condition and the patient's response rather than by strict adherence to formulae that correct adult doses for age or body weight. Carefully observe growth and development in infants and children on prolonged therapy.

Pharmacokinetics

Route	Onset	Peak	Duration
Oral	Varies	1–2 h	1–1½ d

Metabolism: Hepatic, T$_{1/2}$: 3.5 h
Distribution: Crosses placenta; enters breast milk
Excretion: Urine

Adverse effects
- **CNS:** *Vertigo, headache,* paresthesias, insomnia, convulsions, psychosis, cataracts, increased intraocular pressure, glaucoma (long-term therapy)

Adverse effects in *Italics* are most common; those in **Bold** are life-threatening.

- **GI:** Peptic or esophageal ulcer, pancreatitis, abdominal distention, nausea, vomiting, *increased appetite, weight gain* (long-term therapy)
- **CV:** Hypotension, shock, hypertension and CHF secondary to fluid retention, thromboembolism, thrombophlebitis, fat embolism, cardiac arrhythmias
- **MS:** Muscle weakness, steroid myopathy, loss of muscle mass, osteoporosis, spontaneous fractures (long-term therapy)
- **Hypersensitivity:** Hypersensitivity or anaphylactoid reactions
- **Endocrine:** Amenorrhea, irregular menses, growth retardation, decreased carbohydrate tolerance, diabetes mellitus, cushingoid state (long-term effect), increased blood sugar, increased serum cholesterol, decreased T_3 and T_4 levels, HPA suppression with systemic therapy longer than 5 d
- **Electrolyte imbalance:** *Na^+ and fluid retention*, hypokalemia, hypocalcemia
- **Other:** *Immunosuppression, aggravation, or masking of infections; impaired wound healing*; thin, fragile skin; petechiae, ecchymoses, purpura, striae; subcutaneous fat atrophy

Clinically important drug-drug interactions

- Increased therapeutic and toxic effects of prednisone if taken concurrently with troleandomycin, ketoconazole • Increased theraputic and toxic effects of estrogens, including oral contraceptives, if taken concurrently with prednisone • Risk of severe deterioration of muscle strength when given to myasthenia gravis patients who also are receiving ambenonium, edrophonium, neostigmine, pyridostigmine • Decreased steroid blood levels when taken with barbiturates, phenytoin, rifampin • Decreased effectiveness of salicylates when taken with prednisone

Drug-lab test interferences

- False-negative nitroblue-tetrazolium test for bacterial infection • Suppression of skin test reactions

■ Nursing Considerations

Assessment

- *History:* Infections; kidney or liver disease, hypothyroidism, ulcerative colitis with impending perforation, diverticulitis, active or latent peptic ulcer, inflammatory bowel disease, CHF, hypertension, thromboembolic disorders, osteoporosis, convulsive disorders, diabetes mellitus; hepatic disease; lactation
- *Physical:* Body weight, temperature, reflexes and grip strength, affect and orientation, P, BP, peripheral perfusion, prominence of superficial veins, R, adventitious sounds, serum electrolytes, blood glucose

Implementation

- Administer once-a-day doses before 9 AM to mimic normal peak corticosteroid blood levels.
- Arrange for increased dosage when patient is subject to stress.
- Arrange to taper doses when discontinuing high-dose or long-term therapy.
- Do not give live virus vaccines with immunosuppressive doses of corticosteroids.

Drug-specific teaching points

- Do not stop taking the drug without consulting your health care provider.
- Avoid exposure to infections.
- Report unusual weight gain, swelling of the extremities, muscle weakness, black or tarry stools, fever, prolonged sore throat, colds or other infections, worsening of the disorder for which the drug is being taken.

❏ primaquine phosphate

(prim' a kween)

Pregnancy Category C

Drug classes

Antimalarial
8-aminoquinoline

Adverse effects in *Italics* are most common; those in **Bold** are life-threatening.

Therapeutic actions
Disrupts the parasite's mitochondria, creating a major disruption in the metabolic processes; some gametocytes and exoerythrocytic forms are destroyed, and others are rendered incapable of undergoing division; by eliminating exoerythrocytic forms, primaquine prevents development of erythrocytic forms responsible for relapses in vivax malaria.

Indications
- Radical cure of vivax malaria
- Prevention of relapse in vivax malaria or following the termination of chloroquine phosphate suppressive therapy in an area where vivax malaria is endemic

Contraindications/cautions
- Contraindicated in the presence of allergy to primaquine; the acutely ill suffering from systemic disease with hematologic depression.
- Use caution in the presence of pregnancy.

Dosage
Patients should receive a course of chloroquine phosphate to eliminate erythrocytic forms of the parasite.
Adult: Begin treatment during the last 2 wk of, or following, a course of suppression with chloroquine or a comparable drug; 26.3 mg (15 mg base)/d PO for 14 d.
Pediatric: 0.5 mg/kg per day PO (0.3 mg base/kg per day) for 14 d. Maximum 15 mg base/dose.

Pharmacokinetics

Route	Onset	Peak
Oral	Varies	1–3 h

Metabolism: Hepatic, $T_{1/2}$: 4 h
Distribution: Crosses placenta; may enter breast milk
Excretion: Urine

Adverse effects
- **GI:** *Nausea, vomiting, epigastric distress,* abdominal cramps
- **Hematologic:** Leukopenia, hemolytic anemia in patients with G-6-PD deficiency, methhemoglobinemia in NADH methemoglobin reductase deficient individuals

Clinically important drug-drug interactions
- Increased toxicity if taken with quinacrine
- Increased risk of bone marrow depression if taken with hemolytic drugs or drugs that cause bone marrow depression

■ Nursing Considerations
Assessment
- *History:* Allergy to primaquine; acutely ill suffering from systemic disease with hematologic depression
- *Physical:* Abdominal exam; CBC, hemoglobin, G-6-PD in deficient patients

Implementation
- Administer with food if GI upset occurs.
- Administer concurrently with course of chloroquine phosphate.
- Schedule doses for weekly same-day therapy on a calendar.
- Arrange for CBC and hemoglobin determinations before beginning therapy and periodically during therapy.

Drug-specific teaching points
- Take full course of drug therapy as prescribed.
- Take drug with food if GI upset occurs.
- Mark your calendar with the drug days for once-a-week therapy.
- Be aware that this drug may cause stomach pain, loss of appetite, nausea, vomiting, or abdominal cramps; report severe problems.
- Arrange to have regular blood tests while you are on this drug to evaluate drug effects.
- Report darkening of the urine, severe abdominal cramps, GI distress, persistent nausea, vomiting.

❑ primidone

(pri' mi done)
Apo-Primidone (CAN),
Mysoline, Primaclone (CAN)

Pregnancy Category D

Adverse effects in *Italics* are most common; those in **Bold** are life-threatening.

Drug classes
Antiepileptic

Therapeutic actions
Mechanism of action not understood; primidone and its two metabolites, phenobarbital and phenylethylmalonamide, all have antiepileptic activity.

Indications
- Control of grand mal, psychomotor, or focal epileptic seizures, either alone or with other antiepileptics; may control grand mal seizures refractory to other antiepileptics
- Unlabeled use: treatment of benign familial tremor (essential tremor)—750 mg/d

Contraindications/cautions
- Contraindicated in the presence of hypersensitivity to phenobarbital, porphyria, lactation (somnolence and drowsiness may occur in nursing newborns).
- Use caution in the presence of pregnancy (association between use of antiepileptic drugs by women with epilepsy and an elevated incidence of birth defects in children born to these women; however, do not discontinue antiepileptic therapy in pregnant women who are receiving such therapy to prevent major seizures; discontinuing medication is likely to precipitate status epilepticus, with attendant hypoxia and risk to both mother and unborn child; to prevent neonatal hemorrhage, women taking primidone during pregnancy should be given prophylactic vitamin K_1 therapy for 1 mo prior to and during delivery).

Dosage
Adult
- ***Regimen for patients who have received no previous therapy:*** Days 1–3, 100–125 mg PO at bedtime; days 4–6, 100–125 mg bid; days 7–9, 100–125 mg tid; day 10–maintenance, 250 mg tid. The usual maintenance dosage is 250 mg tid–qid. If required, increase dosage to 250 mg five to six times daily, but do not exceed dosage of 500 mg qid (2 g/d).
- ***Regimen for patients already receiving other antiepileptic drugs:*** Start primidone at 100–125 mg PO at bedtime. Gradually increase to maintenance level as the other drug is gradually decreased. Continue this regimen until satisfactory dosage level is achieved for the combination, or the other medication is completely withdrawn. When therapy with primidone alone is the objective, the transition should not be completed in less than 2 wk.

Pediatric
- ***Children > 8 y:*** *Regimen for patients who have received no previous therapy:* Days 1–3, 100–125 mg PO at bedtime; days 4–6, 100–125 mg bid; days 7–9, 100–125 mg tid; day 10–maintenance, 250 mg tid. The usual maintenance dosage is 250 mg tid–qid. If required, increase dosage to 250 mg five to six times daily, but do not exceed dosage of 500 mg qid (2 g/d).
- ***Children < 8 y:*** *Regimen for patients who have received no previous therapy:* Days 1–3, 50 mg PO at bedtime; days 4–6, 50 mg bid; days 7–9, 100 mg bid; day 10–maintenance, 125–250 mg tid. The usual maintenance dosage is 125–250 mg tid or 10–25 mg/kg per day in divided doses.

Pharmacokinetics

Route	Onset	Peak
Oral	Varies	3–7 h

Metabolism: Hepatic, $T_{1/2}$: 3–24 h
Distribution: Crosses placenta; enters breast milk
Excretion: Urine

Adverse effects
- CNS: *Ataxia, vertigo, fatigue, hyperirritability*, emotional disturbances, nystagmus, diplopia, drowsiness, personality deterioration with mood changes and paranoia
- GI: *Nausea, anorexia,* vomiting

- **Hematologic:** Megaloblastic anemia that responds to folic acid therapy
- **GU:** Sexual impotence
- **Other:** Morbiliform skin eruptions

Clinically important drug-drug interactions
- Toxicity when given with phenytoins • Increased CNS effects, impaired hand-eye coordination, and death may occur if acute alcohol ingestion occurs while taking primidone • Increased renal toxicity may occur if taken concurrently with methoxyflurane • Increased pharmacologic effects when given with valproic acid • Decreased serum concentrations of primidone and increased serum concentrations of carbamazepine if taken concurrently • Decreased serum concentrations of primidone if taken concurrently with ethosuximide, methsuximide, phensuximide, phenylbutazone, oxyphenbutazone • Decreased effects of the following drugs given with primidone: oral anticoagulants, corticosteroids, oral contraceptives and estrogens, beta-adrenergic blockers (especially propranolol, metoprolol), theophylline, metronidazole, griseofulvin • Decreased half-life of quinidine, doxycycline when given concomitantly or within 2 wk of primidone

■ Nursing Considerations

Assessment
- *History:* Hypersensitivity to phenobarbital, porphyria, pregnancy, lactation
- *Physical:* Skin—color, lesions; orientation, affect, reflexes, vision exam; bowel sounds, normal output; CBC and a sequential multiple analysis-12 (SMA-12), EEG

Implementation
- Arrange to reduce dosage, discontinue primidone, or substitute other antiepileptic medication gradually; abrupt discontinuation may precipitate status epilepticus.
- Arrange for patient to have CBC and SMA-12 test every 6 mo during therapy.
- Arrange for folic acid therapy if megaloblastic anemia occurs; primidone does not need to be discontinued.
- Arrange for appropriate counseling for women of childbearing age who wish to become pregnant.
- Evaluate for therapeutic serum levels: 5–12 μg/ml for primidone.

Drug-specific teaching points
- Take this drug exactly as prescribed; do not discontinue this drug abruptly or change dosage, except on the advice of your prescriber.
- Arrange for frequent checkups, including blood tests, to monitor your response to this drug. It is very important that you keep all appointments for checkups.
- Use contraception at all times. If you wish to become pregnant while you are taking this drug, you should consult your physician.
- Know that the following side effects may occur: drowsiness, dizziness, muscular incoordination (these symptoms may occur initially but usually disappear with continued therapy; avoid driving a car or performing other tasks requiring alertness if these occur); vision changes (avoid performing tasks that require visual acuity); GI upset (taking the drug with food or milk and eating frequent, small meals may help).
- Wear a medical alert tag at all times so that any emergency medical personnel taking care of you will know that you are an epileptic taking antiepileptic medication.
- Report skin rash, joint pain, unexplained fever, pregnancy.

☐ probenecid

*(proe **ben'** e sid)*
Benemid, Probalan

Pregnancy Category C

Drug classes
Uricosuric
Antigout drug

Adverse effects in *Italics* are most common; those in **Bold** are life-threatening.

Therapeutic actions
Inhibits the renal tubular reabsorption of urate, increasing the urinary excretion of uric acid, decreasing serum uric acid levels, retarding urate deposition, and promoting resorption of urate deposits; also inhibits the renal tubular reabsorption of most penicillins and cephalosporins.

Indications
- Treatment of hyperuricemia associated with gout and gouty arthritis
- Adjuvant to therapy with penicillins or cephalosporins, for elevation and prolongation of plasma levels of the antibiotic

Contraindications/cautions
- Contraindicated in the presence of allergy to probenecid, blood dyscrasias, uric acid kidney stones, acute gouty attack, pregnancy.
- Use caution in the presence of peptic ulcer, acute intermittent porphyria, G-6-PD deficiency, chronic renal insufficiency, lactation.

Dosage
Adult
- ***Gout:*** 0.25 g PO bid for 1 wk; then 0.5 g PO bid. Maintenance: continue dosage that maintains the normal serum uric acid levels. When no attacks occur for 6 mo or more, decrease the daily dosage by 0.5 g every 6 mo.
- ***Penicillin or cephalosporin therapy:*** 2 g/d PO in divided doses.
- ***Gonorrhea treatment:*** Single 1-g dose PO ½ h before penicillin administration.

Pediatric
- ***Penicillin or cephalosporin therapy:*** 2–14 y: 25 mg/kg PO initial dose, then 40 mg/kg per day divided in four doses. Children weighing > 50 kg: adult dosage. Do not use in children younger than 2 y.
- ***Gonorrhea treatment:*** Children weighing < 45 kg: 23 mg/kg PO in one single dose ½ h before penicillin administration.

Geriatric or renal impaired: 1 g/d PO may be adequate. Daily dosage may be increased by 0.5 g every 4 wk. Probenecid may not be effective in chronic renal insufficiency when glomerular filtration rate < 30 ml/min.

Pharmacokinetics

Route	Onset	Peak
Oral	Varies	2–4 h

Metabolism: Hepatic, $T_{1/2}$: 5–8 h
Distribution: Crosses placenta; may enter breast milk
Excretion: Urine

Adverse effects
- **CNS:** *Headache*
- **GI:** *Nausea, vomiting, anorexia,* sore gums
- **Hematologic:** Anemia, hemolytic anemia
- **GU:** *Urinary frequency,* exacerbation of gout and uric acid stones
- **Hypersensitivity:** Reactions including anaphylaxis, dermatitis, pruritus, fever
- **Other:** Blushing, dizziness

Clinically important drug-drug interactions
- Decreased effectiveness of probenecid when taken with salicylates • Decreased renal excretion and increased serum levels of methotrexate, dyphylline, when taken with probenecid • Increased pharmacologic effects of thiopental when taken with probenecid

Drug-lab test interferences
- False-positive test for urine glucose if using Benedict's test, Clinitest (use Clinistix) • Falsely high determination of theophylline levels • Inhibited excretion of urinary 17-ketosteroids, phenolsulfonphthalein, sulfobromophthalein

■ Nursing Considerations

Assessment
- *History:* Allergy to probenecid, blood dyscrasias, uric acid kidney stones, acute gouty attack, peptic ulcer, acute intermittent porphyria, G-6-PD deficiency,

Adverse effects in *Italics* are most common; those in **Bold** are life-threatening.

chronic renal insufficiency, pregnancy, lactation
- *Physical:* Skin—lesions, color; reflexes, gait; liver evaluation, normal output, gums; urinary output; CBC, renal and liver function tests, urinalysis

Implementation
- Administer drug with meals or antacids if GI upset occurs.
- Force fluids—2.5 to 3 L/d—to decrease the risk of renal stone development.
- Check urine alkalinity; urates crystallize in acid urine; sodium bicarbonate or potassium citrate may be ordered to alkalinize urine.
- Arrange for regular medical follow-up and blood tests during the course of therapy.
- Double-check any analgesics ordered for pain; salicylates should be avoided.

Drug-specific teaching points
- Take the drug with meals or antacids if GI upset occurs.
- Know that the following side effects may occur: headache (monitor lighting, temperature, noise; consult with nurse or physician if this becomes severe); dizziness (change position slowly; avoid driving or operating dangerous machinery until you know the effects of the drug); exacerbation of gouty attack or renal stones (drink plenty of fluids while on this drug—2.5–3 L/d); nausea, vomiting, loss of appetite (taking the drug with meals or antacids may help).
- Report flank pain, dark urine or blood in urine, acute gout attack, unusual fatigue or lethargy, unusual bleeding or bruising.

▢ probucol

(proe' byoo kole)
Lorelco
Pregnancy Category B

Drug classes
Antihyperlipidemic agent

Therapeutic actions
Lowers serum cholesterol with little effect on serum triglycerides; increases the rate of breakdown of LDL; inhibits the early stages of cholesterol synthesis; and slightly inhibits absorption of dietary cholesterol.

Indications
- Reduction of elevated serum cholesterol in patients with primary hypercholesterolemia (elevated LDL) in patients who have not responded to diet, weight reduction, control of diabetes

Contraindications/cautions
- Contraindicated in the presence of allergy to probucol; prolonged Q-T interval on ECG, serious ventricular arrhythmias, unexplained syncope; pregnancy; lactation.
- Use caution in the presence of hypokalemia, hypomagnesemia, severe bradycardia, AV block, recent or acute MI or inflammation.

Dosage
Adult: 500 mg PO bid with morning and evening meals. 500 mg PO qd may be just as effective.
Pediatric: Safety and efficacy not established.

Pharmacokinetics

Route	Onset	Peak	Duration
Oral	Varies	20–40 d	6 mo

Metabolism: Hepatic, $T_{1/2}$: 20 d
Distribution: Crosses placenta; enters breast milk
Excretion: Bile and feces

Adverse effects
- CNS: *Headache, dizziness,* paresthesias, peripheral neuritis, conjunctivitis, blurred vision, tearing
- GI: *Diarrhea, flatulence, abdominal pain, nausea, vomiting,* heartburn, indigestion, anorexia

Adverse effects in *Italics* are most common; those in **Bold** are life-threatening.

- **CV:** *Prolongation of the Q-T interval on the ECG*
- **Hematologic:** Eosinophilia, lower Hct, lower hemoglobin levels, thrombocytopenia
- **GU:** Impotence, nocturia
- **Dermatologic:** Rash, pruritus
- **Idiosyncratic responses:** Dizziness, palpitations, syncope, nausea, vomiting, chest pain

Clinically important drug-drug interactions

- Risk of pronounced lowering of HDL levels with little change in total cholesterol or LDL if given concurrently with clofibrate

■ Nursing Considerations

Assessment

- *History:* Allergy to probucol, prolonged Q-T interval on ECG, serious ventricular arrhythmias, unexplained syncope, hypokalemia, hypomagnesemia, severe bradycardia, AV block, recent or acute MI or inflammation, pregnancy, lactation
- *Physical:* Skin—lesions, color, temperature; orientation, affect, reflexes; P, auscultation, baseline ECG, peripheral perfusion; bowel sounds, normal output; lipid studies, CBC, clotting profile

Implementation

- Arrange for screening of lipids before beginning therapy.
- Determine that patient has tried dietary therapy, weight loss, exercise, and so forth before beginning drug therapy.
- Arrange to continue treatment of underlying contributory conditions such as hypothyroidism and diabetes mellitus.
- Administer drug with meals.
- Arrange for regular follow-up during long-term therapy.

Drug-specific teaching points

- Take drug with meals in the morning and evening.
- Know that the following side effects may occur: diarrhea (this may resolve, or other measures may need to be taken to alleviate this problem); nausea, heartburn, loss of appetite (small, frequent meals may help); dizziness, drowsiness, vertigo, fainting (avoid driving and operating dangerous machinery until you know how this drug affects you); headache, muscle and joint aches and pains (these may lessen over time; if they become bothersome, consult with your nurse or physician).
- Arrange to have regular follow-up visits to your doctor for blood tests to evaluate drug effectiveness.
- Report severe diarrhea, severe abdominal pain, persistent nausea, vomiting, palpitations, chest pain.

☐ procainamide HCl

(proe kane a' mide)

Procan SR, Pronestyl, Pronestyl SR

Pregnancy Category C

Drug classes
Antiarrhythmic

Therapeutic actions
Type 1A antiarrhythmic: decreases rate of diastolic depolarization (decreases automaticity) in ventricles, decreases the rate of rise and height of the action potential, increases fibrillation threshold.

Indications
- Treatment of documented ventricular arrhythmias that are judged to be life-threatening

Contraindications/cautions
- Contraindicated in the presence of allergy to procaine, procainamide, or similar drugs; tartrazine sensitivity (tablets marketed as *Pronestyl* contain tartrazine); second- or third-degree heart block (unless electrical pacemaker operative); SLE; torsade de pointes; pregnancy; lactation.
- Use caution in the presence of myasthenia gravis, hepatic or renal disease.

Dosage
Adult
- *Oral:* 50 mg/kg per day PO in divided doses q3h. Maintenance dose of 50

mg/kg per day (sustained release) in divided doses q6h, starting 2–3 h after last dose of standard oral preparation.

To Provide 50 mg/k/day

Body Weight	Standard Preparation	Sustained-Release Preparation
<55 kg	250 mg q3h	500 mg q6h
55–90 kg	375 mg q3h	750 mg q6h
>90 kg	500 mg q3h	1,000 mg q6h

- ***IM administration:*** 0.5–1.0 g q4–8h until oral procainamide can be started.
- ***Direct IV injection:*** Dilute in 5% Dextrose Injection. Give 100 mg q5min at a rate not to exceed 25–50 mg/min (maximum dose 1 g).
- ***IV infusion:*** 500–600 mg over 25–30 min, then 2–6 mg/min. Monitor very closely.

Pediatric
- ***Oral:*** 15–50 mg/kg per day divided every 3–6 h; maximum, 4 g/d.
- ***IM:*** 20–30 mg/kg per day divided every 4–6 h; maximum 4 g/d.
- ***IV:*** Loading dose, 3–6 mg/kg per dose over 5 min; maintenance, 20–80 mg/kg per minute per continuous infusion; maximum, 100 mg/dose or 2 g/d.

Pharmacokinetics

Route	Onset	Peak	Duration
Oral	30 min	60–90 min	3–4 h
IV	Immediate	20–60 min	3–4 h
IM	10–30 min	15–60 min	3–4 h

Metabolism: Hepatic, $T_{1/2}$: 2.5–4.7 h
Distribution: Crosses placenta; enters breast milk
Excretion: Urine

IV facts
Preparation: Dilute the 100 or 500 mg/ml dose in 5% Dextrose in Water.
Infusion: Slowly inject directly into vein or into tubing of actively running IV; maintenance doses should be given by continual IV infusion using a pump to maintain rate.

Adverse effects
- **CNS:** Mental depression, giddiness, convulsions, confusion, psychosis
- **GI:** *Anorexia, nausea,* vomiting, bitter taste, diarrhea
- **CV:** *Hypotension*, cardiac conduction disturbances
- **Hematologic:** Granulocytopenia
- **Dermatologic:** *Rash*, pruritus, urticaria
- **Other:** Lupus syndrome, fever, chills

Clinically important drug-drug interactions
- Increased procainamide levels if given with cimetidine, trimethoprim, amiodarone

■ Nursing Considerations

Assessment
- *History:* Allergy to procaine, procainamide, or similar drugs; tartrazine sensitivity; second- or third-degree heart block (unless electrical pacemaker operative); myasthenia gravis; hepatic or renal disease; SLE; torsade de pointes; pregnancy; lactation
- *Physical:* Body weight, skin—color, lesions; bilateral grip strength; P, BP, auscultation, ECG, edema; bowel sounds, liver evaluation; urinalysis, renal and liver function tests, complete blood count

Implementation
- Monitor patient response carefully, especially when beginning therapy.
- Arrange for reduced dosage in patients under 120 lb.
- Arrange for reduced dosage in patients with hepatic or renal failure.
- Be alert to the fact that dosage adjustment may be necessary when procainamide is given with other antiarrhythmics, antihypertensives, cimetidine, or alcohol.
- Check to see that patients with supraventricular tachyarrhythmias have been digitalized before giving procainamide.
- Take care to differentiate the sustained-release (SR) form from the regular preparation.
- Monitor cardiac rhythm and BP frequently if IV route is used.

Adverse effects in *Italics* are most common; those in **Bold** are life-threatening.

- Arrange for periodic ECG monitoring and determination of ANA titers when on long-term therapy.
- Arrange for frequent monitoring of blood counts during therapy.
- Give dosages at evenly spaced intervals, around the clock; determine a schedule that will minimize sleep interruption.
- Evaluate for safe and effective serum drug levels: 4–8 µg/ml.

Drug-specific teaching points

- Take this drug at evenly spaced intervals, around the clock. Do not double up doses; do not skip doses; take exactly as prescribed. You may need an alarm clock to wake you up to take the drug. The best schedule for you will be determined to decrease sleep interruption as much as possible. *Do not* chew the sustained-release tablets.
- Be aware that you will require frequent monitoring of cardiac rhythm.
- Know that the following side effects may occur: nausea, loss of appetite, vomiting (small, frequent meals may help); small wax cores may be passed in the stool (this is from the sustained-release tablet; do not be concerned); rash (careful skin care is important).
- Do not stop taking this drug for any reason without checking with your health care provider.
- Return for regular follow-up visits to check your heart rhythm and blood counts.
- Report joint pain, stiffness; sore mouth, throat, gums; fever, chills; cold or flulike syndromes; extensive rash, sensitivity to the sun.

⃞ procarbazine hydrochloride

*(proe **kar**' ba zeen)*

MIH, N-methylhydrazine

Matulane, Natulan (CAN)

Pregnancy Category D

Drug classes
Antineoplastic agent

Therapeutic actions
Cytotoxic: inhibits DNA, RNA, and protein synthesis, causing cell death, but the exact mechanism of action is not fully understood.

Indications
- In combination with other antineoplastics for treatment of stage III and IV Hodgkin's disease (part of the MOPP—nitrogen mustard, vincristine, procarbazine, prednisone—therapy)

Contraindications/cautions
- Contraindicated in the presence of allergy to procarbazine, irradiation, other chemotherapy, leukopenia, thrombocytopenia, anemia, inadequate bone marrow reserve (by bone marrow aspiration), pregnancy (teratogenic); lactation.
- Use caution in the presence of impaired hepatic or renal function.

Dosage
Adult: Base dosage on actual body weight: use estimated dry weight if patient is obese or if fluid gain is marked. 2–4 mg/kg per day PO for the first wk in single or divided doses. Maintain at 4–6 mg/kg per day PO until maximum response is obtained or WBC falls below 4,000/mm^3 or platelets fall below 100,000/mm^3. If hematologic toxicity occurs, discontinue drug until satisfactory recovery is made, then resume treatment at 1–2 mg/kg per day. When maximum response is obtained, maintain dose at 1–2 mg/kg per day.
Pediatric: Dosage regimen not established. As a general guide, give 50 mg/d PO for the first week; maintain daily dose at 100 mg/m^2 until hematologic toxicity occurs (see above). Discontinue drug, and when possible resume treatment with 50 mg/d.

Pharmacokinetics

Route	Onset	Peak
Oral	Rapid	30–90 min

Metabolism: Hepatic, $T_{1/2}$: 10–60 min

Distribution: Crosses placenta; enters breast milk
Excretion: Urine

Adverse effects
- **CNS:** Paresthesias, neuropathies, headache, *dizziness*, depression, apprehension, nervousness, insomnia, nightmares, hallucinations, falling, weakness, fatigue, lethargy, *drowsiness, unsteadiness*, ataxia, foot drop, decreased reflexes, tremors, coma, confusion, convulsions
- **GI:** Stomatitis, anorexia, *nausea, vomiting*, diarrhea, constipation, dry mouth, dysphagia
- **Hematologic:** **Bone marrow depression**, bleeding tendencies
- **GU:** Hematuria, urinary frequency, nocturia
- **Dermatologic:** Dermatitis, pruritus, herpes, hyperpigmentation, flushing, alopecia
- **Other:** Fever, chills, malaise, myalgia, arthralgia, pain, sweating, edema, cough, pneumonitis symptoms, cancer

Clinically important drug-drug interactions
- Disulfiram-like reaction if taken with alcohol • Decreased serum levels and therapeutic actions of digoxin if taken concurrently

■ Nursing Considerations

Assessment
- *History:* Allergy to procarbazine, irradiation, chemotherapy, leukopenia, thrombocytopenia, anemia, inadequate bone marrow reserve, impaired hepatic or renal function, pregnancy, lactation
- *Physical:* Weight; temperature; skin—color, lesions; hair; reflexes, orientation, affect, gait; mucous membranes, abdominal exam; CBC, renal and liver function tests, urinalysis

Implementation
- Arrange for laboratory tests (hemoglobin, Hct, WBC, differential, reticulocytes, platelets) before beginning therapy and every 3–4 d during therapy.
- Arrange for baseline and weekly repeat of urinalysis, transaminase, alkaline phosphatase, BUN.
- Discontinue drug therapy, and consult with physician if any of the following occur: CNS signs or symptoms, leukopenia (WBC < 4,000/mm^3), platelets < 100,000/mm^3, stomatitis, hypersensitivity reaction, bleeding tendencies, diarrhea.

Drug-specific teaching points
- Prepare a calendar noting return for specific treatment days, diagnostic tests, and additional courses of drug therapy.
- Know that the following side effects may occur: loss of appetite, nausea, vomiting, mouth sores (frequent mouth care, small frequent meals may help; try to maintain good nutrition if at all possible; an antiemetic also may be ordered); constipation or diarrhea (a bowel program may be established to help out with this problem); disorientation, dizziness, headache (take special precautions to avoid injury if these occur); rash, loss of hair (these are effects of the drug; they should pass when the drug is discontinued; you may wish to arrange for a wig or other suitable head covering before hair loss occurs; it is important to keep head covered in extremes of temperature).
- Arrange to have regular blood tests to monitor the drug's effects.
- Avoid alcoholic beverages or products containing alcohol while you are on this drug; severe reactions can occur.
- Avoid foods high in tyramine (a list will be provided by the dietician) while you are on this drug; severe reactions can occur.
- Use contraceptive methods while on this drug (both men and women); serious fetal harm can occur.
- Report fever, chills, sore throat, unusual bleeding or bruising, vomiting of blood, black or tarry stools, cough, shortness of breath, thick bronchial secretions, pregnancy.

Adverse effects in *Italics* are most common; those in **Bold** are life-threatening.

▢ prochlorperazine

(proe klor per' a zeen)

Rectal suppositories:
Compazine

prochlorperazine edisylate

Oral syrup, injection:
Compazine

prochlorperazine maleate

Oral tablets and sustained-release capsules: Compazine, PMS-Prochlorperazine (CAN), Stemetil (CAN)

Pregnancy Category C

Drug classes
Phenothiazine (piperazine)
Dopaminergic blocking drug
Antipsychotic drug
Antiemetic drug
Antianxiety drug

Therapeutic actions
Mechanism of action not fully understood: antipsychotic drugs block postsynaptic dopamine receptors in the brain, but this may not be necessary and sufficient for antipsychotic activity; depresses the reticular activating system, including the parts of the brain involved with wakefulness and emesis; anticholinergic, antihistaminic (H_1), and alpha-adrenergic blocking activity also may contribute to some of its therapeutic (and adverse) actions.

Indications
- Management of manifestations of psychotic disorders
- Control of severe nausea and vomiting
- Short-term treatment of nonpsychotic anxiety (not drug of choice)

Contraindications/cautions
- Contraindicated in the presence of coma or severe CNS depression, bone marrow depression, blood dyscrasia, circulatory collapse, subcortical brain damage, Parkinson's disease, liver damage, cerebral arteriosclerosis, coronary disease, severe hypotension or hypertension.
- Use caution in the presence of respiratory disorders, glaucoma, prostatic hypertrophy, epilepsy, breast cancer (elevations in prolactin may stimulate a prolactin-dependent tumor), thyrotoxicosis, peptic ulcer, decreased renal function, myelography within previous 24 h or scheduled within 48 h, exposure to heat or phosphorous insecticides, pregnancy, lactation, children younger 12 y, especially those with chickenpox, CNS infections (children are especially susceptible to dystonias that may confound the diagnosis of Reye's syndrome).

Dosage
Adult
- ***Psychiatry:*** Initially, 5–10 mg PO tid or qid. Gradually increase dosage every 2–3 d as necessary up to 50–75 mg/d for mild or moderate disturbances, 100–150 mg/d for more severe disturbances. For immediate control of severely disturbed adults, 10–20 mg IM repeated q2–4h (every hour for resistant cases); switch to oral therapy as soon as possible.
- ***Antiemetic:*** *Control of severe nausea and vomiting:* 5–10 mg PO tid–qid; 15 mg (sustained-release) on arising; 10 mg (sustained-release) q12h; 25 mg rectally bid; or 5–10 mg IM initially, repeated q3–4h up to 40 mg/d.
- ***Surgery, to control nausea, vomiting:*** 5–10 mg IM 1–2 h before anesthesia or during and after surgery (may repeat once in 30 min); 5–10 mg IV 15 min before anesthesia or during and after surgery (may repeat once); or as IV infusion, 20 mg/L of isotonic solution added to infusion 15–30 min before anesthesia.

Pediatric: Generally not recommended for children under 20 lb (9.1 kg) or younger than 2 y; do not use in pediatric surgery.
- ***Children 2–12 y:*** 2.5 mg PO or rectally bid–tid. Do not give more than 10 mg on first day. Increase dosage according to patient response; total daily dose usually does not exceed 20 mg (2–5 y) or 25 mg (6–12 y).
- ***Children younger than 12 y:*** 0.13 mg/kg by deep IM injection. Switch to

prochlorperazine ■ 933

oral dosage as soon possible (usually after one dose).
- **Antiemetic: Control of severe nausea/vomiting in children over 20 lb or older than 2 y**: *Oral or rectal administration*: *9.1–13.2 kg:* 2.5 mg qd–bid, not to exceed 7.5 mg/d. *13.6–17.7 kg:* 2.5 mg bid–tid, not to exceed 10 mg/d. *18.2–38.6 kg:* 2.5 mg tid or 5 mg bid, not to exceed 15 mg/d.
— *IM:* 0.132 mg/kg (usually only one dose).

Pharmacokinetics

Route	Onset	Duration
Oral	30–40 min	3–4 h (10–12 SR)
PR	60–90 min	3–4 h
IM	10–20 min	3–4 h
IV	Immediate	3–4 h

Metabolism: Hepatic, T$_{1/2}$: unknown
Distribution: Crosses placenta; enters breast milk
Excretion: Urine

IV facts
Preparation: Dilute 20 mg in not less than 1 L of isotonic solution.
Infusion: Inject 5–10 mg directly IV 15–30 min before induction (may be repeated once), or infuse dilute solution 15–30 min before induction; do not exceed 5 mg/ml per minute.

Adverse effects
Antipsychotic Drugs
- CNS: *Drowsiness*, insomnia, vertigo, headache, weakness, tremor, ataxia, slurring, cerebral edema, seizures, exacerbation of psychotic symptoms, extrapyramidal syndromes—*pseudoparkinsonism*; *dystonias; akathisia*, tardive dyskinesias, potentially irreversible; **neuroleptic malignant syndrome**
- CV: Hypotension, orthostatic hypotension, hypertension, tachycardia, bradycardia, cardiac arrest, CHF, cardiomegaly, **refractory arrhythmias** (some fatal), pulmonary edema
- Respiratory: Bronchospasm, laryngospasm, dyspnea; suppression of cough reflex and potential for aspiration
- Hematologic: Eosinophilia, leukopenia, leukocytosis, anemia; aplastic anemia; hemolytic anemia; thrombocytopenic or nonthrombocytopenic purpura; pancytopenia
- Hypersensitivity: Jaundice, urticaria, angioneurotic edema, laryngeal edema, photosensitivity, eczema, asthma, anaphylactoid reactions, exfoliative dermatitis
- EENT: Glaucoma, *photophobia, blurred vision*, miosis, mydriasis, deposits in the cornea and lens (opacities), pigmentary retinopathy
- Endocrine: Lactation, breast engorgement in females, galactorrhea; SIADH; amenorrhea, menstrual irregularities; gynecomastia in males; changes in libido; hyperglycemia or hypoglycemia; glycosuria; hyponatremia; pituitary tumor with hyperprolactinemia; inhibition of ovulation, infertility, pseudopregnancy; reduced urinary levels of gonadotropins, estrogens, progestins
- Autonomic: Dry mouth, salivation, nasal congestion, nausea, vomiting, anorexia, fever, pallor, flushed facies, sweating, constipation, paralytic ileus, urinary retention, incontinence, polyuria, enuresis, priapism, ejaculation inhibition, male impotence
- Other: *Urine discolored pink to red-brown*

Clinically important drug-drug interactions
- Additive CNS depression with alcohol
- Additive anticholinergic effects and possibly decreased antipsychotic efficacy with anticholinergic drugs • Increased likelihood of seizures with metrizamide • Increased chance of severe neuromuscular excitation and hypotension if given to patients receiving barbiturate anesthetics (methohexital, thiamylal, phenobarbital, thiopental)
- Decreased antihypertensive effect of guanethidine when taken concurrently

Adverse effects in *Italics* are most common; those in **Bold** are life-threatening.

Drug-lab test interferences
- False-positive pregnancy tests (less likely if serum test is used) • Increase in protein-bound iodine, not attributable to an increase in thyroxine

■ Nursing Considerations
Assessment
- *History:* Coma or severe CNS depression; bone marrow depression; circulatory collapse; subcortical brain damage; Parkinson's disease; liver damage; cerebral arteriosclerosis; coronary disease; severe hypotension or hypertension; respiratory disorders; glaucoma, prostatic hypertrophy; epilepsy; breast cancer; thyrotoxicosis; peptic ulcer, decreased renal function; myelography within previous 24 h or scheduled within 48 h; exposure to heat or phosphorous insecticides; pregnancy; lactation; children younger than 12 y
- *Physical:* Body weight, temperature; reflexes, orientation, intraocular pressure; P, BP, orthostatic BP; R, adventitious sounds; bowel sounds and normal output; liver evaluation; urinary output, prostate size; CBC; urinalysis; thyroid, liver, and kidney function tests

Implementation
- Do not change brand names of oral preparations; bioavailability differences have been documented for different brands.
- Do not allow patient to crush or chew sustained-release capsules.
- Do not administer SC because of local irritation.
- Give IM injections deeply into the upper outer quadrant of the buttock.
- Avoid skin contact with oral solution; contact dermatitis has occurred.
- Arrange for discontinuation of drug if serum creatinine, BUN become abnormal or if WBC count is depressed.
- Monitor elderly patients for dehydration, and institute remedial measures promptly; sedation and decreased sensation of thirst related to CNS effects of drug can lead to severe dehydration.
- Consult physician regarding appropriate warning of patient or patient's guardian about tardive dyskinesias.
- Consult physician about dosage reduction, use of anticholinergic antiparkinsonian drugs (controversial) if extrapyramidal effects occur.

Drug-specific teaching points
- Take drug exactly as prescribed.
- Do not crush or chew sustained-release capsules.
- Avoid skin contact with drug solutions.
- Avoid driving a car or engaging in other dangerous activities if CNS, vision changes occur.
- Avoid prolonged exposure to sun, or use a sunscreen or covering garments if exposure is unavoidable.
- Maintain fluid intake, and use precautions against heatstroke in hot weather.
- Report sore throat, fever, unusual bleeding or bruising, rash, weakness, tremors, impaired vision, dark urine (pink or reddish brown urine is to be expected), pale stools, yellowing of the skin or eyes.

☐ procyclidine

(proe sye' kli deen)
Kemadrin, PMS Procyclidine (CAN), Procyclid (CAN)

Pregnancy Category C

Drug classes
Antiparkinsonism drug (anticholinergic type)

Therapeutic actions
Has anticholinergic activity in the CNS that is believed to help normalize the hypothesized imbalance of cholinergic/dopaminergic neurotransmission created by the loss of dopaminergic neurons in the basal ganglia of the brain of parkinsonism patients; reduces severity of rigidity and reduces the akinesia and tremor that characterize parkinsonism; less effective overall than levodopa; peripheral anticholinergic effects suppress secondary symptoms of parkinsonism, such as drooling.

Indications
- Treatment of parkinsonism (postencephalitic, arteriosclerotic, and idiopathic

types), alone or with other drugs in more severe cases
- Relief of symptoms of extrapyramidal dysfunction that accompany phenothiazine and reserpine therapy
- Control of sialorrhea resulting from neuroleptic medication

Contraindications/cautions
- Contraindicated in the presence of hypersensitivity to procyclidine; glaucoma, especially angle-closure glaucoma; pyloric or duodenal obstruction; stenosing peptic ulcers; achalasia (megaesophagus); prostatic hypertrophy or bladder neck obstructions; myasthenia gravis; lactation.
- Use caution in the presence of tachycardia, cardiac arrhythmias, hypertension, hypotension, hepatic or renal dysfunction, alcoholism, chronic illness, people who work in hot environments, pregnancy.

Dosage
Adult
- **Parkinsonism not previously treated:** Initially 2.5 mg PO tid after meals. If well tolerated, gradually increase dose to 5 mg tid and occasionally before retiring if necessary.
- **Transferring from other therapy:** Substitute 2.5 mg PO tid for all or part of the original drug, then increase procyclidine as required, while withdrawing other drug.
- **Drug-induced extrapyramidal symptoms:** Initially 2.5 mg PO tid. Increase by 2.5-mg increments until patient obtains relief of symptoms. In most cases, results will be obtained with 10–20 mg/d.

Pediatric: Safety and efficacy not established.

Geriatric patients: Strict dosage regulation may be necessary. Patients older than 60 y often develop increased sensitivity to the CNS effects of anticholinergic drugs.

Pharmacokinetics

Route	Onset	Peak
Oral	Varies	1.1–2 h

Metabolism: Hepatic, $T_{1/2}$: 11.5–12.6 h
Distribution: Crosses placenta; enters breast milk
Excretion: Urine

Adverse effects
Peripheral Anticholinergic Effects
- CNS: *Blurred vision, mydriasis*, diplopia, increased intraocular tension, angle-closure glaucoma
- GI: *Dry mouth, constipation*, dilation of the colon, paralytic ileus
- CV: Tachycardia, palpitations
- GU: *Urinary retention*, urinary hesitancy, dysuria, difficulty achieving or maintaining an erection
- General: *Flushing, decreased sweating,* elevated temperature

Effects of Centrally Acting Anticholinergic Drugs
- CNS: *Disorientation, confusion*, memory loss, hallucinations, psychoses, agitation, nervousness, delusions, delirium, paranoia, euphoria, excitement, *lightheadedness, dizziness,* depression, drowsiness, weakness, giddiness, paresthesia, heaviness of the limbs, numbness of fingers
- GI: Acute suppurative parotitis, nausea, vomting, epigastric distress
- CV: Hypotension, orthostatic hypotension
- Dermatologic: Skin rash, urticaria, other dermatoses
- Other: Muscular weakness, muscular cramping

Clinically important drug-drug interactions
- Paralytic ileus, sometimes fatal, when given with phenothiazines • Additive adverse CNS effects, toxic psychosis, with other drugs that have central (CNS) anticholinergic properties, phenothiazines • Possible masking of the development of persistent extrapyramidal symptoms, tardive dyskinesia, in patients on long-term therapy with phenothiazines, haloperidol • Decreased therapeutic efficacy of phenothiazines, haloperidol possibly due to central antagonism

Adverse effects in *Italics* are most common; those in **Bold** are life-threatening.

Nursing Considerations

Assessment
- *History:* Hypersensitivity to procyclidine; glaucoma; pyloric or duodenal obstruction; stenosing peptic ulcers; achalasia; prostatic hypertrophy or bladder neck obstructions; myasthenia gravis; cardiac arrhythmias; hypertension, hypotension; hepatic or renal dysfunction; alcoholism; chronic illness; people who work in hot environment; pregnancy; lactation
- *Physical:* Body weight; body temperature; skin—color, lesions; orientation, affect, reflexes, bilateral grip strength; visual exam including tonometry; P, BP, orthostatic BP, auscultation; bowel sounds, normal output, liver evaluation; urinary output, voiding pattern, prostate palpation; liver and kidney function tests

Implementation
- Arrange to decrease dosage or discontinue drug temporarily if dry mouth is so severe that swallowing or speaking becomes difficult.
- Give with caution, and arrange dosage reduction in hot weather, as appropriate to patient's lifestyle; drug interferes with sweating and ability of body to maintain body heat equilibrium; anhidrosis and fatal hyperthermia have occurred.
- Give with meals if GI upset occurs; give before meals to patients bothered by dry mouth; give after meals if drooling is a problem or if drug causes nausea.
- Ensure that patient voids just before receiving each dose of drug if urinary retention is a problem.

Drug-specific teaching points
- Take this drug exactly as prescribed.
- Know that the following side effects may occur: drowsiness, dizziness, confusion, blurred vision (avoid driving a car or engaging in activities that require alertness and visual acuity if these occur); nausea (frequent, small meals may help); dry mouth (sucking sugarless lozenges or ice chips may help); painful or difficult urination (emptying the bladder immediately before each dose may help); constipation (if maintaining adequate fluid intake, exercising regularly do not help, consult your nurse or physician); use caution in hot weather (this drug makes you more susceptible to heat prostration).
- Report difficult or painful urination, constipation, rapid or pounding heartbeat, confusion, eye pain or rash.

☐ progesterone

*(proe **jess'** ter one)*

progesterone in oil

Parenteral: Gesterol 50, Progestilin (CAN)

Intrauterine system: Progestasert

progesterone aqueous, progesterone powder

Pregnancy Category X

Drug classes
Hormone
Progestin

Therapeutic actions
Endogenous female progestational substance; transforms proliferative endometrium into secretory endometrium; inhibits the secretion of pituitary gonadotropins, which prevents follicular maturation and ovulation; inhibits spontaneous uterine contractions; may have some estrogenic, anabolic, or androgenic activity.

Indications
- Treatment of primary and secondary amenorrhea
- Treatment of functional uterine bleeding
- Contraception in parous and nulliparous women (intrauterine system)
- Unlabeled uses: treatment of premenstrual syndrome, prevention of premature labor and habitual abortion in the first trimester, treatment of menorrhagia (intrauterine system)

Contraindications/cautions
- Contraindicated in the presence of allergy to progestins, thrombophlebitis, thromboembolic disorders, cerebral hemor-

progesterone

rhage or history of these conditions, hepatic disease, carcinoma of the breast or genital organs, undiagnosed vaginal bleeding, missed abortion, diagnostic test for pregnancy, pregnancy (fetal abnormalities, including masculinization of the female fetus have occurred), lactation; pelvic inflammatory disease, venereal disease, postpartum endometritis, pelvic surgery, uterine or cervical carcinoma (intrauterine system).
- Use caution in the presence of epilepsy, migraine, asthma, cardiac or renal dysfunction.

Dosage
Administer parenteral preparation by IM route only.
Adult
- ***Amenorrhea:*** 5–10 mg/d IM for 6–8 consecutive d. Expect withdrawal bleeding 48–72 h after the last injection. Spontaneous normal cycles may follow.
- ***Functional uterine bleeding:*** 5–10 mg/d IM for six doses. Bleeding should cease within 6 d. If estrogen is being given, begin progesterone after 2 wk of estrogen therapy. Discontinue injections when menstrual flow begins.
- ***Contraception:*** Insert a single intrauterine system into the uterine cavity. Contraceptive effectiveness is retained for 1 y. The system must be replaced 1 y after insertion.

Pharmacokinetics

Route	Onset	Peak
IM	Varies	Unknown

Metabolism: Hepatic, $T_{1/2}$: 5 min
Distribution: Crosses placenta; enters breast milk
Excretion: Urine

Adverse effects
Parenteral
- CNS: Sudden, partial or complete loss of vision, proptosis, diplopia, migraine, precipitation of acute intermittent porphyria, mental depression, pyrexia, insomnia, somnolence, *dizziness*
- GI: Cholestatic jaundice, nausea
- CV: Thrombophlebitis, cerebrovascular disorders, retinal thrombosis, pulmonary embolism
- GU: *Breakthrough bleeding, spotting, change in menstrual flow, amenorrhea, changes in cervical erosion and cervical secretions, breast tenderness* and secretion, transient increase in sodium and chloride excretion
- Dermatologic: Rash with or without pruritus, acne, melasma or chloasma, alopecia, hirsutism, *photosensitivity*
- General: Fluid retention, edema, *increase or decrease in weight*, effects similar to those seen with oral contraceptives

Effects of Oral Contraceptives
- GI: Hepatic adenoma
- CV: Increased blood pressure, **thromboembolic and thrombotic disease**
- Endocrine: Decreased glucose tolerance

Intrauterine System
- CV: Bradycardia and syncope related to insertional pain
- GU: Endometritis, spontaneous abortion, septic abortion, septicemia, perforation of the uterus and cervix, pelvic infection, cervical erosion, vaginitis, leukorrhea, amenorrhea, uterine embedment, *complete or partial expulsion of the device*

Drug-lab test interferences
- Inaccurate tests of hepatic and endocrine function

■ Nursing Considerations

Assessment
- *History:* Allergy to progestins, thrombophlebitis, thromboembolic disorders, cerebral hemorrhage, hepatic disease, carcinoma of the breast or genital organs, undiagnosed vaginal bleeding, missed abortion, epilepsy, migraine, asthma, cardiac or renal dysfunction, PID, venereal disease, postpartum endometritis, pelvic surgery, uterine or cervical carcinoma, pregnancy, lactation
- *Physical:* Skin—color, lesions, turgor; hair; breasts; pelvic exam; orientation, affect; ophthalmologic exam; P, auscultation, peripheral perfusion, edema; R,

Adverse effects in *Italics* are most common; those in **Bold** are life-threatening.

adventitious sounds; liver evaluation; liver and renal function tests, glucose tolerance; Pap smear

Implementation
- Arrange for pretreatment and periodic (at least annual) history and physical, which should include BP, breasts, abdomen, pelvic organs, and a Pap smear.
- Arrange for insertion of intrauterine system during or immediately after menstrual period to ensure that the patient is not pregnant; arrange to have patient reexamined after first month menses to ensure that system has not been expelled.
- Caution patient before beginning therapy of the need to prevent pregnancy during treatment, the need for frequent medical follow-up.
- Administer parenteral preparations by IM injection only.
- Arrange to discontinue medication and consult physician if sudden partial or complete loss of vision occur; if papilledema or retinal vascular lesions are present on exam, the drug should be discontinued.
- Arrange to discontinue medication and consult physician at the first sign of thromboembolic disease: leg pain, swelling, peripheral perfusion changes, shortness of breath.

Drug-specific teaching points
- Be aware that this drug can only be given IM; it will be given daily for the specified number of days, or the drug is inserted vaginally and can remain for 1 y (as appropriate).
- Know that the following side effects may occur: sensitivity to light (avoid exposure to the sun; use sunscreen and protective clothing if exposure is necessary); dizziness, sleeplessness, depression (use caution if driving or performing tasks that require alertness if these occur); skin rash, skin color changes, loss of hair; fever; nausea.
- Be aware that this drug should not be taken during pregnancy, serious fetal abnormalities have been reported. If you think that you are pregnant, consult physician immediately.
- Report pain or swelling and warmth in the calves, acute chest pain or shortness of breath, sudden severe headache or vomiting, dizziness or fainting, visual disturbances, numbness or tingling in the arm or leg.

Intrauterine System
- Report excessive bleeding, severe cramping, abnormal vaginal discharge, fever or flulike symptoms.

▢ promazine hydrochloride

(proe' ma zeen)
Prozine-50, Sparine

Pregnancy Category C

Drug classes
Phenothiazine (aliphatic)
Dopaminergic blocking drug
Antipsychotic drug

Therapeutic actions
Mechanism of action not fully understood: antipsychotic drugs block postsynaptic dopamine receptors in the brain, but this may not be necessary and sufficient for antipsychotic activity; depresses the reticular activating system, including the parts of the brain involved with wakefulness and emesis; anticholinergic, antihistaminic (H_1), and alpha-adrenergic blocking activity also may contribute to some of its therapeutic (and adverse) actions.

Indications
- Management of manifestations of psychotic disorders

Contraindications/cautions
- Contraindicated in the presence of coma or severe CNS depression, bone marrow depression, blood dyscrasia, circulatory collapse, subcortical brain damage, Parkinson's disease, liver damage, cerebral arteriosclerosis, coronary disease, severe hypotension or hypertension.
- Use caution in the presence of respiratory disorders, glaucoma, prostatic hy-

pertrophy, epilepsy or history of epilepsy, breast cancer, thyrotoxicosis, allergy to aspirin (the oral 25-mg tablets and the syrup contain tartrazine; many patients with allergy to aspirin also are allergic to tartrazine), peptic ulcer, decreased renal function, myelography within previous 24 h or scheduled within 48 h, exposure to heat or phosphorous insecticides, pregnancy, lactation, children younger than 12 y, especially those with chickenpox, CNS infections (children are especially susceptible to dystonias that may confound the diagnosis of Reye's syndrome).

Dosage

Full clinical effects may require 6 wk–6 mo of therapy.
Adult: Dosage varies with severity of condition.
- ***Severely agitated patients:*** 50–150 mg IM. Repeat if necessary in 30 min (up to 300 mg total dose). *After control is obtained, change to oral (or IM) maintenance dosage:* 10–200 mg PO or IM q4–6h. Do not exceed 1,000 mg/d, because higher doses have not yielded greater results. IV use not recommended; drug is very irritating to vein and tissues.

Pediatric
- ***Children older than 12 y:*** *Acute episodes of psychotic chronic disease:* 10–25 mg PO or IM q4–6h. Generally not recommended for children younger than 12 y.

Geriatric: Use lower doses and increase dosage more gradually than in younger patients.

Pharmacokinetics

Route	Onset	Duration
Oral	30 min	4–6 h
IM	15–30 min	

Metabolism: Hepatic, $T_{1/2}$: unknown
Distribution: Crosses placenta; enters breast milk
Excretion: Urine

Adverse effects
Antipsychotic Drugs
- **CNS:** *Drowsiness*, insomnia, vertigo, headache, weakness, tremor, ataxia, slurring, cerebral edema, seizures, exacerbation of psychotic symptoms, extrapyramidal syndromes—*pseudoparkinsonism; dystonias; akathisia*, tardive dyskinesias, potentially irreversible (no known treatment), **neuroleptic malignant syndrome**
- **CV:** Hypotension, orthostatic hypotension, hypertension, tachycardia, bradycardia, cardiac arrest, CHF, cardiomegaly, **refractory arrhythmias** (some fatal), pulmonary edema
- **Respiratory:** Bronchospasm, laryngospasm, dyspnea; suppression of cough reflex and potential for aspiration
- **Hematologic:** Eosinophilia, leukopenia, leukocytosis, anemia; aplastic anemia; hemolytic anemia; thrombocytopenic or nonthrombocytopenic purpura; pancytopenia
- **EENT:** Glaucoma, *photophobia, blurred vision*, miosis, mydriasis, deposits in the cornea and lens (opacities), pigmentary retinopathy
- **Hypersensitivity:** Jaundice, urticaria, angioneurotic edema, laryngeal edema, photosensitivity, eczema, asthma, anaphylactoid reactions, exfoliative dermatitis
- **Endocrine:** Lactation, breast engorgement in females, galactorrhea; SIADH; amenorrhea, menstrual irregularities; gynecomastia in males; changes in libido; hyperglycemia or hypoglycemia; glycosuria; hyponatremia; pituitary tumor with hyperprolactinemia; inhibition of ovulation, infertility, pseudopregnancy; reduced urinary levels of gonadotropins, estrogens, progestins
- **Autonomic:** Dry mouth, salivation, nasal congestion, nausea, vomiting, anorexia, fever, pallor, flushed facies, sweating, constipation, paralytic ileus, urinary retention, incontinence, polyuria, enuresis, priapism, ejaculation inhibition, male impotence

Adverse effects in *Italics* are most common; those in **Bold** are life-threatening.

promazine hydrochloride

- Other: *Urine discolored pink to red-brown*

Clinically important drug-drug interactions
- Additive CNS depression with alcohol
- Additive anticholinergic effects and possibly decreased antipsychotic efficacy with anticholinergic drugs
- Increased likelihood of seizures with metrizamide
- Increased chance of severe neuromuscular excitation and hypotension if given to patients receiving barbiturate anesthetics (methohexital, thiamylal, phenobarbital, thiopental)
- Decreased antihypertensive effect of guanethidine if taken with antipsychotic drugs

Drug-lab test interferences
- False-positive pregnancy tests
- Increase in protein-bound iodine, not attributable to an increase in thyroxine

■ Nursing Considerations

Assessment
- *History:* Severe CNS depression, blood dyscrasia, circulatory collapse, subcortical brain damage, Parkinson's disease, liver damage, cerebral arteriosclerosis, coronary disease, severe hypotension or hypertension, respiratory disorders, glaucoma, prostatic hypertrophy, epilepsy, breast cancer, thyrotoxicosis, allergy to aspirin or tartrazine, peptic ulcer, decreased renal function, myelography within previous 24 h or scheduled within 48 h, exposure to heat or phosphorous insecticides, pregnancy, lactation, children younger than 12 y
- *Physical:* Body weight, temperature; reflexes, orientation; intraocular pressure; P, BP, orthostatic BP; R, adventitious sounds; bowel sounds and normal output, liver evaluation; urinary output, prostate size; CBC; urinalysis; thyroid, liver, and kidney function tests

Implementation
- Do not change dosage in chronic therapy more often than weekly; drug requires 4–7 d to achieve steady-state plasma levels.
- Reserve parenteral administration for bed ridden patients. If IM injections are given to ambulatory patients, provide proper precautions to prevent orthostatic hypotension.
- Give IM injections deeply into large muscle mass (gluteal region is preferred).
- Reduce initial dose to 50 mg in patients who are acutely inebriated (to avoid additive depressant effects with alcohol).
- Use the syrup for oral administration to patients who refuse the tablets; syrup may be diluted in citrus or chocolate-flavored drinks.
- Avoid skin contact with oral solution; contact dermatitis has occurred.
- Arrange for discontinuation of drug if serum creatinine, BUN become abnormal or if WBC count is depressed.
- Monitor elderly patients for dehydration, and institute remedial measures promptly; sedation and decreased sensation of thirst related to CNS effects of drug can lead to severe dehydration.
- Consult physician regarding appropriate warning of patient or patient's guardian about tardive dyskinesias.
- Consult physician about dosage reduction, use of anticholinergic antiparkinsonian drugs (controversial) if extrapyramidal effects occur.

Drug-specific teaching points
- Take drug exactly as prescribed.
- Avoid skin contact with drug solutions.
- Avoid driving a car or engaging in other dangerous activities if CNS, vision changes occur.
- Avoid prolonged exposure to sun or use a sunscreen or covering garments if this is necessary.
- Maintain fluid intake, and use precautions against heatstroke in hot weather.
- Report sore throat, fever, unusual bleeding or bruising, rash, weakness, tremors, impaired vision, dark urine (pink or reddish brown urine is to be expected), pale stools, yellowing of the skin or eyes.

Adverse effects in *Italics* are most common; those in **Bold** are life-threatening.

promethazine hydrochloride

(proe meth' a zeen)

Anergan, Histanil (CAN), Mallergan, Pentazine, Phenazine, Phencen, Phenergan, Phenoject-50, PMS-Promethazine (CAN), Pro-50, Prometh, Prorex, V-Gan

Pregnancy Category C

Drug classes
Phenothiazine
Dopaminergic blocking drug
Antihistamine
Antiemetic
Antimotion sickness drug
Sedative

Therapeutic actions
Selectively blocks H_1 receptors, diminishing the effects of histamine on cells of the upper respiratory tract and eyes and decreasing the sneezing, mucus production, itching, and tearing that accompany allergic reactions in sensitized people exposed to antigens; blocks cholinergic receptors in the vomiting center that are believed to mediate the nausea and vomiting caused by gastric irritation, by input from the vestibular apparatus (motion sickness, nausea associated with vestibular neuritis), and by input from the chemoreceptor trigger zone (drug- and radiation-induced emesis); depresses the reticular activating system, including the parts of the brain involved with wakefulness.

Indications
- Symptomatic relief of symptoms associated with perennial and seasonal allergic rhinitis, vasomotor rhinitis, allergic conjunctivitis; mild, uncomplicated urticaria and angioedema; amelioration of allergic reactions to blood or plasma; dermatographism, adjunctive therapy (with epinephrine and other measures) in anaphylactic reactions
- Treatment and prevention of motion sickness; prevention and control of nausea and vomiting associated with anesthesia and surgery
- Preoperative, postoperative, or obstetric sedation
- Adjunct to analgesics to control postoperative pain
- Adjunctive IV therapy with reduced amounts of meperidine or other narcotic analgesics in special surgical situations, such as repeated bronchoscopy, ophthalmic surgery, or in poor-risk patients

Contraindications/cautions
- Contraindicated in the presence of hypersensitivity to antihistamines or phenothiazines, coma or severe CNS depression, bone marrow depression, vomiting of unknown cause, concomitant therapy with MAOIs, lactation (lactation may be inhibited).
- Use caution in the presence of lower respiratory tract disorders (drug may cause thickening of secretions and impair expectoration), glaucoma, prostatic hypertrophy, cardiovascular disease or hypertension, breast cancer, thyrotoxicosis, pregnancy (jaundice and extrapyramidal symptoms have been reported in infants whose mothers received phenothiazines during pregnancy; drug may inhibit platelet aggregation in neonate if taken by mother within 2 wk of delivery), children (antihistamine overdosage may cause hallucinations, convulsions, and death), a child with a history of sleep apnea, a family history of sudden infant death syndrome, or Reye's syndrome (drug may mask the symptoms of Reye's syndrome and contribute to its development), the elderly (more likely to cause dizziness, sedation, syncope, toxic confusional states, hypotension, and extrapyramidal effects in the elderly).

Dosage
Adult
- ***Allergy:*** Average dose is 25 mg PO or by rectal suppository, preferably at bedtime. If necessary, 12.5 mg PO before meals and at bedtime; 25 mg IM or IV

for serious reactions. May repeat within 2 h if necessary.
- **Motion sickness:** 25 mg PO bid. Initial dose should be scheduled ½–1 h before travel; repeat in 8–12 h if necessary. Thereafter, give 25 mg on arising and before evening meal.
- **Nausea and vomiting:** 25 mg PO; repeat doses of 12.5–25.0 mg as needed, q4–6h. Give rectally or parenterally if oral dosage is not tolerated. 12.5–25.0 mg IM or IV, not to be repeated more frequently than q4–6h.
- **Sedation:** 25–50 mg PO, IM, or IV.
- **Preoperative use:** 50 mg PO the night before, or 50 mg with an equal dose of meperidine and the required amount of belladonna alkaloid.
- **Postoperative sedation and adjunctive use with analgesics:** 25–50 mg PO, IM, or IV.
- **Labor:** 50 mg IM or IV in early stages. When labor is established, 25–75 mg with a reduced dose of narcotic. May repeat once or twice at 4-h intervals. Maximum dose within 24 h is 100 mg.

Pediatric
- **Allergy:** 25 mg PO at bedtime or 6.25–12.5 mg tid.
- **Motion sickness:** 12.5–25.0 mg PO or rectally bid.
- **Nausea and vomiting:** 1 mg/kg PO q4–6h as needed.
- **Sedation:** 12.5–50.0 mg PO or rectally.
- **Preoperative use:** 1 mg/kg PO in combination with an equal dose of meperidine and the required amount of an atropine-like drug.
- **Postoperative sedation and adjunctive use with analgesics:** 12.5–50.0 mg PO.

Pharmacokinetics

Route	Onset	Duration
Oral	20 min	12 h
IM	20 min	12 h
IV	3–5 min	12 h

Metabolism: Hepatic, $T_{1/2}$: unknown

Distribution: Crosses placenta; enters breast milk
Excretion: Urine

IV facts
Preparation: Dilute to a concentration no greater than 25 mg/ml.
Infusion: Infuse no faster than 25 mg/min.

Adverse effects
- CNS: *Dizziness, drowsiness, poor coordination, confusion, restlessness, excitation,* convulsions, tremors, headache, blurred vision, diplopia, vertigo, tinnitus
- GI: *Epigastric distress*, nausea, vomiting, diarrhea, constipation
- CV: Hypotension, palpitations, bradycardia, tachycardia, extrasystoles
- Respiratory: *Thickening of bronchial secretions*; chest tightness; dry mouth, nose, and throat; respiratory depression; suppression of cough reflex, potential for aspiration
- Hematologic: Hemolytic anemia, hypoplastic anemia, thrombocytopenia, leukopenia, agranulocytosis, pancytopenia
- GU: *Urinary frequency, dysuria*, urinary retention, decreased libido, impotence
- Dermatologic: Urticaria, rash, photosensitivity, chills
- Other: Tingling, heaviness and wetness of the hands

Clinically important drug-drug interactions
• Additive anticholinergic effects when taken concurrently with anticholinergic drugs • Increased likelihood of seizures with metrizamide • Increased frequency and severity of neuromuscular excitation and hypotension in patients receiving methohexital, thiamylal, phenobarbital anesthetic, thiopental • Enhanced CNS depression if taken concurrently with alcohol

■ Nursing Considerations
Assessment
- *History:* Hypersensitivity to antihistamines or phenothiazines, severe CNS de-

pression, bone marrow depression, vomiting of unknown cause, concomitant therapy with MAO inhibitors, lactation, lower respiratory tract disorders, glaucoma, prostatic hypertrophy, cardiovascular disease or hypertension, breast cancer, thyrotoxicosis, pregnancy, history of sleep apnea or a family history of SIDS, child with Reye's syndrome
- *Physical:* Body weight, temperature; reflexes, orientation, intraocular pressure; P, BP, orthostatic BP; R, adventitious sounds; bowel sounds and normal output, liver evaluation; urinary output, prostate size; CBC; urinalysis; thyroid, liver, and kidney function tests

Implementation
- Do not give tablets, rectal suppositories to children younger than 2 y.
- Give IM injections deep into muscle.
- Do not administer SC; tissue necrosis may occur.
- Do not administer intra-arterially; arteriospasm and gangrene of the limb may result.
- Arrange for dosage reduction of barbiturates given concurrently with promethazine by at least half; arrange for dosage reduction of narcotic analgesics given concomitantly by one-fourth to one-half.

Drug-specific teaching points
- Take drug exactly as prescribed
- Avoid using alcohol.
- Avoid driving a car or engaging in other dangerous activities if CNS, vision changes occur.
- Avoid prolonged exposure to sun, or use a sunscreen or covering garments if exposure is necessary.
- Maintain fluid intake, and use precautions against heatstroke in hot weather.
- Report sore throat, fever, unusual bleeding or bruising, rash, weakness, tremors, impaired vision, dark urine, pale stools, yellowing of the skin or eyes.

☐ propafenone hydrochloride

(proe paf' a non)
Rythmol

Pregnancy Category C

Drug classes
Antiarrhythmic

Therapeutic actions
Class IC antiarrhythmic: local anesthetic effects with a direct membrane stablizing action on the myocardial membranes; refractory period is prolonged with a reduction of spontaneous automaticity and depressed trigger activity.

Indications
- Treatment of documented life-threatening ventricular arrhythmias; reserve use for those patients in whom the benefits outweigh the risks
- Unlabeled uses; treatment of supraventricular tachycardias, including atrial fibrillation associated with Wolff-Parkinson-White syndrome

Contraindications/cautions
- Contraindicated in the presence of hypersensitivity to propafenone, uncontrolled CHF, cardiogenic shock, cardiac conduction disturbances in the absence of an artificial pacemaker, bradycardia, marked hypotension, bronchospastic disorders, manifest electrolyte imbalance, pregnancy contraindication (teratogenic in preclinical studies), lactation.
- Use caution in the presence of hepatic, renal dysfunction.

Dosage
Adult: Initially titrate on the basis of response and tolerance. Initiate with 150 mg PO q8h (450 mg/d). Dosage may be increased at a minimum of 3- to 4-d intervals to 225 mg PO q8h (675 mg/d) and if necessary, to 300 mg PO q8h (900 mg/d). Do not exceed 900 mg/d. Decrease dosage in patients with significant widening of the QRS complex or with AV block.
Pediatric: Safety and efficacy not established.
Geriatric: Use with caution; increase the dose of propafenone more gradually during the initial phase of treatment.

Pharmacokinetics

Route	Onset	Peak
Oral	Varies	$3\frac{1}{2}$ h

Metabolism: Hepatic, $T_{1/2}$: 2–10 h
Distribution: Crosses placenta; enters breast milk
Excretion: Urine

Adverse effects

- CNS: *Dizziness, headache, weakness, blurred vision,* abnormal dreams, speech or vision disturbances, coma, confusion, depression, memory loss, numbness, paresthesias, psychosis/mania, seizures, tinnitus, vertigo
- GI: *Unusual taste, nausea, vomiting, constipation,* dyspepsia, cholestasis, gastroenteritis, hepatitis
- CV: *First-degree AV block, intraventricular conduction disturbances,* **CHF**, atrial flutter, AV dissociation, **cardiac arrest**, sick sinus syndrome, sinus pause, sinus arrest, supraventricular tachycardia
- Hematologic: Agranulocytosis, anemia, granulocytopenia, leukopenia, purpura, thrombocytopenia, positive ANA
- MS: Muscle weakness, leg cramps, muscle pain
- Dermatologic: Alopecia, pruritus

Clinically important drug-drug interactions

- Increased serum levels of propafenone and risk of increased toxicity if given concomitantly with quinidine, cimetidine, beta-blockers • Increased serum levels of digoxin, warfarin when given concomitantly

■ Nursing Considerations

Assessment

- *History:* Hypersensitivity to propafenone, uncontrolled CHF, cardiogenic shock, cardiac conduction disturbances in the absence of an artificial pacemaker, bradycardia, marked hypotension, bronchospastic disorders, manifest electrolyte imbalance, hepatic or renal dysfunction, pregnancy, lactation
- *Physical:* Reflexes, affect; BP, P, ECG, peripheral perfusion, auscultation; abdomen, normal function; renal and liver function tests; CBC, Hct, electrolytes; ANA

Implementation

- Monitor patient response carefully, especially when beginning therapy. Increase dosage at minimum of 3- to 4-d intervals only.
- Arrange for reduced dosage in patients with renal or liver dysfunction, patients with marked previous myocardial damage.
- Arrange to increase dosage slowly in patients with renal, liver, or myocardial dysfunction.
- Arrange for periodic ECG monitoring to monitor effects on cardiac conduction.

Drug-specific teaching points

- Take the drug every 8 h around the clock; work with your nurse to determine a schedule that will interrupt sleep the least.
- Be aware that frequent monitoring of ECG will be necessary to change dosage or determine effects of drug on cardiac conduction.
- Know that the following side effects may occur: dizziness, headache (avoid driving a car or performing hazardous tasks if these occur); headache, weakness (medications may be available to help; rest periods may help); nausea, vomiting, unusual taste (proper nutrition is important; taking the drug with meals may help); constipation.
- Do not stop taking this drug for any reason without checking with your health care provider.
- Report swelling of the extremities, difficulty breathing, fainting, palpitations, vision changes, chest pain.

☐ propantheline bromide

*(proe **pan'** the leen)*
Pro-Banthine (CAN)

Pregnancy Category C

Drug classes
Anticholinergic (quaternary)
Antimuscarinic

propantheline bromide ■ 945

Parasympatholytic drug
Antispasmodic

Therapeutic actions
Competitively blocks the effects of acetylcholine at muscarinic cholinergic receptors that mediate the effects of parasympathetic postganglionic impulses, relaxing the GI tract and inhibiting gastric acid secretion.

Indications
- Adjunctive therapy in the treatment of peptic ulcer
- Unlabeled uses: antisecretory and antispasmodic effects

Contraindications/cautions
- Contraindicated in the presence of glaucoma, adhesions between iris and lens, stenosing peptic ulcer, pyloroduodenal obstruction, paralytic ileus, intestinal atony, severe ulcerative colitis, toxic megacolon, symptomatic prostatic hypertrophy, bladder neck obstruction, bronchial asthma, COPD, cardiac arrhythmias, tachycardia, myocardial ischemia, sensitivity to anticholinergic drugs or bromides, impaired metabolic, liver or kidney function, myasthenia gravis, lactation.
- Use caution in the presence of pregnancy, Down syndrome, brain damage, spasticity, hypertension, hyperthyroidism.

Dosage
Adult: 15 mg PO ½ h before meals and at bedtime.
- ***Mild symptoms or person of small stature:*** 7.5 mg PO tid.

Pediatric
- ***Peptic ulcer:*** Safety and efficacy not established.
- ***Antisecretory:*** 1.5 mg/kg per day PO divided into doses tid–qid.
- ***Antispasmodic:*** 2–3 mg/kg per day PO in divided doses q4–6h and at bedtime.

Geriatric: 7.5 mg PO tid.

Pharmacokinetics
Metabolism: Hepatic, $T_{1/2}$: 3–4 h

Distribution: Crosses placenta; enters breast milk
Excretion: Urine

Route	Onset	Peak	Duration
Oral	30–60 min	2–6 h	6 h

Adverse effects
- **CNS:** *Blurred vision*, mydriasis, cycloplegia, photophobia, increased intraocular pressure
- **GI:** *Dry mouth, altered taste perception, nausea, vomiting, dysphagia*, heartburn, constipation, bloated feeling, paralytic ileus, gastroesophageal reflux
- **CV:** Palpitations, tachycardia
- **GU:** *Urinary hesitancy and retention*; impotence
- **Local:** *Irritation at site of IM injection*
- **Other:** Decreased sweating and predisposition to heat prostration, suppression of lactation, nasal congestion

Clinically important drug-drug interactions
• Decreased antipsychotic effectiveness of haloperidol when given concurrently • Decreased pharmacologic/therapeutic effects of phenothiazines if taken concurrently

■ Nursing Considerations

Assessment
- *History:* Adhesions between iris and lens, stenosing peptic ulcer, pyloroduodenal obstruction, intestinal atony, severe ulcerative colitis, symptomatic prostatic hypertrophy, bladder neck obstruction, bronchial asthma, COPD, cardiac arrhythmias, myocardial ischemia, sensitivity to anticholinergic drugs; bromides; impaired metabolic, liver or kidney function, myasthenia gravis, lactation, Down's syndrome, brain damage, spasticity, hypertension, hyperthyroidism
- *Physical:* Bowel sounds, normal output; urinary output, prostate palpation; R, adventitious sounds; pulse, BP; intraocular pressure, vision exam; bilateral grip strength, reflexes; liver palpation, liver and renal function tests.

Adverse effects in *Italics* are most common; those in **Bold** are life-threatening.

Implementation
- Ensure adequate hydration; provide environmental control (temperature) to prevent hyperpyrexia.
- Encourage patient to void before each dose of medication if urinary retention becomes a problem.

Drug-specific teaching points
- Take drug exactly as prescribed.
- Avoid hot environments while taking this drug (you will be heat intolerant, and dangerous reactions may occur).
- Know that the following side effects may occur: constipation (ensure adequate fluid intake, proper diet); dry mouth (sugarless lozenges, frequent mouth care may help; this effect sometimes lessens with time); blurred vision, sensitivity to light (it may help to know that these are drug effects that will go away when you discontinue the drug; avoid tasks that require acute vision; wear sunglasses when in bright light if these occur); impotence (this is a drug effect that will go away when you discontinue the drug; difficulty urinating (it may help to empty the bladder immediately before taking each dose of drug).
- Report skin rash, flushing, eye pain, difficulty breathing, tremors, loss of coordination, irregular heartbeat, palpitations, headache, abdominal distention, hallucinations, severe or persistent dry mouth, difficulty swallowing, difficulty in urination, severe constipation, sensitivity to light.

❒ propoxyphene hydrochloride

(proe pox' i feen)

dextropropoxyphene
Darvon, Dolene

propoxyphene napsylate
Darvocet-N, Darvon-N

Pregnancy Category C
C-IV controlled substance

Drug classes
Narcotic agonist analgesic

Therapeutic actions
Acts as agonist at specific opioid receptors in the CNS to produce analgesia, euphoria, sedation; the receptors mediating these effects are thought to be the same as those mediating the effects of endogenous opioids (enkephalins, endorphins).

Indications
- Relief of mild to moderate pain

Contraindications/cautions
- Contraindicated in the presence of hypersensitivity to narcotics, pregnancy (neonatal withdrawal has occurred in infants born to mothers who used narcotics during pregnancy; safety for use in pregnancy not established), labor or delivery (especially when delivery of a premature infant is expected; administration of narcotics to the mother can cause respiratory depression of neonate; may prolong labor), lactation.
- Use caution in the presence of renal or hepatic dysfunction, emotional depression.

Dosage
Adult
- ***Propoxyphene hydrochloride:*** 65 mg PO q4h as needed. Do not exceed 390 mg/d.
- ***Propoxyphene napsylate:*** 100 mg PO q4h as needed. Do not exceed 600 mg/d.

Pediatric: Not recommended.
Geriatric or impaired adult: Use caution; reduced dosage may be necessary.

Pharmacokinetics

Route	Onset	Peak
Oral	Varies	2–2½ h

Metabolism: Hepatic, $T_{1/2}$: 6–12 h
Distribution: Crosses placenta; enters breast milk
Excretion: Urine

Adverse effects
- **CNS:** *Dizziness, sedation,* lightheadedness, headache, weakness, euphoria, dysphoria, minor visual disturbances
- **GI:** *Nausea, vomiting,* constipation, abdominal pain, liver dysfunction
- **Dermatologic:** Skin rashes
- **Other:** Tolerance and dependence, psychological dependence

Clinically important drug-drug interactions
• Increased likelihood of respiratory depression, hypotension, profound sedation, or coma in patients receiving barbiturate general anesthetics. • Increased serum levels and toxicity of carbamazepine if taken concurrently • Decreased absorption and serum levels of propoxyphene if given with charcoal

■ Nursing Considerations

Assessment
- *History:* Hypersensitivity to narcotics, pregnancy, lactation, renal or hepatic dysfunction, emotional depression
- *Physical:* Skin—color, texture, lesions; orientation, reflexes, affect; bowel sounds, normal output; liver, kidney function tests

Implementation
- Administer to women who are lactating 4–6 h before the next scheduled feeding to minimize the amount in milk.
- Arrange to limit the amount of drug dispensed to depressed, emotionally labile, or potentially suicidal patients; propoxyphene intake alone or with other CNS depressants has been associated with deaths in such patients.
- Provide narcotic antagonist, facilities for assisted or controlled respiration on standby in case respiratory depression occurs.
- Give drug with milk or food if GI upset occurs.
- Reassure patient about addiction liability; most patients who receive opiates for medical reasons do not develop dependence syndromes.

Drug-specific teaching points
- Take drug exactly as prescribed.
- Know that the following side effects may occur: nausea, loss of appetite (taking the drug with food, eating frequent, small meals should minimize these effects); constipation (a laxative may help); dizziness, sedation, drowsiness, impaired visual acuity (avoid driving a car, performing other tasks that require alertness, visual acuity).
- Do not take any leftover medication for other disorders, and do not let anyone else take the prescription.
- Report severe nausea, vomiting, constipation, shortness of breath or difficulty breathing.

❒ propranolol hydrochloride

(proe pran' oh lole)
Apo-Propranolol (CAN),
Inderal, Novopranol (CAN),
PMS-Propranolol (CAN),
Propranolol Intensol

Pregnancy Category C

Drug classes
Beta-adrenergic blocking agent (nonselective beta-blocker)
Antianginal drug
Antiarrhythmic drug
Antihypertensive drug

Therapeutic actions
Competitively blocks beta-adrenergic receptors in the heart and juxtaglomerular apparatus, decreasing the influence of the sympathetic nervous system on these tissues, the excitablity of the heart, cardiac workload and oxygen consumption, and the release of renin and lowering blood pressure; has membrane-stabilizing (local anesthetic) effects that contribute to its antiarrhythmic action; acts in the CNS to reduce sympathetic outflow and vasoconstrictor tone. The mecha-

Adverse effects in *Italics* are most common; those in **Bold** are life-threatening.

propranolol hydrochloride

nism by which it prevents migraine headaches is unknown.

Indications
- Hypertension alone or with other drugs, especially diuretics
- Angina pectoris caused by coronary atherosclerosis
- IHSS to manage associated stress-induced angina, palpitations, and syncope
- Cardiac arrhythmias, especially supraventricular tachycardia, and ventricular tachycardias induced by digitalis or catecholamines
- Prevention of reinfarction in clinically stable patients 1–4 wk after MI
- Pheochromocytoma, an adjunctive therapy after treatment with an alpha-adrenergic blocker to manage tachycardia before or during surgery or if the pheochromocytoma is inoperable.
- Prophylaxis for migraine headache
- Management of acute situational stress reaction (stage fright)
- Treatment of essential tremor, familial or hereditary
- Unlabeled uses: recurrent GI bleeding in cirrhotic patients, schizophrenia, tardive dyskinesia, acute panic symptoms, vaginal contraceptive

Contraindications/cautions
- Contraindicated in the presence of allergy to beta-blocking agents, sinus bradycardia, second- or third-degree heart block, cardiogenic shock, CHF, bronchial asthma, bronchospasm, COPD, pregnancy (neonatal bradycardia, hypoglycemia, and apnea have occurred in human infants whose mothers received propranolol, and low birth weight occurs with chronic maternal use during pregnancy), lactation.
- Use caution in the presence of hypoglycemia and diabetes, thyrotoxicosis, hepatic dysfunction.

Dosage
Adult
- **Oral**
  - *Hypertension:* 40 mg regular propranolol bid *or* 80 mg sustained-release (SR) qd initially; usual maintenance dose, 120–240 mg/d given bid or tid *or* 120–160 mg SR qd (maximum dose, 640 mg/d).
  - *Angina:* 10–20 mg tid or qid *or* 80 mg SR qd initially; gradually increase dosage at 3- to 7-d intervals; usual maintenance dose, 160 mg/d (maximum dose, 320 mg/d).
  - *IHSS:* 20–40 mg tid or qid *or* 80–160 mg SR qd.
  - *Arrhythmias:* 10–30 mg tid or qid.
  - *MI:* 180–240 mg/d given tid or qid (maximum dose, 240 mg/d).
  - *Pheochromocytoma:* Preoperatively, 60 mg/d for 3 d in divided doses; inoperable tumor, 30 mg/d in divided doses.
  - *Migraine:* 80 mg/d qd (SR) or in divided doses; usual maintenance dose, 160–240 mg/d.
  - *Essential tremor:* 40 mg bid; usual maintenance dose, 120 mg/d.
  - *Situational anxiety:* 40 mg, timing based on the usual onset of action.
- **Parenteral**
  - *Life-threatening arrhythmias:* 1–3 mg IV with careful monitoring, not to exceed 1 mg/min; may give second dose in 2 min, but then do not repeat for 4 h. (*Note:* IV dosage is *markedly* less than oral because of "first pass effect" with oral propranolol).

Pediatric: Safety and efficacy not established.

Pharmacokinetics

Route	Onset	Peak	Duration
Oral	20–30 min	60–90 min	6–12 h
IV	Immediate	1 min	4–6 h

Metabolism: Hepatic, $T_{1/2}$: 3–5 h
Distribution: Crosses placenta; enters breast milk
Excretion: Urine

IV facts
Preparation: No further preparation is needed.

Infusion: Inject directly IV or into tubing of running IV; do not exceed 1 mg/min.

propranolol hydrochloride ■ 949

Adverse effects
- **CNS:** Dizziness, vertigo, tinnitus, *fatigue*, emotional depression, paresthesias, sleep disturbances, hallucinations, disorientation, memory loss, slurred speech
- **GI:** *Gastric pain, flatulence, constipation, diarrhea, nausea, vomiting,* anorexia, ischemic colitis, renal and mesenteric arterial thrombosis, retroperitoneal fibrosis, hepatomegaly, acute pancreatitis
- **CV:** *Bradycardia, CHF, cardiac arrhythmias, sinoartial or AV nodal block,* peripheral vascular insufficiency, claudication, CVA, pulmonary edema, hypotension
- **Respiratory:** Bronchospasm, dyspnea, cough, bronchial obstruction, nasal stuffiness, rhinitis, pharyngitis
- **GU:** *Impotence, decreased libido,* Peyronie's disease, dysuria, nocturia, frequency
- **MS:** Joint pain, arthralgia, muscle cramp
- **EENT:** Eye irritation, dry eyes, conjunctivitis, blurred vision
- **Dermatologic:** Rash, pruritus, sweating, dry skin
- **Allergic reactions:** Pharyngitis, erythematous rash, fever, sore throat, laryngospasm, respiratory distress
- **Other:** *Decreased exercise tolerance, development of ANAs,* hyperglycemia or hypoglycemia, elevated serum transaminase, alkaline phosphatase, and LDH

Clinically important drug-drug interactions
- Increased effects of propranolol with verapamil • Decreased effects of propranolol with indomethacin, ibuprofen, piroxicam, sulindac, barbiturates • Prolonged hypoglycemic effects of insulin if taken concurrently with propranolol • Peripheral ischemia possible if propranolol combined with ergot alkaloids • Initial hypertensive episode followed by bradycardia if taken concurrently with epinephrine • Increased "first-dose response" to prazosin when taken concurrently with propranolol • Increased serum levels and toxic effects if taken concurrently with lidocaine, cimetidine • Increased serum levels of propranolol and phenothiazines, hydralazine if the two drugs are taken concurrently • Paradoxical hypertension when clonidine is given with beta-blockers; increased rebound hypertension when clonidine is discontinued in patients on beta-blockers • Decreased serum levels and therapeutic effects if propranolol is taken with methimazole, propylthiouracil • Decreased bronchodilator effects of theophyllines taken with propranolol • Decreased antihypertensive effects of propranolol if taken concurrently with NSAIDs (ie, ibuprofen, indomethacin, piroxicam, sulindac), rifampin

Drug-lab test interferences
- Interference with glucose or insulin tolerance tests, glaucoma screening tests

■ Nursing Considerations

Assessment
- *History:* Allergy to beta-blocking agents, sinus bradycardia, second- or third-degree heart block, cardiogenic shock, CHF, bronchial asthma, bronchospasm, COPD, hypoglycemia and diabetes, thyrotoxicosis, hepatic dysfunction, pregnancy, lactation
- *Physical:* Weight, skin—color, lesions, edema, temperature; reflexes, affect, vision, hearing, orientation; BP, P, ECG, peripheral perfusion; R, auscultation; bowel sounds, normal output, liver evaluation; bladder palpation; liver and thyroid function tests; blood and urine glucose

Implementation
- Do not discontinue drug abruptly after chronic therapy (hypersensitivity to catecholamines may have developed, causing exacerbation of angina, MI, and ventricular dysrhythmias). Taper drug gradually over 2 wk with monitoring.
- Ensure that alpha-adrenergic blocker has been given before giving propranolol when treating patients with pheochromocytoma; endogenous catecholamines secreted by the tumor can cause severe hypertension if vascular beta receptors

are blocked without concomitant alpha blockade.
- Consult with physician about withdrawing drug if patient is to undergo surgery (withdrawal is controversial).
- Provide continual cardiac monitoring and regular BP monitoring for patients on IV propranolol.
- Give oral drug with food to facilitate absorption.

Drug-specific teaching points
- Take this drug with meals. Do not discontinue the medication abruptly; abrupt discontinuation can cause a worsening of the disorder for which you are taking the drug.
- Know that the following side effects may occur: dizziness, drowsiness, light-headedness, blurred vision (avoid driving a car or performing hazardous tasks if these occur); nausea, loss of appetite (frequent, small meals may help); nightmares, depression (notify your health care provider who may be able to change your medication); sexual impotence.
- Report difficulty breathing, night cough, swelling of extremities, slow pulse, confusion, depression, rash, fever, sore throat.
- For diabetic patients: Be aware that the normal signs of hypoglycemia (sweating, tachycardia) may be blocked by this drug; monitor your blood/urine glucose carefully; be sure to eat regular meals, and take your diabetic medication regularly.

☐ propylthiouracil

*(proe pill thye oh **yoor**' a sill)*
PTU, Propyl-Thyracil (CAN)
Pregnancy Category D

Drug classes
Antithyroid drug

Therapeutic actions
Inhibits the synthesis of thyroid hormones; partially inhibits the peripheral conversion of T_4 to T_3, the more potent form of thyroid hormone.

Indications
- Hyperthyroidism

Contraindications/cautions
- Contraindicated in the presence of allergy to antithyroid poroducts, pregnancy (can induce hypothyroidism or cretinism in the fetus; use only if absolutely necessary and when mother has been informed about potential harm to the fetus; if antithyroid drug is needed, this is the drug of choice).
- Use caution if lactating (if antithyroid drug is needed, this is the drug of choice).

Dosage
Administered only PO usually in three equal doses q8h.
Adult: *Initial:* 300 mg/d PO, up to 400–900 mg/d in severe cases. Maintenance, 100–150 mg/d.
Pediatric
- ***6–10 y:*** *Initial:* 50–150 mg/d PO.
- ***> 10 y:*** *Initial:* 150–300 mg/d PO. Maintenance is determined by the needs of the patient.

Pharmacokinetics

Route	Onset
Oral	Varies

Metabolism: Hepatic, $T_{1/2}$: 1–2 h
Distribution: Crosses placenta; enters breast milk
Excretion: Urine

Adverse effects
- CNS: *Paresthesias, neuritis, vertigo, drowsiness,* neuropathies, depression, headache
- GI: *Nausea, vomiting, epigastric distress,* loss of taste, jaundice, hepatitis
- CV: Vasculitis, periarteritis
- Hematologic: **Agranulocytosis,** granulocytopenia, thrombocytopenia, hypoprothrombinemia, bleeding
- GU: Nephritis
- Dermatologic: *Skin rash, urticaria,* pruritus, skin pigmentation, exfoliative dermatitis, lupus-like syndrome, loss of hair

Adverse effects in *Italics* are most common; those in **Bold** are life-threatening.

- **Other:** Arthralgia, myalgia, edema, lymphadenopathy, drug fever

Clinically important drug-drug interactions
- Increased risk of bleeding when taken concurrently with oral anticoagulants
- Alterations in theophylline, metoprolol, propranolol, digitalis glycoside clearance, serum levels and effects as patient moves from hyperthyroid state to euthyroid state

Nursing Considerations

Assessment
- *History:* Allergy to antithyroid poroducts, pregnancy, lactation
- *Physical:* Skin—color, lesions, pigmentation; orientation, reflexes, affect; liver evaluation; CBC, differential, prothrombin time; liver and renal function tests

Implementation
- Administer drug in three equally divided doses at 8-h intervals; try to schedule to allow patient to sleep at his or her regular time.
- Arrange for regular, periodic blood tests to monitor bone marrow depression and bleeding tendencies.
- Advise medical personnel who may be doing surgical procedures with this patient that he or she is on this drug and therefore at greater risk for bleeding problems.

Drug-specific teaching points
- Take this drug around the clock at 8-h intervals.
- Be aware that this drug will need to be taken for a prolonged period to achieve the desired effects.
- Know the following side effects may occur: dizziness, weakness, vertigo, drowsiness (use caution if operating a car or dangerous machinery if these effects occur); nausea, vomiting, loss of appetite (small, frequent meals may help); rash, itching.
- Report fever, sore throat, unusual bleeding or bruising, headache, general malaise.

protamine sulfate

(proe' ta meen)

Pregnancy Category C

Drug classes
Heparin antagonist

Therapeutic actions
Strongly basic proteins found in salmon sperm; protamines form stable salts with heparin, which results in the immediate loss of anticoagulant activity; administered when heparin has not been given; protamine has anticoagulant activity.

Indications
- Heparin overdose

Contraindications/cautions
- Allergy to protamine sulfate or fish products, pregnancy, lactation.

Dosage
Dosage is determined by the amount of heparin in the body and the amount of time that has elapsed since the heparin was given; the longer the interval, the smaller the dose required.

Adult and Pediatric: 1 mg IV neutralizes 90 USP U of heparin derived from lung tissue or 115 USP U of heparin derived from intestinal mucosa.

Pharmacokinetics

Route	Onset	Duration
IV	5 min	2 h

Metabolism: Degraded in body, $T_{1/2}$: unknown
Distribution: Crosses placenta; may enter breast milk

IV facts
Preparation: Administer injection undiluted; if dilution is necessary, use 5% Dextrose in Water or Saline; refrigerate any diluted solution. Do not store diluted solution; no preservatives are added. Reconstitute powder for injection with 5 ml Bacteriostatic Water for Injection with benzyl

alcohol added to the 50-mg vial (25 ml to the 250-mg vial); stable at room temperature for 72 h.

Infusion: Administer very slowly IV; do not exceed 50 mg in any 10-min period; do not give more than 100 mg over a short period of time.

Incompatibilities: Do not mix in lines with incompatible antibiotics, including many penicillins and cephalosporins.

Adverse effects
- GI: *Nausea/vomiting*
- CV: *Hypotension*
- Hypersensitivity: Anaphylactoid reactions—dyspnea, flushing, hypotension, bradycardia, **anaphylaxis** (sometimes fatal)

■ Nursing Considerations

Assessment
- *History:* Allergy to protamine sulfate or fish products, pregnancy, lactation
- *Physical:* Skin—color, temperature; orientation, reflexes; P, BP, auscultation, peripheral perfusion; R, adventitous sounds; plasma thrombin time

Implementation
- Maintain emergency equipment for resuscitation and treatment of shock on standby in case of anaphylactoid reaction.
- Monitor coagulation studies to adjust dosage, and screen for heparin "rebound" and response to drug.

Drug-specific teaching points
- Report shortness of breath, difficulty breathing, flushing, feeling of warmth, dizziness, lack or orientation, numbness, tingling.

❒ protriptyline hydrochloride

*(proe **trip**' ti leen)*
Triptil (CAN), Vivactil

Pregnancy Category C

Drug classes
Tricyclic antidepressant (TCA; secondary amine)

Therapeutic actions
Mechanism of action unknown; the TCAs are structurally related to the phenothiazine antipsychotic drugs (eg, chlorpromazine), but in contrast to the phenothiazines, TCAs inhibit the presynaptic reuptake of the neurotransmitters norepinephrine and serotonin; anticholinergic at CNS and peripheral receptors; the relation of these effects to clinical efficacy is unknown.

Indications
- Relief of symptoms of depression (endogenous depression most responsive; unlike other TCAs, protriptyline is "activating" and may be useful in withdrawn and anergic patients)
- Unlabeled use: treatment of obstructive sleep apnea

Contraindications/cautions
- Contraindicated in the presence of hypersensitivity to any tricyclic drug, concomitant therapy with an MAOI, recent MI, myelography within previous 24 h or scheduled within 48 h, pregnancy (limb reduction abnormalities reported), lactation.
- Use caution in the presence of electroshock therapy; preexisting cardiovascular disorders (eg, severe coronary heart disease, progressive heart failure, angina pectoris, paroxysmal tachycardia); angle-closure glaucoma, increased intraocular pressure, urinary retention, ureteral or urethral spasm; seizure disorders (TCAs lower the seizure threshold); hyperthyroidism (predisposes to CVS toxicity, including cardiac arrhythmias); impaired hepatic, renal function; psychiatric patients (schizophrenic or paranoid patients may exhibit a worsening of psychosis with TCA therapy); manic-depressive patients (may shift to hypomanic or manic phase); elective surgery (TCAs should be discontinued as long as possible before surgery).

Adverse effects in *Italics* are most common; those in **Bold** are life-threatening.

protriptyline hydrochloride ■ 953

Dosage

Adult: 15–40 mg/d PO in three to four divided doses initially. May gradually increase to 60 mg/d if necessary. Do not exceed 60 mg/d. Make increases in dosage in the morning dose.

Pediatric: Not recommended.

Geriatric and adolescents: Initially 5 mg tid PO. Increase gradually if necessary. Monitor cardiovascular system closely if dose exceeds 20 mg/d.

Pharmacokinetics

Route	Onset	Peak
Oral	Slow	24–30 h

Metabolism: Hepatic, $T_{1/2}$: 67–89 h
Distribution: Crosses placenta; enters breast milk
Excretion: Urine

Adverse effects

- CNS: *Sedation and anticholinergic (atropine-like) effects*—dry mouth, blurred vision, disturbance of accommodation for near vision, mydriasis, increased intraocular pressure, *confusion* (especially in elderly), *disturbed concentration*, hallucinations, disorientation, decreased memory, feelings of unreality, delusions, anxiety, nervousness, restlessness, agitation, panic, insomnia, nightmares, hypomania, mania, exacerbation of psychosis, drowsiness, weakness, fatigue, headache, numbness, tingling, paresthesias of extremities, incoordination, motor hyperactivity, akathisia, ataxia, tremors, peripheral neuropathy, extrapyramidal symptoms, *seizures*, speech blockage, dysarthria, tinnitus, altered EEG
- GI: *Dry mouth, constipation*, paralytic ileus, *nausea*, vomiting, anorexia, epigastric distress, diarrhea, flatulence, dysphagia, peculiar taste, increased salivation, stomatitis, glossitis, parotid swelling, abdominal cramps, black tongue
- CV: *Orthostatic hypotension*, hypertension, syncope, tachycardia, palpitations, MI, arrhythmias, heart block, precipitation of CHF, stroke
- Hematologic: Bone marrow depression, including agranulocytosis; eosinophila; purpura; thrombocytopenia; leukopenia
- GU: Urinary retention, delayed micturition, dilation of the urinary tract, gynecomastia, testicular swelling in men; breast enlargement, menstrual irregularity and galactorrhea in women; increased or decreased libido; impotence
- Hypersensitivity: Skin rash, pruritus, vasculitis, petechiae, photosensitization, edema (generalized or of face and tongue), drug fever
- Endocrine: Elevated or depressed blood sugar; elevated prolactin levels; inappropriate ADH secretion
- Withdrawal: Symptoms with abrupt discontinuation of prolonged therapy: nausea, headache, vertigo, nightmares, malaise
- Other: Nasal congestion, excessive appetite, weight gain or loss, sweating, alopecia, lacrimation, hyperthermia, flushing, chills

Clinically important drug-drug interactions

- Increased TCA levels and pharmacologic effects when given with cimetidine, fluoxetine, ranitidine • Increased half-life and therefore increased bleeding if taken with dicumarol • Altered response, including dysrhythmias and hypertension if taken with sympathomimetics • Risk of severe hypertension when taken concurrently with clonidine • Hyperpyretic crises, severe convulsions, hypertensive episodes, and deaths when MAO inhibitors are given with TCAs • Decreased hypotensive activity of guanethidine if taken concurrently

■ Nursing Considerations
Assessment

- *History:* Hypersensitivity to any tricyclic drug; concomitant therapy with an MAOI; recent MI; myelography within previous 24 h or scheduled within 48 h; pregnancy; lactation; electroshock therapy; preexisting cardiovascular disorders; angle-closure glaucoma, increased intraocular pressure, urinary retention,

Adverse effects in *Italics* are most common; those in **Bold** are life-threatening.

ureteral or urethral spasm; seizure disorders; hyperthyroidism; impaired hepatic, renal function; psychiatric patients; manic-depressive patients; elective surgery
- *Physical:* Body weight; temperature; skin—color, lesions; orientation, affect, reflexes, vision and hearing; P, BP, orthostatic BP, perfusion; bowel sounds, normal output, liver evaluation; urine flow, normal output; usual sexual function, frequency of menses, breast and scrotal examination; liver function tests, urinalysis, CBC, ECG

Implementation
- Ensure that depressed and potentially suicidal patients have access to only limited quantities of drug.
- Arrange to reduce dosage if minor side effects develop; arrange to discontinue the drug if serious side effects occur.
- Arrange for CBC if patient develops fever, sore throat, or other sign of infection during therapy.

Drug-specific teaching points
- Take drug exactly as prescribed; do not to stop taking this drug abruptly or without consulting the physician or nurse.
- Avoid alcohol, other sleep-inducing drugs, OTC drugs while on this drug.
- Avoid prolonged exposure to sunlight or sunlamps; use a sunscreen or protective garments if long exposure to sunlight is unavoidable.
- Know that the following side effects may occur: headache, dizziness, drowsiness, weakness, blurred vision (these effects are reversible; safety measures may need to be taken if these become severe; avoid driving an automobile or performing tasks that require alertness while these persist); nausea, vomiting, loss of appetite, dry mouth (small, frequent meals, frequent mouth care and sucking sugarless candies may help); nightmares, inability to concentrate, confusion; changes in sexual function.
- Report dry mouth, difficulty in urination, excessive sedation.

❐ pseudoephedrine hydrochloride

*(soo dow e **fed**' rin)*

d-isoephedrine hydrochloride

Cenafed, Decofed, Dorcol Pediatric Formula, Eltor (CAN), Halofed, Neofed, Novafed (prescription drug), Pediacare, Robidrine (CAN), Sudafed, Sudrin

pseudoephedrine sulfate
Afrin Repetabs (prescription drug)

Pregnancy Category C

Drug classes
Nasal decongestant
Sympathomimetic amine

Therapeutic actions
Effects are mediated by alpha-adrenergic receptors; causes vasoconstriction in mucous membranes of nasal passages, resulting in their shrinkage, which promotes drainage and improves ventilation.

Indications
- Temporary relief of nasal congestion caused by the common cold, hay fever, other respiratory allergies
- Nasal congestion associated with sinusitis
- Promotes nasal or sinus drainage
- Relief of eustachian tube congestion

Contraindications/cautions
- Contraindicated in the presence of allergy or idiosyncrasy to sympathomimetic amines, severe hypertension and coronary artery disease, lactation, pregnancy.
- Use caution in the presence of hyperthyroidism, diabetes mellitus, arteriosclerosis, ischemic heart disease, increased intraocular pressure, prostatic hypertrophy.

Dosage
Adult: 60 mg q4–6h PO (sustained-release, q12h); do not exceed 240 mg in 24 h.

pseudoephedrine hydrochloride ■ 955

Pediatric
- **6–12 y:** 30 mg q4–6h PO; do not exceed 120 mg in 24 h.
- **2–5 y:** 15 mg as syrup q4–6h PO; do not exceed 60 mg in 24 h.
- **1–2 y:** 7 drops (0.02 ml.kg) q4–6h PO; up to four doses per day.
- **3–12 mo:** 3 drops/kg q4–6h PO, up to four doses per day.

Geriatric: These patients are more likely to experience adverse reactions; use with caution.

Pharmacokinetics

Route	Onset	Duration
Oral	30 min	4–6 h

Metabolism: Hepatic, $T_{1/2}$: 7 h
Distribution: Crosses placenta; enters breast milk
Excretion: Urine

Adverse effects

- CNS: *Fear, anxiety, tenseness, restlessness, headache, light-headedness, dizziness, drowsiness, tremors,* insomnia, hallucinations, psychological disturbances, prolonged psychosis, convulsions, CNS depression, weakness, blurred vision, ocular irritation, tearing, photophobia, orofacial dystonia
- GI: *Nausea/vomiting,* anorexia
- CV: *Hypertension, arrhythmias,* cardiovascular collapse with hypotension, palpitations, tachycardia, precordial pain
- **Respiratory:** Respiratory difficulty
- GU: Dysuria
- **Dermatologic:** *Pallor,* sweating

Clinically important drug-drug interactions

- Increased hypertension when taken with MAOIs, guanethidine, furazolidone • Increased duration of action when taken with urinary alkalinizers (potassium citrate, sodium citrate, sodium lactate, tromethamine, sodium acetate, sodium bicaronate) • Decreased therapeutic effects and increased elimination of pseudoephedrine if taken with urinary acidifiers (ammonium chloride, sodium acid phosphate, potassium phosphate) • Decreased antihypertensive effects of methyldopa

■ Nursing Considerations

Assessment

- *History:* Allergy or idiosyncrasy to sympathomimetic amines, severe hypertension and CAD, hyperthyroidism, diabetes mellitus, arteriosclerosis, increased intraocular pressure, prostatic hypertrophy, pregnancy, lactation
- *Physical:* Skin—color, temperature; reflexes, affect, orientation, peripheral sensation, vision; BP, P, auscultation; R, adventitious sounds; urinary output, bladder percussion, prostate palpation

Implementation

- Administer cautiously to patients with cardiovascular disease, diabetes mellitus, hyperthyroidism, increased intraocular pressure, hypertension, and to patients older than 60 y who may have increased sensitivity to sympathomimetic amines.
- Avoid prolonged use; underlying medical problems may be causing the congestion.
- Monitor cardiovascular effect carefully; hypertensive patients who take this drug may experience changes in BP because of the additional vasoconstriction. However, if a nasal decongestant is needed, pseudoephedrine is the drug of choice.

Drug-specific teaching points

- Do not exceed the recommended daily dose; serious overdosage can occur. Use caution when using more than one OTC preparation because many of these drugs contain pseudoephedrine, and unintentional overdose may occur.
- Avoid prolonged use because underlying medical problems can be disguised.
- Know that the following side effects may occur: dizziness, weakness, restlessness, light-headedness, tremors (avoid driving a car or performing hazardous tasks if these occur).
- Report palpitations, nervousness, sleeplessness, sweating.

Adverse effects in *Italics* are most common; those in **Bold** are life-threatening.

☐ pyrantel pamoate

*(pi **ran'** tel)*
Antiminth, Combantrin (CAN), Reese's Pinworm

Pregnancy Category C

Drug classes
Anthelmintic

Therapeutic actions
A depolarizing neuromuscular blocking agent that causes spastic paralysis of *Enterobius vermicularis* and *Ascaris lumbricoides*.

Indications
- Treatment of enterobiasis (pinworm infection)
- Treatment of ascariasis (roundworm infection)

Contraindications/cautions
- Allergy to pyrantel pamoate, pregnancy, lactation.

Dosage
Adult: 11 mg/kg (5 mg/lb) PO as a single oral dose. Maximum total dose of 1 g.
Pediatric: Safety and efficacy not established for children younger than 2 y.

Pharmacokinetics

Route	Onset	Peak
Oral	Slow	1–3 h

Metabolism: Hepatic, $T_{1/2}$: 47–100 h
Distribution: Crosses placenta; may enter breast milk
Excretion: Feces and urine

Adverse effects
- CNS: Headache, dizziness, drowsiness, insomnia
- GI: *Anorexia, nausea, vomiting, abdominal cramps, diarrhea*, gastralgia, tenesmus, transient elevation of SGOT
- Dermatologic: Rash

Clinically important drug-drug interactions
- Pyrantel and piperazine are antagonistic in *Ascaris*; avoid concomitant use

■ Nursing Considerations
Assessment
- *History:* Allergy to pyrantel pamoate, pregnancy, lactation
- *Physical:* Skin—color, lesions; orientation, affect; bowel sounds; SGOT levels

Implementation
- Culture for ova and parasites.
- Administer drug with fruit juice or milk; make sure the entire dose is taken at once.
- Arrange for treatment of all family members (pinworm infestations).
- Arrange for disinfection of toilet facilities after patient use (pinworms).
- Arrange for daily laundering of bed linens, towels, nightclothes, and undergarments (pinworms).

Drug-specific teaching points
- Make sure that you take the entire dose at once. Drug may be taken with fruit juice or milk.
- Be aware that pinworms are easily transmitted; all family members should be treated for complete eradication.
- Be aware that strict handwashing and hygiene measures are important. Launder undergarments, bedlinens, nightclothes daily; disinfect toilet facilities daily and bathroom floors periodically (pinworm).
- Know that the following side effects may occur: nausea, abdominal pain, diarrhea (small, frequent meals may help; ready access to bathroom facilities may be necessary); drowsiness, dizziness, insomnia (if these occur, avoid driving and use of dangerous machinery).
- Report skin rash, joint pain, severe GI upset, severe headache, dizziness.

☐ pyrazinamide

*(peer a **zin'** a mide)*
PMS-Pyrazinamide (CAN), Tebrazid (CAN)

Pregnancy Category C

Adverse effects in *italics* are most common; those in **Bold** are life-threatening.

Drug classes
Antituberculous drug ("second-line")

Therapeutic actions
Bacteriostatic or bacteriocidal against *Mycobacterium tuberculosis*; mechanism of action is unknown.

Indications
- Initial treatment of active tuberculosis in adults and children when combined with other antituberculous agents.
- Treatment of active tuberculosis after treatment failure with primary drugs

Contraindications/cautions
- Contraindicated in the presence of allergy to pyrazinamide, acute hepatic disease, pregnancy, lactation.
- Use caution in the presence of gout, diabetes mellitus, acute intermittent porphyria.

Dosage
Adult/pediatric: 15–30 mg/kg per day PO, given once a day; do not exceed 3 g/d. Always use with up to 4 other antituberculous agents; administer for the first 2 mo of a 6-mo treatment program. 50–70 mg/kg PO twice weekly may increase compliance and is being studied as an alternate dosing schedule.

Pharmacokinetics

Route	Onset	Peak
Oral	Rapid	2 h

Metabolism: Hepatic, $T_{1/2}$: 9–10 h
Distribution: Crosses placenta; enters breast milk
Excretion: Urine

Adverse effects
- **GI:** *Hepatotoxicity, nausea, vomiting,* diarrhea
- **Hematologic:** Sideroblastic anemia, adverse effects on clotting mechanism or vascular integrity
- **Dermatologic:** Rashes, photosensitivity
- **Other:** Active gout

Drug-lab test interferences
- False readings on Acetest, Ketostix urine tests

■ Nursing Considerations
Assessment
- *History:* Allergy to pyrazinamide, acute hepatic disease, gout, diabetes mellitus, acute intermittent porphyria, pregnancy, lactation
- *Physical:* Skin—color, lesions; joint status; body temperature; liver evaluation; liver function tests, serum and urine uric acid levels, blood and urine glucose, CBC

Implementation
- Administer only in conjunction with other antituberculous agents.
- Administer once a day.
- Arrange for follow-up of liver function tests (AST, ALT) prior to and every 2–4 wk during therapy.
- Arrange for discontinuation of drug if liver damage or hyperuricemia in conjunction with acute gouty arthritis occurs.

Drug-specific teaching points
- Take this drug once a day; it will need to be taken with your other TB drugs.
- Take this drug regularly; avoid missing doses. *Do not* discontinue this drug without first consulting your prescriber.
- Know that the following side effects may occur: loss of appetite, nausea, vomiting (taking the drug with food may help); skin rash, sensitivity to sunlight (avoid exposure to the sun).
- Arrange to have regular, periodic medical checkups, which will include blood tests to evaluate the drug effects.
- Report fever, malaise, loss of appetite, nausea, vomiting, darkened urine, yellowing of skin and eyes, severe pain in great toe, instep, ankle, heel, knee, or wrist.

☐ pyridostigmine bromide

*(peer id oh **stig'** meen)*
Mestinon, Regonol

Pregnancy Category C

Adverse effects in *Italics* are most common; those in **Bold** are life-threatening.

Drug classes
Cholinesterase inhibitor
Antimyasthenic drug
Antidote

Therapeutic actions
Increases the concentration of acetylcholine at the sites of cholinergic transmission and prolongs and exaggerates the effects of acetylcholine by reversibly inhibiting the enzyme acetylcholinesterase, thus facilitating transmission at the skeletal neuromuscular junction.

Indications
- Treatment of myasthenia gravis
- Antidote for nondepolarizing neuromuscular junction blockers (eg, tubocurarine) after surgery (parenteral)

Contraindications/cautions
- Contraindicated in the presence of hypersensitivity to anticholinesterases; adverse reactions to bromides; intestinal or urogenital tract obstruction, peritonitis, lactation.
- Use caution in the presence of asthma, peptic ulcer, bradycardia, cardiac arrhythmias, recent coronary occlusion, vagotonia, hyperthyroidism, epilepsy, pregnancy (given IV near term, drug may stimulate uterus and induce premature labor).

Dosage
Adult
- **Symptomatic control of myasthenia gravis**
  - *Oral:* Average dose is 600 mg given over 24 h; range, 60–1,500 mg, spaced to provide maximum relief. Sustained-release tablets, average dose is 180–540 mg qd or bid. Individualize dosage, allowing at least 6 h between doses. Optimum control may require supplementation with the more rapidly acting syrup or regular tablets.
  - *Parenteral:* To supplement oral dosage preoperatively and postoperatively, during labor, during myasthenic crisis, and so forth: give 1/30 the oral dose IM or very slowly IV. May be given 1 h before second stage of labor is complete (enables patient to have adequate strength and protects neonate in immediate postnatal period).
- **Antidote for nondepolarizing neuromuscular blockers:** Give atropine sulfate 0.6–1.2 mg IV immediately before slow IV injection of pyridostigmine 0.1–0.25 mg/kg. 10–20 mg pyridostigmine usually suffices. Full recovery usually occurs within 15 min but may take 30 min.

Pediatric
- **Symptomatic control of myasthenia gravis**
  - *Oral:* 7 mg/kg per day divided into five or six doses.
  - *Parenteral: Neonates of myasthenic mothers who have difficulty swallowing, sucking, breathing:* 0.05–0.15 mg/kg IM. Change to syrup as soon as possible.

Pharmacokinetics

Route	Onset	Duration
Oral	35–45 min	3–6 h
IM	15 min	3–6 h
IV	5 min	3–6 h

Metabolism: Hepatic and tissue, $T_{1/2}$: 1.9–3.7 h
Distribution: Crosses placenta; enters breast milk
Excretion: Urine

IV facts
Preparation: No further preparation is required.
Infusion: Infuse very slowly, directly into vein or into tubing of actively running IV of D5W, 0.9% Sodium Chloride, Lactated Ringer's, or D5/Lactated Ringer's.

Adverse effects
Parasympathomimetic Effects
- GI: *Salivation, dysphagia, nausea, vomiting, increased peristalsis, abdominal cramps,* flatulence, diarrhea
- CV: *Bradycardia, cardiac arrhythmias,* **AV block and nodal rhythm,** cardiac ar-

Adverse effects in *Italics* are most common; those in **Bold** are life-threatening.

rest, decreased cardiac output leading to hypotension, syncope
- **Respiratory:** *Increased pharyngeal and tracheobronchial secretions*, laryngospasm, bronchospasm, bronchiolar constriction, dyspnea
- **GU:** *Urinary frequency and incontinence*, urinary urgency
- **EENT:** *Lacrimation, miosis,* spasm of accommodation, diplopia, conjunctival hyperemia
- **Dermatologic:** Diaphoresis, flushing

Skeletal Muscle Effects
- **CNS:** Convulsions, dysarthria, dysphonia, drowsiness, dizziness, headache, loss of consciousness
- **Respiratory:** Respiratory muscle paralysis, **central respiratory paralysis**
- **Dermatologic:** Skin rash, urticaria, **anaphylaxis**
- **Peripheral:** Skeletal muscle weakness, fasciculations, muscle cramps, arthralgia
- **Local:** Thrombophlebitis after IV use

Clinically important drug-drug interactions
- Decreased effectiveness with profound muscular depression when given concurrently with corticosteroids • Increased and prolonged neuromuscular blockade if given with succinylcholine

■ Nursing Considerations

Assessment
- *History:* Hypersensitivity to anticholinesterases; adverse reactions to bromides; intestinal or urogenital tract obstruction, peritonitis, lactation, asthma, peptic ulcer, cardiac arrhythmias, recent coronary occlusion, vagotonia, hyperthyroidism, epilepsy, pregnancy
- *Physical:* Bowel sounds, normal output; urinary frequency, voiding pattern, normal output; R, adventitious sounds; P, auscultation, BP; reflexes, bilateral grip strength, ECG; thyroid function tests; skin color, texture, lesions

Implementation
- Administer IV slowly.
- Be aware that overdosage with anticholinesterase drugs can cause muscle weakness (cholinergic crisis) that is difficult to differentiate from myasthenic weakness; the administration of atropine may mask the parasympathetic effects of anticholinesterase overdose and further confound the diagnosis.
- Maintain atropine sulfate on standby as an antidote and antagonist to pyridostigmine in case of cholinergic crisis or unusual sensitivity to pyridostigmine.
- Discontinue drug, and consult physician for excessive salivation, emesis, frequent urination, or diarrhea.
- Arrange for decreased dosage of drug if excessive sweating, nausea occur.

Drug-specific teaching points
- Take drug exactly as prescribed (patient and a significant other should receive extensive teaching about the effects of the drug, the signs and symptoms of myasthenia gravis, the fact that muscle weakness may be related both to drug overdosage and to exacerbation of the disease, and that it is important to report muscle weakness promptly to the nurse or physician so that proper evaluation can be made).
- Know that the following side effects may occur: blurred vision, difficulty with far vision, difficulty with dark adaptation (use caution while driving, especially at night, or performing hazardous tasks in reduced light); increased urinary frequency, abdominal cramps; sweating (avoid hot or excessively humid environments while you are taking this drug).
- Report muscle weakness, nausea, vomiting, diarrhea, severe abdominal pain, excessive sweating, excessive salivation, frequent urination, urinary urgency, irregular heartbeat, difficulty in breathing.

❐ pyrimethamine

(peer i meth' a meen)
Pregnancy Category C

Adverse effects in *Italics* are most common; those in **Bold** are life-threatening.

pyrimethamine

Drug classes
Antimalarial
Folic acid antagonist

Therapeutic actions
Folic acid antagonist: selectively inhibits plasmodial dihydrofolate reductase, which is important to cellular biosynthesis of purines, pyrimidines, and certain amino acids; highly selective against plasmodia and *Toxoplasma gondii*.

Indications
- Chemoprophylaxis of malaria due to susceptible strains of plasmodia; fast-acting schizonticides are preferable for treatment of acute attacks, but concurrent use of pyrimethamine will initiate transmission control and suppressive cure
- Treatment of toxoplasmosis with concurrent use of a sulfonamide

Contraindications/cautions
- Contraindicated in the presence of allergy to pyrimethamine, G-6-PD deficiency (may cause hemolytic anemia).
- Use caution in the presence of pregnancy (teratogenic in preclinical studies), lactation.

Dosage
Adult and pediatric older than 10 y
- **Chemoprophylaxis of malaria:** 25 mg PO once weekly for at least 6–10 wk.
- **With fast-acting schizonticides for treatment of acute attack:** 25 mg/d PO for 2 d.
- **Toxoplasmosis:** Initially 50–75 mg/d PO with 1–4 g of a sulfapyrimidine; continue for 1–3 wk. Dosage of each drug may then be decreased by half and continued for an additional 4–5 wk.

Pediatric
- **Chemoprophylaxis of malaria:** *4–10 y*: 12.5 mg PO once weekly for 6–10 wk. *Younger than 4 y*: 6.25 mg PO once weekly for 6–10 wk.
- **With fast-acting schizonticides for treatment of acute attacks:** *4–10 y*: 25 mg/d PO for 2 d.
- **Toxoplasmosis:** 1 mg/kg per day PO divided into two equal daily doses. After 2–4 d, reduce to half and continue for approximately 1 mo.

Pharmacokinetics

Route	Onset	Peak
Oral	Varies	2–6 h

Metabolism: Hepatic, $T_{1/2}$: 4 d
Distribution: crosses placenta; enters breast milk
Excretion: urine

Adverse effects
- **GI:** *Anorexia, vomiting*, atrophic glossitis
- **Hematologic:** *Megaloblastic anemia, leukopenia, thrombocytopenia, pancytopenia*, folic acid deficiency with large doses used to treat toxoplasmosis, hemolytic anemia in patients with G-6-PD deficiency

■ Nursing Considerations

Assessment
- *History:* Allergy to pyrimethamine, G-6-PD deficiency, pregnancy, lactation
- *Physical:* Abdominal exam, mucous membranes; CBC, hemoglobin, G-6-PD in deficient patients

Implementation
- Administer with food if GI upset occurs.
- Schedule dosages for weekly same-day therapy on a calendar.
- Arrange for CBC and hemoglobin determinations before beginning therapy and semiweekly during therapy.
- Arrange for decreased dosage or discontinuation of drug if signs of folic acid deficiency develop; leucovorin may be given in a dose of 3–9 mg/d IM for 3 d to return depressed platelet or WBC counts to safe levels.

Drug-specific teaching points
- Take full course of drug therapy as prescribed; take drug with food or meals if GI upset occurs.
- Mark your calendar with the drug days for once a week therapy.

Adverse effects in *Italics* are most common; those in **Bold** are life-threatening.

- Be aware that this drug may cause stomach pain, loss of appetite, nausea, vomiting or abdominal cramps.
- Arrange to have regular blood tests while you are on this drug to evaluate drug effects.
- Report darkening of the urine, severe abdominal cramps, GI distress, persistent nausea, vomiting.

☐ quazepam

(kwa' ze pam)
Doral

Pregnancy Category X
C-IV controlled substance

Drug classes
Benzodiazepine
Sedative/hypnotic

Therapeutic actions
Exact mechanisms of action not understood; acts mainly at subcortical levels of the CNS, leaving the cortex relatively unaffected; main sites of action may be the limbic system and mesencephalic reticular formation; benzodiazepines potentiate the effects of GABA, an inhibitory neurotransmitter.

Indications
- Insomnia characterized by difficulty in falling asleep, frequent nocturnal awakenings, or early morning awakening
- Recurring insomnia or poor sleeping habits
- Acute or chronic medical situations requiring restful sleep

Contraindications/cautions
- Contraindicated in the presence of hypersensitivity to benzodiazepines, psychoses, acute narrow-angle glaucoma, shock, coma, acute alcoholic intoxication with depression of vital signs, pregnancy (increased risk of congenital malformations, neonatal withdrawal syndrome), labor and delivery ("floppy infant" syndrome reported when mothers were given benzodiazepines during labor), lactation (may cause infants to become lethargic and lose weight).
- Use caution in the presence of impaired liver or kidney function, debilitation, depression, suicidal tendencies.

Dosage
Adult: Initially 15 mg PO until desired response is seen. May reduce to 7.5 mg in some patients.
Pediatric: Not for use in children younger than 18 y.
Geriatric patients or those with debilitating disease: Attempt to reduce nightly dosage after the first one or two nights of therapy.

Pharmacokinetics

Route	Onset	Peak
Oral	Varies	2 h

Metabolism: Hepatic, $T_{1/2}$: 39 h
Distribution: Crosses placenta; enters breast milk
Excretion: Urine

Adverse effects
- **CNS:** *Transient, mild drowsiness initially; sedation; depression; lethargy; apathy; fatigue; lightheadedness; disorientation; restlessness; confusion;* crying; delirium; headache; slurred speech; dysarthria; stupor; rigidity; tremor; dystonia; vertigo; euphoria; nervousness; difficulty in concentration; vivid dreams; psychomotor retardation; extrapyramidal symptoms; *mild paradoxical excitatory reactions during first 2 wk of treatment* (especially in psychiatric patients, aggressive children, and with high dosage); visual and auditory disturbances; diplopia; nystagmus; depressed hearing; nasal congestion
- **GI:** *Constipation, diarrhea,* dry mouth, salivation, nausea, anorexia, vomiting, difficulty in swallowing, gastric disorders, elevations of blood enzymes, hepatic dysfunction, jaundice
- **CV:** *Bradycardia, tachycardia,* cardiovascular collapse, hypertension and hypotension, palpitations, edema

Adverse effects in *Italics* are most common; those in **Bold** are life-threatening.

- **Hematologic:** Decreased hematocrit (primarily with long-term therapy), blood dyscrasias (agranulocytosis, leukopenia, neutropenia)
- **GU:** *Incontinence, urinary retention, changes in libido*, menstrual irregularities
- **Dermatologic:** Urticaria, pruritus, skin rash, dermatitis
- **Other:** Hiccups, fever, diaphoresis, paresthesias, muscular disturbances, gynecomastia
- **Dependence:** *Drug dependence with withdrawal syndrome* when drug is discontinued (more common with abrupt discontinuation of higher dosage used for longer than 4 mo)

Clinically important drug-drug interactions
- Increased CNS depression when taken with alcohol, omeprazole • Increased pharmacologic effects of quazepam when given with cimetidine, disulfiram, oral contraceptives • Decreased sedative effects of quazepam if taken concurrently with theophylline, aminophylline, dyphylline, oxitriphylline

■ Nursing Considerations
Assessment
- *History:* Hypersensitivity to benzodiazepines, psychoses, acute narrow-angle glaucoma, shock, coma, acute alcoholic intoxication, pregnancy, labor and delivery, lactation, impaired liver or kidney function, debilitation, depression, suicidal tendencies
- *Physical:* Skin—color, lesions; body temperature; orientation, reflexes, affect, ophthalmologic exam; P, BP; R, adventitious sounds; liver evaluation, abdominal exam, bowel sounds, normal output; CBC, liver and renal function tests

Implementation
- Arrange to monitor liver and kidney function, CBC at intervals during long-term therapy.
- Arrange to taper dosage gradually after long-term therapy, especially in epileptic patients.

Drug-specific teaching points
- Take drug exactly as prescribed.
- Do not stop taking this drug (long-term therapy) without consulting your health care provider.
- Be aware that the following side effects may occur: drowsiness, dizziness (these may become less pronounced after a few days; avoid driving a car or engaging in other dangerous activities if these occur); GI upset (taking the drug with water may help); depression, dreams, emotional upset, crying; nocturnal sleep may be disturbed for several nights after discontinuing the drug.
- Report severe dizziness, weakness, drowsiness that persists, rash or skin lesions, palpitations, swelling of the extremities, visual changes, difficulty voiding.

☐ quinacrine hydrochloride

(kwin' a kreen)

Pregnancy Category C

Drug classes
Antimalarial
Anthelmintic
Antiprotozoal drug

Therapeutic actions
Couples with and fixes plasmodial DNA, thus inhibiting DNA replication, RNA transcription, and protein synthesis, leading to destruction of the parasite.

Indications
- Treatment and suppression of malaria
- Treatment of giardiasis and cestodiasis
- Unlabeled use: prevention of recurrence of pneumothorax when used intrapleurally as a sclerosing agent in total doses of 100–1,500 mg

Contraindications/cautions
- Contraindicated in the presence of allergy to quinacrine, pregnancy.
- Use caution in the presence of G-6-PD deficiency (hemolysis may occur); psori-

Adverse effects in *Italics* are most common; those in **Bold** are life-threatening.

quinacrine hydrochloride ▪ 963

asis or porphyria; impaired hepatic function.

Dosage
Adult
- ***Treatment of malaria:*** 200 mg PO with 1 g sodium bicarbonate q6h for five doses; then 100 mg tid PO for 6 d.
- ***Suppression of malaria:*** 100 mg per day PO for 1–3 mo.
- ***Treatment of dwarf tapeworm:*** 1 tbsp of sodium sulfate dissolved in water the night before medication. Then 900 mg quinacrine PO on an empty stomach in three portions 20 min apart with a sodium sulfate purge 1½ h later. Take 100 mg tid PO on the following 3 d.
- ***Treatment of tapeworm:*** Bland diet the day before medication with fasting following the evening meal. Administer a saline purge or saline enema before treatment and saline purge 1–2 h later. Four doses of 200 g 10 min apart with 600 mg sodium bicarbonate with each dose.
- ***Treatment of giardiasis:*** 100 mg tid PO for 5–7 d.

Pediatric
- ***Treatment of malaria:*** Older than 8 y: Adult dose. *4–8 y:* 200 mg tid PO the first day, then 100 mg q12h for 6 d. *1–4 y:* 100 mg tid PO the first day, then 100 mg/d for 6 d.
- ***Suppression of malaria:*** 50 mg/d PO.
- ***Treatment of dwarf tapeworm:*** Give ½ tbsp sodium sulfate the night before medication:
  - *4–8 y:* 200 mg PO, then 100 mg PO after breakfast for 3 d.
  - *8–10 y:* 300 mg PO, the 100 mg bid PO after breakfast for 3 d.
  - *11–14 y:* 400 mg PO, then 100 mg tid PO after breakfast for 3 d.
- ***Treatment of tapeworm:*** Administer in three to four divided doses 10 min apart. Give 300 mg sodium bicarbonate with each dose.
  - *5–10 y:* 400 mg PO total dose.
  - *11–14 y:* 600 mg PO total dose.

- ***Treatment of giardiasis:*** 7 mg/kg per day (maximum dose of 300 mg/d) given in three divided doses after meals for 5 d. Examine stool after 2 wk, and repeat course if needed.

Geriatric: Use with caution in patients older than 60 y; risk of transitory psychosis.

Pharmacokinetics

Route	Onset	Peak
Oral	Varies	1–3 h

Metabolism: $T_{1/2}$: 5 d
Distribution: Crosses placenta; enters breast milk
Excretion: Urine, feces

Adverse effects
- **CNS:** *Headache, dizziness*, epileptiform convulsions, toxic psychosis with doses of only 50–100 mg tid for a few days, nervousness, vertigo, irritability, emotional changes, nightmares, transient psychosis (infrequent, reversible), reversible corneal edema or deposits, visual halos, focusing difficulty, blurred vision, retinopathy with high doses given for prolonged period
- **GI:** *Diarrhea, anorexia, nausea, abdominal cramps,* vomiting
- **Dermatologic:** Exfoliative dermatitis, contact dermatitis
- **Other:** *Yellowing of the urine and skin* (temporary effect, not jaundice), hepatitis, aplastic anemia with prolonged therapy

Clinically important drug-drug interactions
- Increased toxicity of primaquine if used concurrently with quinacrine; avoid concurrent use

▪ Nursing Considerations
Assessment
- *History:* Allergy to quinacrine, G-6-PD deficiency, psoriasis or porphyria, impaired hepatic function, pregnancy
- *Physical:* Skin—color, lesions; orientation, affect, reflexes, ophthalmic examination; liver evaluation, bowel sounds;

Adverse effects in *Italics* are most common; those in **Bold** are life-threatening.

CBC, differential; urine; stool for ova and parasites as indicated

Implementation
- Monitor patient's response to therapy; resistant strains of *Plasmodium falciparum* have emerged and should be treated with quinine or other therapy.
- Administer after meals with a full glass of water, tea, or fruit juice for use with malaria; administer on an empty stomach for treatment of giardiasis or cestodiasis.
- Disguise bitter taste of pulverized tablets in honey or jam.
- Arrange for periodic blood tests during prolonged therapy, and discontinue drug at any sign of severe blood disorder.
- Arrange for pretherapy ophthalmologic exam and periodic complete exams during long-term therapy.
- Offer support and encouragement to deal with purge, passage of worms during treatment of cestodiasis; expelled worms will be stained yellow, which allows easy identification.

Drug-specific teaching points
- Take drug after meals with a full glass of water, tea, or fruit juice for treatment of malaria. Drug must be taken on an empty stomach for treatment of giardiasis or cestodiasis; treatment involves purges, enemas, and may involve other medications. Follow orders carefully.
- Know that the following side effects may occur: dizziness, headache, blurred vision (use caution if driving or performing tasks that require alertness if these effects occur); diarrhea, nausea, stomach cramps, vomiting (taking the drug after meals may help); yellowing of the skin and urine (do not be alarmed; this is temporary and is not jaundice).
- Arrange to have periodic blood tests and complete ophthalmologic exams while you are on this drug.
- Report changes in vision—blurring, halos; skin rash; nightmares; emotional changes; severe headache.

quinapril hydrochloride

(kwin' ah pril)
Accupril

Pregnancy Category D

Drug classes
Antihypertensive
Angiotensin-converting enzyme (ACE) inhibitor

Therapeutic actions
Quanpril blocks ACE from coverting angiotensin I to angiotensin II, a powerful vasoconstrictor, leading to decreased blood pressure, decreased aldosterone secretion, a small increase in serum potassium levels, and sodium and fluid loss; increased prostaglandin synthesis also may be involved in the antihypertensive action.

Indications
- Treatment of hypertension alone or in combination with thiazide-type diuretics
- Unlabeled use: treatment of CHF

Contraindications/cautions
- Contraindicated in the presence of allergy to quinapril or other ACE inhibitors.
- Use caution in the presence of impaired renal function, CHF, salt/volume depletion, lactation.

Dosage
Adult: Initial dose 10 mg PO qd. Maintenance dose, 20–80 mg/d PO as a single dose or two divided doses. Patients on diuretics should discontinue the diuretic 2–3 d before beginning benazepril therapy. If blood pressure is not controlled, add diuretic slowly. If diuretic cannot be discontinued, begin quinapril therapy with 5 mg.
Pediatric: Safety and efficacy not established.
Geriatric or renal impaired: Initial dose, 10 mg with Ccr > 60 ml/min, 5 mg with Ccr 30–60 ml/min, 2.5 mg with Ccr 10–30 ml/min.

quinestrol ■ 965

Pharmacokinetics

Route	Onset	Peak	Duration
Oral	1 h	1 h	24 h

Metabolism: Hepatic, $T_{1/2}$: 2 h
Distribution: Crosses placenta; enters breast milk
Excretion: Urine and feces

Adverse effects
- **GI:** *Nausea,* abdominal pain, vomiting, dairrhea
- **CV:** Angina pectoris, orthostatic hypotension in salt/volume depleted patients, palpitations
- **Respiratory:** *Cough,* asthma, bronchitis, dyspnea, sinusitis
- **Dermatologic:** Rash, pruritus, diaphoresis, flushing
- **Other:** Angioedema, asthenia, myalgia, arthralgia

■ Nursing Considerations

Assessment
- *History:* Allergy to quinapril other ACE inhibitors, impaired renal function, CHF, salt/volume depletion, lactation
- *Physical:* Skin—color, lesions, turgor; body temperature; P, BP, peripheral perfusion; mucous membranes, bowel sounds, liver evaluation; urinalysis, renal and liver function tests, CBC and differential

Implementation
- Alert surgeon and mark patient's chart with notice that quinapril is being taken; the angiotensin II formation subsequent to compensatory renin release during surgery will be blocked; hypotension may be reversed with volume expansion.
- Monitor patient closely in any situation that may lead to a fall in blood pressure secondary to reduction in fluid volume (excessive perspiration and dehydration, vomiting, diarrhea) because excessive hypotension may occur.

Drug-specific teaching points
- Do not stop taking the medication without consulting your physician.

- Know that the following side effects may occur: GI upset, loss of appetite (these may be limited effects that will pass with time); lightheadedness (this usually passes after the first few days of therapy; if it occurs, change position slowly and limit your activities to those that do not require alertness and precision); dry cough (this is irritating but not harmful).
- Be careful in any situation that may lead to a drop in blood pressure (diarrhea, sweating, vomiting, dehydration); if lightheadedness or dizziness should occur, consult your nurse or physician.
- Report mouth sores; sore throat, fever, chills; swelling of the hands, feet; irregular heartbeat, chest pains; swelling of the face, eyes, lips, tongue; difficulty breathing; persistent cough.

⌐ quinestrol

(kwin ess' trole)
Estrovis

Pregnancy Category X

Drug classes
Hormone
Estrogen

Therapeutic actions
Estrogens are endogenous female sex hormones important in the development of the female reproductive system and secondary sex characteristics. They affect the release of pituitary gonadotropins and cause capillary dilatation, fluid retention, protein anabolism, and thin cervical mucus; conserve calcium and phosphorus and encourage bone formation; inhibit ovulation and prevent postpartum breast discomfort. They are responsible for the proliferation of the endometrium; absence or decline of estrogen produces signs and symptoms of menopause on the uterus, vagina, breasts, cervix; quinestrol is stored in

Adverse effects in *Italics* are most common; those in **Bold** are life-threatening.

body fat, slowly released over several days and metabolized to ethinyl estradiol.

Indications
- Palliation of moderate to severe vasomotor symptoms, atrophic vaginitis, kraurosis vulvae associated with menopause
- Treatment of female hypogonadism, female castration, primary ovarian failure

Contraindications/cautions
- Contraindicated in the presence of allergy to estrogens, breast cancer (except in specific, selected patients), estrogen-dependent neoplasm, undiagnosed abnormal genital bleeding, active thrombophlebitis or thromboembolic disorders or history of such from previous estrogen use, pregnancy (serious fetal defects; women of childbearing age should be advised of the potential risks and birth control measures suggested), lactation.
- Use caution in the presence of metabolic bone disease, renal insufficiency, CHF.

Dosage
Administer PO only.
Adult
- ***Moderate to severe vasomotor symptoms associated with menopause, atrophic vaginitis, kraurosis vulvae, female hypogonadism, female castration, primary ovarian failure:*** 100 μg/d PO for 7 d. Follow with 100 μg/wk for maintenance starting 2 wk after treatment begins. Increase dosage to 200 μg/week if the therapeutic response is not desirable or optimal.

Pediatric: Not recommended due to effect on the growth of the long bone.

Pharmacokinetics

Route	Onset	Peak
Oral	Slow	4–8 wk

Metabolism: Hepatic, $T_{1/2}$: 120 h
Distribution: Crosses placenta; enters breast milk
Excretion: Urine and bile

Adverse effects
- CNS: Steepening of the corneal curvature with a resultant change in visual acuity and intolerance to contact lenses, *headache*, migraine, dizziness, mental depression, chorea, convulsions
- GI: Gallbladder disease (in postmenopausal women), **hepatic adenoma** (rarely occurs, but may rupture and cause death), *nausea, vomiting, abdominal cramps, bloating*, cholestatic jaundice, colitis, acute pancreatitis
- CV: Increased blood pressure, thromboembolic and thrombotic disease
- Hematologic: Hypercalcemia (in breast cancer patients with bone metastases), decreased glucose tolerance
- GU: Increased risk of endometrial cancer in postmenopausal women, *breakthrough bleeding, change in menstrual flow, dysmenorrhea, premenstrual-like syndrome*, amenorrhea, vaginal candidiasis, cystitis-like syndrome, endometrial cystic hyperplasia
- Dermatologic: *Photosensitivity, peripheral edema, chloasma*, erythema nodosum or multiforme, hemorrhagic eruption, loss of scalp hair, hirsutism, urticaria, dermatitis
- Other: Weight changes, reduced carbohydrate tolerance, aggravation of porphyria, edema, changes in libido, breast tenderness

Clinically important drug-drug interactions
- Increased therapeutic and toxic effects of corticosteroids if taken concurrently • Decreased serum levels of quinestrol if taken with drugs that enhance hepatic metabolism of the drug: barbiturates, phenytoin, rifampin

Drug-lab test interferences
- Increased sulfobromophthalein retention • Increased prothrombin and factors VII, VIII, IX, and X • Decreased antithrombin III • Increased thyroid-binding globulin with increased PBI, T_4 • Increased uptake of free T_3 resin (free T_4 is unaltered) • Impaired glucose toler-

Adverse effects in *Italics* are most common; those in **Bold** are life-threatening.

ance • Decreased pregnanediol excretion • Reduced response to metyrapone test • Reduced serum folate concentration • Increased serum triglycerides and phospholipid concentration

■ Nursing Considerations
Assessment
- *History:* Allergy to estrogens, breast cancer, estrogen-dependent neoplasm, undiagnosed abnormal genital bleeding, active thrombophlebitis or thromboembolic disorders, pregnancy, lactation, metabolic bone disease, renal insufficiency, CHF
- *Physical:* Skin—color, lesions, edema; breast exam; injection site; orientation, affect, reflexes; P, auscultation, BP, peripheral perfusion; R, adventitious sounds; bowel sounds, liver evaluation, abdominal exam; pelvic exam; serum calcium, phosphorus; liver and renal function tests; Pap smear; glucose tolerance test

Implementation
- Arrange for pretreatment and periodic (at least annual) history and physical, which should include BP, breasts, abdomen, pelvic organs, and a Pap smear.
- Caution patient before beginning therapy of the risks involved with estrogen use, the need to prevent pregnancy during treatment, the need for frequent medical follow-up, the need for periodic rests from drug treatment (as appropriate).
- Administer cyclically for short term only when treating postmenopausal conditions because of the risk of endometrial neoplasm; taper to the lowest effective dose, and provide a drug-free week each month if at all possible.
- Arrange for the concomitant use of progestin therapy during chronic estrogen therapy in women; this will mimic normal physiologic cycling and allow for cyclic uterine bleeding, an effect which may decrease the risk of endometrial cancer.

Drug-specific teaching points
- Be aware that the drug must be used in cycles or for short term; prepare a calendar of drug days, rest days, and drug-free periods for the patient; many potentially serious problems have occurred with the use of this drug, including development of cancers, blood clots, liver problems.
- Arrange to have periodic medical exams throughout therapy.
- Be aware that this drug cannot be given to pregnant women because of serious toxic effects to the baby.
- Know that the following side effects may occur: nausea, vomiting, bloating; headache, dizziness, mental depression (use caution if driving or performing tasks that require alertness if this occurs); sensitivity to sunlight (use a sunscreen, and wear protective clothing until your tolerance to this effect of the drug is known); skin rash, loss of scalp hair, darkening of the skin on the face; changes in menstrual patterns.
- Report pain in the groin or calves of the legs, chest pain or sudden shortness of breath, abnormal vaginal bleeding, lumps in the breast, sudden severe headache, dizziness or fainting, changes in vision or speech, weakness or numbness in the arm or leg, severe abdominal pain, yellowing of the skin or eyes, severe mental depression.

☐ quinethazone

(kwin eth' a zone)
Aquamox (CAN), Hydromox

Pregnancy Category C

Drug classes
Thiazide-like diuretic

Therapeutic actions
Inhibits reabsorption of sodium and chloride in distal renal tubule, increasing excretion of sodium, chloride, and water by the kidney.

Indications
- Adjunctive therapy in edema associated with CHF, cirrhosis, corticosteroid and estrogen therapy, renal dysfunction
- Hypertension, as sole therapy or in combination with other antihypertensives

- Unlabeled use: diabetes insipidus, especially nephrogenic diabetes insipidus

Contraindications/cautions
- Contraindicated in the presence of fluid or electrolyte imbalances, pregnancy, lactation.
- Use caution in the presence of renal or liver disease, gout, SLE, glucose tolerance abnormalities, hyperparathyroidism, manic-depressive disorders.

Dosage
Adult: 50–100 mg qd PO. 150–200 mg/d may be needed.
Pediatric: Safety and efficacy not established.

Pharmacokinetics

Route	Onset	Peak	Duration
Oral	2 h	6 h	18–24 h

Metabolism: Hepatic, $T_{1/2}$: unknown
Distribution: Crosses placenta; enters breast milk
Excretion: Urine

Adverse effects
- CNS: *Dizziness, vertigo,* paresthesias, weakness, headache, drowsiness, fatigue, leukopenia, thrombocytopenia, agranulocytosis, aplastic anemia, neutropenia
- GI: *Nausea, anorexia, vomiting, dry mouth,* diarrhea, constipation, jaundice, hepatitis, pancreatitis
- CV: Orthostatic hypotension, venous thrombosis, volume depletion, cardiac arrhythmias, chest pain
- GU: *Polyuria, nocturia,* impotence, loss of libido
- Dermatologic: Photosensitivity, rash, purpura, exfoliative dermatitis, hives
- Other: Muscle cramps and muscle spasms, fever, gouty attacks, flushing, weight loss, rhinorrhea

Clinically important drug-drug interactions
- Risk of hyperglycemia if taken with diazoxide • Decreased absorption of quinethazone if taken with cholestyramine, colestipol • Increased risk of digitalis glycoside toxicity if hypokalemia occurs • Increased risk of lithium toxicity when taken with thiazides • Increased fasting blood glucose, leading to need to adjust dosage of antidiabetic agents.

Drug-lab test interferences
- Decreased PBI levels without clinical signs of thyroid disturbances

■ Nursing Considerations

Assessment
- *History:* Fluid or electrolyte imbalances, renal or liver disease, gout, SLE, glucose tolerance abnormalities, hyperparathyroidism, manic-depressive disorders, pregnancy, lactation
- *Physical:* Orientation, reflexes, muscle strength; pulses, BP, orthostatic BP, perfusion, edema, baseline ECG; R, adventitious sounds; liver evaluation, bowel sounds; CBC, serum electrolytes, blood glucose; liver and renal function tests; serum uric acid, urinalysis

Implementation
- Withdraw drug 2–3 d before elective surgery; reduce dosage of preanesthetic and anesthetic agents if emergency surgery is indicated.
- Administer with food or milk if GI upset occurs.
- Mark calendars or other reminders of drug days for outpatients on every other day or 3- to 5-d/wk therapy.
- Measure and record regular body weights to monitor fluid changes.

Drug-specific teaching points
- Take drug early in the day so sleep will not be disturbed by increased urination.
- Weigh yourself daily, and record weights.
- Protect skin from exposure to sun or bright lights.
- Be aware that increased urination will occur.
- Use caution if dizziness, drowsiness, feeling faint occur.
- Report rapid weight gain or loss, swelling in ankles or fingers, unusual bleeding or bruising, muscle cramps.

quinidine gluconate (contains 62% anhydrous quinidine alkaloid)

(kwin' i deen)

Duraquin, Quinaglute Dura-Tabs, Quinate (CAN), Quinatime, Quin-Release

quinidine polygalacturonate (contains 60% anhydrous quinidine alkaloid)

Cardioquin

quinidine sulfate (contains 83% anhydrous quinidine alkaloid)

Cin-Quin, Novoquindin (CAN), Quinidex Extentabs, Quinora

Pregnancy Category C

Drug classes
Antiarrhythmic

Therapeutic actions
Type 1A antiarrhythmic: decreases automaticity in ventricles, decreases height and rate of rise of action potential, decreases conduction velocity, increases fibrillation threshold.

Indications
- Treatment of atrial arrhythmias, paroxysmal or chronic ventricular tachycardia without heart block
- Maintenance therapy after electrocardioversion of atrial fibrillation or atrial flutter
- Treatment of life-threatening *P. falciperum* infections or when IV therapy (quinidine gluconate) is indicated

Contraindications/cautions
- Contraindicated in the presence of allergy or idiosyncrasy to quinidine, second- or third-degree heart block, myasthenia gravis, pregnancy (neonatal thrombocytopenia has been reported), lactation.
- Use caution in the presence of renal disease, especially renal tubular acidosis, CHF, hepatic insufficiency.

Dosage
Adult: Administer a test dose of one tablet PO or 200 mg IM to test for idiosyncratic reaction. 200–300 mg tid or qid PO or 300–600 mg q8h or q12h if sustained-release form is used.
- **Paroxysmal supraventricular arrhythmias:** 400–600 mg PO q2–3h until paroxysm is terminated.
- *IM:* Acute tachycardia: 600 mg IM quinidine gluconate, followed by 400 mg every 2 h until rhythm is stable.
- *IV:* 330 mg quinidine gluconate injected slowly IV at rate of 1 ml/min of diluted solution (10 ml of quinidine gluconate injection diluted to 50 ml with 5% glucose).

Pediatric: Safety and efficacy not established.

Pharmacokinetics

Route	Onset	Duration
Oral	1–3 h	6–8 h
IM	30–90 min	6–8 h
IV	Rapid	6–8 h

Metabolism: Hepatic, $T_{1/2}$: 6–7 h
Distribution: Crosses placenta; enters breast milk
Excretion: Urine and feces

IV facts
Preparation: Dilute 800 mg quinidine gluconate in 50 ml 5% Dextrose Injection.
Infusion: Inject slowly at rate of 1 ml/min.

Adverse effects
- **CNS:** Vision changes (photophobia, blurring, loss of night vision, diplopia)
- **GI:** *Nausea, vomiting, diarrhea*, liver toxicity
- **CV:** *Cardiac arrhythmias*, cardiac conduction disturbances, including heart block, hypotension
- **Hematologic:** Hemolytic anemia, hypoprothrombinemia, thrombocytopenic purpura, agranulocytosis, lupus erythematosus (resolves after withdrawal)

Adverse effects in *Italics* are most common; those in **Bold** are life-threatening.

970 ■ quinine sulfate

- **Hypersensitivity:** Rash, flushing, urticaria, angioedema, respiratory arrest
- **Other:** *Cinchonism* (ringing in ears, headache, nausea, dizziness, fever, tremor, visual disturbances)

Clinically important drug-drug interactions
- Increased effects and increased risk of toxicity of quinidine if taken with cimetidine, amiodarone, verapamil • Increased cardiac depressant effects if used with sodium bicarbonate, antacids • Decreased quinidine levels if given with phenobarbital, hydantoins, rifampin • Increased neuromuscular blocking effects of depolarizing and nondepolarizing neuromuscular blocking agents, succinylcholine if given with quinidine • Increased digoxin and digitoxin levels and toxicity if given with quinidine • Increased effect of oral anticoagulants and bleeding if given with quinidine

Drug-lab test interferences
- Quinidine serum levels are inaccurate if the patient is also taking triamterene

■ Nursing Considerations

Assessment
- *History:* Allergy or idiosyncrasy to quinidine, second- or third-degree heart block, myasthenia gravis, renal disease, CHF, hepatic insufficiency, pregnancy, lactation
- *Physical:* Skin—color, lesions; orientation, cranial nerves, reflexes, bilateral grip strength; P, BP, auscultation, ECG, edema; bowel sounds, liver evaluation; urinalysis, renal and liver function tests; CBC

Implementation
- Monitor patient response carefully, especially important when beginning therapy.
- Arrange for reduced dosage in patients with hepatic or renal failure.
- Arrange for reduced dosage in patients on digoxin, digitoxin; adjust dosage if phenobarbital, hydantoin, or rifampin is added or discontinued.
- Check to see that patients with atrial flutter or fibrillation have been digitalized before starting quinidine.
- Take care to differentiate the sustained-release form from the regular preparation.
- Monitor cardiac rhythm carefully, and frequently monitor BP if drug is given IV or IM.
- Arrange for periodic ECG monitoring when on long-term therapy.
- Arrange for frequent monitoring of blood counts, liver function tests during long-term therapy.
- Evaluate for safe and effective serum drug levels: 2–6 μg/ml.

Drug-specific teaching points
- Take this drug exactly as prescribed. *Do not chew* the sustained-release tablets. If GI upset occurs, you may take this drug with food.
- Be aware that frequent monitoring of cardiac rhythm, blood tests will be needed.
- Know that the following side effects may occur: nausea, loss of appetite, vomiting (small, frequent meals may help); dizziness, lightheadedness, vision changes (do not drive a car or operate dangerous machinery if these drug effects occur); rash (careful skin care is important).
- Wear a medical alert tag stating that you are on this drug.
- Return for regular follow-up visits to check your heart rhythm and blood counts.
- Report sore mouth, throat, gums, fever, chills, cold or flulike syndromes, ringing in the ears, severe vision disturbances, headache, unusual bleeding or bruising.

❐ quinine sulfate

(kwi' nine)

Formula Q, Legatrin, M-KYA, Quinamm, Quiphile, Q-vel

Pregnancy Category X

Adverse effects in *Italics* are most common; those in **Bold** are life-threatening.

quinine sulfate

Drug classes
Antimalarial
Skeletal muscle relaxant

Therapeutic actions
Believed to act by entering plasmodial DNA molecules, reducing effectiveness of DNA as template; also affects many enzyme systems of the plasmodia, depresses oxygen uptake and carbohydrate metabolism (antimalarial). Increases the refractory period by direct action on the muscle fiber, decreases the excitability of the motor-end plate by a curariform action, and affects intracellular calcium distribution (skeletal muscle relaxant).

Indications
- Treatment of chloroquine-resistant falciparum malaria as an adjunct with pyrimethamine and sulfadiazine or tetracycline
- Prevention and treatment of nocturnal recumbency leg cramps, including those associated with arthritis, diabetes, varicose veins, thrombophlebitis, arteriosclerosis, static foot deformities

Contraindications/cautions
- Contraindicated in the presence of allergy to quinine, G-6-PD deficiency, optic neuritis, tinnitus, history of blackwater fever, pregnancy, lactation.
- Use caution in the presence of cardiac arrhythmias.

Dosage
Adult
- ***Chloroquine resistant malaria:*** 650 mg q8h PO for 5–7 d.
- ***Chloroquine sensitive malaria:*** 600 mg q8h PO for 5–7 d.
- ***Nocturnal leg cramps:*** 260–300 mg PO at bedtime. May be taken after the evening meal and at bedtime.

Pediatric
- ***Chloroquine resistant malaria:*** 25 mg/kg per day given q8h PO for 5–7 d.
- ***Chloroquine sensitive malaria:*** 10 mg/kg PO q8h for 5–7 d.

Pharmacokinetics

Route	Onset	Peak
Oral	Varies	1–3 h

Metabolism: Hepatic, $T_{1/2}$: 4–5 h
Distribution: Crosses placenta; enters breast milk
Excretion: Urine

Adverse effects
- **CNS:** *Visual disturbances*, including disturbed color vision and perception, photophobia, blurred vision with scotomata, night blindness, amblyopia, diplopia, diminished visual fields, mydriasis, optic atrophy; tinnitus, deafness, vertigo; headache; fever; apprehension, restlessness, confusion; syncope, excitement; delirium; hypothermia; convulsions
- **GI:** *Nausea, vomiting,* epigastric pain, hepatitis, diarrhea
- **Hematologic:** Acute hemolysis, hemolytic anemia, thrombocytopenia purpura, agranulocytosis, hypoprothrombinemia
- **Hypersensitivity:** Cutaneous rashes, pruritus, flushing, sweating, facial edema, asthmatic symptoms
- **Other:** *Cinchonism* (tinnitus, headache, nausea, slightly disturbed vision, GI upset, nervousness, cardiovascular effects), anginal symptoms

Clinically important drug-drug interactions
- Increased serum levels of digoxin and digitoxin if taken concurrently with quinidine, possible interaction with quinine
- Increased effectiveness of neuromuscular blocking agents, succinylcholine, and possible respiratory difficulties if taken concurrently
- Increased anticoagulant effect of warfarin, other oral anticoagulants if taken concurrently

Drug-lab test interferences
- Interference with results of 17-hydroxycorticosteroid determinations
- Falsely elevated levels of 17 ketogenic steroids using the Zimmerman method

Adverse effects in *Italics* are most common; those in **Bold** are life-threatening.

Nursing Considerations

Assessment
- *History:* Allergy to quinine, G-6-PD deficiency, optic neuritis, tinnitus, history of blackwater fever, cardiac arrhythmias, pregnancy, lactation
- *Physical:* Skin—color, lesions; body temperature; orientation, affect, reflexes, ophthalmic examination, audiologic examination; P, rhythm; liver evaluation; CBC, differential; prothrombin time; G-6-PD in appropriate patients

Implementation
- Administer with food or meals to decrease GI upset.
- Administer with pyrimethamine and sulfadiazine or tetracycline if given to treat malaria.
- Arrange to discontinue drug at any sign of hypersensitivity or cinchonism.
- Monitor CBC and differential periodically during therapy.

Drug-specific teaching points
- Take drug with food or meals to decrease GI upset. Take at bedtime if used for night-time leg cramps.
- Know that the following side effects may occur: dizziness, fainting, confusion, restlessness, blurred vision (use caution if driving or performing tasks that require alertness if these effects occur); diarrhea, nausea, stomach cramps, vomiting (taking the drug with food or meals may help); blurred vision; decreased hearing; ringing in the ears.
- Be aware that this drug should not be taken during pregnancy; serious birth defects may occur. If you think you are pregnant or are trying to become pregnant, consult your nurse or physician.
- Report severe ringing in the ears, headache, marked changes in vision, unusual bleeding or bruising, marked loss of hearing, fever, chills.

☐ ramipril

(ra mi' prill)
Altace
Pregnancy Category C

Drug classes
Antihypertensive
Angiotensin-converting enzyme (ACE) inhibitor

Therapeutic actions
Ramipril blocks ACE from converting angiotensin I to angiotensin II, a powerful vasoconstrictor, leading to decreased blood pressure, decreased aldosterone secretion, a small increase in serum potassium levels, and sodium and fluid loss; increased prostaglandin synthesis also may be involved in the antihypertensive action.

Indications
- Treatment of hypertension alone or in combination with thiazide-type diuretics

Contraindications/cautions
- Contraindicated in the presence of allergy to ramipril, pregnancy (embryocidal in preclinical studies).
- Use caution in the presence of impaired renal function, CHF, salt/volume depletion, lactation.

Dosage
Adult: Initial dose 2.5 mg PO qd. Adjust dose according to blood pressure response, usually 2.5–20 mg/d as a single dose or in two equally divided doses. Discontinue diuretic 2–3 d before beginning therapy; if not possible, administer initial dose of 1.25 mg.
Pediatric: Safety and efficacy not established.
Geriatric and renal impaired: Excretion is reduced in renal failure; use smaller initial dose, 1.25 mg PO qd in patients with Ccr < 40 ml/min; dosage may be titrated upward until pressure is controlled or a maximum of 5 mg/d.

Pharmacokinetics

Route	Onset	Peak	Duration
Oral	1–2 h	1–4 h	24 h

Metabolism: Hepatic, $T_{1/2}$: 13–17 h
Distribution: Crosses placenta; enters breast milk
Excretion: Urine and feces

Adverse effects
- **GI:** *Gastric irritation, aphthous ulcers, peptic ulcers, dysgeusia,* cholestatic jaundice, hepatocellular injury, anorexia, constipation
- **CV:** *Tachycardia,* angina pectoris, myocardial infarction, Raynaud's syndrome, CHF, hypotension in salt/volume depleted patients
- **Hematologic:** Neutropenia, agranulocytosis, thrombocytopenia, hemolytic anemia, **fatal pancytopenia**
- **GU:** *Proteinuria,* renal insufficiency, renal failure, polyuria, oliguria, urinary frequency
- **Dermatologic:** *Rash, pruritus,* pemphigoid-like reaction, scalded mouth sensation, exfoliative dermatitis, photosensitivity, alopecia
- **Other:** *Cough,* malaise, dry mouth, lymphadenopathy

Clinically important drug-drug interactions
- Decreased absorption of ramipril may occur if taken with food

Drug-lab test interferences
- False-positive test for urine acetone.

■ Nursing Considerations

Assessment
- *History:* Allergy to ramipril, impaired renal function, CHF, salt/volume depletion, pregnancy, lactation
- *Physical:* Skin—color, lesions, turgor; body temperature; P, BP, peripheral perfusion; mucous membranes, bowel sounds, liver evaluation; urinalysis, renal and liver function tests, CBC and differential

Implementation
- Administer 1 h before or 2 h after meals.
- Discontinue diuretic for 2–3 d before beginning ramipril therapy, if possible, to avoid severe hypotensive effect.
- Alert surgeon and mark patient's chart with notice that ramipril is being taken; the angiotensin II formation subsequent to compensatory renin release during surgery will be blocked; hypotension may be reversed with volume expansion.
- Monitor patient closely in any situation that may lead to a fall in blood pressure secondary to reduction in fluid volume (excessive perspiration and dehydration, vomiting, diarrhea) because excessive hypotension may occur.
- Arrange for reduced dosage in patients with impaired renal function.

Drug-specific teaching points
- Take drug 1 h before meals. Do not stop taking the medication without consulting your prescriber.
- Know that the following side effects may occur: GI upset, loss of appetite, change in taste perception (these may be limited effects that will pass with time; mouth sores (frequent mouth care may help); skin rash; fast heart rate; dizziness, lightheadedness (this usually passes after the first few days of therapy; if it occurs, change position slowly, and limit your activities to those that do not require alertness and precision).
- Be careful in any situation that may lead to a drop in blood pressure (diarrhea, sweating, vomiting, dehydration); if lightheadedness or dizziness should occur, consult your nurse or physician.
- Report mouth sores; sore throat, fever, chills; swelling of the hands, feet; irregular heartbeat, chest pains; swelling of the face, eyes, lips, tongue, difficulty in breathing.

❒ ranitidine

(ra nye' te deen)
Zantac

Pregnancy Category B

Drug classes
Histamine$_2$ (H$_2$) antagonist

Therapeutic actions
Competitively inhibits the action of histamine at the histamine$_2$ (H$_2$) receptors

---

Adverse effects in *Italics* are most common; those in **Bold** are life-threatening.

of the parietal cells of the stomach, inhibiting basal gastric acid secretion and gastric acid secretion that is stimulated by food, insulin, histamine, cholinergic agonists, gastrin, and pentagastrin.

Indications
- Short-term treatment of active duodenal ulcer
- Maintenance therapy for duodenal ulcer at reduced dosage
- Short-term treatment of active, benign gastric ulcer
- Short-term treatment of gastroesophageal reflux disease
- Pathologic hypersecretory conditions (eg, Zollinger-Ellison syndrome)
- Treatment of erosive esophagitis

Contraindications/cautions
- Contraindicated in the presence of allergy to ranitidine, lactation.
- Use caution in the presence of impaired renal or hepatic function.

Dosage
Adult
- ***Active duodenal ulcer:*** 150 mg bid PO for 4–8 wk. Alternatively, 300 mg PO once daily at bedtime *or* 50 mg IM or IV q6–8h *or* by intermittent IV infusion, diluted to 100 ml and infused over 15–20 min. Do not exceed 400 mg/d.
- ***Maintenance therapy, duodenal ulcer:*** 150 mg PO at bedtime.
- ***Active gastric ulcer:*** 150 mg bid PO *or* 50 mg IM or IV q6–8h.
- ***Pathologic hypersecretory syndrome:*** 150 mg bid PO. Individualize dose with patient's response. *Do not exceed 6 g/d.*
- ***Gastroesophageal reflux disease, esophagitis, benign gastric ulcer:*** 150 mg bid PO.

Pediatric: Safety and efficacy not established.

Geriatric or impaired renal function: Ccr < 50 ml/min, accumulation may occur; use lowest dose possible, 150 mg q24h PO *or* 50 mg IM or IV q18–24 h. Dosing may be increased to q12h if patient tolerates it and blood levels are monitored.

Pharmacokinetics

Route	Onset	Peak	Duration
Oral	Varies	1–3 h	8–12 h
IM	Rapid	15 min	8–12 h
IV	Immediate	5–10 min	8–12 h

Metabolism: Hepatic, $T_{1/2}$: 2–3 h
Distribution: Crosses placenta; enters breast milk
Excretion: Urine

IV facts
Preparation: For IV injection, dilute 50 mg in 0.9% Sodium Chloride Injection, 5% or 10% Dextrose Injection, Lactated Ringer's Solution, 5% Sodium Bicarbonate Injection to a volume of 20 ml; solution is stable for 48 h at room temperature. For intermittent IV, use as follows: dilute 50 mg in 100 ml of 5% Dextrose Injection or other compatible solution

Infusion: Inject over 5 min or more; for intermittent infusion, infuse over 15–20 min; continuous infusion, 6.25 mg/h

Adverse effects
- CNS: *Headache,* malaise, dizziness, somnolence, insomnia, vertigo
- GI: *Constipation, diarrhea, nausea, vomiting, abdominal pain,* hepatitis, increased SGPT levels
- CV: Tachycardia, bradycardia, PVCs (rapid IV administration)
- Hematologic: Leukopenia, granulocytopenia, thrombocytopenia, pancytopenia
- GU: Gynecomastia, impotence or loss of libido
- Dermatologic: *Rash,* alopecia
- Local: *Pain at IM site, local burning or itching at IV site*
- Other: Arthralgias

Clinically important drug-drug interactions
- Increased effects of warfarin, tricyclic antidepressants taken with ranitidine • Decreased effectiveness of diazepam if taken concurrently • Decreased clearance and

possible increased toxicity of lidocaine, nifedipine if given concurrently

■ Nursing Considerations

Assessment
- *History:* Allergy to ranitidine, impaired renal or hepatic function, lactation
- *Physical:* Skin—lesions; orientation, affect; pulse, baseline ECG; liver evaluation, abdominal exam, normal output; CBC, liver and renal function tests

Implementation
- Administer oral drug with meals and at bedtime.
- Arrange for decreased doses in renal and liver failure.
- Arrange for administration of concurrent antacid therapy to relieve pain.
- Administer IM dose undiluted, deep into large muscle group.
- Arrange for regular follow-up including blood tests to evaluate effects.

Drug-specific teaching points
- Take drug with meals and at bedtime. Therapy may continue for 4–6 wk or longer.
- Be aware that if you also are on an antacid, you should take it exactly as it has been prescribed, being careful of the times of administration.
- Arrange to have regular medical follow-up while you are on this drug to evaluate your response.
- Know that the following side effects may occur: constipation or diarrhea (if this becomes uncomfortable, notify your nurse or physician); nausea, vomiting (taking the drug with meals may help); enlargement of breasts, impotence or loss of libido (these are reversible and will pass when the drug therapy has been discontinued); headache (monitoring lights, temperature, noise levels may help).
- Report sore throat, fever, unusual bruising or bleeding, tarry stools, confusion, hallucinations, dizziness, severe headache, muscle or joint pain.

▢ rauwolfia derivatives

*(rab **wool'** fee a)*

whole root rauwolfia
Raudixin

reserpine (re ser' peen)
Reserfia (CAN)

Pregnancy Category C

Drug classes
Antihypertensive drug
Adrenergic neuron blocking drug

Therapeutic actions
Whole root rauwolfia is a combination of alkaloids; reserpine is one of the alkaloids extracted from whole root rauwolfia and refined; antihypertensive effects depend on depletion of the neurotransmitter norepinephrine from postganglionic sympathetic adrenergic nerve terminals; sedative and tranquilizing effects are thought to depend on depletion of biogenic amines (norepinephrine, serotonin, dopamine) in the CNS.

Indications
- Relief of symptoms in agitated psychotic states (eg, schizophrenia), primarily in patients unable to tolerate phenothiazines or who require antihypertensive medication (seldom used solely for antihypertensive effects)
- Treatment of mild essential hypertension; adjunctive therapy in the treatment of severe hypertension

Contraindications/cautions
- Contraindicated in the presence of hypersensitivity to rauwolfia derivatives, tartrazine (in preparations of whole root rauwolfia marketed as *Raudixin*); history of bronchial asthma or allergy; emotional depression (especially with suicidal tendencies), patients receiving electroconvulsive therapy; active peptic ulcer, ulcerative colitis; pheochromocytoma; pregnancy (neonates born to mothers receiving reserpine near term have shown increased respiratory secretions, nasal

congestion, cyanosis, retractions, lethargy, anorexia); lactation.
- Use caution in the presence of gallstones, renal or hepatic dysfunction.

Dosage
Orally, 200–300 mg of powdered whole root = 0.5 mg reserpine.

Adult
- ***Whole root rauwolfia:*** Average dose is 200–400 mg/d PO, given in two divided doses. Use higher doses cautiously as emotional depression, other adverse effects may increase considerably. Maintenance dosage, 50–300 mg/d PO given as a single dose or as two divided doses.
- ***Reserpine***
 – *Hypertension:* Initial dose of 0.5 mg/d PO for 1 or 2 wk. Reduce to 0.1–0.25 mg/d for maintenance. Use higher doses cautiously; serious emotional depression and other adverse effects may increase considerably.
 – *Psychiatric disorders:* Average initial dose is 0.5 mg/d PO (range 0.1–1 mg/d).

Pediatric: Safety and efficacy not established.

Geriatric or impaired renal or hepatic function: Use caution.

Pharmacokinetics

Route	Onset	Peak
Oral	Slow	3–3½ h

Metabolism: Hepatic, $T_{1/2}$: 4.5–11.3 h
Distribution: Crosses placenta; enters breast milk
Excretion: Urine

Adverse effects
- CNS: *Drowsiness, depression, nervousness, dizziness, headache,* paradoxical anxiety, nightmares, parkinsonian syndrome, extrapyramidal symptoms, deafness, glaucoma, uveitis, optic atrophy, conjunctival reddening
- GI: *Diarrhea, hypersecretion, nausea, vomiting,* anorexia, GI bleeding, dry mouth
- CV: Angina-like symptoms, arrhythmias, bradycardia, syncope, orthostatic hypotension
- Respiratory: *Nasal congestion (frequent),* dyspnea, epistaxis
- Hematologic: Thrombocytopenic purpura, other hematologic reactions
- GU: *Impotence or decreased libido,* dysuria
- Dermatologic: Pruritus, rash
- Other: *Muscle aches,* asthma in asthmatic patients; breast enlargement, pseudolactation, gynecomastia; possibly increased risk of breast carcinoma

Clinically important drug-drug interactions
- Decreased response to indirect-acting sympathomimetic drugs (ephedrine, mephentermine)

Drug-lab test interferences
- Reserpine may interfere with tests for 17-ketosteroids, 17-hydroxycorticosteroids

■ Nursing Considerations

Assessment
- *History:* Hypersensitivity to rauwolfia derivatives, tartrazine; bronchial asthma or allergy; emotional depression; electroconvulsive therapy; active peptic ulcer, ulcerative colitis; pheochromocytoma; gallstones; renal or hepatic dysfunction; pregnancy; lactation
- *Physical:* Body weight; skin—color, lesions; status of nasal mucous membranes; orientation, affect, reflexes; ophthalmologic exam with tonometry; P, BP, orthostatic BP, perfusion, edema, auscultation; R, adventitious sounds; bowel sounds, normal output, liver evaluation; breast exam; liver and kidney function tests, urinalysis; CBC and differential; stool guaiac test

Implementation
- Arrange to discontinue rauwolfia alkaloids, reserpine at the first sign of despondency, early morning insomnia, loss of appetite, impotence, or self-deprecation; drug-induced depression may persist for several months after withdrawal of drug

and may be severe enough to result in suicide.
- Arrange to discontinue rauwolfia/reserpine therapy at least 2 wk before electroshock therapy.

Drug-specific teaching points
- Take this drug exactly as prescribed; do not miss doses.
- Know that the following side effects may occur: drowsiness, dizziness, lightheadedness, headache, weakness (these are often transient symptoms that occur when you begin treatment or when the dosage is increased; avoid driving a car or engaging in tasks that require alertness while you are experiencing these symptoms); GI upset (frequent, small meals may help); dreams, nightmares (it may help to know that these are drug effects that will go away when the drug is discontinued); dizziness, lightheadedness when you get up (get up slowly; use caution when climbing stairs); impotence, failure of ejaculation, decreased libido; breast enlargement, sore breasts; stuffy nose.
- Report bruising, nose bleeds, skin rash, depression or loss of interest in surroundings, habitual early morning awakening, "gnawing" abdominal pain in the middle of the night, painful urination, black or tarry stools, bloody stools.

◻ ribavirin

(rye ba vye' rin)
Virazole

Pregnancy Category X

Drug classes
Antiviral drug

Therapeutic actions
Antiviral activity against respiratory syncytial virus (RSV), influenza virus, and herpes simplex virus; mechnanism of action is not known.

Indications
- Carefully selected hospitalized infants and children with RSV infection of lower respiratory tract
- Orphan drug use: treatment of hemorrhagic fever with renal syndrome
- Unlabeled use for aerosol: treatment of some influenza A and B infections
- Unlabeled uses of oral preparation: treatment of some viral diseases, including acute and chronic hepatitis, herpes genitalis, measles, Lassa fever

Contraindications/cautions
- Allergy to drug product, COPD, pregnancy (causes fetal damage), lactation.

Dosage
For use only with small-particle aerosol generator. Check operating instructions carefully.
Adult or Pediatric: Dilute to 20 mg per ml and deliver for 12–18 h/d for at least 3 but not more than 7 d.

Pharmacokinetics

Route	Onset	Peak
Aerosol	Slow	60–90 min

Metabolism: Cellular, $T_{1/2}$: 9.5 h
Distribution: Crosses placenta; enters breast milk
Excretion: Urine and feces

Adverse effects
- **CV:** Cardiac arrest, hypotension
- **Respiratory:** *Deteriorating respiratory function*, pneuomothorax, apnea, bacterial pneumonia
- **Hematologic:** Anemia
- **Dermatologic:** Skin rash
- **Other:** Conjuctivitis

Clinically important drug-drug interactions
- Increased likelihood of digitalis toxicity if taken concurrently with ribavirin

■ Nursing Considerations
Assessment
- *History:* Allergy to drug product, COPD, pregnancy, lactation

- *Physical:* Skin—rashes, lesions; P, BP, auscultation; R, adventitious sounds; Hct

Implementation
- Ensure proper use of small-particle aerosol generator; check operating instructions carefully.
- Ensure that water used as diluent should not contain any other substance.
- Replace solution in the unit every 24 h.
- Store

- Prepare patient for the reddish-orange coloring of body fluids (urine, sweat, sputum, tears, feces, saliva); soft contact lenses may be permanently stained; patients should be advised not to wear them during drug therapy.
- Arrange for follow-up of evaluation of hematologic profile.

Drug-specific teaching points
- Take drug in a single daily dose. Take on an empty stomach, 1 h before or 2 h after meals.
- Take this drug regularly; avoid missing any doses; *do not* discontinue this drug without first consulting your health care provider.
- Know that the following side effects may occur: reddish-orange coloring of body fluids (tears, sweat, saliva, urine, feces, sputum; this is an expected occurence and is not dangerous; do not be alarmed; stain will wash out of clothing, but soft contact lenses may be permanently stained; do not wear them when on this drug); nausea, vomiting, epigastric distress (the drug dosage may need to be divided).
- Arrange to have periodic medical check-ups, which will include blood tests to evaluate the drug effects.
- Report fever, chills, muscle and bone pain, excessive tiredness or weakness, loss of appetite, nausea, vomiting, yellowing of eyes.

☐ rifampin

(rif am pin)
Rifadin, Rimactane, Rofact (CAN)

Pregnancy Category C

Drug classes
Antituberculous drug ("first-line")
Antibiotic

Therapeutic actions
Inhibits DNA-dependent RNA polymerase activity in susceptible bacterial cells.

Indications
- Treatment of pulmonary tuberculosis in conjunction with at least one other effective antituberculous drug
- Neisseria meningitidis carriers, for asymptomatic carriers to eliminate meningococci from nasopharynx; not for treatment of meningitis
- Unlabeled uses: infections caused by *Staphylococcus aureus* and *Staphylococcus epidermis*, usually in combination therapy; gram-negative bacteremia in infancy; Legionella (*Legionella pneumophilia*), not responsive to erythromycin; leprosy (in combination with dapsone); prophylaxis of meningitis due to *Haemophilus influenzae*

Contraindications/cautions
- Contraindicated in the presence of allergy to any rifamycin, acute hepatic disease, nursing a baby.
- Use caution in pregnancy (teratogenic effects have been reported in preclinical studies; safest antituberculous regimen for use in pregnancy is considered to be rifampin, isoniazid, and ethambutol).

Dosage
Adult
- ***Pulmonary tuberculosis:*** 600 mg in a single daily dose PO or IV (used in conjunction with other antituberculous drugs). Continue therapy until bacterial conversion and maximal improvement occur.
- ***Meningococcal carriers:*** 600 mg PO or IV once daily for 4 consecutive d.

Pediatric (> 5 y)
- ***Pulmonary tuberculosis:*** 10–20 mg/kg per day PO or IV not to exceed 600 mg/d.
- ***Meningococcal carriers:*** 10–20 mg/kg PO or IV once daily for 4 consecutive d, not to exceed 600 mg/d.

Pharmacokinetics

Route	Onset	Peak
Oral	Varies	1–4 h
IV	Rapid	End of infusion

Metabolism: Hepatic, $T_{1/2}$: 3–5.1 h

Distribution: Crosses placenta; enters breast milk
Excretion: Feces and urine

IV facts
Preparation: Reconstitute by transferring 10 ml Sterile Water for Injection to vial containing 600 mg rifampin; swirl gently. Resultant fluid contains 60 mg/ml; stable at room temperature. Further mix with 500–100 ml of Dextrose 5% or Sterile Saline.

Infusion: Infuse over 30–180 min, depending on volume.

Adverse effects
- CNS: *Headache, drowsiness, fatigue, dizziness,* inability to concentrate, mental confusion, generalized numbness, ataxia, muscle weakness, visual disturbances, exudative conjunctivitis
- GI: *Heartburn, epigastric distress,* anorexia, nausea, vomiting, gas, cramps, diarrhea, pseudomembranous colitis, pancreatitis, *elevations of liver enzymes,* hepatitis
- Hematologic: *Eosinophilia, thrombocytopenia, transient leukopenia,* hemolytic anemia, decreased hemoglobin, hemolysis
- GU: Hemoglobinuria, hematuria, renal insufficiency, acute renal failure, menstrual disturbances
- Dermatologic: *Rash,* pruritus, urticaria, pemphigoid reaction, flushing, reddish-orange discoloration of body fluids—tears, saliva, urine, sweat, sputum
- Other: Pain in extremities, osteomalacia, myopathy, fever, *"flulike" syndrome*

Clinically important drug-drug interactions
- Increased incidence of rifampin-related hepatitis if taken with isoniazid • Decreased effectiveness of rifampin if taken with p-aminosalicyclic acid, ketoconazole; give the drugs at least 8–12 h apart • Decreased effectiveness of metoprolol, propranolol, quinidine, corticosteroids, oral contraceptives, methadone, oral anticoagulants, oral sulfonylureas, digitoxin, theophyllines, phenytoin, cyclosporine, ketoconazole, verapamil if taken concurrently with rifampin

Drug-lab test interferences
- Rifampin inhibits the standard assays for serum folate and vitamin B_{12}

■ Nursing Considerations

Assessment
- *History:* Allergy to any rifamycin, acute hepatic disease, pregnancy, lactation
- *Physical:* Skin—color, lesions; temperature; gait, muscle strength; orientation, reflexes, ophthalmologic examination; liver evaluation; CBC, liver and renal function tests, urinalysis

Implementation
- Administer on an empty stomach, 1 h before or 2 h after meals.
- Administer in a single daily dose.
- Consult pharmacist for preparation of rifampin suspension for children and adults who cannot swallow capsules.
- Prepare patient for the reddish-orange coloring of body fluids (urine, sweat, sputum, tears, feces, saliva); soft contact lenses may be permanently stained; patients should be advised not to wear them during drug therapy.
- Arrange for follow-up of liver and renal function tests, CBC, ophthalmologic examinations.

Drug-specific teaching points
- Take drug in a single daily dose. Take on an empty stomach, 1 h before or 2 h after meals.
- Take this drug regularly; avoid missing any doses; *do not* discontinue this drug without first consulting your physician.
- Know that the following side effects may occur: reddish-orange coloring of body fluids (tears, sweat, saliva, urine, feces, sputum; this is an expected occurence and is not dangerous; do not be alarmed; stain will wash out of clothing, but soft contact lenses may be permanently stained; do not wear them when on this

drug); nausea, vomiting, epigastric distress; skin rashes or lesions; numbness, tingling, drowsiness, fatigue (use caution if driving a car or operating dangerous machinery; use precautions to avoid injury).
- Arrange to have periodic medical checkups, which will include an eye examination and blood tests to evaluate the drug effects.
- Report fever, chills, muscle and bone pain, excessive tiredness or weakness, loss of appetite, nausea, vomiting, yellowing of skin or eyes, unusual bleeding or bruising, skin rash or itching.

rimantadine HCl

(ri man' ta deen)
Flumadine

Pregnancy Category C

Drug classes
Antiviral drug

Therapeutic actions
Synthetic antiviral agent that inhibits viral replication, possibly by preventing the uncoating of the virus.

Indications
- Prophylaxis and treatment of illness caused by influenza A virus in adults
- Prophylaxis against influenza A virus in children

Contraindications/cautions
- Allergy to amantadine, rimantadine; lactation.
- Use caution in the presence of seizures, liver or renal disease, pregnancy.

Dosage
Adult and pediatric > 10 y
- ***Prophylaxis:*** 100 mg/d PO bid.
- ***Treatment:*** Same dose as above; start treatment as soon after exposure as possible, continuing for 7 d.
- ***Patients with renal/hepatic disease:*** Dose of 100 mg PO qd is recommended.

Pediatric
- ***Prophylaxis for < 10 y:*** 5 mg/kg PO qd; do not exceed 150 mg/d.

Pharmacokinetics

Route	Onset	Peak
Oral	Slow	6 h

Metabolism: $T_{1/2}$: 25.4 h
Distribution: Crosses placenta; enters breast milk
Excretion: Unchanged in the urine

Adverse effects
- **CNS:** *Lightheadedness, dizziness, insomnia,* confusion, irritability, ataxia, psychosis, depression, hallucinations
- **GI:** *Nausea,* anorexia, constipation, dry mouth
- **CV:** CHF, orthostatic hypotension, dyspnea
- **GU:** Urinary retention

Clinically important drug-drug interactions
- Decreased effectiveness of rimantidine if taken with acetaminophen, aspirin • Increased serum levels and effects of rimantidine if taken with cimetidine

■ Nursing Considerations

Assessment
- *History:* Allergy to amantadine, rimantidine; seizures; liver or renal disease; lactation
- *Physical:* Orientation, vision, speech, reflexes; BP, orthostatic BP, P, auscultation, perfusion, edema; R, adventitious sounds; urinary output; BUN, creatinine clearance

Implementation
- Administer full course of drug to achieve the beneficial antiviral effects.

Drug-specific teaching points
- Know that the following may occur as a result of the drug therapy: drowsiness, blurred vision (use caution in driving or using dangerous equipment while on this drug); dizziness, lightheadedness (avoid sudden position changes); irritability or

Adverse effects in *Italics* are most common; those in **Bold** are life-threatening.

mood changes (this is often an effect of the drug; if this becomes severe, the drug may need to be changed).
- Report swelling of the fingers or ankles, shortness of breath, difficulty urinating, tremors, slurred speech, difficulty walking.

▢ risperidone

*(ris **peer**' i dohn)*
Risperdal

Pregnancy Category C

Drug classes
Antipsychotic drug
Benzisoxazole

Therapeutic actions
Mechanism of action not fully understood: blocks dopamine and serotonin receptors in the brain, depresses the reticular activating system; anticholinergic, antihistaminic, and alpha-adrenergic blocking activity may contribute to some of its therapeutic and adverse actions.

Indications
- Management of the manifestations of psychotic disorders

Contraindications/cautions
- Contraindicated in the presence of allergy to risperidone, lactation.
- Use caution in the presence of cardiovascular disease, pregnancy, renal or hepatic impairment, hypotension.

Dosage
Adult:Initially: 1 mg PO bid; then gradually continue to increase with daily dosage increments of 1 mg/d on the second and third days to a target dose of 3 mg PO bid by the third day. *Reinitiation of treatment:* Follow initial dosage guidelines, using extreme care due to increased risk of severe adverse effects with reexposure. *Switching from other antipsychotics:* minimize the overlap period and discontinue other antipsychotic before beginning risperidone therapy.

Pediatric: Safety and efficacy not established.
Geriatric or renal/hepatic impaired: Initial dose of 0.5 mg PO bid; monitor patient for adverse effects and response.

Pharmacokinetics

Route	Onset	Peak	Duration
Oral	Varies	3–17 h	weeks

Metabolism: Hepatic, $T_{1/2}$: 20 h
Distribution: Crosses placenta; enters breast milk
Excretion: Urine and feces

Adverse effects
- **CNS:** *Insomnia, anxiety, agitation, headache,* somnolence, aggression. dizziness, **tardive dyskinesias**
- **GI:** *Nausea, vomiting, constipation,* abdominal discomfort, dry mouth, increased saliva
- **CV:** Orthostatic hypotension, arrhythmias
- **Respiratory:** Rhinitis, coughing, sinusitis, pharyngitis, dyspnea
- **Dermatologic:** Rash, dry skin, seborrhea, photosensitivity
- **Other:** Chest pain, arthralgia, back pain, fever, **neuroleptic malignant syndrome**

Clinically important drug-drug interactions
- Increased therapeutic and toxic effects of risperidone if taken with clozapine • Decreased therapeutic effect of risperidone if taken with carbamazepine • Decreased effectiveness of levodopa if taken concurrently

■ Nursing Considerations

Assessment
- *History:* Allergy to risperidone, lactation, cardiovascular disease, pregnancy, renal or hepatic impairment, hypotension
- *Physical:* Body temperature, weight; reflexes, orientation; P, BP, orthostatic BP; R, adventitious sounds; bowel sounds, normal output, liver evaluation; CBC, urinalysis, liver and kidney function tests

Adverse effects in *Italics* are most common; those in **Bold** are life-threatening.

Implementation
- Maintain seizure precautions, especially when initiating therapy and increasing dosage.
- Monitor body temperature. If fever occurs, determine that no underlying infection is present, and consult physician for appropriate comfort measures.
- Advise patient to use some form of contraception during drug therapy.
- Follow guidelines for discontinuation or reinstitution of the drug carefully.

Drug-specific teaching points
- Be aware that dosage will be increased gradually to achieve most effective dose. Do not take more than your prescribed dosage. Do not make up missed doses, contact your nurse of physician if this occurs. Do not stop taking this drug suddenly; gradual reduction of dosage is needed to prevent side effects.
- Know that the following effects may occur as a result of drug therapy: drowsiness, dizziness, sedation, seizures (avoid driving a car, operating machinery, or performing tasks that require concentration); dizziness, faintness on arising (change positions slowly; use caution if this occurs); increased salivation (it might help to know that this is a drug effect; constipation; sensitivity to the sun (use a sunscreen or protective clothing if exposure to the sun is unavoidable).
- Know that this drug cannot be taken during pregnancy. If you think you are pregnant or wish to become pregnant, contact your nurse or physician.
- Report lethargy, weakness, fever, sore throat, malaise, mouth ulcers, palpitations.

▢ ritodrine hydrochloride

(ri' toe dreen)
Yutopar

Pregnancy Category B

Drug classes
Sympathomimetic drug
Beta$_2$-selective adrenergic agonist

Tocolytic drug (uterine relaxant): In low doses, acts relatively selectively to relax the pregnant uterus; at higher doses, beta$_2$ selectivity is lost and the drug also acts as beta$_1$ receptors to cause typical sympathomimetic cardiac effects.

Indications
- Management of preterm labor in selected patients; IV ritodrine is used to arrest the acute episode, oral ritodrine to avert relapse

Contraindications/cautions
- Contraindicated in the presence of hypersensitivity to ritodrine or components of preparation (ritodrine injection contains sodium metabisulfite; some patients are allergic to sulfites); pregnancies of shorter duration than 20 wk; antepartum hemorrhage; eclampsia and severe preeclampsia; intrauterine fetal death; chorioamnionitis; maternal cardiac disease; pulmonary hypertension; maternal hyperthyroidism; uncontrolled maternal diabetes mellitus; preexisting maternal medical conditions that would be seriously affected by a beta-adrenergic agonist, such as hypovolemia, cardiac arrhythmias associated with tachycardia or digitalis toxicity, uncontrolled hypertension, pheochromocytoma, bronchial asthma already treated by betamimetics or steroids.

Dosage
Individualize dosage by balancing uterine response and unwanted effects. The following is a guide to safe and effective dosage.
IV: 0.1 mg/min initially (0.33 ml/min or 20 drops/min using a microdrip chamber at the recommended dilution; see below). Gradually increase by 0.05 mg/min (10 drops/min) every 10 min until desired result is attained. Usual effective dosage is between 0.15 and 0.35 mg/min (30–70 drops/min) continued for at least 12 h after uterine contractions cease.
Oral maintenance: 10 mg PO approximately 30 min before terminating IV therapy. Usual dosage for first 24 h of oral therapy is 10 mg q2h; thereafter, 10–20 mg q4–6h. Do not exceed total daily dose of 120 mg.

984 ■ ritodrine hydrochloride

Pharmacokinetics

Route	Onset	Peak
Oral	Varies	30–60 min
IV	Rapid	

Metabolism: Hepatic, $T_{1/2}$: 1.7–2.6 h
Distribution: Crosses placenta; enters breast milk
Excretion: Urine

IV facts

Preparation: Empty the contents of three ampuls (50 mg/ampul; total of 150 mg) into 500 ml of compatible IV diluent to make a solution of 0.3 mg/ml concentration. Compatible diluents are 0.9% Sodium Chloride Solution, 5% Dextrose Solution; 10% Dextran 40 in 0.9% Sodium Chloride Solution, 10% Invert Sugar Solution, Ringer's Solution, Hartmann's Solution. Store at room temperature; protect from excessive heat. Do not use after 48 h. Do not use IV solutions that are discolored or contain any precipitate or particulate matter.

Infusion: Use a controlled infusion device to administer IV infusions; an IV microdrip chamber (60 drops/ml) can provide a convenient range of infusion rates.

Adverse effects
Maternal Effects

- CNS: *Headache, weakness, tremor,* nervousness, restlessness, emotional upset, anxiety, malaise
- GI: *Nausea, vomiting,* ileus, constipation, diarrhea
- CV: *Increase in heart rate, increase in systolic blood pressure, decrease in diastolic blood pressure, palpitations,* chest pain, supraventricular tachycardia, sinus bradycardia with withdrawal of drug
- Respiratory: Dyspnea, hyperventilation, postpartum pulmonary edema (sometimes fatal)
- Hypersensitivity: Anaphylactic shock, rash
- Other: *Erythema,* transient elevation blood glucose, hypokalemia

Fetal Effects
- GI: Ileus
- CV: *Fetal heart rate increase,* hypotension in neonates whose mothers were treated with other beta-adrenergic agonists
- Hematologic: Hypoglycemia, hypocalcemia in neonates whose mothers were treated with other beta-adrenergic agonists

Clinically important drug-drug interactions

- Increased sympathomimetic effects when given with other sympathomimetic drugs
- Decreased therapeutic effects of ritodrine when given with beta-adrenergic blockers
- Potentially fatal pulmonary edema when given to patients who have received corticosteroids

■ Nursing Considerations
Assessment

- *History:* Hypersensitivity to ritodrine or components of preparation, pregnancy, antepartum hemorrhage, eclampsia and severe preeclampsia, intrauterine fetal death, chorioamnionitis, maternal cardiac disease, pulmonary hypertension, maternal hyperthyroidism, uncontrolled maternal diabetes mellitus, hypovolemia, cardiac arrhythmias, uncontrolled hypertension, pheochromocytoma, bronchial asthma already treated by betamimetics or steroids
- *Physical:* Maternal and fetal heart rate, maternal BP and R, plasma glucose and electrolytes (potassium)

Implementation

- Monitor maternal P, R closely; persistent maternal P > 140 beats/min or persistent tachypnea (respiratory rate > 20/min) may be signs of impending pulmonary edema.
- Use care to avoid fluid overload; serial hemograms may be helpful as an indication of the state of hydration.
- Maintain patient in left lateral position during the infusion to minimize hypotension.

Adverse effects in *Italics* are most common; those in **Bold** are life-threatening.

saliva substitute ■ 985

- Give oral drug 1 h before or 2 h after meals; food may interfere with oral absorption.

Drug-specific teaching points
- Take oral drug exactly as prescribed.
- Report chest pain, dizziness, insomnia, weakness, tremor or irregular heart beat.

◻ saliva substitute

(sa lie' vah)

Moi-Stir, Orex, Salivart, Xero-Lube

Pregnancy Category Unknown

Drug classes
Saliva substitute

Therapeutic actions
Contains electrolytes and carboxymethylcellulose as a thickening agent to serve as a substitute for saliva in dry mouth syndromes.

Indications
- Management of dry mouth and throat in xerostomia caused by stroke, medications, radiation therapy, chemotherapy, other illnesses

Contraindications/cautions
- Contraindicated in the presence of hypersensitivity to carboxymethylcellulose, parabens, components of the preparation.
- Use caution in the presence of renal failure, CHF, hypertension.

Dosage
Adult: Spray or apply to oral mucosa as needed.
Pediatric: Safety and efficacy not established.

Pharmacokinetics
Not generally absorbed systemically. Electrolytes may be absorbed and dealt with in normal electrolyte pathways.

Adverse effects
- *Other:* Excessive absorption of electrolytes (elevated magnesium, sodium, potassium)

■ Nursing Considerations

Assessment
- *History:* Allergy to carboxymethylcellulose, parabens, CHF, hypertension, renal failure
- *Physical:* BP, P, auscultation, edema; renal function tests; mucosa evaluation

Implementation
- Administer as needed for dry mouth and throat.
- Have patient try to swish saliva substitute around mouth following application.
- Monitor patient while eating; swallowing may be impaired and additional therapy required.

Drug-specific teaching points
- Apply the drug as instructed; swish it around in your mouth after application.
- Use as needed for dry mouth and throat.
- Take care when eating because swallowing may be difficult; additional therapy may be needed.
- Report swelling, headache, irregular heart beat, leg cramps, failure to relieve discomfort of dry mouth and throat.

◻ salmeterol

(sal mee' ter ol)

Serevent

Pregnancy Category C

Drug classes
Beta$_2$-agonist
Asthmatic drug

Therapeutic actions
Long-acting agonist that binds to beta$_2$ receptors in the lungs, causing bronchodilitation; also inhibits the release of inflammatory mediators in the lung, blocking swelling and inflammation.

Adverse effects in *Italics* are most common; those in **Bold** are life-threatening.

Indications
- Prevention of bronchospasm in select patients with asthma, reversible obstructive airway disease, and exercise-induced asthma

Contraindications/cautions
- Contraindicated in the presence of hypersensitivity to salmeterol, acute asthma attack, worsening or deteriorating asthma (use could be life-threatening), acute airway obstruction.
- Use caution in the presence of pregnancy, lactation.

Dosage
Adult: 2 puffs q12h using pressurized metered-dose inhaler, which delivers 25 μg; 2 puffs 30–60 min before exertion if used only for exercise-induced asthma. Do not exceed 4 puffs/d.
Pediatric: Safety and efficacy not established.

Pharmacokinetics

Route	Onset	Peak	Duration
Inhalation	13–20 m	3–4 h	7.5–17 h

Metabolism: Hepatic, $T_{1/2}$: unknown
Distribution: Crosses placenta; may enter breast milk
Excretion: Feces

Adverse effects
- **CNS:** *Headache, tremor*
- **CV:** *Tachycardia, palpitations*, hypertension
- **Respiratory:** Worsening of asthma, difficulty breathing, bronchospasm

■ Nursing Considerations

Assessment
- *History:* Allergy to salmeterol, pregnancy, acute asthma attack, worsening asthma, lactation
- *Physical:* R, adventitious sounds; P, BP, EKG; orientation, reflexes; liver function tests

Implementation
- Ensure that drug is not used to treat acute asthma or for patients with worsening or deteriorating asthma (deaths have been reported).
- Instruct patient in the proper use of metered inhaler.
- Monitor use of inhaler; patients who use more than 4 puffs/d may experience a worsening of asthma and should be regularly evaluated by their physician.
- Encourage patients who experience exercise-induced asthma to use drug 30–60 min before activity.
- Arrange for periodic evaluation of respiratory condition while on this drug.

Drug-specific teaching points
- Use the pressurized metered-dose inhaler as instructed. Use only twice a day. If drug is to be used periodically for exercise-induced asthma, use 30–60 min before activity.
- Arrange for periodic evaluation of your respiratory problem while on this drug.
- Know that the following side effects may occur: headache (appropriate analgesics may be ordered); tremors (use care in performing dangerous tasks if this occurs); fast heart, palpitations (monitor activity if this occurs; rest frequently).
- Report severe headache, irregular heart beat, worsening of asthma, difficulty breathing.

❒ salsalate

(sal' sa late)

salicylsalicylic acid

Amigesic, Argesic, Artha-G, Disalcid, Mono-Gesic, Salflex, Salsitab

Pregnancy Category C

Drug classes
Antipyretic
Analgesic
Anti-inflammatory
Antirheumatic
Salicylate
NSAID

Adverse effects in *Italics* are most common; those in **Bold** are life-threatening.

Therapeutic actions
Analgesic and antirheumatic effects are attributable to the ability to inhibit the synthesis of prostaglandins, important mediators of inflammation; antipyretic effects are not fully understood, but salicylates probably act in the thermoregulatory center of the hypothalamus to block the effects of endogenous pyrogen by inhibiting the synthesis of the prostaglandin intermediary; after absorption, this drug is hydrolyzed into two molecules of salicylic acid; insoluble in gastric secretions, it is not absorbed in the stomach, but in the small intestine; reported to cause fewer GI adverse effects than aspirin.

Indications
- Relief of mild to moderate pain
- Reduction of fever
- Relief of symptoms of various inflammatory conditions—rheumatic fever, rheumatoid arthritis, osteoarthritis

Contraindications/cautions
- Allergy to salicylates or NSAIDs, bleeding disorders, impaired hepatic or renal function, GI ulceration (less of a problem with salicylates than with some others), lactation, pregnancy.

Dosage
Adult: 3,000 mg/d PO given in divided doses.
Pediatric: Safety and efficacy not established.

Pharmacokinetics

Route	Onset	Peak	Duration
Oral	10–30 min	1–3 h	3–6 h

Metabolism: Hepatic, $T_{1/2}$: 2–3 h (15–30 h with large doses over extended periods)
Distribution: Crosses placenta; enters breast milk
Excretion: Urine

Adverse effects
NSAIDs
- **CNS:** *Headache, dizziness, somnolence, insomnia,* fatigue, tiredness, dizziness, tinnitus, ophthalmologic effects
- **GI:** *Nausea, dyspepsia, GI pain,* diarrhea, vomiting, *constipation,* flatulence
- **Respiratory:** Dyspnea, hemoptysis, pharyngitis, bronchospasm, rhinitis
- **Hematologic:** Bleeding, platelet inhibition with higher doses, neutropenia, eosinophilia, leukopenia, pancytopenia, thrombocytopenia, agranulocytosis, granulocytopenia, aplastic anemia, decreased hemoglobin or hematocrit, bone marrow depression, menorrhagia
- **GU:** Dysuria, renal impairment
- **Dermatologic:** *Rash,* pruritus, sweating, dry mucous membranes, stomatitis
- **Salicylism:** Dizziness, tinnitus, difficulty hearing, nausea, vomiting, diarrhea, mental confusion, lassitude (dose related)
- **Acute salicylate toxicity:** Respiratory alkalosis, hyperpnea, tachypnea, hemmorhage, excitement, confusion, asterixis, pulmonary edema, convulsions, tetany, metabolic acidosis, fever, coma, cardiovascular collapse, renal and respiratory failure
- **Other:** Peripheral edema, anaphylactoid reactions to **fatal anaphylactic shock**

Clinically important drug-drug interactions
- Increased risk of GI ulceration with corticosteroids if taken with salsalate • Increased risk of salicylate toxicity with carbonic anhydrase inhibitors • Increased toxicity of carbonic anhydrase inhibitors, valproic acid if taken concurrently • Decreased serum salicylate levels if taken with corticosteroids, antacids, urine alkalinizers (sodium acetate, sodium bicarbonate, sodium citrate, sodium lactate, tromethamine) • Increased methotrexate levels and toxicity if taken with salsalate • Greater glucose-lowering effect of sulfonylureas, insulin with large doses of salicylates • Decreased uricosuric effect of probenecid, sulfinpyrazone if taken with salsalate • Decreased diuretic effect of spironolactone if taken with salsalate

Adverse effects in *Italics* are most common; those in **Bold** are life-threatening.

Drug-lab test interferences
• Decreased serum protein-bound iodine (PBI) • False-negative readings for urine glucose by glucose oxidase method and copper reduction method • Interference with urine 5-HIAA determinations by fluorescent methods but not by nitrosonaphthol colorimetric method • Interference with urinary ketone determination by ferric chloride method • Falsely elevated urine VMA levels with most tests; false decrease in VMA using the Pisano method

■ Nursing Considerations
Assessment
- *History:* Allergy to salicylates or NSAIDs, bleeding disorders, impaired hepatic or renal function, GI ulceration, lactation, pregnancy
- *Physical:* Skin color and lesions; eighth cranial nerve function, orientation, reflexes, affect; P, BP, perfusion; R, adventitious sounds; liver evaluation and bowel sounds; CBC, urinalysis, stool guiaiac, renal and liver function tests

Implementation
- Administer drug with food or after meals if GI upset occurs.
- Administer drug with a full glass of water to reduce risk of tablet/capsule lodging in the esophagus.
- Institute emergency procedures if overdose occurs: gastric lavage, induction of emesis, activated charcoal, supportive therapy.
- Provide further comfort measures to reduce pain, fever, and inflammation.

Drug-specific teaching points
- Take the drug with food or after meals if GI upset occurs.
- Report ringing in the ears, dizziness, confusion, abdominal pain, rapid or difficult breathing, nausea, vomiting.

❒ sargramostim

(sar gram' oh stim)
granulocyte macrophage colony-stimulating factor, GM-CSF

Leukine, Prokine

Pregnancy Category C

Drug classes
Colony Stimulating Factor

Therapeutic actions
Human GM-CSF produced by recombinant DNA technology; increases the proliferation and differentiation of hematopoietic progenitor cells; can activate mature granulocytes and macrophages.

Indications
- Myeloid reconstitution after autologous bone marrow transplantation
- Bone marrow transplantation failure or engraftment delay
- Unlabeled uses: treatment of myelodysplastic syndrome, decreases nadir of leukopenia related to myelosuppression of chemotherapy, corrects neutropenia in aplastic anemia patients, decreases transplant-associated organ system damage, promotes early grafting, increases the WBC count in AIDS patients receiving zidovudine

Contraindications/cautions
- Contraindicated in the presence of hypersensitivity to yeast products, excessive leukemic myeloid blasts in bone marrow or peripheral blood, pregnancy.
- Use caution in the presence of renal or hepatic failure, lactation.

Dosage
Adult
- **Myeloid reconstitution after autologous bone marrow transplantation:** 250 µg/m^2 per day for 21 d as a 2-h IV infusion beginning 2–4 h after the autologous bone marrow infusion and not less than 24 h after the last dose of chemotherapy.
- **Bone marrow transplantation failure or engraftment delay:** 250 µg/m^2 per day for 14 d as a 2-h IV infusion; can be repeated after 7 d off therapy.

Pediatric: Safety and efficacy not established.

Pharmacokinetics

Route	Peak	Duration
IV	2 h	6 h

Metabolism: Unknown metabolism, $T_{1/2}$: 12–17 min then 2 h
Distribution: Crosses placenta; may enter breast milk

IV facts
Preparation: Reconstitute with 1 ml Sterile Water for Injection; gently swirl contents to avoid foaming; do not shake, and avoid excessive agitation. Resulting solution should be clear, colorless, and isotonic. Do not reenter vial; discard any unused portion. Dilute in 0.9% Sodium Chloirde Injection; administer within 6 h; refrigerate until ready to use.

Infusion: Infuse over 2 h; do not use an in-line membrane filter; do not mix with any other medication or in any other diluent.

Compatabilities: Do not mix with any solution other than 0.9% Sodium Chloride or add to any other medications.

Adverse effects
- CNS: Headache, *fever*, generalized weakness, fatigue, *malaise, asthenia*
- GI: *Nausea, vomiting*, stomatitis, anorexia, *diarrhea*, constipation
- CV: Edema
- Dermatologic: *Alopecia*, rash, mucositis
- Other: *Bone pain*, generalized pain, sore throat, cough

■ Nursing Considerations
Assessment
- *History:* Hypersensitivity to yeast products, pregnancy, lactation, excessive leukemic myeloid blasts in bone marrow or peripheral blood, pregnancy, renal or hepatic failure
- *Physical:* Skin—color, lesions, hair; body temperature; abdominal exam, status of mucous membranes; CBC, platelets; body temperature

Implementation
- Obtain CBC and platelet count prior to and twice weekly during therapy.
- Administer no less than 24 h after cytotoxic chemotherapy and within 2–4 h of bone marrow infusion.
- Administer daily as a 2-h infusion for 14–21 d as ordered.
- Store in refrigerator; allow to warm to room temperature before use; if vial is at room temperature for > 6 h, discard the vial. Use each vial is for one dose; do not reenter the vial; discard any unused drug.
- Do not shake vial before use.

Drug-specific teaching points
- Be aware that this drug must be given daily IV for 2–3 wk.
- Avoid exposure to infection while you are receiving this drug (eg, avoid crowds, visitors with infections).
- Know that the following side effects may occur: nausea and vomiting (small, frequent meals may help); loss of hair (you may want to arrange for appropriate head covering; it is very important to cover head in very cold or very hot temperatures); fever (appropriate medication may help).
- Be aware that frequent blood tests will be needed to evaluate the effects of this drug on your blood.
- Report fever, chills, sore throat, weakness, pain or swelling at injection site, difficulty breathing, chills.

❒ scopolamine hydrobromide

*(skoe **pol'** a meen)*

hyoscine HBr
Parenteral: Scopolamine HBr
Oral OTC preparation: Triptone
Transdermal system: Transderm-Scop
Ophthalmic solution: Isopto Hyoscine Ophthalmic
Pregnancy Category C

Drug classes
Anticholinergic
Antimuscarinic

Adverse effects in *Italics* are most common; those in **Bold** are life-threatening.

scopolamine hydrobromide

Parasympatholytic
Antimotion sickness drug
Diagnostic agent (ophthalmic prep)
Belladonna alkaloid

Therapeutic actions

Mechanism of action as antimotion sickness drug not understood; antiemetic action may be mediated by interference with cholinergic impulses to the vomiting center (CTZ); has sedative and amnesia-inducing properties; blocks the effects of acetylcholine at muscarinic cholinergic receptors that mediate the effects of parasympathetic postganglionic impulses, thus depressing salivary and bronchial secretions, inhibiting vagal influences on the heart, relaxing the GI and GU tracts, inhibiting gastric acid secretion, relaxing the pupil of the eye (mydriatic effect), and preventing accommodation for near vision (cycloplegic effect).

Indications

- Prevention and control of nausea and vomiting due to motion sickness (oral, transdermal, parenteral preparations)
- Adjunctive therapy with antacids and H_2 antihistamines in peptic ulcer supportive treatment of functional GI disorders (diarrhea, pylorospasm, hypermotility, irritable bowel syndrome, spastic colon, acute enterocolitis, pancreatitis, infant colic)
- Treatment of biliary colic in conjunction with narcotic analgesic
- Relief of urinary frequency and urgency, nocturnal enuresis, and ureteral colic (in conjunction with a narcotic analgesic)
- Suppression of vagally mediated bradycardia
- Preanesthetic medication to control bronchial, nasal, pharyngeal, and salivary secretions; prevent bronchospasm and laryngospasm; block cardiac vagal inhibitory reflexes during induction of anesthesia and intubation; produce sedation
- Induction of obstetric amnesia in conjunction with analgesics calming delirium

Ophthalmic Solution

- Diagnostically to produce mydriasis and cycloplegia
- Preoperative and postoperative states in the treatment of iridocyclitis

Contraindications/cautions

- Contraindicated in the presence of hypersensitivity to anticholinergic drugs; glaucoma; adhesions between iris and lens; stenosing peptic ulcer, pyloroduodenal obstruction, paralytic ileus, intestinal atony, severe ulcerative colitis, toxic megacolon, symptomatic prostatic hypertrophy, bladder neck obstruction, bronchial asthma, COPD, cardiac arrhythmias, tachycardia, myocardial ischemia; impaired metabolic, liver or kidney function (increased likelihood of adverse CNS effects); myasthenia gravis, pregnancy (may cause respiratory depression in neonates, contribute to neonatal hemorrhage); lactation.
- Use caution in the presence of Down's syndrome, brain damage, spasticity, hypertension, hyperthyroidism; glaucoma or tendency to glaucoma (ophthalmic solution).

Dosage

Adult

- **Oral**
  - *Motion sickness:* 0.25 mg 1 h before anticipated travel. Repeat in 4 h if needed. Do not exceed 1 mg in 24 h.
- **Transdermal**
  - *Motion Sickness:* Apply one transdermal system to the postauricular skin at least 4 h before antiemetic effect is required. Scopolamine 0.5 mg will be delivered over 3 d. If continued effect is needed, replace system every 3 d.
- **Parenteral:** 0.32–0.65 mg SC or IM. May give IV after dilution in Sterile Water for Injection.
- **Ophthalmic solution**
  - *Refraction:* Instill 1–2 drops into the eye(s) 1 h before refracting.
  - *Uveitis:* Instill 1–2 drops into the eye(s) up to three times daily.

scopolamine hydrobromide ■ 991

Pediatric: Do not use oral scopolamine in children younger than 6 y unless directed by physician. Do not use transdermal system in children.
- *Parenteral:* 0.006 mg/kg SC, IM, or IM; maximum dose is 0.3 mg.

Geriatric: More likely to cause serious adverse reactions, especially CNS reactions.

Pharmacokinetics

Route	Onset	Peak	Duration
Oral, IM, SC	30 min	60 min	4–6 h
IV	10 min	60 min	2–4 h
Transdermal	4–5 h		72 h
Opthalmologic	10–20 min	30–45 min	Days

Metabolism: Hepatic, $T_{1/2}$: 8 h
Distribution: Crosses placenta; enters breast milk
Excretion: Urine

IV facts
Preparation: Dilute in Sterile Water for Injection.
Infusion: Inject directly into vein or into tubing of actively running IV; inject slowly.

Adverse effects
- CNS: *Pupil dilation, photophobia, blurred vision, headache, drowsiness,* dizziness, mental confusion, excitement, restlessness, hallucinations, delirium in the presence of pain
- GI: *Dry mouth, constipation,* paralytic ileus, altered taste perception, nausea, vomiting, dysphagia, heartburn
- CV: Palpitations, tachycardia
- GU: *Urinary hesitancy and retention,* impotence
- Hypersensitivity: Anaphylaxis, urticaria, other dermatologic effects
- Other: Suppression of lactation, flushing, fever, *nasal congestion, decreased sweating*

Clinically important drug-drug interactions
- Decreased antipsychotic effectiveness of haloperidol when given with scopolamine • Decreased effectiveness of phenothiazines given with scopolamine, but increased incidence of paralytic ileus

■ Nursing Considerations
Assessment
- *History:* Hypersensitivity to anticholinergic drugs; glaucoma; adhesions between iris and lens; stenosing peptic ulcer, pyloroduodenal obstruction, intestinal atony, severe ulcerative colitis, symptomatic prostatic hypertrophy, bladder neck obstruction, bronchial asthma, COPD, cardiac arrhythmias, myocardial ischemia; impaired metabolic, liver or kidney function; myasthenia gravis; Down syndrome, brain damage, spasticity; hypertension, hyperthyroidism; pregnancy; lactation
- *Physical:* Skin—color, lesions, texture; body temperature; orientation, reflexes, bilateral grip strength; affect; ophthalmic exam; P, BP; R, adventitious sounds; bowel sounds, normal output; urinary output, prostate palpation; liver and kidney function tests, ECG

Implementation
- Ensure adequate hydration; provide environmental control (temperature) to prevent hyperpyrexia.

Drug-specific teaching points
- Take as prescribed, 30 min before meals. Avoid excessive dosage.
- Avoid hot environments while you are taking this drug. You will be heat intolerant, and dangerous reactions may occur.
- Know that the following side effects may occur: dizziness, sedation, drowsiness (use caution if driving or performing tasks that require alertness if these occur); constipation (ensure adequate fluid intake, proper diet); dry mouth (sugarless lozenges, frequent mouth care may help; this effect sometimes lessens with time); blurred vision, sensitivity to light (it may help to know that these are drug effects that will go away when you discontinue the drug; avoid tasks that require acute vision; wear sunglasses when in bright light if these occur); impotence (this is

Adverse effects in *Italics* are most common; those in **Bold** are life-threatening.

a drug effect that will go away when you discontinue the drug); difficulty urinating (it may help to empty the bladder immediately before taking each dose of drug).
- Avoid alcohol while taking this drug; serious sedation could occur.
- Report skin rash, flushing, eye pain, difficulty breathing, tremors, loss of coordination, irregular heartbeat, abdominal distention, hallucinations, severe or persistent dry mouth, difficulty urinating, constipation, sensitivity to light.

☐ secobarbital

*(see koe **bar'** bi tal)*

secobarbital sodium
Novosecobarb (CAN), Seconal Sodium

Pregnancy Category C
C-II controlled substance

Drug classes
Barbiturate (short-acting)
Sedative
Hypnotic
Anticonvulsant

Therapeutic actions
General CNS depressant; barbiturates inhibit impulse conduction in the ascending reticular activating system, depress the cerebral cortex, alter cerebellar function, depress motor output, and can produce excitation (especially with subanesthetic doses in the presence of pain), sedation, hypnosis, anesthesia, and deep coma; at anesthetic doses, has anticonvulsant activity.

Indications
- Hypnotic, for short-term treatment of insomnia (not effective for more than 14 d), and preanesthetic medication (oral)
- Intermittent use as a sedative, hypnotic, or preanesthetic medication (parenteral)
- In anesthetic doses for the emergency control of convulsive seizures associated with tetanus

Contraindications/cautions
- Contraindicated in the presence of hypersensitivity to barbiturates; manifest or latent porphyria; marked liver impairment; nephritis; severe respiratory distress, respiratory disease with dyspnea, obstruction, or cor pulmonale; previous addiction to sedative-hypnotic drugs (drug may be ineffective, and use may contribute to further addiction); pregnancy (readily crosses placenta and has caused fetal damage, neonatal withdrawal syndrome).
- Use caution in the presence of acute or chronic pain (drug may cause paradoxical excitement or mask important symptoms); seizure disorders (abrupt discontinuation of daily doses of drug can result in status epilepticus); lactation (has caused drowsiness in nursing infants); fever, hyperthyroidism, diabetes mellitus, severe anemia, pulmonary or cardiac disease, status asthmaticus, shock, uremia; impaired liver or kidney function, debilitation.

Dosage
Adult
- **Oral**
- *Preoperative sedation:* 200–300 mg 1–2 h before surgery.
- *Bedtime hypnotic:* 100 mg.
- **Parenteral:** Adjust dosage on basis of age, weight, condition.
- *IM:* Inject deeply into large muscle mass. Do not give more than 250 mg (5 ml) in one injection. *Bedtime hypnotic:* 100–200 mg. *Dentistry (as sedative):* Usual dose is 2.2 mg/kg (1 mg/lb), maximum 100 mg, 10–15 min before the procedure. 1.1–1.6 mg/kg may suffice.
- *IV:* Restrict use of this route to conditions in which other routes are not feasible or in which a rapid effect is imperative. *Anesthetic:* To provide basal hypnosis for general, spinal, or regional anesthesia. To facilitate intubation, administer at a rate ≤50 mg/15 sec. Discontinue administration as soon as desired degree of hypnosis is attained. Do not exceed 250 mg. If hypnosis is inadequate after 250 mg, add a small dose of meperidine.

Dentistry, patients who are to receive nerve blocks: 100–150 mg IV. Patient will awaken in 15 min and can be discharged in 30 min if accompanied. *Convulsions in tetanus:* Initial dose of 5.5 mg/kg (2.5 mg/lb) IV. Repeat q3–4h as needed. Rate of administration should not exceed 50 mg/15 min.

Pediatric: *Use caution:* barbiturates may produce irritability, excitability, inappropriate tearfulness, and aggression.

- *Oral*
- *Preoperative sedation:* 2–6 mg/kg (maximum 100 mg) 1–2 h before surgery.
- ***Rectal (injectable solution):*** Prior to ENT procedures. Dilute with lukewarm tap water to a concentration of 1%–1.5% and administer after a cleansing enema. *< 40 kg (88lb):* 5 mg/kg (2.3 mg/lb). *> 40 kg:* 4 mg/kg (1.8 mg/lb). Hypnosis should follow in 15–20 min.
- ***Parenteral***
- *IM:* 4–5 mg/kg to provide basal hypnosis. *Dentistry (as sedative):* Usual dose is 2.2 mg/kg (1 mg/lb) IM, maximum 100 mg, 10–15 min before the procedure. 1.1–1.6 mg/kg may suffice.

Geriatric patients or those with debilitating disease: Reduce dosage and monitor closely. May produce excitement, depression, confusion.

Pharmacokinetics

Route	Onset	Peak	Duration
Oral	10–15 min	15–30 min	3–4 h
IV	Immediate	1–3 min	15 min
IM	Rapid	7–10 min	1–4 h

Metabolism: Hepatic, $T_{1/2}$: 15–40 h
Distribution: Crosses placenta; enters breast milk
Excretion: Urine

IV facts

Preparation: No further preparation required; refrigerate; protect from light; do not use if solution contains precipitate.

Infusion: Infuse slowly over time periods listed for each use.

Adverse effects

- CNS: *Somnolence, agitation, confusion, hyperkinesia, ataxia, vertigo, CNS depression, nightmares, lethargy, residual sedation (hangover), paradoxical excitement, nervousness, psychiatric disturbance, hallucinations, insomnia, anxiety, dizziness, thinking abnormality*
- GI: *Nausea, vomiting, constipation, diarrhea, epigastric pain*
- CV: *Bradycardia, hypotension, syncope*
- Respiratory: *Hypoventilation, apnea, respiratory depression,* laryngospasm, bronchospasm, circulatory collapse
- Hypersensitivity: Skin rashes, angioneurotic edema, serum sickness, morbiliform rash, urticaria; rarely, exfoliative dermatitis, Stevens-Johnson syndrome, sometimes fatal
- Local: *Pain, tissue necrosis at injection site*, gangrene; arterial spasm with inadvertent intra-arterial injection; thrombophlebitis; permanent neurologic deficit if injected near a nerve
- Other: Tolerance, psychological and physical dependence; **withdrawal syndrome** (sometimes fatal)

Clinically important drug-drug interactions

- Increased CNS depression when taken with alcohol • Increased renal toxicity if methoxyflurane is taken with secobarbital • Decreased effects of the following drugs given with barbiturates: oral anticoagulants, corticosteroids, oral contraceptives and estrogens, metronidazole, metoprolol, propranolol, doxycycline, oxyphenbutazone, phenylbutazone, quinidine • Decreased theophylline serum levels and effectiveness secondary to increased clearance when given with secobarbital

■ Nursing Considerations
Assessment

- *History:* Hypersensitivity to barbiturates; manifest or latent porphyria; marked

liver impairment; nephritis; severe respiratory distress; previous addiction to sedative-hypnotic drugs; pregnancy; acute or chronic pain; seizure disorders; lactation; fever, hyperthyroidism, diabetes mellitus, severe anemia, pulmonary or cardiac disease, shock, uremia; impaired liver or kidney function, debilitation
- *Physical:* Body weight; body temperature; skin—color, lesions; orientation, affect, reflexes; P, BP, orthostatic BP; R, adventitious sounds; bowel sounds, normal output, liver evaluation; liver and kidney function tests, blood and urine glucose, BUN

Implementation

- Monitor patient responses, blood levels (as appropriate) if any of the above interacting drugs are given with secobarbital; suggest alternate means of contraception to women on oral contraceptives for whom secobarbital is prescribed.
- Do not administer intra-arterially; may produce arteriospasm, thrombosis, gangrene.
- Administer IV doses slowly.
- Administer IM doses deep in a muscle mass.
- Do not use discolored parenteral solutions or those that contain a precipitate.
- Remain with children who have received secobarbital rectally.
- Monitor injection sites carefully for irritation, extravasation (IV use); solutions are alkaline and very irritating to the tissues.
- Monitor P, BP, respiration carefully during IV administration.
- Arrange to taper dosage gradually after repeated use, especially in epileptic patients.

Drug-specific teaching points

Preanesthetic Medication or as a Basal Hypnotic

- Be aware that this drug will make you drowsy (or induce sleep) and less anxious.
- Try not to get up after you have received this drug (request assistance if you feel you must sit up or move about for any reason).

Outpatients

- Take this drug exactly as prescribed.
- Be aware that this drug is habit-forming; its effectiveness in facilitating sleep disappears after a short time; do not take this drug longer than 2 wk (for insomnia) and do not increase the dosage without consulting the prescriber.
- Know that the following side effects may occur: drowsiness, dizziness, "hangover," impaired thinking (these effects may become less pronounced after a few days; avoid driving a car or engaging in activities that require alertness if these occur); GI upset (taking the drug with food may help); dreams, nightmares, difficulty concentrating, fatigue, nervousness (it may help to know that these are effects of the drug that will go away when the drug is discontinued).
- Be aware that you should not become pregnant while taking this drug; use a means of contraception other than oral contraceptive preparations while on secobarbital.
- Report severe dizziness, weakness, drowsiness that persists, rash or skin lesions, pregnancy.

☐ selegiline hydrochloride

(se le' ge leen)
L-Deprenyl, Eldepryl

Pregnancy Category C

Drug classes
Antiparkinson agent

Therapeutic actions
Mechanism of action not completely understood; inhibits monoamine oxidase (MAO) type B activity; may have other mechanisms of increasing dopaminergic activity.

Indications
- Adjunct in the management of parkinsonian patients being treated with levodopa/carbidopa who exhibit deterioration in the quality of their response to this therapy

selegiline hydrochloride ■ 995

Contraindications/cautions
- Hypersensitivity to selegiline, pregnancy, lactation.

Dosage
Given to patients receiving levodopa/carbidopa therapy who demonstrate a deteriorating response to their treatment.
Adult: 10 mg/d PO administered as divided doses of 5 mg each taken at breakfast and lunch. Avoid higher doses because of the increased risk of adverse effects. After 2–3 d of treatment, attempt to reduce the dose of levodopa/carbidopa; reduction of 10%–30% appears typical. Further reduction may be possible during continued selegiline therapy.
Pediatric: Safety and efficacy not established.

Pharmacokinetics

Route	Onset	Peak
Oral	Rapid	30–120 min

Metabolism: Hepatic, $T_{1/2}$: 20.5 h
Distribution: Crosses placenta; enters breast milk
Excretion: Urine

Adverse effects
- **CNS:** *Headache, dizziness, lightheadedness, confusion, hallucinations, dyskinesias, vivid dreams,* increased tremor, loss of balance, restlessness, depression, drowsiness, disorientation, apathy
- **GI:** *Nausea,* vomiting, *abdominal pain,* constipation, heartburn, diarrhea, anorexia, *dry mouth,* rectal bleeding
- **CV:** Orthostatic hypotension, hypertension, arrhythmia, palpitations, hypotension, tachycardia
- **GU:** Slow urination, transient nocturia, prostatic hypertrophy, urinary hesistancy, retention
- **Dermatologic:** Increased sweating, diaphoresis, facial hair, hair loss, hematoma, rash, photosensitivity
- **Other:** Asthma, diplopia, blurred vision

Clinically important drug-drug interactions
- Severe adverse effects, even fatalaties have been reported when meperidine is given to patients on MAO inhibitors; because the mechanism of action of selegiline is not clear, avoid the combination of selegiline and meperidine and other narcotic analgesics • Risk of serious toxicity if given with tricyclic antidepressants (TCAs), selective serotonin reuptake inhibitors (SSRIs); avoid this combination.

■ Nursing Considerations
Assessment
- *History:* Hypersensitivity to selegiline, pregnancy, lactation
- *Physical:* Abdominal exam; reflexes, affect; BP, P; urinary output, renal function

Implementation
- Administer only as an adjunct with levodopa/carbidopa therapy to patients whose symptoms are deteriorating.
- Administer twice a day, with breakfast and lunch.
- Ensure that dosage does not exceed 10 mg/d; MAO B selectivity may be lost, and patient will be at risk for severe hypertensive reactions.
- Monitor patient carefully for improvement of Parkinson's symptoms; if symptoms improve after 2–3 d of treatment, arrange to begin reducing the dosage of levodopa/carbidopa. 10%–30% decrease is typical.

Drug-specific teaching points
- Take this drug twice a day, with breakfast and lunch. Continue to take your levodopa/carbidopa. The dosage of the levodopa may need to be decreased after a few days of therapy. Do not stop taking this drug without consulting your presciber. Do not exceed the dose of 10 mg/d; serious reactions could occur.
- Know that the following side effects may occur as a result of drug therapy: dizziness, lightheadedness, confusion (avoid driving a car or performing hazardous tasks if these occur); headache, fatigue, joint pain (medications may be available

Adverse effects in *Italics* are most common; those in **Bold** are life-threatening.

996 ■ sertraline hydrochloride

to help); nausea, vomiting, diarrhea (small, frequent meals may help; proper nutrition is important); dry mouth (frequent mouth care, sucking ice chips or sugarless lozenges may be helpful).
- Report severe headache, confusion, mood changes, sleep disturbances, dizziness on arising, fainting.
- Maintain all of the usual activities and restrictions that apply to your Parkinson's disease. If this becomes difficult, consult with your prescriber.

☐ sertraline hydrochloride

(sir' trah leen)
Zoloft

Pregnancy Category B

Drug classes
Antidepressant
SSRI

Therapeutic actions
Acts as an antidepressant by inhibiting CNS neuronal uptake of serotonin; blocks uptake of serotonin with little effect on norepinephrine, muscarinic, histaminergic, and alpha$_1$-adrenergic or dopaminergic receptors.

Indications
- Treatment of depression
- Unlabeled use: treatment of obsessive-compulsive disorders

Contraindications/cautions
- Contraindicated in the presence of hypersensitivity to sertraline; pregnancy.
- Use caution in the presence of impaired hepatic or renal function, lactation.

Dosage
Adult: Administer once a day, in the morning or in the evening. 50 mg PO qd; may be increased to up to 200 mg/d; dosage increases should not occur at intervals < 1 wk. Current studies indicated efficacy for up to 16 wk; further study is needed to determine dosage needs for extended use.

Pediatric: Safety and efficacy not established.
Geriatric or renal impaired: Administer a lower dose in these patients. Monitor response as a guide for dosage.

Pharmacokinetics

Route	Onset	Peak
Oral	Slow	4½–8.4 h

Metabolism: Hepatic; $T_{1/2}$: 26 h
Distribution: Crosses placenta; may enter breast milk
Excretion: Urine and feces

Adverse effects
- **CNS:** *Headache, nervousness, drowsiness, anxiety, tremor, dizziness, insomnia* lightheadedness, agitation, sedation, abnormal gait, convulsions, *vision changes, fatigue*
- **GI:** *Nausea,* vomiting, *diarrhea, dry mouth,* anorexia, dyspepsia, constipation, taste changes, flatulence, gastroenteritis, dysphagia, gingivitis
- **CV:** Hot flashes, palpitations, chest pain
- **Respiratory:** Upper respiratory infections, pharyngitis, cough, dyspnea, bronchitis, *rhinitis*
- **GU:** *Painful menstruation,* sexual dysfunction, frequency, cystitis, impotence, urgency, vaginitis
- **Dermatologic:** *Sweating,* rash, pruritus, acne, contact dermatitis
- **Other:** Hot flashes, fever, back pain, thirst

Clinically important drug-drug interactions
• Serious, sometimes fatal, reactions if taken with MAO inhibitors

Clinically important drug-food interactions
• Increased rate of absorption if sertraline is taken with food

■ Nursing Considerations

Assessment
- *History:* Hypersensitivity to sertraline, impaired hepatic or renal function, lactation, pregnancy
- *Physical:* Weight; temperature; skin—rash, lesions; reflexes, affect; bowel

Adverse effects in *Italics* are most common; those in **Bold** are life-threatening.

sounds, liver evaluation; P, peripheral perfusion; urinary output, renal and liver function tests

Implementation
- Arrange for lower dose in elderly patients and patients with hepatic or renal impairment.
- Establish suicide precautions for severly depressed patients. Dispense only a small number of capsules at a time to these patients.
- Administer drug once a day, in the morning or in the evening.
- Increase dosage at intervals of not less than 1 wk.
- Counsel patient about the use of nonhormonal contraceptives while on this drug; pregnancy should be avoided because of the possible risk to the fetus.

Drug-specific teaching points
- Take this drug once a day, at the same time each day, in the morning or in the evening; do not exceed the prescribed dose.
- Know that the following side effects may occur: dizziness, drowsiness, nervousness, insomnia (avoid driving a car or performing hazardous tasks); nausea, vomiting (small frequent meals may help); dry mouth (sucking sugarless lozenges and frequent mouth care may help); excessive sweating (monitor temperature; avoid overheating).
- Do not take this drug during pregnancy. If you think that you are pregnant or wish to become pregnant, consult with your physician.
- Report rash, mania, seizures, edema, difficulty breathing.

☐ simethicone

(sigh meth' ih kohn)

Flatulex, Gas Relief, Gas-X, Major-Con, Mylanta Gas, Mylicon, Oval (CAN), Phazyme, Phazyme 55 (CAN)

Pregnancy Category Unknown

Drug classes
Antiflatulent

Therapeutic actions
Defoaming action disperses and prevents the formation of mucus surrounded gas pockets in the GI tract; changes the surface tension of gas bubbles in the stomach and small intestine, enabling the bubbles to coalesce, freeing gas to be more easily freed by belching or flatus.

Indications
- Relief of symptoms and pressure of excess gas in the digestive tract; postoperative gaseous distention and pain, use in endoscopic examination; air swallowing; functional dyspepsia; spastic or irritable colon; diverticulosis
- Unlabeled use: treatment of colic in infants

Contraindications/cautions
- Allergy to components of the product.

Dosage
Adult
- ***Capsules:*** 125 mg PO qid, after each meal and at bedtime.
- ***Tablets:*** 40–125 mg PO qid, after each meal and at bedtime.
- ***Drops:*** 40–80 mg PO qid up to 500 mg/d, after each meal and at bedtime.

Pediatric
- *Younger than 2 y:* 20 mg PO qid after each meal and at bedtime; up to 240 mg/d.
- *2–12 y:* 40 mg PO qid after each meal and at bedtime.

Pharmacokinetics
Not absorbed systemically; excreted unchanged in the feces.

Adverse effects
- GI: Nausea, vomiting, *diarrhea,* constipation, belching, passing of flatus

■ Nursing Considerations
Assessment
- *History:* Hypersensitivity to simethicone
- *Physical:* Bowel sounds, normal output

Adverse effects in *Italics* are most common; those in **Bold** are life-threatening.

Implementation
- Administer drug after each meal and at bedtime.
- Shake drops thoroughly before each use.
- Add drops to 30 ml cool water, infant formula, or other liquid to help facilitate administration to infants.
- Ensure that patient chews chewable tablets thoroughly before swallowing.

Drug-specific teaching points
- Take this drug after each meal and at bedtime; chew chewable tablets thoroughly before swallowing; shake drops bottle thoroughly before administration. Parents may want to add drops to 30 ml cool water, infant formula, or other liquid to ease administration.
- Know that you may experience increased belching and passing of flatus as gas disperses.
- Report extreme abdominal pain, worsening of condition being treated, vomiting.

☐ simvastatin

*(sim va **stah'** tin)*
Zocor

Pregnancy Category X

Drug classes
Antihyperlipidemic agent
HMG CoA inhibitor

Therapeutic actions
Inhibits HMG co-enzyme A, the enzyme that catalyzes the first step in the cholesterol synthesis pathway, resulting in a decrease in serum cholesterol, serum LDLs (associated with increased risk of coronary artery disease), and either an increase or no change in serum HDLs (associated with decreased risk of coronary artery disease).

Indications
- As an adjunct to diet in the treatment of elevated total cholestrol and LDL cholesterol in patients with primary hypercholesterolemia (types IIa and IIb) whose response to dietary restriction of saturated fat and cholesterol and other nonpharmacologic measures has not been adequate

Contraindications/cautions
- Contraindicated in the presence of allergy to simvastatin, fungal byproducts, pregnancy, lactation.
- Use caution in the presence of impaired hepatic function, cataracts.

Dosage
Adult: Initially, 5–10 mg PO qd once daily in the evening. Maximum dose, 50 mg/d.
Pediatric: Safety and efficacy not established.
Geriatric: Starting dose, 5 mg/d PO; increase dose slowly, monitoring response.

Pharmacokinetics

Route	Onset	Peak
Oral	Slow	1.3–2.4 h

Metabolism: Hepatic, $T_{1/2}$: unknown
Distribution: Crosses placenta; enters breast milk
Excretion: Urine and feces

Adverse effects
- CNS: *Headache*, asthenia
- GI: *Flatulence, abdominal pain, cramps, constipation, nausea,* dyspepsia, heartburn

Clinically important drug-drug interactions
- Possible severe myopathy or rhabdomyolysis if taken with gemfibrozil • Increased bleeding effects with warfarin when taken concurrently

■ Nursing Considerations

Assessment
- *History:* Allergy to simvastatin, fungal byproducts; impaired hepatic function; pregnancy; lactation
- *Physical:* Orientation, affect; liver evaluation, abdominal exam; lipid studies, liver function tests

Adverse effects in *Italics* are most common; those in **Bold** are life-threatening.

Implementation
- Ensure that patient has tried a cholesterol-lowering diet regimen for 3–6 mo before beginning therapy.
- Administer drug in the evening; highest rates of cholesterol synthesis are between midnight and 5 AM.
- Arrange for regular follow-up during long-term therapy.

Drug-specific teaching points
- Take drug in the evening.
- Know that the following side effects may occur: nausea (small, frequent meals may help); headache, muscle and joint aches and pains (these may lessen with time).
- Arrange to have periodic blood tests while you are on this drug.
- Report severe GI upset, changes in vision, unusual bleeding or bruising, dark urine or light-colored stools.

◻ sodium bicarbonate

Parenteral: Neut
Prescription and OTC preparations: Bell/ans, Soda Mint
Pregnancy Category C

Drug classes
Electrolyte
Systemic alkalinizer
Urinary alkalinizer
Antacid

Therapeutic actions
Increases plasma bicarbonate; buffers excess hydrogen ion concentration; raises blood pH; reverses the clinical manifestations of acidosis; increases the excretion of free base in the urine, effectively raising the urinary pH; neutralizes or reduces gastric acidity, resulting in an increase in the gastric pH, which inhibits the proteolytic activity of pepsin.

Indications
- Treatment of metabolic acidosis, in conjunction with measures to control the cause of the acidosis
- Adjunctive treatment in severe diarrhea with accompanying loss of bicarbonate
- Treatment of certain drug intoxications, hemolytic reactions that require alkalinization of the urine; prevention of methotrexate nephrotoxicity by alkalinization of the urine
- Minimization of uric acid crystalluria in gout, in conjunction with uricosuric agents
- Minimization of sulfonamide crystalluria
- Symptomatic relief of upset stomach from hyperacidity associated with peptic ulcer, gastritis, peptic esophagitis, gastric hyperacidity, hiatal hernia (oral)
- Prophylaxis of GI bleeding, stress ulcers, aspiration pneumonia (oral)

Contraindications/cautions
- Contraindicated in the presence of allergy to components of preparations; low serum chloride (secondary to vomiting, continuous GI suction, diuretics associated with hypochloremic alkalosis); metabolic and respiratory alkalosis; hypocalcemia (alkalosis may precipitate tetany).
- Use caution in the presence of impaired renal function, CHF, edematous or sodium-retaining states, oliguria or anuria, potassium depletion (may predispose to metabolic alkalosis), pregnancy.

Dosage
Adult
- **Urinary alkalinization:** 325 mg–2 g qid PO. Maximum daily dose, 16 g in patients younger than 60 y, 8 g in patients older than 60 y.
- **Antacid:** 0.3–2 g qd to qid PO. Usually 1 and 3 h after meals and at bedtime.
- **Cardiac arrest:** Adjust dosage based on arterial blood pH, $PaCO_2$, and calculation of base deficit; initial dose, 1 mEq/kg IV followed by 0.5 mEq/kg every 10 min during arrest.
- **Metabolic acidosis:** Initially 2–5 mEq/kg over 4–8 h IV. May be added to IV fluids, with rate and dosage determined by arterial blood gases and estimation of base deficit.

Pediatric
- **Neonates and children younger than 2 y:** Use caution and slow admin-

1000 ■ sodium bicarbonate

istration to prevent hypernatremia, decrease in cerebral spinal fluid pressure, and possible intracranial hemorrhage.
- *Cardiac arrest, infants up to 2 y:* 4.2% solution IV at a rate not to exceed 8 mEq/kg per day. Initially 1–2 mEq/kg given over 1–2 min followed by 1 mEq/kg every 10 min during arrest.
- *Metabolic acidosis:* Older children, follow adult recommendation. Younger children, use caution, and base dosage on blood gases and calculation of base deficit.

Geriatric and renal impaired: Reduce dosage and carefully monitor base deficit and clinical response.

Pharmacokinetics

Route	Onset	Peak	Duration
Oral	Rapid	30 min	1–3 h
IV	Immediate	Rapid	

Metabolism: T$_{1/2}$: unknown
Distribution: Crosses placenta; enters breast milk
Excretion: Urine

IV facts

Preparation: Direct IV push requires no further preparation; continuous infusion may be diluted in saline, dextrose, and dextrose/saline solutions.

Infusion: Administer by IV direct injection slowly; continuous infusion should be regulated with close monitoring of electrolytes and response.

Compatibilities: Avoid solutions containing calcium; precipitation may occur.

Adverse effects

- **GI:** Gastric rupture following ingestion
- **Hematologic:** *Systemic alkalosis* (headache, nausea, irritability, weakness, tetany, confusion), hypokalemia secondary to intracellular shifting of potassium
- **Local:** Chemical cellulitis, tissue necrosis, ulceration and sloughing at the site of infiltration (parenteral)

Clinically important drug-drug interactions

- Increased pharmacologic effects of anorexiants, sympathomimetics when taken with oral sodium bicarbonate • Increased half-lives and duration of effects of amphetamines, ephedrine, pseudoephedrine due to alkalinization of urine by sodium bicarbonate • Decreased pharmacologic effects of lithium, salicylates, sulfonylureas, demeclocycline, doxycycline, methacycline, and other tetracyclines when taken with sodium bicarbonate

■ Nursing Considerations

Assessment

- *History:* Allergy to components of preparations; low serum chloride; metabolic and respiratory alkalosis; hypocalcemia; impaired renal function; CHF, edematous, or sodium-retaining states; oliguria or anuria; potassium depletion; pregnancy
- *Physical:* Skin—color, turgor; injection sites; P, rhythm, peripheral edema; bowel sounds, abdominal exam; urinary output; serum electrolytes, serum bicarbonate, arterial blood gases, urinalysis, renal function tests

Implementation

- Monitor arterial blood gases, and calculate base deficit when administering parenteral sodium bicarbonate. Adjust dosage based on patient response. Administer slowly, and do not attempt complete correction within the first 24 h; risk of systemic alkalosis is increased.
- Administer parenteral preparations by IV route only.
- Check serum potassium levels before IV administration; risk of metabolic acidosis is increased in states of hypokalemia, and the dosage of sodium bicarbonate may need to be reduced. Monitor IV injection sites carefully; if infiltration occurs, promptly elevate the site, apply warm soaks, and if needed, arrange for the local injection of lidocaine or hyaluronidase to prevent sloughing.

Adverse effects in *Italics* are most common; those in **Bold** are life-threatening.

sodium chloride ■ 1001

- Have patient chew oral tablets thoroughly before swallowing, and follow them with a full glass of water.
- Do not administer oral sodium bicarbonate within 1–2 h of other oral drugs to reduce the incidence of drug-drug interactions.
- Monitor cardiac rhythm carefully during IV administration.

Drug-specific teaching points
- Chew oral tablets thoroughly, and follow with a full glass of water. Do not take within 1–2 h of any other drugs to decrease the interactions of these drugs.
- Arrange to have periodic blood tests and medical evaluation while you are on this drug.
- Report irritability, headache, tremors, confusion, swelling of extremities, difficulty breathing, black or tarry stools, pain at IV injection site (parenteral form).

❒ sodium chloride

(klor' ide)

Parenteral: Sodium Chloride Injection (various)

Prescription and OTC oral preparations: Slo-Salt

Pregnancy Category C

Drug classes
Electrolyte

Therapeutic actions
Sodium chloride is the principal salt involved in the maintenance of plasma tonicity; important for maintaining plasma volume, promoting membrane stability and electrolyte balance.

Indications
- Treatment of hyponatremia
- Dilution and reconstitution of parenteral drugs
- Hydration and replacement of fluid loss

Contraindications/cautions
- Contraindicated in the presence of hypernatremia, fluid retention, pregnancy, any condition when increased sodium or chloride could be detrimental.
- Use caution in the presence of impaired renal function, CHF, edematous or sodium-retaining states, lactation, surgical patients.

Dosage
Adult
- ***Oral:*** 1–2 g PO tid.
- ***IV:*** Isotonic (replacement) 1 L administered over 1 h; hypotonic (0.45%; hydration) 1–2 L over 1–2 h; hypertonic (3–5%; treatment of hyponatremia) 100 ml over 1 h.

Pediatric: Safety and efficacy not determined; replacement must be monitored closely and based on clinical response.

Geriatric and renal impaired: Reduce dosage, and carefully monitor base deficit and clinical response.

Pharmacokinetics

Route	Onset	Peak
Oral	Unknown	
IV	Immediate	End of infusion

Metabolism: $T_{1/2}$: unknown
Distribution: Crosses placenta; enters breast milk
Excretion: Urine

IV facts
Preparation: Concentrated sodium chloride must be further diluted before use; other preparations may be given as provided; change infusion q24h; use only if solution is clear.
Infusion: Administer by IV direct injection slowly; continuous infusion should be regulated with close monitoring of electrolytes and response.

Adverse effects
- **GI:** Anorexia, nausea, abdominal distention
- **Hematologic:** Hypernatremia, fluid overload
- **Local:** Chemical cellulitis, tissue necrosis, ulceration and sloughing at the site

Adverse effects in *Italics* are most common; those in **Bold** are life-threatening.

sodium fluoride

of infiltration, pain at site of injection (parenteral)

■ Nursing Considerations

Assessment
- *History:* Hypernatremia, fluid retention, pregnancy, impaired renal function, CHF, edematous or sodium-retaining states, lactation, surgical patients
- *Physical:* Skin—color, turgor; injection sites; P, rhythm, peripheral edema; bowel sounds, abdominal exam; urinary output; serum electrolytes, urinalysis, renal function tests

Implementation
- Monitor serum electrolytes carefully before and during administration. Administer slowly. Rapid infusion can result in pain and irritation at injection site.
- Administer parenteral preparations by IV route only.
- Monitor IV injection sites carefully; if infiltration occurs, promptly elevate the site, apply warm soaks, and if needed, arrange for the local injection of lidocaine or hyaluronidase to prevent sloughing.
- Monitor surgical patients for postoperative salt intolerance (weakness, dehydration, disorientation, nausea, distention, oliguria); if this occurs, discontinue infusion and provide appropriate supportive measures.
- Assess patients taking oral tablets for actual salt loss; excessive use of these tablets can cause hypernatremia.

Drug-specific teaching points
- Take these tablets only as prescribed.
- Arrange to have periodic blood tests and medical evaluation while you are on this drug.
- Report irritability, confusion, tremors, swelling of extremities, difficulty breathing, black or tarry stools.

❏ sodium fluoride

(flor' ide)

Fluor-A-Day (CAN), Fluoritab, Fluotic (CAN), Flura, Flura-Loz, Fluro-Drops, Karidium, Luride Lozi Tablets, PDF (CAN), Pediaflor, Pedident (CAN), Pharmaflur, Phos-Flur

Pregnancy Category C

Drug classes
Mineral

Therapeutic actions
Acts systemically before tooth eruption and topically after tooth eruption to increase tooth resistance to acid dissolution and promote remineralization of teeth and inhibit caries formation by microbes.

Indications
- Prevention of dental caries
- Unlabeled use: prevention of osteoporosis

Contraindications/cautions
- Contraindicated in areas where fluoride content of drinking water exceeds 0.7 ppm, in the presence of low sodium or sodium-free diets, hypersensitivity to fluoride.
- Use caution in the presence of pregnancy, lactation.

Dosage
Adult: Up to 60 mg/d PO with calcium supplements, estrogen, vitamin D to prevent osteoporosis.
- ***Rinse:*** 10 ml; swish around teeth and spit out.

Pediatric: Dosage refers to daily dose.
- ***Fluoride content of drinking water < 0.3 ppm***
- *Younger than 2 y:* 0.25 mg PO.
- *2–3 y:* 0.5 mg PO.
- *3–12 y:* 1 mg PO.
- ***Fluoride content of drinking water 0.3–0.7 ppm***
- *Younger than 2 y:* 0.125 mg PO.
- *2–3 y:* 0.25 mg PO.
- *3–14 y:* 0.25–0.75 mg PO.
- ***Topical rinse***
- *6–12 y:* 5–10 ml/d.
- *Older than 12 y:* 10 ml; swish around teeth and spit out.

Adverse effects in *Italics* are most common; those in **Bold** are life-threatening.

Pharmacokinetics

Route	Onset	Peak
Oral	Unknown	

Metabolism: $T_{1/2}$: unknown
Distribution: Crosses placenta; enters breast milk
Excretion: Urine, sweat glands, feces

Adverse effects

- **Dermatologic:** Eczema, atopic dermatitis, urticaria, rash
- **Other:** Gastric distress, headache, weakness, staining of teeth (with rinse)

Clinically important drug-food interactions

- Milk, dairy products may decrease absorption; avoid simultaneous use

Nursing Considerations

Assessment

- *History:* Fluoride content of drinking water, low sodium or sodium-free diets, hypersensitivity to fluoride, pregnancy, lactation
- *Physical:* Skin—color, turgor; state of teeth and gums

Implementation

- Do not administer with milk or dairy products.
- Inform patient that tablets may be chewed, swallowed whole, added to drinking water or juice.
- Administer drops undiluted, or mix with fluids or food.
- Ensure that patient has brushed and flossed teeth before the use of rinse and that patient expectorates fluid; it should not be swallowed.
- Monitor teeth, and arrange for dental consultation if mottling of teeth occurs.
- Monitor patient for signs of overdose (salivation, nausea, abdominal pain, vomiting, diarrhea, irritability, convulsions, respiratory arrest); forced diuresis, gastric lavage, supportive measures may be required.

Drug-specific teaching points

- Take this drug as prescribed; chew tablets, swallow whole, or add to drinking water or fruit juice.
- Dilute drops in fluids or food, or take undiluted.
- Brush and floss before use of rinse; swish around mouth and spit out liquid; do not eat, drink, or rinse out mouth for 30 min after use.
- Avoid simultaneous use of milk or diary products and this drug.
- Arrange to have regular dental examinations while you are on this drug.
- Report increased salivation, nausea, abdominal pain, diarrhea, irritability, mottling of teeth

☐ sodium polystyrene sulfonate

(pol ee stye' reen)
Kayexalate, SPS

Pregnancy Category C

Drug classes
Potassium-removing resin

Therapeutic actions
An ion exchange resin that releases sodium ions in exchange for potassium ions as it passes along the intestine after oral administration or is retained in the colon after enema, thus reducing elevated serum potassium levels; action is limited and unpredictable.

Indications
- Treatment of hyperkalemia

Contraindications/cautions
- Severe hypertension, severe CHF, marked edema (risk of sodium overload).

Dosage
Adult
- **Oral:** 15–60 g/d, best given as 15 g one to four times per day. May be given as suspension with water or syrup (20–100 ml). Often given with sorbitol to combat constipation.

Adverse effects in *Italics* are most common; those in **Bold** are life-threatening.

sodium polystyrene sulfonate

- **Enema:** 30–50 g q6h given in appropriate vehicle and retained for 30–60 min.

Pediatric: Give lower doses, using the exchange ratio of 1 mEq potassium/g resin as the basis for calculation.

Pharmacokinetics

Route	Onset
Oral	2–12 h
Rectal	Very long

Excretion: Through the feces or expelled as enema

Adverse effects
- GI: *Constipation, fecal impaction, gastric irritation, anorexia, nausea, vomiting*
- Hematologic: *Hypokalemia*, electrolyte abnormalities (particularly decrease in calcium and magnesium)

Clinically important drug-drug interactions
- Risk of metabolic alkalosis when administered with nonabsorbable cation-donating antacids

■ Nursing Considerations

Assessment
- *History:* Severe hypertension, severe CHF, marked edema
- *Physical:* Orientation, reflexes; P, auscultation, BP, baseline ECG, peripheral edema; bowel sounds, abdominal exam; serum electrolytes

Implementation
- Administer resin through plastic stomach tube, if appropriate; may be mixed with a diet appropriate for renal failure patients.
- Administer powder form of resin in an oral suspension in a syrup base to increase palatability.
- Administer as an enema after first giving a cleansing enema; insert a soft, large rubber tube into the rectum for a distance of about 20 cm; with the tip well into the sigmoid colon, tape into place. Suspend the resin in 100 ml sorbitol or 20% Dextrose in Water at body temperature, introduce by gravity, keeping the particles in suspension by stirring. Flush with 50–100 ml fluid and clamp the tube, leaving it in place. If back leakage occurs, elevate hips or have patient assume the knee-chest position. Retain suspension for at least 30–60 min, several hours is preferable, then irrigate the colon with a non–sodium-containing solution at body temperature; 2 qt of solution may be necessary to remove the resin. Drain the return constantly through a Y-tube connection.
- Prepare fresh suspensions for each dose. Do not store beyond 24 h. Do not heat suspensions; this may alter the exchange properties.
- Monitor patient and consider use of other measures (IV calcium, sodium bicarbonate, or glucose and insulin) in cases of severe hyperkalemia, in states of rapid tissue breakdown (eg, burns, renal failure).
- Monitor serum electrolytes (potassium, sodium, calcium, magnesium) regularly during therapy, and arrange for appropriate measures to counteract disturbances.
- Arrange for treatment of constipation with 10–20 ml of 70% sorbitol q2h or as needed to produce two watery stools per day. Establish a bowel training program, as appropriate.

Drug-specific teaching points
- This drug is often used in emergency situations in which case drug teaching should be incorporated into patient teaching about the entire emergency situation.
- Know that the following side effects may occur: GI upset, constipation.
- Be aware that frequent blood tests will be necessary to monitor the effectiveness of this drug.
- Report confusion, irregular heartbeats, constipation, severe GI upset.

Adverse effects in *Italics* are most common; those in **Bold** are life-threatening.

☐ sodium thiosalicylate

(theye o sall i' sill ayte)
Rexolate, Tusal

Pregnancy Category C

Drug classes
Antipyretic
Analgesic (non-narcotic)
Anti-inflammatory
Antirheumatic
Salicylate
NSAID

Therapeutic actions
Analgesic and antirheumatic effects are attributable to the ability to inhibit the synthesis of prostaglandins, important mediators of inflammation; antipyretic effects are not fully understood, but salicylates probably act in the thermoregulatory center of the hypothalamus to block the effects of endogenous pyrogen by inhibiting the synthesis of the prostaglandin intermediary.

Indications
- Active gout
- Muscular pain and musculoskeletal disturbances
- Rheumatic fever

Contraindications/cautions
- Contraindicated in the presence of chickenpox or viral infection in children.
- Use caution in the presence of allergy to salicylates or NSAIDs, bleeding disorders, impaired hepatic or renal function, GI ulceration (less of a problem with this salicylate than with some others); pregnancy, lactation.

Dosage
Adult
- ***Acute gout:*** 100 mg q3–4h IM for 2 d, then 100 mg/d IM.
- ***Muscular pain and musculoskeletal disturbances:*** 50–100 mg/d or on alternate days IM.
- ***Rheumatic fever:*** 100–150 mg q4–6h IM for 3 d, then reduce to 100 mg bid. Continue until patient is asymptomatic.

Pediatric: Dosage schedule not established.

Pharmacokinetics

Route	Onset	Peak
IM	Immediate	15–100 min

Metabolism: Hepatic, $T_{1/2}$: 2–18 h
Distribution: Crosses placenta; enters breast milk
Excretion: Urine

Adverse effects
NSAIDs
- CNS: *Headache, dizziness, somnolence, insomnia,* fatigue, tiredness, dizziness, tinnitus, ophthalmologic effects
- GI: *Nausea, dyspepsia, GI pain,* diarrhea, vomiting, *constipation,* flatulence
- **Respiratory:** Dyspnea, hemoptysis, pharyngitis, bronchospasm, rhinitis
- **Hematologic:** Bleeding, platelet inhibition with higher doses, neutropenia, eosinophilia, leukopenia, pancytopenia, thrombocytopenia, agranulocytosis, granulocytopenia, aplastic anemia, decreased hemoglobin or hematocrit, bone marrow depression, mennorhagia
- **GU:** Dysuria, renal impairment
- **Dermatologic:** *Rash,* pruritus, sweating, dry mucous membranes, stomatitis
- **Other:** Peripheral edema, anaphylactoid reactions to fatal anaphylactic shock; salicylism: dizziness, tinnitus, difficulty hearing, nausea, vomiting, diarrhea, mental confusion, lassitude (dose related); acute salicylate toxicity (respiratory alkalosis, hyperpnea, tachypnea, hemmorhage, excitement, confusion, asterixis, pulmonary edema, convulsions, tetany, metabolic acidosis, fever, coma, cardiovascular collapse, renal and respiratory failure; dose related: 20–25 g in adults)

Clinically important drug-drug interactions
• Increased risk of GI ulceration with corticosteroids if taken with sodium thiosalicylate • Increased risk of salicylate toxicity with carbonic anhydrase inhibitors • In-

creased toxicity of carbonic anhydrase inhibitors, valproic acid if taken concurrently • Decreased serum salicylate levels if taken with corticosteroids, antacids, urine alkalinizers (sodium acetate, sodium bicarbonate, sodium citrate, sodium lactate, tromethamine) • Increased methotrexate levels and toxicity if taken with sodium thiosalicylate • Greater glucose-lowering effect of sulfonylureas, insulin with large doses of salicylates • Decreased uricosuric effect of probenecid, sulfinpyrazone if taken concurrently • Decreased diuretic effect of spironolactone if taken with sodium thiosalicylate

Drug-lab test interferences
• Decreased serum PBI • False-negative readings for urine glucose by glucose oxidase method and copper reduction method • Interference with urine 5-HIAA determinations by fluorescent methods but not by nitrosonaphthol colorimetric method • Interference with urinary ketone determination by ferric chloride method • Falsely elevated urine VMA levels with most tests; false decrease in VMA using the Pisano method

■ Nursing Considerations

Assessment
- *History:* Allergy to salicylates or NSAIDs, bleeding disorders, impaired hepatic or renal function, GI ulceration; lactation; pregnancy; chickenpox or viral infection
- *Physical:* Skin color and lesions; eighth cranial nerve function, orientation, reflexes, affect; P, BP, perfusion; R, adventitious sounds; liver evaluation and bowel sounds; CBC, urinalysis, stool guiaiac; renal and liver function tests.

Implementation
- Administer by IM injection.
- Avoid use of this preparation in patients with sodium restrictions.
- Institute emergency procedures if overdose occurs: gastric lavage, induction of emesis, activated charcoal, supportive therapy.

Drug-specific teaching points
- Report ringing in the ears, dizziness, confusion, abdominal pain, rapid or difficult breathing, nausea, vomiting.

❒ somatrem

(soe' ma trem)
Protropin

Pregnancy Category C

Drug classes
Hormonal agent

Therapeutic actions
Artificial hormone with identical amino acid sequence of pituitary-derived human growth hormone plus one additional amino acid; therapeutically equivalent to human somatotropin; withdrawn from the market because of microbial impurities; stimulates skeletal (linear) growth, growth of internal organs, protein synthesis, many other metabolic processes required for normal growth.

Indications
- Long-term treatment of children who have growth failure due to lack of adequate endogenous growth hormone secretion
- Orphan drug use: treatment of short stature associated with Turner's syndrome

Contraindications/cautions
- Known sensitivity to somatrem, benzyl alcohol, closed epiphyses, underlying cranial lesions.

Dosage
Individualize dosage based on patient response. Up to 0.1 mg/kg IM given three times per week is recommended. Do not exceed this dosage.

Pharmacokinetics

Route	Onset	Peak
IM	Varies	Days to weeks

Metabolism: Hepatic, $T_{1/2}$: 20–30 min
Excretion: Urine

Adverse effects
- **Hematologic:** *Development of antibodies to growth hormone*
- **Endocrine:** Hypothyroidism, insulin resistance

■ Nursing Considerations
Assessment
- *History:* Sensitivity to somatrem, benzyl alcohol, closed epiphyses, underlying cranial lesions
- *Physical:* Height; body weight; thyroid function tests, glucose tolerance tests, growth hormone levels

Implementation
- Reconstitute each 5-mg vial for administration to adults or older children with 1–5 ml of Bacteriostatic Water for Injection (Benzyl Alcohol Preserved) only.
- Reconstitute drug for use in newborns with plain Water for Injection without benzyl alcohol. Benzyl alcohol has been associated with severe toxicity in newborns. Use only one dose per vial and discard the unused portion.
- Prepare the solution by injecting the diluent into the vial, aiming the stream of liquid against the glass wall. Swirl the product vial with a gentle rotary motion until the contents are completely dissolved. *Do not shake.* After reconstitution, contents should be clear without particulate matter. Use a needle that is long enough (at least 1 in) to ensure injection deep into the muscle layer.
- Refrigerate vials; reconstituted vials should be used within 7 d; do not freeze drug.
- Arrange for periodic testing of glucose tolerance, thyroid function, and growth hormone antibodies. Arrange for appropriate treatment if indicated by test results.

Drug-specific teaching points
- Know that this drug must be given IM three times per week.
- Be aware that you may experience sudden growth; increase in appetite; a decrease in thyroid function (replacement hormone can be ordered).
- Report lack of growth, increased hunger, thirst, increased and frequent voiding, fatigue, dry skin, intolerance to cold.

❒ somatropin

*(soe ma **troe**' pin)*
Humatrope, Nutropin

Pregnancy Category C

Drug classes
Hormonal agent

Therapeutic actions
Hormone of recombinant DNA origin; contains the identical amino acid sequence of pituitary-derived human growth hormone; equivalent to human somatotropin from cadaver sources; withdrawn from the market because of microbial impurities; stimulates skeletal (linear) growth, growth of internal organs, protein synthesis, many other metabolic processes required for normal growth.

Indications
- Long-term treatment of children who have growth failure due to lack of adequate endogenous growth hormone secretion
- Treatment of children with growth failure associated with chronic renal failure, chronic renal insufficiency, up to the time of renal transplantation
- Orphan drug uses: enhancement of nitrogen retention in severe burns, treatment of short stature associated with Turner's syndrome

Contraindications/cautions
- Known sensitivity to somatropin, benzyl alcohol, glycerin (*Humatrope*), closed epiphyses, underlying cranial lesions.

Dosage
Individualize dosage based on patient response. Up to 0.06 mg/kg (0.16 IU/kg) IM or SC given three times per week is

1008 ■ sotalol hydrochloride

recommended. The same total dosage can be given in smaller increments six to seven times per week. Do not exceed this dosage.

Pharmacokinetics

Route	Onset	Peak
IM/SC	Varies	3–7½ h

Metabolism: Hepatic, $T_{1/2}$: 15–50 min
Distribution: Crosses placenta; enters breast milk
Excretion: Urine and feces

Adverse effects
- Hematologic: *Development of antibodies to growth hormone* (not as likely as with somatrem)
- Endocrine: Hypothyroidism, insulin resistance

■ Nursing Considerations

Assessment
- *History:* Known sensitivity to somatropin, closed epiphyses, underlying cranial lesions
- *Physical:* Height; body weight; thyroid function tests, glucose tolerance tests, growth hormone levels

Implementation
- Administer drug IM or SC, depending on patient.
- Divide total dose into smaller increments given six to seven times a week for smaller patients unable to tolerate injections.
- Reconstitute drug carefully following manufacturer's instructions; do not shake; do not inject if solution is cloudy or contains particulate matter.
- Refrigerate vials; reconstituted vials should be used within 7 d; do not freeze drug.
- Arrange for periodic testing of glucose tolerance, thyroid function, and growth hormone antibodies. Arrange for appropriate treatment if indicated by test results.

Drug-specific teaching points
- Be aware that the drug must be given IM or SC three times per week. Drug can be given in smaller doses six to seven times a week if needed.
- Know that you may experience sudden growth, increase in appetite, decrease in thyroid function (replacement hormone can be ordered).
- Report lack of growth, increased hunger, thirst, increased and frequent voiding, fatigue, dry skin, intolerance to cold.

☐ sotalol hydrochloride

(sob' tal lole)
Betapace

Pregnancy Category B

Drug classes
Beta-adrenergic blocking agent (beta$_1$ selective)
Antiarrhythmic drug

Therapeutic actions
Blocks beta-adrenergic receptors of the sympathetic nervous system in the heart and juxtaglomerular apparatus (kidney), thus decreasing the excitability of the heart, decreasing cardiac output and oxygen consumption.

Indications
- Treatment of life-threatening ventricular arrhythmias; because of proarrhythmic effects, use for less than life-threatening arrhythmias, even symptomatic ones, is not recommended.

Contraindications/cautions
- Contraindicated in the presence of sinus bradycardia (HR < 45 beats/min), second- or third-degree heart block (PR interval > 0.24 sec), cardiogenic shock, CHF, asthma, COPD, lactation .
- Use caution in the presence of diabetes or thyrotoxicosis, hepatic or renal impairment.

Dosage
Adult: Initial dose, 80 mg PO bid. Adjust dose gradually, evey 2–3 d, until appropriate response occurs; may require 240–320 mg/d.

Adverse effects in *Italics* are most common; those in **Bold** are life-threatening.

Pediatric: Safety and efficacy not established.

Geriatric or renal impaired: CCr > 60 ml/min, 12-h dosing intervals; CCr 30–60 ml/min, 24-h dosing intervals; CCr 10–30 ml/min, 36- to 48-h dosing intervals; CCr < 10 ml/min, individualize dose based on response.

Pharmacokinetics

Route	Onset	Peak
Oral	Varies	3–4 h

Metabolism: $T_{1/2}$: 12 h
Distribution: Crosses placenta; enters breast milk
Excretion: Urine

Adverse effects

- CNS: Dizziness, vertigo, tinnitus, fatigue, emotional depression, paresthesias, sleep disturbances, hallucinations, disorientation, memory loss, slurred speech
- GI: *Gastric pain, flatulence, constipation, diarrhea, nausea, vomiting,* anorexia
- CV: *CHF, cardiac arrhythmias, SA or AV nodal block,* peripheral vascular insufficiency, claudication, CVA, pulmonary edema, hypotension
- Respiratory: Bronchospasm, dyspnea, cough, bronchial obstruction, nasal stuffiness, rhinitis
- GU: *Impotence, decreased libido,* Peyronie's disease, dysuria, nocturia, frequent urination
- MS: Joint pain, arthralgia, muscle cramp
- EENT: Eye irritation, dry eyes, conjunctivitis, blurred vision
- Dermatologic: Rash, pruritus, sweating, dry skin
- Allergic reactions: Pharyngitis, erythematous rash, fever, sore throat, **laryngospasm, respiratory distress**
- Other: *Decreased exercise tolerance, development of antinuclear antibodies,* hyperglycemia or hypoglycemia, elevated serum transaminase

Clinically important drug-drug interactions

• Possible increased effects of sotalol if taken with verapamil • Increased risk of postural hypotension if taken concurrently with prazosin • Possible increased blood pressure lowering effects if taken concurrently with aspirin, bismuth subsalicylate, magnesium salicylate, sulfinpyrazone, oral contraceptives • Decreased antihypertensive effects if taken with NSAIDs, clonidine • Possible increased hypoglycemic effect of insulin if taken concurrently

Drug-lab test interferences

• Possible false results with glucose or insulin tolerance tests (oral)

■ Nursing Considerations

Assessment

- *History:* Sinus bradycardia, second- or third-degree heart block, cardiogenic shock, CHF, asthma, COPD, pregnancy, lactation, diabetes or thyrotoxicosis
- *Physical:* Body weight, skin condition, neurologic status, P, BP, ECG, respiratory status, kidney and thyroid function, blood and urine glucose

Implementation

- May be given with meals.
- Do not administer to patients unless they are not responsive to other antiarrhythmics and have a life-threatening ventricular arrhythmia. Monitor patient response carefully; proarrhythmic effect can be pronounced.
- Do not discontinue drug abruptly after chronic therapy. Taper drug gradually over 2 wk with monitoring (abrupt withdrawal may cause serious beta-adrenergic rebound effects).
- Discontinue other antiarrhythmics gradually, allowing for two to three plasma half-lives of the drug before starting sotalol. After discontinuing amiodarone, do not start sotalol until QT interval is normalized.
- Consult with physician about withdrawing drug if patient is to undergo surgery (withdrawal is controversial).

Adverse effects in *Italics* are most common; those in **Bold** are life-threatening.

Drug-specific teaching points
- Take drug with meals.
- Do not to stop taking this drug unless instructed to do so by a health care provider.
- Avoid driving or dangerous activities if dizziness, weakness occur.
- Know that the following side effects may occur: dizziness, lightheadedness, loss of appetite, nightmares, depression, sexual impotence.
- Report difficulty breathing, night cough, swelling of extremities, slow pulse, confusion, depression, rash, fever, sore throat.

☐ spectinomycin hydrochloride

*(spek ti noe **mye'** sin)*
Trobicin

Pregnancy Category B

Drug classes
Antibiotic

Therapeutic actions
Bactericidal: inhibits protein synthesis of susceptible strains of *Neisseria gonorrhoeae*, causing cell death.

Indications
- Acute gonococcal urethritis and proctitis in males
- Acute gonococcal cervicitis and proctitis in females
- *Not effective* in treating syphilis or pharyngeal infections caused by *N. gonorrhoeae*

Contraindications/cautions
- Contraindicated in the presence of allergy to spectinomycin, lactation.
- Use caution in the presence of pregnancy (safety not established; but drug is recommended treatment for penicillin or probenecid allergic pregnant women with gonococcal infections).

Dosage
Adult: 2 g IM. In geographic areas where antibiotic resistance is prevalent, 4 g IM divided between two gluteal injection sites is preferred.
Pediatric: Not recommended.
CDC recommended treatment for gonorrhea (for penicillin-allergic patients or penicillinase-producing N. gonorrhoeae infections)— uncomplicated infections: 2 g IM.
- *< 45 kg:* 40 mg/kg IM.
- ***Penicillinase-producing N. gonorrhoeae:*** 2 g IM.
- *< 45 kg:* 40 mg/kg IM.
- ***Gonococcal infections in pregnancy:*** 2 g IM.

Pharmacokinetics

Route	Onset	Peak
IM	Varies	1 h

Metabolism: $T_{1/2}$: 1.5–2.8 h
Distribution: Crosses placenta; enters breast milk
Excretion: Urine

Adverse effects
- **CNS:** *Dizziness, chills,* fever, insomnia
- **Hematologic:** Decreased Hct, hemoglobin, creatinine clearance, increased alkaline phosphatase, BUN, SGPT
- **GU:** *Decreased urine output without documented renal toxicity*
- **Dermatologic:** Urticaria
- **Local:** *Soreness at injection site*

■ Nursing Considerations

Assessment
- *History:* Allergy to spectinomycin, pregnancy, lactation
- *Physical:* Site of infection, skin—color, lesions; orientation, reflexes; R, adventitious sounds; CBC, liver and renal function tests

Implementation
- Administer only IM; administer deep into upper outer quadrant of the gluteus to decrease discomfort.

Adverse effects in *Italics* are most common; those in **Bold** are life-threatening.

- Reconstitute with Bacteriostatic Water for Injection with 0.9% benzyl alcohol: 3.2 ml diluent for 2-g vial, 6.2 ml diluent for 4-g vial. Stable for 24 h after being reconstituted.
- Culture site of infection before beginning therapy.
- Monitor for development of resistant strains on prolonged therapy.
- Monitor blood counts, renal and liver function tests on long-term therapy.

Drug-specific teaching points
- Be aware that this drug is available only in the IM form.
- Report worsening of infection, dark urine, yellowing of the skin or eyes, skin rash or itching.

spirapril

(spear' ah pril)
Renormax

Pregnancy Category C

Drug classes
Antihypertensive
Angiotensin converting enzyme inhibitor

Therapeutic actions
Renin, synthesized by the kidneys, is released into the circulation where it acts on a plasma precursor to produce angiotensin I, which is converted by angiotensin converting enzyme to angiotensin II, a potent vasoconstrictor that also causes release of aldosterone from the adrenals. Both of these actions increase blood pressure. Spirapril blocks the conversion of angiotensin I to angiotensin II, leading to decreased blood pressure, decreased aldosterone secretion, a small increase in serum potassium levels, and sodium and fluid loss; increased prostaglandin synthesis may also be involved in the antihypertensive action.

Indications
- Treatment of hypertension—alone or in combination with thiazide-type diuretics

Contraindications/cautions
- Allergy to ACE inhibitors; impaired renal function; CHF; salt/volume depletion, lactation

Dosage
Adult: 3–24 mg PO bid to tid, based on patient response.
Pediatric: Safety and efficacy not established.
Geriatric and renal impaired: Excretion is reduced in renal failure; use smaller initial dose and titrate at smaller doses with 1–2 wk intervals between increases; slowly titrate to smallest effective dose; use of a loop diuretic is preferred with renal dysfunction.

Pharmacokinetics

Route	Onset	Peak
Oral	15 min	0.5–1.5 h

Metabolism: $T_{1/2}$: 2 hours
Distribution: Crosses placenta; passes into breast milk
Excretion: Urine

Adverse effects
- **GI:** *gastric irritation, aphthous ulcers, peptic ulcers, dysgeusia,* cholestatic jaundice, hepatocellular injury, anorexia, constipation
- **CV:** *tachycardia,* angina pectoris, **myocardial infarction**, Raynaud's syndrome, CHF, hypotension in salt/volume depleted patients
- **Hematologic:** neutropenia, agranulocytosis, thrombocytopenia, hemolytic anemia, **fatal pancytopenia**
- **GU:** *proteinuria,* renal insufficiency, renal failure, polyuria, oliguria, urinary frequency
- **Dermatologic:** *rash, pruritus,* pemphigoid-like reaction, scalded mouth sensation, exfoliative dermatitis, photosensitivity, alopecia
- **Other:** *cough,* malaise, dry mouth, lymphadenopathy

Clinically important drug-drug interactions
- Increased risk of hypersensitivity reactions if taken concurrently with allopurinal

Adverse effects in *Italics* are most common; those in **Bold** are life-threatening.

1012 ■ spironolactone

Decreased antihypertensive effects if taken with indomethacin

Drug-lab test interferences
- False-positive test for urine acetone

■ Nursing Considerations

Assessment
- *History*: Allergy to ACE inhibitors; impaired renal function; CHF; salt/volume depletion; pregnancy; lactation
- *Physical*: Skin—color, lesions, turgor; body temperature; P, BP, peripheral perfusion; mucous membranes, bowel sounds, liver evaluation; urinalysis, renal and liver function tests, CBC and differential

Implementation
- Alert surgeon and mark patient's chart with notice that spirapril is being taken; the angiotensin II formation subsequent to compensatory renin release during surgery will be blocked; hypotension may be reversed with volume expansion.
- Monitor patient closely in any situation that may lead to a fall in blood pressure secondary to reduction in fluid volume (excessive perspiration and dehydration, vomiting, diarrhea), as excessive hypotension may occur.
- Arrange for reduced dosage in patients with impaired renal function.

Drug-specific teaching points
- Do not stop taking the medication without consulting your physician
- Know that the following side effects may occur: GI upset, loss of appetite, change in taste perception (these may be limited effects that will pass with time); mouth sores (frequent mouth care may help); skin rash; fast heart rate; dizziness, lightheadedness (this usually passes after the first few days of therapy; if it occurs, change position slowly and limit your activities to those that do not require alertness and precision).
- Be careful in any situation that may lead to a drop in blood pressure (diarrhea, sweating, vomiting, dehydration); if lightheadedness or dizziness occur, consult your nurse or physician.
- Report mouth sores; sore throat, fever, chills; swelling of the hands, feet; irregular heartbeat, chest pains; swelling of the face, eyes, lips, tongue; difficulty in breathing.

⬜ spironolactone

*(speer on oh **lak'** tone)*
Aldactone

Pregnancy Category D

Drug classes
Potassium-sparing diuretic
Aldosterone antagonist

Therapeutic actions
Competitively blocks the effects of aldosterone in the renal tubule, causing loss of sodium and water and retention of potassium.

Indications
- Primary hyperaldosteronism, diagnosis, maintenance
- Adjunctive therapy in edema associated with CHF, nephrotic syndrome, hepatic cirrhosis
- Treatment of hypokalemia or prevention of hypokalemia in patients who would be at high risk if hypokalemia occurred: digitalized patients, patients with cardiac arrhythmias
- Essential hypertension, usually in combination with other drugs
- Unlabeled uses: treatment of hirsutism due to its antiandrogenic properties, palliation of symptoms of PMS syndrome, treatment of familial male precocious puberty, short-term treatment of acne vulgaris

Contraindications/cautions
- Contraindicated in the presence of allergy to spironolactone, hyperkalemia, renal disease, lactation.
- Use caution in the presence of pregnancy.

Dosage
Adult
- ***Edema:*** 100–200 mg/d PO in single or divided doses. Adjust to patient's response.

Alternate-day therapy or intermittent-day therapy may be the most effective treatment.
- ***Diagnosis of hyperaldosteronism:*** 400 mg/d PO for 3–4 wk (long test). Correction of hypokalemia and hypertension are presumptive evidence of primary hyperaldosteronism 400 mg/d PO for 4 d (short test). If serum K+ increases but decreases when drug is stopped, presumptive diagnosis can be made.
- ***Maintenance therapy for hyperaldosteronism:*** 100–400 mg/d PO.
- ***Essential hypertension:*** 50–100 mg/d PO. May be combined with other diuretics.
- ***Hypokalemia:*** 25–100 mg/d PO.

Pediatric
- ***Edema:*** 3.3 mg/kg/d PO adjusted to patient's response.

Pharmacokinetics

Route	Onset	Peak	Duration
Oral	24–48 h	48–72 h	48–72 h

Metabolism: Hepatic, $T_{1/2}$: 20 h
Distribution: Crosses placenta; enters breast milk
Excretion: Urine

Adverse effects
- **CNS:** *Dizziness, headache, drowsiness,* fatigue, ataxia, confusion
- **GI:** *Cramping, diarrhea,* dry mouth, thirst
- **Hematologic:** **Hyperkalemia, hyponatremia**
- **GU:** Impotence, irregular menses, amenorrhea, postmenopausal bleeding
- **Dermatologic:** *Rash,* urticaria
- **Other:** Carcinogenic in animals, *deepening of the voice, hirsutism, gynecomastia*

Clinically important drug-drug interactions
- Increased hyperkalemia if taken with potassium supplements, diets rich in potassium • Decreased diuretic effect of spironolactone if taken with salicylates

Drug-lab test interferences
- Interference with radioimmunoassay for digoxin; false increase in serum digoxin levels

■ Nursing Considerations

Assessment
- *History:* Allergy to spironolactone, hyperkalemia, renal disease, pregnancy, lactation
- *Physical:* Skin—color, lesions, edema; orientation, reflexes, muscle strength; P, baseline ECG, BP; R, pattern, adventitious sounds; liver evaluation, bowel sounds; urinary output patterns, menstrual cycle; CBC, serum electrolytes, renal function tests, urinalysis

Implementation
- Mark calendars of outpatients as reminders of drug days if every other day or 3- to 5-d/wk therapy is most effective for treating edema.
- Administer single daily doses early in the day so that increased urination does not interfere with sleep.
- Make suspension as follows: tablets may be pulverized and given in cherry syrup for young children. This suspension is stable for 1 mo if refrigerated.
- Measure and record regular body weights to monitor mobilization of edema fluid.
- Avoid giving patient foods rich in potassium.
- Arrange for regular evaluation of serum electrolytes, BUN.

Drug-specific teaching points
- Record alternate-day therapy on a calendar, or prepare dated envelopes. Take the drug early in the day because increased urination will occur.
- Weigh yourself on a regular basis, at the same time of the day and in the same clothing, and record the weight on your calendar.
- Avoid foods that are rich in potassium (eg, fruits, Sanka) while you are taking this drug.
- Know that the following side effects may occur: increased volume and frequency

Adverse effects in *Italics* are most common; those in **Bold** are life-threatening.

of urination; dizziness, confusion, feeling faint on arising, drowsiness (if these changes occur, avoid rapid position changes, hazardous activities [like driving a car], and alcohol, which can intensify these problems); increased thirst (sucking on sugarless lozenges may help to alleviate the thirst; frequent mouth care may also help); changes in menstrual cycle, deepening of the voice, impotence, enlargement of the breasts can occur (these are reversible when the drug is stopped).
- Report loss or gain of more than 3 lb in one day, swelling in your ankles or fingers, dizziness, trembling, numbness, fatigue, enlargement of breasts, deepening of voice, impotence, muscle weakness or cramps.

☐ stanozolol

*(stan **ob'** zoe lole)*
Winstrol

Pregnancy Category X
C-III Controlled Substance

Drug classes
Anabolic steroid
Hormonal agent

Therapeutic actions
Synthetic testosterone analog with strong anabolic activity and weak androgenic activity; promotes body tissue-building processes and reverses catabolic or tissue-depleting processes; increases hemoglobin and red cell mass.

Indications
- Prophylactic use to decrease frequency and severity of hereditary angioedema attacks

Contraindications/cautions
- Known sensitivity to anabolic steroids; prostate or breast cancer in males, benign prostatic hypertrophy, breast cancer in females, pituitary insufficiency, MI (effects on cholesterol), nephrosis, liver disease, hypercalcemia, pregnancy (masculinization of the fetus can occur), lactation.

Dosage
Adult: Initially, 2 mg PO tid. After favorable response in terms of prevention of attacks, decrease dosage to 2 mg/d over 2–3 mo.
Pediatric: Long-term therapy is contraindicated because of possibility of serious disruption of growth and development; weigh benefits and risks.

Pharmacokinetics

Route	Onset
Oral	Rapid

Metabolism: Hepatic, $T_{1/2}$: unknown
Distribution: Crosses placenta; enters breast milk
Excretion: Urine

Adverse effects
- CNS: *Excitation, insomnia,* chills, toxic confusion
- GI: Hepatotoxicity, peliosis, **hepatitis with life-threatening liver failure or intra-abdominal hemorrhage**; liver cell tumors, sometimes malignant and fatal, *nausea, vomiting, diarrhea, abdominal fullness, loss of appetite, burning of tongue*
- Hematologic: *Blood lipid changes*—decreased HDL and sometimes increased LDL; iron deficiency anemia, hypercalcemia, altered serum cholesterol levels; *retention of sodium, chloride, water,* potassium, phosphates and calcium
- GU: Possible increased risk of prostatic hypertrophy, carcinoma in geriatric patients
- Endocrine: *Virilization: prepubertal males*—phallic enlargement, hirsutism, increased skin pigmentation; *postpubertal males*—inhibition of testicular function, gynecomastia, testicular atrophy, priapism, baldness, epidiymitis, change in libido; *females* — hirsutism, hoarseness, deepening of the voice, clitoral enlargement, menstrual irregulari-

ties, baldness; decreased glucose tolerance
- **Other:** *Acne,* premature closure of the epiphyses

Clinically important drug-drug interactions

- Potentiation of oral anticoagulants if taken with anabolic steroids • Decreased need for insulin, oral hypoglycemica agents if anabolic steroids are used

Drug-lab test interferences

- Altered glucose tolerance tests • Decrease in thyroid function tests, an effect that may persist for 2–3 wk after therapy • Increased creatinine, creatinine clearance, which may last for 2 wk after therapy

■ Nursing Considerations

Assessment

- *History:* Known sensitivity to anabolic steroids, prostate or breast cancer, benign prostatic hypertrophy, pituitary insufficiency, MI, nephrosis, liver disease, hypercalcemia, pregnancy, lactation
- *Physical:* Skin—color, texture; hair distribution pattern; affect, orientation; abdominal exam, liver evaluation; serum electrolytes, serum cholesterol levels, glucose tolerance tests, thyroid function tests, long-bone x-ray (in children)

Implementation

- Administer with food if GI upset or nausea occurs.
- Monitor patient for occurrence of attacks with stressful or traumatic situations; dosage may need to be increased.
- Monitor effect on children with long-bone x-rays every 3–6 mo during therapy; discontinue drug well before the bone age reaches the norm for the patient's chronologic age because effects may continue for 6 mo after therapy.
- Monitor patient for occurrence of edema; arrange for appropriate diuretic therapy as needed.
- Arrange to monitor liver function, serum electrolytes periodically during therapy, and consult with physician for appropriate corrective measures as needed.
- Arrange to measure cholesterol levels periodically in patients who are at high risk for coronary artery disease.
- Monitor diabetic patients closely because glucose tolerance may change. Adjustments may be needed in insulin, oral hypoglycemic dosage, and diet.

Drug-specific teaching points

- Take drug with food if nausea or GI upset occurs.
- Know that the following side effects may occur: nausea, vomiting, diarrhea, burning of the tongue (small, frequent meals may help); body hair growth, baldness, deepening of the voice, loss of libido, impotence (most of these effects will be reversible when the drug is stopped); excitation, confusion, insomnia (avoid driving, performing tasks that require alertness if these effects occur); swelling of the ankles, fingers (medication may be ordered to help).
- Be aware that diabetic patients need to monitor urine sugar closely as glucose tolerance may change; report any abnormalities to physician, and corrective action can be taken.
- Be aware that these drugs do not enhance athletic ability but do have serious effects and should not be used for increasing muscle strength.
- Report ankle swelling, skin color changes, severe nausea, vomiting, hoarseness, body hair growth, deepening of the voice, acne, menstrual irregularities in women.

❒ stavudine

(stay vew' den)
Zerit

Pregnancy Category C

Drug classes
Antiviral drug

Therapeutic actions
Inhibits replication of some retroviruses, including HIV, HTLV III, LAV, ARV.

Adverse effects in *Italics* are most common; those in **Bold** are life-threatening.

Indications
- Treatment of adults with advanced HIV infection who are intolerant to approved therapies with proven clinical benefit or who have experienced significant clinical or immunologic deterioration while receiving these therapies or for whom these therapies are contraindicated

Contraindications/cautions
- Contraindicated in the presence of life-threatening allergy to any component, pregnancy, lactation.
- Use caution in the presence of compromised bone marrow, impaired renal or hepatic function.

Dosage
Adult: 40 mg q12h PO without regard to meals.
Pediatric: Safety and efficacy not established.

Pharmacokinetics

Route	Onset	Peak
Oral	Varies	$\frac{1}{2}$–$1\frac{1}{2}$ h

Metabolism: Hepatic, $T_{1/2}$: 30–60 min
Distribution: Crosses placenta; may enter breast milk
Excretion: Urine

Adverse effects
- **CNS:** *Headache*, insomnia, myalgia, *asthenia*, malaise, dizziness, paresthesia, somnolence
- **GI:** *Nausea, GI pain, diarrhea*, anorexia, vomiting, dyspepsia
- **Hematologic:** *Agranulocytopenia*, severe anemia requiring transfusions
- **Other:** *Fever*, diaphoresis, dyspnea, *rash*, taste perversion

■ Nursing Considerations

Assessment
- *History:* Life-threatening allergy to any component, compromised bone marrow, impaired renal or hepatic function, pregnancy, lactation
- *Physical:* Skin—rashes, lesions, texture; body temperature; affect, reflexes, peripheral sensation; bowel sounds, liver evaluation; renal and hepatic function tests, CBC and differential

Implementation
- Arrange to monitor hematologic indices every 2 wk during therapy.
- Administer the drug every 12 h, around the clock; schedule dosing so it will not interrupt sleep.

Drug-specific teaching points
- Take drug every 12 h. Do not share this drug; take exactly as prescribed.
- Be aware that stavudine is not a cure for AIDS; opportunisitc infections may occur, and regular medical care should be sought to deal with the disease.
- Arrange for frequent blood tests needed during the course of treatment; results of blood counts may indicate a need for decreased dosage or discontinuation of the drug for a period of time.
- Know that the following side effects may occur as a result of drug therapy: nausea, loss of appetite, change in taste (small, frequent meals may help); dizziness, loss of feeling (take appropriate precautions if these occur); headache, fever, muscle aches.
- Be aware that stavudine does not reduce the risk of transmission of HIV to others by sexual contact or blood contamination; use appropriate precautions.
- Report extreme fatigue, lethargy, severe headache, severe nausea, vomiting, difficulty breathing, skin rash.

☐ streptokinase

*(strep toe **kin'** ase)*
Streptase, Kabikinase

Pregnancy Category C

Drug classes
Thrombolytic enzyme

Therapeutic actions
Enzyme isolated from streptococcal bacteria; converts endogenous plasminogen to the enzyme plasmin (fibrinolysin) which

Adverse effects in *Italics* are most common; those in **Bold** are life-threatening.

degrades fibrin clots, fibrinogen, and other plasma proteins; lyses thrombi and emboli.

Indications
- Coronary artery thrombosis, IV or intracoronary use within 6 h of onset of symptoms of coronary occlusion
- Deep venous thrombosis of the deep veins
- Arterial thrombosis and embolism not originating on the left side of the heart
- Occluded AV cannulae

Contraindications/cautions
- Contraindicated in the presence of allergy to streptokinase (Note: most patients have been exposed to streptococci and to streptokinase and therefore have developed resistance to the drug; however, allergic reactions are relatively rare), active internal bleeding, recent (within 2 mo) CVA, intracranial or intraspinal surgery, intracranial neoplasm, recent major surgery, obstetric delivery, organ biopsy, or rupture of a noncompressible blood vessel.
- Use caution in the presence of recent serious GI bleed, recent serious trauma, including CPR; severe hypertension; SBE; hemostatic defects; cerebrovascular disease; diabetic hemorrhagic retinopathy; septic thrombosis; pregnancy; lactation.

Dosage
Adult
- ***Lysis of coronary artery thrombi:*** Bolus dose of 20,000 IU directly into the coronary artery. Maintenance dose of 2,000 IU/min for 60 min for a total dose of 140,000 IU *or* 1,500,000 IU administered over 60 min in an infusion of the 1,500,000-U vial diluted to a total volume of 45 ml.
- ***Deep vein thrombosis, pulmonary or arterial embolism, arterial thrombosis:*** Loading dose of 250,000 IU infused into a peripheral vein over 30 min. Maintenance dose, 100,000 IU/h for 24–72 h depending on the patient's response and the area being treated. After treatment with streptokinase, treat with continuous infusion heparin, beginning after thrombin time decreases to less than twice the control value.
- ***AV cannula occlusion:*** Slowly instill 250,000 IU in 2 ml IV solution into the occluded cannula; clamp the cannula for 2 h; then aspirate the catheter and flush with saline.

Pediatric: Safety and efficacy not established.

Pharmacokinetics

Route	Onset	Peak
IV	Immediate	30–60 min

Metabolism: $T_{1/2}$: 23 min
Distribution: Crosses placenta; may enter breast milk
Excretion: Unknown

IV facts
Preparation: Reconstitute vial with 5 ml of Sterile Water for Injection or 5% Dextrose Injection; direct diluent at side of the vial, not directly into the streptokinase. Avoid shaking during reconstitution; gently roll or tilt vial to reconstitute. Further dilute the reconstituted solutions slowly to a total of 45 ml. Solution may be filtered through 0.22 or 0.45 filter. Do not add other medications to reconstituted solutions. Discard solutions that contain large amounts of flocculation. Refrigerate reconstituted solution; discard reconstituted solution after 24 h. Reconstitute the contents of 250,000-IU vial with 2 ml Sodium Chloride or 5% Dextrose Injection for use in AV cannulae.

Infusion: Administer as indicated for each specific problem being treated.

Adverse effects
- CNS: Headache
- CV: Angioneurotic edema, arrhythmias (with intracoronary artery infusion)
- Respiratory: Breathing difficulty, bronchospasm
- Hematologic: *Bleeding (minor or surface* to major internal bleeding)
- Dermatologic: Skin rash, urticaria, itching, flushing
- Other: Musculoskeletal pain, *fever*

Adverse effects in *Italics* are most common; those in **Bold** are life-threatening.

Clinically important drug-drug interactions
- Increased risk of hemorrhage if used with heparin or oral anticoagulants, aspirin, indomethacin, phenylbutazone

Drug-lab test interferences
- Marked decrease in plasminogen, fibrinogen • Increases in thrombin time (TT), activated partial thromboplastin (APTT), prothrombin time (PT)

Nursing Considerations
Assessment
- *History:* Allergy to streptokinase; active internal bleeding, recent CVA; intracranial or intraspinal surgery; intracranial neoplasm; recent major surgery; obstetric delivery; organ biopsy; or rupture of a noncompressible blood vesse; recent serious GI bleed; recent serious trauma; severe hypertension; SBE; hemostatic defects; cerebrovascular disease; diabetic hemorrhagic retinopathy; septic thrombosis; pregnancy; lactation
- *Physical:* Skin—color, temperature, lesions; temperature; orientation, reflexes; P, BP, peripheral perfusion, baseline ECG; R, adventitous sounds; liver evaluation; Hct, platelet count, TT, APTT, PT

Implementation
- Discontinue heparin if it is being given, unless ordered specifically for coronary artery infusion.
- Arrange for regular monitoring of coagulation studies.
- Apply pressure or pressure dressings to control superficial bleeding (at invaded or disturbed areas).
- Avoid any arterial invasive procedures during therapy.
- Arrange for typing and cross-matching of blood if serious blood loss occurs and whole blood transfusions are required.
- Institute treatment within 2–6 h of onset of symptoms for evolving MI; within 7 d of other thrombotic event.
- Monitor cardiac rhythm continually during coronary artery infusion.

Drug-specific teaching points
- Be aware that you will need frequent blood tests and IV injections.
- Report rash, difficulty breathing, dizziness, disorientation, numbness, tingling.

☐ streptomycin sulfate

*(strep toe **mye'** sin)*
Pregnancy Category C

Drug classes
Aminoglycoside antibiotic
Antituberculous drug

Therapeutic actions
Bactericidal: inhibits protein synthesis in susceptible strains of gram-negative bacteria; mechanism of lethal action not fully understood, but functional integrity of cell membrane appears to be disrupted.

Indications
- Infections caused by susceptible strains of *Mycobacterium tuberculosis* (in combination with other antituberculous drugs; the fourth drug with isoniazid, rifampin, pyrazinamide)
- Serious infections caused by susceptible strains of *Yersinia pestis, Francisella tularensis, Brucella, Haemophilus ducreyi, Haemophilus influenzae, Klebsiella pneumoniae, Escherichia coli, Proteus, Enterobacter aerogenes, Streptococcus faecalis, Streptococcus viridans,* gram-negative bacilli, when other less toxic drugs are ineffective or contraindicated (use in combination with another agent for *H. influenzae, K. pneumoniae* and in bacteremia)
- Unlabeled use: part of a 3–5 drug regimen in the treatment of *Mycobacterium avium* in AIDS patients (11–13 mg/kg per 24 h)

Contraindications/cautions
- Contraindicated in the presence of allergy to aminoglycosides; pregnancy, lactation, herpes, vaccinia, varicella, fungal infections.
- Use caution in the elderly or patients with diminished hearing, decreased renal function, dehydration, neuromuscular disorders.

Dosage
Adult
- **Tuberculosis:** 15 mg/kg with a maximum of 1 g/d IM with other antituberculous drugs. Ultimately, reduce dosage to 25–30 mg/kg or maximum of 1.5 g two to three times per week. Total treatment period is at least 1 y or until toxic symptoms appear or organisms develop resistance.
- **Tularemia:** 1–2 g/d IM in divided doses for 7–10 d or until patient is afebrile for 5–7 d.
- **Plague:** 2 g/d IM in divided doses for a minimum of 10 d.
- **Bacterial endocarditis due to penicillin-sensitive alpha and nonhemolytic streptococci:** 1 g bid IM for 1 wk with penicillin. Then 0.5 g bid IM for 1 wk with penicillin.
- **Enterococcal endocarditis:** 1 g bid IM for 2 wk then 0.5 g bid IM for 4 wk in combination with penicillin.
- **Other severe infections:** 1–2 g IM in divided doses q6–12h; do not exceed 2 g/d.

Pediatric
- **Tuberculosis:** 20–40 mg/kg per day IM in divided doses q6–12h to a maximum of 1 g/d; reduce to 25–30 mg/kg IM two to three times weekly or a maximum of 1.5 g.
- **Other severe infections:** 20–40 mg/kg per day IM in divided doses q6–12h.

Geriatric or renal failure patients:
Reduce dosage, and monitor patient carefully.

Pharmacokinetics

Route	Onset	Peak
Oral	Rapid	1–2 h

Metabolism: Hepatic, $T_{1/2}$: 2.5 h
Distribution: Crosses placenta; enters breast milk
Excretion: Urine

Adverse effects
- **CNS:** Ototoxicity, vestibular paralysis, confusion, disorientation, depression, lethargy, nystagmus, visual disturbances, headache, *numbness, tingling,* tremor, paresthesias, muscle twitching, convulsions, muscular weakness, neuromuscular blockade
- **GI:** Hepatic toxicity, *nausea, vomiting, anorexia,* weight loss, stomatitis, increased salivation
- **CV:** Palpitations, hypotension, hypertension
- **Hematologic:** *Leukemoid reaction,* agranulocytosis, granulocytosis, leukopenia, leukocytosis, thrombocytopenia, eosinophilia, pancytopenia, anemia, hemolytic anemia, increased or decreased reticulocyte count, electrolyte disturbances
- **GU:** *Nephrotoxicity*
- **Hypersensitivity:** Hypersensitivity reactions: *purpura, rash,* urticaria, exfoliative dermatitis, itching
- **Local:** *Pain, irritation, arachnoiditis at IM injection sites*
- **Other:** Fever, apnea, splenomegaly, joint pain, *superinfections*

Clinically important drug-drug interactions
- Increased ototoxic, nephrotoxic, neurotoxic effects if taken with other aminoglycosides, cephalothin, potent diuretics • Increased neuromuscular blockade and muscular paralysis when given with anesthetics, nondepolarizing neuromuscular blocking drugs, succinylcholine • Increased bactericidal effect if combined with penicillins, cephalopsorins, carbenicillin, ticarcillin

■ Nursing Considerations
Assessment
- *History:* Allergy to aminoglycosides; pregnancy; lactation; herpes, vaccinia, varicella; fungal, mycobacterial infections; decreased hearing; decreased renal function, dehydration, neuromuscular disorders
- *Physical:* Renal functon tests; eighth cranial nerve function; state of hydration; hepatic function, CBC, skin color and lesions, orientation and affect, reflexes,

Adverse effects in *Italics* are most common; those in **Bold** are life-threatening.

bilateral grip strength, body weight, bowel sounds

Implementation
- Arrange culture and sensitivity tests of infection before beginning therapy.
- Use IM route only; give by deep intramuscular injection.
- Ensure adequate hydration of patient before and during therapy.

Drug-specific teaching points
- Be aware that this drug can only be given by injection.
- Know that the following side effects may occur: ringing in ears, headache, dizziness (use appropriate precautions if these occur); nausea, vomiting, loss of appetite (small, frequent meals and frequent mouth care may help).
- Report hearing changes, dizziness, pain at injection site, rash.

⬜ streptozocin

(strep toe zoe' sin)

Zanosar

Pregnancy Category C

Drug classes
Alkylating agent, nitrosourea
Antineoplastic drug

Therapeutic actions
Cytotoxic: inhibits DNA synthesis, leading to cell death partially through the production of intrastrand cross-links in DNA; cell cycle nonspecific.

Indications
- Metastatic islet cell carcinoma of the pancreas

Contraindications/cautions
- Contraindicated in the presence of allergy to streptozocin; hematopoietic depression; pregnancy (teratogenic and embryotoxic in preclinical studies; suggest the use of birth control during therapy); lactation.
- Use caution in the presence of impaired renal or hepatic function.

Dosage
Two different dosage schedules have been used.
Adult: *Daily schedule:* 500 mg/m^2 of body surface area IV for 5 consecutive d every 6 wk. *Weekly schedule:* Initial dose of 1,000 mg/m^2 of body surface area IV at weekly intervals for the first 2 wk. Increase subsequent doses if response and toxicity do not occur, but *do not exceed 1,500 mg/m^2* of body surface area.

Pharmacokinetics

Route	Onset	Duration
IV	Varies	24 h

Metabolism: Hepatic, T$_{1/2}$: 35 min
Distribution: Crosses placenta; enters breast milk
Excretion: Urine

IV facts
Preparation: Reconstitute with 9.5 ml of Dextrose Injection or 0.9% Sodium Chloride Injection. The resultant pale gold solution contains 100 mg/ml streptozocin. Dilute further with diluents listed above, if needed. Refrigerate vials and protect from light; once reconstituted, use within 12 h.
Infusion: Infuse slowly.

Adverse effects
- CNS: Lethargy, confusion, depression
- GI: *Nausea, vomiting,* diarrhea, *hepatotoxicity*
- Hematologic: Hematologic toxicity, glucose intolerance
- GU: *Renal toxicity*
- Other: Infertility, cancer

■ Nursing Considerations

Assessment
- *History:* Allergy to streptozocin, hematopoietic depression, impaired renal or hepatic function, pregnancy, lactation
- *Physical:* Weight; orientation, affect; liver evaluation; CBC, differential; urinal-

ysis; blood glucose, serum electrolytes, liver and renal function tests

Implementation
- Arrange for blood and urine tests to evaluate renal function before beginning therapy and weekly during therapy. Also arrange to monitor liver function tests and CBC during therapy.
- Arrange for reduced dosage or discontinuation of therapy if renal toxicity occurs—proteinuria, elevated BUN, plasma creatinine, serum electrolytes.
- Use special precautions when handling the streptozocin; contact with the skin poses a carcinogenic hazard to the area exposed. Wear rubber gloves; if powder or solution comes in contact with the skin, wash immediately with soap and water.
- Administer IV only; intra-arterial administration causes more rapid toxic renal effects.
- Arrange for pretherapy medicating with antiemetic, if needed, to decrease the severity of nausea and vomiting.
- Monitor urine output and perform frequent urinalysis for any sign of renal failure.

Drug-specific teaching points
- Be aware that this drug can only be given IV. Prepare a calendar with the course of treatment to follow.
- Know that the following side effects may occur: nausea, vomiting, loss of appetite (an antiemetic may be ordered for you; small frequent meals also may help); confusion, depression, lethargy (it sometimes helps to know that this is a drug effect).
- Be aware that this drug can cause severe birth defects; it is advisable to use birth control methods while on this drug.
- Arrange to have regular medical follow-up, including blood and urine tests to follow the effects of the drug on your body and to determine your next dose.
- Report unusual bleeding or bruising, fever, chills, sore throat, stomach or flank pain, changes in urinary output, confusion, depression.

☐ succimer

(sux' i mer)
Chemet

Pregnancy Category C

Drug classes
Antidote
Chelating agent

Therapeutic actions
Forms water-soluble chelates with lead, leading to increased urinary excretion of lead.

Indications
- Treatment of lead poisoning in children with blood levels > 45 μg/dl (not for prophylactic use)
- Unlabeled uses: treatment of other heavy metal poisonings (mercury, arsenic)

Contraindications/cautions
- Contraindicated in the presence of allergy to succimer, pregnancy (teratogenic and embryotoxic in preclinical studies), lactation.
- Use caution in the presence of impaired renal or hepatic function.

Dosage
Pediatric: Starting dose of 10 mg/kg or 350 mg/m^2 q8h PO for 5 d; reduce dosage to 10 mg/kg or 350 mg/m^2 q12h PO for 2 wk (therapy runs for 19 d).

Pharmacokinetics

Route	Onset	Peak
Oral	Varies	1–2 h

Metabolism: Hepatic, T$_{1/2}$: 2 d
Distribution: Crosses placenta; may enter breast milk
Excretion: Feces and urine

Adverse effects
- **CNS:** Drowsiness, dizziness, sleepiness, otitis media, watery eyes

Adverse effects in *Italics* are most common; those in **Bold** are life-threatening.

1022 ■ sucralfate

- **GI:** *Nausea, vomiting*, diarrhea, metal taste in mouth, loss of appetite
- **GU:** Decreased urination, voiding difficulty
- **Dermatologic:** Papular rash, herpetic rash, mucocutaneous eruptions, pruritus
- **General:** *Back, stomach, flank, head, rib pain*, chills, fever, flulike symptoms

Clinically important drug-drug interactions
- High risk of toxicity if taken with other chelating agents (EDTA)

Drug-lab test interferences
- False-positive tests of urine ketones using *Ketostix* • False decrease in serum uric acid, CPK

■ Nursing Considerations

Assessment
- *History:* Allergy to succimer, lactation, pregnancy, renal or hepatic impairment
- *Physical:* Weight; orientation, affect; liver evaluation; urinalysis; liver and renal function tests; serum lead levels

Implementation
- Arrange for testing of serum blood levels before beginning therapy.
- Identify the source of lead in the environment, and facilitate its removal; succimer is not prophylactic to prevent lead poisoning.
- Ensure that patient continues therapy for full 19 d.
- Administer to children who cannot swallow capsules by seperating the capsules and sprinkling the medicated beads on a small amount of soft food or putting them in a spoon and following with a fruit drink.

Drug-specific teaching points
- Administer to children who cannot swallow capsules by seperating the capsules and sprinkling the medicated beads on a small amount of soft food or putting them in a spoon and following with a fruit drink.
- Ensure that child maintains good fluid intake during therapy.

- Know that the following side effects may occur: nausea, vomiting, loss of appetite (small, frequent meals may help); abdominal, back, rib, flank pain (appropriate medications may be ordered).
- Report rash, difficulty breathing, difficulty walking, tremors.

☐ sucralfate

(soo **kral'** fate)
Carafate, Sulcrate (CAN)

Pregnancy Category B

Drug classes
Antipeptic agent

Therapeutic actions
Forms an ulcer-adherent complex at duodenal ulcer sites, protecting the ulcer against acid, pepsin, and bile salts, thereby promoting ulcer healing; also inhibits pepsin activity in gastric juices.

Indications
- Short-term treatment of duodenal ulcers, up to 8 wk
- Maintenance therapy for duodenal ulcer patients at reduced dosage after healing has occurred
- Unlabeled uses: accelerates healing of gastric ulcers, treatment of NSAID- or aspirin-induced GI symptoms and GI damage, prevention of stress ulcers in critically ill patients
- Orphan drug use: treatment of oral and esophageal ulcers due to radiation, chemotherapy, and sclerotherapy

Contraindications/cautions
- Allergy to sucralfate, chronic renal failure/dialysis (buildup of aluminum may occur if taken in conjunction with aluminum-containing products), pregnancy, lactation.

Dosage
Adult
- ***Active duodenal ulcer:*** 1 g PO qid on an empty stomach (1 h before meals

Adverse effects in *Italics* are most common; those in **Bold** are life-threatening.

and at bedtime). Continue treatment for 4–8 wk.
- **Maintenance:** 1 g PO bid.

Pediatric: Safety and efficacy not established.

Pharmacokinetics

Route	Onset	Duration
Oral	30 min	5 h

Metabolism: Hepatic, $T_{1/2}$: 6–20 h
Distribution: Crosses placenta; may enter breast milk
Excretion: Feces

Adverse effects
- **CNS:** Dizziness, sleeplessness, vertigo
- **GI:** *Constipation*, diarrhea, nausea, indigestion, gastric discomfort, dry mouth
- **Dermatologic:** Rash, pruritus
- **Other:** Back pain

Clinically important drug-drug interactions
- Decreased serum levels and effectiveness of phenytoin, ciprofloxacin, norfloxacin, penicillamine when taken with sucralfate; separate administration by 2 h • Risk of aluminum toxicity if taken with aluminum-containing antacids

■ Nursing Considerations

Assessment
- *History:* Allergy to sucralfate, chronic renal failure/dialysis, pregnancy, lactation
- *Physical:* Skin—color, lesions; reflexes, orientation; mucous membranes, normal output

Implementation
- Administer drug on an empty stomach, 1 h before or 2 h after meals and at bedtime.
- Monitor patient's pain; antacids may be ordered to relieve pain.
- Administer antacids between doses of sucralfate, not within ½ h before or after sucralfate doses.

Drug-specific teaching points
- Take the drug on an empty stomach, 1 h before or 2 h after meals and at bedtime.
- Be aware that if you are also taking antacids for pain relief; do not take antacids ½ h before or after taking sucralfate.
- Know that the following side effects may occur: dizziness, vertigo (if this occurs, avoid driving or operating dangerous machinery while you are on this drug); indigestion, nausea (small, frequent meals may help); dry mouth (frequent mouth care, sucking on sugarless candies may help); constipation (appropriate measures may be taken).
- Report severe gastric pain.

❏ sufentanil citrate

(soo *fen' ta* nil)
Sufenta

Pregnancy Category C
C-II Controlled Substance

Drug classes
Narcotic agonist analgesic

Therapeutic actions
Acts at specific opioid receptors, causing analgesia, respiratory depression, physical depression, euphoria.

Indications
- Analgesic adjunct to maintain balanced general anesthesia
- Primary anesthetic with 100% oxygen to induce and maintain anesthesia in patients undergoing major surgical procedures

Contraindications/cautions
- Contraindicated in the presence of known sensitivity to sufentanil, pregnancy.
- Use caution in the presence of obesity, hepatic disease, head injury, diabetes, arrhythmias, lactation, severe debilitation.

Dosage
Individualize dosage; monitor vital signs routinely.

Adverse effects in *Italics* are most common; those in **Bold** are life-threatening.

1024 ■ sufentanil citrate

Adult
- ***Adjunct to general anesthesia:*** 2–8 μg/kg IV initially; 25–50 μg for maintenance.
- ***With oxygen for anesthesia:*** 8–30 μg/kg IV initially; supplement with doses of 25–50 μg IV.

Pediatric (2–12 y)
- ***With oxygen for anesthesia:*** 10–25 μg/kg IV initially; supplement with doses of 25–50 μg IV.

Pharmacokinetics

Route	Onset	Duration
IV	Immediate	5 min

Metabolism: Hepatic, $T_{1/2}$: 2.7 h
Distribution: Crosses placenta; enters breast milk

IV facts
Preparation: Protect vials from light.
Infusion: Administer slowly over 1–2 min by direct injection or into running IV tubing.

Adverse effects
- CNS: *Sedation, clamminess, sweating, headache, vertigo, floating feeling, dizziness, lethary, confusion, lightheadedness,* nervousness, unusual dreams, agitation, euphoria, hallucinations, delirium, insomnia, anxiety, fear, disorientation, impaired mental and physical performance, coma, mood changes, weakness, headache, tremor, convulsions
- GI: *Nausea, vomiting,* dry mouth, anorexia, constipation, biliary tract spasm
- CV: Palpitation, increase or decrease in blood pressure, circulatory depression, **cardiac arrest**, **shock**, tachycardia, bradycardia, arrhythmia, palpitations
- Respiratory: Slow, shallow respiration, apnea, suppression of cough reflex, laryngospasm, bronchospasm
- GU: Ureteral spasm, spasm of vesical sphincters, urinary retention or hesitancy, oliguria, antidiuretic effect, reduced libido or potency
- EENT: Diplopia, blurred vision
- Dermatologic: Rash, hives, pruritus, flushing, warmth, sensitivity to cold
- Local: Phlebitis following IV injection, pain at injection site
- Other: Physical tolerance and dependence, psychological dependence, local skin irritation with transdermal system

Clinically important drug-drug interactions
- Potentiation of effects of sufentanil when given with barbiturate anesthetics

Drug-lab test interferences
- Elevated biliary tract pressure may cause increases in plasma amylase, lipase; determinations of these levels may be unreliable for 24 h after administration of narcotics

■ Nursing Considerations

Assessment
- *History:* Hypersensitivity to sufentanil or narcotics, physical dependence on a narcotic analgesic, pregnancy, lactation, COPD, increased intracranial pressure, acute MI, biliary tract surgery, renal or hepatic dysfunction
- *Physical:* Orientation, reflexes, bilateral grip strength, affect; pupil size, vision; pulse, auscultation, BP; R, adventitious sounds; bowel sounds, normal output; liver and kidney function tests

Implementation
- Administer to women who are lactating 4–6 h before the next scheduled feeding to minimize the amount in milk.
- Provide narcotic antagonist, facilities for assisted or controlled respiration on standby during parenteral administration.

Drug-specific teaching points
- Incorporate teaching about drug into preoperative or postoperative teaching program.
- Know that the following side effects may occur: dizziness, sedation, drowsiness, impaired visual acuity (ask for assistance if you need to move); nausea, loss of appetite (lying quietly, eating frequent, small meals should minimize these ef-

Adverse effects in *Italics* are most common; those in **Bold** are life-threatening.

fects); constipation (a laxative may help).
- Report severe nausea, vomiting, palpitations, shortness of breath or difficulty breathing.

◻ sulfadiazine

(sul fa dye' a zeen)

Pregnancy Category C
Pregnancy Category D (labor and delivery)

Drug classes
Antibiotic
Sulfonamide

Therapeutic actions
Bacteriostatic: competitively antagonizes para-aminobenzoic acid (PABA), an essential component of folic acid synthesis in susceptible gram-negative and gram-positive bacteria; prevents cell replication.

Indications
- Treatment of acute infections caused by susceptible organisms: urinary tract infections, chancroid, inclusion conjunctivitis, trachoma, nocardiosis, toxoplasmosis (with pyrimethamine), malaria (as adjunctive therapy for chloroquine-resistant strains of *P. falciparum*), acute otitis media (due to *H. influenzae* when used with penicillin or erythromycin), *H. influenzae* meningitis (as adjunctive therapy with parenteral streptomycin), meningococcal meningitis, rheumatic fever

Contraindications/cautions
- Contraindicated in the presence of allergy to sulfonamides, sulfonylureas, thiazides; pregnancy (teratogenic in preclinical studies; at term, may bump fetal bilirubin from plasma protein binding sites and cause kernicterus); lactation (risk of kernicterus, diarrhea, rash).
- Use caution in the presence of impaired renal or hepatic function, G-6-PD deficiency, porphyria.

Dosage
Adult: Loading dose, 2–4 g PO. Maintenance dose, 2–4 g/d PO in four to six divided doses.
- ***Prevention of recurrent attacks of rheumatic fever (not for initial therapy of streptococcal infections):*** >30 kg: 1 g/d PO. <30 kg: 0.5 g/d PO.

Pediatric
- ***Older than 2 mo:*** Initial dose, 75 mg/kg PO. Maintenance dose, 120–150 mg/kg per day PO in four to six divided doses with a maximum dose of 6 g/d. Maximum dose, 6 g/d.
- ***<2 mo, not recommended except to treat congenital toxoplasmosis:*** Loading dose, 75–100 mg/kg PO. Maintenance dose, 100–150 mg/kg per day in four divided doses.
- *3–4 wk:* 25 mg/kg PO per dose four times per day.
- *Older than 2 mo:* 25–50 mg/kg PO per dose qid.

Pharmacokinetics

Route	Onset	Peak
Oral	Varies	3–6 h

Metabolism: Hepatic, $T_{1/2}$: unknown
Distribution: Crosses placenta; enters breast milk
Excretion: Urine

Adverse effects
- **CNS:** *Headache*, peripheral neuropathy, mental depression, convulsions, ataxia, hallucinations, tinnitus, vertigo, insomnia, hearing loss, drowsiness, transient lesions of posterior spinal column, transverse myelitis
- **GI:** *Nausea, emesis, abdominal pains*, diarrhea, bloody diarrhea, anorexia, pancreatitis, stomatitis, impaired folic acid absorption, hepatitis, hepatocellular necrosis
- **Hematologic:** *Agranulocytosis*, aplastic anemia, thrombocytopenia, leukopenia, hemolytic anemia, hypoprothrombinemia, methemoglobinemia, megaloblastic anemia

Adverse effects in *Italics* are most common; those in **Bold** are life-threatening.

- **GU:** *Crystalluria, hematuria,* proteinuria, nephrotic syndrome, toxic nephrosis with oliguria and anuria, oligospermia, infertility
- **Dermatologic:** *Photosensitivity,* cyanosis, petechiae, alopecia
- **Hypersensitivity:** Stevens-Johnson syndrome, generalized skin eruptions, epidermal necrolysis, urticaria, serum sickness, pruritus, exfoliative dermatitis, **anaphylactoid reactions,** periorbital edema, conjunctival and scleral redness, photosensitization, arthralgia, allergic myocarditis, transient pulmonary changes with eosinophilia, decreased pulmonary function
- **Other:** Drug fever, chills, periarteritis nodosum

Clinically important drug-drug interactions
- Increased risk of hypoglycemia when tolbutamide, tolazamide, glyburide, glipizide, acetohexamide, chlorpropamide are taken concurrently • Increased risk of phenytoin toxicity when taken with sulfonamides

Drug-lab test interferences
- False-positive urinary glucose tests using Benedict's method

■ Nursing Considerations

Assessment
- *History:* Allergy to sulfonamides, sulfonylureas, thiazides; pregnancy, lactation; impaired renal or hepatic function; G-6-PD deficiency
- *Physical:* Body temperature; skin—color, lesions; culture of infected site; orientation, reflexes, affect, peripheral sensation; R, adventitious sounds; mucous membranes, bowel sounds, liver evaluation; liver and renal function tests, CBC and differential, urinalysis

Implementation
- Arrange for culture and sensitivity tests of infected area before beginning therapy; repeat cultures if response is not as expected.
- Administer drug on an empty stomach, 1 h before or 2 h after meals, with a full glass of water.
- Ensure adequate fluid intake; sulfadiazine is very insoluble and may cause crystalluria if high concentrations occur in the urine; alkalinization of the urine may be necessary.
- Discontinue drug immediately if hypersensitivity reaction occurs.

Drug-specific teaching points
- Complete full course of therapy.
- Take the drug on an empty stomach, 1 h before or 2 h after meals, with a full glass of water.
- Drink eight glasses of water per day.
- Be aware that this drug is specific to this disease; do not use to self-treat any other infection.
- Know that the following side effects may occur: sensitivity to sunlight (use sunscreens; wear protective clothing if exposed to the sun); dizziness, drowsiness, difficulty walking, loss of sensation (avoid driving or performing tasks that require alertness if these occur); nausea, vomiting, diarrhea; loss of fertility.
- Report blood in the urine, rash, ringing in the ears, difficulty breathing, fever, sore throat, chills.

▢ sulfamethizole

*(sul fa **meth'** i zole)*

Pregnancy Category C
Pregnancy Category D (at term)

Drug classes
Antibiotic
Sulfonamide

Therapeutic actions
Bacteriostatic: competitively antagonizes PABA, an essential component of folic acid synthesis in susceptible gram-negative and gram-positive bacteria, preventing cell replication.

Adverse effects in *Italics* are most common; those in **Bold** are life-threatening.

sulfamethizole

Indications
- Treatment of urinary tract infections caused by susceptible organisms

Contraindications/cautions
- Contraindicated in the presence of allergy to sulfonamides, sulfonylureas, thiazides; pregnancy (teratogenic in preclinical studies; at term, may bump fetal bilirubin from plasma protein-binding sites and cause kernicterus); lactation (risk of kernicterus, diarrhea, rash).
- Use caution in the presence of impaired renal or hepatic function, G-6-PD deficiency, porphyria.

Dosage
Adult: 0.5–1 g tid–qid PO.
Pediatric (older than 2 mo): 30–45 mg/kg per day PO in four divided doses.

Pharmacokinetics

Route	Onset	Peak
Oral	Varies	3–6 h

Metabolism: Hepatic, $T_{1/2}$: unknown
Distribution: Crosses placenta; enters breast milk
Excretion: Urine

Adverse effects
- **CNS:** *Headache,* peripheral neuropathy, mental depression, convulsions, ataxia, hallucinations, tinnitus, vertigo, insomnia, hearing loss, drowsiness, transient lesions of posterior spinal column, transverse myelitis
- **GI:** *Nausea, emesis, abdominal pains,* diarrhea, bloody diarrhea, anorexia, pancreatitis, stomatitis, impaired folic acid absorption, hepatitis, hepatocellular necrosis
- **Hematologic:** **Agranulocytosis,** aplastic anemia, thrombocytopenia, leukopenia, hemolytic anemia, hypoprothrombinemia, methemoglobinemia, megaloblastic anemia
- **GU:** *Crystalluria, hematuria,* proteinuria, nephrotic syndrome, toxic nephrosis with oliguria and anuria, oligospermia, infertility
- **Dermatologic:** *Photosensitivity,* cyanosis, petechiae, alopecia
- **Hypersensitivity:** Stevens-Johnson syndrome, generalized skin eruptions, epidermal necrolysis, urticaria, serum sickness, pruritus, exfoliative dermatitis, anaphylactoid reactions, periorbital edema, conjunctival and scleral redness, photosensitization, arthralgia, allergic myocarditis, transient pulmonary changes with eosinophilia, decreased pulmonary function
- **Other:** Drug fever, chills, periarteritis nodosum

Clinically important drug-drug interactions
- Increased risk of hypoglycemia when tolbutamide, tolazamide, glyburide, glipizide, acetohexamide, chlorpropamide are taken concurrently • Increased risk of phenytoin toxicity when taken with sulfonamides

Drug-lab test interferences
- Possible false-positive urinary glucose tests using Benedict's method

■ Nursing Considerations

Assessment
- *History:* Allergy to sulfonamides, sulfonylureas, thiazides; pregnancy; lactation; impaired renal or hepatic function; G-6-PD deficiency
- *Physical:* Body temperature; skin—color, lesions; culture of infected site; orientation, reflexes, affect, peripheral sensation; R, adventitious sounds; mucous membranes, bowel sounds, liver evaluation; liver and renal function tests, CBC and differential, urinalysis

Implementation
- Arrange for culture and sensitivity tests of infected area before beginning therapy; repeat cultures if response is not as expected.
- Administer drug on an empty stomach, 1 h before or 2 h after meals, with a full glass of water.
- Ensure adequate fluid intake; sulfamethizole is very insoluble and may cause crystalluria if high concentrations occur

Adverse effects in *Italics* are most common; those in **Bold** are life-threatening.

in the urine; alkalinization of the urine may be necessary.
- Discontinue drug immediately if hypersensitivity reaction occurs.

Drug-specific teaching points
- Complete full course of therapy.
- Take the drug on an empty stomach, 1 h before or 2 h after meals, with a full glass of water.
- Drink eight glasses of water per day.
- Be aware that this drug is specific to this disease; do not use to self-treat any other infection.
- Know that the following side effects may occur: sensitivity to sunlight (use sunscreens, wear protective clothing if exposed to the sun); dizziness, drowsiness, difficulty walking, loss of sensation (avoid driving or performing tasks that require alertness if these occur); nausea, vomiting, diarrhea; loss of fertility.
- Report blood in the urine, rash, ringing in the ears, difficulty breathing, fever, sore throat, chills.

☐ sulfamethoxazole

(sul fa meth ox' a zole)
Gantanol, Urobak

Pregnancy Category C
Pregnancy Category D (at term)

Drug classes
Antibiotic
Sulfonamide

Therapeutic actions
Bacteriostatic: competitively antagonizes PABA, an essential component of folic acid synthesis in susceptible gram-negative and gram-positive bacteria, preventing cell replication.

Indications
- Treatment of acute infections caused by susceptible organisms: urinary tract infections, chancroid, inclusion conjunctivitis, trachoma, nocardiosis, toxoplasmosis (with pyrimethamine), malaria (as adjunctive therapy for chloroquine-resistant strains of *P. falciparum*), acute otitis media (due to *H. influenzae* when used with penicillin or erythromycin)
- Meningococcal meningitis

Contraindications/cautions
- Contraindicated in the presence of allergy to sulfonamides, sulfonylureas, thiazides; pregnancy (teratogenic in preclinical studies; at term, may bump fetal bilirubin from plasma protein-binding sites and cause kernicterus); lactation (risk of kernicterus, diarrhea, rash).
- Use caution in the presence of impaired renal or hepatic function, G-6-PD deficiency, porphyria.

Dosage
Adult
- ***Mild to moderate infections:*** Loading dose, 2 g PO. Maintenance dose, 1 g PO morning and evening.
- ***Severe infections:*** 2 g PO initially, then 1 g tid PO.

Pediatric (older than 2 mo): 50–60 mg/kg PO followed by 25–30 mg/kg morning and evening. Do not exceed 75 mg/kg per day *or* 50–60 mg/kg per day divided q12h, not to exceed 3 g/d.

Pharmacokinetics

Route	Onset	Peak
Oral	30–60 min	2 h

Metabolism: Hepatic, $T_{1/2}$: 7–12 h
Distribution: Crosses placenta; enters breast milk
Excretion: Urine

Adverse effects
- **CNS:** *Headache*, peripheral neuropathy, mental depression, convulsions, ataxia, hallucinations, tinnitus, vertigo, insomnia, hearing loss, drowsiness, transient lesions of posterior spinal column, transverse myelitis
- **GI:** *Nausea, emesis, abdominal pains*, diarrhea, bloody diarrhea, anorexia, pancreatitis, stomatitis, impaired folic acid

Adverse effects in *Italics* are most common; those in **Bold** are life-threatening.

absorption, hepatitis, hepatocellular necrosis
- **Hematologic:** *Agranulocytosis,* aplastic anemia, thrombocytopenia, leukopenia, hemolytic anemia, hypoprothrombinemia, methemoglobinemia, megaloblastic anemia
- **GU:** *Crystalluria, hematuria,* proteinuria, nephrotic syndrome, toxic nephrosis with oliguria and anuria, oligospermia, infertility
- **Dermatologic:** *Photosensitivity,* cyanosis, petechiae, alopecia
- **Hypersensitivity:** Stevens-Johnson syndrome, generalized skin eruptions, epidermal necrolysis, urticaria, serum sickness, pruritus, exfoliative dermatitis, anaphylactoid reactions, periorbital edema, conjunctival and scleral redness, photosensitization, arthralgia, allergic myocarditis, transient pulmonary changes with eosinophilia, decreased pulmonary function
- **Other:** Drug fever, chills, periarteritis nodosum

Clinically important drug-drug interactions
- Increased risk of hypoglycemia when tolbutamide, tolazamide, glyburide, glipizide, acetohexamide, chlorpropamide are taken concurrently • Decreased immunosuppressive effect of cyclosporine and increased risk of nephrotoxicity if given with sulfamethoxazole

Drug-lab test interferences
- Possible false-positive urinary glucose tests using Benedict's method

■ Nursing Considerations

Assessment
- *History:* Allergy to sulfonamides, sulfonylureas, thiazides; pregnancy; lactation; impaired renal or hepatic function; G-6-PD deficiency; porphyria
- *Physical:* Body temperature; skin—color, lesions; culture of infected site; orientation, reflexes, affect, peripheral sensation; R, adventitious sounds; mucous membranes, bowel sounds, liver evaluation; liver and renal function tests, CBC and differential, urinalysis

Implementation
- Arrange for culture and sensitivity tests of infected area before beginning therapy; repeat cultures if response is not as expected.
- Administer drug on an empty stomach, 1 h before or 2 h after meals, with a full glass of water.
- Ensure adequate fluid intake; sulfamethoxazole is very insoluble and may cause crystalluria if high concentrations occur in the urine; alkalinization of the urine may be necessary.
- Discontinue drug immediately if hypersensitivity reaction occurs.

Drug-specific teaching points
- Complete full course of therapy.
- Take the drug on an empty stomach, 1 h before or 2 h after meals, with a full glass of water.
- Drink eight glasses of water per day.
- Be aware that this drug is specific to this disease; do not use to self-treat any other infection.
- Know that the following side effects may occur: sensitivity to sunlight (use sunscreens, wear protective clothing if exposed to the sun); dizziness, drowsiness, difficulty walking, loss of sensation (avoid driving or performing tasks that require alertness if these occur); nausea, vomiting, diarrhea; loss of fertility.
- Report blood in the urine, rash, ringing in the ears, difficulty breathing, fever, sore throat, chills.

▢ sulfasalazine

*(sul fa **sal'** a zeen)*
Azulfidine

Pregnancy Category C
Pregnancy Category D (at term)

Drug classes
Antibiotic
Sulfonamide

Adverse effects in *Italics* are most common; those in **Bold** are life-threatening.

Therapeutic actions
Bacteriostatic: competitively antagonises PABA, an essential component of folic acid synthesis in susceptible gram-negative and gram-positive bacteria; one-third of the oral dose is absorbed from the small intestine; remaining two-thirds passes into the colon where it is split into 5-aminosalicylic acid and sulfapyridine; most of the sulfapyridine is absorbed; the 5-aminosalicylic acid acts locally as an anti-inflammatory agent.

Indications
- Treatment of ulcerative colitis
- Unlabeled uses: management of rheumatoid arthritis, collagenous colitis, Crohn's disease

Contraindications/cautions
- Contraindicated in the presence of allergy to sulfonamides, sulfonylureas, thiazides; pregnancy (teratogenic in preclinical studies); at term, may bump fetal bilirubin from plasma protein-binding sites and cause kernicterus); lactation (risk of kernicterus, diarrhea, rash).
- Use caution in the presence of impaired renal or hepatic function, G-6-PD deficiency, porphyria.

Dosage
Administer around the clock; dosage intervals should not exceed 8 h. Give after meals.
Adult: Initial therapy, 3–4 g/d PO in evenly divided doses. Initial doses of 1–2 g/d PO may lessen adverse GI effects. Doses > 4 g/d increase risk of toxicity. Maintenance, 2 g/d PO in evenly spaced doses (500 mg qid).
Pediatric (older than 2 y): Initial therapy, 40–60 mg/kg per 24 h PO in four to six divided doses. Maintenance therapy, 20–30 mg/kg per 24 h PO in four equally divided doses. Maximum dosage, 2 g/d.

Pharmacokinetics

Route	Onset	Peak
Oral	Varies	1½–6 h, 6–24 h metabolite

Metabolism: Hepatic, $T_{1/2}$: 5–10 h

Distribution: Crosses placenta; enters breast milk
Excretion: Urine

Adverse effects
- **CNS:** Headache, peripheral neuropathy, mental depression, convulsions, ataxia, hallucinations, tinnitus, vertigo, insomnia, hearing loss, drowsiness, transient lesions of posterior spinal column, transverse myelitis
- **GI:** *Nausea, emesis, abdominal pains,* diarrhea, bloody diarrhea, anorexia, pancreatitis, stomatitis, impaired folic acid absorption, hepatitis, hepatocellular necrosis
- **Hematologic:** Agranulocytosis, aplastic anemia, thrombocytopenia, leukopenia, hemolytic anemia, hypoprothrombinemia, methemoglobinemia, megaloblastic anemia
- **GU:** *Crystalluria, hematuria,* proteinuria, nephrotic syndrome, toxic nephrosis with oliguria and anuria, oligospermia, infertility
- **Dermatologic:** Photosensitivity, cyanosis, petechiae, alopecia
- **Hypersensitivity:** Stevens-Johnson syndrome, generalized skin eruptions, epidermal necrolysis, urticaria, serum sickness, pruritus, exfoliative dermatitis, anaphylactoid reactions, periorbital edema, conjunctival and scleral redness, photosensitization, arthralgia, allergic myocarditis, transient pulmonary changes with eosinophilia, decreased pulmonary function
- **Other:** Drug fever, chills, periarteritis nodosum

Clinically important drug-drug interactions
- Increased risk of hypoglycemia when tolbutamide, tolazamide, glyburide, glipizide, acetohexamide, chlorpropamide are taken concurrently • Increased risk of folate deficiency if taking sulfasalazine, monitor patients receiving folic acid carefully for signs of folate deficiency

Adverse effects in *Italics* are most common; those in **Bold** are life-threatening.

Drug-lab test interferences
- Possible false-positive urinary glucose tests using Benedict's method

■ Nursing Considerations
Assessment
- *History:* Allergy to sulfonamides, sulfonylureas, thiazides; pregnancy; lactation; impaired renal or hepatic function; G-6-PD deficiency; porphyria
- *Physical:* Body temperature; skin—color, lesions; culture of infected site; orientation, reflexes, affect, peripheral sensation; R, adventitious sounds; mucous membranes, bowel sounds, liver evaluation; liver and renal function tests, CBC and differential, urinalysis

Implementation
- Arrange for culture and sensitivity tests of infected area before beginning therapy; repeat cultures if response is not as expected.
- Administer drug after meals or with food to prevent GI upset. Administer the drug around the clock.
- Ensure adequate fluid intake; sulfasalazine is very insoluble and may cause crystalluria if high concentrations occur in the urine; alkalinization of the urine may be necessary.
- Discontinue drug immediately if hypersensitivity reaction occurs.

Drug-specific teaching points
- Complete full course of therapy.
- Take the drug with food or meals to decrease GI upset.
- Drink eight glasses of water per day.
- Be aware that this drug is specific to this disease; do not use to self-treat any other infection.
- Know that the following side effects may occur: sensitivity to sunlight (use sunscreens, wear protective clothing if exposed to the sun); dizziness, drowsiness, difficulty walking, loss of sensation (avoid driving or performing tasks that require alertness if these occur); nausea, vomiting, diarrhea; loss of fertility; yellow-orange urine
- Report blood in the urine, rash, ringing in the ears, difficulty breathing, fever, sore throat, chills.

❐ sulfinpyrazone

*(sul fin **peer'** a zone)*
Anturan (CAN), Anturane

Pregnancy Category C

Drug classes
Uricosuric
Antigout drug
Antiplatelet drug

Therapeutic actions
Inhibits the renal tubular reabsorption of uric acid, increasing the urinary excretion of uric acid, decreasing serum uric acid levels, retarding urate deposition, and promoting the resorption of urate deposits. Inhibits prostaglandin synthesis, which prevents platelet aggregation, but lacks analgesic and anti-inflammatory activity.

Indications
- Chronic gouty arthritis
- Intermittent gouty arthritis
- Unlabeled uses: post-MI therapy to decrease incidence of sudden death; in rheumatic mitral stenosis to decrease the frequency of systemic embolism

Contraindications/cautions
- Contraindicated in the presence of allergy to sulfinpyrazone, phenylbutazone, or other pyrazoles; blood dyscrasias; peptic ulcer or symptoms of GI inflammation.
- Use caution in the presence of renal failure, pregnancy, lactation.

Dosage
Adult
- ***Gout:*** 200–400 mg/d PO in two divided doses with meals or milk, gradually increase to maintenance dose over 1 wk. Maintenance, 400 mg/d PO in two divided doses. May increase to 800 mg/d if needed or reduce to 200 mg/d. Regulate dose by monitoring serum uric acid levels.
- ***Inhibition of platelet aggregation:*** 200 mg PO tid or qid.

Pediatric: Safety and efficacy not established.

1032 ■ sulfisoxazole

Pharmacokinetics

Route	Onset	Peak	Duration
Oral	Varies	1–2 h	4–6 h

Metabolism: $T_{1/2}$: 2.2–3 h
Distribution: Crosses placenta; may enter breast milk
Excretion: Urine

Adverse effects
- GI: *Upper GI disturbances*
- Hematologic: Blood dyscrasias
- GU: Exacerbation of gout and uric acid stones, renal failure
- Dermatologic: Rash

Clinically important drug-drug interactions
- Decreased effectiveness of sulfinpyrazone when taken with salicylates • Increased pharmacologic effects of tolbutamide, glyburide, warfarin taken concurrently • Increased risk of hepatotoxicity if taken concurrently with acetaminophen

■ Nursing Considerations

Assessment
- *History:* Allergy to sulfinpyrazone, phenylbutazone, or other pyrazoles; blood dyscrasias; peptic ulcer or symptoms of GI inflammation; renal failure; pregnancy; lactation
- *Physical:* Skin—lesions, color; liver evaluation, normal output, gums; urinary output; CBC, renal and liver function tests, urinalysis

Implementation
- Administer drug with meals or antacids to prevent GI upset.
- Force fluids (2.5 to 3 L/d) to decrease the risk of renal stone development.
- Check urine alkalinity (urates crystallize in acid urine) sodium bicarbonate or potassium citrate may be ordered to alkalinize urine.
- Arrange for regular medical follow-up and blood tests during the course of therapy.
- Double-check any analgesics ordered for pain; salicylates, acetaminophen should be avoided.

Drug-specific teaching points
- Take the drug with meals or antacids to prevent GI upset.
- Know that the following side effects may occur: exacerbation of gouty attack or renal stones (drink plenty of fluids while on this drug, 2.5–3 L/d); nausea, vomiting, loss of appetite (taking the drug with meals or antacids may help).
- Report flank pain, dark urine or blood in urine, acute gout attack, unusual fatigue or lethargy, unusual bleeding or bruising.

❒ sulfisoxazole

(sul fi sox' a zole)

Gantrisin, Novosoxazole (CAN)

Pregnancy Category C
Pregnancy Category D (at term)

Drug classes
Antibiotic
Sulfonamide

Therapeutic actions
Bacteriostatic: competitively antagonizes PABA, an essential component of folic acid synthesis in susceptible gram-negative and gram-positive bacteria, preventing cell replication.

Indications
- Treatment of acute infections caused by susceptible organisms: urinary tract infections, chancroid, inclusion conjunctivitis, trachoma, nocardiosis, toxoplasmosis (with pyrimethamine), malaria (as adjunctive therapy for chloroquine-resistant strains of *P. falciparum*), acute otitis media (due to *H. influenzae* when used with penicillin or erythromycin), *H. influenzae* meningitis (as adjunctive therapy with parenteral streptomycin), meningicoccal meningitis
- Conjunctivitis, corneal ulcer, superficial ocular infections due to susceptible microorganisms

Adverse effects in *Italics* are most common; those in **Bold** are life-threatening.

sulfisoxazole ■ 1033

- Adjunctive treatment with systemic sulfonamide therapy for trachoma (ophthalmic preparations)
- CDC recommended for treatment of sexually transmitted diseases
- Unlabeled use: chemoprophylaxis for recurrent otitis media

Contraindications/cautions
- Contraindicated in the presence of allergy to sulfonamides, sulfonylureas, thiazides; pregnancy (teratogenic in preclinical studies; at term, may bump fetal bilirubin from plasma protein-binding sites and cause kernicterus); lactation (risk of kernicterus, diarrhea, rash).
- Use caution in the presence of impaired renal or hepatic function, G-6-PD deficiency, porphyria.

Dosage
Adult
- ***Oral:*** Loading dose, 2–4 g PO. Maintenance dose, 4–8 g/d PO in four to six divided doses.
- ***CDC recommended treatment of sexually transmitted diseases***
  – *Lymphogranuloma venereum:* As an alternative regimen to doxycycline, 500 mg PO qid for 21 d.
  – *Treatment of uncomplicated urethral, endocervical, or rectal Chlamydia trachomatis infections:* As an alternative regimen to doxycycline or tetracycline (if erythromycin is not tolerated), 500 mg PO qid for 10 d.
- ***Ophthalmic solution:*** 1–2 drops into the lower conjunctival sac q2–3h.
- ***Ophthalmic ointment:*** Apply a small amount in the lower conjunctival sac one to four times per day and at bedtime.

Pediatric (older than 2 mo)
- ***Oral:*** Initial dose, 75 mg/kg PO. Maintenance dose, 120–150 mg/kg per day PO in four to six divided doses with a maximum dose of 6 g/d.

Pharmacokinetics

Route	Onset	Peak
Oral	Varies	2–4 h

Metabolism: Hepatic, $T_{1/2}$: 4.5–7.8 h
Distribution: Crosses placenta; enters breast milk
Excretion: Urine

Adverse effects
Systemic
- CNS: *Headache*, peripheral neuropathy, mental depression, convulsions, ataxia, hallucinations, tinnitus, vertigo, insomnia, hearing loss, drowsiness, transient lesions of posterior spinal column, transverse myelitis
- GI: *Nausea, emesis, abdominal pains*, diarrhea, bloody diarrhea, anorexia, pancreatitis, stomatitis, impaired folic acid absorption, hepatitis, hepatocellular necrosis
- Hematologic: **Agranulocytosis,** aplastic anemia, thrombocytopenia, leukopenia, hemolytic anemia, hypoprothrombinemia, methemoglobinemia, megaloblastic anemia
- GU: *Crystalluria, hematuria,* proteinuria, nephrotic syndrome, toxic nephrosis with oliguria and anuria, oligospermia, infertility
- Dermatologic: *Photosensitivity,* cyanosis, petechiae, alopecia
- Hypersensitivity: Stevens-Johnson syndrome, generalized skin eruptions, epidermal necrolysis, urticaria, serum sickness, pruritus, exfoliative dermatitis, anaphylactoid reactions, periorbital edema, conjunctival and scleral redness, photosensitization, arthralgia, allergic myocarditis, transient pulmonary changes with eosinophilia, decreased pulmonary function
- Other: Drug fever, chills, periarteritis nodosum

Ophthalmic
- CNS: *Blurred vision, headache, browache, local irritation,* burning and stinging, epithelial keratitis, reactive hyperemia

Clinically important drug-drug interactions
- Increased risk of hypoglycemia when tolbutamide, tolazamide, glyburide, glipizide,

Adverse effects in *Italics* are most common; those in **Bold** are life-threatening.

acetohexamide, chlorpropamide are taken concurrently • Ophthalmic solutions of sulfonamide are incompatible with silver preparations

Drug-lab test interferences

• False-positive urinary glucose tests using Benedict's method • False-positive results with Urobilistix test and sulfosalicylic acid tests for urinary protein

■ Nursing Considerations

Assessment

- *History:* Allergy to sulfonamides, sulfonylureas, thiazides; impaired renal or hepatic function; G-6-PD deficiency; porphyria; pregnancy; lactation
- *Physical:* Body temperature; skin—color, lesions; culture of infected site; orientation, reflexes, affect, peripheral sensation; R, adventitious sounds; mucous membranes, bowel sounds, liver evaluation; liver and renal function tests, CBC and differential, urinalysis

Implementation

- Arrange for culture and sensitivity tests of infected area before beginning therapy; repeat cultures if response is not as expected.
- Administer oral drug on an empty stomach, 1 h before or 2 h after meals, with a full glass of water.
- Administer ophthalmic solution by having patient lie down or tilt the head back and look at the ceiling; hold dropper above eye; do not touch eye; drop medicine inside the lower lid. Release lower lid, and have patient keep eye open and refrain from blinking for 30 sec. Apply gentle pressure to the bridge of the nose for about 1 min to decrease systemic absorption. Tell patient not to close eyes tightly or blink more than normal. Do not administer other eye drops within 5 min of sulfisoxazole.
- Do not administer ophthalmic solution if it is discolored dark brown.
- Administer ophthalmic ointment as follows: Hold tube in the hand to warm it up; have patient lie down or tilt head backward and look at ceiling. Squeeze small amount of ointment inside lower lid; do not touch tip of tube or cap to eye, fingers, or any surface. Have patient close eye gently and roll eyeball in all directions while eye is closed. Do not administer any other ophthalmic ointment for 10 min.
- Discontinue drug immediately if hypersensitivity reaction occurs.
- Monitor CBC, differential, urinalysis before beginning therapy and periodically during therapy.

Drug-specific teaching points

- Take complete full course of therapy. Take the drug on an empty stomach, 1 h before or 2 h after meals, with a full glass of water. For ophthalmic use, hold tube in the hand to warm it up; lie down or tilt head backward and look at ceiling. Squeeze small amount of ointment inside lower lid; do not touch tip of tube or cap to eye, fingers, or any surface. Close eye gently and roll eyeball in all directions while eye is closed. Do not administer any other ophthalmic ointment for 10 min.
- Be aware that this drug is specific to this disease. Do not use to self-treat any other infection.
- Know that the following side effects may occur: sensitivity to sunlight (use sunscreens, wear protective clothing if exposed to the sun); dizziness, drowsiness, difficulty walking, loss of sensation (avoid driving or performing tasks that require alertness if these occur); nausea, vomiting, diarrhea; loss of fertility.
- Report blood in the urine; rash; ringing in the ears; difficulty breathing; fever; sore throat; chills; worsening of condition, pain, itching, swelling of eye (ophthalmic preparations).

❐ sulindac

*(sul **in'** dak)*
Clinoril

Pregnancy Category B

Drug classes
NSAID

Therapeutic actions
Anti-inflammatory, analgesic, and antipyretic activities largely related to inhibition of prostaglandin synthesis; exact mechanisms of action are not known.

Indications
- Acute or long-term use to relieve signs and symptoms of osteoarthritis, rheumatoid arthritis, ankylosing spondylitis, acute painful shoulder (acute subacromial bursitis/supraspinatus tendinitis), acute gouty arthritis

Contraindications/cautions
- Contraindicated in the presence of pregnancy, lactation.
- Use caution in the presence of allergies, renal, hepatic, cardiovascular, and GI conditions.

Dosage
Do not exceed 400 mg/d.
Adult
- **Rheumatoid arthritis/osteoarthritis, ankylosing spondylitis:** Initial dose of 150 mg bid PO. Individualize dosage.
- **Acute painful shoulder, acute gouty arthritis:** 200 mg bid PO. After adequate response, reduce dosage. Acute painful shoulder usually requires 7–14 d of therapy. Acute gouty arthritis, 7 d.

Pediatric: Safety and efficacy not established.

Pharmacokinetics

Route	Onset	Peak	Duration
Oral	Varies	2–4 h	10–12 h

Metabolism: Hepatic, $T_{1/2}$: 8–10 h
Distribution: Crosses placenta; enters breast milk
Excretion: Urine and feces

Adverse effects
NSAIDs
- CNS: *Headache, dizziness, somnolence, insomnia*, fatigue, tiredness, dizziness, tinnitus, ophthamological effects
- GI: *Nausea, dyspepsia, GI pain,* diarrhea, vomiting, *constipation*, flatulence
- Respiratory: Dyspnea, hemoptysis, pharyngitis, bronchospasm, rhinitis
- Hematologic: Bleeding, platelet inhibition with higher doses, neutropenia, eosinophilia, leukopenia, pancytopenia, thrombocytopenia, agranulocytosis, granulocytopenia, aplastic anemia, decreased hemoglobin or hematocrit, bone marrow depression, mennorrhagia
- GU: Dysuria, renal impairment
- Dermatologic: *Rash*, pruritus, sweating, dry mucous membranes, stomatitis
- Other: Peripheral edema, anaphylactoid reactions to **fatal anaphylactic shock**

Clinically important drug-drug interactions
- Increased serum lithium levels and risk of toxicity if taken concurrently with sulindac. • Decreased antihypertensive effects of beta-blockers if taken concurrently • Decreased therapeutic effects of bumetanide, furosemide, ethacrynic acid taken concurrently

Clinically important drug-food interactions
- Decreased rate but not extent of absorption when taken with food

■ Nursing Considerations
Assessment
- *History:* Allergies, renal, hepatic, cardiovascular, and GI conditions; pregnancy; lactation
- *Physical:* Skin—color and lesions; orientation, reflexes, ophthalmologic and audiometric evaluation, peripheral sensation; P, edema; R, adventitious sounds; liver evaluation; CBC, clotting times, renal and liver function tests; serum electrolytes, stool guaiac

Implementation
- Administer drug with food or milk if GI upset occurs.
- Arrange for periodic ophthalmologic examination during long-term therapy.

Adverse effects in *Italics* are most common; those in **Bold** are life-threatening.

1036 ■ sumatriptan succinate injection

- Institute emergency procedures if overdose occurs: gastric lavage, induction of emesis, supportive therapy.

Drug-specific teaching points
- Take drug with food or meals if GI upset occurs.
- Take only the prescribed dosage.
- Be aware that dizziness, drowsiness can occur (avoid driving or the use of dangerous machinery while on this drug).
- Report sore throat, fever, rash, itching, weight gain, swelling in ankles or fingers; changes in vision; black, tarry stools.

❑ sumatriptan succinate injection

*(sew mah **trip'** tan)*
Imitrex

Pregnancy Category C

Drug classes
Antimigraine agent
Serotonin selective agonist

Therapeutic actions
Binds to serotonin receptors to cause vascular constrictive effects on cranial bood vessels, causing the relief of migraine in selective patients.

Indications
- Treatment of acute migraine attacks with or without aura
- Unlabeled use: treatment of cluster headaches

Contraindications/cautions
- Contraindicated in the presence of allergy to sumatriptan, active coronary artery disease, uncontrolled hypertension, hemiplegic migraine, pregnancy.
- Use caution in the presence of the elderly, lactation.

Dosage
Adult: 6 mg SC with a maximum of 12 mg/24 h; two 6-mg injections separated by at least 1 h.

Pediatric: Safety and efficacy not established.

Pharmacokinetics

Route	Onset	Peak
SC	Varies	5–20 min

Metabolism: Hepatic, $T_{1/2}$: 115 min
Distribution: Crosses placenta; may enter breast milk
Excretion: Urine

Adverse effects
- **CNS:** *Dizziness, vertigo,* headache, anxiety, malaise/fatigue, *weakness, myalgia*
- **GI:** Abdominal discomfort, dysphagia
- **CV:** *Blood pressure alterations, tightness or pressure in chest*
- **Local:** *Injection site discomfort*
- **Other:** *Tingling, warm/hot sensations, burning sensation, feeling of heaviness, pressure sensation, numbness, feeling of tightness,* feeling strange, cold sensation

Clinically important drug-drug interactions
- Prolonged vasoactive reactions with taken concurrently with ergot-containing drugs

■ Nursing Considerations

Assessment
- *History:* Allergy to sumatriptan, active coronary artery disease, uncontrolled hypertension, hemiplegic migraine, pregnancy, lactation
- *Physical:* Skin—color and lesions; orientation, reflexes, peripheral sensation; P, BP; renal and liver function tests

Implementation
- Administer to relieve acute migraine, not as a prophylactic measure.
- Administer as SC injection just below the skin as soon as possible after symptoms begin.
- Repeat injection in not less than 1 h if relief is not obtained; only two injections may be given each 24 h.
- Monitor BP of patients with possible coronary artery disease; discontinue suma-

Adverse effects in *Italics* are most common; those in **Bold** are life-threatening.

- triptan at any sign of angina, prolonged high blood pressure.

Drug-specific teaching points
- Learn to use the autoinjector; injection may be repeated in not less than 1 h if relief is not obtained; do not administer more than two injections in 24 h.
- Inject just below the skin as soon as possible after the beginning of a migraine; this drug is for an acute attack only, not for use to prevent attacks.
- Be aware that this drug should not be taken during pregnancy; if you suspect that you are pregnant, contact physician and refrain from using drug.
- Be aware that the following side effects may occur: dizziness, drowsiness (avoid driving or the use of dangerous machinery while on this drug); numbness, tingling, feelings of tightness or pressure.
- Contact physician immediately if you experience chest pain or pressure that is severe or does not go away.
- Report feelings of heat, flushing, tiredness, feelings of sickness, swelling of lips or eyelids.

☐ tacrine hydrochloride

(tay' krin)
tetrahydroaminoacridine
THA, Cognex

Pregnancy Category C

Drug classes
Cholinesterase inhibitor
Alzheimer's drug

Therapeutic actions
Centrally acting reversible cholinesterase inhibitor, leading to elevated acetylcholine levels in the cortex, which slows the neuronal degradation that occurs in Alzheimer's disease.

Indications
- Treatment of mild to moderate dementia of the Alzheimer's type

Contraindications/cautions
- Contraindicated in the presence of allergy to tacrine or acridine derivatives, previous tacrine-associated jaundice, pregnancy.
- Use caution in the presence of renal or hepatic disease; bladder obstruction; seizure conditions; sick sinus syndrome; GI bleed; anesthesia.

Dosage
Adult: 10 mg PO qid; maintain this dose for 6 wk with regular monitoring of transaminase levels; after 6 wk, increase dose to 20 mg PO qid; if patient is tolerant to drug and transaminase levels are WNL, increase at 6-wk intervals at 10-mg increases to a total of 120–160 mg/d.
Pediatric: Safety and efficacy not established.

Pharmacokinetics

Route	Onset	Peak
Oral	Varies	1–2 h

Metabolism: Hepatic, $T_{1/2}$: 2–4 h
Distribution: Crosses placenta; may enter breast milk
Excretion: Urine

Adverse effects
- **CNS:** *Headache, fatigue, dizziness, confusion,* ataxia, insomnia, somnolence, tremor, agitation, depression, anxiety, abnormal thinking
- **GI:** *Nausea, vomiting, diarrhea, dyspepsia, anorexia, abdominal pain,* flatulence, constipation, **hepatoxicity**
- **Respiratory:** *Rhinitis,* upper respiratory infections, coughing
- **GU:** Urinary frequency, urinary tract infections
- **Dermatologic:** *Skin rash,* flushing, purpura

Clinically important drug-drug interactions
- Increased effects and risk of toxicity of theophylline, cholinesterase inhibitors taken concurrently • Decreased effects of anticholinergics taken concurrently • Increased effects of tacrine if taken concurrently with cimetidine

Clinically important drug-food interactions

- Decreased absorption and serum levels of tacrine if taken with food

Nursing Considerations

Assessment

- *History:* Allergy to tacrine or acridine derivatives, previous tacrine-associated jaundice; pregnancy; renal or hepatic disease; bladder obstruction; seizure conditions; sick sinus syndrome; GI bleed; anesthesia
- *Physical:* Orientation, affect, reflexes; BP, P; R, adventitious sounds; urinary output; abdominal exam; renal and liver function tests; serum transaminase levels

Implementation

- Arrange for regular transaminase level determination before and during therapy.
- Administer around the clock at regular intervals for best results.
- Administer on an empty stomach, 1 h before or 2 h after meals.
- Administer with meals only if severe GI upset occurs.
- Arrange to decrease dose and slowly discontinue drug if side effects become severe.
- Notify surgeons that patient is on tacrine; exaggerated muscle relaxation may occur if succinylcholine-type drugs are used.
- Do not suddenly discontinue high doses of drug.
- Monitor patient for any signs of neurologic change or deterioration; drug does not stop the disease but slows the degeneration.

Drug-specific teaching points

- Take drug exactly as prescribed, around the clock. Work with your nurse to establish a schedule that is least disruptive for you. Do not take more than the prescribed dose.
- Take drug on an empty stomach, 1 h before or 2 h after meals. If severe GI upset occurs, drug may be taken with meals.
- Be aware that this drug does not cure the disease but is thought to slow down the degeneration associated with the disease.
- Arrange for regular blood tests and follow-up visits while adjusting to this drug.
- Know that the following side effects may occur: nausea, vomiting (small, frequent meals may help); dizziness, confusion, lightheadedness (use caution if driving or performing tasks that require alertness if these occur).
- Report nausea, vomiting, changes in stool or urine color, diarrhea, rash, changes in neurologic functioning, yellowing of eyes or skin.

☐ tacrolimus

(tack row' lim us)
FK506, Prograf

Pregnancy Category C

Drug classes
Immunosuppressant

Therapeutic actions
Immunosuppressant; inhibits T-lymphocyte activation; exact mechanism of action not known but binds to intracellular protein, which may prevent the generation of nuclear factor of activated T cells and suppresses the immune activation and response of T cells.

Indications

- Prophylaxis for organ rejection in liver transplants in conjunction with adrenal corticosteroids
- Unlabeled use: prophylaxis in kidney, bone marrow, cardiac, pancreas, pancreatic island cell, and small bowel transplantation; treatment of autoimmune disease; recalcitrant psoriasis

Contraindications/cautions

- Contraindicated in the presence of allergy to tacrolimus, hypersensitibity to HCO-60 polyoxyl 60 hydrogenated castor oil, pregnancy, lactation.
- Use caution in the presence of impaired renal function, hypokalemia, malabsorption.

Dosage
Adult
- ***Oral:*** 0.15–0.3 mg/kg per day; administer inital dose no sooner than 6 h after transplant; divide into two doses given q12h. If transferring from IV, give first dose 8–12 h after discontinuing IV infusion. Titrate dose based on clinical assessment of rejection tolerance of drug.
- ***Parenteral:*** Patients unable to take capsules; 0.05–0.1 mg/kg per day as continuous IV infusion begun no sooner than 6 h after transplant. Switch to oral drug as soon as possible.

Pediatric: Children require the larger dose; begin treatment at higher end of recommended adult dose.

Pharmacokinetics

Route	Onset	Peak
Oral	Varies	1½–3½ h
IV	Rapid	1–2 h

Metabolism: Hepatic, $T_{1/2}$: 5.7 h, then 11.7 h

Distribution: Crosses placenta; enters breast milk

Excretion: Bile and urine

IV facts
Preparation: Dilute IV solution immediately before use; use 0.9% Sodium Chloride Injection or 5% Dextrose Injection to a concentration of 0.004 and 0.02 mg/ml. Do not store in a PVC container; discard after 24 h.

Infusion: Give by continuous IV infusion.

Adverse effects
- CNS: *Tremor, headache, insomnia*, paresthesias
- GI: **Hepatotoxicity**, *constipation, diarrhea, nausea, vomiting*, anorexia
- CV: Hypertension
- Hematologic: Leukopenia, anemia, hyperkalemia, hypokalemia, hyperglycemia
- GU: *Renal dysfunction*, nephrotoxicity, UTI, oliguria
- Other: Abdominal pain, pain, fever, asthenia, back pain, ascites, neoplasias

Clinically important drug-drug interactions
• Increased risk of nephrotoxicity if taken with other nephrotoxic agents (erythromycin) • Risk of severe myopathy or rhabdomyolysis if taken with lovastatin • Increased risk of toxicity if taken with diltiazem, metoclopramide, nicardipine, cimetidine, clarithromycin, calcium channel-blockers • Decreased therapeutic effect of tacrolimus if taken with carbamazeine, phenobarbital, phenytoin, rifamycins

■ Nursing Considerations

Assessment
- *History:* Allergy to tacrolimus or polyoxyethylated castor oil, impaired renal function, malabsorption, lactation
- *Physical:* Body temperature; skin—color, lesions; BP, peripheral perfusion; liver evaluation, bowel sounds, gum evaluation; renal and liver function tests, CBC

Implementation
- Use parenteral administration only if patient is unable to take the oral solution; transfer to oral solution as soon as possible.
- Monitor renal and liver function tests before and periodically during therapy; marked decreases in function could require changes in dosage or discontinuation of the drug.
- Monitor liver function and hematologic tests to determine titration dosage as appropriate.

Drug-specific teaching points
- Avoid infection while you are on this drug; avoid crowds or people who have infections. Notify your health care provider at once if you injure yourself.
- Know that the following side effects may occur: nausea, vomiting (taking the drug with food may help); diarrhea; headache (analgesics may be ordered).
- Be aware that this drug should not be taken during pregnancy. If you think that you are pregnant or you want to

Adverse effects in *Italics* are most common; those in **Bold** are life-threatening.

become pregnant, discuss this with your prescriber.
- Arrange to have periodic blood tests to monitor your response to this drug and its effects on your body.
- Do not discontinue this medication without your prescriber's advice.
- Report unusual bleeding or bruising, fever, sore throat, mouth sores, tiredness.

☐ tamoxifen citrate

*(ta **mox**' i fen)*
Alpha-Tamoxifen (CAN), Apo-Tamoxifen (CAN), Nolvadex, Novo-Tamoxifen (CAN), Tamofen (CAN), Tamone (CAN), Tamoplex (CAN)

Pregnancy Category D

Drug classes
Antiestrogen

Therapeutic actions
Potent antiestrogenic effects: competes with estrogen for binding sites in target tissues, such as the breast.

Indications
- Adjunct with cytotoxic chemotherapy following radical or modified radical mastectomy to delay recurrence of surgically curable breast cancer in postmenopausal women or women older than 50 y with positive axillary nodes
- Treatment of advanced, metastatic breast cancer in women and men; alternative to oophorectomy or ovarian radiation in premenopausal women
- Unlabeled uses: treatment of mastalgia; useful for decreasing size and pain of gynecomastia; preventive therapy for women at high risk of breast cancer; treatment of pancreatic carcinoma

Contraindications/cautions
- Allergy to tamoxifen, pregnancy, lactation.

Dosage
Adult: 10–20 mg bid PO given morning and evening.

Pharmacokinetics

Route	Onset	Peak
Oral	Varies	4–7 h

Metabolism: Hepatic, $T_{1/2}$: 7–14 h
Distribution: Crosses placenta; enters breast milk
Excretion: Feces

Adverse effects
- **CNS:** Depression, lightheadedness, dizziness, headache, corneal opacity, decreased visual acuity, retinopathy
- **GI:** *Nausea, vomiting,* food distaste
- **Hematologic:** Hypercalcemia, especially in patients with bone metastases, thrombocytopenia, leukopenia, anemia
- **GU:** *Vaginal bleeding, vaginal discharge, menstrual irregularities,* pruritus vulvae
- **Dermatologic:** *Hot flashes, skin rash*
- **Other:** Peripheral edema; increased bone and tumor pain and local disease (initially seen with a good tumor response, usually subsides); cancer in animal studies

Clinically important drug-drug interactions
- Increased risk of bleeding if taken with oral anticoagulants • Increased serum levels of tamoxifen if taken with bromocriptine

Drug-lab test interferences
- Possible increase in calcium levels, T_4 levels without hyperthyroidism

■ Nursing Considerations

Assessment
- *History:* Allergy to tamoxifen, pregnancy, lactation
- *Physical:* skin—lesions, color, turgor; pelvic exam; orientation, affect, reflexes; ophthalmologic exam; peripheral pulses, edema; liver function tests, CBC and differential, estrogen receptor evaluation of tumor cells

Adverse effects in *Italics* are most common; those in **Bold** are life-threatening.

Implementation
- Administer bid, in the morning and the evening.
- Arrange for periodic blood counts during therapy.
- Arrange for initial ophthalmologic exam and periodic exams if visual changes occur.
- Counsel patient about the need to use contraception to avoid pregnancy while taking this drug; inform patient that serious fetal harm could occur.
- Arrange for decrease in dosage if adverse effects become severe.

Drug-specific teaching points
- Take the drug twice a day, in the morning and evening.
- Know that the following side effects may occur: bone pain; hot flashes (staying in cool temperatures may help); nausea, vomiting (small, frequent meals may help); weight gain; menstrual irregularities; dizziness, headache, lightheadedness (use caution if driving or performing tasks that require alertness if these occur).
- Be aware that this drug can cause serious fetal harm and must not be taken during pregnancy. Contraceptive measures should be used while you are taking this drug. If you become pregnant or decide that you would like to become pregnant, consult with your health care provider immediately.
- Report marked weakness, sleepiness, mental confusion, pain or swelling of the legs, shortness of breath, blurred vision.

▢ temazepam

*(te **maz**' e pam)*
Restoril

Pregnancy Category X
C-IV controlled substance

Drug classes
Benzodiazepine
Sedative/hypnotic

Therapeutic actions
Exact mechanisms of action not understood; acts mainly at subcortical levels of the CNS, leaving the cortex relatively unaffected; main sites of action may be the limbic system and mesencephalic reticular formation; benzodiazepines potentiate the effects of gamma-aminobutyrate (GABA), an inhibitory neurotransmitter.

Indications
- Insomnia characterized by difficulty falling asleep, frequent nocturnal awakenings, or early morning awakening
- Recurring insomnia or poor sleeping habits
- Acute or chronic medical situations requiring restful sleep

Contraindications/cautions
- Contraindicated in the presence of hypersensitivity to benzodiazepines, psychoses, acute narrow-angle glaucoma, shock, coma, acute alcoholic intoxication with depression of vital signs, pregnancy (risk of congenital malformations, neonatal withdrawal syndrome), labor and delivery ("floppy infant" syndrome reported when mothers were given benzodiazepines during labor), lactation (infants may become lethargic and lose weight).
- Use caution in the presence of impaired liver or kidney function, debilitation, depression, suicidal tendencies.

Dosage
Adult: 15–30 mg PO before retiring.
Pediatric: Not for use in children younger than 18 y.
Geriatric patients or those with debilitating disease: Initially 15 mg PO; adjust dosage until individual response is determined.

Pharmacokinetics

Route	Onset	Peak
Oral	Varies	2–4 h

Metabolism: Hepatic, $T_{1/2}$: 9.5–12.4 h
Distribution: Crosses placenta; enters breast milk
Excretion: Urine

Adverse effects
- CNS: *Transient, mild drowsiness initially; sedation, depression, lethargy, apathy, fatigue, lightheadedness, disorientation, restlessness, confusion,* crying, delirium, headache, slurred speech, dysarthria, stupor, rigidity, tremor, dystonia, vertigo, euphoria, nervousness, difficulty concentrating, vivid dreams, psychomotor retardation, extrapyramidal symptoms, *mild paradoxical excitatory reactions during first 2 wk of treatment* (especially in psychiatric patients, aggressive children, and with high dosage), visual and auditory disturbances, diplopia, nystagmus, depressed hearing, nasal congestion
- GI: *Constipation, diarrhea,* dry mouth, salivation, nausea, anorexia, vomiting, difficulty in swallowing, gastric disorders, elevations of blood enzymes: hepatic dysfunction, jaundice
- CV: *Bradycardia, tachycardia,* cardiovascular collapse, hypertension and hypotension, palpitations, edema
- Hematologic: Decreased hematocrit (primarily with long-term therapy), blood dyscrasias
- GU: *Incontinence, urinary retention, changes in libido,* menstrual irregularities
- Dermatologic: Urticaria, pruritus, skin rash, dermatitis
- Dependence: *Drug dependence with withdrawal syndrome* when drug is discontinued
- Other: Hiccups, fever, diaphoresis, paresthesias, muscular disturbances, gynecomastia

Clinically important drug-drug interactions
- Increased CNS depression when taken with alcohol • Decreased sedative effects of temazepam if taken concurrently with theophylline, aminophylline, dyphylline, oxitriphylline

■ Nursing Considerations
Assessment
- *History:* Hypersensitivity to benzodiazepines, psychoses, acute narrow-angle glaucoma, shock, coma, acute alcoholic intoxication, pregnancy, lactation, impaired liver or kidney function, debilitation, depression, suicidal tendencies
- *Physical:* Skin—color, lesions; body temperature; orientation, reflexes, affect, ophthalmologic exam; P, BP; R, adventitious sounds; liver evaluation, abdominal exam, bowel sounds, normal output; CBC, liver and renal function tests

Implementation
- Arrange to taper dosage gradually after long-term therapy, especially in epileptic patients.

Drug-specific teaching points
- Take drug exactly as prescribed.
- Do not stop taking this drug (long-term therapy) without consulting your health care provider.
- Avoid pregnancy while taking this drug; use of contraceptive measures is advised; serious fetal harm could occur.
- Know that the following side effects may occur: drowsiness, dizziness (these may become less pronounced after a few days; avoid driving a car or engaging in other dangerous activities if these occur); GI upset (taking the drug with water may help); depression, dreams, emotional upset, crying.
- Be aware that nocturnal sleep may be disturbed for several nights after discontinuing the drug.
- Report severe dizziness, weakness, drowsiness that persists, rash or skin lesions, palpitations, swelling of the extremities, visual changes, difficulty voiding.

☐ teniposide

*(teh **nip'** oh side)*
VM-23, Vumon

Pregnancy Category D

Adverse effects in *Italics* are most common; those in **Bold** are life-threatening.

Drug classes
Mitotic inhibitor
Antineoplastic agent

Therapeutic actions
Late S_2 and early G_2 specific cell toxic: lyses cells entering mitosis; inhibits cells from entering prophase; inhibits DNA synthesis, leading to cell death.

Indications
- In combination with other anticancer drugs for induction therapy in patients with refractory childhood acute lymphoblastic leukemia

Contraindications/cautions
- Allergy to teniposide, *Cremophor EL*, bone marrow suppression, pregnancy, lactation.

Dosage
Modify dosage based on myelosuppression
Pediatric: 165 mg/m^2 teniposide in combination with 300 mg/m^2 cytarabine IV twice weekly for eight to nine doses or 250 mg/m^2 teniposide in combination with 1.5 mg/m^2 vincristine IV weekly for 4–8 wk and prednisone 40 mg/m^2 orally for 28 d.
- ***Renal/hepatic impairment:*** Reduced dosage may be necessary.
- ***Down's syndrome:*** Reduce initial dosings; give the first course at half the usual dose.

Pharmacokinetics

Route	Onset	Peak
IV	30 min	60 min

Metabolism: Hepatic, $T_{1/2}$: 5 h
Distribution: Crosses placenta; enters breast milk
Excretion: Urine and bile

IV facts
Preparation: Dilute with 5% Dextrose Injection or 0.9% Sodium Chloride Injection to give a concentration of 0.1, 0.2, 0.4, or 1 mg/ml. Use of glass or polyolefin plastic bags is recommended; PVC containers may crack or break; diluted solutions are stable for 24 h at room temperature.

Infusion: Administer slowly over 30–60 min or longer. *Do not give by rapid IV infusion.*

Compatibilities: Heparin may cause precipitation; do not mix with other drugs or in other solutions.

Adverse effects
- **CNS:** *Somnolence, fatigue,* peripheral neuropathy
- **GI:** *Nausea, vomiting, anorexia, diarrhea,* stomatitis, aftertaste, liver toxicity
- **CV:** Hypotension (after rapid IV administration)
- **Hematologic:** *Myelosuppression*
- **Dermatologic:** *Alopecia*
- **Hypersensitivity:** Chills, fever, tachycardia, bronchospasm, dyspnea, anaphylactic-like reaction
- **Other:** Potentially, carcinogenesis

■ Nursing Considerations

Assessment
- *History:* Allergy to teniposide, *Cremophor EL*; bone marrow suppression; pregnancy; lactation
- *Physical:* Temperature; weight; hair; orientation, reflexes; BP, P; mucous membranes, abdominal exam; CBC

Implementation
- Do not administer IM or SC because severe local reaction and tissue necrosis occur.
- Avoid skin contact with this drug. The use of rubber gloves is suggested while using this drug; if contact occurs, immediately wash with soap and water.
- Monitor blood pressure during administration; if hypotension occurs, discontinue dose and consult with physician. Fluids and other supportive therapy may be needed.
- Monitor patient's response to therapy before starting therapy and prior to each dose: platelet count, hemoglobin, WBC count, differential. If severe response occurs, discontinue therapy and consult with physician.

Adverse effects in *Italics* are most common; those in **Bold** are life-threatening.

Drug-specific teaching points
- Prepare a calendar showing need to return for specific treatment days and additional courses of drug therapy.
- Know that the following side effects may occur: loss of appetite, nausea, vomiting, mouth sores (frequent mouth care, small, frequent meals may help; try to maintain good nutrition if at all possible; an antiemetic may be ordered); loss of hair (you might want to arrange for a wig or other suitable head covering before the hair loss occurs; it is important to keep the head covered in extremes of temperature).
- Arrange to have regular blood tests to monitor the drug's effects.
- Report severe GI upset, diarrhea, vomiting, unusual bleeding or bruising, fever, chills, sore throat, difficulty breathing.

☐ terazosin hydrochloride

(ter ay' zoe sin)
Hytrin

Drug classes
Antihypertensive drug
Alpha-adrenergic blocking drug

Therapeutic actions
Selectively blocks postsynaptic alpha$_1$-adrenergic receptors, decreasing sympathetic tone on the vasculature, dilating arterioles and veins, and lowering supine and standing blood pressure; unlike conventional alpha-adrenergic blocking agents (eg, phentolamine), it does not also block alpha$_2$ presynaptic receptors, does not cause reflex tachycardia.

Indications
- Treatment of hypertension
- Treatment of symptomatic benign prostatic hyperplasia (BPH)

Contraindications/cautions
- Contraindicated in the presence of hypersensitivity to terazosin, lactation.
- Use caution in the presence of CHF, renal failure, pregnancy.

Dosage
Adjust dosage at 12- or 24-h intervals.
Adult
- **Hypertension:** 1 mg PO at bedtime. Do not exceed 1 mg; strictly adhere to this regimen to avoid severe hypotensive reactions. Slowly increase dose to achieve desired BP response. Usual range, 1–5 mg PO qd. Up to 20 mg/d has been beneficial. Monitor BP 2–3 h after dosing to determine maximum effect. If response is diminished after 24 h, consider increasing dosage. If drug is not taken for several days, restart with initial 1-mg dose.
- **BPH:** Initial dose, 1 mg PO at bedtime. Increase to 2, 5, or 10 mg PO qd. 10 mg/d for 4–6 wk may be required to assess benefit.

Pediatric: Safety and efficacy not established.

Pharmacokinetics

Route	Onset	Peak
Oral	Varies	1–2 h

Metabolism: Hepatic, $T_{1/2}$: 9–12 h
Distribution: Crosses placenta; enters breast milk
Excretion: Feces and urine

Adverse effects
- CNS: *Dizziness, headache, drowsiness, lack of energy, weakness, somnolence,* nervousness, vertigo, depression, paresthesia
- GI: *Nausea,* vomiting, diarrhea, constipation, abdominal discomfort or pain
- CV: *Palpitations,* sodium and water retention, increased plasma volume, *edema,* syncope, tachycardia, orthostatic hypotension, angina
- Respiratory: *Dyspnea, nasal congestion, sinusitis*
- GU: Urinary frequency, incontinence, impotence, priapism
- EENT: Blurred vision, reddened sclera, epistaxis, tinnitus, dry mouth, nasal congestion

Adverse effects in *Italics* are most common; those in **Bold** are life-threatening.

- **Dermatologic:** Rash, pruritus, alopecia, lichen planus
- **Other:** Diaphoresis, lupus erythematosus

■ Nursing Considerations

Assessment
- *History:* Hypersensitivity to terazosin, CHF, renal failure, pregnancy, lactation
- *Physical:* Body weight; skin—color, lesions; orientation, affect, reflexes; ophthalmologic exam; P, BP, orthostatic BP, supine BP, perfusion, edema, auscultation; R, adventitious sounds, status of nasal mucous membranes; bowel sounds, normal output; voiding pattern, urinary output; kidney function tests, urinalysis

Implementation
- Arrange to administer, or have patient take, first dose just before bedtime to lessen likelihood of first dose effect, syncope, believed due to excessive postural hypotension.
- Place patient in recumbent position, and treat supportively if syncope occurs; condition is self-limiting.
- Monitor patient for orthostatic hypotension, which is most marked in the morning, is accentuated by hot weather, alcohol, exercise.
- Monitor edema, body weight in patients with incipient cardiac decompensation, and arrange to add a thiazide diuretic to the drug regimen if sodium and fluid retention, signs of impending CHF occur.

Drug-specific teaching points
- Take this drug exactly as prescribed. Take the first dose just before bedtime. Do not drive a car or operate machinery for 4 h after the first dose.
- Know that the following side effects may occur: dizziness, weakness (these are more likely to occur when you change position, in the early morning, after exercise, in hot weather, and when you have consumed alcohol; some tolerance may occur after you have taken the drug for a while, but you should avoid driving a car or engaging in tasks that require alertness while you are experiencing these symptoms; change position slowly, and use caution when climbing stairs; lie down for a while if dizziness persists); GI upset (frequent, small meals may help); impotence; dry mouth (sucking on sugarless lozenges, ice chips may help); stuffy nose. Most of these effects will gradually disappear with continued therapy.
- Report frequent dizziness or faintness.

☐ terbutaline sulfate

*(ter **byoo'** ta leen)*
Brethaire, Brethine, Bricanyl

Pregnancy Category B

Drug classes
Sympathomimetic drug
Beta$_2$-selective adrenergic agonist
Bronchodilator
Antiasthmatic drug
Tocolytic drug (uterine relaxant)

Therapeutic actions
In low doses, acts relatively selectively at beta$_2$-adrenergic receptors to cause bronchodilation and relax the pregnant uterus; at higher doses, beta$_2$ selectivity is lost and the drug acts at beta$_1$ receptors to cause typical sympathomimetic cardiac effects.

Indications
- Prophylaxis and treatment of bronchial asthma and reversible bronchospasm that may occur with bronchitis and emphysema
- Unlabeled oral and IV use: inhibition of premature labor

Contraindications/cautions
- Contraindicated in the presence of hypersensitivity to terbutaline; tachyarrhythmias, tachycardia caused by digitalis intoxication; general anesthesia with halogenated hydrocarbons or cyclopropane, which sensitize the myocardium to catecholamines; unstable vasomotor system disorders; hypertension; preg-

terbutaline sulfate

nancy; labor and delivery (may inhibit labor; parenteral use of beta-adrenergic agonists can accelerate fetal heart beat, cause hypoglycemia, hypokalemia, and pulmonary edema in the mother and hypoglycemia in the neonate); lactation.
- Use caution in the presence of coronary insufficiency, coronary artery disease, history of stroke, COPD patients who have developed degenerative heart disease, hyperthyroidism, history of seizure disorders, psychoneurotic individuals.

Dosage
Adult
- **Oral:** 5 mg at 6-h intervals tid during waking hours. If side effects are pronounced, reduce to 2.5 mg tid. Do not exceed 15 mg/d.
- ***Parenteral***
  - *Bronchospasm:* 0.25 mg SC into lateral deltoid area. If no significant improvement in 15 min, give another 0.25-mg dose. Do not exceed 0.5 mg/4 h. If patient fails to respond to second 0.25-mg dose within 15–30 min, other therapeutic measures should be considered.
  - *Delay premature labor:* Initiate IV administration at 10 μg/min. Titrate upward to a maximum of 80 μg/min. Maintain at minimum effective dosage for 4 h. Oral doses of 2.5 mg q4–6h have been used as maintenance therapy until term.
- ***Inhalation (each actuation of aerosol dispenser delivers 0.2 mg terbutaline):*** Two inhalations separated by 60 sec q4–6h. Do not repeat more often than q4–6h.

Pediatric
- *Older than 12 y:* Same as adult.
- *Younger than 12 y:* Safety and efficacy not established.

Geriatric: Patients older than 60 y are likely to experience adverse effects. Avoid use in these patients, or use with extreme caution.

IV facts
Preparation: Use of a volume delivery system is suggested; dilute as required in D_5W.

Infusion: Infuse at rate of up to 80 μg/min for up to 4 h.

Adverse effects
- **CNS:** *Restlessness, apprehension, anxiety, fear,* CNS stimulation, hyperkinesia, insomnia, tremor, drowsiness, irritability, weakness, vertigo, headache
- **GI:** *Nausea,* vomiting, heartburn, unusual or bad taste
- **CV:** *Cardiac arrhythmias, palpitations,* anginal pain (less likely with bronchodilator doses of this drug than with bronchodilator doses of a nonselective beta-agonist (isoproterenol), changes in BP (increases or decreases)
- **Respiratory:** *Respiratory difficulties, pulmonary edema, coughing,* bronchospasm, paradoxical airway resistance with repeated, excessive use of inhalation preparations
- **Other:** Sweating, pallor, flushing

Clinically important drug-drug interactions
- Increased likelihood of cardiac arrhythmias when given with halogenated hydrocarbon anesthetics (halothane), cyclopropane

■ Nursing Considerations
Assessment
- *History:* Hypersensitivity to terbutaline; tachyarrhythmias; general anesthesia with halogenated hydrocarbons or cyclopropane; unstable vasomotor system disorders; hypertension; CAD; history of stroke; COPD patients who have developed degenerative heart disease; hyperthyroidism; history of seizure disorders; psychoneurotic individuals; pregnancy; labor and delivery; lactation
- *Physical:* Body weight; skin—color, temperature, turgor; orientation, reflexes; P, BP; R, adventitious sounds; blood and urine glucose; serum electrolytes; thyroid function tests; ECG

Implementation
- Use minimal doses for minimal periods of time; drug tolerance can occur with prolonged use.

Adverse effects in *Italics* are most common; those in **Bold** are life-threatening.

terfenadine ■ 1047

- Maintain a beta-adrenergic blocker (a cardioselective beta-blocker, such as atenolol, should be used in patients with respiratory distress) on standby in case cardiac arrhythmias occur.
- Do not exceed recommended dosage; administer aerosol during second half of inspiration, because the airways are open wider, and the aerosol distribution is more extensive.

Drug-specific teaching points
- Do not exceed recommended dosage; adverse effects or loss of effectiveness may result. Read the instructions that come with the aerosol product, and ask your health care provider or pharmacist if you have any questions.
- Know that the following side effects may occur: weakness, dizziness, inability to sleep (use caution when driving or performing acitivies that require alertness if these effects occur); nausea, vomiting (small, frequent meals may help); fast heart rate, anxiety.
- Report chest pain, dizziness, insomnia, weakness, tremor or irregular heartbeat, failure to respond to usual dosage.

☐ terfenadine

(ter fen' a deen)
Seldane

Pregnancy Category C

Drug classes
Antihistamine (nonsedating)

Therapeutic actions
Competitively blocks the effects of histamine at peripheral H_1 receptor sites; has anticholinergic (atropine-like) and antipruritic effects.

Indications
- Symptomatic relief of symptoms associated with perennial and seasonal allergic rhinitis; vasomotor rhinitis; allergic conjunctivitis; mild, uncomplicated urticaria and angioedema
- Amelioraton of allergic reactions to blood or plasma
- Dermatographism
- Adjunctive therapy in anaphylactic reactions
- Unlabeled uses: lower respiratory conditions, such as histamine-induced bronchoconstriction in asthmatics and exercise and hyperventilation-induced bronchospasm

Contraindications/cautions
- Contraindicated in the presence of allergy to any antihistamines, pregnancy, lactation.
- Use caution in the presence of narrow-angle glaucoma, stenosing peptic ulcer, symptomatic prostatic hypertrophy, asthmatic attack, bladder neck obstruction, pyloroduodenal obstruction.

Dosage
Adult and pediatric older than 12 y: 60 mg PO bid.
Pediatric
- ***6–12 y:*** 30–60 mg PO bid.
- ***3–5 y:*** 15 mg PO bid.

Geriatric: More likely to cause dizziness, sedation, syncope, toxic confusional states, and hypotension in elderly patients; use with caution.

Pharmacokinetics

Route	Onset	Peak	Duration
Oral	1–2 h	3–4 h	12 h

Metabolism: Hepatic, $T_{1/2}$: 20 h
Distribution: Crosses placenta; enters breast milk
Excretion: Feces and urine

Adverse effects
- CNS: *Depression, nightmares,* sedation (terfenadine is less sedating than other antihistamines)
- GI: *Dry mouth, GI upset,* anorexia, increased appetite, nausea, vomiting, diarrhea
- CV: Arrhythmia, increase in QTC intervals
- **Respiratory**: *Bronchospasm, cough, thickening of secretions*

Adverse effects in *Italics* are most common; those in **Bold** are life-threatening.

1048 ■ terpin hydrate

- **GU:** Galactorrhea, menstrual disorders, dysuria, hesitancy
- **Dermatologic:** *Alopecia*, angioedema, skin eruption and itching
- **Other:** Musculoskeletal pain, mild to moderate transaminase elevations

Clinically important drug-drug interactions

- Altered terfenadine metabolism if taken concurrently with ketoconazole, troleandomycin

■ Nursing Considerations

Assessment

- *History:* Allergy to any antihistamines, narrow-angle glaucoma, stenosing peptic ulcer, symptomatic prostatic hypertrophy, asthmatic attack, bladder neck obstruction, pyloroduodenal obstruction, pregnancy, lactation
- *Physical:* Skin—color, lesions, texture; orientation, reflexes, affect; vision exam; R, adventitious sounds; prostate palpation; serum transaminase levels

Implementation

- Administer with food if GI upset occurs.

Drug-specific teaching points

- Avoid excessive dosage.
- Take with food if GI upset occurs.
- Know that the following side effects may occur: dizziness, sedation, drowsiness (use caution if driving or performing tasks that require alertness if these occur); dry mouth (frequent mouth care, sucking sugarless lozenges may help); thickening of bronchial secretions, dryness of nasal mucosa (use of a humidifier may help if this becomes a problem); menstrual irregularities.
- Avoid alcohol while on this drug; serious sedation could occur.
- Report difficulty breathing, hallucinations, tremors, loss of coordination, unusual bleeding or bruising, visual disturbances, irregular heartbeat.

❒ terpin hydrate

(ter' pin)

Pregnancy Category C

Drug classes
Antitussive
Expectorant

Therapeutic actions
Directly stimulates the respiratory tract secretory glands, increasing the production of respiratory fluids; used mainly as an ingredient in cough medications.

Indications
- Symptomatic relief of dry, nonproductive cough

Contraindications/cautions
- Contraindicated in the presence of diabetes, peptic ulcer, pregnancy, lactation.
- Use caution in the presence of history of alcohol dependence.

Dosage
Adult: 85–170 mg PO tid–qid.
Pediatric
- *1–4 y:* 20 mg PO tid–qid.
- *5–9 y:* 40 mg PO tid–qid.
- *10–12 y:* 85 mg PO tid–qid.

Pharmacokinetics
Not reported.

Adverse effects
- **CNS:** *Drowsiness, dizziness*
- **GI:** Nausea, vomiting, abdominal pain

■ Nursing Considerations

Assessment
- *History:* Diabetes, peptic ulcer, alcohol abuse, pregnancy, lactation
- *Physical:* R, adventitious sounds; abdominal exam

Implementation
- Administer with food if severe GI upset occurs.
- Do not give patient water after administration to make the most of soothing effects.

Adverse effects in *Italics* are most common; those in **Bold** are life-threatening.

- Ensure that patient is well hydrated during treatment; humidifier may be helpful in increasing bronchial secretions.

Drug-specific teaching points
- Take this drug with food if severe GI upset occurs.
- Do not exceed recommended dose.
- Know that the following side effects may occur: drowsiness, dizziness (do not drive a car or operate dangerous machinery if these occur).
- Drink plenty of fluids, and consider the use of a humidifier to help facilitate relief of bronchial irritation.
- Report vomiting, worsening of condition being treated, abdominal pain.

testolactone

*(tess toe **lak**' tone)*
Teslac

Pregnancy Category C

Drug classes
Androgen
Hormonal agent
Antineoplastic agent

Therapeutic actions
Synthetic androgen; endogenous androgens are responsible for growth and development of male sex organs and the maintenance of secondary sex characteristics; administration of androgen derivatives increases the retention of nitrogen, sodium, potassium, phosphorus, and decreases urinary excretion of calcium; increases protein anabolism and decreases protein catabolism; stimulates the production of red blood cells; exact mechanism by which antineoplastic effects are exerted is not known.

Indications
- Palliative treatment of advanced disseminated metastatic breast carcinoma in postmenopausal women when hormonal therapy is indicated
- Disseminated breast carcinoma in premenopausal women in whom ovarian function has been subsequently terminated

Contraindications/cautions
- Contraindicated in the presence of known sensitivity to androgens, pregnancy, lactation, carcinoma of the breast in males.
- Use caution in the presence of liver disease, cardiac disease, nephritis, nephrosis.

Dosage
Adult: 250 mg PO qid. Continue therapy for a minimum of 3 mo unless there is active disease progression.
Pediatric: Safety and efficacy not established.

Pharmacokinetics

Route	Onset
Oral	Rapid

Metabolism: Hepatic, $T_{1/2}$: unknown
Distribution: Crosses placenta; enters breast milk
Excretion: Urine

Adverse effects
- **CNS:** *Paresthesias*
- **GI:** *Nausea, vomiting, anorexia, glossitis,* diarrhea, loss appetite, swelling of the tongue
- **CV:** Hypertension
- **Hematologic:** Hypercalcemia
- **Dermatologic:** Rash, dermatitis, aches of the extremities, edema
- **Virilization:** Hirsutism, hoarseness, deepening of the voice, clitoral enlargement, facial hair growth, affected libido

■ Nursing Considerations

Assessment
- *History:* Known sensitivity to androgens, liver or cardiac disease, nephritis, nephrosis, carcinoma of the breast, pregnancy, lactation
- *Physical:* Skin—color, lesions, texture; hair distribution pattern; P, auscultation; abdominal exam, liver evaluation, mu-

Adverse effects in *Italics* are most common; those in **Bold** are life-threatening.

cous membranes; serum electrolytes, liver and renal function tests

Implementation
- Monitor tumor progression through periodic exams.
- Monitor patient for occurrence of edema; arrange for appropriate diuretic therapy as needed.
- Arrange for periodic monitoring of urine and serum calcium during treatment of disseminated breast carcinoma, and arrange for appropriate treatment or discontinuation of the drug if hypercalcemia occurs.

Drug-specific teaching points
- Be aware that this drug will need to be taken for long term to evaluate effects.
- Know that the following side effects may occur: body hair growth, baldness, deepening of the voice, loss of appetite, edema or swelling, redness of the tongue.
- Be aware that this drug is not intended to be taken during pregnancy; serious fetal effects can occur. Contraceptive measures should be used during drug treatment.
- Report numbness or tingling of the fingers, toes, face; significant swelling; severe GI upset.

☐ testosterone (short-acting)

(tess toss' ter one)

Andro-cyp 100, Andronaq, Histerone, Testamone, Testoject-50

Transdermal patch: Testoderm

testosterone cypionate (long-acting)

Andro-Cyp, Andronate, Andronaq LA, dep Andro, Depotest, Depo-Testosterone, Duratest-100, Testa-C, Testoject-LA

testosterone enanthate (long-acting)

Andro L.A., Andropository, Andryl 200, Delatest, Delatestryl, Durathate-200, Everone, Testone LA, Testrin PA

testosterone propionate (short-acting)

Testex

Pregnancy Category X

Drug classes
Androgen
Hormonal agent

Therapeutic actions
Primary natural androgen; responsible for growth and development of male sex organs and the maintenance of secondary sex characteristics; administration of exogenous testosterone increases the retention of nitrogen, sodium, potassium, phosphorus; decreases urinary excretion of calcium; increases protein anabolism and decreases protein catabolism; stimulates the production of red blood cells.

Indications
- Replacement therapy in hypogonadism—primary hypogonadism, hypogonadotropic hypogonadism, delayed puberty (men)
- Metastatic cancer, breast cancer in women who are 1–5 y postmenopausal
- Postpartum breast pain/engorgement

Contraindications/cautions
- Contraindicated in the presence of known sensitivity to androgens, prostate or breast cancer in males, pregnancy, lactation.
- Use caution in the presence of MI, liver disease.

Dosage
Eunuchoidism, eunuchism, postpubertal cryptorchidism for male climacteric symptoms, impotence due to androgen deficiency: 25–50 mg IM two to three times per week (testosterone, testosterone propionate).
Postpartum breast pain/engorgement: 25–50 mg/d IM for 3–4 d (testosterone propionate).

Carcinoma of the breast: 50–100 mg IM three times per week (testosterone, testosterone propionate).
Male hypogonadism (replacement therapy): 50–400 mg IM every 2–4 wk (testosterone enanthate, cypionate).
Males with delayed puberty: 50–200 mg IM every 2–4 wk for a limited duration (testosterone enanthate, cypionate).
Primary hypogonadism, hypogonadotropic hypogonadism in males: Testosterone patch, 4–6 mg/d applied to scrotal skin.
Palliation of mammary cancer in women: 200–400 mg IM every 2–4 wk (testosterone enanthate, cypionate).

Pharmacokinetics

Route	Onset	Duration
IM	Slow	1–3 d
IM cypionate	Slow	2–4 wk
IM enanthate	Slow	2–4 wk
IM propionate	Slow	1–3 d
Dermal	Rapid	24 h

Metabolism: Hepatic, $T_{1/2}$: 10–100 min; up to 8 d cypionate
Distribution: Crosses placenta; enters breast milk
Excretion: Urine and feces

Adverse effects
- CNS: *Dizziness, headache, sleep disorders, fatigue,* tremor, sleeplessness, generalized paresthesia, sleep apnea syndrome, CNS hemorrhage
- GI: *Nausea,* hepatic dysfunction; **hepatocellular carcinoma**
- Hematologic: *Polycythemia, leukopenia,* hypercalcemia, altered serum cholesterol levels, retention of sodium, chloride, water, potassium, phosphates and calcium
- GU: Fluid retention, decreased urinary output
- Dermatologic: *Rash*, dermatitis, anaplylactoid reactions
- Endocrine: *Androgenic effects* (acne, edema, mild hirsutism, decrease in breast size, deepening of the voice, oily skin or hair, weight gain, clitoral hypertrophy or testicular atrophy), *hypoestrogenic effects* (flushing, sweating, vaginitis, nervousness, emotional lability)
- Other: Chills, premature closure of the epiphyses

Drug-lab test interferences
- Altered glucose tolerance tests • Decrease in thyroid function tests, which may persist for 2–3 wk after therapy • Increased creatinine, creatinine clearance, which may last for 2 wk after therapy

■ Nursing Considerations

Assessment
- *History:* Known sensitivity to androgens, prostate or breast cancer in males, MI, liver disease, pregnancy, lactation
- *Physical:* Skin—color, lesions, texture; hair distribution pattern; injection site; affect, orientation, peripheral sensation; abdominal exam, liver evaluation; serum electrolytes, serum cholesterol levels, liver function tests, glucose tolerance tests, thyroid function tests, long-bone x-ray (in children)

Implementation
- Apply dermal patch to clean, dry scrotal skin that has been dry shaved. Do not apply elsewhere, and do not use chemical depilatories.
- Inject testosterone deeply into gluteal muscle.
- Shake vials well before use; crystals will redissolve.
- Do not administer frequently; these drugs are absorbed slowly; testosterone enanthate and cypionate are long acting and provide therapeutic effects for about 4 wk.
- Monitor effect on children with long-bone x-rays every 3–6 mo during therapy; discontinue drug well before the bone age reaches the norm for the patient's chronologic age.
- Monitor patient for occurrence of edema; arrange for appropriate diuretic therapy as needed.

Adverse effects in *Italics* are most common; those in **Bold** are life-threatening.

- Arrange to monitor liver function, serum electrolytes periodically during therapy, and consult with physician for appropriate corrective measures as needed.
- Arrange to periodically measure cholesterol levels in patients who are at high risk for coronary artery disease.
- Monitor diabetic patients closely because glucose tolerance may change; adjustments may be needed in insulin, oral hypoglycemic dosage, and diet.
- Arrange for periodic monitoring of urine and serum calcium during treatment of disseminated breast carcinoma, and arrange for appropriate treatment or discontinuation of the drug.
- Monitor geriatric males for prostatic hypertrophy and carcinoma.
- Discontinue drug, and arrange for appropriate consultation if abnormal vaginal bleeding occurs.

Drug-specific teaching points
- Be aware that this drug can only be given IM. Mark calendar indicating days to come for injection. Patient receiving the dermal patch must apply the patch to dry, clean scrotal skin that has been dry shaved; do not use chemical depilatories.
- Know that the following side effects may occur: body hair growth, baldness, deepening of the voice, loss of libido, impotence (most of these effects will be reversible when the drug is stopped); excitation, confusion, insomnia (avoid driving, performing tasks that require alertness if these effects occur); swelling of the ankles, fingers (medication may be ordered to help).
- Be aware that this drug can not be taken during pregnancy; serious fetal effects could occur. Women: use contraceptive measures when taking this drug.
- Diabetic patients: Monitor urine sugar closely because glucose tolerance may change; report any abnormalities to prescriber, so corrective action can be taken.
- Report ankle swelling; nausea; vomiting; yellowing of skin or eyes; unusual bleeding or bruising; penile swelling or pain; hoarseness, body hair growth, deepening of the voice, acne, menstrual irregularities, pregnancy (women).

❒ tetracycline hydrochloride

(tet ra sye' kleen)

Achromycin Ophthalmic, Achromycin V, Cefracycline (CAN), Medicycline (CAN), Neo-Tetrine (CAN), Nor-Tet, Novotetra (CAN), Panmycin, Robitet, Sumycin, Tetracap, Tetralan, Tetralean (CAN), Tetram, Topicycline

Pregnancy Category D

Drug classes
Antibiotic
Tetracycline

Therapeutic actions
Bacteriostatic: inhibits protein synthesis of susceptible bacteria, preventing cell replication.

Indications
Systemic Administration
- Infections caused by rickettsiae; *Mycoplasma pneumoniae;* agents of psittacosis, ornithosis, lymphogranuloma venereum and granuloma inguinale; *Borrelia recurrentis, Haemophilus ducreyi, Pasteurella pestis, Pasteurella tularensis, Bartonella bacilliformis, Bacteroides, Vibrio comma, Vibrio fetus, Brucella, Escherichia coli, Enterobacter aerogenes, Shigella, Acinetobacter calcoaceticus, Haemophilus influenzae, Klebsiella, Diplococcus pneumoniae, Staphylococcus aureus*
- When penicillin is contraindicated, infections caused by *Neisseria gonorrhoeae, Treponema pallidum, Treponema pertenue, Listeria monocytogenes, Clostridium, Bacillus anthracis, Fusobacterium fusiforme, Actinomyces, Neisseria meningitidis*
- Adjunct to amebicides in acute intestinal amebiasis
- Treatment of acne (oral)

tetracycline hydrochloride ■ 1053

- Uncomplicated urethral, endocervical or rectal infections in adults caused by *Chlamydia trachomatis*
- Instilled in a chest tube, unlabeled use: pleural sclerosing agent in malignant pleural effusions

Ophthalmic Administration
- Treatment of superficial ocular infections due to susceptible strains of microorganisms (ophthalmic preparations)
- Prophylaxis of ophthalmia neonatorum due to *N. gonorrrhoeae* or *C. trachomatis* (ophthalmic preparations)

Topical Administration
- Treatment of acne vulgaris (topical dermatologic solution)
- Treatment and prophylaxis of minor skin infections due to susceptible organisms (topical dermatologic ointment)

Contraindications/cautions
- Systemic administration and dermatologic solution: Contraindicated in the presence of allergy to any of the tetracyclines; allergy to tartrazine (in 250-mg tetracycline capsules marketed under brand name *Panmycin*); pregnancy (toxic to the fetus); lactation (causes damage to the teeth of infant).
- Use caution in the presence of hepatic or renal dysfunction.
- Ophthalmic preparations: Contraindicated in the presence of ocular viral, mycobacterial or fungal infections.

Dosage
Systemic administration
- ***Adult:*** 1–2 g/d PO in two to four equal doses. Up to 500 mg PO qid.
- *Brucellosis:* 500 mg PO qid for 3 wk with 1 g streptomycin bid IM the first week and qd the second wk.
- *Syphilis:* 30–40 g PO in divided doses over 10–15 d.
- *Uncomplicated gonorrhea:* 1.5 g initially, then 500 mg q6h PO to a total of 9 g.
- *Gonococcal urethritis:* 1.5 g PO initially, then 500 mg q4–6h for 4–6 d.
- *Severe acne:* 1 g/d PO in divided doses; then 125–500 mg/d.

- ***Pediatric***
- *Older than 8 y:* 25–50 mg/kg per day PO in four equal doses.

Ophthalmic suspension
- *Acute infections:* 1–2 drops in the affected eye q15–30 min, then decrease frequency as infection resolves.
- *Moderate infections:* 1–2 drops two to six times daily.
- *Acute and chronic trachoma:* 2 drops in each eye bid or qid, continuing for 1–2 mo or longer, with oral tetracycline.

Ophthalmic ointment: ½-in ribbon bid–qid, depending on severity of infection.
Topical dermatologic solution: Apply generously to affected areas bid.
Topical dermatologic ointment: Apply to infected area one to five times daily.

Pharmacokinetics

Route	Onset	Peak
Oral	Varies	2–4 h

Topical, ophthalmic; not generally absorbed systemically

Metabolism: $T_{1/2}$: 6–12 h
Distribution: Crosses placenta; enters breast milk
Excretion: Urine

Adverse effects
Systemic Administration
- **GI:** *Discoloring and inadequate calcification of primary teeth of fetus if used by pregnant women, discoloring and inadequate calcification of permanent teeth if used during period of dental development,* fatty liver, liver failure, *anorexia, nausea, vomiting, diarrhea, glossitis, dysphagia,* enterocolitis, esophageal ulcers
- **Hematologic:** Hemolytic anemia, thrombocytopenia, neutropenia, eosinophilia, leukocytosis, leukopenia
- **Dermatologic:** *Phototoxic reactions, rash,* exfoliative dermatitis
- **Hypersensitivity:** Reactions from urticaria to anaphylaxis, including intracranial hypertension

Adverse effects in *Italics* are most common; those in **Bold** are life-threatening.

- **Other:** *Superinfections*, local irritation at parenteral injection sites

Ophthalmic Preparations

- **Local:** *Transient irritation, stinging, itching*, angioneurotic edema, urticaria, dermatitis, superinfections

Topical Dermatologic Solutions

- **Local:** *Stinging, burning during application; skin irritation*; dermatitis; yellowing of areas of application

Clinically important drug-drug interactions

- Decreased absorption of tetracycline if used with calcium salts, magnesium salts, zinc salts, aluminum salts, bismuth salts, iron, urinary alkalinizers, food, dairy products, charcoal • Increased digoxin toxicity if taken with tetracyclines • Increased nephrotoxicity if taken with methoxyflurane • Decreased effectiveness of oral contraceptives, though rare, has been reported with a risk of breakthrough bleeding or pregnancy if taken with tetracyclines • Decreased activity of penicillins if taken with tetracyclines

■ Nursing Considerations

Assessment

- *History:* Systemic administration and dermatologic solution: allergy to any of the tetracyclines, tartrazine; hepatic or renal dysfunction, pregnancy, lactation. Ophthalmic preparations: ocular viral, mycobacterial, or fungal infections
- *Physical:* Systemic administration, topical dermatologic solution: site of infection, skin—color, lesions; R, adventitious sounds; bowel sounds, output, liver evaluation; urinalysis, BUN, liver and renal function tests. Ophthalmic preparations, dermatologic ointment: site of infection

Implementation

- Administer oral medication on an empty stomach, 1 h before or 2–3 h after meals. Do not give with antacids. If antacids must be used, give them 3 h after the dose of tetracycline.
- Culture infected area before beginning drug therapy.
- Do not use outdated drugs; degraded drug is highly nephrotoxic and should not be used.
- Do not give oral drug with meals, antacids, or food.
- Arrange for regular renal function tests if long-term therapy is used.
- Use topical preparations of this drug only when clearly indicated. Sensitization from the topical use of this drug may preclude its later use in serious infections. Topical preparations containing antibiotics that are not ordinarily given systemically are preferable.

Drug-specific teaching points

Oral Preparations

- Take the drug throughout the day for best results. The drug should be taken on an empty stomach, 1 h before or 2–3 h after meals, with a full glass of water. Do not take the drug with food, dairy products, iron preparations, or antacids.
- Finish your complete prescription; if any is left, discard it immediately. Never take an outdated tetracycline product.
- Be aware that there have been reports of pregnancy occurring when taking tetracycline with oral contraceptives. To be absolutely confident of avoiding pregnancy, the use of an additional type of contraceptive is advised while on this drug.
- Know that the following side effects may occur: stomach upset, nausea (this will pass when the drug therapy is finished); superinfections in the mouth, vagina (frequent washing may help this problem; if it becomes severe, medication may be available to help); sensitivity of the skin to sunlight (use protective clothing and a sunscreen when exposed to the sun).
- Report severe cramps, watery diarrhea, rash or itching, difficulty breathing, dark urine or light-colored stools, yellowing of the skin or eyes.

tetrahydrozoline hydrochloride ■ 1055

Ophthalmic Preparations
- Administer eye drops as follows: lie down or tilt head backward, and look at the ceiling. Drop suspension inside lower eyelid while looking up. Close eye and apply gentle pressure to inner corner of the eye for 1 min.
- Apply ointment inside lower eyelid; close eyes and roll eyeball in all directions.
- Be aware that this drug may cause temporary blurring of vision or stinging after application.
- Take the full course of therapy prescribed; discard any leftover medication immediately.

Topical Dermatologic Solution
- Apply generously until skin is wet.
- Avoid the eyes, nose, and mouth.
- Be aware that you may experience transient stinging or burning; this will subside quickly; skin in the treated area may become yellow; this will wash off.
- Know that you may use cosmetics as you usually do.

Topical Dermatologic Ointment
- Wash area before applying (unless contraindicated); this drug may stain clothing.
- Report worsening of condition, rash, irritation.

❒ tetrahydrozoline hydrochloride

*(tet rah hi **draz'** oh leen)*
Tyzine, Tyzine Pediatric

OTC ophthalmic preparation: Collyrium Fresh Eye Drops, Eyesine, Mallazine Eye Drops, Murine, Optigene 3, Tetrasine, Visine, Collyrium Fresh Eye Drops

Pregnancy Category C

Drug classes
Nasal decongestant
Ophthlamic vasoconstrictor/mydriatic

Therapeutic actions
Acts directly on alpha receptors to produce vasoconstriction of arterioles in nasal passages, which produces a decongestant response; no effect on beta receptors; dilates pupils; increases flow of aqueous humor, vasoconstricts in eyes.

Indications
- Symptomatic relief of nasal and nasopharyngeal mucosal congestion due to the common cold, hay fever, or other respiratory allergies (topical)
- Relief of redness of eyes due to minor irritations (ophthalmic)
- Temporary relief of burning and irritation due to dryness of the eye or discomfort due to minor irritations or to exposure to wind or sun (ophthalmic)

Contraindications/cautions
- Contraindicated in the presence of allergy to tetrahyrozolozine, angle-closure glaucoma, anesthesia with cyclopropane or halothane, thyrotoxicosis, diabetes, hypertension, cardiovascular disorders, women in labor whose BP > 130/80.
- Use caution in the presence of angina, arrhythmias, prostatic hypertrophy, unstable vasomotor syndrome, lactation.

Dosage
Adult
- ***Nasal:*** 2–4 drops of 0.1% solution in each nostril three to four times a day; 3–4 sprays in each nostril q4h as needed.
- ***Opthalmic:*** Instill 1–2 drops into eye(s) up to four times a day.

Pediatric
- ***Nasal***
– *Older than 6 y:* Adult dosage.
– *2–6 y:* 2–3 drops of 0.05% solution in each nostril q4–6h as needed.
- ***Ophthalmic:*** Safety and efficacy not established.

Pharmacokinetics

Route	Onset	Duration
Nasal	5–10 min	6–10 h

Ophthalmic; not generally absorbed systemically.

Metabolism: Hepatic, $T_{1/2}$: unknown
Distribution: Crosses placenta; may enter breast milk
Excretion: Urine

Adverse effects
- CNS: *Fear, anxiety, tenseness, restlessness, headache, lightheadedness, dizziness,* drowsiness, tremor, insomnia, hallucinations, psychological disturbances, convulsions, CNS depression, weakness, blurred vision, ocular irritation, tearing, photophobia, symptoms of paranoid schizophrenia
- GI: *Nausea,* vomiting, anorexia
- CV: Arrhythmias, hypertension resulting in intracranial hemorrhage, cardiovascular collapse with hypotension, palpitations, tachycardia, precordial pain in patients with ischemic heart disease
- GU: Constriction of renal blood vessels, *dysuria, vesical sphincter spasm,* resulting in difficult and painful urination, urinary retention in males with prostatism
- Local: *Rebound congestion* with topical nasal application
- Other: *Pallor,* respiratory difficulty, orofacial dystonia, sweating

Clinically important drug-drug interactions
- Severe hypertension when taken with monoamine oxidase inhibitors (MAOI), tricyclic antidepressants, furazolidone • Additive effects and increased risk of toxicity if taken with urinary alkalinizers • Decreased vasopressor response if taken with reserpine, methyldopa, urinary acidifiers • Decreased hypotensive action of guanethidine if taken concurrently

■ Nursing Considerations

Assessment
- *History:* Allergy to tetrahydrozoline; angle-closure glaucoma; anesthesia with cyclopropane or halothane; thyrotoxicosis, diabetes, hypertension, cardiovascular disorders; prostatic hypertrophy, unstable vasomotor syndrome; lactation
- *Physical:* Skin—color, temperature; orientation, reflexes, peripheral sensation, vision; P, BP, auscultation, peripheral perfusion; R, adventitious sounds; urinary output pattern, bladder percussion, prostate palpation; nasal mucous membrance evaluation

Implementation
- Do not administer ophthalmic solution if it is cloudy or changes color.
- Monitor cardiovascular effects carefully; patients with hypertension who take this drug may experience changes in blood pressure because of the additional vasoconstriction. If a nasal decongestant is needed, pseudoephedrine is the drug of choice.

Drug-specific teaching points
- Do not exceed recommended dose. Demonstrate proper administration technique for topical nasal application and administration of eye drops. Avoid prolonged use because underlying medical problems can be disguised.
- Know that the following side effects may occur: dizziness, weakness, restlessness, lightheadedness, tremor (avoid driving or operating dangerous equipment when these effects occur); urinary retention (emptying the bladder before taking the drug may help).
- Be aware that a rebound congestion may occur when this drug is stopped; drink plenty of fluids, use a humidifier, avoid smoke-filled areas to help decrease problems.
- Report nervousness, palpitations, sleeplessness, sweating.

▢ theophylline

*(thee **off** i lin)*

Immediate-release capsules, tablets: **Bronkodyl, Elixophyllin, Quibron-T Dividose, Slo-Phyllin, Theolair**

Timed-release capsules: **Aerolate, Elixophyllin SR, Slo-bid Gyrocaps, Slo-Phyllin Gyrocaps, Theo-24, Theobid, Theoclear L.A., Theo-Dur Sprinkle, Theospan-SR, Theovent Long-Acting**

Adverse effects in *Italics* are most common; those in **Bold** are life-threatening.

Timed-release tablets:
Constant-T, Quibron-T/SR Dividose, Respbid, Theochron, Theo-Dur, Theolair-SR, Uniphyl

Liquids: Accurbron, Aerolate, Aquaphyllin, Asmalix, Elixomin, Elixophyllin, Lanophyllin, Slo-Phyllin, Theoclear-80, Theolair, Theostat 80

theophylline sodium glycinate

Elixir: Acet-Amp (CAN)

Pregnancy Category C

Drug classes
Bronchodilator
Xanthine

Therapeutic actions
Relaxes bronchial smooth muscle, causing bronchodilation and increasing vital capacity that has been impaired by bronchospasm and air trapping; actions may be mediated by inhibition of phosphodiesterase, which increases the concentration of cyclic adenosine monophosphate; in concentrations that may be higher than those reached clinically, it also inhibits the release of slow-reacting substance of anaphylaxis and histamine.

Indications
- Symptomatic relief or prevention of bronchial asthma and reversible bronchospasm associated with chronic bronchitis and emphysema
- Unlabeled use of 2 mg/kg per day to maintain serum concentrations between 3 and 5 μg/ml: treatment of apnea and bradycardia of prematurity

Contraindications/cautions
- Contraindicated in the presence of hypersensitivity to any xanthines, peptic ulcer, active gastritis, status asthmaticus, pregnancy (tachycardia, jitteriness, and withdrawal apnea have been observed in neonates whose mothers received xanthines up until delivery).
- Use caution in the presence of cardiac arrhythmias, acute myocardial injury, CHF, cor pulmonale, severe hypertension, severe hypoxemia, renal or hepatic disease, hyperthyroidism, alcoholism, labor (may inhibit uterine contractions), lactation.

Dosage
Maintain serum levels in the therapeutic range of 10–20 μg/ml; base dosage on lean body mass.

Adult
- *Theophylline*
- *Acute symptoms requiring rapid theophyllinization in patients not receiving theophylline:* An initial loading dose is required, as indicated below:

Patient Group	Oral Loading	Followed by	Maintenance
Young adult smokers	6 mg/kg	3 mg/kg q4h × 3 doses	3 mg/kg q6h
Non-smoking adults, otherwise healthy	6 mg/kg	3 mg/kg q6h × 2 doses	3 mg/kg q8h

- *Acute symptoms requiring rapid theophyllinization in patients receiving theophylline:* A loading dose is required; each 0.5 mg/kg PO administered as a loading dose will result in about a 1 μg/ml increase in serum theophylline. Ideally, defer loading dose until serum theophylline determination is made. Otherwise, base loading dose on clinical judgment and the knowledge that 2.5 mg/kg of a rapidly absorbed preparation will increase serum theophylline levels by about 5 μg/ml and is unlikely to cause dangerous adverse effects if the patient is not experiencing theophylline toxicity before this dose; maintenance doses are as above.
- *Chronic therapy:* Initial dose of 16 mg/kg per 24 h PO or 400 mg/24 h, whichever is less, in divided doses q6–8h for immediate-release preparations or liquids, q8–12 or 24h for timed-release

preparations (consult manufacturer's recommendations for specific dosage interval). Increase dosage based on serum theophylline levels, or if these are unavailable, increase in 25%-increments at 2- to 3-d intervals as long as drug is tolerated or until maximum dose of 13 mg/kg per day or 900 mg, whichever is less, is reached.

Dosage adjustment based on serum theophylline levels during chronic therapy

Serum Theophylline	Directions
Too low	5–7.5 µg/ml: Increase dose by about 25%, recheck serum level; may need to increase dose again.
	7.5–10 µg/ml: Increase dose by 25%; may need to give total daily dose at more frequent intervals; recheck level at 6 to 12 mo intervals.
Within normal limits	10–20 µg/ml: Maintain dosage; recheck level at 6 to 12 mo intervals.
Too high	20–25 µg/ml: Decrease doses by about 10%; recheck level at 6 to 12 mo intervals.
	25–30 µg/ml: Skip next dose, and decrease subsequent doses by about 25%; recheck serum levels.
	Over 30 µg/ml: Skip next two doses, and decrease subsequent doses by 50%; recheck serum level.

- Measure serum theophylline in blood sample drawn 1–2 h after administration of immediate-release preparations, 4 h after administration of most sustained-release products.
- *Rectal:* 500 mg q6–8h by rectal suppository or retention enema.
- **Theophylline sodium glycinate (44.5%–47.3% theophylline):** 330–660 mg PO q6–8h after meals.

Pediatric: Use in children younger than 6 mo not recommended. Use of timed-release products in children younger than 6 y not recommended.

- **Theophylline**
- *Acute symptoms requiring rapid theophyllinization in patients not receiving theophylline:* An initial loading dose is required, as follows:

Patient Group	Oral Loading	Followed by	Maintenance
6 mo–9 y	6 mg/kg	4 mg/kg q4h × 3 doses	4 mg/kg q6h
9–16 y	6 mg/kg	3 mg/kg q4h × 3 doses	3 mg/kg q3h

- *Infants preterm to younger than 6 mo:* Initial and maintenance doses need to be reduced because elimination of theophylline appears to be delayed in these patients:

Infant	Loading Dose	Maintenance Dose
Preterm (≤40 wk postconception)	1 mg/kg for each 2 µg/ml serum concentration desired	1 mg/kg q12h
Term (birth or 40 wk postconception)		
Up to 4 wk postnatal		1–2 mg/kg q12h
4–8 wk		1–2 mg/kg q8h
> 8 wk		1–3 mg/kg q6h

- *Chronic therapy:* Initial dose of 16 mg/kg per 24 h PO or 400 mg/24 h, whichever is less, in divided doses q6–8h for immediate-release preparations or liquids, q8–12 or 24h for timed-release preparations in children younger than 6 y (consult manufacturer's recommendations for specific dosage interval). Increase dosage based on serum theophylline levels, or if these are unavailable, increase in 25%-increments at 2- to 3-d intervals as long as drug is tolerated or until maximum dose given below is reached:

Age	Maximum Daily Dose
Younger than 9 y	24 mg/kg/day
9–12 y	20 mg/kg/day
12–16 y	18 mg/kg/day
Older than 16 y	13 mg/kg/day

theophylline ■ 1059

- ***Theophylline sodium glycinate***
  - *6–12 y:* 220–330 mg q6–8h PO after meals.
  - *3–6 y:* 110–165 mg q6–8h PO after meals.
  - *1–3 y:* 55–110 mg q6–8h PO after meals.

Geriatric or impaired adult: Use caution, especially in elderly men, and in patients with cor pulmonale, CHF.

- *Acute symptoms requiring rapid theophyllinization in patients not receiving theophylline:* An initial loading dose is required, as follows:

Patient Group	Oral Loading	Followed by	Maintenance
Older patients and patients with cor pulmonale	6 mg/kg	2 mg/kg q6h for two doses	2 mg/kg q8h
Patients with CHF	6 mg/kg	2 mg/kg q8h for two doses	1–2 mg/kg q12h

Pharmacokinetics

Route	Onset	Peak
Oral	Varies	2 h

Metabolism: Hepatic, $T_{1/2}$: 3–15 h (nonsmoker) or 4–5 h (smokers)
Distribution: Crosses placenta; may enter breast milk
Excretion: Urine

Adverse effects

- **Serum theophylline levels < 20 μg/ml:** Adverse effects uncommon.
- **Serum theophylline levels > 20–25 μg/ml:** *Nausea, vomiting, diarrhea, headache, insomnia, irritability* (75% of patients)
- **Serum theophylline levels > 30–35 μg/ml:** Hyperglycemia, hypotension, cardiac arrhythmias, tachycardia (> 10 μg/ml in premature newborns); **seizures, brain damage, death**
- CNS: *Irritability (especially children); restlessness,* dizziness, muscle twitching, convulsions, severe depression, stammering speech; abnormal behavior characterized by withdrawal, mutism and unresponsiveness alternating with hyperactive periods
- GI: *Loss of appetite*, hematemesis, epigastric pain, gastroesophageal reflux during sleep
- CV: Palpitations, sinus tachycardia, ventricular tachycardia, **life-threatening ventricular arrhythmias, circulatory failure**
- Respiratory: Tachypnea, **respiratory arrest**
- GU: Proteinuria, increased excretion of renal tubular cells and RBCs; diuresis (dehydration), urinary retention in men with prostate enlargement
- Other: Fever, flushing, hyperglycemia, SIADH, rash, increased SGOT

Clinically important drug-drug interactions

- Increased effects and toxicity when given with cimetidine, erythromycin, troleandomycin, ciprofloxacin, norfloxacin, enoxacin, ofloxacin, oral contraceptives, ticlopidine, ranitidine • Possibly increased effects when given with rifampin • Increased serum levels and risk of toxicity in hypothyroid patients, decreased levels in patients who are hyperthyroid; monitor patients on thioamines, thyroid hormones for changes in serum levels as patients becomes euthyroid • Increased cardiac toxicity when given with halothane • Decreased effects in patients who are cigarette smokers (1–2 packs/day); theophylline dosage may need to be increased 50%–100% • Decreased effects when given with barbiturates, charcoal • Decreased effects of phenytoins, benzodiazepines, and theophylline preparations when given concomitantly • Decreased effects of nondepolarizing neuromuscular blockers given concurrently • Mutually antagonistic effects of beta-blockers and theophylline preparations.

Adverse effects in *Italics* are most common; those in **Bold** are life-threatening.

Clinically important drug-food interactions
- Theophylline elimination is increased by a low-carbohydrate, high-protein diet and by charcoal broiled beef • Theophylline elimination is decreased by a high-carbohydrate, low-protein diet • Food may alter bioavailability, absorption of timed-release theophylline preparations; these may rapidly release their contents in the presence of food and cause toxicity. Timed-release forms should be taken on an empty stomach.

Drug-lab test interferences
- Interference with spectrophotometric determinations of serum theophylline levels by furosemide, phenylbutazone, probenecid, theobromine; coffee, tea, cola beverages, chocolate, acetaminophen cause falsely high values • Alteration in assays of uric acid, urinary catecholamines, plasma free fatty acids

■ Nursing Considerations

Assessment
- *History:* Hypersensitivity to any xanthines, peptic ulcer, active gastritis, status asthmaticus, cardiac arrhythmias, acute myocardial injury, CHF, cor pulmonale, severe hypertension, severe hypoxemia, renal or hepatic disease, hyperthyroidism, pregnancy, lactation
- *Physical:* Skin—color, texture, lesions; reflexes, bilateral grip strength, affect; P, auscultation, BP, perfusion; R, adventious sounds; bowel sounds, normal output; frequency, voiding pattern, normal urinary output; ECG; EEG; thyroid, liver, kidney function tests

Implementation
- Caution patient not to chew or crush enteric-coated timed-release preparations.
- Give immediate release, liquid dosage forms with food if GI effects occur.
- Do not give timed-release preparations with food; these should be given on an empty stomach, 1 h before or 2 h after meals.
- Monitor results of serum theophylline level determinations carefully, and arrange for reduced dosage if serum levels exceed therapeutic range of 10–20 μg/ml.
- Monitor patient carefully for clinical signs of adverse effects, particularly if serum theophylline levels are not available.
- Maintain diazepam on standby to treat seizures.

Drug-specific teaching points
- Take this drug exactly as prescribed. If a timed-release product is prescribed, you should take this drug on an empty stomach, 1 h before or 2 h after meals. Do not chew or crush timed-release preparations; it may be necessary for you to take this drug around the clock for adequate control of asthma attacks.
- Avoid excessive intake of coffee, tea, cocoa, cola beverages, chocolate. These contain substances related to theophylline that may increase the side effects you experience.
- Be aware that smoking cigarettes or other tobacco products may markedly influence the effects of theophylline. It is preferable not to smoke while you are taking this drug. Notify your nurse or physician if you change your smoking habits while you are taking this drug; it may be necessary to change your drug dosage.
- Arrange to have frequent blood tests to monitor the effect of this drug and ensure safe and effective dosage.
- Know that the following side effects may occur: nausea, loss of appetite (taking this drug with food may help; applies only to immediate-release or liquid dosage forms); difficulty sleeping, depression, emotional lability (it may be reassuring to know that these are drug effects).
- Report nausea, vomiting, severe GI pain, restlessness, convulsions, irregular heartbeat.

❐ thiabendazole

*(thye a **ben**' da zole)*
Mintezol

Pregnancy Category C

thiabendazole ■ 1061

Drug classes
Anthelmintic

Therapeutic actions
Suppresses egg or larva production of helminths and may inhibit the subsequent development of eggs and larvae that are passed in the feces; inhibits a helminth-specific enzyme.

Indications
- Treatment of strongyloidiasis (threadworm infection), cutaneous larva migrans (creeping eruption), and visceral larva migrans. Not a primary therapy, but no additional agent is usually needed if patient is infected with enterobiasis (pinworm infection) while being treated for one of the above.
- When more specific therapy cannot be used or when a second agent is desirable, for the treatment of ascariasis (roundworm infection), uncinariasis (hookworm infection), trichuriasis (whipworm infection)
- Alleviation of symptoms of invasive trichinosis

Contraindications/cautions
- Contraindicated in the presence of allergy to thiabendazole, pregnancy.
- Use caution in the presence of renal or hepatic dysfunction, anemia, malnourishment or dehydration.

Dosage
Adult and pediatric (> 30 lb)
- **< 150 lb:** 10 mg/lb per dose PO.
- **> 150 lb:** 1.5 g/dose PO. Maximum daily dose is 3 g. Clinical experience in children weighing < 30 lb is limited.

Indication	Regimen
Enterobiasis	two doses/d for 1 d, repeat in 7 d to reduce risk of reinfection (or 2 doses/d for 2 successive d)
Strongyloidiasis Ascariasis Uncinariasis Trichuriasis	two doses per day for 2 successive d (or one single dose of 20 mg/lb)
Cutaneous larva migrans	two doses/d for 2 successive d (repeat treatment if

Indication	Regimen (cont'd)
	lesions still present 2 d after therapy)
Trichinosis	two doses/d for 2–4 successive d as needed

Pharmacokinetics

Route	Onset	Peak
Oral	Rapid	1–2 h

Metabolism: Hepatic, $T_{1/2}$: unknown
Distribution: Crosses placenta; may enter breast milk
Excretion: Urine

Adverse effects
- **CNS:** *Dizziness, drowsiness, giddiness, weariness, headache,* tinnitus, hyperirritability, numbness, abnormal sensation in eyes, blurred vision, xanthopsia
- **GI:** *Anorexia, nausea,* vomiting, epigastric distress, diarrhea, perianal rash, jaundice, cholestasis, parenchymal liver damage
- **CV:** Hypotension, collapse
- **Hematologic:** Rise in SGOT, hyperglycemia, leukopenia
- **GU:** Enuresis, *malodor of urine,* crystalluria, hematuria
- **Hypersensitivity:** Reactions ranging from rash, fever, chills, angioedema, lymphadenopathy, anaphylaxis, **Stevens-Johnson syndrome** (sometimes fatal)

■ Nursing Considerations
Assessment
- *History:* Allergy to thiabendazole, renal or hepatic dysfunction, anemia, malnourishment or dehydration, pregnancy, lactation
- *Physical:* Skin—color, lesions, turgor; orientation, affect; bowel sounds, output; liver and renal function tests, urinalysis, CBC

Implementation
- Culture for ova and parasites.
- Administer drug with food; have patient chew tablets before swallowing them.

Adverse effects in *Italics* are most common; those in **Bold** are life-threatening.

- Discontinue drug, and consult with physician if hypersensitivity reactions occur.
- Arrange for treatment of all family members (pinworm infestations).
- Arrange for disinfection of toilet facilities after patient use (pinworms).
- Arrange for daily laundry of bed linens, towels, nightclothes, and undergarments (pinworms).

Drug-specific teaching points

- Take drug with food to decrease GI upset. Tablets should be chewed before swallowing.
- Be aware that pinworms are easily transmitted; all family members should be treated for complete eradication.
- Be aware that strict handwashing and hygiene measures are important; launder undergarments, bedlinens, nightclothes daily; disinfect toilet facilities daily and bathroom floors periodically (pinworms).
- Know that the following side effects may occur: nausea, abdominal pain, diarrhea (small, frequent meals may help; ready access to bathroom facilities may be necessary); drowsiness, dizziness, insomnia (if these occur, avoid driving and use of dangerous machinery); strange odor may develop in the urine (do not be concerned; this is an effect of the drug).
- Report skin rash, joint pain, severe GI upset, fever, chills, swelling of feet or hands, yellow color to skin or eyes.

▢ thiethylperazine maleate

*(thye eth il **per'** a zeen)*
Torecan

Pregnancy Category X

Drug classes
Antiemetic drug
Antivertigo drug

Therapeutic actions
Mechanism of action not fully understood: acts directly on the CTZ and the vomiting center to suppress nausea and vomiting.

Indications
- Relief of nausea and vomiting
- Unlabeled use: treatment of vertigo

Contraindications/cautions
- Allergy to phenothiazines, comatose or severely depressed states, pregnancy, lactation, intracardiac or intracranial surgery.

Dosage
Adult
- ***Oral and rectal:*** 10–30 mg/d in divided doses.
- ***IM:*** 2 ml, one to three times per day.

Pediatric: Safety and efficacy not determined for children younger than 12 y.

Pharmacokinetics

Route	Onset	Duration
Oral, PR	60 min	4 h
IM	30 min	4 h

Metabolism: Hepatic, $T_{1/2}$: unknown
Distribution: Crosses placenta; enters breast milk
Excretion: Urine

Adverse effects
- CNS: *Drowsiness, insomnia, vertigo,* headache, weakness, tremors, ataxia, slurring, cerebral edema, seizures, exacerbation of psychotic symptoms, *extrapyramidal syndromes*; neuroleptic malignant syndrome
- GI: *Dry mouth, salivation, nausea, vomiting, anorexia, constipation*, paralytic ileus, incontinence
- CV: *Hypotension, otrhostatic hypotension,* hypertension, tachycardia, bradycardia, cardiac arrest, CHF, cardiomegaly, refractory arrhythmias, pulmonary edema
- Respiratory: Bronchospasm, laryngospasm, dyspnea, suppression of cough reflex and potential aspiration
- Hematologic: **Eosinophilia, leukopenia, leukocytosis,** *anemia*, aplas-

Adverse effects in *italics* are most common; those in **Bold** are life-threatening.

tic anemia, hemolytic anemia, thrombocytopenic or nonthrombocytopenic purpura, pancytopenia, elevated serum cholesterol
- **GU:** *Urinary retention,* polyuria, incontinence
- **EENT:** Nasal congestion, glaucoma, *photophobia, blurred vision,* miosis, mydriasis, deposits in the cornea and lens, pigmentary retinopathy
- **Hypersensitivity:** Jaundice, *urticaria,* angioneurotic edema, laryngeal edema, photosensitivity, eczema, asthma, anaphylactoid reactions, exfoliative dermatitis
- **Endocrine:** Lactation, breast engorgement in females, galactorrhea, SIADH secretion, amenorrhea
- **Other:** Fever, heatstroke, pallor, flushed facies, sweating, *photosensitivity*

Clinically important drug-drug interactions
- Additive CNS depression, hypotension if given preoperatively with barbiturate anesthetics, alcohol, meperidine • Additive effects of both drugs if concurrently with beta-blockers • Increased risk of tachycardia, hypotension if given concurrently with epinephrine, norepinephrine • Increased risk of seizure if taken with metrizamide

Drug-lab test interferences
- False-positive pregnancy tests (less likely if serum test is used) • Increase in protein-bound iodine, not attributable to an increase in thyroxine

■ Nursing Considerations

Assessment
- *History:* Allergy to phenothiazines, comatose or severely depressed states, lactation, pregnancy, intracranial or intracardiac surgery
- *Physical:* Body temperature, body weight, skin—color, turgor; reflexes, orientation; P, BP, orthostatic BP, ECG; R, adventitious sounds; bowel sounds, normal output, liver evaluation; prostate palpation, normal urine output; CBC; urinalysis

Implementation
- Protect the rectal suppositories from light; refrigerate.
- For use after surgery; give slowly by deep IM injection into upper outer quadrant of buttock at or shortly before the termination of anesthesia.
- Keep the patient recumbent for $\frac{1}{2}$ h after injection to avoid orthostatic hypotension.
- Be alert to potential for aspiration because of suppressed cough reflex.

Drug-specific teaching points
- Know that the following side effects may occur: drowsiness (avoid driving a car or operating dangerous machinery if this occurs; avoid alcohol, which will increase the drowsiness); faintness, dizziness (change position slowly, use caution climbing stairs).
- Report sore throat, fever, unusual bleeding or bruising, rash, weakness, tremors, impaired vision, dark urine, pale stools, yellowing of the skin and eyes.

❒ thioguanine

*(thye oh **gwah**' neen)*
TG, 6-Thioguanine
Lanvis (CAN)

Pregnancy Category D

Drug classes
Antimetabolite
Antineoplastic drug

Therapeutic actions
Tumor-inhibiting properties, probably due to interference with a number of steps in the synthesis and use of purine nucleotides, which are normally incorporated into DNA and RNA.

Indications
- Remission induction, consolidation and maintenance therapy of acute leukemias (lymphatic, myelogenous, and acute myelomonocytic) alone and in combination therapy
- Palliative treatment of chronic myelogenous leukemia

Adverse effects in *Italics* are most common; those in **Bold** are life-threatening.

Contraindications/cautions
- Contraindicated in the presence of allergy to thioguanine, prior resistance to thioguanine, hematopoietic depression, pregnancy (potential mutagen and teratogen), lactation.
- Use caution in the presence of impaired hepatic function.

Dosage
Adult and Pediatric: Initial dosage, 2 mg/kg per day PO daily for 4 wk. If no clinical improvement is seen and there are no toxic effects, increase dose to 3 mg/kg per day. If complete hematologic remission is obtained, institute maintenance therapy. No adjustment of dosage is needed if used as part of combination therapy.

Pharmacokinetics

Route	Onset	Peak
Oral	Slow	8 h

Metabolism: Hepatic, $T_{1/2}$: 11 h
Distribution: Crosses placenta; enters breast milk
Excretion: Urine

Adverse effects
- **GI:** Hepatotoxicity, *nausea, vomiting, anorexia,* diarrhea, stomatitis
- **Hematologic:** **Bone marrow depression, immunosuppression, hyperuricemia** due to rapid lysis of malignant cells
- **Other:** Fever, weakness, cancer, chromosomal aberrations

■ Nursing Considerations

Assessment
- *History:* Allergy to thioguanine, prior resistance to thioguanine, hematopoietic depression, impaired hepatic function, pregnancy, lactation
- *Physical:* Skin—color; mucous membranes, liver evaluation, abdominal exam; CBC, differential, hemoglobin, platelet counts; liver function tests; serum uric acid

Implementation
- Arrange for tests to evaluate hematopoietic status before beginning therapy and frequently during therapy.
- Arrange for discontinuation of drug therapy if platelet count < 50,000; polymorphonuclear granuloctye count < 1,000; consult physician for dosage adjustment.
- Arrange for discontinuation of this drug at any sign of hematologic or hepatic toxicity; consult physician.
- Ensure that patient is well hydrated before therapy and during therapy to minimize adverse effects of hyperuricemia; allopurinal and drugs to alkalinize the urine are sometimes prescribed.
- Administer as a single daily dose.

Drug-specific teaching points
- Drink adequate fluids while you are on this drug; drink at least 8–10 glasses of fluid each day.
- Know that the following side effects may occur: mouth sores (frequent mouth care will be needed); nausea, vomiting, loss of appetite (small, freqent meals may help); increased susceptibility to infection (avoid crowded areas and exposure to disease as much as possible).
- Be aware that this drug may cause miscarriages and birth defects. It is advisable to use birth control while on this drug; men also should use birth control measures while on this drug and for a time afterwards.
- Arrange to have frequent, regular medical follow-up, including frequent blood tests to follow the effects of the drug on your body.
- Report fever, chills, sore throat, unusual bleeding or bruising, yellow discoloration of the skin or eyes, abdominal pain, flank pain, joint pain, swelling of the feet or legs.

❒ thioridazine hydrochloride

*(thye oh **rid'** a zeen)*
Apo-Thioridazine (CAN), Mellaril

Pregnancy Category C

Adverse effects in *Italics* are most common; those in **Bold** are life-threatening.

thioridazine hydrochloride ■ 1065

Drug classes
Phenothiazine (piperidine)
Dopaminergic blocking drug
Antipsychotic drug
Antianxiety agent

Therapeutic actions
Mechanism of action not fully understood: blocks postsynaptic dopamine receptors in the brain, but this may not be necessary and sufficient for antipsychotic activity; depresses the reticular activating system, including the parts of the brain involved with wakefulness and emesis; anticholinergic, antihistaminic (H_1), and alpha-adrenergic blocking activity also may contribute to some of its effects.

Indications
- Management of manifestations of psychotic disorders and short-term treatment of moderate to marked depression with anxiety in adults
- Treatment of multiple symptoms, such as agitation, anxiety, depressed mood, tension, sleep disturbances, and fears in geriatric patients
- Treatment of severe behavioral problems in children marked by combativeness or by explosive hyperexcitable behavior
- Short-term treatment of hyperactive children with accompanying conduct disorders consisting of some or all of the following symptoms: impulsivity, difficulty sustaining attention, aggressivity, mood lability, poor frustration tolerance

Contraindications/cautions
- Contraindicated in the presence of coma or severe CNS depression, bone marrow depression, blood dyscrasia, circulatory collapse, subcortical brain damage, Parkinson's disease, liver damage, cerebral arteriosclerosis, coronary disease, severe hypotension or hypertension.
- Use caution in the presence of respiratory disorders ("silent pneumonia" may develop); glaucoma, prostatic hypertrophy; epilepsy or history of epilepsy (drug lowers seizure threshold); breast cancer; thyrotoxicosis (severe neurotoxicity may develop); peptic ulcer, decreased renal function; myelography within previous 24 h or scheduled within 48 h; exposure to heat or phosphorous insecticides; pregnancy; lactation; children younger than 12 y, especially those with chickenpox, CNS infections (children are especially susceptible to dystonias that may confound the diagnosis of Reye's syndrome).

Dosage
Full clinical effects may require 6 wk–6 mo of therapy.
Adult
- **Psychotic manifestations:** 50–100 mg PO tid. Increase gradually to a maximum of 800 mg/d if necessary to control symptoms and then gradually reduce to minimum effective dose. Total daily dose ranges from 200–800 mg divided into two to four doses.

Pediatric
- **2–12 y:** 0.5–3.0 mg/kg per day PO.
- **Moderate disorders:** Initially, 10 mg PO bid–tid.
- **Hospitalized, severely disturbed children:** Initially, 25 mg PO bid–tid.

Geriatric
- **Short-term treatment of depression with anxiety in geriatric patients:** Initially, 25 mg PO tid. Dosage ranges from 10 mg bid–qid in milder cases to 50 mg tid–qid for more severely disturbed patients.

Pharmacokinetics

Route	Onset	Peak	Duration
Oral	Varies	2–4 h	8–12 h

Metabolism: Hepatic, $T_{1/2}$: 10–20 h
Distribution: Crosses placenta; enters breast milk
Excretion: Urine

Adverse effects
Antipsychotic Drugs
- CNS: *Drowsiness,* insomnia, vertigo, headache, weakness, tremor, ataxia, slurring, cerebral edema, seizures, exacerbation of psychotic symptoms, extrapyramidal syndromes—*pseudoparkinsonism;*

Adverse effects in *Italics* are most common; those in **Bold** are life-threatening.

dystonias; akathisia, tardive dyskinesias, potentially irreversible **neuroleptic malignant syndrome** (NMS)
- CV: Hypotension, orthostatic hypotension, hypertension, tachycardia, bradycardia, cardiac arrest, CHF, cardiomegaly, **refractory arrhythmias** (some fatal), pulmonary edema
- Respiratory: Bronchospasm, laryngospasm, dyspnea; suppression of cough reflex and potential for aspiration
- Hematologic: Eosinophilia, leukopenia, leukocytosis, anemia; aplastic anemia; hemolytic anemia; thrombocytopenic or nonthrombocytopenic purpura; pancytopenia
- EENT: Glaucoma, *photophobia, blurred vision*, miosis, mydriasis, deposits in the cornea and lens (opacities), pigmentary retinopathy
- Hypersensitivity: Jaundice, urticaria, angioneurotic edema, laryngeal edema, photosensitivity, eczema, asthma, anaphylactoid reactions, exfoliative dermatitis
- Endocrine: Lactation, breast engorgement, galactorrhea; SIADH secretion; amenorrhea, menstrual irregularities; gynecomastia in males; changes in libido; hyperglycemia or hypoglycemia; glycosuria; hyponatremia; pituitary tumor with hyperprolactinemia; inhibition of ovulation, infertility, pseudopregnancy; reduced urinary levels of gonadotropins, estrogens, progestins
- Autonomic: *Dry mouth, salivation, nasal congestion, nausea*, vomiting, anorexia, fever, pallor, flushed facies, sweating, constipation, paralytic ileus, urinary retention, incontinence, polyuria, enuresis, priapism, ejaculation inhibition, male impotence
- Other: *Urine discolored pink to red-brown*

Clinically important drug-drug interactions

- Additive CNS depression with alcohol
- Additive anticholinergic effects and possibly decreased antipsychotic efficacy with anticholinergic drugs
- Increased likelihood of seizures with metrizamide
- Increased effects from both drugs in given in combination with propranolol
- Decreased antihypertensive effect of guanethidine when taken concurrently

Drug-lab test interferences
- False-positive pregnancy tests (less likely if serum test is used)
- Increase in protein-bound iodine not attributable to an increase in thyroxine

■ Nursing Considerations

Assessment
- *History:* Coma or severe CNS depression; blood dyscrasia; circulatory collapse; subcortical brain damage; Parkinson's disease; liver damage; cerebral arteriosclerosis; coronary disease; severe hypotension or hypertension; respiratory disorders; glaucoma, prostatic hypertrophy; epilepsy; breast cancer; thyrotoxicosis; peptic ulcer, decreased renal function; myelography within previous 24 h or scheduled within 48 h; exposure to heat or phosphorous insecticides; pregnancy; lactation; chickenpox; CNS infections
- *Physical:* Body weight, temperature; reflexes, orientation, intraocular pressure; P, BP, orthostatic BP; R, adventitious sounds; bowel sounds and normal output, liver evaluation; urinary output, prostate size, CBC, urinalysis, thyroid, liver and kidney function tests

Implementation
- Arrange for ophthalmologic (slit lamp) examination before and during drug therapy.
- Do not change brand names; bioavailability differences have been documented for different brands.
- Be aware that the oral concentrate may be administered in distilled or acidified tap water or suitable juices, or use the flavored suspension.
- Do not change dosage in chronic therapy more often than weekly; drug requires 4–7 d to achieve steady-state plasma levels.

- Avoid skin contact with oral solution; contact dermatitis has occurred.
- Arrange for discontinuation of drug if serum creatinine, BUN become abnormal or if WBC count is depressed.
- Monitor elderly patients for dehydration, and institute remedial measures promptly; sedation and decreased sensation of thirst related to CNS effects of drug can lead to severe dehydration.
- Consult physician regarding appropriate warning of patient or patient's guardian about tardive dyskinesias.
- Consult physician about dosage reduction, use of anticholinergic antiparkinsonian drugs (controversial) if extrapyramidal effects occur.

Drug-specific teaching points
- Take drug exactly as prescribed.
- Avoid skin contact with drug solutions.
- Avoid driving a car or engaging in other dangerous activities if CNS, vision changes occur.
- Avoid prolonged exposure to sun, or use a sunscreen or covering garments if exposure is necessary.
- Maintain fluid intake and use precautions against heatstroke in hot weather.
- Arrange for ophthalmologic exams periodically during therapy.
- Report sore throat, fever, unusual bleeding or bruising, rash, weakness, tremors, impaired vision, dark urine (pink or reddish brown urine is to be expected), pale stools, yellowing of the skin or eyes.

☐ thiotepa

*(thye oh **tep'** ah)*
triethylenethiophosphoramide, ESPA, TSPA

Pregnancy Category D

Drug classes
Alkylating agent
Antineoplastic drug

Therapeutic actions
Cytotoxic: disrupts the bonds of DNA, causing cell death; cell cycle nonspecific.

Indications
- Treatment of adenocarcinoma of the breast, ovary
- Superficial papillary carcinoma of the urinary bladder
- Controlling intracavity effusions secondary to diffuse or localized neoplastic disease of various serosal cavities
- Treatment of lymphoma, including Hodgkin's disease; no longer a drug of choice
- Unlabeled use: prevention of pterygium recurrences following surgery

Contraindications/cautions
- Contraindicated in the presence of allergy to thiotepa, hematopoietic depression, pregnancy, lactation.
- Use caution in the presence of impaired hepatic or renal function, concomitant therapy with other alkylating agents or irradiation.

Dosage
Adult
- ***IV administration:*** 0.3–0.4 mg/kg at 1- to 4-wk intervals.
- ***Intratumor administration:*** Drug is diluted in sterile water to a concentration of 10 mg/ml, then 0.6–0.8 mg/kg is injected directly into the tumor after a local anesthetic is injected through the same needle. Maintainance doses of 0.07–0.8 mg/kg every 1–4 wk depending on the condition of the patient.
- ***Intracavity administration:*** 0.6–0.8 mg/kg through the same tube that is used to remove fluid from the cavity.
- ***Intravesical administration:*** Dehydrate patient with papillary carcinoma of the bladder for 8–12 h prior to treatment. Then instill 60 mg in 30–60 ml of distilled water into the bladder by catheter. Retain for 2 h. If patient is unable to retain 60 ml, give the dose in 30 ml. Repeat once a week for 4 wk.

Pharmacokinetics

Route	Onset
IV	Gradual

Metabolism: Hepatic, $T_{1/2}$: unknown

1068 ■ thiothixene

Distribution: Crosses placenta; enters breast milk
Excretion: Urine

IV facts

Preparation: Reconstitute powder with Sterile Water for Injection. 1.5 ml of diluent gives a drug concentration of 5 mg/0.5 ml of solution. May be further diluted with Sodium Chloride Injection, Dextrose Injection, Dextrose and Sodium Chloride Injection, Ringer's Injection, Lactated Ringer's Injection. Powder should be stored in the refrigerator, reconstituted solution is stable for 5 d if refrigerated. Use of Sterile Water for Injection produces an isotonic solution, other diluents may produce a hypertonic solution that may cause mild to moderate discomfort on injection. Check solution before use; solution should be clear to slightly opaque; grossly opaque solutions or solutions with precipitates should not be used.
Infusion: Administer IV dose directly and rapidly. There is no need for slow IV drip or the use of large volumes of fluid.

Adverse effects

- CNS: *Dizziness,* headache
- GI: *Nausea, vomiting,* anorexia
- Hematologic: *Hematopoietic toxicity*
- GU: *Amenorrhea, interference with spermatogenesis*
- Dermatologic: Hives, skin rash, weeping from subcutaneous lesions
- Other: Febrile reactions, cancer

■ Nursing Considerations

Assessment

- *History:* Allergy to thiotepa, hematopoietic depression, impaired renal or hepatic function, concomitant therapy with other alkylating agents or irradiation, pregnancy, lactation
- *Physical:* Weight; skin—color, lesions; temperature; orientation, reflexes; CBC, differential; urinalysis; liver and renal function tests

Implementation

- Arrange for blood tests to evaluate bone marrow function before beginning therapy, weekly during therapy and for at least 3 wk after therapy.
- Arrange to mix solution with 2% procaine HCl, 1:1,000 epinephrine HCl, or both for local use into single or multiple sites.
- Arrange for reduced dosage in cases of renal or hepatic impairment and for bone marrow depression.

Drug-specific teaching points

- Be aware that this drug can be given only parenterally. Prepare a calendar with the courses of treatment outlined for the patient.
- Know that the following side effects may occur: nausea, vomiting, loss of appetite (an antiemetic may be ordered for you; small frequent meals also may help); dizziness, headache (special safety precautions will be used to help to prevent falls or injury if this occurs); amenorrhea in women, change in sperm production in men (this effect on fertility can be upsetting).
- Be aware that this drug should not be taken during pregnancy, some means of birth control should be used while you are on this drug. If you become pregnant, consult with your physician.
- Arrange to have regular medical follow-up, including blood tests to follow the effects of the drug.
- Report unusual bleeding or bruising, fever, chills, sore throat, stomach or flank pain, severe nausea and vomiting, skin rash or hives.

▢ thiothixene

*(thye oh **thix**' een)*

thiothixene hydrochloride
Navane

Pregnancy Category C

Drug classes

Dopaminergic blocking drug
Antipsychotic drug
Thioxanthene, not a phenothiazine

Adverse effects in *Italics* are most common; those in **Bold** are life-threatening.

Therapeutic actions
Mechanism of action not fully understood: blocks postsynaptic dopamine receptors in the brain, but this may not be necessary and sufficient for antipsychotic activity.

Indications
- Management of manifestations of psychotic disorders

Contraindications/cautions
- Contraindicated in the presence of coma or severe CNS depression, blood dyscrasia, circulatory collapse, subcortical brain damage, Parkinson's disease, liver damage, cerebral arteriosclerosis, coronary disease, severe hypotension or hypertension, pregnancy, lactation.
- Use caution in the presence of respiratory disorders ("silent pneumonia" may develop); glaucoma, prostatic hypertrophy; epilepsy or history of epilepsy (drug lowers seizure threshold); breast cancer; thyrotoxicosis (severe neurotoxicity may develop); peptic ulcer, decreased renal function; myelography within previous 24 h or scheduled within 48 h; exposure to heat or phosphorous insecticides; children younger than 12 y, especially those with chickenpox, CNS infections (children are especially susceptible to dystonias that may confound the diagnosis of Reye's syndrome).

Dosage
Full clinical effects may require 6 wk–6 mo of therapy.

Adult
- ***Oral:*** Initially 2 mg tid (mild conditions) or 5 mg bid (more severe conditions). Increase dose as needed; the usual optimum dose is 20–30 mg/d. May increase to 60 mg/d, but further increases rarely increase beneficial response.
- ***IM (for more rapid control and when oral dosage is not feasible):*** Usual dose is 4 mg bid–qid. Most patients are controlled on 16–20 mg/d. Maximum dosage is 30 mg/d. Institute oral medication as soon as feasible; dosage adjustment may be necessary when changing to oral forms.

Pediatric: Not recommended for children younger than 12 y.

Geriatric and debilitated patients: Use lower doses and increase dosage more gradually.

Pharmacokinetics

Route	Onset	Duration
Oral	Slow	12 h
IM	1–6 h	12 h

Metabolism: Hepatic, $T_{1/2}$: 34 h
Distribution: Crosses placenta; enters breast milk
Excretion: Bile and feces

Adverse effects
Antipsychotic Drugs
- **CNS:** *Drowsiness*, insomnia, vertigo, headache, weakness, tremor, ataxia, slurring, cerebral edema, seizures, exacerbation of psychotic symptoms, extrapyramidal syndromes—*pseudoparkinsonism; dystonias; akathisia*, tardive dyskinesias, potentially irreversible NMS; extrapyramidal symptoms, hyperthermia, autonomic disturbances (rare, but 20% fatal)
- **CV:** Hypotension, orthostatic hypotension, hypertension, tachycardia, bradycardia, cardiac arrest, CHF, cardiomegaly, **refractory arrhythmias** (some fatal), pulmonary edema
- **Respiratory:** Bronchospasm, laryngospasm, dyspnea, suppression of cough reflex and potential for aspiration
- **Hematologic:** Eosinophilia, leukopenia, leukocytosis, anemia; aplastic anemia; hemolytic anemia; thrombocytopenic or nonthrombocytopenic purpura; pancytopenia
- **EENT:** Glaucoma, *photophobia, blurred vision*, miosis, mydriasis, deposits in the cornea and lens (opacities), pigmentary retinopathy
- **Hypersensitivity:** Jaundice, urticaria, angioneurotic edema, laryngeal edema, photosensitivity, eczema, asthma, anaphylactoid reactions, exfoliative dermatitis

Adverse effects in *Italics* are most common; those in **Bold** are life-threatening.

- **Endocrine:** Lactation, breast engorgement in females, galactorrhea; SIADH secretion; amenorrhea, menstrual irregularities; gynecomastia in males; changes in libido; hyperglycemia or hypoglycemia; glycosuria; hyponatremia; pituitary tumor with hyperprolactinemia; inhibition of ovulation, infertility, pseudopregnancy; reduced urinary levels of gonadotropins, estrogens, progestins
- **Autonomic:** *Dry mouth, salivation, nasal congestion, nausea,* vomiting, anorexia, fever, pallor, flushed facies, sweating, constipation, paralytic ileus, urinary retention, incontinence, polyuria, enuresis, priapism, ejaculation inhibition, male impotence
- **Other:** *Urine discolored pink to red-brown*

Drug-lab test interferences
- False-positive pregnancy tests (less likely if serum test is used) • Increase in protein-bound iodine not attributable to an increase in thyroxine

■ Nursing Considerations
Assessment
- **History:** Severe CNS depression; blood dyscrasia; circulatory collapse; subcortical brain damage; Parkinson's disease; liver damage; cerebral arteriosclerosis; coronary disease; severe hypotension or hypertension; respiratory disorders; glaucoma, prostatic hypertrophy; epilepsy; breast cancer; thyrotoxicosis; peptic ulcer, decreased renal function; myelography within previous 24 h or scheduled within 48 h; exposure to heat or phosphorous insecticides; pregnancy; lactation; chickenpox; CNS infections
- **Physical:** Body weight, temperature; reflexes, orientation, intraocular pressure; P, BP, orthostatic BP; R, adventitious sounds; bowel sounds and normal output, liver evaluation; urinary output, prostate size. Arrange for CBC, urinalysis, thyroid, liver and kidney function tests.

Implementation
- Reconstitute the powder for injection with 2.2 ml of Sterile Water for Injection. Store at room temperature for up to 48 h and then discard any unused solution.
- Avoid skin contact with oral solution; contact dermatitis has occurred.
- Arrange for discontinuation of drug if serum creatinine, BUN become abnormal or if WBC count is depressed.
- Monitor elderly patients for dehydration, and institute remedial measures promptly; sedation and decreased sensation of thirst related to CNS effects of drug can lead to severe dehydration.
- Consult physician regarding appropriate warning of patient or patient's guardian about tardive dyskinesias.
- Consult physician about dosage reduction, use of anticholinergic antiparkinsonian drugs (controversial) if extrapyramidal effects occur.

Drug-specific teaching points
- Take drug exactly as prescribed.
- Avoid skin contact with drug solutions.
- Avoid driving a car or engaging in other dangerous activities if CNS, vision changes occur.
- Avoid prolonged exposure to sun or use a sunscreen or covering garments if exposure is necessary.
- Maintain fluid intake, and use precautions against heatstroke in hot weather.
- Report sore throat, fever, unusual bleeding or bruising, rash, weakness, tremors, impaired vision, dark urine (pink or reddish brown urine is to be expected), pale stools, yellowing of the skin or eyes.

❒ thyroid desiccated

(thye' roid)

Armour Thyroid, S-P-T, Thyrar, Thyroid Strong

Pregnancy Category A

Drug classes
Thyroid hormone preparation (contains T_3 and T_4 in their natural state and ratio)

Therapeutic actions
Increases the metabolic rate of body tissues, increasing oxygen consumption, respira-

tory and heart rate; rate of fat, protein, and carbohydrate metabolism; and growth and maturation; exact mechanism of action is not known.

Indications
- Replacement therapy in hypothyroidism
- Pituitary TSH suppression, in the treatment and prevention of euthyroid goiters and management of thyroid cancer
- Thyrotoxicosis in conjunction with antithyroid drugs and prevention of goitrogenesis, hypothyroidism, and thyrotoxicosis during pregnancy

Contraindications/cautions
- Contraindicated in the presence of allergy to active or extraneous constituents of drug (preparations marketed as *Thyrar* are derived from bovine thyroids; preparations marketed as *S-P-T* are derived from porcine thyroids); thyrotoxicosis and acute MI uncomplicated by hypothyroidism.
- Use caution in the presence of Addison's disease (treatment of hypoadrenalism with corticosteroids should precede thyroid therapy), pregnancy.

Dosage
Adult
- ***Myxedema:*** Initial dosage, 16 mg/d PO for 2 wk, followed by 32 mg/d PO for 2 or more wk, then 65 mg/d. Assess after 1 and 2 mo of therapy with the 65-mg dose, and increase dosage if needed up to 130 mg/d for 2 mo. Reassess, and increase to 195 mg/d if needed; make further increases, if needed, in 32- or 65-mg/d increments. Maintenance, 65–195 mg/d.
- ***Hypothyroidism without myxedema:*** Initial dosage, 65 mg/d PO, increased by 65 mg q30 d PO until desired result is obtained. Maintenance, same as above.

Pediatric: Initial dosage, 16 mg/d PO for 2 wk, followed by 32 mg/d PO for 2 or more wk, then 65 mg/d. Assess in 2 mo, and increase dosage if needed up to 130 mg/d for 2 mo. Maintenance, 65–195 mg/d. Actually, dosage may be greater during periods of growth; monitor clinical condition and laboratory tests to determine correct dose (sleeping pulse and basal morning temperature are guides to treatment).

Pharmacokinetics

Route	Onset	Peak
Oral	Varies	4 h

Metabolism: Liver, kidney, and tissue, $T_{1/2}$: 1–2 d (T_3), 6–7 d (T_4)
Distribution: Crosses placenta; enters breast milk
Excretion: Urine and feces

Adverse effects
All rare at therapeutic doses.
- **Dermatologic:** Partial loss of hair in first few months of therapy in children
- **Endocrine:** Hyperthyroidism (palpitations, elevated pulse pressure, tachycardia, arrhythmias, angina pectoris, cardiac arrest; tremors, headache, nervousness, insomnia; nausea, diarrhea, changes in appetite; weight loss, menstrual irregularities, sweating, heat intolerance, fever)
- **Hypersensitivity:** Allergic skin reactions

Clinically important drug-drug interactions
- Decreased absorption if taken concurrently with cholestyramine • Increased risk of bleeding if taken with warfarin, dicumarol • Decreased effectiveness of digitalis glycosides if taken with thyroid replacement • Alterations in theophylline clearance occur in hypothyroid patients; if thyroid state changes during therapy, monitor patient carefully

■ Nursing Considerations
Assessment
- *History:* Allergy to active or extraneous constituents of drug, bovine, or porcine products; thyrotoxicosis; acute MI uncomplicated by hypothyroidism; Addison's disease; lactation
- *Physical:* Skin—lesions, color, temperature, texture; temperature; muscle tone,

Adverse effects in *Italics* are most common; those in **Bold** are life-threatening.

orientation, reflexes; P, auscultation, baseline ECG, BP; R, adventitious sounds; thyroid function tests

Implementation
- Monitor patient response carefully when beginning therapy, and adjust dosage accordingly.
- Administer as a single daily dose before breakfast.
- Arrange for regular, periodic blood tests of thyroid function.
- Monitor cardiac response throughout therapy.

Drug-specific teaching points
- Take as a single dose before breakfast.
- Be aware that this drug replaces a very important hormone and will need to be taken for life. Do not discontinue this drug for any reason without consulting your nurse or physician; serious problems can occur.
- Wear or carry a medical alert tag to alert medical personnel who may take care of you in an emergency that you are on this drug.
- Know that nausea and diarrhea may occur (dividing the dose may help).
- Arrange to have periodic blood tests and medical evaluations while you are on this drug. It is important to keep your scheduled appointments.
- Report headache, chest pain, palpitations, fever, weight loss, sleeplessness, nervousness, irritability, unusual sweating, intolerance to heat, diarrhea.

☐ thyrotropin

(thye roe troe' pin)
thyroid-stimulating hormone, TSH

Thytropar

Pregnancy Category C

Drug classes
Hormone
Diagnostic agent

Therapeutic actions
Produces increased uptake of iodine by the thyroid, increased formation of thyroid hormone, increased release of thyroid hormone, and cellular hyperplasia of the thyroid on prolonged stimulation.

Indications
- Diagnostic agent to differentiate thyroid failure and to establish a diagnosis of decreased thyroid reserve
- Used for PBI and I^{131} uptake determinations

Contraindications/cautions
- Contraindicated in the presence of allergy to thyrotrophin, beef products, coronary thrombosis, untreated Addison's disease.
- Use caution in the presence of cardiac disease, pregnancy.

Dosage
Adult: 10 U IM or SC for 1–3 d. Follow by a radioiodine study 24 h after the last injection. No response occurs with thyroid failure; substantial response will occur in pituitary failure.
Pediatric: Safety and efficacy not established.

Pharmacokinetics

Route	Onset
SC, IM	Days

Metabolism: $T_{1/2}$: 30–35 min
Distribution: Crosses placenta; enters breast milk
Excretion: Urine

Adverse effects
- CNS: *Headache*
- GI: *Nausea, vomiting*
- CV: Transitory hypotension, tachycardia
- **Hypersensitivity:** Reactions including anaphylaxis
- Other: Thyroid gland swelling, *urticaria*

■ Nursing Considerations

Assessment
- *History:* Allergy to thyrotropin, beef products, untreated Addison's disease, cardiac disease, pregnancy

- *Physical:* Skin—color, lesions; thyroid gland exam; BP, P; R, adventitious sounds; thyroid function tests

Implementation
- Store reconstituted solution in refrigerator; do not store longer than 2 wk.
- Administer by IM or SC routes only.

Drug-specific teaching points
- Be aware that injections will be made on 3 consecutive d. 24 h following the last injection, a radioiodine study will be performed to determine the effects of this drug on your thyroid gland.
- Know that the following side effects may occur: nausea, vomiting, rash, swelling on the thyroid gland.
- Report dizziness, palpitations, difficulty breathing.

☐ ticarcillin disodium

*(tye kar **sill**' in)*
Ticar

Pregnancy Category B

Drug classes
Antibiotic
Penicillin with extended spectrum

Therapeutic actions
Bactericidal: inhibits synthesis of cell wall of action-sensitive organisms, causing cell death.

Indications
- Severe infections caused by sensitive organisms, particularly *Pseudomonas aeruginosa, Proteus, E. coli*
- Infections caused by anaerobic bacteria
- GU infections caused by the above or *Enterobacter, Streptococcus faecalis*

Contraindications/cautions
- Contraindicated in the presence of allergies to penicillins, cephalosporins or other allergens.
- Use caution in the presence of renal disorders, pregnancy, lactation (may cause diarrhea or candidiasis in the infant).

Dosage
Maximum recommended dosage, 24 g/d. Maximum dose of single IM injection, 2 g.

Adult
- **UTIs:** 1 g IM *or* direct IV q6h, up to 150–200 mg/kg per day IV in divided doses q4–6h in severe cases.
- **Other infections:** 200–300 mg/kg per day IV in divided doses q3, 4, or 6h.

Geriatric or renal insufficiency: Initial dose of 3 g IV followed by the following doses:

Creatinine Clearance (ml/min)	Dosage
>60	3 g q4h IV
30–60	2 g q4h IV
10–30	2 g q8h IV
<10	2 g q12h IV or 1 g q6h IM
<10 with hepatic dysfunction	2 g qd or 1 g q12h IM
Patients on peritoneal dialysis	3 g q12h IV
Patients on hemodialysis	2 g q12h with 3 g after each dialysis

Pediatric
- **UTIs (< 40 kg):** 50–100 mg/kg per day IM *or* direct IV in divided doses q6–8h up to 150–200 mg/kg per day in divided doses q4–6h IV.
- **Other infections (< 40 kg):** 200–300 mg/kg per day q4–6h IV.

Neonates: May be given IM or over 10–20 min IV.
- **< 2 kg, 0–7 d:** 75 mg/kg q12h initially; after 7 d old, 75 mg/kg q8h.
- **> 2 kg, 0–7 d:** 75 mg/kg q8h; after 7 d old, 100 mg/kg q8h.

Pharmacokinetics

Route	Onset	Peak
IM	Rapid	30–75 min
IV	Rapid	End of infusion

Metabolism: Hepatic, $T_{1/2}$: 0.8–1.4 h
Distribution: Crosses placenta; enters breast milk
Excretion: Urine

1074 ■ ticarcillin disodium

IV facts

Preparation: Reconstitute each gm of ticarcillin for IV use with 4 ml of Sodium Chloride Injection, 5% Dextrose Injection, or Lactate Ringer's Injection. Each 1 ml of solution will contain approximately 200 mg. Date reconstituted solution. Reconstituted solution (10–50 mg/ml) is stable for 72 h at room temperature if diluted with Sodium Chloride or 5% Dextrose; 48 h if diluted with Lactated Ringer's; 14 d if refrigerated. Do not store for more than 72 h if for multidose purposes.

Infusion: Direct injection: administer as slowly as possible to avoid vein irritation. Infusion should be run by continuous drip or intermittently over a 30-min to 2-h period.

Compatibilities: Do not mix in the same solution as gentamicin, tobramycin, amikacin.

Adverse effects

- CNS: Lethargy, hallucinations, seizures
- GI: *Glossitis, stomatitis, gastritis, sore mouth,* furry tongue, black "hairy" tongue, *nausea, vomiting, diarrhea,* abdominal pain, bloody diarrhea, enterocolitis, pseudomembranous colitis, nonspecific hepatitis
- **Hematologic:** Anemia, thrombocytopenia, leukopenia, neutropenia, prolonged bleeding time
- GU: Nephritis—oliguria, proteinuria, hematuria, casts, azotemia, pyuria
- Hypersensitivity reactions: *Rash, fever, wheezing,* anaphylaxis
- Local: *Pain, phlebitis,* thrombosis at injection site
- Other: *Superinfections*—oral and rectal moniliasis, vaginitis, sodium overload

Clinically important drug-drug interactions

- Decreased effectiveness of ticarcillin if taken concurrently with tetracyclines
- Inactivation of parenteral aminoglycosides (amikacin, gentamicin, kanamycin, neomycin, metilmicin, streptomycin, tobramycin) if taken concurrently

Drug-lab test interferences

- False-positive Coombs' test with IV use

■ Nursing Considerations

Assessment

- *History:* Allergies to penicillins, cephalosporins, other allergens; renal disorders; pregnancy; lactation
- *Physical:* Culture infected area; skin—color, lesion; R, adventitious sounds; bowel sounds; CBC, liver and renal function tests, serum electrolytes, Hct, urinalysis

Implementation

- Culture infected area before beginning treatment; reculture area if response is not as expected.
- Arrange to continue therapy for at least 2 d after signs of infection have disappeared, usually 7–10 d.
- Administer by IM or IV routes only.
- Reconstitute each gram for IM use with 2 ml Sodium Chloride Injection, 5% Dextrose Injection, Lactated Ringer's Injection, or 1% lidocaine HCl without epinephrine. Each 2.6 ml will contain 1 g ticarcillin. Inject deep into a large muscle.
- Maintain epinephrine, IV fluids, vasopressors, bronchodilators, oxygen, and emergency equipment on standby in case of serious hypersensitivity reaction.

Drug-specific teaching points

- Be aware that this drug is given by injection.
- Know that upset stomach, nausea, diarrhea (small, frequent meals may help); mouth sores (frequent mouth care may help); pain or discomfort at injection sites may occur.
- Report difficulty breathing, rashes, severe diarrhea, severe pain at injection site, mouth sores.

Adverse effects in *Italics* are most common; those in **Bold** are life-threatening.

☐ ticlopidine hydrochloride

*(tye **klob'** pih deen)*
Ticlid

Pregnancy Category B

Drug classes
Antiplatelet drug

Therapeutic actions
Interferes with platelet membrane function by inhibiting fibrinogen binding and platelet-platelet interactions; inhibits platelet aggregation and prolongs bleeding time; effect is irreversible for life of the platelet.

Indications
- Reduction of the risk of thrombotic stroke in patients who have experienced stroke precursors and in patients who have had a completed thrombotic stroke; reserve for use in patients who are intolerant to aspirin therapy because side effects of drug may be life-threatening
- Unlabeled uses: intermittent claudication, chronic arterial occlusion, subarachnoid hemmorhage, uremic patients with AV shunts or fistulas, open heart surgery, coronary artery bypass grafts, primary glomerulonephritis, sickle cell disease

Contraindications/cautions
- Contraindicated in the presence of allergy to ticlopidine, neutropenia, thrombocytopenia, hemostatic disorders, bleeding ulcer, intracranial bleeding, severe liver disease, lactation.
- Use caution in the presence of renal disorders, pregnancy, elevated cholesterol, recent trauma.

Dosage
Adult: 250 mg PO bid with food.
Pediatric: Safety and efficacy not established for children younger than 18 y.

Pharmacokinetics

Route	Onset	Peak
Oral	Rapid	2 h

Metabolism: Hepatic, $T_{1/2}$: 12.6 h, then 4–5 d
Distribution: Crosses placenta; enters breast milk
Excretion: Urine and feces

Adverse effects
- **CNS:** Dizziness
- **GI:** *Diarrhea, nausea, vomiting, abdominal pain,* flatulence, dyspepsia, anorexia
- **Hematologic:** *Neutropenia,* bleeding
- **Local:** *Pain, phlebitis,* thrombosis at injection site
- **Other:** Rash, purpura

Clinically important drug-drug interactions
- Decreased effectiveness of digoxin if taken concurrently • Increased serum levels and effects of theophylline, aspirin taken concurrently • Increased effects of ticlopodine if taken concurrently with cimetidine • Decreased absorption of ticlopodine if taken with antacids

Clinically important drug-food interactions
- Increased availability of toclopidine if taken with food

■ Nursing Considerations

Assessment
- *History:* Allergy to ticlopidine, neutropenia, thrombocytopenia, hemostatic disorders, bleeding ulcer, intracranial bleeding, severe liver disease, lactation, renal disorders, pregnancy, elevated cholesterol, recent trauma
- *Physical:* Skin—color, lesions; orientation; bowel sounds, normal output; CBC, liver and renal function tests, serum cholesterol

Implementation
- Monitor WBC count before use and frequently while initiating therapy; if neuto-

Adverse effects in *Italics* are most common; those in **Bold** are life-threatening.

penia is present or occurs, discontinue drug immediately.
- Administer drug with food or just after eating to minimize GI irritation and increase absorption.
- Maintain IV methylprednisolone (20 mg) on standby in case excessive bleeding occurs.
- Monitor patient for any sign of excessive bleeding (eg, bruises, dark stools), and monitor bleeding times.
- Provide increased precautions against bleeding during invasive procedures; bleeding will be prolonged.
- Mark chart of any patient receiving ticlopidine to alert medical personnel of potential for increased bleeding in cases of surgery or dental surgery.

Drug-specific teaching points
- Take drug with meals or just after eating.
- Be aware that you will require regular blood tests to monitor your response to this drug.
- Be aware that it may take longer than normal to stop bleeding while on this drug; avoid contact sports, use electrical razors, and so forth; apply pressure for extended periods to bleeding sites.
- Know that upset stomach, nausea, diarrhea, loss of appetite (small, frequent meals may help) may occur.
- Notify any dentist or surgeon that you are on this drug before invasive procedures.
- Report fever, chills, sore throat, skin rash, bruising, bleeding, dark stools or urine.

▢ timolol maleate

(tye moe' lole)
Blocadren, Timoptic

Pregnancy Category C

Drug classes
Beta-adrenergic blocking agent
Antihypertensive agent
Antiglaucoma agent

Therapeutic actions
Competitively blocks beta-adrenergic receptors in the heart and juxtaglomerular apparatus, decreasing the influence of the sympathetic nervous system on these tissues and decreasing the excitability of the heart, decreasing cardiac output and oxygen consumption, decreasing the release of renin, and lowering blood pressure; reduces intraocular pressure by decreasing the production of aqueous humor and possibly by increasing aqueous humor outflow.

Indications
- Hypertension, used alone or in combination with other antihypertensives, especially thiazide-type diuretics
- Prevention of reinfarction in MI patients who are hemodynamically stable
- Prophylaxis of migraine
- Reduction of intraocular pressure in chronic open-angle glaucoma, some patients with secondary glaucoma, aphakic patients with glaucoma (ophthalmic solution)

Contraindications/cautions
- Contraindicated in the presence of sinus bradycardia (HR < 45 beats/min), second- or third-degree heart block (PR interval > 0.24 sec), cardiogenic shock, CHF, asthma, COPD, pregnancy, lactation.
- Use caution in the presence of diabetes or thyrotoxicosis (timolol can mask the usual cardiac signs of hypoglycemia and thyrotoxicosis).

Dosage
Adult
- **Oral**
  - *Hypertension:* Initially, 10 mg bid. Increase dosage at 1-wk intervals to a maximum of 60 mg/d divided into two doses, as necessary. Usual maintenance dose is 20–40 mg/d.
  - *Prevention of reinfarction in MI (long-term prophylaxis in patients who survived the acute phase):* 10 mg bid PO.
  - *Migraine:* 10 mg PO bid; during maintenance, the 20 mg/d may be given as a single dose. May be increased to a maximum of 30 mg/d in divided doses or decreased to 10 mg/d. Discontinue if

satisfactory response is not obtained after 6–8 wk.
- **Ophthalmic administration:** Initially 1 drop of 0.25% solution bid into the affected eye(s). Adjust dosage on basis of resonse to 1 drop of 0.5% solution bid or 1 drop of 0.25% solution qd. When replacing other agents, make change gradually and individualize dosage.

Pediatric: Safety and efficacy not established.

Pharmacokinetics

Route	Onset	Peak
Oral	Varies	1–2 h
Ophthalmologic	Rapid	1–5 h

Metabolism: Hepatic, $T_{1/2}$: 3–4 h
Distribution: Crosses placenta; enters breast milk
Excretion: Urine

Adverse effects
Oral
- **CNS:** Dizziness, vertigo, tinnitus, fatigue, emotional depression, paresthesias, sleep disturbances, hallucinations, disorientation, memory loss, slurred speech
- **GI:** *Gastric pain, flatulence, constipation, diarrhea, nausea, vomiting,* anorexia, ischemic colitis, renal and mesenteric arterial thrombosis, retroperitoneal fibrosis, hepatomegaly, acute pancreatitis
- **CV:** *CHF, cardiac arrhythmias, sinoatrial or AV nodal block,* peripheral vascular insufficiency, claudication, CVA, pulmonary edema, hypotension
- **Respiratory:** Bronchospasm, dyspnea, cough, bronchial obstruction, nasal stuffiness, rhinitis, pharyngitis (less likely than with propranolol)
- **GU:** *Impotence, decreased libido,* Peyronie's disease, dysuria, nocturia, frequent urination
- **MS:** Joint pain, arthralgia, muscle cramp
- **EENT:** Eye irritation, dry eyes, conjunctivitis, blurred vision
- **Dermatologic:** Rash, pruritus, sweating, dry skin
- **Allergic reactions:** Pharyngitis, erythematous rash, fever, sore throat, laryngospasm, respiratory distress
- **Other:** *Decreased exercise tolerance, development of antinuclear antibodies* (ANA), hyperglycemia or hypoglycemia, elevated serum transaminase, alkaline phosphatase

Ophthalmic
- **Local:** Ocular irritation, decreased corneal sensitivity, visual refractive changes, diplopia, ptosis

Clinically important drug-drug interactions
- Increased effects of timolol if taken with verapamil • Increased risk of postural hypotension if taken concurrently with prazosin • Decreased antihypertensive effects if taken with NSAIDs, clonidine • Decreased elimination of theophyllines with resultant decrease in expected actions of both drugs when taken concurrently • Peripheral ischemia and possible gangrene if taken with ergotamine, methysergide, dihydroergotamine • Increased risk of hypoglycemia and masked signs of hypoglycemia if taken with insulin • Hypertension followed by severe bradycardia if given concurrently with epinephrine • All of the above apply because ophthalmic timolol has been shown to be absorbed systemically. In addition, use caution in the following: • Additive effects are possible when taken with oral beta-blockers.

Drug-lab test interferences
- Possible false results with glucose or insulin tolerance tests (oral)

■ Nursing Considerations

Assessment
- *History:* Sinus bradycardia, second- or third-degree heart block, cardiogenic shock, CHF, asthma, COPD, pregnancy, lactation, diabetes or thyrotoxicosis
- *Physical:* Body weight, skin condition, neurologic status, P, BP, ECG, respiratory status, kidney and thyroid function, blood and urine glucose

Adverse effects in *Italics* are most common; those in **Bold** are life-threatening.

Implementation
- Do not discontinue drug abruptly after chronic therapy (hypersensitivity to catecholamines may have developed, causing exacerbation of angina, MI, and ventricular dysrhythmias). Taper drug gradually over 2 wk with monitoring.
- Consult with physician about withdrawing drug if patient is to undergo surgery (withdrawal is controversial).

Drug-specific teaching points
- Do not to stop taking this drug unless instructed to do so by a health care provider.
- Avoid driving or dangerous activities if CNS effects occur.
- Report difficulty breathing, night cough, swelling of extremities, slow pulse, confusion, depression, rash, fever, sore throat.
- Ophthalmic: Administer eye drops properly to minimize systemic absorption.

☐ tiopronin

*(tye oh **pro**' nin)*
Thiola

Pregnancy Category C

Drug classes
Thiol compound

Therapeutic actions
Active reducing and complexing compound, which undergoes thiol-disulfide exchange with cystine during urine formation to form a water-soluble mixed disulfide, reducing cystine and leading to a reduction in the formation of cystine (kidney) stone formation.

Indications
- Prevention of cystine (kidney) stone formation in patients with severe homozygous cystinuria with urinary cystine greater than 500 mg/d and who are resistant to treatment with conservative measures

Contraindications/cautions
- Contraindicated in the presence of hypersensitivity to tiopronin; history of agranulocytosis, aplastic anemia, thrombocytopenia; pregnancy; lactation.
- Use caution in the presence of history of severe reaction to penicillamine.

Dosage
Use only after more conservative measures have been tried and failed.
Adult: Initially 800 mg/d PO. Average dose is 1,000 mg/d. Give in divided doses three times per day at least 1 h before or 2 h after meals. Measure urinary cystine 1 mo after treatment and every 3 mo thereafter. Readjust dosage depending on urinary cystine levels.
Pediatric: Safety and efficacy in children younger than 9 y not established.
- ***Older than 9 y:*** Initial dosage based on 15 mg/kg per day PO with adjustments based on patient response.

Pharmacokinetics

Route	Onset	Peak	Duration
Oral	Varies	4 h	72 h

Metabolism: Renal, $T_{1/2}$: unknown
Distribution: Crosses placenta; enters breast milk
Excretion: Urine

Adverse effects
- Hematologic: Leukopenia, eosinophilia, thrombocytopenia
- GU: Proteinuria
- Dermatologic: *Erythematous, maculopapular* or *morbilliform rash*, lupus erythematosus-like reaction, wrinkling and friability of skin
- General: *Fever*

■ Nursing Considerations
Assessment
- *History:* Hypersensitivity to tiopronin, agranulocytosis, aplastic anemia, thrombocytopenia, severe reaction to penicillamine, pregnancy, lactation
- *Physical:* Temperature; skin—color, lesions; urinary output; urinalysis, urinary

Adverse effects in *Italics* are most common; those in **Bold** are life-threatening.

cystine levels, 24 h urinary protein, liver function tests, CBC, Hct, electrolytes

Implementation
- Attempt conservative measures to decrease stone formation before beginning drug therapy: Provide at least 3 L of fluid, including two glasses with each meal and at bedtime. Advise patient to get up at night to void and to drink two more glasses of fluid before returning to bed. Additional fluids should be added if sweating, diarrhea occur. A minimum urinary output of 2 L/d should be maintained. Alkali therapy may be used to keep urinary pH in a range of 6.5–7. If cystine stones continue to be formed, tiopronin therapy can be used.
- Arrange to initiate therapy at a lower than normal dose in patients with a history of severe penicillamine reaction.
- Administer in divided doses, tid at least 1 h before or 2 h after meals.
- Arrange to measure urinary cystine levels 1 mo after treatment and every 3 mo thereafter. Adjust dosage based on amount needed to keep cystine concentration below its solubility limit (generally < 250 mg/L).
- Monitor blood counts before and periodically during therapy.
- Monitor patient for any abnormal urinary findings. Discontinue drug if abnormalities occur.
- Discontinue drug if fever occurs; reinstate at a smaller dose, gradually increasing dosage until desired effect is achieved.

Drug-specific teaching points
- Take this drug three times a day, 1 h before or 2 h after meals. Arrange for periodic blood and urine tests to determine the effects of the drug on your blood count and urine and to determine the appropriate dosage needed. It is important that you keep appointments for these tests.
- Continue to drink at least 3 L of fluid each day. Get up to void during the night, and drink more fluid before returning to bed.
- Know that the following side effects may occur: skin rash, easy breaking of skin (proper skin care will be very important).
- Report fever, sore throat, chills, bleeding, easy bruising.
- Maintain all of the dietary and other treatments being prescribed for your chronic kidney stone condition.

tobramycin sulfate

(toe bra mye' sin)

Nebcin (parenteral), Tobrex Ophthalmic

Pregnancy Category B

Drug classes
Aminoglycoside antibiotic

Therapeutic actions
Bactericidal: inhibits protein synthesis in susceptible strains of gram-negative bacteria; mechanism of lethal action is not fully understood, but functional integrity of bacterial cell membrane appears to be disrupted.

Indications
- Serious infections caused by susceptible strains of *P. aeruginosa, E. coli*, indole-positive *Proteus* species, *Providencia* species, *Klebsiella-Enterobacter-Serratia* group, *Citrobacter* species, and staphylococci (including *S. aureus*; parenteral)
- Staphylococcal infections when penicillin is contraindicated or when the bacteria are not susceptible
- Serious, life-threatening gram-negative infections when susceptibility studies have not been completed (sometimes concurrent penicillin or cephalosporin therapy)
- Treatment of superficial ocular infections due to susceptible strains of organisms (ophthalmic solution)

Contraindications/cautions
- Contraindicated in the presence of allergy to aminoglycosides; pregnancy, lactation.
- Use caution in the presence of the elderly or to any patient with diminished hearing, decreased renal function, dehydra-

1080 ■ tobramycin sulfate

tion, neuromuscular disorders (myasthenia gravis, parkinsonism, infant botulism); herpes, vaccinia, varicella, mycobacterial infections, fungal infections (ophthalmic solutions).

Dosage

IM or IV

- **Adult:** 3 mg/kg per day in three equal doses q8h. Up to 5 mg/kg per day in three to four equal doses can be used in life-threatening infections, but reduce to 3 mg/kg per day as soon as possible. Do not exceed 5 mg/kg per day unless serum levels are monitored.
- **Pediatric:** 6–7.5 mg/kg per day divided into three to four equal doses q6–8h.
- *Prematures or neonates younger than 1 wk:* Up to 4 mg/kg per day in two equal doses q12h.
- **Geriatric or renal failure patients:** Reduce dosage, and carefully monitor serum drug levels and renal function tests throughout treatment. Reduced dosage nomogram is available; consult manufacturer's information.

Eye solution

- *Mild to moderate disease:* 1–2 drops into conjunctival sac of affected eye(s) q4h.
- *Severe disease:* 2 drops into conjunctival sac of affected eye(s) hourly until improvement occurs.

Ophthalmic ointment: $\frac{1}{2}$-in ribbon bid–tid. Severe infection, $\frac{1}{2}$-in q3–4h.

Pharmacokinetics

Route	Onset	Peak
IM/IV	Rapid	30–90 min
Ophthalmologic	Rapid	

Metabolism: Minimal hepatic, $T_{1/2}$: 2–3 h
Distribution: Crosses placenta; enters breast milk
Excretion: Urine

IV facts

Preparation: Dilute vials of solution for injection. Usual volume of diluent is 50–100 ml of 9% Sodium Chloride Injection or 5% Dextrose Injection (less for children). Reconstitute powder for injection with Sterile Water for Injection according to manufacturer's instructions.

Infusion: Infuse over 20–60 min.
Compatibilities: Do not premix with other drugs; administer other drugs seperately.

Adverse effects

- **CNS:** Ototoxicity, vestibular paralysis, confusion, disorientation, depression, lethargy, nystagmus, visual disturbances, headache, *numbness, tingling,* tremor, paresthesias, muscle twitching, convulsions, muscular weakness, neuromuscular blockade
- **GI:** Hepatic toxicity, *nausea, vomiting, anorexia,* weight loss, stomatitis, increased salivation
- **CV:** Palpitations, hypotension, hypertension
- **Hematologic:** *Leukemoid reaction,* agranulocytosis, granulocytosis, leukopenia, leukocytosis, thrombocytopenia, eosinophilia, pancytopenia, anemia, hemolytic anemia, increased or decreased reticulocyte count, electrolyte disturbances
- **GU:** *Nephrotoxicity*
- **EENT:** Localized ocular toxicity and hypersensitivity reactions; *lid itching, swelling;* conjunctival erythema; punctate keratitis
- **Hypersensitivity:** Hypersensitivity reactions: *purpura, rash,* urticaria, exfoliative dermatitis, itching
- **Local:** *Pain, irritation, arachnoiditis at IM injection sites*
- **Other:** Fever, apnea, splenomegaly, joint pain, *superinfections*

Clinically important drug-drug interactions

- Increased ototoxic, nephrotoxic, neurotoxic effects if taken with other aminoglycosides, cephalothin, potent diuretics • Increased neuromuscular blockade and muscular paralysis when given with anesthetics, nondepolarizing neuromuscular blocking drugs, succinylcholine • Poten-

Adverse effects in *Italics* are most common; those in **Bold** are life-threatening.

tial inactivation of both drugs if mixed with beta-lactam-type antibiotics. Increased bactericidal effect if combined with penicillins, cephalopsorins, carbenicillin, ticarcillin

■ Nursing Considerations

Assessment
- *History:* Allergy to aminoglycosides; diminished hearing, decreased renal function, dehydration, neuromuscular disorders, lactation, pregnancy; infections (ophthalmic solutions)
- *Physical:* Body weight; renal function, eighth cranial nerve function; state of hydration; hepatic function, CBC, skin—color and lesions; orientation and affect; reflexes; bilateral grip strength; body weight; bowel sounds

Implementation
- Arrange culture and sensitivity tests of infection before beginning therapy.
- Limit duration of treatment to short term to reduce the risk of toxicity; usual duration of treatment is 7–14 d.
- Use ophthalmologic tobramycin only when indicated by sensitivity tests; use of opthalmologic tobramycin may cause sensitization that will contraindicate the systemic use of tobramycin or other aminoglycosides in serious infections.
- Monitor total serum concentration of tobramycin if ophthalmologic solution is used concurrently with parenteral aminoglycosides.
- Administer IM dose by deep intramuscular injection.
- Assure that patient is well hydrated before and during therapy.

Drug-specific teaching points

Parenteral
- Report hearing changes, dizziness, pain at injection site.

Ophthalmic Solution
- Tilt head back; place medication into conjunctival sac, and close eye; apply light finger pressure on lacrimal sac for 1 min.
- Know that solution may cause blurring of vision or stinging on administration.
- Report severe stinging, itching, or burning.

❒ tocainide hydrochloride

(toe kay' nide)
Tonocard

Pregnancy Category C

Drug classes
Antiarrhythmic

Therapeutic actions
Type 1B antiarrhythmic: decreases the excitability of myocardial cells by a dose-dependent decrease in Na^+ and K^+ conductance.

Indications
- Treatment of life-threatening ventricular arrhythmias
- Unlabeled uses: treatment of myotonic dystrophy, trigeminal neuralgia

Contraindications/cautions
- Contraindicated in the presence of allergy to tocainide or amide-type local anesthetics, cardiac conduction abnormalities (heart block in the absence of an artificial ventricular pacemaker), pregnancy (abortions and stillbirths have occurred), lactation.
- Use caution in the presence of CHF, atrial fibrillation or atrial flutter, renal or hepatic disease, potassium imbalance, bone marrow failure, cytopenia.

Dosage
Careful patient assessment and evaluation with close monitoring of cardiac response are necessary for determining the correct dosage for each patient.
Adult: 400 mg PO q8h. 1,200–1,800 mg/d in three divided doses is the suggested therapeutic range.
Pediatric: Safety and efficacy not established.
Geriatric or renal/hepatic impairment: Lower doses required; < 1,200 mg/d may suffice.

Pharmacokinetics

Route	Onset	Peak
Oral	Varies	30–120 min

Metabolism: Hepatic, $T_{1/2}$: 15 h
Distribution: Crosses placenta; enters breast milk
Excretion: Urine

Adverse effects
- **CNS:** *Lightheadedness, dizziness,* fatigue, drowsiness, disorientation, hallucinations, *numbness, paresthesias,* visual disturbances,*tremor*
- **GI:** *Nausea,* vomiting, abdominal pain, diarrhea
- **CV:** CHF, cardiac arrhythmias
- **Respiratory:** Pulmonary fibrosis, **pneumonitis**
- **Hematologic:** Leukopenia, agranulocytosis, hypoplastic anemia, thrombocytopenia
- **Dermatologic:** Sweating, hot flashes, night sweats

Clinically important drug-drug interactions
- Decreased pharmacologic effects of tocainide if taken concurrently with rifampin

■ Nursing Considerations

Assessment
- *History:* Allergy to tocainide or amide-type local anesthetics, CHF, cardiac conduction abnormalities, atrial fibrillation or atrial flutter, hepatic or renal disease, potassium imbalance, pregnancy, lactation
- *Physical:* Body weight; orientation, reflexes; P, BP, auscultation, ECG, edem; R, adventitious sounds; bowel sounds, liver evaluation; urinalysis, CBC, serum electrolytes, renal and liver function tests

Implementation
- Carefully monitor patient response, especially when beginning therapy.
- Reduce dosage in patients with renal or hepatic disease.
- Check serum K^t levels before administration.
- Carefully monitor cardiac rhythm.
- Arrange for regular follow-up of blood counts.
- Evaluate for safe and effective serum levels (4–10 μg/ml).

Drug-specific teaching points
- Be aware that you will require frequent monitoring of cardiac rhythm.
- Know that the following side effects may occur: drowsiness, dizziness, numbness (avoid driving or working with dangerous machinery until you know your response to the drug); nausea, vomiting, diarrhea (small, frequent meals may help); sweating, night sweats, hot flashes.
- Do not stop taking this drug for any reason without checking with your health care provider.
- Return for regular follow-up visits to check your heart rhythm and blood cell counts.
- Report cough, wheezing, difficulty breathing, unusual bleeding or bruising, fever, chills, sore throat, tremors, visual changes, palpitations.

☐ tolazamide

*(tole **az'** a mide)*
Tolinase

Pregnancy Category C

Drug classes
Antidiabetic agent
Sulfonylurea, first generation

Therapeutic actions
Stimulates insulin release from functioning beta cells in the pancreas; may improve binding between insulin and insulin receptors or increase the number of insulin receptors; has significant uricosuric activity.

Indications
- Adjunct to diet to lower blood glucose in patients with non–insulin-dependent diabetes mellitus (type II)

Adverse effects in *Italics* are most common; those in **Bold** are life-threatening.

tolazamide ■ 1083

- Adjunct to insulin therapy in the stabilization of certain cases of insulin-dependent maturity-onset diabetes, reducing the insulin requirement and decreasing the chance of hypoglycemic reactions

Contraindications/cautions

- Contraindicated in the presence of allergy to sulfonylureas; diabetes complicated by fever, severe infections, severe trauma, major surgery, ketosis, acidosis, coma (insulin is indicated in these conditions); type I or juvenile diabetes; serious hepatic or renal impairment; pregnancy.
- Use caution in the presence of uremia, thyroid or endocrine impairment, glycosuria, hyperglycemia associated with primary renal disease, lactation.

Dosage

Adult: 100 mg/d PO if fasting blood sugar (FBS) is < 200 mg%, or 250 mg/d if FBS is > 200 mg%. Adjust dose accordingly. If dose is larger than 500 mg/d, give in divided doses bid. Dosage greater than 1 g/d not recommended.

Pediatric: Safety and efficacy not established.

Geriatric: Geriatric patients tend to be more sensitive to the drug. Start with a lower initial dose; monitor for 24 h, and gradually increase dose as needed.

Pharmacokinetics

Route	Onset	Peak	Duration
Oral	Varies	4–6 h	12–24 h

Metabolism: Hepatic, $T_{1/2}$: 7 h
Distribution: Crosses placenta; enters breast milk
Excretion: Urine

Adverse effects

- **GI:** *Anorexia, nausea, vomiting, epigastric discomfort, heartburn*
- **Hematologic:** *Hypoglycemia*, leukopenia, thrombocytopenia, anemia
- **Dermatologic:** Allergic skin reactions, eczema, pruritus, erythema, urticaria, photosensitivity
- **Hypersensitivity:** Fever, eosinophilia, jaundice
- **Other:** Possible increased risk of cardiovascular mortality

Clinically important drug-drug interactions

- Increased risk of hypoglycemia if tolazamide is taken concurrently with insulin, sulfonamides, chloramphenicol, fenfluramine, oxyphenbutazone, phenylbutazone, salicylates, clofibrate, monoamine oxidase inhibitors • Decreased effectiveness of both tolazamide and diazoxide if taken concurrently • Increased risk of hyperglycemia if tolazamide is taken with thiazides, other diuretics • Risk of hypoglycemia and hyperglycemia if tolazamide is taken with ethanol; "disulfiram reaction" also has been reported.

■ Nursing Considerations

Assessment

- *History:* Allergy to sulfonylureas; diabetes complicated by fever, severe infections, severe trauma, major surgery, ketosis, acidosis, coma; type I or juvenile diabetes; serious hepatic or renal impairment; uremia; thyroid or endocrine impairment; glycosuria; hyperglycemia associated with primary renal disease; pregnancy; lactation
- *Physical:* Skin—color, lesions; body temperature; orientation, reflexes, peripheral sensation; R, adventitious sounds; liver evaluation, bowel sounds; urinalysis, BUN, serum creatinine, liver function tests, blood glucose, CBC

Implementation

- Administer drug in the morning before breakfast. If severe GI upset occurs or if dosage is > 500 g/d, dose may be divided with one dose before breakfast and one before the evening meal.
- Monitor urine and serum glucose levels frequently to determine effectiveness of drug and dosage.
- Arrange for transfer to insulin therapy during periods of high stress, infections, surgery, trauma, and so forth.
- Arrange for use of IV glucose if severe hypoglycemia occurs as a result of overdose.

Adverse effects in *Italics* are most common; those in **Bold** are life-threatening.

Drug-specific teaching points

- Do not discontinue this medication without consulting physician.
- Monitor urine or blood for glucose and ketones as prescribed,
- Be aware that the drug is not to be used during pregnancy.
- Avoid alcohol while on this drug.
- Report fever, sore throat, unusual bleeding or bruising, skin rash, dark urine, light-colored stools, hypoglycemic or hyperglycemic reactions.

▢ tolazoline hydrochloride

(toe laz' a leen)

Priscoline

Pregnancy Category C

Drug classes
Vasodilator
Antihypertensive

Therapeutic actions
Weak alpha-adrenergic blocker; increases cardiac output and heart rate, increases GI motility, stimulates GI secretions, and causes peripheral vasodilation.

Indications
- Persistent pulmonary hypertension of the newborn when systemic arterial oxygenation cannot be maintained by the usual methods
- Unlabeled uses: to improve blood flow in peripheral vascular diseases, to improve visualization of vessels during arteriography

Contraindications/cautions
- Allergy to tolazoline.

Dosage
Adult
- ***Vascular disorders:*** 10–50 mg SC, IM, IV qid.
- ***Improve visualization of vessels:*** 12.5–50 mg prior to arteriography

Pediatric: 1–2 mg IV through scalp needle over 10 min; follow with an infusion of 1–2 mg/kg per hour for 36–48 h.

Pharmacokinetics

Route	Onset	Peak	Duration
IV, IM, SC	Varies	30–60 min	3–4 h

Metabolism: Hepatic, $T_{1/2}$: 1.5–41 h
Distribution: May cross placenta or enter breast milk
Excretion: Urine

IV facts
Preparation: No further preparation is required.
Infusion: Initial injection over 10 min; then use metered delivery system and dilute into an infusion of dextrose, saline, Lactated Ringer's or combination of these.
Compatiblities: Do not mix with other drugs.

Adverse effects
- GI: Nausea, vomiting, diarrhea, hepatitis, **GI hemorrhage**
- CV: Hypotension, tachycardia, arrhythmias, hypertension, **pulmonary hemmorhage**
- Hematologic: Leukopenia, thrombocytopenia
- Dermatologic: Flushing, pilomotor acitivity, rash
- Renal: Edema, oliguria, hematuria

Clinically important drug-drug interactions
- Risk of severe hypotension when given with epinephrine

■ Nursing Considerations

Assessment
- *History:* Allergy to tolazoline; hypotension, pregnancy, lactation
- *Physical:* Skin—color, lesions; body temperature; orientation, reflexes, peripheral sensation; R, adventitious sounds; BP, P, peripheral perfusion; renal and liver function tests

Implementation
- Store in refrigerator and protect from light.
- Administer antacid before tolazoline dose to decrease problems associated with increased gastric secretions.
- Monitor blood pressure closely during administration; arrange for supportive therapy as needed.
- Monitor acid–base balance, oxygenation, vital signs, and electrolytes carefully during administration.
- Assess patients for signs of bleeding: bruising, dark stools, petechiae, vomiting.

Drug-specific teaching points
- Incorporate teaching about this drug into the overall teaching plan for the parents of the affected newborn.

◻ tolbutamide

(tole byoo' ta mide)
Mobenol (CAN),
Novobutamide (CAN),
Oramide, Orinase

Pregnancy Category C

Drug classes
Antidiabetic agent
Sulfonylurea, first generation

Therapeutic actions
Stimulates insulin release from functioning beta cells in the pancreas; may improve binding between insulin and insulin receptors or increase the number of insulin receptors.

Indications
- Adjunct to diet to lower blood glucose in patients with non–insulin-dependent diabetes mellitus (type II)
- Adjunct to insulin therapy in the stabilization of certain cases of insulin-dependent maturity-onset diabetes, reducing the insulin requirement and decreasing the chance of hypoglycemic reactions

Contraindications/cautions
- Contraindicated in the presence of allergy to sulfonylureas; diabetes complicated by fever, severe infections, severe trauma, major surgery, ketosis, acidosis, coma (insulin is indicated in these conditions); type I or juvenile diabetes; serious hepatic or renal impairment, uremia; thyroid or endocrine impairment; glycosuria, hyperglycemia associated with primary renal disease, pregnancy, lactation.

Dosage
Adult: 0.25–3 g/d PO in single morning or divided doses. Maintenance dosage, > 2 g/d is seldom required.
Pediatric: Safety and efficacy not established.
Geriatric: Geriatric patients tend to be more sensitive to the drug. Start with a lower initial dose, monitor for 24 h, and gradually increase dose as needed.

Pharmacokinetics

Route	Onset	Peak	Duration
Oral	1 h	4–6 h	6–12 h

Metabolism: Hepatic, $T_{1/2}$: 7 h
Distribution: Crosses placenta; enters breast milk
Excretion: Urine

Adverse effects
- **GI:** *Anorexia, nausea, vomiting, epigastric discomfort, heartburn*
- **Hematologic:** *Hypoglycemia*, leukopenia, thrombocytopenia, anemia
- **Dermatologic:** Allergic skin reactions, eczema, pruritus, erythema, urticaria, photosensitivity
- **Hypersensitivity:** Fever, eosinophilia, jaundice
- **Other:** Possible increased risk of cardiovascular mortality

Clinically important drug-drug interactions
- Increased risk of hypoglycemia if tolbutamide is taken concurrently with insulin, sulfonamides, chloramphenicol, fenfluramine, oxyphenbutazone, phenylbutazone, salicylates, clofibrate, MAOIs, dicumarol, ri-

fampin • Decreased effectiveness of both tolbutamide and diazoxide if taken concurrently • Increased risk of hyperglycemia if tolbutamide is taken with thiazides, other diuretics • Risk of hypoglycemia and hyperglycemia if tolbutamide is taken with ethanol

Drug-lab test interferences
- False-positive reaction for urine albumin if measured with acidification-after-boiling-test; no interference has been reported using sulfosalicylic acid test

■ Nursing Considerations

Assessment
- *History:* Allergy to sulfonylureas; diabetes complicated by fever, severe infections, severe trauma, major surgery, ketosis, acidosis, coma; type I or juvenile diabetes; serious hepatic or renal impairment; uremia; thyroid or endocrine impairment; glycosuria, hyperglycemia associated with primary renal disease; pregnancy; lactation
- *Physical:* Skin—color, lesions; body temperature; orientation, reflexes, peripheral sensation; R, adventitious sounds; liver evaluation, bowel sounds; urinalysis, BUN, serum creatinine, liver function tests, blood glucose, CBC

Implementation
- Administer drug in the morning before breakfast; if severe GI upset occurs, dose may be divided.
- Monitor urine and serum glucose levels frequently to determine effectiveness of drug and dosage.
- Transfer patients from one oral hypoglycemic agent to another with no transitional period or priming dose.
- Arrange for transfer to insulin therapy during periods of high stress (eg, infections, surgery, trauma).
- Arrange for use of IV glucose if severe hypoglycemia occurs as a result of overdose.

Drug-specific teaching points
- Take this drug early in the morning before breakfast. If GI upset occurs, drug may be taken with food or in divided doses. Do not discontinue this medication without consulting your health care provider.
- Know that the following side effects may occur: nausea, GI upset, vomiting (taking the drug with food may help); diarrhea; rash, delays in healing (use good skin care; try to avoid injury).
- Be aware that this drug is not to be used during pregnancy. If you become pregnant or want to become pregnant, consult your prescriber.
- Avoid alcohol while on this drug; serious reactions can occur.
- Report fever, sore throat, unusual bleeding or bruising, skin rash, dark urine, light-colored stools, hypoglycemic or hyperglycemic reactions.

🗋 tolmetin sodium

(tole' met in)
Tolectin, Tolectin DS

Pregnancy Category C

Drug classes
NSAID

Therapeutic actions
Anti-inflammatory, analgesic, and antipyretic activities largely related to inhibition of prostaglandin synthesis; exact mechanisms of action are not known.

Indications
- Treatment of acute flares and long-term management of rheumatoid arthritis
- Treatment of juvenile rheumatoid arthritis

Contraindications/cautions
- Contraindicated in the presence of pregnancy, lactation.
- Use caution in the presence of allergies, renal, hepatic, cardiovascular, and GI conditions.

Dosage
Do not exceed 2,000 mg/d (rheumatoid arthritis) or 1,600 mg/d (osteoarthritis).
Adult
- ***Rheumatoid arthritis/osteoarthritis:*** Initial dose, 400 mg PO tid

(1,200 mg/d) preferably including doses on arising and at bedtime. Maintenance dose, 600–1,800 mg/d in three to four divided doses for rheumatoid arthritis, 600–1,600 mg/d in three to four divided doses for osteoarthritis.
Pediatric (> 2 y): 20 mg/kg per day PO in three to four divided doses; when control has been achieved, the usual dose is 15–30 mg/kg per day. Do not exceed 30 mg/kg per day.

Pharmacokinetics

Route	Onset	Peak
Oral	Varies	30–60 min

Metabolism: Hepatic, $T_{1/2}$: 1–1.5 h
Distribution: Crosses placenta; enters breast milk
Excretion: Urine

Adverse effects

- CNS: *Headache, dizziness, somnolence, insomnia*, fatigue, tiredness, dizziness, tinnitus, ophthalmologic effects
- GI: *Nausea, dyspepsia, GI pain, diarrhea*, vomiting, constipation, flatulence
- **Respiratory:** Dyspnea, hemoptysis, pharyngitis, bronchospasm, rhinitis
- **Hematologic:** Bleeding, platelet inhibition with higher doses, neutropenia, eosinophilia, leukopenia, pancytopenia, thrombocytopenia, agranulocytosis, granulocytopenia, aplastic anemia, decreased hemoglobin or hematocrit, bone marrow depression, mennorhagia
- GU: Dysuria, renal impairment, including renal failure, interstitial nephritis, hematuria
- **Dermatologic:** *Rash*, pruritus, sweating, dry mucous membranes, stomatitis
- **Other:** Peripheral edema, anaphylactoid reactions to fatal anaphylactic shock

Drug-lab test interferences

- False-positive tests for proteinuria using acid precipitation tests; no interference has been reported with dye-impregnated reagent strips.

■ Nursing Considerations

Assessment
- *History:* Allergies, renal, hepatic, cardiovascular, and GI conditions; pregnancy, lactation
- *Physical:* Skin—color and lesions; orientation, reflexes, ophthalmologic and audiometric evaluation, peripheral sensation; P, edema; R, adventitious sounds; liver evaluation; CBC, clotting times, renal and liver function tests; serum electrolytes, stool guaiac

Implementation
- Administer with milk or food; bioavailability is decreased by up to 16%.
- Use antacids other than sodium bicarbonate if GI upset occurs.
- Arrange for periodic ophthalmologic examination during long-term therapy.
- Institute emergency procedures if overdose occurs—gastric lavage, induction of emesis, supportive therapy.

Drug-specific teaching points
- Take drug with food.
- Take only the prescribed dosage.
- Know that dizziness, drowsiness can occur (avoid driving or the use of dangerous machinery while on this drug).
- Report sore throat, fever, rash, itching, weight gain, swelling in ankles or fingers; changes in vision; black, tarry stools.

☐ torsemide

(tor' seh myde)
Demadex

Pregnancy Category B

Drug classes
Loop (high-ceiling) diuretic

Therapeutic actions
Inhibits the reabsorption of sodium and chloride from the proximal and distal renal tubules and the loop of Henle, leading to a natriuretic diuresis.

Adverse effects in *Italics* are most common; those in **Bold** are life-threatening.

Indications
- Treatment of hypertension and edema associated with CHF, hepatic disease, renal disease

Contraindications/cautions
- Allergy to torsemide; electrolyte depletion; anuria, severe renal failure; hepatic coma; SLE; gout; diabetes mellitus; lactation

Dosage
Do not exceed 200 mg/d.
Adult
- ***CHF:*** 10–20 mg PO or IV qd. Dose may be titrated upward until desired results are seen.
- ***Chronic renal failure:*** 20 mg PO or IV qd. Dose may be titrated upward until desired results are seen.
- ***Hepatic failure:*** 5–10 mg PO or IV qd. Do not exceed 40 mg/d.
- ***Hypertension:*** 5 mg PO qd. May be increased to 10 mg if response is not sufficient.

Pediatric: Safety and efficacy not established.

Pharmacokinetics

Route	Onset	Peak	Duration
Oral	60 min	60–120 min	6–8 h
IV	10 min	60 min	6–8 h

Metabolism: $T_{1/2}$: 210 min
Distribution: Crosses placenta; may enter breast milk
Excretion: Unchanged in the urine

IV facts
Preparation: May be given direct IV or diluted in solution with 5% Dextrose in Water, 0.9% Sodium Chloride, Lactated Ringer's Solution. Discard unused solution after 24 h.

Infusion: Give by direct injection slowly, over 1–2 min. Further diluted in solution, give slowly.

Adverse effects
- CNS: *Asterixis, dizziness,* vertigo, paresthesias, confusion, fatigue, nystagmus, *weakness, headache, drowsiness,* fatigue, blurred vision, tinnitus, irreversible hearing loss
- GI: *Nausea, anorexia, vomiting, diarrhea,* gastric irritation and pain, dry mouth, acute pancreatitis, jaundice
- CV: *Orthostatic hypotension,* volume depletion, cardiac arrhythmias, thrombophlebitis
- GU: *Polyuria, nocturia,* glycosuria, renal failure
- Hematologic: *Hypokalemia,* leukopenia, anemia, thrombocytopenia
- Local: *Pain, phlebitis at injection site*
- Other: Muscle cramps and muscle spasms, weakness, arthritic pain, fatigue, hives, photosensitivity, rash, pruritus, sweating, nipple tenderness

Clinically important drug-drug interactions
- Decreased diuresis and natriuresis with NSAIDs • Increased risk of cardiac glycoside toxicity (secondary to hypokalemia)
- Increased risk of ototoxicity if taken with aminoglycoside antibiotics, cisplatin

■ Nursing Considerations
Assessment
- *History:* Allergy to torsemide, electrolyte depletion, anuria, severe renal failure, hepatic coma, SLE, gout, diabetes mellitus, lactation
- *Physical:* Skin—color, lesions; edema; orientation, reflexes, hearing; pulses, baseline ECG, BP, orthostatic BP, perfusion; R, pattern, adventitious sounds; liver evaluation, bowel sounds; urinary output patterns; CBC, serum electrolytes, blood sugar, liver and renal function tests, uric acid, urinalysis

Implementation
- Administer with food or milk to prevent GI upset.
- Mark calendars or other reminders of drug days for outpatients if intermittent therapy is the most effective for treating edema.
- Administer single daily doses early in the day so increased urination will not disturb sleep.

Adverse effects in *Italics* are most common; those in **Bold** are life-threatening.

- Avoid IV use if oral use is at all possible.
- Measure and record regular body weights to monitor fluid changes.
- Arrange to monitor serum electrolytes, hydration, liver function during long-term therapy.
- Provide diet rich in potassium or supplemental potassium.

Drug-specific teaching points
- Record alternate-day or intermittent therapy on a calendar or dated envelopes.
- Take the drug early in the day so increased urination will not disturb sleep.
- Take the drug with food or meals to prevent GI upset.
- Weigh yourself on a regular basis, at the same time of the day and in the same clothing, and record the weight on your calendar.
- Know that the following side effects may occur: increased volume and frequency of urination (have ready access to a bathroom when drug effect is greatest); dizziness, feeling faint on arising, drowsiness (if these changes occur, avoid rapid position changes and hazardous activities [like driving a car] and alcohol consumption, which can intensify these problems); sensitivity to sunlight (use sunglasses, wear protective clothing, or use a sunscreen when outdoors); increased thirst (sucking on sugarless lozenges may help to alleviate the thirst; frequent mouth care also may help); loss of body potassium (a potassium-rich diet, or even a potassium supplement, will be necessary).
- Report loss or gain of more than 3 lb in one day; swelling in your ankles or fingers; unusual bleeding or bruising; nausea, dizziness, trembling, numbness, fatigue; muscle weakness or cramps.

▢ tranylcypromine sulfate

*(tran ill **sip**' roe meen)*

Parnate

Pregnancy Category C

tranylcypromine sulfate ■ 1089

Drug classes
Antidepressant
MAOIs, hydrazine derivative

Therapeutic actions
Irreversibly inhibits MAO, an enzyme that breaks down biogenic amines, such as epinephrine, norepinephrine, and serotonin, allowing these biogenic amines to accumulate in neuronal storage sites; according to the "biogenic amine hypothesis," this accumulation of amines is responsible for the clinical efficacy of MAOIs as antidepressants.

Indications
- Treatment of adult outpatients with reactive depression; efficacy in endogenous depression has not been established
- Unlabeled use: treatment of bulimia having characteristics of atypical depression

Contraindications/cautions
- Contraindicated in the presence of hypersensitivity to any MAOI; pheochromocytoma, CHF; history of liver disease or abnormal liver function tests; severe renal impairment; confirmed or suspected cerebrovascular defect; cardiovascular disease, hypertension; history of headache (headache is an important indicator of hypertensive reaction to drug); myelography within previous 24 h or scheduled within 48 h; lactation.
- Use caution in the presence of seizure disorders; hyperthyroidism; impaired hepatic, renal function; psychiatric patients (agitated or schizophrenic patients may show excessive stimulation; manic-depressive patients may shift to hypomanic or manic phase); patients scheduled for elective surgery (MAOIs should be discontinued 10 d before surgery); pregnancy or in women of childbearing age.

Dosage
Improvement should be seen within 48 h to 3 wk.
Adult: Usual effective dose is 30 mg/d PO in divided doses. If no improvement is seen within 2 wk, increase dosage in 10 mg/d in increments of 1 to 3 wk. May be increased to a maximum of 60 mg/d.

Pediatric: Not recommended for children younger than 16 y.
Geriatric: Patients older than 60 y are more prone to develop adverse effects; use with caution.

Pharmacokinetics

Route	Onset	Duration
Oral	Rapid	10 d

Metabolism: Hepatic, $T_{1/2}$: unkown
Distribution: Crosses placenta; enters breast milk
Excretion: Urine

Adverse effects

- **CNS:** *Dizziness, vertigo, headache, overactivity, hyperreflexia, tremors, muscle twitching, mania, hypomania, jitteriness, confusion, memory impairment, insomnia, weakness, fatigue, drowsiness, restlessness, overstimulation, increased anxiety, agitation, blurred vision, sweating,* akathisia, ataxia, coma, euphoria, neuritis, repetitious babbling, chills, glaucoma, nystagmus
- **GI:** *Constipation, diarrhea, nausea, abdominal pain, edema, dry mouth, anorexia, weight changes*
- **CV:** Hypertensive crises, sometimes fatal, sometimes with intracranial bleeding, usually attributable to ingestion of contraindicated food or drink containing tyramine (see ''Drug-Food Interactions'' below); symptoms include some or all of the following: occipital headache, which may radiate frontally; palpitations; neck stiffness or soreness; nausea; vomiting; sweating (sometimes with fever, cold and clammy skin); dilated pupils; photophobia; tachycardia or bradycardia; chest pain; *orthostatic hypotension, sometimes associated with falling; disturbed cardiac rate and rhythm,* palpitations, tachycardia
- **GU:** Dysuria, incontinence, urinary retention, sexual disturbances
- **Dermatologic:** Minor skin reactions, spider telangiectases, photosensitivity
- **Other:** Hematologic changes, black tongue, hypernatremia

Clinically important drug-drug interactions

- Increased sympathomimetic effects (hypertensive crisis) when given with sympathomimetic drugs (norepinephrine, epinephrine, dopamine, dobutamine, levodopa, ephedrine), amphetamines, other anorexiants, local anesthetic solutions containing sympathomimetics • Hypertensive crisis, coma, severe convulsions when given with tricyclic antidepressants (eg, imipramine, desipramine) • Additive hypoglycemic effect when given with insulin, oral sulfonylureas (eg, tolbutamide) • Increased risk of adverse interactive actions if taken concurrently with meperidine

Clinically important drug-food interactions

- Tyramine (and other pressor amines) contained in foods are normally broken down by MAO enzymes in the GI tract; in the presence of MAOIs, these vasopressors may be absorbed in high concentrations; in addition, tyramine releases accumulated norepinephrine from nerve terminals; thus, hypertensive crisis may occur when the following foods that contain tyramine or other vasopressors are ingested by a patient on an MAOI: dairy products (blue, camembert, cheddar, mozzarella, parmesan, romano, roquefort, Stilton cheeses; sour cream; yogurt); meats, fish (liver, pickled herring, fermented sausages [bologna, pepperoni, salami], caviar, dried fish, other fermented or spoiled meat or fish); undistilled beverages (imported beer, ale; red wine, especially Chianti; sherry; coffee, tea, colas containing caffeine; chocolate drinks); fruit/vegetables (avocado, fava beans, figs, raisins, bananas, yeast extracts, soy sauce, chocolate)

■ Nursing Considerations

Assessment

- *History:* Hypersensitivity to any MAOI; pheochromocytoma, CHF; abnormal liver function tests; severe renal impairment; confirmed or suspected cerebrovascular defect; cardiovascular disease, hypertension; history of headache, myelography

Adverse effects in *Italics* are most common; those in **Bold** are life-threatening.

within previous 24 h or scheduled within 48 h; lactation; seizure disorders; hyperthyroidism; impaired hepatic, renal function; psychiatric patients; patients scheduled for elective surgery; pregnancy
- *Physical:* Body weight; temperature; skin—color, lesions; orientation, affect, reflexes, vision; P, BP, orthostatic BP, perfusion; bowel sounds, normal output, liver evaluation; urine flow, normal output; liver, kidney function tests, urinalysis, CBC, ECG, EEG

Implementation
- Limit amount of drug that is available to suicidal patients.
- Monitor BP and orthostatic BP carefully; arrange for more gradual increase in dosage initially in patients who show tendency for hypotension.
- Arrange for periodic liver function tests during therapy; arrange for discontinuation of drug at first sign of hepatic dysfunction or jaundice.
- Arrange to monitor BP carefully (and if appropriate, discontinue drug) if patient reports unusual or severe headache.
- Provide phentolamine or another alpha-adrenergic blocking drug on standby in case of hypertensive crisis.

Drug-specific teaching points
- Take drug exactly as prescribed.
- Do not stop taking drug abruptly or without consulting the physician or nurse.
- Avoid the ingestion of tyramine-containing foods or beverages while on this drug and for 10 d afterward (patient and significant other should receive a list of such foods and beverages).
- Know that the following side effects may occur: dizziness, weakness or fainting when arising from a horizontal or sitting position (change position slowly; these effects usually disappear after a few days of therapy); drowsiness, blurred vision (these effects are reversible; safety measures may need to be taken if these become severe; avoid driving an automobile or performing tasks that require alertness while these persist); nausea, vomiting, loss of appetite (small, frequent meals, frequent mouth care may help); nightmares, confusion, inability to concentrate, emotional changes; changes in sexual function.
- Report headache, skin rash, darkening of the urine, pale stools, yellowing of the eyes or skin, fever, chills, sore throat, or any other unusual symptoms.

☐ trazodone hydrochloride

(traz' oh done)
Desyrel

Pregnancy Category C

Drug classes
Antidepressant
SSRI

Therapeutic actions
Mechanism of action unknown; differs from other antidepressants in that it is a triazolopyridine compound, not a tricyclic antidepressant, not an amphetamine-like CNS stimulant, and not an MAOI; inhibits the presynaptic reuptake of the neurotransmitter serotonin and potentiates the behavioral effects of the serotonin precursor; the relation of these effects to clinical efficacy is unknown.

Indications
- Treatment of depression in inpatient and outpatient settings and for depressed patients with and without anxiety
- Unlabeled uses: treatment of aggressive behavior, cocaine withdrawal

Contraindications/cautions
- Contraindicated in the presence of hypersensitivity to trazodone, electroshock therapy, recent MI, pregnancy (congenital abnormalities have occurred).
- Use caution in the presence of preexisting cardiac disease (arrhythmias, including ventricular tachycardia, may be more likely), lactation.

Dosage
Adult: Initially 150 mg/d PO. May be increased by 50 mg/d every 3–4 d. Maximum dose for outpatients should not exceed

trazodone hydrochloride

400 mg/d in divided doses. Maximum dose for inpatients or those severely depressed should not exceed 600 mg/d in divided doses. Use lowest effective dosage for maintenance.

Pediatric: Safety and efficacy not established for children younger than 18 y.

Pharmacokinetics

Route	Onset	Peak
Oral	Varies	1–2 h

Metabolism: Hepatic, $T_{1/2}$: 3–6 h and then 5–9 h
Distribution: Crosses placenta; may enter breast milk
Excretion: Urine and feces

Adverse effects

- **CNS:** *Anger, hostility, agitation, nightmares/vivid dreams, hallucinations, delusions, hypomania, confusion, disorientation, decreased concentration, impaired memory, impaired speech, dizziness, incoordination, drowsiness, fatigue,* excitement, insomnia, nervousness, paresthesia, tremors, akathisia, headache, grand mal seizures, tinnitus, blurred vision, red eyes, nasal/sinus congestion, *malaise*
- **GI:** *Abdominal/gastric disorder, decreased/increased appetite, bad taste in mouth, dry mouth, hypersalivation, nausea, vomiting, diarrhea, flatulence, constipation*
- **CV:** *Hypertension, hypotension, shortness of breath, syncope, tachycardia, palpitations,* chest pain, myocardial infarction, ventricular ectopic activity, occasional sinus bradycardia with long-term use
- **Hematologic:** Anemia, neutropenia, leukopenia, liver enzyme alterations
- **GU:** *Decreased libido,* impotence, priapism, retrograde ejaculation, early menses, missed periods, hematuria, delayed urine flow, increased urinary frequency
- **MS:** Musculoskeletal aches and pains, muscle twitches
- **Hypersensitivity:** *Allergic skin conditions, edema,* rash
- **Other:** Sweating, clamminess

■ Nursing Considerations

Assessment

- *History:* Hypersensitivity to trazodone, electroshock therapy, recent MI, preexisting cardiac disease, pregnancy, lactation
- *Physical:* Skin—color, lesions; orientation, affect, reflexes, vision and hearing; P, BP, orthostatic BP, perfusion; bowel sounds, normal output, liver evaluation; urine flow, normal output; usual sexual function, frequency of menses; liver function tests, urinalysis, CBC, ECG

Implementation

- Ensure that depressed and potentially suicidal patients have access to only limited quantities of drug.
- Administer shortly after a meal or light snack to enhance absorption.
- Administer major portion of dose at bedtime if drowsiness occurs.
- Anticipate symptomatic relief during the first week of therapy with optimal effects within 2 wk (some patients require 2–4 wk to respond).
- Monitor patient for orthostatic hypotension during therapy.
- Arrange to discontinue therapy immediately if priapism occurs.
- Arrange for CBC if patient develops fever, sore throat, or other signs of infection during therapy.

Drug-specific teaching points

- Take drug with food or a snack to enhance absorption and decrease likelihood of dizziness.
- Avoid alcohol, other sleep-inducing drugs, over-the-counter OTC drugs while you are on this drug.
- Know that the following side effects may occur: ringing in the ears, headache, dizziness, drowsiness, weakness (these effects are reversible; safety measures may need to be taken if these become severe; avoid driving an automobile or per-

Adverse effects in *Italics* are most common; those in **Bold** are life-threatening.

forming tasks that require alertness while these persist); nausea, vomiting, loss of appetite (small, frequent meals, frequent mouth care may help); dry mouth (sucking sugarless candies may help); changes in sexual function and abilities; nightmares, dreams, confusion, inability to concentrate (it may help to know that these are effects of the drug and they may lessen with time).
- Report dizziness, lightheadedness, faintness, blood in urine, fever, chills, sore throat, skin rash, prolonged or inappropriate penile erection (discontinue drug immediately).

☐ triamcinolone

(trye am sin' oh lone)
Oral: Kenacort

triamcinolone acetonide

IM, intra-articular, or soft-tissue injection; respiratory inhalant; dermatologic ointment, cream, lotion, aerosol: Aristocort, Azmacort, Cenocort A-40, Flutex, Kenaject, Kenalog, Triacet, Triamonide, Triderm

triamcinolone diacetate

IM, intra-articular, intrasynovial, intralesional injection: Amcort, Aristocort Intralesional, Articulose, Cenocort Forte, Triam Forte, Triamolone 40, Trilone, Tristoject

triamcinolone hexacetonide

Intra-articular, intralesional injection: Aristospan Intra-articular, Aristospan Intralesional

Pregnancy Category C

Drug classes

Corticosteroid (intermediate acting)
Glucocorticoid
Hormonal agent

Therapeutic actions

Enters target cells and binds to cytoplasmic receptors, thereby initiating many complex reactions that are responsible for its anti-inflammatory and immunosuppressive effects.

Indications

- Hypercalcemia associated with cancer (systemic)
- Short-term management of various inflammatory and allergic disorders, such as rheumatoid arthritis, collagen diseases (eg, SLE), dermatologic diseases (eg, pemphigus), status asthmaticus, and autoimmune disorders
- Hematologic disorders: thrombocytopenia purpura, erythroblastopenia
- Ulcerative colitis, acute exacerbations of mutiple sclerosis, and palliation in some leukemias and lymphomas
- Trichinosis with neurologic or myocardial involvement
- Pulmonary emphysema with bronchial spasm or edema; diffuse interstitial pulmonary fibrosis; with diuretics in CHF with refractory edema and in cirrhosis with refractory ascites
- Postoperative dental inflammatory reactions
- Arthritis, psoriatic plaques, and so forth (intra-articular, soft-tissue administration)
- Control of bronchial asthma requiring corticosteroids in conjunction with other therapy (respiratory inhalant)
- To relieve inflammatory and pruritic manifestations of dermatoses that are steroid responsive (dermatologic preparations)

Contraindications/cautions

- Contraindicated in the presence of infections, especially tuberculosis, fungal infectons, amebiasis, vaccinia and varicella, and antibiotic-resistant infections; lactation; allergy to tartrazine in 8-mg oral tablets marketed under the brand name *Kenacort*.
- Use caution in the presence of pregnancy (teratogenic in preclinical studies); kidney or liver disease, hypothyroidism, ulcerative colitis with impending perfora-

tion, diverticulitis, active or latent peptic ulcer, inflammatory bowel disease, CHF, hypertension, thromboembolic disorders, osteoporosis, convulsive disorders, diabetes mellitus.

Dosage

Systemic
- **Adult:** Individualize dosage, depending on the severity of the condition and the patient's response. Administer daily dose before 9 AM to minimize adrenal suppression. If long-term therapy is needed, alternate-day therapy should be considered. After long-term therapy, withdraw drug slowly to avoid adrenal insufficiency. For maintenance therapy, reduce initial dose in small increments at intervals until the lowest dose that maintains satisfactory clinical response is reached.
- **Pediatric:** Individualize dosage, depending on the severity of the condition and the patient's response rather than by strict adherence to formulae that correct adult doses for age or body weight. Carefully observe growth and development in infants and children on prolonged therapy.

Oral (triamcinolone)
– *Adrenal insufficiency:* 4–12 mg/d, plus a mineralocorticoid.
– *Rheumatic, dermatologic, allergic, opthtbalmologic, hematologic disorders and asthma:* 8–60 mg/d.
– *Tuberculosis meningitis:* 32–48 mg/d.
– *Acute leukemia: Adult:* 16–40 mg up to 100 mg/d. *Pediatric:* 1–2 mg/kg per day.

IM (triamcinolone acetonide): 2.5–60.0 mg/d.

IM (triamcinolone diacetate): 40 mg/wk. A single parenteral dose four to seven times the oral daily dose provides control for 4 d–4 wk.

Intra-articular, intralesional (dose will vary with joint or soft tissue site to be injected)
– *Triamcinolone acetonide:* 2.5–15.0 mg.
– *Triamcinolone diacetate:* 5–40 mg.
– *Triamcinolone hexacetonide:* 2–20 mg.

Respiratory inhalant (triamcinolone acetonide): 200 μg released with each actuation delivers about 100 μg to the patient.
- **Adult:** 2 inhalations tid–qid, not to exceed 16 inhalations/d.
- **Pediatric (6–12 y):** 1–2 inhalations tid–qid, not to exceed 12 inhalations/d.

Topical dermatologic preparations: Apply sparingly to affected area bid–qid.

Pharmacokinetics

Route	Onset	Peak	Duration
Oral	24–48 h	1–2 h	2.25 d
IM	24–48 h	8–10 h	1–6 wk

Metabolism: Hepatic, $T_{1/2}$: 2–5 h
Distribution: Crosses placenta; enters breast milk
Excretion: Urine

Adverse effects

Effects depend on dose, route, and duration of therapy.
- **CNS:** *Vertigo, headache,* paresthesias, insomnia, convulsions, psychosis, cataracts, increased intraocular pressure, glaucoma (long-term therapy)
- **GI:** Peptic or esophageal ulcer, pancreatitis, abdominal distention, nausea, vomiting, *increased appetite, weight gain* (long-term therapy)
- **CV:** Hypotension, shock, hypertension and CHF secondary to fluid retention, thromboembolism, thrombophlebitis, fat embolism, cardiac arrhythmias
- **MS:** Muscle weakness, steroid myopathy, loss of muscle mass, osteoporosis, spontaneous fractures (long-term therapy)
- **Hypersensitivity:** Hypersensitivity or anaphylactoid reactions
- **Endocrine:** Amenorrhea, irregular menses, growth retardation, decreased carbohydrate tolerance, diabetes mellitus, cushingoid state (long-term effect), increased blood sugar, increased serum cholesterol, decreased T_3 and T_4 levels,

hypothalamic-pituitary-adrenal (HPA) suppression with systemic therapy longer than 5 d
- Electrolyte imbalance: *Na+ and fluid retention*, hypokalemia, hypocalcemia
- Other: *Immunosuppression, aggravation, or masking of infections; impaired wound healing*; thin, fragile skin; petechiae, ecchymoses, purpura, striae; subcutaneous fat atrophy

Intra-articular
- Local: Osteonecrosis, tendon, rupture, infection

Intralesional (face and head)
- Local: Blindness (rare)

Respiratory Inhalants
- Local: Oral, laryngeal, and pharyngeal irritation; fungal infections

Topical Dermatologic Ointments, Creams, Sprays
- Local: Local burning, irritation, acneiform lesions, striae, skin atrophy

Systemic absorption of dermatologic preparations can lead to HPA suppression (see above), growth retardation in children, and other systemic adverse effects. Children may be at special risk of systemic absorption because of their larger skin surface to body weight ratio.

Clinically important drug-drug interactions
- Increased therapeutic and toxic effects of triamcinolone if taken with troleandomycin
- Risk of severe deterioration of muscle strength when given to myasthenia gravis patients who are also receiving ambenonium, edrophonium, neostigmine, pyridostigmine
- Decreased steroid blood levels when taken with barbiturates, phenytoin, rifampin
- Decreased effectiveness of salicylates when taken with triamcinolone

Drug-lab test interferences
- False-negative nitroblue-tetrazolium test for bacterial infection
- Suppression of skin test reactions

■ Nursing Considerations

Assessment
- *History:* Infections; kidney or liver disease; hypothyroidism; ulcerative colitis with impending perforation; diverticulitis; active or latent peptic ulcer; inflammatory bowel disease; CHF; hypertension; thromboembolic disorders; osteoporosis; convulsive disorders; diabetes mellitus; pregnancy; lactation; allergy to tartrazine
- *Physical:* Body weight, temperature, reflexes and grip strength, affect and orientation, P, BP, peripheral perfusion, prominence of superficial veins, R, adventitious sounds, serum electrolytes, blood glucose.

Implementation
- Administer once-a-day doses before 9 AM to mimic normal peak corticosteroid blood levels.
- Arrange for increased dosage when patient is subject to stress.
- Arrange to taper doses when discontinuing high-dose or long-term therapy.
- Do not give live virus vaccines with immunosuppressive doses of corticosteroids.
- Arrange to taper systemic steroids carefully during transfer to inhalational steroids; deaths caused by adrenal insufficiency have occurred.
- Use caution when occlusive dressings, tight diapers, and so forth cover affected area; these can increase systemic absorption of the drug when using topical preparations.
- Avoid prolonged use of topical preparations near the eyes, in genital and rectal areas, and in skin creases.

Drug-specific teaching points
- Do not stop taking the drug without consulting your health care provider.
- Avoid exposure to infections.
- Report unusual weight gain, swelling of the extremities, muscle weakness, black or tarry stools, fever, prolonged sore throat, colds or other infections, worsening of the disorder for which the drug is being taken.

Intra-articular Administration
- Do not overuse joint after therapy, even if pain is gone.

Adverse effects in *Italics* are most common; those in **Bold** are life-threatening.

Respiratory Inhalant
- Do not use during an acute asthmatic attack or to manage status asthmaticus.
- Do not use with systemic fungal infections.
- Do not use this drug more often than prescribed.
- Do not stop using this drug without consulting your health care provider.
- Administer inhalational bronchodilator drug first, if receiving concomitant bronchodilator therapy.

Topical Dermatologic Preparations
- Apply drug sparingly, avoid contact with eyes.
- Report irritation or infection at the site of application.

▢ triamterene

(trye am' ter een)
Dyrenium

Pregnancy Category B

Drug classes
Potassium-sparing diuretic

Therapeutic actions
Inhibits sodium reabsorption in the renal distal tubule, causing loss of sodium and water and retention of potassium.

Indications
- Edema associated with CHF, nephrotic syndrome, hepatic cirrhosis; steroid-induced edema, edema from secondary hyperaldosteronism (alone or with other diuretics for added diuretic or antikaliuretic effects)

Contraindications/cautions
- Contraindicated in the presence of allergy to triamterene, hyperkalemia, renal disease (except nephrosis), liver disease, lactation.
- Use caution in the presence of diabetes mellitus, pregnancy.

Dosage
Adult: 100 mg bid PO if used alone. Reduce dosage if added to other diuretic therapy. Maintenance dosage should be individualized, may be as low as 100 mg every other day. Do not exceed 300 mg/d.
Pediatric: Safety and efficacy not established.

Pharmacokinetics

Route	Onset	Peak	Duration
Oral	2–4 h	6–8 h	12–16 h

Metabolism: Hepatic, $T_{1/2}$: 3 h
Distribution: Crosses placenta; enters breast milk
Excretion: Urine

Adverse effects
- **CNS:** *Headache*, drowsiness, fatigue, weakness
- **GI:** *Nausea, anorexia, vomiting, dry mouth*, diarrhea
- **Hematologic:** Hyperkalemia, blood dyscrasias
- **GU:** Renal stones, intersititial nephritis
- **Dermatologic:** Rash, photosensitivity

Clinically important drug-drug interactions
- Increased hyperkalemia if taken with potassium supplements, diets rich in potassium, ACE inhibitors
- Increased serum levels of triamterene and possible toxicity if taken with cimetidine, indomethacin
- Increased risk of amantadine toxicity if taken concurrently

Drug-lab test interferences
- Interference with fluorescent measurement of serum quinidine levels

■ Nursing Considerations

Assessment
- *History:* Allergy to triamterene, hyperkalemia, renal or liver disease, diabetes mellitus, pregnancy, lactation
- *Physical:* Skin color, lesions, edema; orientation, reflexes, muscle strength; pulses, baseline ECG, BP; R, pattern, adventitious sounds; liver evaluation, bowel sounds; urinary output patterns; CBC,

serum electrolytes, blood sugar, liver and renal function tests, urinalysis

Implementation
- Administer with food or milk if GI upset occurs.
- Mark calendars or provide some other reminder of drug days for outpatients if every other day or 3- to 5-d/wk therapy is the most effective for treating edema.
- Administer early in the day so that increased urination does not disturb sleep.
- Measure and record regular body weights to monitor mobilization of edema fluid.
- Arrange for regular evaluation of serum electrolytes, BUN.

Drug-specific teaching points
- Record alternate-day therapy on a calendar, or make dated envelopes. Take the drug early in the day as increased urination will occur. The drug may be taken with food or meals if GI upset occurs.
- Weigh yourself on a regular basis, at the same time of the day and in the same clothing, and record the weight on your calendar.
- Know that the following side effects may occur: increased volume and frequency of urination (have ready access to a bathroom when drug effect is greatest); drowsiness (avoid rapid position changes; do not engage in hazardous activities [like driving a car] if this change occurs; this problem is often made worse by the use of alcohol); avoid foods that are rich in potassium (eg, fruits, Sanka); sensitivity to sunlight and bright lights (wear sunglasses, and use sunscreens and protective clothing when outdoors).
- Report loss or gain of more than 3 lb in one day, swelling in your ankles or fingers, fever, sore throat, mouth sores, unusual bleeding or bruising, dizziness, trembling, numbness, fatigue.

▢ triazolam

(trye ay' zoe lam)
Halcion

Pregnancy Category X
C-IV controlled substance

Drug classes
Benzodiazepine
Sedative/hypnotic

Therapeutic actions
Exact mechanisms of action not understood; acts mainly at subcortical levels of the CNS, leaving the cortex relatively unaffected; main sites of action may be the limbic system and mesencephalic reticular formation; benzodiazepines potentiate the effects of GABA, an inhibitory neurotransmitter.

Indications
- Insomnia characterized by difficulty falling asleep, frequent nocturnal awakenings, or early morning awakening
- Recurring insomnia or poor sleeping habits
- Acute or chronic medical situations requiring restful sleep

Contraindications/cautions
- Contraindicated in the presence of hypersensitivity to benzodiazepines; pregnancy (risk of congenital malformations, neonatal withdrawal syndrome); labor and delivery ("floppy infant" syndrome reported when mothers were given benzodiazepines during labor); lactation (infants may become lethargic and lose weight).
- Use caution in the presence of impaired liver or kidney function, debilitation, depression, suicidal tendencies.

Dosage
Adult: 0.125–0.5 mg PO before retiring.
Pediatric: Not for use in children younger than 18 y.
Geriatric patients or those with debilitating disease: Initially, 0.125–0.25 mg PO. Adjust as needed and tolerated.

Pharmacokinetics

Route	Onset	Peak
Oral	Varies	½–2 h

Metabolism: Hepatic, $T_{1/2}$: 1.5–5.5 h
Distribution: Crosses placenta; enters breast milk
Excretion: Urine

Adverse effects
- CNS: *Transient, mild drowsiness initially; sedation, depression, lethargy, apathy, fatigue, lightheadedness, disorientation, restlessness, confusion,* crying, delirium, headache, slurred speech, dysarthria, stupor, rigidity, tremor, dystonia, vertigo, euphoria, nervousness, difficulty in concentration, vivid dreams, psychomotor retardation, extrapyramidal symptoms; *mild paradoxical excitatory reactions, during first 2 wk of treatment* (especially in psychiatric patients, aggressive children, and with high dosage), visual and auditory disturbances, diplopia, nystagmus, depressed hearing, nasal congestion
- GI: *Constipation, diarrhea,* dry mouth, salivation, nausea, anorexia, vomiting, difficulty in swallowing, gastric disorders, elevations of blood enzymes: hepatic dysfunction, jaundice
- CV: *Bradycardia, tachycardia,* cardiovascular collapse, hypertension and hypotension, palpitations, edema
- Hematologic: Decreased hematocrit, blood dyscrasias
- GU: *Incontinence, urinary retention, changes in libido,* menstrual irregularities
- Dermatologic: Urticaria, pruritus, skin rash, dermatitis
- Dependence: *Drug dependence with withdrawal syndrome* when drug is discontinued (more common with abrupt discontinuation of higher dosage used for longer than 4 mo)
- Other: Hiccups, fever, diaphoresis, paresthesias, muscular disturbances, gynecomastia

Clinically important drug-drug interactions
- Increased CNS depression and sedation when taken with alcohol, cimetidine, omeprazole, disulfiram, oral contraceptives • Decreased sedative effects of triazolam if taken concurrently with theophylline, aminophylline, dyphylline, oxitriphylline

■ Nursing Considerations
Assessment
- *History:* Hypersensitivity to benzodiazepines, pregnancy, lactation, impaired liver or kidney function, debilitation, depression, suicidal tendencies
- *Physical:* Skin—color, lesions; body temperature; orientation, reflexes, affect, ophthalmologic exam; P, BP; R, adventitious sounds; liver evaluation, abdominal exam, bowel sounds, normal output; CBC, liver and renal function tests

Implementation
- Arrange for periodic blood counts, urinalyses, and blood chemistry analyses with protracted treatment.
- Arrange to taper dosage gradually after long-term therapy, especially in epileptic patients.

Drug-specific teaching points
- Take drug exactly as prescribed.
- Do not stop taking this drug (long-term therapy) without consulting your health care provider.
- Avoid alcohol, sleep-inducing, or OTC drugs while on this drug.
- Avoid pregnancy while taking this drug; use of contraceptive measures is advised; serious fetal harm could occur.
- Know that the following side effects may occur: drowsiness, dizziness (these may become less pronounced after a few days; avoid driving a car or engaging in other dangerous activities if these occur); GI upset (taking the drug with food may help); depression, dreams, emotional upset, crying; disturbance of nocturnal sleep for several nights after discontinuing the drug.
- Report severe dizziness, weakness, drowsiness that persists, rash or skin lesions, palpitations, swelling of the extremities, visual changes, difficulty voiding.

❒ trichlormethiazide

(trye klor meth eye' a zide)
Diurese, Metahydrin, Naqua

Pregnancy Category C

Adverse effects in *Italics* are most common; those in **Bold** are life-threatening.

trichlormethiazide

Drug classes
Thiazide diuretic

Therapeutic actions
Inhibits reabsorption of sodium and chloride in distal renal tubule, thereby increasing excretion of sodium, chloride, and water by the kidney.

Indications
- Adjunctive therapy in edema associated with CHF, cirrhosis, corticosteroid and estrogen therapy, renal dysfunction
- Hypertension, as sole therapy or in combination with other antihypertensives
- Unlabeled uses: calcium nephrolithiasis alone or with amiloride or allopurinol to prevent recurrences in hypercalciuric or normal calciuric patients, diabetes insipidus, especially nephrogenic diabetes insipidus

Contraindications/cautions
- Contraindicated in the presence of fluid or electrolyte imbalances, pregnancy, lactation, allergy to tartrazine or aspirin (tartrazine contained in tablets marketed under the name *Metahydrin*).
- Use caution in the presence of renal or liver disease, gout, SLE, glucose tolerance abnormalities, hyperparathyroidism, manic-depressive disorders.

Dosage
Adult
- ***Edema, hypertension:*** 2–4 mg PO qd.
- ***Calcium nephrolithiasis:*** 4 mg/d PO.

Pediatric: Safety and efficacy not established.

Pharmacokinetics

Route	Onset	Peak	Duration
Oral	2 h	6 h	24 h

Metabolism: Hepatic, $T_{1/2}$: 2.3–7.3 h
Distribution: Crosses placenta; enters breast milk
Excretion: Urine

Adverse effects
- **CNS:** *Dizziness, vertigo,* paresthesias, weakness, headache, drowsiness, fatigue, leukopenia, thrombocytopenia, agranulocytosis, aplastic anemia, neutropenia
- **GI:** *Nausea, anorexia, vomiting, dry mouth,* diarrhea, constipation, jaundice, hepatitis, pancreatitis
- **CV:** Orthostatic hypotension, venous thrombosis, volume depletion, cardiac arrhythmias, chest pain
- **GU:** *Polyuria, nocturia,* impotence, loss of libido
- **Dermatologic:** Photosensitivity, rash, purpura, exfoliative dermatitis, hives
- **Other:** Muscle cramps and muscle spasms, fever, gouty attacks, flushing, weight loss, rhinorrhea

Clinically important drug-drug interactions
- Risk of hyperglycemia if taken with diazoxide • Decreased absorption of trichlormethiazide if taken with cholestyramine, colestipol • Increased risk of digitalis glycoside toxicity if hypokalemia occurs • Increased risk of lithium toxicity when taken with thiazides • Increased fasting blood glucose leading to need to adjust dosage of antidiabetic agents

Drug-lab test interferences
- Decreased PBI levels without clinical signs of thyroid disturbances

■ Nursing Considerations

Assessment
- *History:* Fluid or electrolyte imbalances, renal or liver disease, gout, SLE, glucose tolerance abnormalities, hyperparathyroidism, manic-depressive disorders, pregnancy, lactation, allergy to tartrazine or aspirin
- *Physical:* Skin—color and lesions; orientation, reflexes, muscle strength; pulses, BP, orthostatic BP, perfusion, edema, baseline ECG; R, adventitious sounds; liver evaluation, bowel sounds; CBC, serum electrolytes, blood glucose, liver and renal function tests, serum uric acid, urinalysis

Implementation
- Administer with food or milk if GI upset occurs.

Adverse effects in *Italics* are most common; those in **Bold** are life-threatening.

- Mark calendars or provide other reminders of drug days for outpatients on every other day or 3- to 5-d/wk therapy.
- Administer early in the day so increased urination will not disturb sleep.

Drug-specific teaching points
- Take drug early in the day so sleep will not be disturbed by increased urination.
- Weigh yourself daily, and record weights on your calendar.
- Protect skin from exposure to sun or bright lights.
- Know that increased urination will occur (stay close to bathroom facilities).
- Use caution if dizziness, drowsiness, feeling faint occur.
- Report rapid weight gain or loss, swelling in ankles or fingers, unusual bleeding or bruising, muscle cramps.

▢ trientine hydrochloride

(trye' en teen)
Syprine

Pregnancy Category C

Drug classes
Chelating agent for removal of copper from the body

Therapeutic actions
Chelating agent that combines with copper in the body, making it a more soluble compound that is excreted in the urine.

Indications
- Treatment of patients with Wilson's disease who are intolerant of penicillamine

Contraindications/cautions
- Allergy to trientine, pregnancy, lactation.

Dosage
Warning: interruptions of daily therapy for even a few days have been followed by sensitivity reactions when the drug is reinstituted.

Adult: Initially, 750–1250 mg/d PO in divided doses bid, tid, or qid. May increase to a maximum of 2 g/d. Must be given on an empty stomach.
Pediatric
- ***Younger than 12 y:*** Initially, 500–750 mg/d PO in divided doses bid, tid, qid. May increase to a maximum of 1,500 mg/d.

Pharmacokinetics

Route	Onset	Peak
Oral	Varies	60 min

Metabolism: Hepatic, $T_{1/2}$: unknown
Distribution: Crosses placenta; enters breast milk
Excretion: Urine

Adverse effects
- General: *Iron deficiency*, SLE
- Hypersensitivity: Reactions such as asthma, bronchitis, *dermatitis*

■ Nursing Considerations

Assessment
- *History:* Allergy to trientine, pregnancy, lactation
- *Physical:* Skin—color, lesions; body temperature; R, adventitious sounds (to detect hypersensitivity reactions); CBC, hemoglobin levels, titer for ANA, serum and 24-h urine copper levels

Implementation
- Arrange for monitoring of CBC, hemoglobin, and serum and 24-h urinary copper levels before beginning therapy and periodically (every 6–12 mo) during therapy.
- Administer drug on an empty stomach, 1 h before or 2 h after meals and at least 1 h apart from any other drug, food, or milk.
- Ensure that patient swallows capsules whole with water; do not open or chew.
- Wash any area that comes in contact with the capsule contents carefully because of the risk of contact dermatitis.
- Monitor body temperature nightly during first month of treatment.

Adverse effects in *Italics* are most common; those in **Bold** are life-threatening.

trifluoperazine hydrochloride ■ 1101

- Arrange for nutritional consultation; if iron supplements are needed, ensure that they are given at least 2 h apart from trientine.
- Evaluate for 24-h urinary copper levels of 0.5–1 mg.

Drug-specific teaching points
- Do not open or chew capsules. Take on an empty stomach, 1 h before or 2 h after meals and at least 1 h apart from any other drug, food, or milk.
- Know that the following side effects may occur: iron deficiency (you will need to have periodic blood tests to evaluate this and may need take iron supplements).
- Be aware that this drug is not to be used during pregnancy. If you become pregnant or want to become pregnant, consult your prescriber.
- Report skin rash, difficulty breathing, cough or wheezing, fever, chills.

☐ trifluoperazine hydrochloride

*(trye floo oh **per'** a zeen)*
Apo-Trifluoperazine (CAN), Stelazine

Pregnancy Category C

Drug classes
Phenothiazine (piperazine)
Dopaminergic blocking drug
Antipsychotic drug
Antianxiety agent

Therapeutic actions
Mechanism of action not fully understood: antipsychotic drugs block postsynaptic dopamine receptors in the brain, but this may not be necessary and sufficient for antipsychotic activity; depresses the reticular activating system, including the parts of the brain involved with wakefulness and emesis; anticholinergic, antihistaminic (H_1), and alpha-adrenergic blocking activity also may contribute to some of its therapeutic (and adverse) actions.

Indications
- Management of manifestations of psychotic disorders
- Treatment of nonpsychotic anxiety (not drug of choice)

Contraindications/cautions
- Contraindicated in the presence of coma or severe CNS depression, bone marrow depression, blood dyscrasia, circulatory collapse, subcortical brain damage, Parkinson's disease, liver damage, cerebral arteriosclerosis, coronary disease, severe hypotension or hypertension.
- Use caution in the presence of respiratory disorders ("silent pneumonia" may develop); glaucoma, prostatic hypertrophy; epilepsy or history of epilepsy (drug lowers seizure threshold); breast cancer; thyrotoxicosis (severe neurotoxicity may develop); peptic ulcer, decreased renal function; myelography within previous 24 h or scheduled within 48 h; exposure to heat or phosphorous insecticides; pregnancy; lactation; children younger than 12 y, especially those with chickenpox, CNS infections (children are especially susceptible to dystonias that may confound the diagnosis of Reye's syndrome).

Dosage
Adult
- ***Psychotic disorders***
  – ***Oral:*** 2–5 mg bid. Start small or emaciated patients on the lower dosage. Most patients will show optimum response with 15 or 20 mg/d. Optimum dosage should be reached within 2–3 wk.
  – ***IM:*** For prompt control of severe symptoms, 1–2 mg by deep IM injection q4–6h, as needed. Do not give more often than q4h. More than 6 mg/d is rarely needed. More than 10 mg/d should be given only in exceptional cases.

Pediatric: Adjust dosage to weight of child and severity of symptoms. The following dosages are for hospitalized or closely supervised children 6–12 y.
- ***Oral:*** Initially, 1 mg qd–bid. It is usually not necessary to exceed 15 mg/d. Older children with severe symptoms may require higher dosage.

1102 ■ trifluoperazine hydrochloride

- *IM:* For prompt control of severe symptoms, 1 mg qd–bid.

Geriatric: Use lower doses, and increase dosage more gradually than in younger patients.

- ***Nonpsychotic disorders:*** Usual dose 1–2 mg bid. Do not administer more than 6 mg/d or for longer than 12 wk.

Pharmacokinetics

Route	Onset	Peak	Duration
Oral	Varies	2–4 h	< 12 h
IM	Rapid	1–2 h	< 12 h

Metabolism: Hepatic, $T_{1/2}$: 47–100 h
Distribution: Crosses placenta; enters breast milk
Excretion: Bile and feces

Adverse effects

- CNS: *Drowsiness*, insomnia, vertigo, headache, weakness, tremor, ataxia, slurring, cerebral edema, seizures, exacerbation of psychotic symptoms, extrapyramidal syndromes—*pseudoparkinsonism; dystonias; akathisia;* tardive dyskinesias, potentially irreversible (no known treatment), neuroleptic malignant syndrome
- CV: Hypotension, orthostatic hypotension, hypertension, tachycardia, bradycardia, cardiac arrest, CHF, cardiomegaly, **refractory arrhythmias**, pulmonary edema
- Respiratory: Bronchospasm, laryngospasm, dyspnea, suppression of cough reflex and potential for aspiration
- Hematologic: Eosinophilia, leukopenia, leukocytosis, anemia; aplastic anemia; hemolytic anemia; thrombocytopenic or nonthrombocytopenic purpura; pancytopenia
- EENT: glaucoma, *photophobia, blurred vision*, miosis, mydriasis, deposits in the cornea and lens (opacities), pigmentary retinopathy
- Hypersensitivity: Jaundice, urticaria, angioneurotic edema, laryngeal edema, photosensitivity, eczema, asthma, anaphylactoid reactions, exfoliative dermatitis
- Endocrine: Lactation, breast engorgement in females, galactorrhea; SIADH; amenorrhea, menstrual irregularities; gynecomastia in males; changes in libido; hyperglycemia or hypoglycemia; glycosuria; hyponatremia; pituitary tumor with hyperprolactinemia; inhibition of ovulation, infertility, pseudopregnancy; reduced urinary levels of gonadotropins, estrogens, progestins
- Autonomic: *Dry mouth, salivation, nasal congestion, nausea*, vomiting, anorexia, fever, pallor, flushed facies, sweating, constipation, paralytic ileus, urinary retention, incontinence, polyuria, enuresis, priapism, ejaculation inhibition, male impotence
- Other: *Urine discolored pink to red-brown*

Clinically important drug-drug interactions

- Additive CNS depression with alcohol • Additive anticholinergic effects and possibly decreased antipsychotic efficacy with anticholinergic drugs • Increased likelihood of seizures with metrizamide • Increased frequency and severity of neuromuscular excitation and hypotension in patients who are premedicated with trifluoperazine and are given barbiturate anesthetics (methohexital, thiamylal, phenobarbital, thiopental) • Decreased antihypertensive effect of guanethidine when taken with trifluoperazine

Drug-lab test interferences

- False-positive pregnancy tests (less likely if serum test is used) • Increase in protein-bound iodine, not attributable to an increase in thyroxine

■ Nursing Considerations
Assessment

- *History:* Coma or severe CNS depression; bone marrow depression; blood dyscrasia; circulatory collapse; subcortical brain damage; Parkinson's disease; liver damage; cerebral arteriosclerosis; coronary disease; severe hypotension or hypertension; respiratory disorders; glaucoma,

Adverse effects in *Italics* are most common; those in **Bold** are life-threatening.

prostatic hypertrophy; epilepsy; breast cancer; thyrotoxicosis; peptic ulcer, decreased renal function; myelography within previous 24 h or scheduled within 48 h; exposure to heat or phosphorous insecticides; pregnancy; lactation; chickenpox; CNS infections
- *Physical:* Body weight, temperature; reflexes, orientation, intraocular pressure; P, BP, orthostatic BP; R, adventitious sounds; bowel sounds and normal output, liver evaluation; urinary output, prostate size; CBC; urinalysis; thyroid, liver, and kidney function tests

Implementation
- Do not change brand names; bioavailability differences have been documented for different brands.
- Dilute oral concentrate (for institutional use only) immediately before use by adding the dose to 60 ml of one of the following: tomato or fruit juice, milk, simple syrup, orange syrup, carbonated beverages, coffee, tea, or water; semisolid foods (soup, pudding) also may be used.
- Avoid skin contact with drug solution; contact dermatitis has occurred.
- Arrange for discontinuation of drug if serum creatinine, BUN become abnormal or WBC count depressed.
- Monitor elderly patients for dehydration, and institute remedial measures promptly; sedation and decreased sensation of thirst related to CNS effects of drug can lead to severe dehydration.
- Consult physician regarding appropriate warning of patient or patient's guardian about tardive dyskinesias.
- Consult physician about dosage reduction, use of anticholinergic antiparkinsonian drugs (controversial) if extrapyramidal effects occur.

Drug-specific teaching points
- Take drug exactly as prescribed.
- Avoid skin contact with drug solutions.
- Avoid driving a car or engaging in other dangerous activities if CNS, vision changes occur.
- Avoid prolonged exposure to sun, or use a sunscreen or covering garments if exposure is necessary.
- Maintain fluid intake, and use precautions against heatstroke in hot weather.
- Report sore throat, fever, unusual bleeding or bruising, rash, weakness, tremors, impaired vision, dark urine (pink or reddish brown urine is to be expected), pale stools, yellowing of the skin or eyes.

☐ triflupromazine hydrochloride

(trye flu proe' ma zeen)
Vesprin

Pregnancy Category C

Drug classes
Phenothiazine
Dopaminergic-blocking drug
Antipsychotic drug
Antiemetic drug
Antianxiety drug

Therapeutic actions
Mechanism of action not fully understood: blocks postsynaptic dopamine receptors in the brain; depresses the parts of the brain involved with wakefulness and emesis; anticholinergic, antihistaminic (H_1), and alpha-adrenergic blocking.

Indications
- Management of manifestations of psychotic disorders, excluding psychotic depressive reactions
- Control of severe nausea and vomiting

Contraindications/cautions
- Contraindicated in the presence of allergy to triflupromazine, comatose or severely depressed states, bone marrow depression, circulatory collapse, subcortical brain damage.
- Use caution in the presence of Parkinson's disease; liver damage; cerebral or coronary arteriosclerosis; severe hypotension or hypertension; respiratory disorders; glaucoma; epilepsy or history of epilepsy; peptic ulcer or history of peptic ulcer; decreased renal function; prostate hypertrophy; breast cancer; thyrotoxicosis; myelography within 24 h or scheduled within 48 h; lactation; exposure to

1104 ■ triflupromazine hydrochloride

heat, phosphorous insecticides; children with chickenpox, CNS infections (such children are more susceptible to dystonias, which may confound the diagnosis of Reye's syndrome or other encephalopathy; may mask symptoms of Reye's syndrome, encephalopathies)

Dosage
Adult
- ***Psychotic disorders:*** 60 mg IM up to a maximum of 150 mg/d.
- ***Nausea and vomiting:*** 5–15 mg IM q4h, up to a maximum of 60 mg/d. 1 mg IV up to a maximum of 3 mg/d.

Pediatric (older than 2 y)
- ***Psychiatric disorders:*** 0.2–0.25 mg/kg IM up to a maximum of 10 mg/d.
- ***Nausea and vomiting:*** 0.2–0.25 mg/kg IM up to a maximum of 10 mg/d. Do not give IV.

Pharmacokinetics

Route	Onset	Peak	Duration
IM	10–15 min	15–20 min	4–6 h

Metabolism: Hepatic, $T_{1/2}$: 10–20 h
Distribution: Crosses placenta; enters breast milk
Excretion: Urine

IV facts
Preparation: No further preparation required.
Infusion: Inject slowly into tubing of actively running IV.

Adverse effects
- CNS: *Drowsiness, insomnia, vertigo,* headache, weakness, tremors, ataxia, slurring, cerebral edema, seizures, exacerbation of psychotic symptoms, *extrapyramidal syndromes*; neuroleptic malignant syndrome
- GI: *Dry mouth, salivation, nausea, vomiting, anorexia, constipation*, paralytic ileus, incontinence
- CV: *Hypotension, otrhostatic hypotension,* hypertension, tachycardia, bradycardia, cardiac arrest, CHF, cardiomegaly, refractory arrhythmias, pulmonary edema
- Respiratory: Bronchospasm, laryngospasm, dyspnea, suppression of cough reflex and potential aspiration
- Hematologic: **Eosinophilia, leukopenia, leukocytosis,** *anemia*, aplastic anemia, hemolytic anemia, thrombocytopenic or nonthrombocytopenic purpura, pancytopenia, elevated serum cholesterol
- GU: *Urinary retention,* polyuria, incontinence, priapism, ejaculation inhibition, male impotence, urine discolored pink to red-brown
- EENT: Nasal congestion, glaucoma, *photophobia, blurred vision*, miosis, mydriasis, deposits in the cornea and lens, pigmentary retinopathy
- Hypersensitivity: Jaundice, *urticaria,* angioneurotic edema, laryngeal edema, photosensitivity, eczema, asthma, anaphylactoid reactions, exfoliative dermatitis, contact dermatitis with drug solutions
- Endocrine: Lactation, breast engorgement in females, galactorrhea, SIADH secretion, amenorrhea, menstrual irregularities, gynecomastia in males, changes in libido, hyperglycemia, inhibition of ovulation, infertility, pseudopregnancy, reduced urinary levels of gonadotropins, estrogens and progestins
- Other: Fever, heatstroke, pallor, flushed facies, sweating, *photosensitivity*

Clinically important drug-drug interactions
- Additive anticholinergic effects and possibly decreased antipsychotic efficacy if taken concurrently with anticholinergic drugs • Additive CNS depression, hypotension if given preoperatively with barbiturate anesthetics, alcohol, meperidine • Additive effects of both drugs if concurrently with beta-blockers • Increased risk of tachycardia, hypotension if given concurrently with epinephrine, norepinephrine • Increased risk of seizure if taken with metrizamide

Adverse effects in *Italics* are most common; those in **Bold** are life-threatening.

triflupromazine hydrochloride ■ 1105

- Decreased hypotension effect if taken concurrently with guanethidine

Drug-lab test interferences
- False-positive pregnancy tests (less likely if serum test is used) • Increase in protein-bound iodine, not attributable to an increase in thyroxine

■ Nursing Considerations

Assessment
- *History:* Allergy to triflupromazine; comatose or severely depressed states; bone marrow depression; circulatory collapse; subcortical brain damage, Parkinson's disease; liver damage; cerebral or coronary arteriosclerosis; severe hypotension or hypertension; respiratory disorders; glaucoma; epilepsy; peptic ulcer; decreased renal function; prostate hypertrophy; breast cancer; thyrotoxicosis; myelography within 24 h or scheduled within 48 h; lactation; exposure to heat, phosphorous insecticides; chickenpox, CNS infections
- *Physical:* Body temperature, body weight, skin—color, turgor; reflexes, orientation, intraocular pressure, ophthalmologic exam; P, BP, orthostatic BP, ECG; R, adventitious sounds; bowel sounds, normal output, liver evaluation; prostate palpation, normal urine output; CBC; urinalysis; thyroid, liver, and kidney function tests; EEG (as appropriate)

Implementation
- Do not give by SC injection; give slowly by deep IM injection into upper outer quadrant of buttock.
- Reserve IV use for situations when IM use is not possible. Do not use IV in children.
- Keep the patient recumbent for ½ h after injection to avoid orthostatic hypotension.
- Avoid skin contact with drug solutions because of the possibility of contact dermatitis.
- Consult with physician regarding warning patient or the patient's guardian about the possibility of tardive dyskinesias developing with continued use.
- Be alert to potential for aspiration because of suppressed cough reflex.
- Monitor renal function tests and arrange for discontinuation of drug if serum creatinine, BUN become abnormal.
- Monitor CBC and arrange for discontinuation of drug if WBC count is depressed.
- Consult with physician about dosage reduction or use of anticholinergic antiparkinsonian drugs (controversial) if extrapyramidal effects occur.
- Arrange to withdraw drug gradually after high-dose therapy; gastritis, nausea, dizziness, headache, tachycardia, insomnia have occurred after abrupt withdrawal.
- Monitor elderly patients for dehydration: sedation and decreased sensation of thirst due to CNS effects can lead to dehydration, hemoconcentration, and reduced pulmonary ventilation; promptly institute remedial measures.
- Avoid use of epinephrine as vasopressor if drug-induced hypotension occurs.

Drug-specific teaching points
- Be aware that this drug can be given only by injection.
- Know that the following side effects may occur: drowsiness (avoid driving a car or operating dangerous machinery if this occurs; avoid alcohol, which will increase the drowsiness); sensitivity to the sun (avoid prolonged sun exposure, and wear garments that cover you or use a sunscreen if you must be out in the sun); pink or reddish-brown urine (this is an expected drug effect that does not indicate blood in your urine or that anything is wrong); faintness, dizziness (change position slowly; use caution climbing stairs; this effect usually goes away after several weeks of therapy).
- Use caution in hot weather; you may be prone to heatstroke while on this drug; keep up fluid intake, and do not exercise unduly in a hot climate.
- Report sore throat, fever, unusual bleeding or bruising, rash, weakness, tremors, impaired vision, dark urine, pale stools, yellowing of the skin and eyes.

☐ trihexyphenidyl hydrochloride

*(trye hex ee **fen'** i dill)*
Apo-Trihex (CAN), Artane, Trihexy

Pregnancy Category C

Drug classes
Antiparkinsonism drug (anticholinergic type)

Therapeutic actions
Has anticholinergic activity in the CNS that is believed to help normalize the hypothesized imbalance of cholinergic/dopaminergic neurotransmission created by the loss of dopaminergic neurons in the basal ganglia of the brain of parkinsonism patients; reduces severity of rigidity and reduces to a lesser extent the akinesia and tremor that characterise parkinsonism; less effective overall than levodopa; peripheral anticholinergic effects suppress secondary symptoms of parkinsonism, such as drooling.

Indications
- Adjunct in the treatment of parkinsonism (postencephalitic, arteriosclerotic, and idiopathic)
- Adjuvant therapy with levodopa
- Control of drug-induced extrapyramidal disorders

Contraindications/cautions
- Contraindicated in the presence of hypersensitivity to trihexyphenidyl; glaucoma, especially angle-closure glaucoma; pyloric or duodenal obstruction, stenosing peptic ulcers, achalasia (megaesophagus); prostatic hypertrophy or bladder neck obstructions; myasthenia gravis; lactation.
- Use caution in the presence of cardiac arrhythmias, hypertension, hypotension, hepatic or renal dysfunction, alcoholism, chronic illness, people who work in hot environment, pregnancy.

Dosage
Adult
- ***Parkinsonism:*** 1–2 mg PO the first day. Increase by 2-mg increments at 3- to 5-d intervals until a total of 6–10 mg is given daily. Postencephalitic patients may require 12–15 mg/d. Tolerated best if daily dose is divided into three (or four) doses administered at mealtimes (and bedtime).
- ***Concomitant use with levodopa:*** Usual dose of each may need to be reduced; however, trihexyphenidyl has been shown to decrease bioavailability of levodopa. Adjust dosage on basis of response. 3–6 mg/d PO of trihexyphenidyl is usually adequate.
- ***Concomitant use with other anticholinergics:*** Gradually substitute trihexyphenidyl for all or part of the other anticholinergic and reduce dosage of the other anticholinergic gradually.
- ***Drug-induced extrapyramidal symptoms:*** Initially 1 mg PO. If reactions are not controlled in a few hours, progressively increase subsequent doses until control is achieved. Dose of tranquilizer may need to be reduced temporarily to expedite control of extrapyramidal symptoms. Adjust dosage of both drugs subsequently to maintain ataractic effect without extrapyramidal reactions.
- ***Sustained-release preparations:*** Do not use for initial therapy. Substitute on a milligram for milligram of total daily dose basis after patient is stabilized on conventional dosage forms. A single PO dose after breakfast or two divided doses 12 h apart may be given.

Pediatric: Safety and efficacy not established.

Geriatric patients: Patients older than 60 y often develop increased sensitivity to the CNS effects of anticholinergic drugs.

Pharmacokinetics

Route	Onset	Peak
Oral	Varies	1–1.3 h

Metabolism: Hepatic, $T_{1/2}$: 5.6–10.2 h
Distribution: Crosses placenta; enters breast milk
Excretion: Urine

Adverse effects
Peripheral Anticholinergic Effects
- CNS (some CNS effects are characteristic of centrally acting anticholinergic drugs): *Disorientation, confusion,* memory loss, hallucinations, psychoses, agitation, nervousness, delusions, delirium, paranoia, euphoria, excitement, *lightheadedness, dizziness,* depression, drowsiness, weakness, giddiness, paresthesia, heaviness of the limbs, numbness of fingers, *blurred vision, mydriasis,* diplopia, increased intraocular tension, angle-closure glaucoma
- GI: *Dry mouth, constipation,* dilation of the colon, paralytic ileus
- CV: Tachycardia, palpitations, hypotension, orthostatic hypotension, acute suppurative parotitis, nausea, vomiting, epigastric distress
- GU: *Urinary retention,* urinary hesitancy, dysuria, difficulty achieving or maintaining an erection
- Dermatologic: Skin rash, urticaria, other dermatoses
- General: *Flushing, decreased sweating,* elevated temperature
- Other: Muscular weakness, muscular cramping

Clinically important drug-drug interactions
- Additive adverse CNS effects; toxic psychosis when given with phenothiazines • Possible masking of the development of persistent extrapyramidal symptoms, tardive dyskinesia, in patients on long-term therapy with antipsychotic drugs, such as phenothiazines, haloperidol • Decreased therapeutic efficacy of antipsychotic drugs (phenothiazines, haloperidol)

■ Nursing Considerations
Assessment
- *History:* Hypersensitivity to trihexyphenidyl, glaucoma, pyloric or duodenal obstruction, stenosing peptic ulcers, achalasia, prostatic hypertrophy or bladder neck obstructions, myasthenia gravis, tachycardia, cardiac arrhythmias, hypertension, hypotension, hepatic or renal dysfunction, alcoholism, chronic illness, people who work in hot environments, pregnancy, lactation
- *Physical:* Body weight; body temperature; skin—color, lesions; orientation, affect, reflexes, bilateral grip strength, visual exam, including tonometry; P, BP, orthostatic BP, auscultation; bowel sounds, normal output, liver evaluation; urinary output, voiding pattern, prostate palpation; liver and kidney function tests

Implementation
- Arrange to decrease dosage or discontinue drug temporarily if dry mouth is so severe that swallowing or speaking becomes difficult.
- Give with caution and arrange dosage reduction in hot weather as appropriate to patient's lifestyle; drug interferes with sweating and ability of body to maintain body heat equilibrium; anhidrosis and fatal hyperthermia have occurred.
- Ensure that patient voids just before receiving each dose of drug if urinary retention is a problem.

Drug-specific teaching points
- Take this drug exactly as prescribed.
- Know that the following side effects may occur: drowsiness, dizziness, confusion, blurred vision (avoid driving a car or engaging in activities that require alertness and visual acuity if these occur); nausea (frequent, small meals may help); dry mouth (sucking sugarless lozenges or ice chips may help); painful or difficult urination (emptying the bladder immediately before each dose may help); constipation (if maintaining adequate fluid intake, exercising regularly do not help, consult your nurse or physician).
- Use caution in hot weather (this drug makes you more susceptible to heat prostration).
- Report difficult or painful urination, constipation, rapid or pounding heartbeat, confusion, eye pain or rash.

Adverse effects in *Italics* are most common; those in **Bold** are life-threatening.

☐ trimeprazine tartrate

*(trye **mep**' ra zeen)*
Panectyl (CAN), Temaril

Pregnancy Category C

Drug classes
Phenothiazine
Dopaminergic-blocking drug
Antihistamine

Therapeutic actions
Selectively blocks H_1 histamine receptors, diminishing the effects of histamine on cells of the upper respiratory tract and eyes and decreasing the sneezing, mucus production, itching, and tearing that accompany allergic reactions in sensitized people exposed to antigens.

Indications
- Symptomatic relief of symptoms associated with perennial and seasonal allergic rhinitis, vasomotor rhinitis, allergic conjunctivitis; mild, uncomplicated urticaria and angioedema
- Amelioration of allergic reactions to blood or plasma
- Dermatographism
- Adjunctive therapy (with epinephrine and other measures) in anaphylactic reactions

Contraindications/cautions
- Contraindicated in the presence of hypersensitivity to antihistamines or phenothiazines, coma or severe CNS depression, bone marrow depression, blood dyscrasia, vomiting of unknown cause, lactation (lactation may be inhibited).
- Use caution in the presence of respiratory disorders ("silent pneumonia" may develop); glaucoma, prostatic hypertrophy; cardiovascular disease or hypertension; breast cancer; thyrotoxicosis (severe neurotoxicity may develop); pregnancy; children (antihistamine overdosage amy cause hallucinations, convulsions, and death; special caution in children with history of sleep apnea or a family history of sudden infant death syndrome, or in a child with Reye's syndrome; children are especially susceptible to dystonias that may confound the diagnosis of Reye's syndrome); the elderly (more likely to cause dizziness, sedation, syncope, toxic confusional states, hypotension, and extrapyramidal effects in the elderly).

Dosage
Adult: 2.5 mg PO qid *or* one 5-mg sustained-release capsule q12h.
Pediatric
- **> 6 y:** One 5-mg sustained-release capsule per day PO.
- **Older than 3 y:** 2.5 mg PO hs or tid, if needed.
- **6 mo–3 y:** 1.25 mg PO hs or tid, if needed.

Pharmacokinetics

Route	Onset	Peak	Duration
Oral	Varies	30–60 min	4–6 h

Metabolism: Hepatic, $T_{1/2}$: 10–12 h
Distribution: Crosses placenta; enters breast milk
Excretion: Urine

Adverse effects
- **CNS:** *Drowsiness,* insomnia, vertigo, headache, weakness, tremor, ataxia, slurring, cerebral edema, seizures, tinnitus, vertigo, tingling and heaviness in the hands
- **CV:** Hypotension, orthostatic hypotension, hypertension, tachycardia, bradycardia
- **Respiratory:** Bronchospasm, laryngospasm, dyspnea; suppression of cough reflex; *thickening of bronchial secretions,* tightness of the chest; potential for aspiration
- **Hematologic:** Eosinophilia, leukopenia, leukocytosis, anemia; aplastic anemia; hemolytic anemia; thrombocytopenic or nonthrombocytopenic purpura; pancytopenia
- **EENT:** Glaucoma, photophobia, *blurred vision,* diplopia, miosis

- **Autonomic:** *Dry mouth, salivation, nasal congestion, nausea*, vomiting, anorexia, fever, pallor, flushed facies, sweating, constipation, paralytic ileus, urinary retention, incontinence, polyuria, enuresis, priapism, ejaculation inhibition, male impotence
- **Other:** Infrequently, typical phenothiazine adverse effects, including extrapyramidal syndromes, hyperprolactinemia

Clinically important drug-drug interactions

- Additive CNS depression with alcohol
- Additive anticholinergic effects with anticholinergic drugs • Increased likelihood of seizures with metrizamide • Increased frequency and severity of neuromuscular excitation and hypotension in patients who are premedicated with trimeprazine and are given barbiturate anesthetics (methohexital, thiamylal, phenobarbital, thiopental)

■ Nursing Considerations

Assessment

- *History:* Hypersensitivity to antihistamines or phenothiazines, severe CNS depression, blood dyscrasia, vomiting of unknown cause, lactation, respiratory disorders, glaucoma, prostatic hypertrophy, cardiovascular disease or hypertension, breast cancer, thyrotoxicosis, pregnancy, history of sleep apnea or a family history of sudden infant death syndrome, Reye's syndrome
- *Physical:* Body weight, temperature; reflexes, orientation, intraocular pressure; P, BP, orthostatic BP; R, adventitious sounds; bowel sounds and normal output, liver evaluation; urinary output, prostate size. Arrange for CBC, urinalysis, thyroid, liver, and kidney function tests

Implementation

- Maintain fluid intake, and protect patient from exposure to heat.

Drug-specific teaching points

- Take drug exactly as prescribed.
- Avoid driving a car or engaging in other dangerous activities if CNS, vision changes occur.
- Avoid prolonged exposure to sun, or use a sunscreen or covering garments if exposure is necessary.
- Maintain fluid intake, and use precautions against heatstroke in hot weather.
- Report sore throat, fever, unusual bleeding or bruising, rash, weakness, tremors, impaired vision, dark urine (pink or reddish brown urine is to be expected), pale stools, yellowing of the skin or eyes.

❑ trimethadione

*(trye meth a **dye**' one)*
Tridione

Pregnancy Category D

Drug classes
Anticonvulsant

Therapeutic actions
Increases seizure threshold; sedative effects that may progress to ataxia.

Indications
- Control of absence (petit mal) seizures refractory to treatment with other drugs

Contraindications/cautions
- Contraindicated in the presence of hypersensitivity to oxazolidinediones; pregnancy, lactation.
- Use caution in the presence of hepatic, renal abnormalities.

Dosage
Adult: 300 mg PO tid; may increase by 300 mg/d at weekly intervals; maximum dose, 2.4 g/d.
Pediatric
- *Older than 6 y:* 300–900 mg/d PO in three to four divided doses.

Pharmacokinetics

Route	Onset	Peak	Duration
Oral	15–30 min	½–2 h	5–10 d

Metabolism: Hepatic, $T_{1/2}$: 16–24 h
Distribution: Crosses placenta; enters breast milk
Excretion: Urine

Adverse effects in *Italics* are most common; those in **Bold** are life-threatening.

Adverse effects
- CNS: *Drowsiness, ataxia, dizziness,* sedation, headache, paresthesias
- GI: GI distress, abnormal liver function tests, hepatitis
- Hematologic: Aplastic anemia
- Dermatologic: *pruritus,* **exfoliative dermatitis**
- Other: Vaginal bleeding, **lupus-like syndrome**, fetal malformations, *photosensitivity*

■ Nursing Considerations

Assessment
- *History:* Hypersensitivity to oxazolidineodiones; hepatic, renal abnormalities; lactation, pregnancy
- *Physical:* Skin—color, lesions; orientation, affect, reflexes, bilateral grip strength, vision exam; bowel sounds, normal output, liver evaluation; liver and kidney function tests, urinalysis, CBC with differential, EEG

Implementation
- Administer with food if GI upset occurs.
- Arrange to reduce dosage, discontinue trimethadione, or substitute other antiepileptic medication gradually; abrupt discontinuation may precipitate absence (petit mal) status.
- Arrange to discontinue drug if skin rash, depression of blood count, lupus-like syndrome occur.
- Advise patient to avoid pregnancy while on this drug; contraceptive counseling should be advised.

Drug-specific teaching points
- Take this drug exactly as prescribed; may be taken with meals if GI upset occurs.
- Do not discontinue this drug abruptly or change dosage, except on the advice of your prescriber.
- Arrange for frequent checkups to monitor your response to this drug.
- Know that the following side effects may occur: drowsiness, dizziness, confusion, blurred vision (avoid driving a car or performing other tasks requiring alertness or visual acuity if these occur); GI upset (taking the drug with food or milk and eating frequent, small meals may help); sensitivity to sunlight (avoid exposure to sunlight; use a sunscreen and wear protective clothing if exposure is unavoidable).
- Wear a medical alert tag at all times so that any emergency medical personnel taking care of you will know that you are an epileptic taking antiepileptic medication.
- Be aware that this drug has caused serious birth defects; avoid pregnancy while on this drug.
- Report skin rash, joint pain, unexplained fever, sore throat, unusual bleeding or bruising, drowsiness, dizziness, blurred vision, bruising, pregnancy.

❒ trimethaphan camsylate

(trye meth' a fan)
Arfonad

Pregnancy Category C

Drug classes
Antihypertensive drug (hypertensive emergencies)
Ganglionic blocker

Therapeutic actions
Occupies cholinergic receptors of autonomic postganglionic neurons, blocking the effects of acetylcholine released from preganglionic nerve terminals, decreasing the effects of the sympathetic (and parasympathetic) nervous systems on effector organs; reduces sympathetic tone on the vasculature, causing vasodilation and decreased BP; decreases sympathetic cardioaccelerator impulses to the heart; decreases the release of catecholamines from the adrenal medulla; has short duration of action (10–30 min).

Indications
- Controlled hypotension during surgery
- Short-term control of BP in hypertensive emergencies

trimethaphan camsylate ■ 1111

- Emergency treatment of pulmonary edema in patients with pulmonary hypertension associated with systemic hypertension
- Unlabeled use: dissecting aortic aneurysm or ischemic heart disease when other agents cannot be used

Contraindications/cautions
- Contraindicated in the presence of hypersensitivity to trimethaphan, when hypotension may subject the patient to undue risk (eg, uncorrected anemia, hypovolemia, shock [incipient and frank], asphyxia, or uncorrected respiratory insufficiency), when IV fluid replacement and blood replacement are unavailable, pregnancy (hypotension may have serious consequences to the fetus).
- Use caution in the presence of arteriosclerosis, cardiac disease, hepatic or renal disease, degenerative CNS disease, Addison's disease, diabetes, patients taking steroids, allergic individuals (drug liberates histamine, which may precipitate asthmatic attack in sensitive individuals).

Dosage
This is a potent hypotensive drug that should be administered only by physicians trained in the techniques of producing controlled hypotension.
Adult: Position patient to avoid cerebral anoxia. Start IV drip at a rate of 3–4 ml/min (3–4 mg/min), then individualize. Rates vary from 0.3–6 mg/min. Determine BP frequently; when used during surgery, stop administration prior to wound closure to permit BP to return to normal. A systolic BP of 100 mm Hg will usually be attained within 10 min after discontinuation.
Pediatric: As adult, but start IV drip at 50–150 μg/kg per minute. Use great caution.
Geriatric or debilitated: Use with caution. The elderly may be more sensitive to the hypotensive effects.

Pharmacokinetics
Metabolism: Plasmal, $T_{1/2}$: unknown
Excretion: Urine

Route	Onset	Peak	Duration
IV	Immediate	End of infusion	10–30 min

IV facts
Preparation: Dilute 500 mg (10 ml) of trimethaphan to 500 ml (1 mg/ml) with 5% Dextrose Injection (do not use any other vehicle).
Infusion: Administer only by continuous IV infusion.
Compatibilities: Do not add any other drug to infusion or infuse through the same line.

Adverse effects
- CNS: Blurred vision
- GI: Dry mouth, constipation
- CV: *Orthostatic hypotension*
- GU: Urinary retention

Clinically important drug-drug interactions
- Prolonged apnea may occur if given concurrently with atracurium, gallamine triethiodide, pancuronium, tubocurarine, vecuronium, metocurine iodide • Prolonged neuromuscular blockade if given concurrently with succinylcholine

■ Nursing Considerations

Assessment
- *History:* Hypersensitivity to trimethaphan; uncorrected anemia, hypovolemia, shock, asphyxia or uncorrected respiratory insufficiency; arteriosclerosis, cardiac disease, hepatic or renal disease, degenerative CNS disease, Addison's disease, diabetes, patients taking steroids; history of allergies; pregnancy
- *Physical:* Orientation, affect, reflexes, pupil size (note: pupillary dilation may not indicate anoxia; the drug appears to have a specific effect on the pupil); P, BP, orthostatic BP, supine BP, perfusion, edema, auscultation; normal urinary output; renal, hepatic function tests; blood and urine glucose

Adverse effects in *Italics* are most common; those in **Bold** are life-threatening.

Implementation
- Do not use the infusion fluid for administration of any other drugs.
- Always dilute trimethaphan before use; prepare solutions immediately before use, and discard unused portion.
- Ensure adequate oxygenation during treatment, especially with regard to coronary and cerebral circulation.

Drug-specific teaching points
In most situations in which this drug is used, the patient will be totally unaware of the use of the drug and will not need drug-related teaching. However, if the patient is conscious during trimethaphan therapy, the following points should be covered:
- Be aware that you will need frequent monitoring of BP, blood tests, checks of IV dosage rate.
- Request assistance if you need to sit up for any reason; you should not try to move around while you are receiving this drug.
- Know that the following side effects may occur: dry mouth (you may have sugarless lozenges, ice to suck, as appropriate); blurred vision (this is an annoying effect that will go away when the drug is discontinued).
- Report pain at the injection site, difficulty breathing, skin rash or itching.

☐ trimethobenzamide hydrochloride

*(trye meth oh **ben**' za mide)*
Oral preparations: Tigan, Trimazide
Suppositories: Tebamide, T-Gen, Tigan, Trimazide
Parenteral preparations: Arrestin, Ticon, Tigan, Tiject-20

Pregnancy Category C

Drug classes
Antiemetic drug (anticholinergic)

Therapeutic actions
Mechanism of action not understood; antiemetic action may be mediated through the chemoreceptor trigger zone (CTZ); impulses to the vomiting center do not appear to be affected.

Indications
- Control of nausea and vomiting

Contraindications/cautions
- Contraindicated in the presence of allergy to trimethobenzamide, benzocaine, or similar local anesthetics; uncomplicated vomiting in children (drug may contribute to development of Reye's syndrome or unfavorably influence its outcome; extrapyramidal effects of drugs may obscure diagnosis of Reye's syndrome); pregnancy.
- Use caution in the presence of lactation; acute febrile illness, encephalitides, gastroenteritis, dehydration, electrolyte imbalance, especially when these occur in children, the elderly, or debilitated; narrow-angle glaucoma; stenosing peptic ulcer; symptomatic prostatic hypertrophy; bronchial asthma; bladder neck obstruction; pyloroduodenal obstruction; cardiac arrhythmias.

Dosage
Adult
- **Oral:** 250 mg tid–qid.
- **Rectal suppositories:** 200 mg tid–qid.
- **Parenteral:** 200 mg IM tid–qid.

Pediatric: Do not administer parenterally to children.
- *30–90 lb (13.6–40.9 kg):* Oral: 100–200 mg tid–qid. Rectal suppositories: 100–200 mg tid–qid.
- *< 30 lb:* Rectal suppositories: 100 mg tid–qid.
- *Premature and newborn:* Not recommended.

Geriatric: More likely to cause serious adverse reactions in elderly patients; use with caution.

Pharmacokinetics

Route	Onset	Duration
Oral	10–40 min	3–4 h
IM	15 min	2–3 h

Metabolism: Hepatic, $T_{1/2}$: unknown

Distribution: Crosses placenta; enters breast milk
Excretion: Urine

Adverse effects
- CNS: Parkinsonlike symptoms, **coma, convulsions, opisthotonus, depression,** disorientation, *dizziness, drowsiness, headache, blurred vision*
- GI: Diarrhea
- CV: Hypotension
- Hematologic: Blood dyscrasias, jaundice
- Hypersensitivity: Allergic-type skin reactions
- Local: *Pain following IM injections*

■ Nursing Considerations

Assessment
- *History:* Allergy to trimethobenzamide, benzocaine, or similar local anesthetics; uncomplicated vomiting in children; pregnancy; lactation; acute febrile illness, encephalitides, gastroenteritis, dehydration, electrolyte imbalance; narrow-angle glaucoma; stenosing peptic ulcer; symptomatic prostatic hypertrophy; bronchial asthma; bladder neck obstruction; pyloroduodenal obstruction; cardiac arrhythmias
- *Physical:* Skin—color, lesions, texture; body temperature; orientation, reflexes, affect; vision exam; P, BP; R, adventitious sounds; bowel sounds; prostate palpation; CBC, serum electrolytes

Implementation
- Administer IM injections deep into upper outer quadrant of the gluteal region.
- Teach patient technique of administering rectal suppositories, as appropriate.
- Ensure adequate hydration.

Drug-specific teaching points
- Take as prescribed. Use proper technique for administering rectal suppositories. Avoid excessive dosage.
- Know that the following side effects may occur: dizziness, sedation, drowsiness (use caution if driving or performing tasks that require alertness if these occur); diarrhea; blurred vision (it may help to know that this is a drug effect that will go away when you discontinue the drug).
- Avoid alcohol while taking this drug; serious sedation could occur.
- Report difficulty breathing, tremors, loss of coordination, sore muscles or muscle spasms, unusual bleeding or bruising, sore throat, visual disturbances, irregular heartbeat, yellowing of the skin or eyes.

☐ trimethoprim

*(trye **meth'** oh prim)*

TMP
Proloprim, Trimpex

Pregnancy Category C

Drug classes
Antibacterial

Therapeutic actions
Inhibits the synthesis of nucleic acids and proteins in susceptible bacteria; the bacterial enzyme involved in this reaction is more readily inhibited than the mammalian enzyme.

Indications
- Uncomplicated urinary tract infections caused by susceptible strains of *E. coli, Proteus mirabilis, Klebsiella pneumoniae, Enterobacter* species, and coagulase-negative *Staphylococcus* species, including *Staphylococcus saprophyticus*

Contraindications/cautions
- Contraindicated in the presence of allergy to trimethoprim, pregnancy (teratogenic in preclinical studies), megaloblastic anemia due to folate deficiency.
- Use caution in the presence of hepatic or renal dysfunction, lactation.

Dosage
Adult: 100 mg PO q12h *or* 200 mg q24h for 10 d.
Pediatric: Effectiveness for children younger than 12 y has not been established.
Geriatric or renal impaired: Creatinine clearance of 15–30 ml/min, 50 mg PO q12h; creatinine clearance of < 15 ml/min, not recommended.

Adverse effects in *Italics* are most common; those in **Bold** are life-threatening.

trimetrexate glucuronate

Pharmacokinetics

Route	Onset	Peak
Oral	Varies	1–4 h

Metabolism: Hepatic, $T_{1/2}$: 8–10 h
Distribution: Crosses placenta; enters breast milk
Excretion: Urine

Adverse effects
- **GI:** *Epigastric distress*, nausea, vomiting, glossitis
- **Hematologic:** Thrombocytopenia, leukopenia, neutropenia, megoblastic anemia, methemoglobinemia, elevated serum transaminase and bilirubin, increased BUN and serum creatinine levels
- **Dermatologic:** *Rash*, pruritus, exfoliative dermatitis
- **Other:** Fever

■ Nursing Considerations

Assessment
- *History:* Allergy to trimethoprim, megaloblastic anemia due to folate deficiency, renal or hepatic dysfunction, pregnancy, lactation
- *Physical:* Skin—color, lesions; temperature; status of mucous membranes; CBC; liver and renal function tests

Implementation
- Perform culture and sensitivity tests before beginning drug therapy.
- Protect the 200-mg tablets from exposure to light.
- Arrange for regular, periodic blood counts during therapy.
- Discontinue drug, consult with physician if any significant reduction in any formed blood element occurs.

Drug-specific teaching points
- Take the full course of the drug; take all the tablets prescribed.
- Know that the following side effects may occur: epigastric distress, nausea, vomiting (small, frequent meals may help); skin rash (consult with your nurse or physician for appropriate skin care).
- Arrange to have medical checkups, including blood tests, periodically during the drug treatment.
- Report fever, sore throat, unusual bleeding or bruising, dizziness, headaches, skin rash.

☐ trimetrexate glucuronate

*(tri me **trex'** ate)*
Neutrexin

Pregnancy Category D

Drug classes
Antineoplastic
Folate antagonist

Therapeutic actions
Inhibits the enzyme responsible for folate activity and DNA, RNA, and protein production, leading to cell death.

Indications
- Alternate therapy with leucovorin for the treatment of moderate-to-severe *Pneumocystis carinii* pneumonia in immunocompromised patients, including patients with AIDS, who are intolerant to or refractory to trimethoprim-sulfamethoxazole therapy
- Unlabeled use: treatment of non–small cell lung, prostate, and colorectal cancer

Contraindications/cautions
- Contraindicated in the presence of allergy to trimetrexate, leucovorin, or methotrexate; pregnancy (teratogenic in preclinical studies); lactation.
- Use caution in the presence of hepatic or renal dysfunction, myelosuppression.

Dosage
Adult: 45 mg/m^2 IV once a day over 60–90 min with leucovorin IV at a dose of 20 mg/m^2 over 5–10 min q6h or orally as four doses of 20 mg/m^2. Treatment course is 21 d of trimetrexate and 24 d of leucovorin.

Adverse effects in *Italics* are most common; those in **Bold** are life-threatening.

trimipramine maleate ■ 1115

Pediatric: Effectiveness for children younger than 18 y has not been established.
Geriatric, renal/hepatic, or hematologically impaired: Reduce dosage, and monitor blood tests before proceeding to next dose.

Pharmacokinetics

Route	Onset
IV	Rapid

Metabolism: Hepatic, $T_{1/2}$: 7–15 h
Distribution: Crosses placenta; enters breast milk
Excretion: Urine

IV facts
Preparation: Reconstitute with 2 ml of 5% Dextrose Injection or Sterile Saline for a concentration of 12.5 mg/ml; solution should appear pale greenish-yellow with no particulate matter; may be further diluted with 5% Dextrose to a concentration of 0.25–2 mg/ml; store at room temperature, protect from light; stable for up to 24 h; discard after that time.
Infusion: Flush IV line with 10 ml of 5% Dextrose Injection before and after infusing trimetrexate; infuse diluted solution over 60 min; leucovorin must be administered seperately.

Adverse effects
- CNS: Confusion
- GI: Nausea, vomiting
- Hematologic: Hyponatremia, hypocalcemia; increased AST, ALT, alkaline phosphatase, bilirubin, serum creatinine, *neutropenia, thrombocytopenia*, anemia
- Other: *Fever*, rash, fatigue

■ Nursing Considerations

Assessment
- *History:* Allergy to trimetrexate, leucovorin, or methotrexate; pregnancy, lactation; use caution in the presence of hepatic or renal dysfunction, myelosuppression
- *Physical:* Skin—color, lesions; temperature; CBC; liver and renal function tests; serum electrolytes

Implementation
- Avoid contact with drug solution; if drug comes in contact with skin, flush with soap and water.
- Arrange for proper disposal of drug, using disposal techniques for cytotoxic drugs.
- Ensure that leucovorin is administered as scheduled while on this drug; it is essential for safe use of trimetrexate.
- Arrange for regular, periodic blood counts and liver function tests during therapy.
- Protect patient from exposure to infection while on this therapy.
- Consult with physician for changes in drug dose or timing if any significant reduction in any formed blood elements occur.
- Monitor for signs of electrolyte disturbances, and arrange for replacement therapy as appropriate.

Drug-specific teaching points
- Be aware that this drug must be given IV in conjunction with another drug, leucovorin. The treatment will last for 21 and 24 d.
- Know that the following side effects may occur: nausea, vomiting (small, frequent meals may help); skin rash.
- Be aware that you will need regular blood tests during the drug treatment.
- Avoid exposure to infections while you are on this drug; you may be more susceptible to infections.
- Report fever, sore throat, unusual bleeding or bruising, extreme fatigue.

☐ trimipramine maleate

*(trye **mi'** pra meen)*
Surmontil

Pregnancy Category C

Adverse effects in *Italics* are most common; those in **Bold** are life-threatening.

trimipramine maleate

Drug classes
Tricyclic antidepressant (TCA; tertiary amine)

Therapeutic actions
Mechanism of action unknown; the TCAs are structurally related to the phenothiazine antipsychotic drugs (eg, chlorpromazine); TCAs inhibit the presynaptic reuptake of the neurotransmitters norepinephrine and serotonin; anticholinergic at CNS and peripheral receptors; the relation of these effects to clinical efficacy is unknown.

Indications
- Relief of symptoms of depression (endogenous depression most responsive); sedative effects of tertiary amine TCAs may be helpful in patients whose depression is associated with anxiety and sleep disturbance
- Unlabeled uses: treatment of peptic ulcer disease, dermatologic disorders

Contraindications/cautions
- Contraindicated in the presence of hypersensitivity to any tricyclic drug, concomitant therapy with an MAOI, recent MI, myelography within previous 24 h or scheduled within 48 h, pregnancy (limb reduction abnormalities reported), lactation.
- Use caution in the presence of electroshock therapy; preexisting cardiovascular disorders (eg, severe coronary heart disease, progressive heart failure, angina pectoris, paroxysmal tachycardia); angle-closure glaucoma, increased intraocular pressure; urinary retention, ureteral or urethral spasm (anticholinergic effects of TCAs may exacerbate these conditions); seizure disorders (TCAs lower the seizure threshold); hyperthyroidism (predisposes to CVS toxicity, including cardiac arrhythmias); impaired hepatic, renal function; psychiatric patients (schizophrenic or paranoid patients may exhibit a worsening of psychosis); manic-depressive patients (may shift to hypomanic or manic phase); elective surgery (TCAs should be discontinued as long as possible before surgery).

Dosage
Adult
- **Hospitalized patients:** Initially, 100 mg/d PO in divided doses. Gradually increase to 200 mg/d as required. If no improvement in 2–3 wk, increase to a maximum dose of 250–300 mg/d.
- **Outpatients:** Initially 75 mg/d PO in divided doses. May increase to 150 mg/d. Do not exceed 200 mg/d. Total daily dosage may be administered at bedtime. Maintenance dose is 50–150 mg/d given as a single bedtime dose. After satisfactory response, reduce to lowest effective dosage. Continue therapy for 3 mo or longer to lessen possibility of relapse.

Pediatric (adolescent): 50 mg/d PO with gradual increases up to 100 mg/d. Not recommended for use if younger than 12 y.

Geriatric: 50 mg/d PO with gradual increases up to 100 mg/d PO.

Pharmacokinetics

Route	Onset	Peak
Oral	Varies	2 h

Metabolism: Hepatic, $T_{1/2}$: 7–30 h
Distribution: Crosses placenta; enters breast milk
Excretion: Urine and feces

Adverse effects
- CNS: *Sedation and anticholinergic (atropine-like) effects; confusion* (especially in elderly), *disturbed concentration*, hallucinations, disorientation, decreased memory, feelings of unreality, delusions, anxiety, nervousness, restlessness, agitation, panic, insomnia, nightmares, hypomania, mania, exacerbation of psychosis, drowsiness, weakness, fatigue, headache, numbness, tingling, paresthesias of extremities, incoordination, motor hyperactivity, akathisia, ataxia, tremors, peripheral neuropathy, extrapyramidal symptoms, *seizures*,

Adverse effects in *Italics* are most common; those in **Bold** are life-threatening.

speech blockage, dysarthria, tinnitus, altered EEG
- **GI:** *Dry mouth, constipation,* paralytic ileus, *nausea,* vomiting, anorexia, epigastric distress, diarrhea, flatulence, dysphagia, peculiar taste, increased salivation, stomatitis, glossitis, parotid swelling, abdominal cramps, black tongue, hepatitis, jaundice (rare), elevated transaminase, altered alkaline phosphatase
- **CV:** *Orthostatic hypotension,* hypertension, syncope, tachycardia, palpitations, MI, arrhythmias, heart block, precipitation of CHF, **stroke**
- **Hematologic:** Bone marrow depression including **agranulocytosis;** eosinophila, purpura, thrombocytopenia, leukopenia
- **GU:** Urinary retention, delayed micturition, dilation of the urinary tract, gynecomastia, testicular swelling in men; breast enlargement, menstrual irregularity and galactorrhea in women; increased or decreased libido; impotence
- **Hypersensitivity:** Skin rash, pruritus, vasculitis, petechiae, photosensitization, edema (generalized or of face and tongue), drug fever
- **Endocrine:** Elevated or depressed blood sugar, elevated prolactin levels, SIADH secretion
- **Withdrawal:** Symptoms with abrupt discontinuation of prolonged therapy: nausea, headache, vertigo, nightmares, malaise
- **Other:** Nasal congestion, excessive appetite, weight gain or loss, sweating, alopecia, lacrimation, hyperthermia, flushing, chills

Clinically important drug-drug interactions

- Increased TCA levels and pharmacologic (especially anticholinergic) effects when given with cimetidine, fluoxetine, ranitidine • Increased bleeding effects if taken concurrently with dicumarol • Risk of dysrhythmias and hypertension if taken with sympathomimetics • Risk of severe hypertension when taken concurrently with clonidine • Hyperpyretic crises, severe convulsions, hypertensive episodes and deaths when MAOIs are given with TCAs • Decreased hypotensive activity of guanethidine if taken with trimipramine • *Note:* MAOIs and tricyclic antidepressants have been used successfully in some patients resistant to therapy with single agents; however, case reports indicate that the combination can cause serious and potentially fatal adverse effects.

■ Nursing Considerations

Assessment

- *History:* Hypersensitivity to any tricyclic drug; concomitant therapy with an MAOI; recent MI; myelography within previous 24 h or scheduled within 48 h; pregnancy; lactation; electroshock therapy; preexisting cardiovascular disorders; angle-closure glaucoma, increased intraocular pressure; urinary retention, ureteral or urethral spasm; seizure disorders; hyperthyroidism; impaired hepatic, renal function; psychiatric patients; manic-depressive patients; elective surgery
- *Physical:* Body weight; temperature; skin—color, lesions; orientation, affect, reflexes, vision and hearing; P, BP, orthostatic BP, perfusion; bowel sounds, normal output, liver evaluation; urine flow, normal output; usual sexual function, frequency of menses, breast and scrotal examination; liver function tests, urinalysis; CBC, ECG.

Implementation

- Ensure that depressed and potentially suicidal patients have access to limited quantities of the drug.
- Administer major portion of dose at bedtime if drowsiness, severe anticholinergic effects occur.
- Arrange to reduce dosage if minor side effects develop; arrange to discontinue the drug if serious side effects occur.
- Arrange for CBC if patient develops fever, sore throat, or other sign of infection during therapy.

Adverse effects in *Italics* are most common; those in **Bold** are life-threatening.

Drug-specific teaching points
- Take drug exactly as prescribed.
- Do not stop taking this drug abruptly or without consulting the physician or nurse.
- Avoid alcohol, other sleep-inducing drugs, OTC drugs while on this drug.
- Avoid prolonged exposure to sunlight or sunlamps; use a sunscreen or protective garments if long exposure to sunlight is unavoidable.
- Know that the following side effects may occur: headache, dizziness, drowsiness, weakness, blurred vision (these effects are reversible; safety measures may need to be taken if these become severe; avoid driving an automobile or performing tasks that require alertness while these persist); nausea, vomiting, loss of appetite, dry mouth (small, frequent meals, frequent mouth care, sucking sugarless candies may help); nightmares, inability to concentrate, confusion; changes in sexual function.
- Report dry mouth, difficulty in urination, excessive sedation.

▢ tripelennamine hydrochloride

*(tri pel **enn**' a meen)*
PBZ

Pregnancy Category C

Drug classes
Antihistamine (ethylenediamine type)

Therapeutic actions
Competitively blocks the effects of histamine at H_1 receptor sites; has anticholinergic (atropine-like), antipruritic, and sedative effects.

Indications
- Symptomatic relief of symptoms associated with perennial and seasonal allergic rhinitis, vasomotor rhinitis, allergic conjunctivitis, mild, uncomplicated urticaria and angioedema
- Amelioraton of allergic reactions to blood or plasma
- Dermatographism
- Adjunctive therapy in anaphylactic reactions

Contraindications/cautions
- Contraindicated in the presence of allergy to any antihistamines, pregnancy, lactation.
- Use caution in the presence of narrow-angle glaucoma, stenosing peptic ulcer, symptomatic prostatic hypertrophy, asthmatic attack, bladder neck obstruction, pyloroduodenal obstruction.

Dosage
Adult: 25–50 mg PO q4–6h. Up to 600 mg/d has been used. Sustained-release preparation: 100 mg PO in the morning and the evening; 100 mg q8h may be needed.
Pediatric: 5 mg/kg per day PO or 150 mg/m^2 per day PO divided into four to six doses. Maximum total dose of 300 mg/d. Do not use sustained-release preparations with children.
Geriatric: More likely to cause dizziness, sedation, syncope, toxic confusional states and hypotension in elderly patients; use with caution.

Pharmacokinetics

Route	Onset	Peak	Duration
Oral	15–30 min	1–2 h	4–6 h

Metabolism: Hepatic, $T_{1/2}$: unknown
Distribution: Crosses placenta; enters breast milk
Excretion: Urine

Adverse effects
- **CNS:** *Drowsiness, sedation, dizziness, disturbed coordination,* fatigue, confusion, restlessness, excitation, nervousness, tremor, headache, blurred vision, diplopia, vertigo, tinnitus, acute labyrinthitis, hysteria, tingling, heaviness and weakness of the hands
- **GI:** *Epigastric distress*, anorexia, increased appetite and weight gain, nausea, vomiting, diarrhea or constipation

Adverse effects in *Italics* are most common; those in **Bold** are life-threatening.

triprolidine hydrochloride 1119

- **CV:** Hypotension, palpitations, bradycardia, tachycardia, extrasystoles
- **Respiratory:** *Thickening of bronchial secretions*, chest tightness, wheezing, nasal stuffiness, dry mouth, dry nose, dry throat, sore throat
- **Hematologic:** Hemolytic anemia, hypoplastic anemia, thrombocytopenia, leukopenia, agranulocytosis, pancytopenia
- **GU:** Urinary frequency, dysuria, urinary retention, early menses, decreased libido, impotence
- **Dermatologic:** Urticaria, rash, anaphylactic shock, photosensitivity, excessive perspiration, chills
- **Other:** Drug abuse when used with pentazocine ("Ts and Blues") as a heroin substitute

■ Nursing Considerations

Assessment
- *History:* Allergy to any antihistamines, narrow-angle glaucoma, stenosing peptic ulcer, symptomatic prostatic hypertrophy, asthmatic attack, bladder neck obstruction, pyloroduodenal obstruction, pregnancy, lactation
- *Physical:* Skin—color, lesions, texture; orientation, reflexes, affect; vision exam; P, BP; R, adventitious sounds; bowel sounds; prostate palpation; CBC with differential

Implementation
- Administer with food if GI upset occurs.
- Administer elixir form if patient is unable to take tablets.
- Caution patient not to crush or chew sustained-release tablets.

Drug-specific teaching points
- Avoid excessive dosage.
- Take with food if GI upset occurs.
- Do not crush or chew sustained-release tablets.
- Know that the following side effects may occur: dizziness, sedation, drowsiness (use caution if driving or performing tasks that require alertness if these occur); epigastric distress, diarrhea, or constipation (taking the drug with meals may help; dry mouth (frequent mouth care, sucking sugarless lozenges may help); thickening of bronchial secretions, dryness of nasal mucosa (use of a humidifier may help if this becomes a problem).
- Avoid alcohol while on this drug; serious sedation could occur.
- Report difficulty breathing, hallucinations, tremors, loss of coordination, unusual bleeding or bruising, visual disturbances, irregular heartbeat.

☐ triprolidine hydrochloride

*(trye **proe**' li deen)*
Prescription preparation:
Myidil
Pregnancy Category B

Drug classes
Antihistamine (alkylamine type)

Therapeutic actions
Competitively blocks the effects of histamine at H_1 receptor sites; has anticholinergic (atropine-like), antipruritic, and sedative effects.

Indications
- Symptomatic relief of symptoms associated with perennial and seasonal allergic rhinitis, vasomotor rhinitis, allergic conjunctivitis, mild, uncomplicated urticaria and angioedema
- Amelioraton of allergic reactions to blood or plasma
- Dermatographism
- Adjunctive therapy in anaphylactic reactions

Contraindications/cautions
- Contraindicated in the presence of allergy to any antihistamines, pregnancy, lactation.
- Use caution in the presence of narrow-angle glaucoma, stenosing peptic ulcer, symptomatic prostatic hypertrophy, asthmatic attack, bladder neck obstruction, pyloroduodenal obstruction.

Adverse effects in *Italics* are most common; those in **Bold** are life-threatening.

1120 ■ tromethamine

Dosage
Adult and pediatric older than 12 y: 2.5 mg q4–6h PO. Do not exceed four doses in 24 h.
Pediatric
- **6–12 y:** 1.25 mg q4–6h PO. Do not exceed four doses in 24 h.
- **Younger than 6 y:** Consult physician.

Geriatric: More likely to cause dizziness, sedation, syncope, toxic confusional states, and hypotension in elderly patients; use with caution.

Pharmacokinetics

Route	Onset	Peak	Duration
Oral	15–30 min	1–2 h	4–6 h

Metabolism: Hepatic, $T_{1/2}$: unknown
Distribution: Crosses placenta; enters breast milk
Excretion: Urine

Adverse effects
- CNS: *Drowsiness, sedation, dizziness, disturbed coordination,* fatigue, confusion, restlessness, excitation, nervousness, tremor, headache, blurred vision, diplopia, vertigo, tinnitus, acute labyrinthitis, hysteria, tingling, heaviness and weakness of the hands
- GI: *Epigastric distress,* anorexia, increased appetite and weight gain, nausea, vomiting, diarrhea or constipation
- CV: Hypotension, palpitations, bradycardia, tachycardia, extrasystoles
- Respiratory: *Thickening of bronchial secretions,* chest tightness, wheezing, nasal stuffiness, dry mouth, dry nose, dry throat, sore throat
- Hematologic: Hemolytic anemia, hypoplastic anemia, thrombocytopenia, leukopenia, agranulocytosis, pancytopenia
- GU: Urinary frequency, dysuria, urinary retention, early menses, decreased libido, impotence
- Dermatologic: Urticaria, rash, anaphylactic shock, photosensitivity, excessive perspiration, chills

■ Nursing Considerations
Assessment
- *History:* Allergy to any antihistamines, narrow-angle glaucoma, stenosing peptic ulcer, symptomatic prostatic hypertrophy, asthmatic attack, bladder neck obstruction, pyloroduodenal obstruction, pregnancy, lactation
- *Physical:* Skin—color, lesions, texture; orientation, reflexes, affect; vision exam; P, BP; R, adventitious sounds; bowel sounds; prostate palpation; CBC with differential

Implementation
- Administer with food if GI upset occurs.
- Administer syrup form if patient is unable to take tablets.

Drug-specific teaching points
- Avoid excessive dosage.
- Take with food if GI upset occurs.
- Do not crush or chew sustained-release tablets.
- Know that the following side effects may occur: dizziness, sedation, drowsiness (use caution if driving or performing tasks that require alertness if these occur); epigastric distress, diarrhea, or constipation (taking the drug with meals may help); dry mouth (frequent mouth care, sucking sugarless lozenges may help); thickening of bronchial secretions, dryness of nasal mucosa (use of a humidifier may help if this becomes a problem).
- Avoid alcohol while on this drug; serious sedation could occur.
- Report difficulty breathing, hallucinations, tremors, loss of coordination, unusual bleeding or bruising, visual disturbances, irregular heartbeat.

▢ tromethamine

*(troe **meth'** a meen)*
Tham, Tham-E

Pregnancy Category C

Drug classes
Systemic alkalinizer

Therapeutic actions
Sodium-free organic amine that acts as a buffer, preventing the occurrence of

*Adverse effects in Italics are most common; those in **Bold** are life-threatening.*

acidosis; acts as a weak osmotic diuretic; may be preferable to sodium bicarbonate in the treatment of metabolic acidosis when sodium restriction is important.

Indications
- Prevention or correction of systemic acidosis; metabolic acidosis associated with coronary artery bypass surgery; correction of acidity of acid dextrose blood in cardiac bypass surgery; cardiac arrest

Contraindications/cautions
- Contraindicated in the presence of anuria, uremia, pregnancy.
- Use caution in the presence of respiratory depression, impaired renal function.

Dosage
Adult and pediatric older than 12 y
- ***Acidosis during cardiac bypass surgery:*** Single dose of 500 ml IV is usually sufficient; 9 ml/kg IV; do not exceed 500 mg/kg per hour.
- ***Acidity of ACD blood:*** 0.5–2.5 g (15–77 ml) IV added to each 500 ml of ACD blood.
- ***Acidosis of cardiac arrest:*** Inject 2–6 g directly into ventricular cavity if chest is open; Inject 3.6–10.8 g IV into a large peripheral vein if chest is not open.

Pharmacokinetics

Route	Onset	Duration
IV	Rapid	8 h

Metabolism: $T_{1/2}$: unknown
Distribution: Crosses placenta; enters breast milk
Excretion: Urine

IV facts
Preparation: Use as provided by manufacturer.
Infusion: Infuse slowly into pump oxygenator, ACD blood, priming fluid or ventricular cavity; infuse slowly into peripheral vein.

Adverse effects
- **GI:** Hemorrhagic hepatic necrosis
- **Respiratory:** Respiratory depression
- **Hematologic:** Decreased blood glucose
- **Local:** Phlebitis, infection of injection site

■ Nursing Considerations
Assessment
- *History:* Anuria, uremia, pregnancy, respiratory depression, impaired renal function.
- *Physical:* P, BP; R, adventitious sounds; CBC, blood gases, electrolytes, glucose

Implementation
- Monitor blood pH, pCO_2, bicarbonate, glucose, electrolytes before and during administration.
- Provide supportive or replacement therapy as needed for hematologic changes.
- Use a large needle in the biggest vein available for peripheral use; alkalinity is very irritating to tissues.

Drug-specific teaching points
Patients receiving this drug will be unconscious and unaware of its use. If local irritation occurs after use, incorporate some information about the drug into the wound care of the injection site.

☐ uracil mustard

(yoor' a sill)
Uracil Mustard
Pregnancy Category X

Drug classes
Alkylating agent
Nitrogen mustard
Antineoplastic drug

Therapeutic actions
Cytotoxic: exact mechanism of action is not known, but it alkylates DNA and interferes with normal replication processes in susceptible cells.

Adverse effects in *Italics* are most common; those in **Bold** are life-threatening.

uracil mustard

Indications
- Palliative treatment of chronic lymphocytic leukemia, non-Hodgkin's lymphomas, chronic myelogenous leukemia
- Palliation of early stages of polycythemia vera before the development of leukemia or myelofibrosis
- Palliative therapy in mycosis fungoides

Contraindications/cautions
- Contraindicated in the presence of allergy to uracil mustard; allergy to tartrazine (in tablets marketed as Uracil Mustard [Upjohn]); leukopenia, thrombocytopenia, aplastic anemia; pregnancy (teratogenic); lactation.
- Use caution in the presence of radiation therapy, chemotherapy, tumor cell infiltration of the bone marrow.

Dosage
Individualize dosage based on hematologic profile and response.
Adult: Single weekly dose of 0.15 mg/kg PO for 4 wk.
Pediatric: Single weekly dose of 0.30 mg/kg PO for 4 wk. If therapeutic response occurs, continue the same weekly dose until relapse occurs.

Pharmacokinetics

Route	Onset	Duration
Oral	Varies	90–120 min

Metabolism: Hepatic, $T_{1/2}$: 1 h
Distribution: Crosses placenta; enters breast milk
Excretion: Urine

Adverse effects
- CNS: Nervousness, irritability, depression
- GI: *Nausea, vomiting, diarrhea,* hepatotoxicity
- Hematologic: **Severe thrombocytopenia, granulocytic and lymphocytic leukopenia, initially;followed by depression of the erythrocyte count and hemoglobin levels** immunosuppression, increased serum uric acid levels due to lysis of cells
- GU: Amenorrhea, azoospermia
- Dermatologic: *Pruritus*, dermatitis, hair loss
- Other: Secondary neoplasia

■ Nursing Considerations
Assessment
- *History:* Allergy to uracil mustard, tartrazine; radiation therapy; chemotherapy; leukopenia, thrombocytopenia, aplastic anemia; tumor cell infiltration of the bone marrow; pregnancy; lactation
- *Physical:* Temperature; weight; skin—color, lesions; hair; orientation, affect; CBC, differential; serum uric acid; liver function tests

Implementation
- Arrange for blood tests to evaluate hematopoietic function before beginning therapy, once or twice weekly during therapy, and for 4 wk after therapy.
- Do not give full dosage within 2–3 wk after a full course of radiation therapy or chemotherapy because of the risk of severe bone marrow depression; reduced dosage may be needed.
- Arrange for increase in dosage in antigout medication, if appropriate.
- Ensure that patient is well hydrated before treatment and maintains hydration during treatment.

Drug-specific teaching points
- Know that the following side effects may occur: nausea, vomiting, loss of appetite (small, frequent meals may help); diarrhea; rash, itching, some hair loss; nervousness, irritability, depression (it may help to know that this is caused by the drug).
- Maintain your fluid intake and nutrition while on this drug. Drink at least 10–12 glassses of fluid a day.
- Be aware that this drug has the potential to cause severe birth defects. It is advisable to use birth control methods while on this drug. The drug also can cause amenorrhea in women and lack of sperm production in men; this effect is usually reversible.

Adverse effects in *Italics* are most common; those in **Bold** are life-threatening.

- Report unusual bleeding or bruising, fever, chills, sore throat, swelling of the feet or hands, stomach or flank pain.

❑ urea

(yoor ee' a)
Ureaphil

Pregnancy Category C

Drug classes
Osmotic diuretic

Therapeutic actions
Elevates the osmolarity of the glomerular filtrate, hindering the reabsorption of water and leading to a loss of water, sodium, and chloride; creates an osmotic gradient in the eye between plasma and ocular fluids, reducing intraocular pressure.

Indications
- Reduction of intracranial pressure and treatment of cerebral edema
- Reduction of elevated intraocular pressure
- Unlabeled use: induction of abortion when used by intra-amniotic injection

Contraindications/cautions
- Active intracranial bleeding (except during craniotomy), marked dehydration, severe renal or hepatic disease, pregnancy, lactation.

Dosage
Adult: Slow IV infusion of 30% solution only: 1–1.5 g/kg. Do not exceed 120 g/d.
Pediatric: 0.5–1.5 g/kg, IV. As little as 0.1 g/kg may be adequate in children younger than 2 y.

Pharmacokinetics

Route	Onset	Peak	Duration
IV	30–45 min	60 min	5–6 h

Metabolism: T$_{1/2}$: unknown
Distribution: Crosses placenta; enters breast milk
Excretion: Urine

IV facts
Preparation: For 135 ml of a 30% solution of sterile urea, mix one 40-g vial with 105 ml of 5% or 10% Dextrose Injection or 10% Invert Sugar in Water; each ml of a 30% solution provides 300 mg of urea; use only fresh solution; discard any solution within 24 h after reconstitution.
Infusion: Administer 30% solution by slow IV infusion; do not exceed 4 ml/min.
Compatibilities: Do not administer urea through the same IV set as blood or blood products.

Adverse effects
- CNS: *Dizziness, headache*, syncope, disorientation
- GI: *Nausea, vomiting*
- Hematologic: Hyponatremia, hypokalemia
- Local: Tissue necrosis if extravasation occurs at IV site
- Other: Thrombophlebitis, febrile response, hypervolemia if improperly administered

■ Nursing Considerations

Assessment
- *History:* Active intracranial bleeding, marked dehydration, hepatic or renal disease, pregnancy, lactation
- *Physical:* Skin—color, edema; orientation, reflexes, muscle strength, pupillary reflexes; pulses, BP, perfusion; R, pattern, adventitious sounds; urinary output patterns; serum electrolytes, urinalysis, renal and liver function tests

Implementation
- Do not infuse in veins of lower extremities of elderly patients.
- Monitor urinary output carefully.
- Monitor BP regularly and carefully.
- Monitor serum electrolytes periodically with prolonged therapy.
- Use an indwelling catheter in comatose patients.

Drug-specific teaching points
- Be aware that this drug can only be given by IV route of administration.

Adverse effects in *Italics* are most common; those in **Bold** are life-threatening.

1124 ■ urofollitropin

- Know that the following side effects may occur: increased urination (bathroom facilities will be made readily available), GI upset (small, frequent meals may help), dry mouth (sugarless lozenges to suck may help this problem), headache, blurred vision (use caution when moving around; ask for assistance).
- Report pain at the IV site, severe headache, chest pain.

❏ urofollitropin

(you' ro fol i tro' pin)
Metrodin

Pregnancy Category X

Drug classes
Hormonal agent
Fertility drug

Therapeutic actions
Gonadotropin extracted from the urine of postmenopausal women; stimulates ovarian follicular growth and maturation in women who do not have primary ovarian failure; to cause ovulation, human chorionic gonadotropin (HCG) must be given when the follicles are sufficiently mature.

Indications
- Urofollitropin and HCG are given sequentially for induction of ovulation in patients with polycystic ovarian disease who have an elevated LH/FSH ratio and who have failed to respond to clomiphene citrate therapy

Contraindications/cautions
- Contraindicated in the presence of known sensitivity to urofollitropin; high levels of FSH, LH, indicating primary ovarian failure; overt thyroid or adrenal dysfunction; organic cranial lesion; abnormal uterine bleeding of undetermined origin; ovarian cysts or enlargement not due to polycystic ovary syndrome; pregnancy (fetal defects have occurred).
- Use caution in the presence of lactation.

Dosage
Individualize dose to the smallest, effective dose. Must be given only by physicians who are thoroughly familiar with infertility problems; must be given with great care.
Initial dose: 75 IU/d IM urofollitropin for 7–12 d followed by 5,000–10,000 U of HCG 1 d after the last urofollitropin dose. May be repeated for two more courses before increasing dose to 150 IU of FSH/d for 7–12 d followed by 5,000–10,000 U HCG 1 d after the last urofollitropin dose. If evidence of ovulation is present, but pregnancy does not occur, repeat the same dose for two more courses.

Pharmacokinetics

Route	Onset
IM	Slow

Metabolism: Hepatic, $T_{1/2}$: unknown
Distribution: Crosses placenta; enters breast milk
Excretion: Urine

Adverse effects
- **CNS:** Headache
- **GI:** *Abdominal discomfort*, distention, bloating, nausea, vomiting, diarrhea
- **CV:** Arterial thromboembolism
- **GU:** Uterine bleeding, *ovarian enlargement*, breast tenderness, ectopic pregnancy, *ovarian overstimulation* (abdominal distention, pain, accompanied in more serious cases by ascites, pleural effusion), multiple births, birth defects in resulting pregnancies
- **Local:** *Pain, rash, swelling or irritation at injection site*
- **Other:** Febrile reaction—fever, chills, musculoskeletal aches or pain, malaise, fatigue

■ Nursing Considerations

Assessment
- *History:* Known sensitivity to urofollitropin; high levels of FSH, LH; overt thyroid or adrenal dysfunction; organic cranial lesion; abnormal uterine bleeding of undetermined origin; ovarian cysts or

Adverse effects in *Italics* are most common; those in **Bold** are life-threatening.

enlargement not due to polycystic ovary syndrome; pregnancy; lactation
- *Physical:* Skin—color, temperature; body temperature; injection site; abdominal exam, pelvic exam; urinary pregnanadiol and gonadotropin; abdominal ultrasound

Implementation
- Arrange for a complete pelvic exam before each course of treatment to rule out ovarian enlargement, pregnancy, other uterine difficulties.
- Caution patient of the risks of multiple births, drug effects, and need for medical evaluation and follow-up.
- Dissolve contents of 1 ampule in 1–2 ml of Sterile Saline. Administer IM immediately; discard any unused reconstituted material.
- Discontinue drug at any sign of ovarian overstimulation, and arrange to have patient admitted to the hospital for observation and supportive measures.
- Examine patient at least every other day for signs of excessive ovarian stimulation during treatment and during a 2-wk post-treatment period.
- Provide women with calendar of treatment days and explanations about the signs of ovulation. Caution patient that 24-h urine collections or abdominal ultrasound will be needed periodically to determine drug effects on the ovaries, that timing of intercourse is important for achieving pregnancy. Patient should engage in intercourse daily beginning on the day prior to HCG administration until ovulation is apparent from determination of progestational activity.

Drug-specific teaching points
- Prepare a calendar showing the treatment schedule and plotting out ovulation.
- Know that the following side effects may occur: abdominal distention, flushing, breast tenderness, pain, rash, swelling at injection site.
- Be aware that there is an increased incidence of multiple births in women using this drug.
- Report bloating, stomach pain, fever, chills, muscle aches or pains, abdominal swelling, back pain, swelling or pain in the legs, pain at injection sites.

❒ urokinase

(yoor oh kin' ase)

Abbokinase, Abbokinase Open-Cath

Pregnancy Category B

Drug classes
Thrombolytic enzyme

Therapeutic actions
Enzyme isolated from human urine; converts plasminogen to the enzyme plasmin (fibrinolysin), which degrades fibrin clots, fibrinogen, and other plasma proteins; lyses thrombi and emboli.

Indications
- Pulmonary emboli for lysis
- Coronary artery thrombosis within 6 h of onset of symptoms of coronary occlusion
- IV catheter clearance

Contraindications/cautions
- Contraindicated in the presence of hypersensitivity to urokinase, active internal bleeding, recent (within 2 mo) CVA, intracranial or intraspinal surgery, intracranial neoplasm.
- Use caution in the presence of recent major surgery, obstetric delivery, organ biopsy, or rupture of a noncompressible blood vessel; recent serious GI bleed; recent serious trauma, including CPR; severe hypertension; SBE; hemostatic defects; cerebrovascular disease; diabetic hemorrhagic retinopathy; septic thrombosis; pregnancy; lactation.

Dosage
Adult
- **IV infusion:** *Give through constant infusion pump:* Priming dose of 4,400 U/kg as an admixture with 5% Dextrose Injection or 0.9% Sodium Chloride at a rate of 90 ml/h over 10 min. Then give 4,400 U/kg per hour at a rate of 15

ml/h for 12 h. At end of infusion, flush the tubing with 0.9% Sodium Chloride or 5% Dextrose Injection equal to the volume of the tubing. At the end of the infusion, treat with continuous heparin IV infusion, beginning heparin when the thrombin time has decreased to less than twice the normal control.
– *Lysis of coronary artery thrombi:* Before therapy, administer heparin bolus of 2,500–10,000 U IV; infuse urokinase into occluded artery at rate of 6,000 U/min for up to 2 h. Continue infusion until the artery is maximally opened, usually 15–30 min after initial opening.
– *IV catheter clearance:* For clearing a central venous catheter; have patient exhale and hold his or her breath any time catheter is not connected to IV tubing. Disconnect catheter and after determining amount of occlusion, attach tuberculin syringe with urokinase solution and inject amount equal to volume of catheter. Wait 5 min and aspirate; repeat aspirations every 5 min for up to 1 h. A repeat infusion of urokinase may be necessary in severe cases. When patency is restored, aspirate 4–5 ml of blood to ensure removal of drug and residual clot. Irrigate gently with 0.9% Sodium Chloride in fresh 10 ml syringe and reconnect IV tubing.
Pediatric: Safety and efficacy not established.

Pharmacokinetics

Route	Onset	Peak
IV	Immediate	End of infusion

Metabolism: Plasma, $T_{1/2}$: unknown
Distribution: Crosses placenta; enters breast milk
Excretion: Unknown

IV facts
Preparation: Reconstitute vial with 5.2 ml of Sterile Water for Injection without preservatives. Avoid shaking during reconstitution; gently roll or tilt vial to reconstitute; consult manufacturer's directions for further dilution. Solution may be filtered through 0.45 or smaller cellulose membrane filter in administration set. Use immediately and discard any unused portion of drug; do not store. Refrigerate vials.
Infusion: Maintain infusion via an infusion pump to ensure accurate delivery.
Compatibilities: Do not add other medications to reconstituted solutions.

Adverse effects
- **CNS:** Headache
- **CV:** angioneurotic edema, arrhythmias (with intracoronary artery infusion)
- **Respiratory:** Breathing difficulty, bronchospasm
- **Hematologic:** **Bleeding** (*minor or surface* to major internal bleeding)
- **Dermatologic:** Skin rash, urticaria, itching, flushing
- **Other:** Musculoskeletal pain, *fever*

Clinically important drug-drug interactions
- Increased risk of hemorrhage if used with heparin or oral anticoagulants, aspirin, indomethacin, phenylbutazone

Drug-lab test interferences
- Marked decrease in plasminogen, fibrinogen; increases in thrombin time, activated partial thromboplastin (APTT), prothrombin time (PT)

■ Nursing Considerations
Assessment
- *History:* Hypersensitivity to urokinase; active internal bleeding; recent CVA, intracranial or intraspinal surgery; intracranial neoplasm; recent major surgery, obstetric delivery, organ biopsy, or rupture of a noncompressible blood vessel; GI bleed; recent serious trauma; severe hypertension; SBE; hemostatic defects; cerebrovascular disease; diabetic hemorrhagic retinopathy; septic thrombosis; pregnancy; lactation
- *Physical:* Skin—color, temperature, lesions; temperature; orientation, reflexes; P, BP, peripheral perfusion, baseline

ECG; R, adventitous sounds; liver evaluation; Hct, platelet count, thrombin time, APTT, PT

Implementation
- Discontinue heparin if it is being given, unless ordered specifically for coronary artery infusion.
- Arrange for regular monitoring of coagulation studies.
- Apply pressure or pressure dressings to control superficial bleeding (at invaded or disturbed areas).
- Avoid any arterial invasive procedures during therapy.
- Arrange for typing and cross-matching of blood if serious blood loss occurs and whole blood transfusions are required.
- Institute treatment within 6 h of onset of symptoms for evolving myocardial infarction; within 7 d of other thrombotic event.
- Monitor cardiac rhythm continually during coronary artery infusion.

Drug-specific teaching points
- Be aware that you will require frequent blood tests; this drug can be given only by IV administration.
- Report rash, difficulty breathing, dizziness, disorientation, numbness, tingling.

ursodiol

(ur soe dye' ole)

ursodeoxycholic acid
Actigall, Ursofalk (CAN)

Pregnancy Category B

Drug classes
Gallstone solubilizing agent

Therapeutic actions
A naturally occurring bile acid that suppresses hepatic synthesis of cholesterol and inhibits intestinal absorption of cholesterol, leading to a decreased cholesterol concentration in the bile and a bile that is cholesterol solubilizing and not cholesterol precipitating.

Indications
- Treatment of selected patients with radiolucent, noncalcified gallstones in gallbladders in whom elective surgery is contraindicated

Contraindications/cautions
- Contraindicated in the presence of allergy to bile salts, hepatic dysfunction, calcified stones, radiopaque stones or radiolucent bile pigment stones, unremitting acute cholecystitis, cholangitis, biliary obstruction, gallstone pancreatitis, biliary-gastrointestinal fistula (cholecystectomy required), pregnancy.
- Use caution in the presence of lactation.

Dosage
Adult: 8–10 mg/kg per day PO given in two to three divided doses. Resolution of the gallstones requires months of therapy; condition needs to be monitored with ultrasound at 6-mo and 1-y intervals.
Pediatric: Safety and efficacy not established.

Pharmacokinetics

Route	Onset	Peak
Oral	Varies	Days

Metabolism: Hepatic, $T_{1/2}$: unknown
Distribution: Crosses placenta; may enter breast milk
Excretion: Feces

Adverse effects
- **CNS:** Headache, fatigue, anxiety, depression, sleep disorder
- **GI:** *Diarrhea,* cramps, heartburn, constipation, nausea, vomiting, anorexia, epigastric distress, dyspepsia, flatulence, abdominal pain
- **Respiratory:** Rhinitis, cough
- **Dermatologic:** Pruritus, rash, urticaria, dry skin, sweating, hair thinning
- **Other:** Back pain, arthralgia, myalgia

Clinically important drug-drug interactions
- Absorption of ursodiol is decreased if taken with bile acid sequestering agents

Adverse effects in *Italics* are most common; those in **Bold** are life-threatening.

(cholestyramine, colestipol), aluminum-based antacids

■ Nursing Considerations
Assessment
- *History:* Allergy to bile salts, hepatic dysfunction, calcified stones, radiopaque stones or radiolucent bile pigment stones, unremitting acute cholecystitis, cholangitis, biliary obstruction, gallstone pancreatitis, biliary-gastrointestinal fistula, pregnancy, lactation
- *Physical:* Liver evaluation, abdominal exam; affect, orientation; skin—color, lesions; liver function tests, hepatic and biliary radiological studies, biliary ultrasound

Implementation
- Assess patient carefully for suitability of ursodiol therapy. Alternative therapy should be reviewed before beginning ursodiol
- Administer drug in two to three divided doses.
- Do not adminster drug with aluminum-based antacids. If such drugs are needed, administer 2–3 h after ursodiol.
- Arrange for patient to be scheduled for periodic oral cholecystograms or ultrasonograms to evaluate drug effectiveness at 6-mo intervals until resolution, then every 3 mo to monitor stone formation. Recurrence of stones within 5 y occurs in more than 50% of patients. If gallstones appear to have dissolved, continue treatment for 3 mo and perform follow-up ultrasound.
- Monitor liver function tests periodically. Carefully assess patient if any change in liver function occurs.

Drug-specific teaching points
- Take drug two to three times a day. Continue to take the drug as long as prescribed. This drug may be needed for a prolonged period.
- Be aware that this drug may dissolve the gallstones that you have now; it does not "cure" the problem that caused the stones in the first place, and in many cases, the stones can recur; medical follow-up is important.
- Arrange to receive periodic x-rays or ultrasound tests of your gallbladder; you also will need periodic blood tests to evaluate your response to this drug. These tests are very important, and you should make every effort to keep follow-up appointments.
- Know that the following side effects may occur: diarrhea; skin rash (proper skin care may help); headache, fatigue (analgesics may help).
- Do not take this drug with any aluminum-based antacids.
- Report gallstone attacks (abdominal pain, nausea, vomiting), yellowing of the skin or eyes.

☐ valproic acid (and derivatives)

*(val **proe'** ik)*
Capsules: Depakene

sodium valproate
Syrup: Depakene

divalproex sodium
Tablets, enteric coated: Depakote, Epival (CAN)

Pregnancy Category D

Drug classes
Antiepileptic

Therapeutic actions
Mechanism of action not understood: antiepileptic activity may be related to the metabolism of the inhibitory neurotransmitter, gamma-aminobutyric acid (GABA); divalproex sodium is a compound containing equal proportions of valproic acid and sodium valproate.

Indications
- Sole and adjunctive therapy in simple (petit mal) and complex absence seizures
- Adjunctive therapy in patients with multiple seizure types, including absence seizures
- Unlabeled uses: sole and adjunctive therapy in atypical absence, myoclonic and grand mal seizures; possibly effective

valproic acid (and derivatives) ▪ 1129

therapy in atonic, complex partial, elementary partial, and infantile spasm seizures; prophylaxis for recurrent febrile seizures in children

Contraindications/cautions
- Contraindicated in the presence of hypersensitivity to valproic acid, hepatic disease or significant hepatic dysfunction.
- Use caution in the presence of children younger than 18 mo; children younger than 2 y, especially those receiving multiple antiepileptic drugs, those with congenital metabolic disorders, those with severe seizures accompanied by severe mental retardation, those with organic brain disorders (higher risk of developing fatal hepatotoxicity); pregnancy (incidence of neural tube defects in the fetus may be increased in mothers receiving valproic acid during the first trimester of pregnancy; do not discontinue antiepileptic therapy in pregnant women who are receiving such therapy to prevent major seizures; discontinuing medication is likely to precipitate status epilepticus, with attendant hypoxia and risk to both mother and unborn child); lactation.

Dosage
Adult: Dosage is expressed as valproic acid equivalents. Initial dose is 15 mg/kg per day PO, increasing at 1-wk intervals by 5–10 mg/kg per day until seizures are controlled or side effects preclude further increases. Maximum recommended dosage is 60 mg/kg per day PO. If total dose > 250 mg/d, give in divided doses.
Pediatric: Use extreme caution. Fatal hepatotoxicity has occurred. Children younger than 2 y are especially susceptible. Monitor all children carefully.

Pharmacokinetics

Route	Onset	Peak
Oral	Varies	1–4 h

Metabolism: Hepatic, $T_{1/2}$: 6–16 h
Distribution: Crosses placenta; enters breast milk
Excretion: Urine

Adverse effects
- CNS: *Sedation*, tremor (may be dose-related), emotional upset, depression, psychosis, aggression, hyperactivity, behavioral deterioration, weakness
- GI: *Nausea, vomiting, indigestion*, diarrhea, abdominal cramps, constipation, anorexia with weight loss, increased appetite with weight gain
- Hematologic: Slight elevations in SGOT, SGPT, LDH; increases in serum bilirubin, abnormal changes in other liver function tests, **hepatic failure,** altered bleeding time; thrombocytopenia; bruising; hematoma formation; frank hemorrhage; relative lymphocytosis; hypofibrinogenemia; leukopenia, eosinophilia, anemia, bone marrow suppression
- GU: Irregular menses, secondary amenorrhea
- Dermatologic: Transient increases in hair loss, skin rash, petechiae

Clinically important drug-drug interactions
- Increased serum phenobarbital, primidone levels if taken concurrently • Complex interactions with phenytoin; breakthrough seizures have occurred with the combination of valproic acid and phenytoin • Increased valproic acid serum levels and toxicity if given concurrently with salicylates • Decreased valproic acid effects if given concurrently with carbamazepine • Decreased serum levels of valproic acid if given concurrently with charcoal

Drug-lab test interferences
- False interpretation of urine ketone test

▪ Nursing Considerations

Assessment
- *History:* Hypersensitivity to valproic acid, hepatic dysfunction, pregnancy, lactation
- *Physical:* Body weight; skin—color, lesions; orientation, affect, reflexes; bowel sounds, normal output; CBC and differential, bleeding time tests, hepatic function tests, serum ammonia level, exocrine pancreatic function tests, EEG

Adverse effects in *Italics* are most common; those in **Bold** are life-threatening.

1130 ■ vancomycin hydrochloride

Implementation

- Give drug with food if GI upset occurs; substitution of the enteric-coated formulation also may be of benefit.
- Arrange to reduce dosage, discontinue valproic acid, or substitute other antiepileptic medication gradually; abrupt discontinuation of all antiepileptic medication may precipitate absence status.
- Arrange for frequent liver function tests; arrange to discontinue drug immediately in the presence of significant hepatic dysfunction, suspected or apparent; hepatic dysfunction has progressed in spite of drug discontinuation.
- Arrange for patient to have platelet counts, bleeding time determination before initiating therapy, at periodic intervals during therapy, and prior to surgery. Monitor patient carefully for signs of clotting defect (eg, bruising, blood tinged toothbrush). Arrange to discontinue drug if there is evidence of hemorrhage, bruising, or disorder of hemostasis.
- Arrange for monitoring of ammonia levels, and arrange to discontinue drug in the presence of clinically significant elevation in levels.
- Arrange for frequent monitoring of serum levels of valproic acid and other antiepileptic drugs given concomitantly, especially during the first few weeks of therapy. Arrange to adjust dosage as appropriate on the basis of these data and clinical response.
- Arrange for appropriate counseling for women of childbearing age who wish to become pregnant.
- Evaluate for therapeutic serum levels—usually 50–100 μg/ml.

Drug-specific teaching points

- Take this drug exactly as prescribed. Do not chew tablets or capsules before swallowing them. Swallow them whole to prevent local irritation of mouth and throat.
- Do not discontinue this drug abruptly or change dosage, except on the advice of your physician.
- Avoid alcohol, sleep-inducing, or OTC drugs while you are on this drug. These could cause dangerous effects.
- Arrange to have frequent checkups, including blood tests, to monitor your response to this drug. It is very important that you keep all appointments for checkups.
- Use contraceptive techniques at all times. If you wish to become pregnant while you are taking this drug, you should consult your physician.
- Know that the following side effects may occur: drowsiness (avoid driving a car or performing other tasks requiring alertness if this occurs; taking the drug at bedtime may minimize this effect); GI upset (taking the drug with food or milk and eating frequent, small meals may help; if this problem persists, substitution of an enteric-coated preparation may be possible and helpful); transient increase in hair loss.
- Wear a medical alert tag at all times so that any emergency medical personnel taking care of you will know that you are an epileptic taking antiepileptic medication.
- Be aware that this drug may interfere with urine tests for ketones (diabetic patients).
- Report bruising, pink stain on the toothbrush, yellowing of the skin or eyes, pale feces, skin rash, pregnancy.

❒ vancomycin hydrochloride

*(van koe **mye'** sin)*
Vancocin, Vancoled

Pregnancy Category C

Drug classes
Antibiotic

Therapeutic actions
Bactericidal: inhibits cell wall synthesis of susceptible organisms, causing cell death.

vancomycin hydrochloride 1131

Indications
- Potentially life-threatening infections not treatable with other less toxic antibiotics (parenteral)
- Severe staphylococci infections in patients who cannot receive or have failed to respond to penicillins and cephalosporins
- Prevention of bacterial endocarditis in penicillin-allergic patients undergoing dental, upper respiratory, GI, or GU surgery or invasive procedures
- Staphylococcal enterocolitis and antibiotic-associated pseudomembranous colitis caused by *Clostridium difficile* (oral)

Contraindications/cautions
- Contraindicated in the presence of allergy to vancomycin.
- Use caution in the presence of hearing loss, renal dysfunction, pregnancy, lactation.

Dosage
Adult: 500 mg PO q6h *or* 1 g PO q12h. 500 mg IV q6h *or* 1 g IV q6h.
Pediatric: 40 mg/kg per day PO in four divided doses. 40 mg/kg per day IV in divided doses added to fluids. Do not exceed 2 g/d.
Neonates: Premature and full-term neonates, use with caution because of incompletely developed renal function. Initial dose of 15 mg/kg q12h PO in first week of life, up to age of 1 mo, then q8h thereafter.
Pseudomembranous colitis caused by C. difficile: Adult: 500 mg to 2 g/d PO in three to four divided doses for 7–10 d. *Pediatric:* 40 mg/kg per day in four divided doses PO. *Neonates:* 10 mg/kg per day PO in divided doses.
Prevention of bacterial endocarditis in penicillin-allergic patients undergoing dental or upper respiratory procedures: Adult and pediatric > 27 kg: 1 g IV slowly over 1 h, beginning 1 h before the procedure. May repeat in 8–12 h. *< 27 kg:* 20 mg/kg IV slowly over 1 h beginning 1 h before the procedure. May repeat in 8–12 h.
Prevention of bacterial endocarditis in patients undergoing GI or GU procedures: Adult and pediatric > 27 kg: 1 g IV slowly over 1 h plus 1.5 mg/kg gentamicin IM or IV concurrently 1 h before the procedure. May repeat in 8–12 h. *< 27 kg:* 20 mg/kg IV slowly over 1 h and 2 mg/kg gentamicin IM or IV concurrently 1 h before the procedure. May repeat in 8–12 h.
Geriatric or renal failure patients: Monitor dosage and serum levels very carefully. Dosage nomogram is available for determining the dose according to creatinine clearance (see manufacturer's insert).

Pharmacokinetics

Route	Onset	Peak
Oral	Varies	
IV	Rapid	End of infusion

Metabolism: Hepatic, $T_{1/2}$: 4–6 h
Distribution: Crosses placenta; may enter breast milk
Excretion: Urine

IV facts
Preparation: *Not* for IM administration. Reconstitute with 10 ml Sterile Water for Injection; 500 mg/ml concentration results. Dilute reconstituted solution with 100–200 ml of 0.9% Sodium Chloride Injection or 5% Dextrose in Water for intermittent infusion. For continuous infusion (use only if intermittent therapy is not possible), add 2–4 (1–2 g) vials reconstituted solution to sufficiently large volume of 0.9% Sodium Chloride Injection or 5% Dextrose in Water to permit slow IV drip of the total daily dose over 24 h. Refrigerate reconstituted solution; stable over 14 d. Further diluted solution is stable for 24 h.

Infusion: For intermittent infusion, infuse q6h, over at least 60 min to avoid irritation, hypotension, throbbing back and neck pain. Administer continuous infusion slowly over 24 h.

Adverse effects
- CNS: *Ototoxicity*
- GI: *Nausea*
- CV: Hypotension (IV administration)
- Hematologic: Eosinophilia

Adverse effects in *Italics* are most common; those in **Bold** are life-threatening.

1132 ■ vasopressin

- GU: *Nephrotoxicity*
- Dermatologic: *Urticaria*, macular rashes
- Other: Superinfections; "**red neck or red man syndrome**" (sudden and profound fall in BP, fever, chills, paresthesias, erythema of the neck and back)

Clinically important drug-drug interactions
- Increased neuromuscular blockade if given with atracurium, galamine triethiodide, metocurine, pancuronium, rucuronium, tubocurarine, vecuronium

■ Nursing Considerations

Assessment
- *History:* Allergy to vancomycin, hearing loss, renal dysfunction, pregnancy, lactation
- *Physical:* Site of infection, skin—color, lesions; orientation, reflexes, auditory function; BP, perfusion; R, adventitious sounds; CBC, renal and liver function tests, auditory tests

Implementation
- Oral solution: Add 115 ml distilled water to contents of 10-g container. Each 6 ml of solution will contain 500 mg vancomycin. Alternatively, dilute the contents of 500-mg vial for injection in 30 ml of water for oral or nasogastric tube administration.
- Observe the patient very closely when giving parenteral solution, particularly the first doses; "red neck" syndrome can occur (see adverse effects); slow administration decreases the risk of adverse effects.
- Culture site of infection before beginning therapy.
- Monitor renal function tests with prolonged therapy.
- Evaluate for safe serum levels; concentrations of 60–80 μg/ml are toxic.

Drug-specific teaching points
- Be aware that this drug is available only in the IV and oral forms.
- Do not stop taking this drug without notifying your nurse or physician.
- Take the full prescribed course of this drug.
- Know that the following side effects may occur: nausea (small, frequent meals may help); changes in hearing; superinfections in the mouth, vagina (frequent hygiene measures will help).
- Report ringing in the ears, loss of hearing, difficulty voiding, rash, flushing.

☐ vasopressin

*(vay soe **press**' in)*

8-arginine-vasopressin
Pitressin Synthetic

Pregnancy Category C

Drug classes
Hormonal agent

Therapeutic actions
Purified form of posterior pituitary having pressor and antidiuretic hormone activities; promotes resorption of water in the renal tubular epithelium, causes contraction of vascular smooth muscle, increases GI motility and tone.

Indications
- Neurogenic diabetes insipidus
- Prevention and treatment of postoperative abdominal distention
- To dispel gas interfering with abdominal roentgenography

Contraindications/cautions
- Contraindicated in the presence of allergy to vasopressin or any components, chronic nephritis.
- Use caution in the presence of vascular disease (may precipitate angina or MI), epilepsy, migraine, asthma, CHF, pregnancy, lactation.

Dosage
5–10 U IM or SC. Repeat at 3- to 4-h intervals as needed.

Adverse effects in *Italics* are most common; those in **Bold** are life-threatening.

Adult
- **Diabetes insipidus**
  - *Intranasal:* Administer on cotton pledgets by nasal spray or dropper *or* 5–10 U bid or tid, IM or SC.
- **Abdominal distention:** 5 U IM initially. Increase to 10 U at subsequent injections given IM at 3- to 4-h intervals.
- **Abdominal roentgenography:** Administer two injections of 10 U IM or SC each. Give 2 h and ½ h before films are exposed. An enema may be given prior to first dose.

Pediatric: Decrease dose proportionately for children.

Pharmacokinetics

Route	Onset	Duration
IM/SC	Varies	2–6 h

Metabolism: Hepatic, $T_{1/2}$: 10–20 min
Distribution: Crosses placenta; enters breast milk
Excretion: Urine

Adverse effects
- CNS: *Tremor, sweating, vertigo,* circumoral pallor, "pounding" in the head
- GI: Abdominal cramps, passage of gas, nausea, vomiting
- Hypersensitivity: Reactions ranging from urticaria, bronchial constriction to anaphylaxis
- Other: *Water intoxication* (drowsiness, lightheadedness, headache, coma, convulsions), local tissue necrosis

■ Nursing Considerations

Assessment
- *History:* Allergy to vasopressin or any components, vascular disease, chronic nephritis, epilepsy, migraine, asthma, CHF, pregnancy
- *Physical:* Skin—color, lesions; nasal mucous membranes (if used intranasally); injection site; orientation, reflexes, affect; P, BP, rhythm, edema, baseline ECG; R, adventitous sounds; bowel sounds, abdominal exam; urinalysis, renal function tests, serum electrolytes

Implementation
- Administer injection by IM route; SC may be used if necessary.
- Monitor condition of nasal passages during long-term intranasal therapy; inappropriate administration can lead to nasal ulceration.
- Monitor patients with cardiovascular diseases very carefully for cardiac reactions.
- Monitor fluid volume for signs of water intoxication and excess fluid load; arrange to decrease dosage if this occurs.

Drug-specific teaching points
- Administer nasally on cotton pledgets, by nasal spray, or dropper. (Watch patient administer drug, and review drug administration periodically with patient.) Other routes must be IM or SC.
- Know that the following side effects may occur: GI cramping, passing of gas; anxiety, tinnitus, vision changes (safety precautions will be taken to help you if these occur; avoid driving or performing tasks that require alertness if these occur); nasal irritation (proper administration will decrease these problems).
- Report swelling, difficulty breathing, chest tightness or pain, palpitations, running nose, painful nasal passages (intranasal).

☐ venlafaxine

*(vin lah **facks' in**)*
Effexor

Pregnancy Category C

Drug classes
Antidepressant

Therapeutic actions
Potentiates the neurotransmitter activity in the CNS; inhibits serontonin, norephinphrine, and dopamine reuptake leading to prolonged stimulation at neuroreceptors.

Adverse effects in *Italics* are most common; those in **Bold** are life-threatening.

Indications
- Treatment of depression

Contraindications/cautions
- Allergy to venlafaxine, use of MAOIs, pregnancy, lactation.

Dosage
Adult: Starting dose, 75 mg/d PO in two to three divided doses taken with food. May be increased slowly up to 225 mg/d to achieve desired effect.
- ***Transfer to or from MAO inhibitor:*** At least 14 d should elapse from the discontinuation of the MAOI and the starting of venlafaxine; allow at least 7 d to elapse from the stopping of venlafaxine to the starting of an MAOI.

Pediatric: Safety and efficacy not established.
Geriatric: No dosage adjustment required.
Hepatic/renal impairment: Reduce total daily dose by 50%, and increase very slowly to achieve desired effect.

Pharmacokinetics

Route	Onset	Duration
PO	Slow	48 h

Metabolism: Hepatic, $T_{1/2}$: 1.3–2 h
Distribution: Crosses placenta; may enter breast milk
Excretion: Urine

Adverse effects
- CNS: *Somnolence, dizziness, insomnia, nervousness,* anxiety, tremor, dreams
- GI: *Nausea, constipation, anorexia,* diarrhea, vomiting, dyspepsia, *dry mouth,* flatulence
- CV: Vasodilation, hypertension, tachycardia
- GU: *Abnormal ejaculation,* impotence, urinary frequency
- Dermatologic: *Sweating,* rash, pruritus
- Other: *Headache, asthenia,* infection, chills, chest pain

Clinically important drug-drug interactions
- Increased serum levels and risk of toxicity if taken concurrently with MAOIs, cimetidine

■ Nursing Considerations
Assessment
- *History:* Allergy to venlafaxine, use of MAOIs, pregnancy, lactation
- *Physical:* Skin—color, temperature, lesions; reflexes, gait, sensation, cranial nerve evaluation; mucous membranes, abdominal exam, normal output; P, BP, peripheral perfusion

Implementation
- Administer drug with food to decrease GI effects.
- Advise patient to use contraceptive measures while on this drug.

Drug-specific teaching points
- Take this drug with food to decrease GI upset.
- Know that the following side effects may occur as a result of drug therapy: loss of appetite, nausea, vomiting, dry mouth (frequent mouth care, small, frequent meals may help; sucking sugarless lozenges may help dry mouth); constipation (a bowel program may be established to help out with this problem); dizziness, drowsiness, tremor (avoid driving a car or operating dangerous machinery while on this drug).
- Avoid alcohol while on this drug.
- Be aware that this drug cannot be taken during pregnancy; it is advisable to use birth control while you are taking this drug. If you become pregnant, consult with your health care provider.
- Report rash, hives, increased depression, pregnancy.

❐ verapamil hydrochloride

*(ver **ap**' a mill)*
Calan, Calan SR, Isoptin, Verelan

Pregnancy Category C

Adverse effects in *Italics* are most common; those in **Bold** are life-threatening.

verapamil hydrochloride ■ 1135

Drug classes
Calcium channel-blocker
Antianginal drug
Antiarrhythmic drug
Antihypertensive

Therapeutic actions
Inhibits the movement of calcium ions across the membranes of cardiac and arterial muscle cells; calcium is involved in the generation of the action potential in specialized automatic and conducting cells in the heart, in arterial smooth muscle, and in excitation-contraction coupling in cardiac muscle cells; inhibition of transmembrane calcium flow results in the depression of impulse formation in specialized cardiac pacemaker cells, slowing of the velocity of conduction of the cardiac impulse, the depression of myocardial contractility, and the dilation of coronary arteries and arterioles and peripheral arterioles; these effects lead to decreased cardiac work, decreased cardiac energy consumption, and in patients with vasospastic (Prinzmetal's) angina, increased delivery of oxygen to myocardial cells.

Indications
- Angina pectoris due to coronary artery spasm (Prinzmetal's variant angina)
- Effort-associated angina
- Chronic stable angina in patients who cannot tolerate or do not respond to beta-adrenergic blockers or nitrates
- Unstable, crescendo, preinfarction angina
- Essential hypertension (sustained-release oral)
- Treatment of supraventricular tachyarrhythmias (parenteral)
- Temporary control of rapid ventricular rate in atrial flutter or atrial fibrillation (parenteral)
- Unlabeled oral uses: paroxysmal supraventricular tachycardia, migraine headache, nocturnal leg cramps, hypertrophic cardiomyopathy

Contraindications/cautions
- Contraindicated in the presence of allergy to verapamil; sick sinus syndrome, except in presence of ventricular pacemaker; heart block (second- or third-degree); hypotension; pregnancy; lactation.
- Use caution in the presence of idiopathic hypertrophic subaortic stenosis, cardiogenic shock, severe CHF, impaired renal or hepatic function.

Dosage
Adult
- ***Oral:*** Initial dose of 80–120 mg tid; increase dose every 1–2 d to achieve optimum therapeutic effects. Usual maintenance dose, 320–480 mg/d.
  – *Hypertension:* 240 mg PO qd, sustained-release form in morning. 80 mg tid.
- ***Parenteral:*** IV use only. Initial dose, 5–10 mg over 2 min; may repeat dose of 10 mg 30 min after first dose if initial response is inadequate.

Pediatric
- ***IV***
  – *Up to 1 y:* Initial dose, 0.1–0.2 mg/kg over 2 min.
  – *1–15 y:* Initial dose, 0.1–0.3 mg/kg over 2 min. Do not exceed 5 mg. Repeat above dose 30 min after initial dose if response is not adequate.

Geriatric or renal impaired: Reduce dosage, and monitor patient response carefully. Give IV doses over 3 min to reduce risk of serious side effects. Administer IV doses very slowly, over 2 min.

Pharmacokinetics

Route	Onset	Peak	Duration
Oral	30 min	1–2.2 h	3–7 h
IV	1–5 min	3–5 min	2 h

Metabolism: Hepatic, $T_{1/2}$: 3–7 h
Distribution: Crosses placenta; enters breast milk
Excretion: Urine

IV facts
Preparation: No further preparation required.
Infusion: Infuse very slowly over 2–3 min.

Adverse effects
- CNS: *Dizziness*, vertigo, emotional depression, sleepiness, *headache*
- GI: *Nausea*, constipation
- CV: *Peripheral edema*, *hypotension*, arrhythmias, bradycardia; **AV heart block**
- Other: Muscle fatigue, diaphoresis

Clinically important drug-drug interactions
- Increased cardiac depression if taken concurrently with beta-adrenergic blocking agents • Additive effects of verapamil and digoxin to slow AV conduction • Increased serum levels of digoxin, carbamazepine, prazosin, quinidine given concurrently • Increased respiratory depression if given to patients receiving atracurium, gallamine, metocurine, pancuronium, rucuronium, tubocurarine, vecuronium • Risk of serious cardiac effects if given with IV beta-adrenergic blocking agents; do not give these drugs within 48 h before or 24 h after IV verapamil • Decreased effects of verapamil if taken with calcium, rifampin

■ Nursing Considerations

Assessment
- *History:* Allergy to verapamil, sick sinus syndrome, heart block, IHSS, cardiogenic shock, severe CHF, hypotension, impaired hepatic or renal function, pregnancy, lactation
- *Physical:* Skin—color, edema; orientation, reflexes; P, BP, baseline ECG, peripheral perfusion, auscultation; R, adventitious sounds; liver evaluation, normal output; liver function tests, renal function tests, urinalysis

Implementation
- Monitor patient carefully (BP, cardiac rhythm, and output) while drug is being titrated to therapeutic dose. Dosage may be increased more rapidly in hospitalized patients under close supervision.
- Monitor BP very carefully if patient is on concurrent doses of antihypertensive drugs.
- Monitor cardiac rhythm regularly during stabilization of dosage and periodically during long-term therapy.
- Administer sustained-release form in the morning with food to decrease GI upset.
- Protect IV solution from light.
- Monitor patients with renal or hepatic impairment very carefully for possible drug accumulation and adverse reactions.

Drug-specific teaching points
- Take sustained-release form in the morning with food.
- Know that the following side effects may occur: nausea, vomiting (small, frequent meals may help); headache (monitor the lighting, noise, and temperature; medication may be ordered if this becomes severe); dizziness, sleepiness (avoid driving or operating dangerous equipment while on this drug); emotional depression (it may help to know that this is a drug effect and should pass when the drug is stopped; constipation (measures may need to be taken to alleviate this problem).
- Report irregular heart beat, shortness of breath, swelling of the hands or feet, pronounced dizziness, constipation.

❑ vidarabine

*(vye **dare**' a been)*

adenine arabinoside, Ara-A
Vira-A

Pregnancy Category C

Drug classes
Antiviral drug

Therapeutic actions
Antiviral activity against herpes simplex types 1 and 2; mechanism of action has not been established; probably interferes with DNA synthesis.

Indications
- Herpes simplex virus encephalitis (parenteral administration)
- Neonatal herpes simplex virus infections (parenteral administration)

Adverse effects in *Italics* are most common; those in **Bold** are life-threatening.

Drug-specific teaching points
- Prepare a calendar of dates to return for specific treatment days and additional courses of drug therapy.
- Know that the following side effects may occur as a result of drug therapy: loss of appetite, nausea, vomiting, mouth sores (frequent mouth care, small frequent meals may help; maintain good nutrition if at all possible; an antiemetic also may be ordered); constipation (a bowel program may be established to help out with this problem); sensitivity to light (wear sunglasses if exposed to the sun; avoid bright lights in general); numbness, tingling, change in style of walking (these are drug related and should pass when the drug therapy is finished, though neuromuscular difficulties sometimes persist for 6 wk); hair loss (you may wish to arrange for a wig or other suitable head covering; it is important to keep the head covered at extremes of temperature; hair loss is usually a temporary situation).
- Be aware that this drug cannot be taken during pregnancy; it is advisable to use birth control while you are taking this drug. If you become pregnant, consult with your physician.
- Arrange to have regular blood tests to monitor the drug's effects.
- Report change in frequency of voiding; swelling of ankle, fingers, and so forth; changes in vision; severe constipation, abdominal pain.

▢ vinorelbine tartrate

(vin oh rel' been)
Navelbine

Pregnancy Category D

Drug classes
Mitotic inhibitor
Antineoplastic agent

Therapeutic actions
Affects cell energy production required for mitosis and interferes with nucleic acid synthesis; has antimitotic effect, prevents the formation of microtubules and leads to cell death; cell cycle specific.

Indications
- First line treatment of ambulatory patients with unresectable advanced non-small cell lung cancer
- Treatment of stage IV non-small cell lung cancer as a single agent or in combination with cisplatin
- Treatment of stage III non-small cell lung cancer in combination with cisplatin

Contraindications/cautions
- Contraindicated in the presence of allergy to vinca alkaloids, pretreatment granulocyte counts <1000 cells/mm^3, pregnancy, lactation.
- Use caution in the presence of liver disease.

Dosage
Do not administer more than once a week because of leukopenic response.
Adult: Initial dose: 30 mg/m^2 as a single IV dose; repeat once a week until progression of disease or toxicity limits use.*In combination with cisplatin*: 120mg/m^2 cisplatin on days 1 and 29 and then every 6 wk. *Hepatic impairment:* Reduce dose.

Pharmacokinetics

Route	Onset
IV	Slow

Metabolism: Hepatic metabolism; T$_{1/2}$: 22–66 h
Distribution: Crosses placenta; passes into breast milk
Excretion: Bile and feces

IV facts
Preparation: Dilute as indicated for 50 or 10 mg solution. Supplied as single use vials only. Discard after withdrawing solution.

Infusion: Inject into tubing of a running IV or directly into the vein over 6–10 min period. Rinse syringe and needle with venous blood prior to withdrawing needle from vein (to minimize extravasation). Do

1142 ■ warfarin sodium

not inject into an extremity with poor circulation or repeatedly into the same vein.

Adverse effects
- **CNS:** numbness, paresthesias (less common with this drug than with other vinca alkaloids); headache, weakness, dizziness
- **GI:** nausea, vomiting, pharyngitis, vesiculation of the mouth, ileus, diarrhea, constipation, anorexia, abdominal pain, *increased liver enzymes*
- **Hematologic:** *granuloctytopenia, leukopenia*
- **Dermatologic:** topical epilation (loss of hair), vesication of the skin
- **Local:** local cellulitis, phlebitis, sloughing of the skin if extravasation occurs
- **Other:** myalgia, arthralgia

Clinically important drug-drug interactions
- Acute pulmonary reactions if given concomitantly with mitomycin • Increased risk of granulocytopenia if given with cisplatin

■ Nursing Considerations

Assessment
- *History:* Allergy to vinca alkaloids, leukopenia, acute infection, liver disease, pregnancy, lactation
- *Physical:* Weight; hair; temperature; reflexes, gait, sensation, orientation, affect; mucous membranes, abdominal exam; CBC, liver function tests, serum albumin

Implementation
- Do not administer IM or SC—severe local reaction and tissue necrosis occur.
- Take care to avoid extravasation; if it should occur, discontinue injection immediately and give remainder of dose in another vein. Consult physician to arrange for hyaluronidase injection into local area, after which apply moderate heat to disperse drug and minimize pain.
- Avoid contact with the eyes; should contact occur, thoroughly wash immediately with water.
- Consult with physician if antiemetic is needed for severe nausea and vomiting.
- Arrange for and check CBC before administration of each dose of drug.

Drug-specific teaching points
- Prepare a calendar for dates to return for specific treatment days and additional courses of drug therapy.
- Know that the following side effects may occur: loss of appetite, nausea, vomiting, mouth sores (frequent mouth care, small frequent meals may help; you will need to try to maintain good nutrition if at all possible; an antiemetic may be ordered); constipation (a bowel program may be established to help this problem); malaise, weakness, dizziness, numbness and tingling (take special precautions to avoid injury if these occur); loss of hair, skin rash (you may wish to obtain a wig if hair loss occurs; it is important to keep the head covered in extremes of temperature).
- Be aware that this drug should not be used during pregnancy. It is advisable to use birth control while taking this drug. If you become pregnant, consult your physician.
- Arrange to have regular blood tests to monitor the drug's effects.
- Report severe nausea, vomiting, pain or burning at injection site, abdominal pain, rectal bleeding, fever, chills, acute infection.

❑ warfarin sodium

(war' far in)

Coumadin, Panwarfin, Sofarin, Warfilone (CAN), Warnerin (CAN)

Pregnancy Category D

Drug classes
Oral anticoagulant
Coumarin derivative

Therapeutic actions
Interferes with the hepatic synthesis of vitamin K-dependent clotting factors (factors

Adverse effects in *Italics* are most common; those in **Bold** are life-threatening.

warfarin sodium ■ 1143

II-prothrombin, VII, IX, and X), resulting in their eventual depletion and prolongation of clotting times.

Indications
- Venous thrombosis and its extension, treatment, and prophylaxis
- Treatment of atrial fibrillation with embolization
- Pulmonary embolism, treatment, and prophylaxis
- Prophylaxis of systemic emobization after acute MI
- Unlabeld uses: prevention of recurrent transient ischemic attacks, prevention of recurrent myocardial infarction, adjunt to therapy in small-cell carcinoma of the lung

Contraindications/cautions
- Contraindictated in the presence of allergy to warfarin or tartrazine (contained in the 7.5-mg tablet marketed as *Panwarfin*); SBE; hemorrhagic disorders; tuberculosis; hepatic diseases; GI ulcers; renal disease; indwelling catheters, spinal puncture; aneurysm; diabetes; visceral carcinoma; uncontrolled hypertension; severe trauma (including recent or contemplated CNS, eye surgery; recent placement of IUD); threatened abortion, menometrorrhagia; pregnancy (known to cause fetal damage and death); lactation (suggest using heparin if anticoagulation is required).
- Use caution in the presence of CHF, diarrhea, fever; thyrotoxicosis; senile, psychotic, or depressed patients.

Dosage
Adjust dosage according to the one-stage prothrombin time to achieve and maintain 1.5–2.5 times the control value or prothrombin activity 20%–30% of normal.
Adult: Initially: 10–15 mg/d PO. Adjust dose according to PT response. *Maintenance:* 2–10 mg/d PO based on PT time.
Geriatric: Lower doses are usually needed; begin dosage lower than adult recommended and closely monitor PT.

Pharmacokinetics

Route	Peak	Duration
Oral	1½–3 d	2–5 d

Metabolism: Hepatic, $T_{1/2}$: 1–2.5 d
Distribution: Crosses placenta; enters breast milk
Excretion: Feces and urine

Adverse effects
- **GI:** *Nausea*, vomiting, anorexia, abdominal cramping, diarrhea, retroperitoneal hematoma, hepatitis, jaundice, mouth ulcers
- **Hematologic:** Granulocytosis, leukopenia, eosinophilia
- **GU:** Priapism, nephropathy, red-orange urine
- **Dermatologic:** *Alopecia, urticaria, dermatitis*
- **Bleeding:** *Hemorrhage*; GI or urinary tract bleeding (hematuria, dark stools; paralytic ileus, intestinal obstruction from hemorrhage into GI tract); petechiae and purpura, bleeding from mucous membranes; hemorrhagic infarction, vasculitis, skin necrosis of female breast; adrenal hemorrhage and resultant adrenal insufficiency; compressive neuropathy secondary to hemorrhage near a nerve
- **Other:** Fever, "purple toes" syndrome

Clinically important drug-drug interactions
- Increased bleeding tendencies if taken concurrently with salicylates, chloral hydrate, phenylbutazone, clofibrate, disulfiram, chloramphenicol, metronidazole, cimetidine, ranitidine, co-trimoxazole, sulfinpyrazone, quinidine, quinine, oxyphenbutazone, thyroid drugs, glucagon, danazol, erythromycin, androgens, amiodarone, cefamandole, cefoperazone, cefotetan, moxalactam, cefazolin, cefoxitin, ceftriaxone, meclofenamate, mefenamic acid, famotidine, nizatidine, nalidixic acid
- Decreased anticoagulation effect may occur if taken concurrently with barbiturates, griseofulvin, rifampin, phenytoin, glutethi-

Adverse effects in *Italics* are most common; those in **Bold** are life-threatening.

mide, carbamazepine, vitamin K, vitamin E, cholestyramine, aminoglutethimide, ethchlorvynol • Altered effects of warfarin if taken concurrently with methimazole, propylthiouracil • Increased activity and toxicity of phenytoin when taken with oral anticoagulants

Drug-lab test interferences
- Red-orange discoloration of alkaline urine may interfere with some lab tests

■ Nursing Considerations

Assessment
- *History:* Allergy to warfarin or tartrazine; SBE; hemorrhagic disorders; tuberculosis; hepatic diseases; GI ulcers; renal disease; indwelling catheters, spinal puncture; aneurysm; diabetes; visceral carcinoma; uncontrolled hypertension; severe trauma; threatened abortion, menometrorrhagia; pregnancy; lactation; CHF, diarrhea, fever; thyrotoxicosis; senile, psychotic or depressed patients
- *Physical:* Skin—lesions, color, temperature; orientation, reflexes, affect; P, BP, peripheral perfusion, baseline ECG; R, adventitious sounds; liver evaluation, bowel sounds, normal output; CBC, urinalysis, guaiac stools, prothrombin time, renal and hepatic function tests

Implementation
- Monitor prothrombin times regularly to adjust dosage.
- Do not change brand names once stabilized; bioavailability problems have been documented.
- Evaluate patient regularly for signs of blood loss (eg, petechiae, bleeding gums, bruises, dark stools, dark urine).
- Do not give patient any IM injections while on warfarin.
- Double check any other drug that is ordered for the patient for potential drug-drug interaction; dosage of both drugs may need to be adjusted.
- Use caution when discontinuing any other medication; dosage of warfarin may need to be adjusted; carefully monitor PT values.
- Maintain vitamin K on standby in case of overdose.
- Arrange for frequent follow-up, including blood tests to evaluate drug effects.
- Evaluate for therapeutic effects: prothrombin time $1\frac{1}{2}$–$2\frac{1}{2}$ times the control value.

Drug-specific teaching points
- Be aware that many factors may change your body's response to this drug—fever, change of diet, change of environment, other medications. The dosage of the drug may have to be changed on several occasions. Be sure to write down any change of dose that is prescribed.
- Do not change any medication that you are taking (adding or stopping another drug) without consulting your nurse or physician. Many other drugs affect the way that your anticoagulant works; starting or stopping another drug can cause excessive bleeding or interfere with the desired effects of the drug.
- Carry or wear a medical alert tag stating that you are on this drug. This will alert any medical personnel who might take care of you in an emergency that you are taking this drug.
- Avoid situations in which you could be easily injured (eg, contact sports, shaving with a straight razor).
- Know that the following side effects may occur: stomach bloating, cramps (this often passes with time); loss of hair, skin rash; orange-red discoloration to the urine (this may be upsetting because it can be mistaken for blood; add vinegar to your urine and the color should disappear).
- Arrange to have periodic blood tests to check on the action of the drug. It is very important that you have these tests.
- Use contraceptive measures while taking this drug; it is important that you do not become pregnant.
- Report unusual bleeding (such as when you are brushing your teeth, excessive bleeding from injuries, excessive bruising), black or bloody stools, cloudy or dark urine, sore throat, fever, chills, severe headaches, dizziness, suspected pregnancy.

xylometazoline hydrochloride

(zye low met az' oh leen)
Otrivin Nasal Drops or Spray,
Otrivin Pediatric Nasal Drops,
Otrivin with M-D Pump (CAN),
Sinutab Sinus Spray (CAN)

Pregnancy Category C

Drug classes
Nasal decongestant

Therapeutic actions
Acts directly on alpha-receptors to produce vasoconstriction of arterioles in nasal passages, which produces a decongestant response; no effect on beta receptors.

Indications
- Symptomatic relief of nasal and nasopharyngeal mucosal congestion due to the common cold, hay fever, or other respiratory allergies (topical)

Contraindications/cautions
- Contraindicated in the presence of allergy to xylometalozine, angle-closure glaucoma, anesthesia with cyclopropane or halothane, thyrotoxicosis, diabetes, hypertension, cardiovascular disorders, women in labor whose BP > 130/80.
- Use caution in the presence of angina, arrhythmias, prostatic hypertrophy, unstable vasomotor syndrome, lactation.

Dosage
Adult: 2–3 sprays or 2–3 drops in each nostril q8–10h.
Pediatric
- **2–12 y:** 2–3 drops of 0.05% solution in each nostril q8–12h.

Pharmacokinetics

Route	Onset	Duration
Nasal	5–10 min	5–6 h

Metabolism: Hepatic, $T_{1/2}$: unknown
Distribution: Crosses placenta; may enter breast milk
Excretion: Urine

Adverse effects
Systemic effects are less likely with topical administration than with systemic administration, but because systemic absorption can take place, the systemic effects should be considered.
- **CNS:** *Fear, anxiety, tenseness, restlessness, headache, lightheadedness, dizziness,* drowsiness, tremor, insomnia, hallucinations, psychological disturbances, convulsions, CNS depression, weakness, blurred vision, ocular irritation, tearing, photophobia, symptoms of paranoid schizophrenia
- **GI:** *Nausea,* vomiting, anorexia
- **CV:** Arrhythmias, hypertension, resulting in intracranial hemorrhage, cardiovascular collapse with hypotension, palpitations, tachycardia, precordial pain in patients with ischemic heart disease
- **GU:** Constriction of renal blood vessels, *dysuria, vesical sphincter spasm,* resulting in difficult and painful urination, urinary retention in males with prostatism
- **Local:** *Rebound congestion* with topical nasal application
- **Other:** *Pallor,* respiratory difficulty, orofacial dystonia, sweating

Clinically important drug-drug interactions
- Severe hypertension when taken with MAOI, tricyclic antidepressants, furazolidone • Additive effects and increased risk of toxicity if taken with urinary alkalinizers • Decreased vasopressor response if taken with reserpine, methyldopa, urinary acidifiers • Decreased hypotensive action of guanethidine if taken concurrently

■ Nursing Considerations
Assessment
- *History:* Allergy to xylometazoline; angle-closure glaucoma; anesthesia with cyclopropane or halothane; thyrotoxicosis, diabetes, hypertension, cardiovascular disorders; prostatic hypertrophy, unstable vasomotor syndrome; lactation.
- *Physical:* Skin—color, temperature; orientation, reflexes, peripheral sensation,

Adverse effects in *Italics* are most common; those in **Bold** are life-threatening.

vision; P, BP, auscultation, peripheral perfusion; R, adventitious sounds; urinary output pattern, bladder percussion; prostate palpation; nasal mucous membrance evaluation

Implementation
- Monitor cardiovascular effects carefully, patients with hypertension who take this drug may experience changes in blood pressure because of the additional vasoconstriction. If a nasal decongestant is needed, pseudoephedrine is the drug of choice.

Drug-specific teaching points
- Do not exceed recommended dose. Demonstrate proper administration technique for topical nasal application. Avoid prolonged use because underlying medical problems can be disguised.
- Know that the following side effects may occur: dizziness, weakness, restlessness, lightheadedness, tremor (avoid driving or operating dangerous equipment when these effects occur); urinary retention (emptying the bladder before taking the drug may help).
- Be aware that a rebound congestion may occur when this drug is stopped; drink plenty of fluids, use a humidifier, avoid smoke-filled areas to help decrease problems.
- Report nervousness, palpitations, sleeplessness, sweating.

☐ zalcitabine

(zal' cye tay been)

dideoxycytidine, ddC
Hivid

Pregnancy Category C

Drug classes
Antiviral drug

Therapeutic actions
Synthetic purine nucleoside, which is active against HIV, inhibits cell protein synthesis, and leads to cell death without viral replication.

Indications
- Combination therapy with zidovudine in advanced HIV infection

Contraindications/cautions
- Contraindicated in the presence of life-threatening allergy to any component, pregnancy, lactation.
- Use caution in the presence of compromised bone marrow, impaired renal or hepatic function.

Dosage
Adult
- **Combination therapy with zidovudine:** 0.75 PO mg administered with 200 mg zidovudine PO q8h.

Pediatric: Safety and efficacy not established for children younger than 13 y.
Geriatric or renal impaired: Ccr of 10–40 ml/min, reduce the dose to 0.75 mg q12h PO; Ccr < 10, reduce dose to 0.75 mg q24h PO.

Pharmacokinetics

Route	Onset	Peak
Oral	Varies	0.8–1.6 h

Metabolism: Hepatic, $T_{1/2}$: 1–3 h
Distribution: Crosses placenta; may enter breast milk
Excretion: Urine and feces

Adverse effects
- CNS: *Headache*, insomnia, myalgia, *asthenia*, malaise, dizziness, paresthesia, somnolence, **peripheral neuropathy**
- GI: *Nausea*, *GI pain*, *diarrhea*, anorexia, vomiting, dyspepsia, oral ulcers
- Hematologic: *Agranulocytopenia*, severe anemia requiring transfusions
- Other: *Fever*, diaphoresis, dyspnea, *rash*, taste perversion

■ Nursing Considerations
Assessment
- *History:* Life-threatening allergy to any component, compromised bone marrow,

impaired renal or hepatic function, pregnancy, lactation
- *Physical:* Skin—rashes, lesions, texture; body temperature; affect, reflexes, peripheral sensation; bowel sounds, liver evaluation; renal and hepatic function tests; CBC and differential

Implementation
- Arrange to monitor hematologic indices every 2 wk during therapy.
- Monitor patient for any signs of peripheral neuropathy (eg, numbness, tingling), and arrange to reduce drug dose by 50% until sensation returns; gradually reintroduce drug. Permanently discontinue drug in patients who experience severe discomfort and loss of sensation.
- Administer the drug every 8 h, around the clock with zidovudine; appropriate rest periods may be needed during the day because of interrupted sleep.

Drug-specific teaching points
- Take drug every 8 h, around the clock. You will need to have an alarm clock to wake you up during the night; rest periods during the day may be necessary. Do not share this drug; take exactly as prescribed.
- Be aware that zalcitabine and zidovudine do not cure AIDS or ARC; opportunisitc infections may occur, and regular medical care should be sought to deal with the disease.
- Arrange for frequent blood tests, needed during the course of treatment; results of blood counts may indicate a need for decreased dosage or discontinuation of the drug for a period of time.
- Know that the following side effects may occur as a result of drug therapy: nausea, loss of appetite, change in taste (small, frequent meals may help); dizziness, loss of feeling (take appropriate precautions if these occur); headache, fever, muscle aches.
- Be aware that these drugs do not reduce the risk of transmission of HIV to others by sexual contact or blood contamination; use appropriate precautions.
- Report extreme fatigue, lethargy, severe headache, severe nausea, vomiting, difficulty breathing, skin rash, numbness, tingling, pain in extremities.

❐ zidovudine

(zid o vew' den)
azidothymidine, AZT, Compound S
Retrovir

Pregnancy Category C

Drug classes
Antiviral drug

Therapeutic actions
Thymidine analogue isolated from the sperm of herring; drug is activated to a triphosphate form that inhibits replication of some retroviruses, including HIV, HTLV III, LAV, ARV.

Indications
- Management of certain adult patients with symptomatic HIV infection (AIDS and advanced ARC) who have a history of cytologically confirmed *P. carinii* pneumonia or an absolute CD4 (T4 helper/inducer) lymphocyte count of less than 200/mm^3 in the peripheral blood before therapy is begun (parenteral)
- Management of patients with HIV infection who have evidence of impaired immunity (CD$_4$ cell count of < 500/mm^3) (oral)
- HIV-infected children older than 3 mo who have HIV-related symptoms or who are asymptomatic with abnormal laboratory values indicating significant HIV-related immunosuppression

Contraindications/cautions
- Contraindicated in the presence of life-threatening allergy to any component, pregnancy, lactation.
- Use caution in the presence of compromised bone marrow, impaired renal or hepatic function.

Dosage
Adult
- ***Symptomatic HIV infection:*** *Initially:* 200 mg q4h (2.9 mg/kg q4h) PO,

around the clock. Monitor hematologic indices every 2 wk. If significant anemia (hemoglobin < 7.5 g/dl, reduction of > 25%) or reduction of granulocytes > 50% below baseline occurs, dose interruption is necessary until evidence of bone marrow recovery is seen. If less severe bone marrow depression occurs, a dosage reduction may be adequate; *or* 1–2 mg/kg q4h IV.

- ***Asymptomatic HIV infection:*** 100 mg q4h PO while awake (500 mg/d).

Pediatric
- ***3 mo–12 y:*** Initial dose, 180 mg/m^2 q6h PO or IV (720 mg/m^2 per day, not to exceed 200 mg q6h).

Pharmacokinetics

Route	Onset	Peak
Oral	Varies	½–1 h½
IV	Rapid	End of infusion

Metabolism: Hepatic, T$_{1/2}$: 30–60 min
Distribution: Crosses placenta; may enter breast milk
Excretion: Urine

IV facts
Preparation: Remove desired dose from vial, and dilute in 5% Dextrose in Water to a concentration no greater than 4 mg/ml.
Infusion: Administer over 60 min; avoid rapid infusion.

Adverse effects
- CNS: *Headache*, insomnia, myalgia, *asthenia*, malaise, dizziness, paresthesia, somnolence
- GI: *Nausea, GI pain, diarrhea*, anorexia, vomiting, dyspepsia
- Hematologic: *Agranulocytopenia*, severe anemia requiring transfusions
- Other: *Fever*, diaphoresis, dyspnea, *rash*, taste perversion

■ Nursing Considerations
Assessment
- *History:* Life-threatening allergy to any component, compromised bone marrow, impaired renal or hepatic function, pregnancy, lactation
- *Physical:* Skin—rashes, lesions, texture; body temperature; affect, reflexes, peripheral sensation; bowel sounds, liver evaluation; renal and hepatic function tests, CBC and differential

Implementation
- Arrange to monitor hematologic indices every 2 wk during therapy.
- Administer the drug every 4 h, around the clock; appropriate rest periods may be needed during the day because of interrupted sleep.

Drug-specific teaching points
- Take drug every 4 h, around the clock. You will need to have an alarm clock to wake you up during the night; rest periods during the day may be necessary. Do not share this drug; take exactly as prescribed.
- Be aware that zidovudine is not a cure for AIDS or ARC; opportunisitc infections may occur, and regular medical care should be sought to deal with the disease.
- Arrange for frequent blood tests, needed during the course of treatment; results of blood counts may indicate a need for decreased dosage or discontinuation of the drug for a period of time.
- Know that the following side effects may occur as a result of drug therapy: nausea, loss of appetite, change in taste (small, frequent meals may help); dizziness, loss of feeling (take appropriate precautions if these occur); headache, fever, muscle aches.
- Be aware that zidovudine does not reduce the risk of transmission of HIV to other by sexual contact or blood contamination; use appropriate precautions.
- Report extreme fatigue, lethargy, severe headache, severe nausea, vomiting, difficulty breathing, skin rash.

☐ zinc

zinc sulfate OTC and prescription drug
Orazinc, Verazinc, Zincate

Adverse effects in *Italics* are most common; those in **Bold** are life-threatening.

zinc gluconate
Pregnancy Category C

Drug classes
Mineral

Therapeutic actions
Natural element that is essential for growth and tissue repair; acts as an integral part of essential enzymes in protein and carbohydrate metabolism.

Indications
- Dietary supplement to treat or prevent zinc deficiencies
- Unlabeled uses: acrodermatitis enteropathica and delayed wound healing associated with zinc deficiency; treatment of acne, rheumatoid arthritis, Wilson's disease; treatment of the common cold

Contraindications/cautions
- Contraindicated in the presence of pregnancy and lactation (recommended dietary allowance is needed, but not supplemental replacement).

Dosage
Adult
- **Recommended dietary allowance (RDA):** 12–15 mg/d PO; pregnancy RDA, 15 mg/d PO; lactation RDA, 6 mg/d PO for the first 6 mo; then 4 mg/d for the next 6 mo.
- **Dietary supplement:** 25–50 mg zinc/d PO.

Pediatric
- **RDA:** 5–10 mg/d PO.

Pharmacokinetics

Route	Onset	Peak
Oral	Slow	Delayed

Metabolism: Hepatic, $T_{1/2}$: unknown
Distribution: Crosses placenta; may enter breast milk
Excretion: Feces

Adverse effects
- **GI:** Vomiting, *nausea*

■ Nursing Considerations
Assessment
- *History:* Lactation, pregnancy
- *Physical:* Bowel sounds, normal output; serum zinc levels

Implementation
- Administer the drug with food if GI upset occurs; avoid bran and other high-fiber foods, calcium, and phosphates that may interfere with absorption.
- Ensure that patient receives only the prescribed dosage. Avoid overdose.

Drug-specific teaching points
- Take this drug exactly as prescribed. Do not exceed prescribed dosage.
- Take the drug with food, but avoid taking it with bran and other high-fiber foods and dairy products that may interfere with absorption.
- Know that nausea and vomiting may occur; taking the drug with food will help.
- Report severe nausea and vomiting, restlessness, fatigue, lethargy.

zolpidem tartrate

(zol' pih dem)
Ambien

Pregnancy Category B
C-IV controlled substance

Drug classes
Sedative/hypnotic (nonbarbiturate)

Therapeutic actions
Modulates GABA receptors to cause suppression of neurons, leading to sedation, anticonvulsant, anxiolytic, and relaxant properties.

Indications
- Short-term treatment of insomnia

Contraindications/cautions
- Contraindicated in the presence of hypersensitivity to zolpidem.
- Use caution in the presence of acute intermittent porphyria, impaired hepatic

Adverse effects in *Italics* are most common; those in **Bold** are life-threatening.

zolpidem tartrate

or renal function, addiction-prone patients, pregnancy, lactation.

Dosage
Adult: Usual dosage is 10 mg PO at bedtime.
Pediatric: Safety and efficacy not established.
Geriatric: Increased chance of confusion, acute brain syndrome; initiate treatment with 5 mg PO.

Pharmacokinetics

Route	Onset	Peak
Oral	45 min	1.6 h

Metabolism: Hepatic, $T_{1/2}$: 2.6 h
Distribution: Crosses placenta; may enter breast milk
Excretion: Urine

Adverse effects
- **CNS:** Convulsions, hallucinations, ataxia, EEG changes, pyrexia, *morning drowsiness, hangover, headache, dizziness,* vertigo, acute brain syndrome and confusion; paradoxical excitation, anxiety, depression, nightmares, dreaming, diplopia, blurred vision, *suppression of REM sleep*; REM rebound when drug is discontinued
- **GI:** Esophagitis, vomiting, *nausea*, diarrhea, constipation
- **Hypersensitivity:** Generalized allergic reactions; pruritus, rash
- **Other:** Influenza-like symptoms, dry mouth, infection

■ Nursing Considerations
Assessment
- *History:* Hypersensitivity to zolpidem, acute intermittent porphyria, impaired hepatic or renal function, addiction-prone patients, lactation, pregnancy
- *Physical:* Body temperature, skin—color, lesions; orientation, affect, reflexes, vision exam; P, BP; bowel sounds, normal output, liver evaluation; CBC with differential; hepatic and renal function tests

Implementation
- Dispense least amount of drug feasible to patients who are depressed or suicidal.
- Withdraw drug gradually if patient has used drug long-term or if patient has developed tolerance. Supportive therapy similar to that for withdrawal from barbiturates may be necessary to prevent dangerous withdrawal symptoms.

Drug-specific teaching points
- Take this drug exactly as prescribed. Do not exceed prescribed dosage. Long-term use is not recommended.
- Know that the following side effects may occur: drowsiness, dizziness, blurred vision (avoid driving a car or performing other tasks requiring alertness or visual acuity if these occur); GI upset (frequent, small meals may help).
- Report skin rash, sore throat, fever, bruising.

Adverse effects in *Italics* are most common; those in **Bold** are life-threatening.

APPENDIX A
Drug Tables

Anorexiants

The anorexiants are primarily phenethylamines, similar to amphetamine. They act in the CNS to release norepinephrine from nerve terminals. The mechanism of action that leads to appetite-suppression is not known; they may directly stimulate the satiety center in the hypothalamus. The drugs are of limited usefulness and this fact should be weighed against the risks involved in their use.

Indications
Exogenous obesity as short-term (8–12 week) adjunct to caloric restriction in a weight-reduction program.

Controlled substances; Pregnancy Category C
Contraindicated in cases of allergy to these drugs, cardiovascular disease, hypertension, hyperthyroidism, glaucoma, history of drug abuse, diabetes mellitus, epilepsy, nursing a baby. Not recommended for children <12 yr of age.

Adverse Effects
Palpitations, tachycardia, arrhythmias, dyspnea, pulmonary hypertension, hypertension, *overstimulation, restlessness, dizziness, insomnia, weakness, fatigue, drowsiness,* malaise, euphoria, *dry mouth, unpleasant taste, nausea,* vomiting, diarrhea, rash, menstrual irregularities, dependence.

Clinically Important Interactions
Do not give to patients who have recently (14 days) or are now taking *MAO inhibitors;* use caution with anyone on *antihypertensives,* the effect may be blocked.

Drug-Specific Teaching Points
Take this drug on an empty stomach, 1 h before meals; the drug can only be used for a short time and then it loses its effectiveness; take the drug early in the day to avoid interference with sleep; drug must be used in conjunction with a caloric reduction, weight loss program; avoid driving a car or operating dangerous machinery when on this drug, drug causes drowsiness; do not become pregnant while taking this drug, drug can harm the fetus; report nervousness, palpitations, chest pain, dizziness, bruising, sore throat.

Anorexiants

Drug	Brand Names	Dosage	Special Considerations
diethylpropion hydrochloride	*Nobesin* (CAN) *Propiont* (CAN) *Regibon* (CAN) *Tenuate* *Tepanil*	25 mg PO tid; sustained capsules–75 mg qd PO in AM	Do not chew or crush sustained release tablets. Eye pain is common, advise the use of sunglasses in bright light. C-IV controlled substance
fenfluramine hydrochloride	*Ponderal* (CAN) *Pondimin*	20 mg PO tid; maximum dose is 120 mg/d	Dry mouth common–use of ice chips may help; headache–analgesic may be ordered. C-IV controlled substance

(continued)

Adverse effects in *Italics* are most common; those in **Bold** are life-threatening.

Amy M. Karch: Lippincott's Nursing Drug Guide. ©1996 J. B. Lippincott Company

Anorexiants (Continued)

Drug	Brand Names	Dosage	Special Considerations
mazindol	*Mazanor* *Sanorex*	1 mg PO tid 1 h before meals or 2 mg PO qd, 1 h before lunch	Eye pain common—advise the use of sunglasses in bright light. Headache—analgesics may help. C-IV controlled substance
phendimetrazine titrate	*Adipost* *Anorex* *Bontril* *Dyrexan-OD* *Obalan* *Plegina* *Pre-lu 2* *Web-less*	35 mg PO tid; sustained release—105 mg PO qd in AM	Eye pain common—advise the use of sunglasses in bright light; headache—analgesics may help. C-III controlled substance
phentermine hydrochloride	*Adipex-P* *Fastin* *Ionamin* *Obe-Nix* *Obephen*	8 mg PO tid, 1/2 h before meals; or 15–37.5 mg PO qd as a single daily dose in the AM	Drug is most effective 1/2 h before meals; eye pain common—advise the use of sunglasses in bright light; headache—analgesics may be helpful. C-IV controlled substance

General Anesthetics

General anesthetics are central nervous system depressants that depress the reticular activating system and cerebral cortex, and can produce sedation, hypnosis, anesthesia, and deep coma; these drugs should *only* be given by medical personnel (*eg,* anesthesiologists) trained in resuscitative techniques, including the establishment of an airway. Nursing care related to these drugs involves patient support, teaching, and evaluation. (see table starting on p. 1153)

Pregnancy Category C
Contraindicated in cases of status asthmaticus; absence of suitable veins for IV administration. Caution should be used in cases of severe cardiovascular disease, hypotension or shock, conditions in which hypnotic effects may be prolonged or potentiated, increased intracranial pressure, myasthenia gravis, asthma.

Adverse Effects
Circulatory depression, thrombophlebitis, myocardial depression, cardiac arrhythmias; *respiratory depression including apnea, laryngospasm, bronchospasm,* hiccups, sneezing, coughing; *emergence delirium, headache,* prolonged somnolence and recovery; *nausea,* emesis, salivation.
Patients receiving these drugs will need to be intubated or have immediate access to ventilation to assure adequate ventilation.

Drug-Specific Teaching Points
What to expect (rapid onset of sleep), what they will feel (with rectal, IV administration), and how they will feel when they wake up.

(text continues on page 1156)

Adverse effects in *Italics* are most common; those in **Bold** are life-threatening.

Appendix A — 1153

General Anesthetics

Drug	Brand Names	Dosage	Special Considerations	Onset/Recovery	Postanesthesia Concerns
Barbiturates					
thiopental sodium	*Pentothal*	Test dose: 50–75 mg IV 50–75 mg IV q20–40 sec. Maintenance: 25–50 mg IV	Do not administer in concentrations less than 2% in Sterile Water. C-III controlled substance.	Rapid/ultrashort	Not analgesic, post-op pain common.
thiamylal sodium	*Surital*	Test dose; 2 ml IV. 1 ml q5sec of 2.5% solution.	Prepare with Sterile Water for Injection. Do not mix with atropine, tobocurarine or succinylcholine.	Rapid/ultrashort	Cough, respiratory depression, not analgesic, post-op pain common.
methohexital sodium	*Brevital*	5–12 ml of 1% solution. Maintenance; 2–4 ml of 1% solution q4–7 min.	Short acting. Do not mix with bacteriostatic water or acid solutions. Should not come in contact with silicone. Avoid contact with rubber stoppers or disposable syringes with silicone.	Rapid/ultra, ultrashort	Respiratory depression and apnea; not analgesic, post-op pain common.
Gases					
nitrous oxide			Frequently causes nausea. Nonexplosive gas. Malignant hypothermia can occur. Monitor. Supplied in blue cylinders.	1–2 min/rapid	Hypoxia; monitor for chest pain, hypertension, stroke.
cyclopropane			Rapid onset. Malignant hypothermia may occur. Very explosive. Supplied in orange cylinders.	1–2 min/rapid	Headache, nausea and vomiting; delirium during recovery.
ethylene			Rapid onset and recovery. Nontoxic. Very explosive. Supplied in red cylinders.	Rapid/rapid	Unpleasant taste, headache.

(continued)

General Anesthetics (Continued)

Drug	Brand Names	Dosage	Special Considerations	Onset/Recovery	Postanesthesia Concerns
Volatile liquids					
desflurane	*Suprane*	3%–1% concentrations, inhaled	Not recommended for induction of pediatric patients. May be used as adjunct for maintenance. Can cause respiratory irritation.	Rapid/rapid	Coughing, laryngospasm, increased secretions.
enflurane	*Enthrane*	2%–4.5% produces anesthesia in 7–10 min.	Causes muscle relaxation. May cause renal toxicity.	Rapid/rapid	Cardiac arrhythmias, respiratory depression.
halothane	*Fluothane*	Administered by nonrebreathing technique, partial rebreathing or closed technique.	Associated with hepatic toxicity. Monitor for malignant hyperthermia.	Rapid/rapid	Hypotension, cardiac arrhythmias.
isoflurane	*Forane*	Inspired 1.5%–3% concentration causes anesthesia in 7–10 min. Maintenance with 1%–2% with nitrous oxide.	Rapid onset and recovery. Causes muscle relaxation. Monitor for hypotension, hypercapnia.	Rapid/rapid	Muscle soreness, bad taste, hypotension
methoxyflurane	*Penthrane*	0.3%–0.8% for anesthesia 0.1%–2% for maintenance.	May cause renal toxicity. Used with oxygen or nitrous oxide.	Slow/prolonged	Respiratory depression; hypotension

Other

droperidol	*Inapsine*	2.5–10 mg IM or IV	Use caution with renal or hepatic failure. Monitor for hypotension.	3–10 min/2–4 h	Drowsiness, chills, hypotension, hallucinations during recovery
etomidate	*Amidate*	0.2–0.6 mg/kg IV over 30–60 sec.	Not recommended in children <10 y. Used for sedation for ventilator patients.	1 min/3–5 min	Myoclonic, tonic movements, nausea and vomiting.
ketamine	*Ketalar*	1–4.5 mg/kg for 5–10 min of anesthesia	Administer slowly over 60 sec. Monitor for severe emergence reactions: dreams, hallucinations, etc. Manage with small dose of hypnotic.	Rapid/45 min	Dissociation, hallucinations; hypertension, increased heart rate
midazolam hydrochloride	*Versed*	0.07–0.06 mg/kg	Onset in 15 min, peaks in 30–60 min. Administer slowly. Monitor for respiratory depression.	Rapid/rapid	Respiratory depression, cough, hiccoughs, nausea and vomiting
propofol	*Diprivan*	100 mcg/kg–2.5 mg/kg	Short-acting. Local burning on injection. Monitor for sedation before discharge; monitor for pulmonary edema.	Rapid/rapid	Hypotension, bradycardia, movement

Local Anesthetics

Local anesthetics prevent the conduction of sensory (pain) impulses by reducing sodium permeability of the nerve membrane, thus decreasing the height and rate of rise of the nerve action potential. The loss of nerve function depends on the nerve involved and the effects of the anesthetic. Progression of nerve function loss is pain, temperature, touch, proprioception, skeletal muscle tone. (see table starting on p. 1158)

Indications
Infiltration anesthesia, peripheral nerve block, spinal anesthesia, relief of local pain.

Pregnancy Category C
Contraindicated in cases of hypersensitivity to local anesthetics, para-aminobenzoic acid (PABA), or to parabens; heart block; shock; septicemia; reduced levels of plasma esterases.

Adverse Effects
Occurrence varies with route of administration: *headache, backache,* septic meningitis, *restlessness, anxiety, dizziness, tinnitus, blurred vision,* pupil constriction, tremors, convulsion, drowsiness, nausea, vomiting, *peripheral vasodilation,* myocardial depression, hypotension or hypertension, decreased cardiac output, heart block, bradycardia, ventricular arrhythmias, **cardiac arrest,** fetal bradycardia, **respiratory arrest,** chills, allergic reactions of delayed onset (urticaria, pruritus, erythema, angioneurotic edema, sneezing, syncope, excessive sweating, elevated temperature, anaphylactoid symptoms), urinary retention, urinary or fecal incontinence, loss of perineal sensation and sexual function, persistent analgesia/anesthesia, paresthesia, weakness, paralysis of lower extremities and loss of sphincter tone, persistent motor or sensory autonomic deficit of lower spinal segments with slow (months) or incomplete recovery, slowing of labor, *sympathetic block and hypotension.*

Dosage
Dosage is determined by the degree of anesthesia desired and the nerve involved; these drugs are often administered by anesthesiologists or others trained in this specific administration.

Clinically Important Interactions
Increased and prolonged neuromuscular blockade produced by succinylcholine if given concurrently with various local anesthetics.

Important Interventions
Assure that resuscitative equipment (airway, oxygen, facilities for positive pressure breathing) is on standby, that drugs for managing seizures, hypotension, cardiac arrest are on standby (thiopental, thiamylal, diazepam, IV fluids, vasopressors), assure that patients receiving spinal anesthetics are well hydrated and remain lying down for up to 12 h after the anesthetic to minimize likelihood of "spinal headache," establish appropriate safety precautions to prevent injury during the time patient has lost sensation.

Drug-Specific Teaching Points
Route of administration, reason for establishing IV line (as appropriate), what feelings to anticipate and what will be experienced, the need to remain lying down after spinal anesthesia; to report burning, pain, headache, difficulty breathing, lack of function in anticipated time frame.

Adverse effects in *Italics* are most common; those in **Bold** are life-threatening.

Commonly Used Biologicals

❐ diptheria and tetanus toxoids, combined, absorbed (DT, Td) (available in adult and pediatric preparations)

Therapeutic Actions
Contains reduced dose of inactivated diphtheria toxin and full dose of inactivated tetanus toxin to provide adequate immunization in adults without the severe sensitivity reactions caused when full pediatric doses of diphtheria toxoid are given to adults.

Indications
Active immunization of adults and children ≥7 y against diphtheria and tetanus.

Adverse Effects
Fretfulness; drowsiness; anorexia; vomiting; transient fever; malaise; generalized aches and pains; edema of injection area with redness, swelling, induration, pain (may persist for a few days); hypersensitivity reactions.

Dosage
2 primary IM doses of 0.5 ml each given at 4–8 wk intervals, followed by a third 0.5 ml IM dose given in 6–12 mo. Routine booster of 0.5 ml IM every 10 y for maintenance of immunity.

Nursing Considerations
- Use caution in pregnant women—**Pregnancy Category C,** safety not established.
- Defer administration of routine immunizing or booster doses in case of acute infection.
- Arrange to interrupt immunosuppressive therapy if emergency booster doses of Td are required due to injury.
- **Not** for treatment of acute tetanus or diphtheria infections.
- Administer by IM injection only, avoid SC or IV injection; deltoid muscle is the preferred site. Do not administer into the same site more than once.
- Arrange for epinephrine 1:1000 to be immediately available at time of injection because of hypersensitivity reactions.
- Provide comfort measures to help the patient cope with the discomforts of the injection: analgesics, warm soaks for injection site, small meals, environmental control—temperature, stimuli.
- Provide patient with written record of immunization and reminder of when booster injection is needed.

❐ diphtheria and tetanus toxoids and whole cell pertussis vaccine, adsorbed (DTwP)

Tri-Immunol

Therapeutic Actions
Provides detoxified diphtheria and tetanus toxins and pertussis vaccine to stimulate an immunologic response in children leading to an active immunity against these diseases.

Indications
Active immunization of infants and children through 6 y of age (between 6 wk and 7 y) against diphtheria, tetanus, pertussis—for primary immunization and routine recall; start immunization at once if whooping cough is present in the community.

(text continues on page 1160)

Local Anesthetics

Drug	Brand-Names	Pharmacokinetics	Uses	Special Considerations
benzocaine	Dermoplast Foile Unguentine Lanacane	Onset: 1 min Duration: 30–60 min	Skin Mucous membrane	Protect patient from injury; alert patient using skin prep to avoid tight bandages.
bupivacaine	Marcaine Sensorcaine	Onset: 5–20 min Duration: 2–7 h	Local Epidural Subarachnoid Caudal Retrobulbar Sympathetic Dental	Do not use for Bier Block–deaths have occurred; do not use .75% solution for obstetric anesthesia
butamben picrate	Butesin Picrate	Onset: slow Duration: 30–60 min	Skin Mucous membr.	Protect patient from injury; advise patient that swallowing may be difficult with throat use.
chloroprocaine	Nesacaine	Onset: 6–15 min Duration: 15–75 min	Nerve block Caudal Epidural	Do not use with subarachnoid administration
dibucaine	Nupercainal	Onset: <15 min Duration: 3–4 h	Skin disorders Mucous membranes	Monitor for local reaction; advise patient to use care not to injure themselves.
etidocaine	Duranest HCl	Onset: 3–15 min Duration: 2–5 h	Peripheral block OB, pelvic, abd. surgery; alveolar block	Monitor for skin breakdown; offer support for lower limb paralysis
lidocaine	Caine-2 Xylocaine Octocaine Dilocaine Nervocaine Nulicaine	Onset: 5–15 min Duration: .5–1.5 h	Caudal Epidural Dental Spinal Cervical Peripheral	Caution patient to avoid injury; shorter acting than many other anesthetics.

	Solarcaine		Skin Mucous membranes
mepivocaine	*Carbocaine* *Isocaine* *Polocaine*	Onset: 3–15 min Duration: .75–1.5 h	Nerve block OB use Caudal Epidural Dental Local infiltrate	Use caution in patients with renal impairment.
prilocaine	*Citanest*	Onset: 1–15 min Duration: 5–3 h	Nerve block Dental	Advise dental patients not to bite themselves.
procaine	*Novocain*	Onset: 2–25 min Duration: 15–75 min	Infiltration Peripheral Spinal	Assure patient that feeling will return; monitor skin condition; keep patient supine to avoid headache.
promaxine	*Tronothane* *PrameGel* *Prax* *Itch-X* *Phicon*	Onset: 3–5 min Duration: <60 min	Skin Mucous membr.	Protect patient from injury; advise patient to limit use; do not cover with tight bandages
tetracaine	*Pontocaine*	Onset: 15–30 min Duration: 2–2.5 h	Spinal Prolonged spinal Skin	Protect patient from skin breakdown; offer reassurance with long periods of lower limb paralysis; keep patient supine to avoid headache

Adverse Effects
Hypersensitivity reactions; erythema, induration, redness, pain, swelling of the injection area; nodule at the injection site which may persist for several weeks; temperature elevations, malaise, chills, irritability, fretfulness, drowsiness, anorexia, vomiting, persistent crying; rarely—fatal reactions.

Dosage
- Primary immunization: For children 6 wk to 6 y (ideally, beginning at age 2–3 mo or at the 6 wk check up): 0.5 ml IM on 3 occasions at 4–8 wk intervals with a reinforcing dose administered 1 y after the third injection.
- Booster doses: 0.5 ml IM when the child is 4–6 y old (preferably before beginning kindergarten or elementary school). If 4th dose was given after the 4 y birthday, however, the preschool dose may be omitted. Booster injections every 10 y should be given after this using the adult diphtheria and tetanus toxoids combination; do not give pertussis vaccine to person ≥7 y.

Nursing Considerations
- Do not use for treatment of acute tetanus, diphtheria or whooping cough infections.
- Do not administer to children >7 y or to adults.
- Do not attempt routine immunization with DTP if the child has a personal history of CNS disease or convulsions.
- Do not administer DTP after recent blood transfusions or immune globulin, in immunodeficiency disorders or with immunosuppressive therapy, or to patients with malignancy.
- Question the parent concerning occurrence of any symptoms or signs of adverse reactions after previous dose before administering repeat dose of the vaccine—if fever >39°C (103°F), convulsions with or without fever, alterations of consciousness, focal neurologic signs, screaming episodes, shock, collapse, somnolence, or encephalopathy have occurred, DTP is contraindicated and diphtheria and tetanus toxoids without pertussis should be used for immunization.
- Administer by IM injection only; avoid SC or IV injection. Midlateral muscle of the thigh is preferred site for infants, deltoid muscle is the preferred site for older children. Do not administer into the same site more than once.
- Arrange for epinephrine 1:1000 to be immediately available at time of injection because of risk of hypersensitivity reactions.
- Provide comfort measures and teach parents to provide comfort measures to help the patient cope with the discomforts of the injection: analgesics, warm soaks for injection site, small meals, environmental control—temperature, stimuli.
- Provide patient with written record of immunization and reminder of when booster injection is needed.

❑ diphtheria and tetanus toxoids and acellular pertussis vaccine, adsorbed (DTaP)

Acel-Imune, Tripedia

Therapeutic Actions
Provides detoxified diphtheria and tetanus toxins and acellular pertussis vaccine to stimulate an immunologic response in children leading to an active immunity against these diseases in children who have received 3–4 doses of DTwP vaccine. Use as the 4th or 5th doses only.

Indications
Induction of immunity against diphthera, tetanus, and pertussis as the fourth and fifth dose in children from ages 15 mo (*Tripedia*) or 17 mo (*Acel-Immune*) through the 7th

birthday). Children must have been previously immunized with 3 or 4 doses of whole cell DTP. Use in children as young as 15 mo if the child is not expected to return at 18 mo for the fourth dose. Being considered for immunization of adults against pertussis.

Adverse Effects

Hypersensitivity reactions; erythema, induration, redness, pain, swelling of the injection area; nodule at the injection site which may persist for several weeks; temperature elevations, malaise, chills, irritability, fretfulness, drowsiness, anorexia, vomiting, persistent crying; rarely—fatal reactions.

Dosage
- Fourth dose: 0.5 ml IM at 18 mo of age, at least 6 mo after last dose of DTwP.
- Fifth dose: 0.5 ml IM at 4–6 years of age or preferably before entry into school. If 4th dose was given after the 4 y birthday, however, the preschool dose may be omitted. Booster injections every 10 y should be given after this using the adult diphtheria and tetanus toxoids combination; do not give pertussis vaccine to person ≥7 y.

Nursing Considerations
- Do not use for treatment of acute tetanus, diphtheria, or whooping cough infections.
- Do not administer to children >7 y or to adults.
- Do not attempt routine immunization with DTaP if the child has a personal history of CNS disease or convulsions.
- Administer only if patient has already received at least 3 doses of DTwP.
- Do not administer DTaP after recent blood transfusions or immune globulin, in immunodeficiency disorders or with immunosuppressive therapy, or to patients with malignancy.
- Question the parent concerning occurrence of any symptoms or signs of adverse reactions after the previous dose before administering a repeat dose of the vaccine—if fever >39°C (103°F), convulsions with or without fever, alterations of consciousness, focal neurologic signs, screaming episodes, shock, collapse, somnolence, or encephalopathy have occurred, DTP is contraindicated and diphtheria and tetanus toxoids without pertussis should be used for immunization.
- Administer by IM injection only; avoid SC or IV injection. Midlateral muscle of the thigh is preferred site for infants, deltoid muscle is the preferred site for older children. Do not administer into the same site more than once.
- Arrange for epinephrine 1:1000 to be immediately available at time of injection because of risk of hypersensitivity reactions.
- Provide comfort measures and teach parents to provide comfort measures to help the patient cope with the discomforts of the injection: analgesics, warm soaks for injection site, small meals, environmental control—temperature, stimuli.
- Provide parent with written record of immunization and reminder of when booster injection is needed.

☐ diphtheria and tetanus toxoids and pertussis vaccine, adsorbed with haemophilus b conjugated vaccine

ACTHIB-DTP

Therapeutic Actions

Provides detoxified diphtheria and tetanus toxins and pertussis vaccine and *Haemophilus influenzae* b conjugate vaccine to stimulate an immunologic response in children leading to an active immunity against these diseases.

Indications
Active immunization of infants and children (2 mo–5 y) against diphtheria, tetanus, pertussis, and *Haemophilus influenzae* b for primary immunization and routine recall.

Adverse Effects
Hypersensitivity reactions; erythema, induration, redness, pain swelling of the injection area; nodule at the injection site which may persist for several weeks; temperature elevations, malaise, chills, irritability, fretfulness, drowsiness, anorexia, vomiting, persistent crying; rarely—fatal reactions.

Dosage
- Primary immunization: For children 2 mo to 5 y, 0.5 ml IM ideally, beginning at age 2 mo; then repeat dose at 4 mo, 6 mo and 15–18 mo).
- Booster dose: Subsequent DTP or DTaP vaccination is needed at 4–6 y.

Nursing Considerations
- Do not use for treatment of acute tetanus, diphtheria, or whooping cough or *H. flu* b infections.
- Do not administer to children over the age of 5 y or to adults.
- Do not attempt routine immunization if the child has a personal history of CNS disease or convulsions.
- Do not administer after recent blood transfusions or immune globulin, in immunodeficiency disorders or with immunosuppressive therapy, or to patients with malignancy.
- Question the parent concerning occurrence of any symptoms or signs of adverse reactions after the previous dose before administering a repeat dose of the vaccine—if fever >39°C (103°F), convulsions with or without fever, alterations of consciousness, focal neurologic signs, screaming episodes, shock, collapse, somnolence, or encephalopathy have occurred, DTP is contraindicated and diphtheria and tetanus toxoids without pertussis should be used for immunization.
- Administer by IM injection only; avoid SC or IV injection. Midlateral muscle of the thigh is preferred site for infants, deltoid muscle is the preferred site for older children. Do not administer into the same site more than once.
- Arrange for epinephrine 1:1000 to be immediately available at time of injection because of risk of hypersensitivity reactions.
- Provide comfort measures and teach parents to provide comfort measures to help the patient cope with the discomforts of the injection: analgesics, warm soaks for injection site, small meals, environmental control—temperature, stimuli.
- Provide parent with written record of immunization and reminder of when booster injection is needed.

☐ diphtheria and tetanus toxoids and whole cell pertussis vaccine with haemophilus influenzae b conjugates vaccine (DTwP-HIB)

Tetramune

Therapeutic Actions
Provides detoxified diphtheria and tetanus toxins and whole cell pertussis vaccine and *Haemophilus influenzae* b conjugate vaccine to stimulate an immunologic response in children leading to an active immunity against these diseases.

Indications
Active immunization of infants and children (2 mo—5 y) against diphtheria, tetanus, pertussis, and *Haemophilus influenzae* b for primary immunization and routine recall.

(Not recommended for children who experienced active *Haemophilus influenzae* b infection ≥24 mo.)

Adverse Effects
Hypersensitivity reactions; erythema, induration, redness, pain, swelling of the injection area; nodule at the injection site which may persist for several weeks; temperature elevations, malaise, chills, irritability, fretfulness, drowsiness, anorexia, vomiting, persistent crying; rarely—fatal reactions.

Dosage
- Primary immunization: For children 2 mo: three doses of 0.5 ml IM at 2 mo intervals with a fourth dose at 15 mo of age.
- Booster dose: Subsequent DTP or DTaP vaccination is needed at 4–6 y.

Nursing Considerations
- Do not use for treatment of acute tetanus, diphtheria, whooping cough, or *H. flu* b infections.
- Do not administer to children >5 y or to adults.
- Do not attempt routine immunization if the child has a personal history of CNS disease or convulsions.
- Do not administer after recent blood transfusions or immune globulin, in immunodeficiency disorders or with immunosuppressive therapy, or to patients with malignancy.
- Question the parent concerning occurrence of any symptoms or signs of adverse reactions after the previous dose before administering a repeat dose of the vaccine—if fever >39°C (103°F), convulsions with or without fever, alterations of consciousness, focal neurologic signs, screaming episodes, shock, collapse, somnolence, or encephalopathy have occurred, DTP is contraindicated and diphtheria and tetanus toxoids without pertussis should be used for immunization.
- Administer by IM injection only; avoid SC or IV injection. Midlateral muscle of the thigh is preferred site for infants, deltoid muscle is the preferred site for older children. Do not administer into the same site more than once.
- Arrange for epinephrine 1:1000 to be immediately available at time of injection because of risk of hypersensitivity reactions.
- Provide comfort measures and teach parents to provide comfort measures to help the patient cope with the discomforts of the injection: analgesics, warm soaks for injection site, small meals, environmental control—temperature, stimuli.
- Provide parent with written record of immunization and reminder of when booster injection is needed.

hemophilus b conjugate vaccine

HibTITER, PedvaxHIB, ProHIBiT

Therapeutic Actions
Vaccine prepared from the purified capsular polysaccharide of the *Hemophilus influenzae* type b (Hib) bacterium bound to an inactive noninfective diphtheria toxoid; stimulates long-lived, non-boostable antibody response that prevents Hib diseases.

Indications
Immunization of children 2 mo–5 y (*Hib TITER*), 18 mo–5 y (*PedvaxHIB* and *ProHIBit*) against diseases caused by *H influenzae* type b.

Adverse Reactions
Erythema and induration at the injection site, fever, acute febrile reactions.

Dosage
PedvaxHIB, ProHIBIT: 0.5 ml IM
HibTITER:
- 2–6 mo old: three separate IM injections of 0.5 ml each given at approximately 2 mo intervals.
- 7–11 mo old: two separate IM injections of 0.5 ml each given at approximately 2 mo intervals.
- 12–14 mo old: one IM injection of 0.5 ml.

All vaccinated children receive a single booster dose at ≥15 mo of age, but not less than 2 mo after the previous dose. Previously unvaccinated children 15–60 mo of age receive a single 0.5 ml IM injection.

Nursing Considerations
- Do not administer to patient with any history of hypersensitivity to any component of the vaccine.
- Do not administer to any patient with febrile illness or active infection; delay vaccine until patient has recovered.
- Have epinephrine 1:1000 immediately available at time of injection in case of severe anaphylactoid reaction.
- Provide comfort measures—analgesics, antipyretics—or instruct parent to provide comfort measures to help the patient cope with any discomfort from the injection.
- Provide parent with a written record of immunization; identify the particular vaccine that is being used; *HibTITER* requires repeat injections, *PedvaxHIB* and *ProHIBit* require no repeat injections.

❐ hepatitis B immune globulin (HBIG)

H-BIG, Hep-B-Gammagee, Hyperhep

Therapeutic Actions
Globulin contains a high titer of antibody to hepatitis B surface (HBsAg), providing a passive immunity to hepatitis B surface antigen.

Indications
- Postexposure prophylaxis following parental exposure (accidental "needle-stick"), direct mucous membrane contact (accidental splash), or oral ingestion (pipetting accident) involving HBsAg-positive materials such as blood, plasma, serum.
- Prophylaxis of infants born to HBsAG-positive mothers.
- Adjunct to hepatitis B vaccine when rapid achievement of protective levels of antibodies is desirable.

Adverse Effects
Hypersensitivity reactions; tenderness, muscle stiffness at the injection site; urticaria, angioedema; fever, chills, nausea, vomiting, chest tightness.

Dosage
- Perinatal exposure: 0.5 ml, IM within 12 h of birth; repeat dose at 3 mo and 6 mo after initial dose.
- Percutaneous exposure: 0.06 ml/kg IM, immediately (within 7 d) and repeat 28–30 d after exposure.

- Individuals at high risk of infection: 0.06 ml/kg IM at same time (but at a different site) as hepatitis B vaccine is given.

Nursing Considerations
- Do not administer to patients with history of allergic response to gamma globulin or with anti-immunoglobulin A antibodies.
- Use caution in pregnant women, **Pregnancy Category C;** safety not established, use only if benefits outweigh potential unknown risks to the fetus.
- HBIG may be administered at the same time or up to 1 mo preceding hepatitis B vaccination without impairing the active immune response from the vaccination.
- Administer IM in the gluteal or deltoid region; do not administer IV.
- Administer the appropriate dose as soon after exposure as possible (within 7 days is preferable); and repeat 28–30 days after exposure.
- Have epinephrine 1:1000 immediately available at time of injection in case of anaphylactic reaction.
- Provide comfort measures to help patient to deal with discomfort of drug therapy—analgesics, antipyretics, environmental control, etc.

hepatitis B vaccine

Engerix-B, Recombivax-HB

Therapeutic Actions
Provides inactivated human hepatitis B surface antigen particles to stimulate active immunity and production of antibodies against hepatitis B surface antigens using surface antigen produced by yeast.

Indications
- Immunization against infection caused by all known subtypes of hepatitis B virus, especially those at high risk for infection—health care personnel, military personnel identified to be at risk, prisoners, users of illicit drugs, populations with high incidence (Eskimos, Indochinese refugees, Haitian refugees), morticians and embalmers, persons at increased risk because of their sexual practices (repeated sexually transmitted diseases, homosexually active males, prostitutes), patients in hemodialysis units, patients requiring frequent blood transfusions, residents of mental institutions, household contacts of people with persistent hepatitis B antigenemia.
- Treatment of choice for infants born to HBsAG-positive mothers.

Adverse Effects
- Soreness, swelling, erythema, warmth, induration at injection site; malaise, fatigue, headache, nausea, vomiting, dizziness, myalgia, arthralgia, rash, low grade fever, pharyngitis, rhinitis, cough, lymphadenopathy, hypotension, dysuria.

Dosage
- Pediatric (birth–10 y): Initial dose–0.5 ml, IM; followed by 0.5 ml IM at 1 mo and 6 mo after initial dose (*Engerix B*); 0.25 ml IM, followed by 0.25 ml IM at 1 mo and 6 mo after initial dose (*Recombivax –HB*).
- Older children (11–19 y): Initial dose–1 ml, IM; followed by 1 ml IM at 1 mo and 6 mo after initial dose (*Engerix B*); 0.5 ml, IM; followed by 0.5 ml IM at 1 mo and 6 mo after initial dose (*Recombivax –HB*).
- Adults: Initial dose–1 ml, IM; followed by 1 ml IM at 1 mo and 6 mo after initial dose, all types.

- Dialysis or immunocompromised patients: Initial dose—two 1 ml injections at different sites, IM; followed by two 1 ml injections, IM at 1 mo and at 6 mo after initial dose (*Engerix B*).
- Revaccination (a booster dose should be considered if anti-HBs levels <10 mIU/ml 1–2 mo after third dose): Children ≤10 y of age: 10 mcg. Adults and children >10 y: 20 mcg. Hemodialysis patients (when antibody testing indicates need): give two 20 mcg doses.

Nursing Considerations
- Do not administer to any patient with known hypersensitivity to any component of the vaccine; allergy to yeast.
- Use caution in pregnant or nursing women—**Pregnancy Category C;** safety not established; use only if clearly needed and benefits outweigh potential unknown effects.
- Use caution with any patient with active infection; delay use of vaccine if at all possible; use with caution in any patient with compromised cardiopulmonary status or patients in whom a febrile or systemic reaction could present a significant risk.
- Administer IM, preferably in the deltoid muscle in adults, the anterolateral thigh muscle in infants and small children. Do not administer IV or intradermally; SC route may be used in patients who are at high risk for hemorrhage following IM injection, but increased incidence of local effects has been noted.
- Shake vaccine container well before withdrawing solution; no dilution is needed, use vaccine as supplied. Vaccine will appear as a slightly opaque, white suspension. Refrigerate vials, do not freeze.
- Have epinephrine 1:1000 immediately available at time of injection in case of severe anaphylactic reaction.
- Provide comfort measures—analgesics, antipyretics, care of injection site—to help patient to cope with the effects of the drug.
- Provide patient or parent with a written record of the immunization and dates that repeat injections and antibody tests are needed.

immunue globulin intramuscular (IG; Gamma Globulin; ISG)

Gamastan, Gammar, Immune Globulin

immune globulin intravenous (IGIV)

Gamimune, Gammagard, Gammar-IV, Iveegam, N, Sandoglobulin, Venoglubulin-I

Therapeutic Actions
Contains human globulin (16.5% IM, 5% IV) which provides passive immunity through the presence of injected antibodies; IM gamma globulin involves a 2–5 day delay before adequate serum levels are obtained, IV gamma globulin provides immediate antibody levels; mechanism of action in idiopathic thrombocytopenic purpura not determined.

Indications
- Prophylaxis after exposure to hepatitis A, measles (rubeola), varicella, rubella—IM route preferred.
- Prophylaxis for patients with immunoglobulin deficiency—IM, IV if immediate increase in antibodies is necessary.

- Idiopathic thrombocytopenic purpura—IV route has produced temporary increase in platelets in emergency situations.
- B-cell chronic lymphocytic leukemia (CLL) (*Gammagard*).

Adverse Effects
Tenderness, muscle stiffness at injection site; urticaria, angioedema, nausea, vomiting, chills, fever, chest tightness; anaphylactic reactions, precipitous fall in blood pressure—more likely with IV administration.

Dosage
- Hepatitis A: 0.02 ml/kg, IM for household and institutional contacts; persons traveling to areas where hepatitis A is common—0.02 ml/kg IM if staying <2 mo, 0.06 ml/kg IM repeated every 5 mo for prolonged stay.
- Measles (rubeola): 0.2 ml/kg IM if exposed <6 days previously; immunocompromised child exposed to measles—0.5 ml/kg to a maximum of 15 ml IM given immediately.
- Varicella: 0.6–1.2 ml/kg IM given promptly if zoster immune globulin is unavailable.
- Rubella: 0.55 ml/kg IM given to those pregnant women who have been exposed to rubella and will not consider a therapeutic abortion may decrease likelihood of infection and fetal damage.
- Immuno globulin deficiency: Initial dosage of 1.3 ml/kg IM followed in 3–4 wk by 0.66 ml/kg IM every 3–4 wk; some patients may require more frequent injections.
- *Sandoglobulin:* 200 mg/kg IV, once a month by IV infusion; if insufficient response, increase dose to 300 mg/kg by IV infusion or repeat more frequently. Idiopathic thrombocytopenic purpura—400 mg/kg IV for 5 consecutive days.
- *Gamimune:* 100 mg/kg IV once a month by IV infusion. May be increased to 200 mg/kg IV or infusion may be repeated more frequently.
- *Gammagard:* 200–400 mg/kg IV, monthly doses of at least 100 mg/kg are recommended. B-cell CLL: 400 mg/kg IV every 3–4 wk. Idiopathic thrombocytopenic purpura: 1000 mg/kg IV, base dose on clinical response. Give up to 3 doses on alternate days if required.
- *Gammar-IV:* 100–200 mg/kg IV every 3–4 wk.
- *Venoglobulin-I:* 200 mg/kg IV administered monthly. Idiopathic thrombocytopenic purpura: 500 mg/kg/day for 2–7 consecutive days.
- *Iveegam:* 200 mg/kg IV per mo.

Nursing Considerations
- Do not administer to patients with history of allergy to gamma globulin or anti-immunoglobulin A antibodies.
- Use IM gamma globulin with caution in patients with thrombocytopenia or any coagulation disorder that would contraindicate IM injections—use only if benefits outweigh risks.
- Use with caution in pregnant women—**Pregnancy Category C;** safety not established.
- Administer 2 wk before or 3 mo after immune globulin administration because antibodies in the globulin preparation may interfere with the immune response to the vaccination.
- Have epinephrine 1:1000 immediately available at time of injection in case of anaphylactic reaction, more likely with IV immune globulin, large IM doses, and repeated injections.
- Refrigerate drug, do not freeze, discard partially used vials.
- Administer IM preparation by IM injection only, do not administer SC or intradermally.
- Administer IV preparation with extreme caution as follows:

   Sandoglobulin: Give the first infusion as a 3% solution (reconstitute by inverting the 2 bottles so that solvent flows into the IV bottle). Start with a flow rate of 0.5–1 ml/min; after 15–30 min increase infusion rate to 1.5–2.5 ml/min. Administer subsequent infusions at a rate of 2–2.5 ml/min; if high doses must be administered repeatedly after the first infusion of 3% solution, use a 6% solution (reconstitute 1 g vial with 16.5 ml diluent, 3 g vial with 50 ml diluent, 6 g vial with 100 ml diluent) with an initial infusion rate of 1–1.5 ml/min, increased after 15–30 min to a maximum of 2.5 ml/min.

Gamimune: May be diluted with 5% dextrose, infusion rate of 0.01–0.02 ml/kg/min for 30 min. If patient does not experience any discomfort, the rate may be increased to 0.02–0.04 ml/kg/min. If side effects occur, reduce the rate or interrupt the infusion until the symptoms subside and resume at a rate tolerable to the patient.

Gammagard: Initially administer at a rate of 0.5 ml/kg/h. If rate causes no distress, may be gradually increased, not to exceed 4 ml/kg/h.

Gammar-IV: Administer at 0.01 ml/kg/min, increasing to 0.02 ml/kg/min after 15–30 min. If adverse reactions occur, slow the infusion rate.

Venoglobulin-I: Infuse at a rate of 0.01–0.02 ml/kg/min for the first 30 min. If patient experiences no distress, may be increased to 0.04 ml/kg/min.

Iveegam: Infuse at rate of 1 ml/min up to a maximum of 2 ml/min of the 5% solution. Drug may be further diluted with 5% dextrose or saline.

- Do not mix immune globulin with any other medications.
- Monitor the patient's vital signs continuously and observe for any symptoms during IV administration—adverse effects appear to be related to the rate of infusion.
- Provide comfort measures or teach patient to provide comfort measures—analgesics, antipyretics, warm soaks to injection site—to help patient to cope with the discomforts of drug therapy.
- Provide patient with written record of injection and dates for follow-up injections as needed.

☐ influenza virus vaccine

Flu-Immune, Fluogen, Fluzone, Flu-Shield

Therapeutic Effects
Inactivated influenza virus antigens stimulate an active immunity through the production of antibodies specific to the antigens used; the antigens used vary from year to year depending on which influenza virus strains are anticipated to be prevalent.

Indications
Prophylaxis for people at high risk of developing complications from infection with influenza virus—adults and children with chronic cardiovascular or pulmonary disorders, chronic metabolic disorders, renal dysfunction, anemia, immunosuppression, asthma; residents of chronic care facilities; medical personnel with extensive contact with high-risk patients, to prevent their transmitting the virus to these patients; children on chronic aspirin therapy who are at high risk of developing Reye's syndrome; people who provide essential community services (to decrease the risk of disruption of services).

Adverse Effects
Tenderness, redness and induration at the injection site; fever, malaise, myalgia; allergic responses—flare, wheal, respiratory symptoms; Guillain-Barré syndrome.

Dosage
- 6–35 mo—split virus or purified surface antigen only—0.25 ml IM repeated in 4 wk.
- 3–6 y—split virus or purified surface antigen only—0.5 ml IM repeated in 4 wk.
- ≥9 y—whole or split virus or purified surface antigen—0.5 ml IM.

Nursing Considerations

- Do not administer to patients with sensitivities to eggs, chicken, chicken feathers, or chicken dander. If an allergic condition is suspected, administer a scratch test or an intradermal injection (0.05–0.1 ml) of vaccine diluted 1:100 in sterile saline—a wheal greater than 5 mm justifies withholding immunization.
- Do not administer to patient with a hypersensitivity to any component of the vaccine; history of Guillain-Barré syndrome.
- Do not administer to infants and children at the same time as diphtheria, tetanus toxoid, and pertussis vaccine (DTP) or within 14 days after Measles Virus Vaccine.
- Delay administration in the presence of acute respiratory disease or other active infection or acute febrile illness.
- Use caution in pregnant women; **Pregnancy Category C;** safety not established, delay use until the second or third trimester to minimize concern over possible teratogenicity.
- Monitor patient for enhanced drug effects and possible toxicity of *theophylline, warfarin sodium* for as long as 3 wk after vaccine injection.
- Administer IM only; the deltoid muscle is preferred for adults and older children, the anterolateral aspect of the thigh for infants and younger children.
- Consider the possible need for amantadine for therapeutic use for patients in high risk groups who develop illness compatible with influenza during a period of known influenza A activity in the community.
- Have epinephrine 1:1000 immediately available at time of injection in case of anaphylactic reaction.
- Provide comfort measures or teach patient to provide comfort measures—analgesics, antipyretics, warm soaks to injection site—to help patient cope with effects of the drug.
- Provide patient with written record of vaccination and dates of second injection as appropriate.

measles (rubeola) virus vaccine, live, attenuated

Attenuvax

Therapeutic Actions

Attenuated measles virus produces a modified measles infection and stimulates an active immune reaction with antibodies to the measles virus.

Indications

- Immunization against measles (rubeola) immediately after exposure to natural measles, more effective if given before exposure—children ≥15 mo (immunization with trivalent MMR vaccine is the preferred product for routine vaccinations).
- Revaccination for children immunized before the age of 12 mo or vaccinated with inactivated vaccine alone.
- Prophylaxis for high school or college age persons in epidemic situations or for adults in isolated communities where measles is not endemic.

Adverse Effects

Moderate fever, rash; high fever—less common; febrile convulsions, **Guillain-Barré syndrome**, ocular palsies—less common; burning or stinging wheal or flare at injection site.

Adverse effects in *Italics* are most common; those in **Bold** are life-threatening.

Dosage
Inject the total volume of the reconstituted vaccine or 0.5 ml of multi-dose vial SC into the outer aspect of the upper arm; the dosage is the same for all patients.

Nursing Considerations
- Do not administer to patients with a history of anaphylactic hypersensitivity to neomycin (contained in injection), to patients with immune deficiency conditions (immunosuppressive therapy with corticosteroids, antineoplastics; neoplasms; immunodeficiency states), to patients receiving immune serum globulin.
- Do not administer to pregnant women, **Pregnancy Category C;** advise patients to avoid pregnancy for 3 mo following vaccination. If measles exposure occurs during pregnancy, provide passive immunity with immune serum globulin.
- Use caution if administering to children with history of febrile convulsions, cerebral injury, or other conditions in which stress due to fever should be avoided.
- Use caution if administering to patient with a history of sensitivity to eggs, chicken, chicken feathers.
- Do not administer within one mo of immunization with other *live virus vaccines;* may be administered concurrently with *monovalent or trivalent polio vaccine, rubella vaccine, mumps vaccine.*
- Do not administer for at least 3 mo following blood or plasma transfusions or administration of serum immune globulin.
- Monitor for possible depression of *tuberculin skin sensitivity;* administer the test before or simultaneously with the vaccine.
- Administer with a sterile syringe free of preservatives, antiseptics, and detergents for each injection (these may inactivate the live virus vaccine); use a 23 gauge, ⅝" needle.
- Refrigerate unreconstituted vial; protect from exposure to light. Use only the diluent supplied with the vaccine and reconstitute just before using; discard reconstituted vaccine if not used within 8 h.
- Have epinephrine 1:1000 immediately available at time of injection in case of anaphylactic reaction.
- Provide comfort measures or teach patient or parent to provide comfort measures to help patient to cope with the discomforts of drug therapy—analgesics, antipyretics, warm soaks to injection site, etc.
- Provide patient or parent with a written record of immunization.

▢ measles, mumps, rubella vaccine, live

MMR-II

Therapeutic Actions
Attenuated measles, mumps, and rubella viruses produce a modified infection and stimulate an active immune reaction with antibodies to these virus.

Indications
Immunization against measles, mumps, rubella in children >15 mo and adults.

Adverse Effects
Moderate fever, rash; high fever—less common; febrile convulsions, **Guillain-Barré syndrome, ocular palsies**—less common; burning or stinging wheal or flare at injection site.

Adverse effects in *Italics* are most common; those in **Bold** are life-threatening.

Dosage
0.5 ml reconstituted vaccine SC into the outer aspect of the upper arm; the dosage is the same for all patients. Booster dose is recommended on entry into school and again at entry into junior high school.

Nursing Considerations
- Do not administer to patients with a history of anaphylactic hypersensitivity to neomycin (contained in injection), to patients with immune deficiency conditions (immunosuppressive therapy with corticosteroids, antineoplastics; neoplasms; immunodeficiency states), to patients receiving immune serum globulin.
- Do not administer to pregnant women, **Pregnancy Category C;** advice patients to avoid pregnancy for 3 mo following vaccination. If measles exposure occurs during pregnancy, provide passive immunity with immune serum globulin.
- Use caution if administering to children with history of febrile convulsions, cerebral injury, or other conditions in which stress due to fever should be avoided.
- Use caution if administering to patient with a history of sensitivity to eggs, chicken, chicken feathers.
- Do not administer within one mo of immunization with other *live virus vaccines;* may be administered concurrently with *monovalent or trivalent polio vaccine, rubella vaccine, mumps vaccine.*
- Do not administer for at least 3 mo following blood or plasma transfusions or administration of serum immune globulin.
- Monitor for possible depression of *tuberculin skin sensitivity;* administer the test before or simultaneously with the vaccine.
- Administer with a sterile syringe free of preservatives, antiseptics, and detergents for each injection (these may inactivate the live virus vaccine); use a 25-gauge, ⅝″ needle.
- Refrigerate unreconstituted vial; protect from exposure to light. Use only the diluent supplied with the vaccine and reconstitute just before using; discard reconstituted vaccine if not used within 8 h.
- Have epinephrine 1:1000 immediately available at time of injection in case of anaphylactic reaction.
- Provide comfort measures or teach patient or parent to provide comfort measures to help patient to cope with the discomforts of drug therapy—analgesics, antipyretics, warm soaks to injection site, etc.
- Provide patient or parent with a written record of immunization.
- MMR is the vaccination of choice for routine vaccinations. Other combinations that are available—rubella and mumps vaccine (*Biavax II*), and measles and rubella (*MR Vax-II*)—are used for specific situations.

☐ mumps virus vaccine, live

Mumpsvax

Therapeutic Actions
Viral antigen stimulates active immunity through production of antibodies to the mumps virus.

Indications
Immunization against mumps in children >12 mo and adults. (Trivalent MMR vaccine is the drug of choice for routine vaccinations.)

Adverse Effects
Fever; parotitis, orchitis; purpura and allergic reactions such as wheal and flare at injection site; febrile seizures, unilateral nerve deafness, encephalitis—rare; anaphylactic reactions.

Dosage
Inject total volume (0.5 ml) of reconstituted vaccine SC into the outer aspect of the upper arm; each dose contains not less than 5000 $TCID_{50}$ (Tissue Culture Infectious Doses) of mumps virus vaccine (vaccine is available only in single dose vials of diluent).

Nursing Considerations
- Do not administer to patients with history of hypersensitivity to neomycin (each single dose vial of vaccine contains 25 mcg neomycin); immune deficiency conditions; **Pregnancy Category C**—advise patient to avoid pregnancy for 3 mo after vaccination.
- Use caution if administering to patient with history of allergy to eggs, chicken, chicken feathers.
- Delay administration in the presence of active infection.
- Do not administer within one month of immunization with other *live virus vaccines* except may be administered concurrently with *live monovalent or trivalent polio vaccine, live rubella vaccine, live measles vaccine.*
- Do not administer for at least 3 mo following blood or plasma transfusions or administration of serum immune globulin.
- Monitor for possible depression of *tuberculin skin sensitivity;* administer the test before or simultaneously with the vaccine.
- Administer with a sterile syringe free of preservatives, antiseptics, and detergents for each injection (these may inactivate the live virus vaccine); use a 25 gauge, ⅝″ needle.
- Refrigerate unreconstituted vial; protect from exposure to light. Use only the diluent supplied with the vaccine and reconstitute just before using; discard reconstituted vaccine if not used within 8 h.
- Have epinephrine 1:1000 immediately available at time of injection in case of anaphylactic reaction.
- Provide comfort measures or teach patient or parent to provide comfort measures to help patient to cope with the discomforts of drug therapy—analgesics, antipyretics, warm soaks to injection site, etc.
- Provide patient or parent with a written record of vaccination.

pneumococcal vaccine, polyvalent

Pneumovax 23, Pnu-Imune 23

Therapeutic Actions
Polysaccharide capsules of the 23 most prevalent or invasive pneumoccocal types stimulate active immunity through antipneumococcal antibody production against the capsule types contained in the vaccine.

Indications
- Immunization against pneumococcal pneumonia and bacteremia caused by the types of pneumococci included in the vaccine—specifically in children over 2 y and adults with chronic illnesses or who are immunocompromised and at increased risk for pneumococcal infections.
- Prophylaxis in children ≥2 y with asymptomatic or symptomatic HIV infections.
- Prevention of pneumococcal otitis media in children >2 y.
- Prophylaxis in community groups at high risk for pneumococcal infections—institutionalized persons, groups in an area of outbreak, patients at high risk of influenza complications including pneumococcal infection.

Adverse Effects
Erythema, induration, soreness at injection site; fever, myalgia; acute febrile reactions, rash, arthralgia—less common; paresthesias, acute radiculoneuropathy—rare; anaphylactic reaction.

Dosage
One 0.5 ml dose SC or IM. Not recommended for children <2 y.

Nursing Considerations
- Do not administer to patients with hypersensitivity to any component of the vaccine or with previous immunization with any polyvalent pneumococcal vaccine.
- Do not administer less than 10 days prior to or during treatment for Hodgkin's disease.
- Use caution if administering to patients who are pregnant—**Pregnancy Category C,** safety not established; or patients who are nursing—safety not established.
- Use caution if administering to patients with cardiac, pulmonary disorders—systemic reaction could pose a significant risk.
- May be administered concomitantly with influenza virus vaccine.
- Administer SC or IM only, preferably in the deltoid muscle or lateral mid-thigh; do not give IV.
- Refrigerate vials. Use directly as supplied, do not dilute (reconstitution is not necessary).
- Have epinephrine 1:1000 immediately available at time of injection in case of anaphylactic reaction.
- Provide or teach patient to provide appropriate comfort measures—analgesics, antipyretics, warm soaks to injection site—to help patient to cope with effects of the drug therapy.
- Provide patient with written record of immunization and caution patient not to have another polyvalent pneumococcal vaccine injection.

❒ poliovirus vaccine, live, oral, trivalent (OPV, TOPV; Sabin)

Orimune

Therapeutic Actions
Live, attenuated virus stimulates active immunity by simulating the natural infection without producing symptoms of the disease.

Indications
Prevention of poliomyelitis caused by Poliovirus Types 1, 2, and 3—routine immunization of infants and children through the age of 18 y.

Adverse Effects
Paralytic diseases in vaccine recipients and their close contacts (risk extremely small).

Dosage
- Infants: 0.5 ml PO at 2 mo, 4 mo, and 18 mo; an optional dose may be given at 6 mo in areas where polio is endemic. A booster dose is recommended at time of entry into elementary school.
- Older children through 18 yrs: 2 doses of 0.5 ml PO 8 wk apart and a third dose 6–12 mo later.
- Adults: Not usually needed in adults in this country; if unimmunized adult is exposed, is traveling to a high risk area, or is a household contact of children receiving TOPV, IPV (inactivated polio virus vaccine; Salk vaccine) is recommended or immunization using the same schedule as older children.

Nursing Considerations

- Do not administer to patients with known hypersensitivity to streptomycin or neomycin (each dose contains <25 mcg of each).
- Defer administration in the presence of persistent vomiting or diarrhea and in patients with acute illness or any advanced debilitating condition.
- Do not administer to any patient with immune deficiency conditions; do not administer shortly after immune serum globulin unless absolutely necessary because of travel or exposure; if given with or shortly after ISG, dose should be repeated after 3 mo.
- Use caution if administering to pregnant patients, **Pregnancy Category C,** safety not established, use only if clearly needed and benefits outweigh unknown effects on the fetus; if immediate protection is needed, TOPV is the recommended therapy.
- Do not administer parenterally; administer directly PO or mix with distilled water, tap water free of chlorine, simple syrup or milk; alternately, it may be adsorbed on bread, cake, or cube sugar.
- Store vaccine frozen or refrigerated; thaw before use; vaccine may go through 10 freeze-thaw cycles if temperature does not exceed 46°F and cumulative thaw does not exceed 24h; if it does, vaccine must be refrigerated and used within 30 days.
- Caution unimmunized adults or adults whose immunological status is not known about the risk of paralytic diseases and polio when they are household contacts of children receiving TOPV; risk can be minimized by giving them 3 doses of IPV a month apart before the children receive TOPV.
- Provide patient or parent with a written record of the vaccination and information on when additional doses are needed.

☐ poliovirus vaccine, inactivated (IPV, Salk)

IPOL, Poliovax

Therapeutic Actions
Inactivated, attenuated sterile suspension of three types of polio virus used to produce antibody response against poliomyelitis infection.

Indications
Prevention of poliomyelitis caused by Poliovirus Types 1, 2, and 3 in adults and children who refuse TOPV or in whom TOPV is contraindicated.

Adverse Effects
Paralytic diseases in vaccine recipients and their close contacts (risk extremely small).

Dosage
- Children: 0.5 ml SC at 2 mo, 4 mo, and 18 mo. A booster dose is needed at time of entry into elementary school.
- Adults: Not usually needed in adults in this country; if unimmunized adult is exposed, is traveling to a high risk area, or is a household contact of children receiving TOPV, IPV (inactivated polio virus vaccine; Salk vaccine) immunization is recommended. 0.5 ml SC—two doses given at 1–2 mo interval and a third dose given 6–12 mo later. Previously vaccinated adults at risk for exposure should receive a 0.5 ml dose of this drug or TOPV.

Nursing Considerations
- Do not administer to patients with known hypersensitivity to streptomycin or neomycin (each dose contains <25 mcg of each).

Appendix A ■ 1175

- Defer administration in the presence of persistent vomiting or diarrhea and in patients with acute illness or any advanced debilitating condition.
- Do not administer to any patient with immune deficiency conditions; do not administer shortly after immune serum globulin unless necessary because of travel or exposure; if given with or shortly after ISG, dose should be repeated after 3 mo.
- Use caution if administering to pregnant patients, **Pregnancy Category C,** safety not established, use only if clearly needed and benefits outweigh potential unknown effects on the fetus; if immediate protection is needed, TOPV is the recommended therapy.
- Refrigerate vaccine. Do not freeze.
- Provide patient or parent with a written record of the vaccination and information on when additional doses are needed.

☐ RH$_o$ (D) immune globulin

Gamulin Rh, HypRho-D, Rhesonativ, RhoGAM

☐ RH$_o$ (D) immune globulin micro-dose

HypRho-D Mini-Dose, MICRhoGAM, Mini-Gamulin Rh

Therapeutic Actions
Suppresses the immune response of nonsensitized Rh$_o$-negative individuals who receive Rh$_o$-positive blood as the result of a fetomaternal hemorrhage or a transfusion accident; each vial of RH$_o$-immune globulin completely suppresses immunity to 15 ml of Rh-positive packed RBCs (about 30 ml whole blood); each vial RH$_o$ immune globulin micro-dose suppresses immunity to 2.5 ml Rh-positive packed RBCs.

Indications
- Prevention of sensitization to the Rh$_o$ factor.
- To prevent hemolytic disease of the newborn (erythroblastosis fetalis) in a subsequent pregnancy—mother must be Rh$_o$ negative, mother must not be previously sensitized to Rh$_o$ factor, infant must be Rh$_o$ positive and direct antiglobulin negative—used at full term delivery, for incomplete pregnancy, for antepartum prophylaxis in case of abortion or ectopic pregnancy.
- To prevent Rh$_o$ sensitization in Rh$_o$-negative patients accidentally transfused with Rh$_o$-positive blood.

Adverse Effects
Pain and soreness at injection site.

Dosage
- Postpartum prophylaxis: 1 vial, IM within 72 h of delivery.
- Antepartum prophylaxis: 1 vial, IM at 28 wk gestation and one vial within 72 h after an Rh-incompatible delivery to prevent Rh isoimmunization during pregnancy.
- Following amniocentesis, miscarriage, abortion, ectopic pregnancy at or beyond 13 wk gestation: 1 vial, IM.
- Transfusion accidents: Multiply the volume in ml of Rh-positive whole blood administered by the hematocrit of the donor unit and divide this volume (in ml) by 15 to obtain the number of vials to be administered. If results of calculation are a fraction, administer the next whole number of vials.

- Spontaneous abortion or induced abortion or termination of ectopic pregnancy up to and including 12 wk gestation (unless the father is Rh negative): 1 vial micro-dose IM given as soon as possible after termination of pregnancy.

Nursing Considerations
- Rh$_o$ globulin is not needed in Rh$_o$-negative mothers if the father can be determined to be Rh$_o$ negative.
- Do not administer to the Rh$_o$-positive postpartum infant, to a Rh$_o$-positive individual, to a Rh$_o$-negative individual previously sensitized to the Rh$_o$ antigen (if it is not known if a woman is Rh$_o$ sensitized, administer the Rh$_o$ globulin).
- Before administration, determine the infant's blood type and arrange for a direct antiglobulin test using umbilical cord, venous, or capillary blood; confirm that the mother is Rh$_o$ negative.
- Do not administer IV; administer IM within 72 h after Rh$_o$-incompatible delivery, miscarriage, abortion or transfusion.
- Prepare one vial dose by withdrawing entire contents of vial; inject entire contents IM.
- Prepare two or more vial dose using 5–10 ml syringes—withdraw contents from the vials to be administered at one time and inject IM; contents of the total number of vials may be injected as a divided dose at different injection sites at the same time, or the total dosage may be divided and injected at intervals, provided the total dose is administered with 72 h postpartum or after a transfusion accident.
- Refrigerate vials; do not freeze.
- Provide appropriate comfort measures if injection sites are painful.
- Reassure patient and explain what has been given and why; the patient will need to know what was given in the event of future pregnancies.

rubella virus vaccine, live

Meruvax II

Therapeutic Actions
Live virus stimulates active immunity through development of antibodies against the rubella virus.

Indications
- Immunization against rubella—children 12 mo of age to puberty, adolescent and adult males, nonpregnant adolescent and adult females, rubella-susceptible women in the postpartum period, leukemia patients in remission whose chemotherapy has been terminated for at least 3 mo, susceptible persons traveling abroad.
- Revaccination of children vaccinated when <12 mo.

Adverse Effects
Burning, stinging at injection site; regional lymphadenopathy, urticaria, rash, malaise, sore throat, fever, headache, polyneuritis—symptoms similar to natural rubella; arthritis, arthralgia—often 2–4 wk after receiving the vaccine.

Dosage
Inject total volume of reconstituted vaccine SC, into the outer aspect of the upper arm; each dose contains not less than 1000 TCID$_{50}$ of rubella.

Nursing Considerations
- Do not administer to patients with a history of anaphylactic hypersensitivity to neomycin (each dose contains 25 mcg neomycin), to patients with immune deficiency conditions, to patients receiving immune serum globulin or blood transfusions.

- Do not administer to pregnant women, **Pregnancy Category C;** advise patients to avoid pregnancy for 3 mo following vaccination.
- Defer administration in the presence of acute respiratory or other active infections; susceptible children with mild illnesses may be vaccinated.
- Do not administer within one mo of immunization with other *live virus vaccines,* except that rubella vaccine may be administered concurrently with *live monovalent or trivalent polio vaccine live measles virus vaccine, live mumps vaccine.*
- Do not administer for at least 3 mo following blood or plasma transfusions or administration of serum immune globulin.
- Monitor for possible depression of *tuberculin skin sensitivity;* administer the test before or simultaneously with the vaccine.
- Refrigerate vials and protect from light. Reconstitute using only the diluent supplied with the vial, use as soon as possible after reconstitution; discard reconstituted vaccine if not used within 8 h.
- Provide or instruct patient to provide appropriate comfort measures to help patient to cope with the adverse effects of the drug—analgesics, antipyretics, fluids, rest, etc.
- Provide patient or parent with a written record of immunization, inform that revaccination is not necessary.

Other Biologicals

For other biologicals, please see the table starting on p.1178.

Chemotherapeutic Regimens

Combinations of therapeutic agents are preferable to single agents in the management of many diseases, leading to increased rates and duration of remissions. Common combinations are based on drug action, cell site specificity, responsiveness, and toxic effects. (see table starting on p.1181)

Commonly Used Fixed-Combination Drugs: Dosages

Analgesics

❑ **acetaminophen with codeine**

CIII Controlled Substance
Tylenol with Codeine

Tablets No. 1: 7.5 mg codeine, 300 mg acetaminophen
Tablets No. 2: 15 mg codeine, 300 mg acetaminophen
Tablets No. 3: 30 mg codeine, 300 mg acetaminophen

(text continues on page 1191)

Other Biologicals

Name	Brand Names	Indications	Dosage	Special Considerations
Immunoglobulins				
cytomegalovirus immunglobulin	*Cytomegalovirus Immune Globulin Intravenous*	Attenuation of CMV associated with kidney transplantation.	150 mg/kg within 72 h; 100 mg/kg at 2, 4, 6, and 8 wk post-transplant; 50 mg/kg at 12 and 16 wks	Given IV. Given to seronegative recipient of seropositive kidney.
lymphocyte, immune globulin, antithymocyte globulin	*Atgam*	Management of allograft rejection in renal transplants; treatment of aplastic anemia.	10–30 mg/kg/day IV adult transplant; 5–25 mg/kg/day IV pediatric transplant. 10–20 mg/kg/day IV for 8–14 days for aplastic anemia.	Possibly useful for other transplants; refrigerate, stable for up to 12 h after reconstitution.
rabies immune globulin	*Hyperab Imogam*	Passive protection against rabies in nonimmunized patients with exposure to rabies.	20 IU/kg IM	Refrigerate vial. Infuse wound area if possible. Give in conjunction with rabies vaccine.
tetanus immune globulin	*Hyper-tet*	Passive immuniz. against tetanus, useful at time of injury.	250 units IM	Do not give IV. Arrange proper medical care of wound. Reduce pediatric dosage based on weight.
varicella-zoster immune globulin	*Varicella-Zoster Immune Globulin*	Passive immunity for immunosuppressed patients with significant exposure to varicella.	125 units/10 kg IM to a max. of 625 units	Administer within 96 h of exposure to chicken pox. Not for use in nonimmunosuppressed individuals.
Antitoxins and antivenins				
diphtheria antitoxin		Prevention or treatment of diphtheria.	20,000–120,000 units IM or by slow IV infusion	Warm before use. Give immediately at first sign of symptoms.
tetanus antitoxin		Prophylactic use in patients who have untended wound for 24 h; treatment of active tetanus.	1500–5000 units IM or SC. Treatment of active tetanus–use 50,000–100,000 units partly IV and rest IM	Perform sensitivity test to equine products. Use only if immune globulin is unavailable.

Appendix A ■ 1179

antivenin (crotalidae) polyvalent	Neutralize the venom of pit vipers; inc. rattlesnakes, copperheads, etc.	20–40 ml IV; up to 100–150 ml IV in severe cases	Removal of venom should be done at once; antivenin to rare breeds of snake may be available from the CDC.
antivenin (micrurus fulvius)	Neutralize the venom of coral snakes in the US	30–50 ml by slow IV injection	Flush with IV fluids after antivenin has been infused. May require up to 100 ml.
Black Widow spider species antivenin	Treatment of symptoms of Black Widow spider bites.	2.5 ml IM; may be given IV in 10–50 ml saline over 15 min	Assure supportive therapy and use of muscle relaxants.
Bacterial vaccines			
BCG *TICE BCG*	Exposure to TB of skin-test negative infants and children; treatment of groups with high rates or TB; travel to areas with high rates of endemic TB.	0.2–0.3 ml percutaneous	Refrigerate, protect from light; keep the vaccination site clean until reaction disappears.
meningococcal polysaccharide vaccine *Menomune-A/C/Y/W-135*	Prevention of meningitis in patients at risk in epidemic or highly endemic areas.	0.5 ml SC	Reconstitute with diluent provided.
cholera vaccine	Immunization against cholera for travelers to areas endemic or epidemic in cholera.	0.2–0.3 ml SC, IM with a booster of 0.5 ml at 10 y	Do not give within 3 wk of yellow fever vaccine.
plague vaccine	Immunization of persons at risk for exposure to plague.	3 doses IM–1 ml followed by 0.2 ml 4 wk later; and 0.2 ml 5 mo later	Use of vaccine increases chances of recovery in epidemic situations.

(continued)

Other Biologicals (Continued)

Name	Brand Names	Indications	Dosage	Special Considerations
Viral vaccines				
Japanese encephalitis vaccine	*JE-VAX*	Active immunization in persons >1 y who will reside or travel in areas where it is endemic or epidemic.	3 SC doses of 1 ml given at days 0, 7, and 30	Refrigerate vial; do not remove rubber stopper; do not travel within 10 days of vaccination.
rabies vaccine	*HDCV* *Imovax Rabies*	Preexposure rabies immunization for patients in high risk area; postexposure antirabies regimen in conjunction with rabies immunoglobulin.	Preexposure; 1 ml IM on days 0, 7, 21, and 28. Postexposure: 1 ml IM on days 0, 3, 7, 21, and 28	Refrigerate. If titers are low, booster may be needed.
yellow fever vaccine	*YF-Vax*	Immunization of travelers to endemic areas.	0.5 ml SC; booster dose suggested q10 yr	Caution with allergy to chicken or egg products.

Chemotherapeutic Regimens

Regimen	Use	Drugs Used
ABDIC	Hodgkin's disease	doxorubicin 45 mg/m^2 IV, day 1 bleomycin 5 mg/m^2 IV, days 1 and 5 dacarbazine 200 mg/m^2/d IV, days 1–5 CCNU 50 mg/m^2 PO day 1 prednisone 40 mg/m^2/d PO, days 1–5 Repeat at 4 wk intervals.
ABVD	Hodgkin's disease	doxorubicin 25 mg/m^2/d IV, days 1 and 14 bleomycin 10 units/m^2 IV, days 1 and 14 vinblastine at 6 mg/m^2/d IV, days 1 and 14 dacarbazine 375 mg/m^2/d IV, days 1 and 14 Repeat twice monthly until remission and continue for 2 more sessions.
ACe	Breast cancer metastatic or recurrent disease	cyclophosphamide 200 mg/mw/d PO, days 3–6 doxorubicin 40 mg/m^2 IV, day 1 Repeat every 21 or 28 d.
A-COPP	Hodgkin's disease (induction in children)	doxorubicin 60 mg/m^2 IV, day 1 cyclophosphamide 300 mg/m^2/d IV, days 14 and 20 vincristine 1.5 mg/m^2 IV, days 14 and 20 procarbazine 100 mg/m^2/d PO, days 14–28 prednisone 40 mg/m^2/d PO, days 1–27, 1st & 4th cycles prednisone 40 mg/m^2/d PO, days 14–27, 2nd, 3rd, 5th, 6th cycles Repeat every 42 days for 6 cycles.
Adria + BCNU	Multiple myeloma	doxorubicin 30 mg/m^2 IV, day 1 carmustine 30 mg/m^2 IV, day 1 Repeat every 21 or 28 d.

(continued)

Chemotherapeutic Regimens (Continued)

Regimen	Use	Drugs Used
Ara-C + ADR	Acute myelocytic leukemia (induction)	cytarabine 100 mg/m^2/d by continuous 24h infusion for 7–10 d prednisone 40 mg/m^2/d PO doxorubicin 30 mg/m^2/d IV for 3 d
Ara-C + DNR + PRED + MP	Acute myelocytic leukemia (children only)	daunorubicin 25 mg/m^2 IV for 1 d cytarabine 80 mg/m^2/d IV for 3 d prednisone 40 mg/m^2/d PO mercaptopurine 100 mg/m^2/d PO. Repeat weekly until remission, then repeat every month or 28 d
Ara-C + 6-TG	Acute myelocytic leukemia	cytarabine 100 mg/m^2/12 h IV for 10d thioguanine 100 mg/m^2/12 h PO for 10d Repeat q30d until remission. cytarabine 100 mg/m^2/12h IV for 5d thioguanine 100 mg/m^2/12h PO for 5d Repeat every month as maintenance.
B-CAVe	Hodgkin's disease (resistant to MOPP)	bleomycin 5 mg/m^2 IV days 1, 28, 35 CCNU 100 mg/m^2 PO, day 1 doxorubicin 60 mg/m^2 IV, day 1 vinblastine 5 mg/m^2 IV, day 1 Continue until patient no longer tolerates dosage
BCVPP	Hodgkin's disease induction	carmustine 100 mg/m^2 IV, day 1 cyclophosphamide 600 mg/m^2 IV, day 1 vinblastine 5 mg/m^2 IV, day 1 procarbazine 50 mg/m^2/d PO, day 1 procarbazine 100 mg/m^2/d PO, days 2–10 prednisone 60 mg/m^2/d PO, days 1–10 Repeat every 28 d for 6 cycles.

CAF	Breast cancer, metastatic disease	cyclophosphamide 100 mg/m²/d PO, day 1–14 doxorubicin 30 mg/m²/d IV, days 1 and 8 fluorouracil 500 mg/m²/d IV, days 1 and 8 Repeat every 4 wk, until a total cumulative mg/m² doxorubicin is given, then substitute methotrexate 40 mg/m² IV and increase flu mg/m² IV.
CAMP	Lung cancer, non-oat cell carcinomas	cyclophosphamide 300 mg/m²/d IV, days 1 and 8 doxorubicin 20 mg/m²/d IV, days 1 and 8 methotrexate 15 mg/m²/d IV, days 1 and 8 procarbazine 100 mg/m²/d PO, days 1–10 Repeat every 28 d.
CAP	Non-small cell carcinoma of the lung	cyclophosphamide 400 mg/m² IV, day 1 doxorubicin 40 mg/m² IV, day 1 cisplatin 40 mg/m² IV, day 1 Repeat every 4 wk.
CAV	Small cell lung cancer (induction)	cyclophosphamide 750 mg/m² IV q3wk doxorubicin 50 mg/m²/IV q3wk vincristine 2 mg IV q3wk
CAVe	Hodgkin's disease (resistant to MOPP)	lomustine 100 mg/m² PO, day 1 doxorubicin 50 mg/m² IV, day 1 vinblastine 5 mg/m² IV, day 1 Repeat every 6 wk for 9 cycles.
CHL + PRED	Chronic lymphocytic leukemia	chlorambucil 0.4 mg/kg/d PO, 1 day every other week prednisone 100 mg/d PO for 2d, every other wk Adjust dosage based on blood counts.
CHOP	Non-Hodgkin's lymphoma or lymphomas with unfavorable histology	cyclophosphamide 750 mg/m²/d IV, day 1 doxorubicin 50 mg/m² IV, day 1 vincristine 1.4 mg/m² IV, day 1

(continued)

Chemotherapeutic Regimens (Continued)

Regimen	Use	Drugs Used
CHOR	Lung cancer, small cell carcinoma	prednisone 60 mg/day PO, days 1–5 Repeat every 21–28 days for 6 cycles. cyclophosphamide 750 mg/m^2/d IV, days 1 and 22 doxorubicin 50 mg/m^2/d IV, days 1 and 22 vincristine 1 mg IV days 1, 8, 15, and 22 Radiation total dose 3000 rad, 10 daily fractions over a 2-wk period beginning with day 36
CISCA	Urinary tract, metastatic disease	cyclophosphamide 650 mg/m^2 IV, day 1 doxorubicin 50 mg/m^2 IV, day 1 cisplatin 100 mg/m^2 IV infusion over, 2h, day 2 Repeat every 21d. Discontinue doxrubicin when total dose is 450 mg/m^2, increase cyclophosphamide to 100 mg/m^2 IV
CISCA/VBiv	Germ cell tumors, advanced	cyclophosphamide 1 g/m^2 IV, days 1 and 2 doxorubicin 80–90 mg/m^2 IV, days 1 and 2 cisplatin 100–120 mg/m^2 IV, day 3 alternating with vinblastine 3 mg/m^2 IV continuous infusion bleomycin 30 mg/d IV continuous infusion
CMC-High dose	Lung cancer, small cell carcinoma	cyclophosphamide 1000 mg/m^2/d IV, days 1 and 29 methotrexate 15 mg/m^2/d IV twice weekly for 6 wk lomustine 100 mg/m^2 PO, day 1
CMF	Breast cancer, metastatic or recurrent disease	cyclophosphamide 100 mg/m^2/d PO, days 1–14 methotrexate 40–60 mg/m^2/d IV, days 1 and 8 fluorouracil 600 mg/m^2/day IV, days 1 and 8 Repeat every 28 d.
CMFP	Breast cancer, metastatic disease	cyclophosphamide 100 mg/m^2/d PO, days 1–14 methotrexate 60 mg/m^2/d IV, days 1 and 8

		fluorouracil 700 mg/m²/d IV, days 1 and 8 prednisone 40 mg/m²/d PO, days 1–14 Repeat every 28 d.
CMFVP (Cooper's regimen)	Breast cancer, metastatic or recurrent disease	cyclophosphamide 2 mg/kg/d PO methotrexate 0.75 mg/kg IV weekly fluorouracil 12 mg/kg IV weekly vincristine 0.025 mg/kg IV weekly prednisone 0.75 mg/kg PO, days 1–21 then taper off
COMLA	Non-Hodgkin's lymphoma	cyclophosphamide 1.5 mg/m² IV, day 1 vincristine 1.4 mg/m² IV, days 1, 8, 15 cytarabine 300 mg/m² IV, days 22, 29, 36, 43, 50, 57, 64, and 71 methotrexate 120 mg/m² IV, days 22, 29, 36, 45, 50, 57, 64, and 71 leucovorin 25 mg/m² PO q6h ×4 beginning 24h after methotrexate
COP	Non-Hodgkin's lymphoma with favorable histology	cyclophosphamide 800–1000 mg/m² IV, day 1 vincristine 1.4 mg/m² IV, day 1 prednisone 60 mg/m²/d PO, days 1–5 Repeat every 21 d for 6 cycles.
COP-BLAM	Non-Hodgkin's lymphoma advanced	cyclophosphamide 400 mg/m² IV, day 1 vincristine 1 mg/m² IV, day 1 prednisone 40 mg/m²/d PO, days 1–10 bleomycin 15 mg/IV, day 14 doxorubicin 40 mg/m² IV, day 1 procarbazine 100 mg/m² PO, days 1–10
COPP or "C"MOPP	Non-Hodgkin's lymphoma, lymphomas with unfavorable histology, Hodgkin's disease	cyclophosphamide 650 mg/m²/d IV, days 1 and 8 vincristine 1.4 mg/m²/d IV, days 1 and 8 procarbazine 100 mg/m²/d PO, days 1–14 prednisone 40 mg/m²/d PO, days 1–14 Repeat every 28 d for 6 cycles.

(continued)

Chemotherapeutic Regimens *(Continued)*

Regimen	Use	Drugs Used
CVP	Non-Hodgkin's lymphoma, lymphomas with favorable histology	cyclophosphamide 400 mg/m^2/d PO, days 2–6 vincristine 1.4 mg/m^2 IV, day 1 prednisone 100 mg/m^2/d PO, days 2–6 Repeat every 21 d for 6 cycles.
CY-VA-DIC	Soft tissue sarcomas, adult sarcomas	cyclophosphamide 500 mg/m^2 IV, day 1 vincristine 1.4 mg/m^2/d IV, days 1 and 5 doxorubicin 50 mg/m^2 IV, day 1 dacarbazine 250 mg/m^2 IV, days 1–5 Repeat every 21 d.
FAC	Breast cancer, metastatic disease	fluorouracil 500 mg/m^2 IV, days 1 and 8 doxorubicin 50 mg/m^2 IV, day 1 cyclophosphamide 500 mg/m^2 IV, day 1 Repeat every 3 wk.
FAM	Lung cancer, non-oat cell carcinomas	fluorouracil 600 mg/m^2/d IV, days 1, 8, 28, 36 doxorubicin 30 mg/m^2 IV, days 1 and 28 mitomycin 10 mg/m^2 IV, day 1 Repeat every 8 wk.
	Gastric carcinoma advanced disease	fluorouracil 600 mg/m^2/d IV, days 1, 8, 29, 36 doxorubicin 30 mg/m^2/d IV, days 1 and 29 mitomycin 10 mg/m^2 IV, day 1 Repeat every 8 wk.
	Pancreatic carcinoma advanced disease	fluorouracil 600 mg/m^2/wk IV, weeks 1, 2, 5, 6, and 9 doxorubicin 30 mg/m^2/wk IV, weeks 1, 5, and 9 mitomycin 10 mg/m^2/wk IV, weeks 1 and 9
FOMi	Non-small cell carcinoma carcinoma of the lung	5FU 300 mg/m^2/d IV, days 1–4 vincristine 2 mg IV, day 1

M-2 Protocol	Multiple myeloma	vincristine 0.03 mg/kg IV, day 1 carmustine 0.5 mg/kg IV, day 1 cyclophosphamide 10 mg/kg IV, day 1 melphalan 0.25 mg/kg/d PO, days 1–4 prednisone 1.0 mg/kg/d PO, days 1–7 then taper to day 21. Continue throughout remission period.
MAC	Ovarian carcinoma, advanced	mitomycin C7 mg/m^2 IV doxorubicin 45 mg/m^2 IV cyclophosphamide 450 mg/m^2 IV Repeat at 3 wk intervals.
MACC	Lung cancer, non-oat cell carcinoma	mitomycin C 40 mg/m^2 IV, day 1 doxorubicin 40 mg/m^2 PO, day 1 cyclophosphamide 400 mg/m^2 IV, day 1 lomustine 30 mg/m^2 PO, day 1 Repeat every 21 d.
MOPP	Hodgkin's disease, induction	mechlorethamine 6 mg/m^2/d IV, days 1 and 8 vincristine 2 mg/m^2/d IV, days 1 and 8 procarbazine 50 mg/m^2/d PO, day 1 procarbazine 100 mg/m^2/d PO, days 2–14 prednisone 40 mg/m^2/d PO, days 1–14 Repeat every 28 d for 6 cycles.
MOPP/ABVD	Hodgkin's disease, advanced	mechlorethamine 6 mg/m^2/d IV, days 1 and 8 vincristine 1.4 mg/m^2/d IV, days 1 and 8 procarbazine 100 mg/m^2/d PO, days 1–14 prednisone 40 mg/m^2/d PO, days 1–14 alternating every other month with:

(continued)

Chemotherapeutic Regimens (Continued)

Regimen	Use	Drugs Used
MOPP-LO BLEO	Hodgkin's disease, induction	doxorubicin 25 mg/m² IV, days 1 and 15 bleomycin 10 mg/m² IV, days 1 and 15 vinblastine 6 mg/m² IV, days 1 and 15 dacarbazine 375 mg/m² IV, days 1 and 15 mechlorethamine 6 mg/m²/d IV, days 1 and 8 vincristine 1.5 mg/m²/d IV, days 1 and 8 procarbazine 100 mg/m²/d PO, days 2–7 and 9–12 prednisone 40 mg/m²/d PO, days 2–7 and 9–12 bleomycin 2 units/m² IV, days 1 and 8 Repeat monthly for 6 cycles.
MPL + PRED (MP)	Multiple myeloma	melphalan 8 mg/m²/d PO, days 1–14 prednisone 75 mg/m²/d PO, days 1–7 Repeat every 28 d for 6 cycles.
MTX + MP	Acute lymphocytic leukemia	methotrexate 20 mg/m²/wk IV mercaptopurine 50 mg/m²/d PO Continue both until relapse or after 3 years of remission.
MTX + MP + CTX	Acute lymphocytic leukemia maintenance therapy	methotrexate 20 mg/m²/wk IV mercaptopurine 50 mg/m²/d PO cyclophosphamide 200 mg/m²/wk IV Continue until relapse or after 3 yr of remission.
M-VAC	Transitional cell carcinoma of the bladder	methotrexate 30 mg/m² IV, day 1 vinblastine 3 mg/m² IV, days 2, 15, 22 doxorubicin 30 mg/m² IV, days 2, 15, 22 cisplatin 70 mg/m² IV, day 2
POCC	Lung cancer, small cell carcinoma	procarbazine 100 mg/m²/d PO, days 1–14 vincristine 2 mg/d IV, days 1 and 8

PVB	Testicular carcinoma

cyclophosphamide 600 mg/m²/d IV, days 1 and 8
lomustine 60 mg/m² PO, day 1
Repeat every 28 d.

cisplatin 20 mg/m²/d IV, days 1–5 every 3 wk for 4 courses
vinblastine 0.2–0.4 mg/kg IV, day 1 every 3 wk for 4 courses
bleomycin 30 units IV day 1 weekly for 12 consecutive weeks

T-2 Protocol — Ewing's sarcoma

Cycle #1: Month 1:
dactinomycin 0.45 mg/m²/d IV, days 1–5
doxorubicin 20 mg/m²/d IV, days 20–22
Radiation days 1–21, then 2 wk rest. Month 2: doxorubicin 20 mg/m²/d IV, days 8–10
vincristine 1.5–2 mg/m² IV, day 24
cyclophosphamide 1200 mg/m² IV, day 24
Radiation days 8–24
Month 3: vincristine 1.5–2 mg/m²/d IV, days 3, 9, and 15
cyclophosphamide 1200 mg/m² IV, day 9
Cycle #2: Repeat Cycle #1 without radiation
Cycle #3: Month 1:
dactinomycin 0.45 mg/m²/d IV, days 1–5
doxorubicin 20 mg/m²/d IV, days 20–22
Month 2: vincristine 1.5–2 mg/m²/d IV, days 8, 15, 22, and 28
cyclophosphamide 1200 mg/m²/d IV, days 8 and 22
Cycle #4: Repeat cycle #3.

VAB-6 — Testicular carcinoma

Induction (q3–4 wk for 2 courses)
cyclophosphamide 600 mg/m² IV, day 1
dactinomycin 1 mg/m² IV, day 1
vinblastine 4 mg/m² IV, day 1
bleomycin 30 mg IV, day 1
bleomycin 20 mg/m²/d by continuous IV infusion over 24h, days 1–3

(continued)

Chemotherapeutic Regimens *(Continued)*

Regimen	Use	Drugs Used
VAC Pulse	Soft tissue sarcomas, rhabdomyosarcoma	cisplatin 120 mg/m² IV, day 4 Maintenance (q3wk for 12 mo) vinblastine 6 mg/m² IV dactinomycin 1 mg/m² IV vincristine 2 mg/m²/wk IV, weeks 1–12 dactinomycin 0.015 mg/kg/d IV for 5 days, week 1 and 13. Continue day courses q3mo for 5–6 courses (maximum daily dose 0.5 mg/d) cyclophosphamide 10 mg/kg/d IV or PO. Continue q6wk for 2 y
VAC Standard	Soft tissue sarcomas, rhabdomyosarcoma, undifferentiated sarcoma	vincristine 2 mg/m²/wk IV, weeks 1–12 dactinomycin 0.015 mg/kg/d IV for 5 days, for 5–6 courses. cyclophosphamide 2.5 mg/kg/d PO. Continue daily for 2 y.
VAD	Refractory multiple myeloma	vincristine 0.4 mg/d IV by continuous infusion doxorubicin 9 mg/m²/d IV by continuous infusion, days 1–4 dexamethasone 40 mg PO every morning for 4 days
VBP	Disseminated testicular cancer	vinblastine 0.2 mg/kg/d IV, days 1 and 2 q3wk for 5 courses cisplatin 20 mg/m²/d IV infusion over vinblastine, days 1–5 courses. bleomycin 30 units/wk IV 6h after vinblastine day of each week for 360 units
VP	Acute lymphocytic leukemia, induction	vincristine 2 mg/m²/wk IV, for 4–6 wk (maximum dose 2 mg) prednisone 60 mg/m²/d PO in divided dose. Taper weeks 5–7.
VP-L-Asparaginase	Acute lymphocytic leukemia, induction	vincristine 2 mg/m²/wk IV for 4–6 wk (maximum dose 2 mg) prednisone 60 mg/m²/d PO in divided doses for 4–6 L-asparaginase 10,000 units/m²/d IV for 14 days

Tablets No. 4: 60 mg codeine, 300 mg acetaminophen
   Usual adult dosage: 1–2 tablets q 4–6 h as needed for pain.

Fioricet with Codeine

Capsules: 30 mg codeine, 325 mg acetaminophen, 40 mg caffeine, 50 mg butabarbital
   Usual adult dosage: 1–2 capsules q4h, up to 6/day.

aspirin with codeine

CIII Controlled Substance
Empirin with Codeine

Tablets No. 2: 15 mg codeine, 325 mg aspirin
Tablets No. 3: 30 mg codeine, 325 mg aspirin
Tablets No. 4: 60 mg codeine, 325 mg aspirin
   Usual adult dosage: 1–2 tablets q 4–6 h as needed for pain.

Fiorinal with Codeine

Capsules: 30 mg codeine, 325 mg aspirin, 40 mg caffeine, 50 mg butabarbital
   Usual adult dosage: 1–2 capsules as needed for pain; up to 6/day

oxycodone with acetaminophen

CII Controlled Substance
Percocet

Tablets: 5 mg oxycodone, 325 mg acetaminophen
   Usual adult dosage: 1–2 tablets q 4–6 h as needed for pain.

oxycodone with aspirin

CII Controlled Substance
Percodan

Tablets: 4.5 mg oxycodone, 325 mg aspirin
   Usual adult dosage: 1–2 tablets q6h as needed for pain.

Antibacterials

Augmentin

Tablets
'250'—250 mg amoxicillin, 125 mg clavulanic acid

'500'—500 mg amoxicillin, 125 mg clavulanic acid
Powder for oral suspension
'125' powder—125 mg amoxicillin, 31.25 mg clavulanic acid
'250' powder—250 mg amoxicillin, 62.5 mg clavulanic acid
Chewable tablets
'125'—125 mg amoxicillin, 31.25 mg clavulanic acid
'250'—250 mg amoxicillin, 62.5 mg clavulanic acid

Usual adult dosage: 1 '250' to 1 '500' tablet q8h.

Usual pediatric dosage: <40 kg: 20–40 mg amoxicillin/kg/d in divided doses q8h (pediatric dosage is based on amoxicillin content).

Also see **amoxicillin;** clavulanic acid protects amoxicillin from breakdown by bacterial β-lactamase enzymes and is given only in combination with certain antibodies that are broken down by β-lactamase.

☐ carbapenem

Primaxin

Powder for injection
250 mg imipenem and 250 mg cilastatin
500 mg imipenem and 500 mg cilastatin

- Follow manufacturer's instructions for reconstituting and diluting the drug.
- Administer each 250–500 mg dose by IV infusion over 20–30 min; infuse each 1 g dose over 40–60 min.
- Dosage recommendations represent the amount of imipenem to be given. Initial dosage should be individualized on the basis of the type and severity of infection. Subsequent dosage is individualized on the basis of the severity of the patient's illness, the degree of susceptibility of the pathogen(s), the patient's age, weight, and creatinine clearance; dosage for adults with normal renal function ranges from 250 mg 1 g q 6–8 h. Dosage should not exceed 50 mg/kg/d or 4 g/d, whichever is less.
- Dosage for patients with **renal impairment:**

	Type of infection:	
CCr (ml/min)	Less severe	Life-threatening
30–70	500 mg q8h	500 mg q6h
20–30	500 mg q12h	500 mg q8h
5–20	250 mg q12h	500 mg q12h
or 0–5 with hemodialysis	250 mg q12h	500 mg q12h

- Imipenem is an antibiotic that inhibits cell wall synthesis in susceptible bacteria; cilastatin inhibits the renal enzyme that metabolizes imipenem; these drugs are commercially available only in the combined formulation.

☐ co-trimoxazole

TMP-SMZ; *Bactrim, Cotrim, Septra, Sulfamethoprim, Sulfatrim, Uroplus*

Tablets
80 mg trimethoprim (TMP) and 400 mg sulfamethoxazole (SMZ)
160 mg trimethoprim and 800 mg sulfamethoxazole

Oral suspension
40 mg trimethoprim and 200 mg sulfamethoxazole per 5 ml
IV infusion
84 mg trimethoprim and 400 mg sulfamethoxazole per 5 ml

Usual adult dosage
- Urinary tract infections, shigellosis and acute otitis media: 160 mg TMP/800 mg sulfamethoxazole, PO q12h; 8–10 mg/kg/d (based on TMP component) in 2–4 divided doses q6, 8, or 12h, IV. Treat for up to 14 days (UTIs) or for 5 days (shigellosis).
- Acute exacerbations of chronic bronchitis: 160 mg TMP/800 mg SMZ PO q12h for 14 days.
- *Pneumocystis carinii* pneumonitis: 20 mg/kg TMP and 100 mg/kg SMZ q24h PO in divided doses q6h; 15–20 mg/kg/d (based on TMP component) in 3–4 divided doses q6–8h, IV. Treat for 14 days.

Usual pediatric dose
- Urinary tract infections, shigellosis, acute otitis media: 8 mg/kg/d TMP and 40 mg/kg/d SMZ PO in 2 divided doses q12h; 8–10 mg/kg/d (based on TMP component) in 2–4 divided doses q6, 8, or 12h, IV. Treat for 10–14 days (UTIs and acute otitis media) or for 5 days (shigellosis).
- *Pneumocystis carinii* pneumonitis: 20 mg/kg TMP and 100 mg/kg SMZ q24h PO in divided doses q6h; 15–20 mg/kg/d (based on TMP component) in 3–4 divided doses q6–8h, IV. Treat for 14 days.

Impaired Renal Function

Creatinine clearance (ml/min)	Dosage
>30 ml/min	Use standard dosage.
15–30 ml/min	Use 1/2 standard dosage.
<15 ml/min	Not recommended.

- Administer IV over 60–90 min. Thoroughly flush IV line after each use, do not refrigerate. IV solution must be diluted before use—see manufacturer's instructions. Do *not* give IM.
- Also see **trimethoprim** and **sulfamethoxazole**.

Pediazole

Granules for oral suspension: erythromycin ethylsuccinate (equivalent of 200 mg erythromycin activity) and 600 mg sulfisoxazole per 5 ml when reconstituted according to manufacturer's directions.
- Usual dosage for acute otitis media: 50 mg/kg/d erythromycin and 150 mg/kg/d sulfisoxazole in divided doses qid for 10 days.
- Administer without regard to meals.
- Refrigerate after reconstitution; use within 14 days.
- Also see **erythromycin** and **sulfisoxazole**.

❏ **piperacillin sodium** and **tazobactam sodium**

Tazobactam is a beta-lactamase inhibitor used in combination with the broad-spectrum penicillin.
- Recommended for appendicitis, peritonitis, postpartum endometritis and PID, community acquired pneumonia, if agent is responsive in sensitivity testing.
- Usual daily adult dose: 12 mg/1.5g IV given as 3.375 g q6h.

- Reduced dosage required for renal impairment or dialysis.
- Administer by IV infusion over 30 min. Reconstitute with 5 ml of suitable diluent per 1g piperacillin. Discard after 24h.

See also **piperacillin.**

Timentin

Powder for injection
3.1 g vial—3 g ticarcillin, 0.1 g clavulanic acid
3.2 g vial—3 g ticarcillin, 0.2 g clavulanic acid

- Administer by IV infusion over 30 min.
- Dosage for 60 kg adults: 3.1 g (3 g ticarcillin and 0.1 g clavulanic acid) q4–6h. <60 kg adults: 200–300 mg ticarcillin/kg/d in divided doses q4–6h.
- Urinary tract infections: 3.2 g (3g ticarcillin and 0.2 g clavulanic acid) q8h.
- Pediatric dosage (children <12y): Not established.
- Geriatric or renal failure patients: Initial loading dose of 3.1 g, then as follows:

Creatinine clearance	Dosage
>60	3.1 g q4h
30–60	2 g q4h
10–30	2 g q8h
<10	2 g q12h
<10 with hepatic disease	3.1 g q12h
On hemodialysis	2 g q12h, supplemented with 3.1 g after each dialysis

- Continue treatment for 2 days after signs and symptoms of infection have disappeared. (Usual duration of therapy: 10–14 days).
- Also see **ticarcillin;** clavulanic acid protects ticarcillin from breakdown by bacterial β-lactamase enzymes and is given only in combination with certain antibiotics that are broken down by β-lactamase.

Unasyn

Available as 1 g sulbactam to every 2 g ampicillin.
- Usual adult dosage: 0.5–1 g sulbactam with 1–2 g ampicillin IM or IV q 6–8 h.
- Also see **ampicillin;** sulbactam inhibits many bacterial penicillinase enzymes, thus broadening the spectrum of ampicillin; sulbactam is also weakly antibacterial alone.

Antidepressants

Etrafon, Triavil

Tablets
2 mg perphenazine, 10 mg amitriptyline
2 mg perphenazine, 25 mg amitriptyline
4 mg perphenazine, 25 mg amitriptyline
4 mg perphenazine, 50 mg amitriptyline (*Triavil* only)

- Usual adult dosage: 2–4 mg perphenazine with 10–50 mg amitriptyline tid–qid. Reduce dosage after initial response.
- Also see **amitriptyline** and **perphenazine.**

Limbitrol

Tablets
5 mg chlordiazepoxide, 12.5 mg amitriptyline
10 mg chlordiazepoxide, 25 mg amitriptyline

- Usual adult dosage: 10 mg chlordiazepoxide with 25 mg amitriptyline tid–qid up to 6 times daily. 5 mg chlordiazepoxide with 12.5 mg amitriptyline tid–qid for patients who do not tolerate the higher doses. Reduce dosage after initial response.
- Also see **amitriptyline** and **chlordiazepoxide.**

Antidiarrheal drug

diphenoxylate HCl with atropine sulfate

CV Controlled Substance

Logen, Lomanate, Lomotil, Lonox

Tablets: 2.5 mg diphenoxylate HCl, 0.025 mg atropine sulfate
Liquid: 2.5 mg diphenoxylate HCl, 0.025 mg atropine sulfate/5 ml

- Individualized dosage; usual adult dosage; 5 mg qid.
- Pediatric initial dosage (use only liquid in children 2–12 y of age): 0.3 mg/kg daily in 4 divided doses.

Age (years)	Weight (kg)	Dose	Frequency
2–5	13–20	2 mg, 4 ml	3 times daily
5–8	20–27	2 mg, 4 ml	4 times daily
8–12	27–36	2 mg, 4 ml	5 times daily

- Reduce dosage as soon as initial control of symptoms is achieved. Maintenance dosage may be as low as $1/4$ of the initial dosage.
- Also see **atropine sulfate** and **meperidine;** diphenoxylate is chemically and pharmacologically related to meperidine, but lacks analgesic activity.

Antihypertensives

Capozide

Tablets
25 mg hydrochlorothiazide and 50 or 25 mg captopril
15 mg hydrochlorothiazide and 50 or 25 mg captopril

- Usual adult dosage: 1–2 tablet qd PO taken in the morning.
- Dosage should be titrated with the individual products, switching to this combination product when patient is stabilized on the dosage of each drug that is available in this combination.
- See also **hydrochlorothiazide, captopril.**

Combipres

Tablets: 15 mg chlorthalidone with 0.1, 0.2, or 0.3 mg clonidine HCl

- Usual adult dosage: 1–2 tablet qd PO taken in the morning.
- Dosage should be titrated with the individual products, switching to this combination product when patient is stabilized on the dosage of each drug that is available in this combination.
- See also **chlorthalidone, clonidine.**

Inderide

Tablets
50 mg hydrochlorothiazide with 160, 120, or 80 mg propranolol HCl
25 mg hydrochlorothiazide with 80 or 40 mg propranolol HCl

- Usual adult dosage: 1–2 tablet qd PO taken in the morning.
- Dosage should be titrated with the individual products, switching to this combination product when patient is stabilized on the dosage of each drug that is available in this combination.
- See also **hydrochlorothiazide, propranolol.**

Vaseretic

Tablets: 10 mg enalapril maleate and 25 mg hydrochlorothiazide

- Usual adult dosage: 1–2 tablet qd PO taken in the morning.
- Dosage should be titrated with the individual products, switching to this combination product when patient is stabilized on the dosage of each drug that is available in this combination.
- See also **enalapril maleate** and **hydrochlorothiazide.**

Ziac

Tablets: 2.5, 6.25 or 10 mg bisoprolol and 6.25 mg hydrochlorothiazide

- Usual adult dosage: 1 tablet/day PO taken in the morning.
- Dosage should be titrated within 1 wk, optimal antihypertensive effect may require 2–3 wk.
- See also **bisoprolol** and **hydrochlorothiazide**

Antimalarials

Aralen Phosphate with Primaquine Phosphate

Tablets: 500 mg chloroquine phosphate (300 mg base) and 79 mg primaquine phosphate (45 mg base)

- Usual adult dosage: start at least 1 day before entering the endemic area. Take 1 tablet weekly on the same day each wk, continuing for 8 wk after leaving endemic area.
- Pediatric dosage: prepare a suspension in chocolate syrup using one tablet (300 mg chloroquine base + 45 mg primaquine base) in 40 ml liquid; dosage is as follows:

Body Weight		Chloroquine	Primaquine	Dose
lb	kg	base (mg)	base (mg)	(ml)
10–15	4.5–6.8	20	3	2.5
16–25	7.3–11.4	40	6	5
26–35	11.8–15.9	60	9	7.5
36–45	16.5–20.5	80	12	10
46–55	20.9–25	100	15	12.5
56–100	25.4–45.4	150	22.5	1/2 tab
>100	>45.4	300	45	1 tab

- See also **chloroquine phosphate** and **primaquine phosphate**.

Fansidar

Tablets: 500 mg sulfadoxine and 25 mg pyrimethamine

- Usual adult dosage: Prophylaxis: 1 tablet, PO once/wk.
- Presumptive treatment: 3 tablets, PO as a single dose.

Prophylaxis	Presumptive Treatment
2–11 months: 1/8 tablet PO, once/wk	2–11 months: 1/4 tablet PO as a single dose
1–3 yrs: 1/4 tablet PO, once/wk	1–3 yrs: 1/2 tablet PO as a single dose
4–8 yrs: 1/2 tablet PO, once/wk	4–8 yrs: 1 tablet PO as a single dose
9–14 yrs: 3/4 tablet PO, once /wk	9–14 yrs: 2 tablets PO as a single dose
>14 yrs: 1 tablet/wk	>14 yrs: 3 tablets PO as a single dose

- Usual pediatric dosage:

Note: Fatalities have occurred in association with this drug, due to Stevens-Johnson syndrome and toxic epidermal necrolysis; drug should be discontinued at first sign of skin rash, depressed blood count, or active bacterial or fungal infection.

- See also **pyrimethamine**.

Antimigraine drugs

Cafergot

Tablets: 1 mg ergotamine tartrate, 100 mg caffeine
- Usual adult dosage: 2 tablets at first sign of attack. Follow with 1 tablet q1/2h, if needed. Maximum dose is 6 tablets/attack. Do not exceed 10 tablets/wk.

Suppositories: 2 mg ergotamine tartrate, 100 mg caffeine
- Usual adult dosage: 1 at first sign of attack; follow with second dose after 1h, if needed. Maximum dose is 2/attack. Do not exceed 5/wk.
- Also see **ergotamine**.

Antiparkinsonism drugs

Sinemet

Tablets
10 mg carbidopa, 100 mg levodopa
25 mg carbidopa, 100 mg levodopa
25 mg carbidopa, 250 mg levodopa

- Usual adult dosage: Starting dose for patients not presently receiving levodopa: one tablet of 10 mg carbidopa/100 mg levodopa or 25 mg carbidopa/100 mg levodopa tid. For patients receiving levodopa: start combination therapy with the morning dose, at least 8 h after the last dose of levodopa, and choose a daily dosage of carbidopa/levodopa that will provide 25% of the previous levodopa daily dosage. Dosage must titrated for each individual, based on the patient's clinical response. See manufacturer's directions for titrating the combination and single agent drugs.
- See also **levodopa;** carbidopa is available alone only by a specific request to the manufacturer from physicians who have a patient who needs a different dosage of carbidopa than is provided by the fixed combination drug; carbidopa is a peripheral inhibitor of dopa decarboxylase, an enzyme that converts dopa to dopamine, which cannot penetrate the CNS; the addition of carbidopa to the levodopa regimen reduces the dose of levodopa needed and decreases the incidence of certain adverse reactions to levodopa.

Diuretics

Aldactazide

Tablets: 25 mg spironolactone, 25 mg hydrochlorothiazide
- Usual adult dosage: 1–8 tablets daily.

Tablets: 50 mg spironolactone, 50 mg hydrochlorothiazide
- Usual adult dosage: 1–4 tablets daily.
- Also see **hydrochlorothiazide** and **spironolactone.**

Dyazide

Capsules: 50 mg triamterene, 25 mg hydrochlorothiazide
- Usual adult dosage: 1 tablet qd or bid after meals.
- Also see **hydrochlorothiazide** and **triamterene.**

Maxzide

Tablets: 75 mg triamterene, 50 mg hydrochlorothiazide
- Usual adult dosage: 1 tablet qd.
- Also see **hydrochlorothiazide** and **triamterene.**

Moduretic

Tablets: 5 mg amiloride, 50 mg hydrochlorothiazide
- Usual adult dosage: 1–2 tablets/d with meals.
- Also see **amiloride** and **hydrochlorothiazide.**

Spirozide

Tablets: 25 mg spironolactone, 25 mg hydrochlorothiazide
- Usual adult dosage: 1–8 tablets daily.
- Also see **hydrochlorothiazide** and **spironolactone.**

Oral contraceptives

- Usual dosage: Take 1 tablet PO daily for 21 d, beginning on day 5 of the cycle (day 1 of the cycle is the first day of menstrual bleeding). Inert tablets or no tablets are taken for the next 7 days. Then start a new course of 21 days.
- Suggested measures for missed doses: one tablet missed—take it as soon as possible, or take 2 tablets the next day; two consecutive tablets missed—take 2 tablets daily for the next 2 days, then resume the regular schedule; three consecutive tablets missed—begin a new cycle of tablets 7 days after the last tablet was taken; use an additional method of birth control until the start of the next menstrual period.

Monophasic

Brevicon, Modicon, Genova 0.5/35, Nelova 0.5/35

Tablets: 35 mg ethinyl estradiol (estrogen) and 0.5 mg norethindrone (progestin)
- See also **ethinyl estradiol, norethindrone.**

Demulen 1/50

Tablets: 50 mg ethinyl estradiol (estrogen) and 1 mg ethynodiol diacetate (progestin)

Demulen 1/35

Tablets: 35 mg ethinyl estradiol (estrogen) and 1 mg ethynodiol diacetate (progestin)
- See also **ethinyl estradiol, progesterone, norgestrel.**

Desogen, Ortho-Cept

Tablets: 30 mcg ethinyl estradiol and 0.5 mg desogestrel
- See also **estrogen, progesterone.**

Enovid-E 21

Tablets: 100 mg mestranol (estrogen) and 2.5 mg norethynodrel (progestin)

Enovid 5 mg

Tablets: 75 mg mestranol (estrogen) and 5 mg norethynodrel (progestin)
- See also **estrogen, progesterone, norgestrel.**

Levlen, Levora, Nordette

Tablets: 30 mg ethinyl estradiol (estrogen) and 0.15 mg levonorgestrel (progestin)
- See also **ethinyl estradiol, progesterone, norgestrel.**

Loestrin 21 1.5/30

Tablets: 30 mg ethinyl estradiol (estrogen) and 1.5 mg norethindrone acetate (progestin)

Loestrin 21 1/20

Tablets: 20 mg ethinyl estradiol (estrogen) and 1 mg norethindrone (progestin)
- See also **ethinyl estradiol, norethindrone.**

Lo/Ovral

Tablets: 30 mg ethinyl estadiol (estrogen) and 0.3 mg norgestrel
- See also **ethinyl estradiol, norgestrel.**

Norinyl 1 + 50, Genora 1/50, Norethrin 1/50, Nelova 1/50M

Tablets: 50 mg mestranol (estrogen) and 1 mg norethindrone (progestin)

Norinyl 1 + 35, Genora 1/35, N.E.E. 1/35, Nelova 35, Norethin 1/35E

Tablets: 35 mg ethinyl estradiol (estrogen) and 1 mg norethindrone (progestin)
- See also **ethinyl estradiol, norethindrone.**

Norlestrin 21 2.5/50

Tablets: 50 mg ethinyl estradiol (estrogen) and 2.5 mg norethindrone acetate (progestin)
- See also **ethinyl estradiol, norethindrone.**

Ortho-Novum 1/50

Tablets: 50 mg ethinyl estradiol (estrogen) and 1 mg norethindrone acetate (progestin)

Ortho-Novum 1/35

Tablets: 35 mg ethinyl estradiol (estrogen) and 1 mg norethindrone (progestin)
- See also **ethinyl estradiol, norethindrone.**

Ovcon-35

Tablets: 35 mg ethinyl estradiol (estrogen) and 1 mg ethynodiol diacetate (progestin)
- See also **ethinyl estradiol, progestin.**

Ovral

Tablets: 50 mg ethinyl estradiol (estrogen) and 0.5 mg norgestrel (progestin) course of 21 d
- See also **ethinyl estradiol, norgestrel.**

Biphasic

Jenest-28, Nevlova 10/11, Ortho-Novum 10/11

Tablets: phase 1–10 tablets, 0.5 mg norethindrone (progestin), and 35 mcg ethinyl estradiol (estrogen); phase 2–11 tablets, 1 mg norethindrone (progestin), and 35 mcg ethinyl estradiol (estrogen).

- See also **ethinyl estradiol, norethindrone.**

Tri-phasic

Ortho Novum 7/7/7

Tablets: phase 1–7 tablets, 0.5 mg norethindrone (progestin), and 35 mcg ethinyl estradiol (estrogen); phase 2–7 tablets, 0.75 mg norethindrone (progestin), and 35 mcg ethinyl estradiol (estrogen); phase 3–7 tablets, 1 mg norethindrone (progestin), and 35 mcg ethinyl estradiol (estrogen).

- See also **norethindrone, ethinyl estradiol.**

Ortho Tri-cyclen

Tablets: phase 1–7 tablets, 0.18 mg norgestimate, 35 mch ethinyl estradiol phase 2–7 tablets, 0.215 mg norgestimate, 35 mch ethinyl estradiol phase 3–0.25 mg norgestimate, 35 mcg ethinyl estradiol

- See also **norethindrone, ethinyl estradiol.**

Tri-Levlen

Tablets: phase 1–6 tablets, 0.05 mg levonorgestrel (progestin), and 30 mcg ethinyl estradiol (estrogen); phase 2–5 tablets, 0.075 mg levonorgestrel (progestin), and 40 mcg ethinyl estradiol (estrogen); phase 3–10 tablets, 0.125 mg levonorgestrel (progestin), and 30 mg ethinyl estradiol (estrogen)

- See also **ethinyl estradiol, norgestrel.**

Tri-Norinyl

Tablets: phase 1–7 tablets, 0.5 mg norethindrone (progestin), and 35 mcg ethinyl estradiol (estrogen); phase 2–9 tablets, 1 mg norethindrone (progestin), and 35 mcg ethinyl estradiol (estrogen); phase 3–5 tablets, 0.5 mg norethindrone (progestin), and 35 mcg ethinyl estradiol (estrogen)

- See also **ethinyl estradiol, norethindrone.**

Triphasil

Tablets: phase 1–6 tablets, 0.05 mg levonorgestrel (progestin), and 30 mcg ethinyl estradiol (estrogen); phase 2–5 tablets, 0.075 mg levonorgestrel (progestin), and 40 mcg ethinyl estradiol (estrogen); phase 3–10 tablets, 0.125 mg levonorgestrel (progestin), and 30 mg ethinyl estradiol (estrogen)

- See also **ethinyl estradiol, norgestrel.**

Respiratory Drugs

Tavist-D

Tablets: 75 mg phenylpropanolamine HCl and 1.34 mg clemastine fumarate
- Usual adult dose: 1 tablet q12h.
- See also **clemastine.**

Trinalin Repetabs

Tablets: 1 mg azatidine maleate and 120 mg pseudoephedrine sulfate
- Usual adult dosage: 1 tablet q 12 h for relief of upper respiratory symptoms of colds, allergies, etc.
- See also **pseudoephedrine;** azatidine is an antihistamine.

Laxatives

The laxatives are used less frequently than they once were in clinical practice. The use of proper diet and exercise has eliminated the need for laxatives in many situations. Most laxatives are available in OTC preparations and are often abused by people who then become dependent on them for GI movement and can develop chronic intestinal disorders. (see table starting on p.1203)

Indications
Short-term relief of constipation; to prevent straining when it is clinically undesirable (post-op abdominal surgery, post-MI, etc.); to evacuate the bowel for diagnostic procedures; to remove ingested poisons from the lower GI tract; as adjunct in anthelmic therapy.

Pregnancy Category C
Contraindicated in cases of allergy to these drugs, third trimester of pregnancy, acute abdominal disorders including appendicitis, diverticulitis, and ulcerative colitis.

Adverse Effects
Excessive bowel activity, perianal irritation, abdominal cramps, weakness, dizziness, fainting, sweating, palpitations, fluid and electrolyte imbalance, *cathartic dependence.*

Drug-Specific Teaching Points
Use as a temporary measure; swallow tablets whole, do not chew; do not take this drug within 1h of antacids, other drugs; increase dietary fiber and fluid intake and maintain daily exercise program to stimulate normal bowel activity; be aware that diarrhea, weakness, and dizziness may occur (do not drive or operate dangerous machinery if this occurs); report sweating, flushing, muscle cramps, excessive thirst.

Peripheral Vasodilators

The peripheral vasodilators are direct-acting, vascular smooth muscle relaxants with no adrenergic stimulating or blocking actions. They are labeled as *"Possibly effective"* for

(text continues on page 1206)

Adverse effects in *Italics* are most common; those in **Bold** are life-threatening.

Laxatives

Drug	Brand Names	Dosage	Type	Onset	Special Considerations
bisacodyl	*Dulcolax* *Fleet lax.* *Dulcagen* *Bisco-Lax*	10–15 mg PO 2.5 g in water via enema	Stimulant	6–10 h Rapid	Allergy to tartrazine in *Dulcolax* tablets; may discolor urine.
cascara		325–650 mg PO	Stimulant	6–10 h	
castor oil	*Neoloid* *Alphamid* *Purge* *Fleet-Flavored Castor* *Emulsoil*	15–30 ml	Stimulant	2–6 h	May be very vigorous; abdominal cramping.
docusate	*Regutol* *Colace* *Disonate* *DOK* *DOS Softgel* *D-S-S* *Modane Soft* *Pro-Sof* *Disonate* *Doxinate* *Dioctoc*	50–240 mg	Detergent Softener	24–72 h	Gentle; beneficial with anorectal conditions that are painful and with dry or hard feces
glycerin	*Sani-Supp* *Fleet Babylex*	Suppository; 4 ml liquid	Hyperosmolar	15–30 min	Insert suppository high into rectum, retain 15 min; insert liquid dispenser and apply gentle, *(continued)*

Laxatives

Drug	Brand Names	Dosage	Type	Onset	Special Considerations
lactulose	*Cephulac* *Cholac* *Chronulac* *Constilac* *Constulose* *Duphalac* *Enulose*	51–30 ml PO	Hyperosmolar	24–48 h	steady pressure until all liquid is gone, then remove. Also used for treatment of portal-system encephalopathy. May be more palatable mixed with fruit juice, water, or milk.
magnesium citrate	*Citrate of Magnesia* *Citro-Nesin*	1 glassful	Saline	0.5–3 h	Reduce pediatric dosage by 1/2.
magnesium hydroxide	*Milk of Magnesia,* *MOM* *Philip's MOM*	15–30 ml	Saline	0.5–3 h	Take with liquids; flavored varieties available.
magnesium sulfate	*Epsom Salts*	10–25 g	Saline	0.5–3 h	Take mixed with glass of water; reduce pediatric dose to 5–10 g in glass of water.
mineral oil	*Agoral Plain* *Kondremul Plain* *Milkinol* *Neo-Cultol*	5–45 ml PO	Emollient	6–8 h	Reduce pediatric dose to 5–20 ml. May decrease absorption of fat-soluble vitamins. Use caution to avoid lipid pneumonia with aspiration.
phenolphthalein	*Alophen Pills* *Ex-Lax* *Lax Pills* *Espotabs*	60–194 mg PO at bedtime	Stimulant	6–10 h	Yellow phenolphthalein is 2–3 times more potent than phenolphthalein; keep away from pets, may be neurotoxic.

	Feen-a-mint Modane Prolet Evan-U-Gen Medilax Phenolax			
polycarbophil	FiberCon Equalactin Mitrolan Fiber-Lax Fiberall	1 g PO 1–4 times/d as needed; do not exceed 6 g/d in adults or 3 g/d in children	Bulk	12–24 h	Good with irritable bowel syndrome, diverticulitis. Abdominal fullness may occur. Smaller doses more frequently may alleviate discomfort.
psyllium	Fiberall Natural Hydrocil Instant Konsyl Metamucil	1 tsp or packet in cool water or juice, 1–3 times/d in children	Bulk	12–24 h	Safest and most physiological. Assure that patient has sufficient water to completely swallow dose.
senna	Senokot Senna-Gen Senokotxtra Black-Draught Gentlax Fletcher's Castoria Dr. Caldwell Senna	1–8 tablets/d at bedtime; suppository; syrup—10–25 ml	Stimulant	6–10 h	May be very aggressive; abdominal cramps and discomfort may occur.

adjunctive treatment of intermittent claudication, arteriosclerosis obliterans, thrombophlebitis, nocturnal leg cramps, Raynaud's phenomenon, and selected cases of ischemic cerebral vascular disease. Although many other drugs that have proven efficacy and therapeutic value are now available for these conditions, these drugs are still available and may be used in some situations.

Pregnancy Category C
Contraindicated in cases of allergy to the drug, severe obliterative coronary artery disease, severe obliterative cerebral vascular disease, glaucoma, active bleeding, bleeding tendency.

Adverse Effects
Heartburn, abdominal pain, eructation; *flushing, headache,* feeling of weakness; *tachycardia;* orthostatic hypotension, dizziness.

Drug-Specific Teaching Points
Take drug with meals or antacids (if prescribed) if GI upset occurs. Report severe headache, chest pain, shortness of breath, loss of consciousness, numbness, tingling in the extremities.

Drug	Brand Name	Dosage	Special Considerations
cyclandelate	*Cyclan* *Cyclospasmol*	1.2–1.6 g/d PO in divided doses after meals and at bedtime. With improvement, decrease in 200 mg intervals. Maintenance: 400–800 mg/d PO in 2–4 divided doses.	Short-term use is rarely beneficial.
ethaverine	*Ethaquin* *Ethatab* *Ethavex*	100 mg PO tid. May increase to 200 mg PO tid.	Long-term therapy is needed. Do not use early in disease.
isoxsuprine hydrochloride	*Isovex* *Vasodilan* *Voxsuprine*	10–20 mg PO 3–4 times/d	Has been used to inhibit premature labor. Can cause serious problems. Not recommended. Rash may occur. Stop drug if rash appears.
nylidrin hydrochloride	*Adrin* *Arlidin*	3–12 mg PO 3–4 time/d	May cause orthostatic hypotension. Change position slowly.
papaverine hydrochloride	*Cerespan* *Genabid* *Pavabid* *Pavased* *Pavasule* *Pavatine*	100–300 mg PO 3–5 times/d 150 mg q12h PO timed release 30–120 mg q3h IM or IV injected slowly over 1–2 min.	IV route may be used for acute vasospasm. Do not mix IV with Lactate Ringer's Solution.

Vitamins

Vitamins are substances that the body requires for carrying out essential metabolic reactions. The body cannot synthesize enough of these components to meet all of its needs. Therefore, vitamins must be obtained from animal and vegetable tissues taken as food. Vitamins are needed only in small amounts because they function as coenzymes

Adverse effects in *Italics* are most common; those in **Bold** are life-threatening.

that activate the protein portion enzymes, which catalyze a great deal of biochemical activity. Vitamins are either water soluble and excreted in the urine, or fat soluble and capable of being stored in adipose tissue. (see table starting on p.1208)

Indications
Treatment of vitamin deficiency; dietary supplement when needed; specific therapeutic uses related to vitamin activity.

Pregnancy Category C
Contraindicated in cases of allergy to these drugs, colorants, additives, or preservatives.

Adverse Effects
Vitamin-specific.

Drug-Drug Interactions
Pyrodoxine interferes with effectiveness of levodopa; fat-soluble vitamins may not be absorbed if given concurrently with mineral oil, cholestyramine, colestipol.

Drug-Specific Teaching Points
Use only in the dosage prescribed; avoid use of OTC drugs that may also contain vitamins in combination.

Topical Agents

Topical agents are drugs that are intended for surface use, not ingestion or injection. They may be very toxic if absorbed into the system, but serve several purposes when used topically. (see table starting on p.1212)

Pregnancy Category C
Contraindicated in cases of allergy to these drugs, open wounds or abrasions.

Adverse Effects
Local irritation, stinging, burning, dermatitis, toxic effects if absorbed systemically.

Drug-Specific Teaching Points
Apply sparingly as directed. Do not use with open wounds or broken skin. Avoid contact with eyes. Report any local irritation, allergic reaction, worsening of condition being treated.

Topical Corticosteroids

Drug Classes
Hormonal agents
Corticosteroids
Glucocorticoids/mineralcorticoids

(text continues on page 1217)

Adverse effects in *Italics* are most common; those in **Bold** are life-threatening.

Vitamins

Vitamin	Brand Names	Type	RDA (PO)	Therapeutic Uses/Special Consideration
A	*Aquasol A* *Del-Vi-A*	Fat soluble	1000 mcg (males) 800 mcg (females) 1300 mcg (nursing) 375–700 mcg (ped.)	Severe deficiency—500,000 IU/d–3 days; then 50,000 IU/d for 2 wk PO or IM. Protect IM vial from light. Hypervitaminosis A can occur—cirrhotic-like liver syndrome with CNS effects, GI drying, rash, liver changes. Treat by discontinuing vitamin; saline, prednisone, calcitonin IV. Liver damage may be permanent.
ascorbic acid (C)	*Flavorcee* *Cebid* *Cetane* *Cevi-Bid* *N'Ice Vitamin C drops* *Dull-C* *Vita-C* *Cevalin*	Water soluble	50–60 mg (males) 50–60 mg (females) 70–90 mg (nursing) 70 mg (pregnancy) 30–45 mg (ped.)	May be given PO, IM, IV (slowly), SC. Treatment of scurvy—300 mg–1 g daily; enhanced wound healing—300–500 mg/d for 7–10 d; burns—1–2 g/d. Also being studied for treatment of common cold, asthma, CAD, wound healing, cancer, schizophrenia.
calcifediol (D³)	*Calcedrol*	Fat soluble		Management of metabolic bone disease or hypocalcemia in patients on chronic renal dialysis: 300–350 mcg/wk given daily or on alternate days. Discontinue if hypercalcemia occurs.
calcitriol (D₃)	*Calcijex* *Rocaltrol*	Fat soluble		Management of hypocalcemia in patients on renal dialysis: 0.25 mcg/d. Reduction of elevated parathyroid hormone: 0.25 mcg/d in the morning as an initial dose then 0.5–2 mcg/d. May be effective in the treatment of psoriasis.
cholecalciferol (D₃)	*Delta-D*	Fat soluble	200–400 IU (males) 200–400 IU (females) 400 IU (nursing) 400 IU (pregnancy) 300–400 IU (ped.)	Vitamin D deficiency—400–1000 IU/d. May be useful for treatment of hypocalcemic tetany and hypoparathyroidism.

cyanocobalamin (B$_{12}$)	*Ener-B*	Water soluble	2 mcg (males) 2 mcg (females) 2.6 mcg (nursing) 2.2 mcg (pregnancy) 0.3–1.4 mcg (ped.)	Deficiency—25–250 mcg/d. Note: not for the treatment of pernicious anemia.
D		Fat soluble	200–400 IU (males) 200–400 IU (females) 400 IU (nursing) 400 IU (pregnancy) 300–400 IU (ped.)	Vitamin D deficiency—400–1000 IU/d. May be useful for treatment of hypocalcemic tetany and hypoparathyroidism. Encourage balanced diet and exposure to sunlight. Do not use with mineral oil.
dihydrotachysterol (DHT; D$_2$)	*Hytakerol* *DHT*	Fat soluble		Treatment of postoperative tetany, idiopathic tetany, hypoparathyroidism: Initial dose 0.8–2.4 mg/d for several days, then 0.2–1 mg/d to achieve normal serum calcium. May supplement with oral calcium.
E	*Aquasol E* *Vita-Plus E Softgels* *E Complex* *Amino-Opti E*	Fat soluble	15 IU (males) 12 IU (females) 16–18 IU (nursing) 15 IU (pregnancy) 4–10 IU (ped.)	Used in certain premature infants to reduce the toxic effects of oxygen on the lung and retina; do not give IV; report—fatigue, weakness, nausea, headache, blurred vision, diarrhea.
ergocalciferol (D$_2$)	*Drisdol drops* *Deltalin Gelseals*	Fat soluble	200–400 IU (males) 200–400 IU (females) 400 IU (nursing) 400 IU (pregnancy) 300–400 IU (ped.)	Give IM in GI, biliary, liver disease. Refractory rickets—12,000–500,000 IU/d Hypoparathyroidism—50,000–200,000 IU/d Familial hypophosphatemia—10,000–80,000 IU/d plus 1–2 g phosphorus.
menadiol sodium diphosphate (K$_4$)	*Synkayvite*	Fat soluble	45–80 mcg (males) 45–65 mcg (females) 65 mcg (nursing) 65 mcg (pregnancy) 5–50 mcg (ped.)	Hypoprothrombinemia due to obstructive jaundice—5 mg/d PO, IM, SC, IV. Hypoprothrombinemia due to antibiotics or salicylates—5–10 mg/d.

(continued)

Vitamins (Continued)

Vitamin	Brand Names	Type	RDA (PO)	Therapeutic Uses/Special Consideration
niacin (B_3)	Nicotinic acid Niacor Nicolar	Water soluble	15–20 mg (males) 13–15 mg (females) 20 mg (nursing) 17 mg (pregnancy) 5–13 mg (ped.)	Prevention and treatment of pellagra: up to 500 mg/d; niacin deficiency: up to 100 mg/d, also used for treatment of hyperlipidemia in patients who do not respond to diet and exercise—1–2 g tid. Do not exceed 6 g/d. Feelings of warmth, flushing may occur with administration but usually pass within 2h.
nicotinamide (B_3)		Water soluble	15–20 mg (males) 13–15 mg (females) 20 mg (nursing) 17 mg (pregnancy) 5–13 mg (ped.)	Prevention and treatment of pellagra: up to 50 mg 3–10 times/d.
P (Bioflavonoids)	Citro-Flav 2000 Pan C-500 Amino-Opti-C Peridin C Span C Flavons-500 Bio Acerola C	Water soluble	None known	Used to treat bleeding, abortion, poliomyelitis, arthritis, diabetes, etc. There is little evidence that these uses have any clinical efficacy.
phytonadione	Mephyton	Fat soluble	45–80 mcg (males) 45–65 mcg (females) 65 mcg (nursing) 65 mcg (pregnancy) 5–30 mcg (ped.)	Hypoprothrombinemia due to anticoagulants—2.5–10 mg PO, IM. Hemorrhagic disease of the newborn: 0.5–1 mg IM within 1h of birth, 1–5 mg IM may be given to the mother before delivery; hypoprothrombinemia in adults 2.5–25 mg PO or IM.
pyridoxine HCl (B_6)	Nestrex Beesix	Water soluble	1.7–2 mg (males) 1.4–1.6 mg (females) 2.1 mg (nursing) 2.2 mg (pregnancy) 0.3–1.4 mg (ped.)	Deficiency: 10–20 mg/d PO or IM for 3 wk. Vitamin B_6 deficiency syndrome: up to 600 mg/day for life. INH poisoning—give an equal amount of pyridoxine: 4 g IV followed by 1g IM q30min. Reduces effectiveness of *levodopa* and leads to serious toxic effects—avoid this combination.

riboflavin (B$_2$)		Water soluble	1.4–1.8 mg (males) 1.2–1.3 mg (females) 1.7–1.8 mg (nursing) 1.6 mg (pregnancy) 0.4–1.2 mg (ped.)	Treatment of deficiency; 5–25 mg/day. May cause a yellow/orange discoloring of the urine.
thiamine HCl (B$_1$)	*Thiamilate* *Biamine*	Water soluble	1.2–1.5 mg (males) 1–1.1 mg (females) 1.6 mg (nursing) 1.5 mg (pregnancy) 0.3–1 mg (ped.)	Treatment of wet beriberi: 10–30 mg IV tid; treatment of beriberi: 10–20 mg IM tid for 2 wk with an oral multivitamin containing 5–10 mg/d for 1 mo. Do not mix in alkaline solutions. Used orally as a mosquito repellant, alters body sweat composition. Feeling of warmth and flushing may occur with administration.

Topical Agents

Drug	Brand Names	Dosage	Special Considerations
Emollients			
boric acid ointment	Borofax	Apply as needed	Relieves burns, itching, irritation.
dexpanthenol	Pantboderm	Apply qd–bid.	Relieves itching and aids in healing for mild skin irritations.
glycerin		Combined with other ingredients—rose water	Moisturizing effect
lanolin		Ointment base, applied generously	Allergy to sheep or sheep products—use caution; base for many ointments
urea	Aquacare Nutraplus Carmol Gormel Lanaphilic Ureacin	2–4 times/d to area affected	Rub in completely. Used to restore nails—cover with plastic wrap; keep dry and remove in 3, 7, 10, or 14 d.
vitamin A and D		Apply locally with gentle massage bid-qid.	Relieves minor burns, chafing, skin irritations. Consult physician if not improved within 7 d.
zinc oxide		Apply as needed.	Relieves burns, abrasion, diaper rash.
Lotions and Solutions			
Burow's solution aluminum acetate	Bluboro Powder Boropak Powder Domeboro Powder Pedi-Boro Soak Paks	Dissolve one packet in a pint of water; apply q15–30 min for 4–8h	Astringent wet dressing for relief of inflammatory conditions, insect bites, athlete's foot, bruise, etc; do not use occlusive dressing.
calamine lotion	Calamax Resinol Calamatum	Apply to affected area tid-qid.	Relieves itching, pain of poison ivy, poison sumac and oak, insect bites, and minor skin irritations.
hamamelis water	Witch Hazel Tucks A-E-R	Apply locally up to 6 times/d.	Relieves itching and irritation of vaginal infection, hemorrhoids, postepisiotomy discomfort, post hemorrhoidectomy care.

Appendix A ■ 1213

Antiseptics

Benzalkonium chloride	*BAC* *Benza* *Zephiran*	Mix in solution as needed; spray for preoperative use; storage of instruments in solution	Thoroughly rinse detergents and soaps from skin before use; add anti-rust tablets for instruments stored in solution; dilute solution as indicated for use.
chlorhexidine gluconate	*Hibiclens* *Dyna-Hex* *Exidine* *Hibistat*	Scrub or rinse; leave on for 15 seconds; for surgical scrub—3 min.	Use for surgical scrub, preoperative skin prep, wound cleansing; preop bathing and showering.
hexachlorophene	*pHisoHex* *Septisol*	Apply as wash.	Surgical wash, scrub; do not use with burns or on mucous membranes; rinse thoroughly.
iodine		Wash affected area with solution.	Highly toxic; avoid occlusive dressings; stains skin and clothing.
povidone iodine	*Betadine* *Aerodine* *ACU-dyne* *Betagen* *Iodex*	Apply as needed.	Treated areas may be bandaged. HIV is inactivated in this solution; causes less irritation than iodine; less toxic.
sodium hypochlorite	*Dakin's*	Apply as antiseptic.	Caution—chemical burns can occur.
thimersol	*Mersol* *Aeroaid*	Apply qd-tid.	Contains mercury compound; used preop and as first aid for abrasions, wounds.

Antibiotics

mupirocin	*Bactroban*	Apply small amt. to affected area tid. May be covered with a gauze dsg.	Use to treat impetigo caused by *Staph. aureus*, *Streptococcus* and *S pyogens*. Monitor for signs of superinfection; reevaluate if no clinical response in 3–5 d.

Antipsoriatics

ammoniated mercury	*Emersal*	Apply qd-bid.	Protect from light; potential sensitizer provoking severe allergic reactions.
anthralin	*Anthra-Derm* *Lasan* *Drithocreme*	Apply qd only to psoriatic lesions	May stain fabrics, skin, hair, fingernails; use protective dressing.

(continued)

Topical Agents (Continued)

Drug	Brand Names	Dosage	Special Considerations
Antiseborrheics			
selenium sulfide	Selsun Blue Excel	Massage 5–10 ml into scalp; rest 2–3 min., rinse	May damage jewelry, remove before use; discontinue if local irritation occurs
chloroxine	Capitrol	Massage into wet scalp; leave lather on for 3 min	May discolor blond, gray, bleached hair. Do not use on active lesions.
Antifungals			
clotrimazole	Lotrimin Mycelex	Gently massage into affected area bid.	Cleanse area before applying; use for up to 4 wk. Discontinue if irritation, worsening of condition occurs.
econazole nitrate	Spectazole	Apply locally qd–bid.	Cleanse area before applying; treat for 2–4 wk. Discontinue if irritation, burning or worsening of condition occurs. For athlete's foot, change socks and shoes at least once a day.
gentian violet		Apply locally bid.	May stain skin and clothing; do not apply to active lesions.
naftifine HCl	Naftin	Gently massage into affected area bid.	Avoid occlusive dressings; wash hands thoroughly after application. Do not use longer than 4 wk.
oxiconazole	Oxistat	Apply qd–bid.	May be needed for up to 1 mo.
terbinafine	Lamisil	Apply to area bid until clinical signs are improved; 1–4 wk	Do not use occlusive dressings; report local irritation; discontinue if local irritation occurs.
tolnaftate	Tinactin Genaspor Ting Aftate	Apply small amount bid for 2–3 wk; 4–6 wk may be needed if skin is very thick	Cleanse skin with soap and water before applying drug, dry thoroughly, wear loose, well-fitting shoes, change socks at least qid.

Pediculocides/scabicides

lindane	*Kwell, Scabene, G-Well*	Apply thin layer to entire body, leave on 8–12h, then wash thoroughly. Shampoo 1–2 oz. into dry hair and leave in place 4 min.	For external use only. Single application is usually sufficient, reapply after 7 d at signs of live lice. Teach hygiene and prevention; treat all contacts. Assure parents this is a readily communicable disease.
crotamiton	*Eurax*	Thoroughly massage into skin of entire body; repeat in 24h. Take a cleansing bath or shower 48h after last application.	For external use only. Change bed linens and clothing the next day. Contaminated clothing can be dry cleaned or washed on hot cycle. Shake well before using.
permethrin	*Nix, Elimite*	Thoroughly massage into all skin areas (30g/adult); wash off after 8–14h. Shampoo into freshly washed, rinsed and towel dried hair. Leave on for 10 min.; rinse.	For external use only. Single application is usually curative. Notify health care provider if rash, itching become worse.

Keratolytics

cantharidin	*Cantharone, Verr-Canth*	Apply to lesion; cover with tape; remove in 24h.	Replace tape with loose bandage; may cause itching and burning, may be tender for 2–6 d; if spilled on skin, wipe off with acetone or tape remover; if contacts eyes, flush immediately and contact physician.
podophyllum resin	*Pod-Ben-25, Podocon-25, Podofin*	Applied only by physician.	Do not use if wart is inflamed or irritated. Very toxic, minimum amount possible is used to avoid absorption.
podofilox	*Condylox*	Apply q12h for 3 consecutive d.	Allow to dry before using area; dispose of used applicator, may cause burning and discomfort.

Topical hemostatics

absorbable gelatin	*Gelfoam*	Smear or press paste to cut surface; when bleeding stops, remove excess. Apply sponge and allow to remain in place, will be absorbed.	Prepare paste by adding 3–4 ml sterile saline to contents of jar. Apply sponge dry or saturated with saline. Assess continually for any sign of infection, agent may act as site of infection or abscess formation. Do not use in presence of infection.

(continued)

Topical Agents (Continued)

Drug	Brand Names	Dosage	Special Considerations
Microfibrillar collagen	*Avitene*	Use dry. Apply directly to the source of bleeding; apply pressure, time will vary from 3–5 min depending on the site. Discard any unused product.	Monitor for infection; do not use in the presence of infection. Remove any excess material once bleeding has been controlled.
thrombin	*Thrombinar, Thrombostat*	Prepare in Sterile Distilled Water of Isotonic Saline; 100–1000 units/ml. Mix freely with blood on the surface of injury.	Contraindicated in presence of any bovine allergies. Watch for any sign of severe allergic reaction in sensitive individuals.
Pain Relief			
capsaicin	*Zostrix*	Apply not more than 3–4 times/day.	Applied locally, provides temporary relief from the pain of osteoarthritis, rheumatoid arthritis, neuralgias. Do not bandage tightly; stop use and seek health care if condition worsens or persists after 14–28 d.
Burn Preparations			
mafenide	*Sulfamylon*	Apply to a clean, debrided wound, 1–2 times/d with a gloved hand. Cover burn at all times with drug, reapply as needed.	Bathe patient in a whirlpool daily to aid debridement. Continue until healing occurs; monitor for infection and toxicity—acidosis. May cause marked discomfort on application.
nitrofurazone	*Furacin*	Apply directly to burn or place on gauze; reapply qd.	Flushing the dressing with sterile saline will facilitate removal. Monitor for signs of superinfections; treat supportively. Rash frequently occurs.
silver sulfadiazine	*Silvadene, Thermazene SSD Cream*	Apply qd–bid to a clean, debrided would; use a 1/16 in thickness.	Bathe patient in a whirlpool to aid debridement. Dressings are not necessary but may be used; reapply whenever necessary. Monitor for fungal superinfections.

Therapeutic Actions
Enters cells and binds cytoplasmic receptors, thereby initiating complex reactions that are responsible for the anti-inflammatory, antipruritic, and antiproliferative effects.

Indications
- Relief of inflammatory and pruritic manifestations of corticosteroid-sensitive dermatoses
- Temporary relief of minor skin irritations, itching and rashes—nonprescription products

Adverse Effects
- CNS: glaucoma, cataracts after prolonged periorbital use that allows the drug to enter the eyes
- Systemic: systemic absorption can occur leading to the adverse effects experienced with systemic use; growth retardation and suppression of the HPA (more likely to occur with occlusive dressings, in patients with liver failure, and with children who have a larger skin-surface-to-body-weight ratio)
- Local: burning, irritation, acneiform lesions, skin atrophy, secondary infection

Dosage
Apply sparingly to affected area bid–tid.

Drug-Specific Teaching Points
- Apply sparingly in a light film, rub in gently. Washing the area before application may increase drug penetration.
- Do not use occlusive dressings, tight-fitting diapers, or plastic pants, unless otherwise indicated. This may increase systemic aborption.
- Avoid prolonged use, especially near the eyes, in genital or rectal areas, on the face and in skin creases. Avoid any direct contact with eyes.
- Use this drug only for the purpose indicated. Do not apply to open lesions.
- Notify nurse or physician if condition becomes worse or persists; if burning or irritation occurs; if infection occurs in the area.

❑ aclometasone dipropionate

Aclovate

Ointment, cream: 0.05% concentration

- Occlusive dressings may be used for the management of refractory lesions of psoriasis and deep-seated dermatoses.

❑ amcinoide

Cyclocort

Ointment, cream, lotion: 0.1% concentration

❑ betamethasone benzoate

Uticort, Bepen (CAN)

Cream, lotion, gel: 0.025% concentration

betamethasone dipropionate

Alphatres, Diprosone, Maxivate, Rhoprosone (CAN), *Taro-Stone* (CAN), *Teledar*

Ointment, cream, lotion, aerosol: 0.05% concentration

betamethasone dipropionate, augmented

Diprolene

Ointment, cream, lotion: 0.05% concentration

betamethasone valerate

Betacort (CAN), *Betaderm* (CAN), *Betatrex, Beta-Val, Betnovate* (CAN), *Celestoderm* (CAN), *Dermabet, Prevex, B*(CAN), *Rholosone* (CAN), *Valisone*

Ointment, cream, lotion: 0.1% concentration

clobetasol propionate

Dermovate (CAN), *Temovate*

Ointment, cream: 0.05% concentration

clocortolone pivalate

Cloderm

Cream: 0.1% concentration

desonide

DesOwen, Tridesiolon

Ointment, cream: 0.05% concentration

desoximetasone

Topicort

Ointment, cream: 0.25% concentration
Gel: 0.05% concentration

dexamethasone

Decaderm

Gel: 0.1% concentration

Aeroseb-Dex

Aerosol: 0.01% concentration

Decaspray

Aerosol: 0.04% concentration

dexamethasone sodium phosphate

Decadron phosphate

Cream: 0.1% concentration

diflorasone diacetate

Florone, Maxiflor, Psorcon

Ointment, cream: 0.05% concentration

Florone E

Cream: 0.5% concentration

fluocinolone acetonide

Flurosyn, Synalar

Ointment: 0.025% concentration
Cream: 0.01% concentration

Flurosyn, Synalar, Synemol

Cream: 0.025% concentration

Fluonid, Flurosyn, Synalar

Solution: 0.01% concentration

◻ fluocinonide

Lidex

Ointment: 0.05% concentration

Fluonex, Lidex, Lyderm Cream (CAN), *Vasoderm*

Cream: 0.05% concentration

Lidex, Topsyn Gel (CAN)

Solution, gel: 0.05% concentration

◻ flurandrenolide

Cordran

Ointment, cream: 0.025% concentration
Ointment, cream, lotion: 0.05% concentration
Tape: 4 mcg/cm^2

◻ fluticasone propionate

Cutivate

Cream: 0.05% concentration
Ointment: 0.005% concentration

◻ halcinonide

Halog

Ointment, cream, solution: 0.1% concentration
Cream: 0.025% concentration

◻ halobetasol propionate

Ultravate

Ointment, cream: 0.05% concentration

◻ hydrocortisone
Lotion: 0.25%

Cortizone 5, Bactine Hydrocortisone, Cort-Dome, Dermolate, Dermtex HC, Hydrotex

Cream, lotion, ointment, aerosol: 0.5%

Cortizone 10, Hycort, Tegrin-HC

Cream, lotion, ointment, solution: 1%

Hytone

Cream, lotion, ointment: 2.5%

❏ hydrocortisone acetate

Cortaid, Lanacort-5 OTC preparations

Ointment: 0.5% concentration

Corticaine (R$_x$), FoilleCort, Gynecort, Lanacort 5 (OTC preparations)

Cream: 0.5% concentration

Anusol-HC, U-Cort

Cream: 1% concentration

Caldecort, Cortaid with Aloe OTC preparations

Cream: 0.5% concentration

CortaGel

OTC preparation
Gel: 0.5% concentration

❏ hydrocortisone butyrate

Locoid

Ointment, cream: 0.1% concentration

❏ hydrocortisone valerate

Westcort

Ointment, cream: 0.2% concentration

❏ mometasone furoate

Elocon

Ointment, cream, lotion: 0.1% concentration

☐ prednicarbate

Dermatop

Cream: 0.1% concentration: preservative free

☐ triamcinolone acetonide

Flutex, Kenalog

Ointment: 0.025% concentration

Aristocort, Flutex, Kenalog

Ointment: 0.1% concentration and 0.5% concentration
Cream: 0.025% concentration and 0.5% concentration

Aristocort, Flutex, Kenalog, Triacet, Triderm

Cream: 0.1% concentration

Kenalog

Lotion: 0.025% and 0.1% concentration

APPENDIX B

Recommended Immunization Schedule*

Immunization	2 mo	4 mo	6 mo	18 mo	4–6 y	10 y
Polio	x	x		x	x	
DPT	x	x	x			
Measles/mumps/rubella					x	
Tetanus/diphtheria booster						x
Hemophilus influenza	x	x	x	x		
Hepatitis B	x	x	x			

*Suggested by the American Academy of Pediatrics, 1994.

APPENDIX C

Formulae for calculating pediatric dosages

Children often require different doses of drugs than adults because childrens' bodies often handle drugs very differently from adults' bodies. The "standard" drug dosages listed in package inserts and references such as the PDR refer to the adult dosage. In some cases, a pediatric dosage is suggested, but in many cases it will need to be calculated based on the child's age, weight, or body surface. The following are some standard formulae for calculating the pediatric dose.

Fried's rule

$$\text{infant's dose } (<1 \text{ y}) = \frac{\text{infant's age (in mo)}}{150 \text{ mo}} \times \text{average adult dose}$$

Young's rule

$$\text{child's dose } (1-12 \text{ y}) = \frac{\text{child's age (in yrs)}}{\text{child's age (in yrs)} + 12} \times \text{average adult dose}$$

Clark's rule

$$\text{child's dose} = \frac{\text{weight of child (lb)}}{150 \text{ lb}} \times \text{average adult dose}$$

Surface area rule

$$\text{child's dose} = \frac{\text{surface area of child (in square meters)}}{1.73} \times \text{average adult dose}$$

The surface area of a child is determined using a nomogram which determines surface area based on height and weight measurements.

Pediatric dosage calculations should be checked by two persons. Many institutions have procedures for double checking the dosage calculation of those drugs (eg, digoxin) used most frequently in the pediatric area.

Appendix C ■ 1225

Nomogram for estimating surface area of infants and young children. To determine the surface area of the patient, draw a straight line between the point representing the height on the left vertical scale and the point representing the weight on the right vertical scale. The point at which this line intersects the middle vertical scale represents the patient's surface area in square meters. (Courtesy of Abbott Laboratories.)

APPENDIX D

FDA Pregnancy Categories

The Food and Drug Administration has established five categories to indicate the potential for a systemically absorbed drug to cause birth defects. The key differentiation among the categories rests upon the degree (reliability) of documentation and the risk-benefit ratio.

Category A: Adequate studies in pregnant women have not demonstrated a risk to the fetus in the first trimester of pregnancy, and there is no evidence of risk in later trimesters.

Category B: Animal studies have not demonstrated a risk to the fetus but there are no adequate studies in pregnant women. *or* Animal studies have shown an adverse effect, but adequate studies in pregnant women have not demonstrated a risk to the fetus during the first trimester of pregnancy, and there is no evidence of risk in later trimesters.

Category C: Animal studies have shown an adverse effect on the fetus but there are no adequate studies in humans; the benefits from the use of the drug in pregnant women may be acceptable despite its potential risks. *or* There are no animal reproduction studies and no adequate studies in humans.

Category D: There is evidence of human fetal risk, but the potential benefits from the use of the drug in pregnant women may be acceptable despite its potential risks.

Category X: Studies in animals or humans demonstrate fetal abnormalities or adverse reaction; reports indicate evidence of fetal risk. The risk of use in a pregnant woman clearly outweighs any possible benefit.

Regardless of the designated Pregnancy Category or presumed safety, *no* drug should be administered during pregnancy unless it is clearly needed.

APPENDIX E
DEA Schedules of Controlled Substances

The Controlled Substances Act of 1970 regulates the manufacturing, distribution, and dispensing of drugs which are known to have abuse potential. The Drug Enforcement Agency (DEA) is responsible for the enforcement of these regulations. The controlled drugs are divided into five DEA schedules based on their potential for abuse and physical and psychological dependence.

Schedule I *(C-I)*: High abuse potential and no accepted medical use (heroin, marijuana, LSD)

Schedule II *(C-II)*: High abuse potential with severe dependence liability (narcotics, amphetamines, and barbiturates)

Schedule III *(C-III)*: Less abuse potential than Schedule II drugs and moderate dependence liability (nonbarbiturate sedatives, nonamphetamine stimulants, limited amounts of certain narcotics)

Schedule IV *(C-IV)*: Less abuse potential than Schedule III and limited dependence liability (some sedatives, antianxiety agents, and nonnarcotic analgesics)

Schedule V *(C-V):* Limited abuse potential. Primarily small amounts of narcotics (codeine) used as antitussives or antidiarrheals. Under federal law, limited quantities of certain Schedule V drugs may be purchased without a prescription directly from a pharmacist. The purchaser must be at least 18 years of age and must furnish suitable identification. All such transactions must be recorded by the dispensing pharmacist.

Prescribing physicians and dispensing pharmacists must be registered with the DEA, which also provides forms for the transfer of Schedule I and II substances and establishes criteria for the inventory and prescribing of controlled substances. State and local laws are often more stringent than federal law. In any given situation, the more stringent law applies.

APPENDIX F

NANDA-Approved Nursing Diagnoses

This list represents the NADA approved nursing diagnoses for clinical use and testing (1994).

Pattern 1: Exchanging
1.1.2.1 Altered Nutrition: More than body requirements
1.1.2.2 Altered Nutrition: Less than body requirements
1.1.2.3 Altered Nutrition: Potential for more than body requirements
1.2.1.1 Risk for Infection
1.2.2.1 Risk for Altered Body Temperature
1.2.2.2 Hypothermia
1.2.2.3 Hyperthermia
1.2.2.4 Ineffective Thermoregulation
1.2.3.1 Dysreflexia
1.3.1.1 Constipation
1.3.1.1.1 Perceived Constipation
1.3.1.1.2 Colonic Constipation
1.3.1.2 Diarrhea
1.3.1.3 Bowel Incontinence
1.3.2 Altered Urinary Elimination
1.3.2.1.1 Stress Incontinence
1.3.2.1.2 Reflex Incontinence
1.3.2.1.3 Urge Incontinence
1.3.2.1.4 Functional Incontinence
1.3.2.1.5 Total Incontinence
1.3.2.2 Urinary Retention
1.4.1.1 Altered (Specify Type) Tissue Perfusion (Renal, cerebral, cardiopulmonary, gastrointestinal, peripheral)
1.4.1.2.1 Fluid Volume Excess
1.4.1.2.2.1 Fluid Volume Deficit
1.4.1.2.2.2 Risk for Fluid Volume Deficit
1.4.2.1 Decreased Cardiac Output
1.5.1.1 Impaired Gas Exchange
1.5.1.2 Ineffective Airway Clearance
1.5.1.3 Ineffective Breathing Pattern
1.5.1.3.1 Inability to Sustain Spontaneous Ventilation
1.5.1.3.2 Dysfunctional Ventilatory Weaning Response (DVWR)
1.6.1 Risk for Injury
1.6.1.1 Risk for Suffocation
1.6.1.2 Risk for Poisoning
1.6.1.3 Risk for Trauma
1.6.1.4 Risk for Aspiration
1.6.1.5 Risk for Disuse Syndrome
1.6.2 Altered Protection
1.6.2.1 Impaired Tissue Integrity
1.6.2.1.1 Altered Oral Mucous Membrane

1.6.2.1.2.1 Impaired Skin Integrity
1.6.2.1.2.2 Risk for Impaired Skin Integrity
#1.7.1 Decreased Adaptive Capacity: Intracranial
#1.8 Energy Field Disturbance
Pattern 2: Communicating
2.1.1.1 Impaired Verbal Communication
Pattern 3: Relating
3.1.1 Impaired Social Interaction
3.1.2 Social Isolation
#3.1.3 Risk for Loneliness
3.2.1 Altered Role Performance
3.2.1.1.1 Altered Parenting
3.2.1.1.2 Risk for Altered Parenting
#3.2.1.1.2.1 Risk for Altered Parent/Infant/Child Attachment
3.2.1.2.1 Sexual Dysfunction
3.2.2 Altered Family Processes
3.2.2.1 Caregiver Role Strain
3.2.2.2 Risk for Caregiver Role Strain
#3.2.2.3.1 Altered Family Process: Alcoholism
3.2.3.1 Parental Role Conflict
3.3 Altered Sexuality Patterns
Pattern 4: Valuing
4.1.1 Spiritual Distress (distress of the human spirit)
#4.2 Potential for Enhanced Spiritual Well Being
Pattern 5: Choosing
5.1.1.1 Ineffective Individual Coping
5.1.1.1.1 Impaired Adjustment
5.1.1.1.2 Defensive Coping
5.1.1.1.3 Ineffective Denial
5.1.2.1.1 Ineffective Family Coping: Disabling
5.1.2.1.2 Ineffective Family Coping: Compromised
#5.1.3.1 Potential for Enhanced Community Coping
#5.1.3.2 Ineffective Community Coping
5.1.2.2 Family Coping: Potential for Growth
5.2.1 Ineffective Management of Therapeutic Regimen (Individuals)
5.2.1.1 Noncompliance (Specify)
#5.2.2 Ineffective Management of Therapeutic Regimen: Families
#5.2.3 Ineffective Management of Therapeutic Regimen: Community
#5.2.4 Ineffective Management of Therapeutic Regimen: Individual
5.3.1.1 Decisional Conflict (Specify)
5.4 Health Seeking Behaviors (Specify)
Pattern 6: Moving
6.1.1.1 Impaired Physical Mobility
6.1.1.1.1 Risk for Peripheral Neurovascular Dysfunction
#6.1.1.1.2 Risk for Perioperative Positioning Injury
6.1.1.2 Activity Intolerance
6.1.1.2.1 Fatigue
6.1.1.3 Risk for Activity Intolerance
6.2.1 Sleep Pattern Disturbance
6.3.1.1 Diversional Activity Deficit
6.4.1.1 Impaired Home Maintenance Management
6.4.2 Altered Health Maintenance

6.5.1 Feeding Self Care Deficit
6.5.1.1 Impaired Swallowing
6.5.1.2 Ineffective Breastfeeding
6.5.1.2.1 Interrupted Breastfeeding
6.5.1.3 Effective Breastfeeding
6.5.1.4 Ineffective Infant Feeding Pattern
6.5.2 Bathing/Hygiene Self Care Deficit
6.5.3 Dressing/Grooming Self Care Deficit
6.5.4 Toileting Self Care Deficit
6.6 Altered Growth and Development
6.7 Relocation Stress Syndrome
#6.8.1 Risk for Disorganized Infant Behavior
#6.8.2 Disorganized Infant Behavior
#6.8.3 Potential for Enhanced Organized Infant Behavior

Pattern 7: Perceiving

7.1.1 Body Image Disturbance
7.1.2 Self Esteem Disturbance
7.1.2.1 Chronic Low Self Esteem
7.1.2.2 Situational Low Self Esteem
7.1.3 Personal Identity Disturbance
7.2 Sensory/Perceptual Alterations (Specify) (Visual, auditory, kinesthetic, gustatory, tactile, olfactory)
7.2.1.1 Unilateral Neglect
7.3.1 Hopelessness
7.3.2 Powerlessness

Pattern 8: Knowing

8.1.1 Knowledge Deficit (Specify)
#8.2.1 Impaired Environmental Interpretation Syndrome
#8.2.2 Acute Confusion
#8.2.3 Chronic Confusion
8.3 Altered Thought Processes
#8.3.1 Impaired Memory

Pattern 9: Feeling

9.1.1 Pain
9.1.1.1 Chronic Pain
9.2.1.1 Dysfunctional Grieving
9.2.1.2 Anticipatory Grieving
9.2.2 Risk for Violence: Self-directed or directed at others
9.2.2.1 Risk for Self-Mutilation
9.2.3 Post-Trauma Response
9.2.3.1 Rape-Trauma Syndrome
9.2.3.1.1 Rape-Trauma Syndrome: Compound Reaction
9.2.3.1.2 Rape-Trauma Syndrome: Silent Reaction
9.3.1 Anxiety
9.3.2 Fear

#New diagnoses added in 1994

APPENDIX G

Narcotic Equianalgesic Dosages

The following are dosages for equal relief of pain when used in the acute care setting for the narcotic drugs below. Chronic administration or abuse of these drugs may alter the pharmacokinetics of the drugs, resulting in varying equivalents.

Drug	Duration	Half-life	Route	Equianalgesic Dosage
Buprenorphine	4–6 h	2–3 h	IM PO	0.4 mg 0.8 mg
Butorphanol	3–4 h	2.5–3.5 h	IM	2 mg
Codeine	4–6 h	3 h	IM PO	120 mg 200 mg
Dezocine	3–6 h	2.4 h	IM	10 mg
Fentanyl	1–2 h	1.5–6 h	IM PO	0.1 mg NA
Hydrocodone	4–8 h	3.3–4.5 h	NA	NA
Levorphanol	6–8 h	12–16 h	IM PO	2 mg 4 mg
Meperidine	2–4 h	3–4 h	IM PO	75 mg 300 mg
Methadone	4–6 h	15–30 h	IM PO	10 mg 20 mg
Morphine	3–7 h	1.5–2 h	IM PO	10 mg 60 mg
Nalbuphine	4–6 h	5 h	IM	10 mg
Oxycodone	4–6 h	NA	PO	30 mg
Oxymorphone	3–6 h	NA	IM PO	1 mg 10 mg
Pentazocine	4–7 h	2–3 h	IM PO	60 mg 180 mg
Propoxyphene	4–6 h	6–12 h	PO	130/200 mg
Sufentanil	NA	2.5 h	IM	0.02 mg

APPENDIX H

Injections Information

Type	Needle gauge	Needle length	Syringe	Comments
Intradermal	26	3/8 in	Tuberculin	Area must be marked or mapped if repeated tests done.
Subcutaneous	25	1/2 in	Tuberculin, insulin	Rotate sites.
Intramuscular	20–23	1–3 in	2–3 ml	Rapid insertion and slow injection help to decrease pain.
Intravenous	20, 21		Bag with tubing.	Monitor site and needle-placement.
Blood	16, 18		Bag with tubing.	Check equipment, needle placement, and injection site regularly.

Injection Procedures

Intradermal injection: Inject directly below the surface of the skin. The injection should produce a wheal or fluid-filled bump that can be seen beneath the skin at the injection site. Skin on the back of the forearm is the usual site for these injections. The area should be marked or mapped for reading tests in 24–48h.

Subcutaneous injection: Inject into the loose connective tissue underneath the skin; do not inject more than 2 ml at a time. Areas of the body that can be "pinched up" are best suited—abdomen, upper thigh, upper arm. The needle is inserted at 45

Subcutaneous injection sites. (Earnest, V.V. [1992]. Clinical skills in nursing practice, 2nd ed. [p. 864]. Philadelphia: J.B. Lippincott.)

Amy M. Karch: Lippincott's Nursing Drug Guide. ©1996 J. B. Lippincott Company

Chart for rotating subcutaneous sites. **A.** Nurse using arm and abdomen. **B.** Client using abdomen and thighs. (Earnest, V.V. [1992]. Clinical skills in nursing practice, 2nd ed. [p. 864]. Philadelphia: J.B. Lippincott.)

degrees; the plunger is pulled back to assure that no blood returns and the needle is not in a vein; if no blood returns, inject solution. Subcutaneous sites should be rotated for frequent injections. Monitor sites for signs of abscess or necrotic tissue. Do not use this method for patients in shock, and monitor patients with poor perfusion or low blood pressure, as the drug may not be absorbed or may be absorbed very slowly.

(text continues on page 1235)

Intramuscular injection sites. ***A.*** Landmarks for the dorsogluteal injection site. ***B.*** Landmarks for the ventrogluteal injection site. *(continued)*

Intramuscular injection sites *(continued)*. ***C.*** Landmarks for the deltoid injection site. ***D.*** Landmarks for the vastus lateralis injection site. *(continued)*

Intramuscular injection: Insert needle quickly into big muscle; pull the plunger back to assure that no blood returns and the needle is not in a vein; if no blood returns, inject slowly. Position the patient to relax the muscle, which will increase blood flow, aid absorption, and decrease pain. Vastus lateralis muscle of the thigh is site of choice for children up to 3 y; ventrogluteal muscle is the site of choice for older children and adults; deltoid muscle and gluteus maximus are other possible sites in special situations.

Intramural injection sites *(continued)*. **E.** Landmarks for the rectus femoris injection site. (Earnest, V.V. [1992]. Clinical skills in nursing practice, 2nd ed. [pp. 865–866]. Philadelphia: JB Lippincott)

Z-Track: Very irritating or staining solutions may be given by Z-track technique. The skin is prepped and pulled very tightly to one side; the needle is inserted into the muscle; the drug is injected as the needle is withdrawn slowly, and the skin released. This procedure allows the various overlapping layers of tissue to slide back into position in a Z formation, sealing off the injected material.

APPENDIX I

Patient Teaching Guide

Instructions:

1. The name of your drug is _____.
2. The dose of the drug that is ordered for you is _____.
3. Special storage instructions for your drug include _____.
4. The drug should be taken _____ times a day. The best time to take your drug is _____, _____, etc.
5. The drug should (not) be taken with meals, because food will affect the way the drug is absorbed.
6. Special activities that should be considered when taking this drug include _____.
7. Some effects of this drug that you may experience include:
8. Do not take this drug with other drugs, including over-the-counter medications without first checking with your health care provider.
9. Tell any nurse, physician, or dentist who is taking care of you that you are taking this drug.
10. Keep this and all medications out of the reach of children.

Notify your nurse of physician if any of the following occur:

1. (specific signs or symptoms associated with drug toxicity)
2. Abrupt stoppage of this drug can cause _____.

Whenever a patient is given the responsibility for drug administration, there are certain facts to which the patient should have ready access. Some states require that patients be given written information about their drugs. Nursing care always includes patient teaching activities. This teaching guide is a sample of one that can be redesigned for individual needs, then copied for distribution to the patient, and just the specific information about each drug—which is found in the patient teaching section of each drug monograph—can be added for a quick, precise teaching aid. The patient needs to know: what the drug is and the dosage prescribed, especially if the patient sees more then one physician or travels; special storage information; how many times a day and *when* the drug should be taken; how to take the drug in relation to meals; specific adverse effects that are expected with this drug; special precautions or activities that are related to the use of this drug, including follow-up visits or tests; signs and symptoms to report to the health care provider; and dangers of abrupt stoppage of the drug. Good practice also requires reminding the patient to avoid all other medications (including OTC drugs) until checking first with his or her health care provider; keep drugs away from children; and report to any other health care provider that he or she is taking this drug.

APPENDIX J
Adjuncts to Anesthetics

Neuromuscular junction (NMJ) blocking agents (nondepolarizing type) and depolarizing agents are used as adjuncts to general anesthetics to produce paralysis.

Therapeutic Actions
NMJ blockers interfere with neuromuscular transmission and cause flaccid paralysis by blocking acetylcholine receptors at the skeletal neuromuscular junction; succinylcholine is a depolarizing agent that blocks the cholinergic receptors of the motor endplate and causes paralysis of short duration.

Indications
These drugs are used as adjuncts to general anesthetics, to facilitate endotracheal intubation and relax skeletal muscle and to relax skeletal muscle in order to facilitate mechanical ventilation.

Contraindications/Cautions: Pregnancy Category C
These drugs are contraindicated in the presence of allergy to NMJ drug; myasthenia gravis; Eaton-Lambert syndrome; labor and delivery (drug has been used safely during cesarean section, but the dose may need to be lowered in patients receiving magnesium sulfate to manage pre-eclampsia. Caution should be used in the presence of carcinoma, renal or hepatic disease, respiratory depression, or altered fluid/electrolyte balance.

Dosage
Primarily administered by anesthesiologists who are skilled in administering artificial respiration and oxygen under positive pressure; facilities for these procedures must be on standby.

Adverse Effects
Depressed respiration, *apnea, histamine release causing wheezing,* bronchospasm; *increased or decreased P, hypotension, vasodilitation—flushing;* profound and prolonged muscle paralysis.

Important Drug-Drug Interactions
- Increased intensity and duration of neuromuscular block with some anesthetics (isoflurane, enflurane, halothane, diethyl ether, methoxyflurane), some parenteral antibiotics (aminoglycosides, clindamycin, capreomycin, vancomycin, lincomycin, bacitracin, polymyxin B, and sodium colistimethate), ketamine, quinine, quinidine, trimethaphan, carbamazepine, diazepam, azathioprine, mercaptopurine, calcium channel-blocking drugs (verapamil, etc.), Mg2+ salts, and in hypokalemia (produced by K+ depleting diuretics).
- Decreased intensity of block with acetylcholine, cholinesterase inhibitors, K+ salts., phenytoin
- Reversal of neuromuscular blockage if taken with aminophylline, dyphylline, oxtriphylline, theophylline

Implementation
- Have on standby, neostigmine, pyridostigmine, or edrophonium (cholinesterase inhibitors) to overcome excessive neuromuscular block; atropine or glycopyrrolate, to prevent parasympathomimetic effects of cholinesterase inhibitors.

Adverse effects in *Italics* are most common; those in **Bold** are life-threatening.

- Change patient's position frequently and provide skin care to prevent decubitus ulcer formation when drug is used for other than brief periods.
- Monitor conscious patient for pain, distress that patient may not be able to communicate, and frequently reassure patient.

Drug Specific Teaching Points

When a patient is conscious during the use of this drug (ventilator, etc.) include the following points:
- Tell patient drug is being used to paralyze muscles to facilitate treatment.
- Carefully explain all procedures; remember that the patient is not capable of verbal communication but can hear and see.

Adjuncts to Anesthetics

atracurium besylate	*Tracrium*	NMJ blocker	Has no effect on pain threshold or consciousness; do not use before induction of unconsciousness; bradycardia during anesthesia is more common with this drug.
doxacurium chloride	*Nuromax*	NMJ blocker	Contains benzyl alcohol and should not be used with premature infants; monitor patient for recovery, prolongation of blockade may occur requiring supportive care.
gallamine triethiodide	*Flaxedil*	NMJ blocker	May be used long-term to manage ventilator patients; monitor patients for increased heart rate.
metocurine iodide		NMJ blocker	Do not give IM; used as adjunct to electroshock therapy.
mivacurium chloride	*Mivacron*	NMJ blocker	Has no effect on pain threshold or consciousness; do not use before unconsciousness has been induced.
pancuronium bromide	*Pavulon*	NMJ blocker	Used long-term to manage patients on mechanical ventilators; monitor patients for prolongation of neuromuscular effects beyond the time needed or anticipated by drug use; supportive care may be needed.
pipecuronium bromide	*Arduan*	NMJ blocker	Recommended only for procedures anticipated to last ≤90 min. Monitor patient for prolongation of neuromuscular blockade; provide supportive care.
rocuronium bromide	*Zemuron*	NMJ blocker	1–2 min onset; short-acting; relatively new drug.
succinylcholine chloride	*Anectine, Quelicin, Sucostrin*	Depolarizer	Used as adjunct to ECT and for prolonged use on mechanical ventilators; monitor patient for histamine release and resulting hypotension and flushing; monitor patient during recovery for prolonged paralysis and provide supportive care.
tubocurarine chloride		NMJ blocker	Used for diagnosis of myasthenia gravis and for electroshock therapy. Do not use any solution that has developed a faint color.
vecuronium bromide	*Norcuron*	NMJ blocker	Has no effect on pain threshold or consciousness; do not use before unconsciousness has been induced. Prolongation of neuromuscular blockade has been reported; monitor patient during recovery and provide supportive care.

APPENDIX K

Ophthalmic Agents

Ophthalmic agents are drugs that are intended for direct administration into the conjunctiva of the eye. These drugs are used to treat glaucoma (miotics constrict the pupil and decrease the resistance to aqueous flow), to aid in diagnosis of eye problems (mydriatics—dilate the pupil for examination of the retina; cyclopegics paralyze the muscles that control the lens to aid refraction), or treat local ophthalmic infections or inflammation; and to provide relief from the signs and symptoms of allergic reactions.

Pregnancy Category C
Contraindicated in cases of allergy to these drugs. These drugs are seldom absorbed systemically, but caution should be taken with any patient who would have problems with the systemic effects of the drug if it were absorbed systemically.

Adverse Effects
Local irritation, stinging, burning, blurring of vision (prolonged when using ointment), tearing; headache.

Dosage
1–2 drops to each eye bid to qid or .25–.5 in of ointment to each eye is the usual dosage.

Solution/drops
Wash hands thoroughly before administering; do not touch dropper to eye or to any other surface; have patient tilt head backward or lie down, stare upward; gently grasp lower eyelid and pull the eyelid away from the eyeball; instill drop(s) into pouch formed by eyelid; release lid slowly; have patient close eye and look downward; apply gentle pressure to the inside corner of the eye for 3–5 min to retard drainage; do not rub eyes; do not rinse eyedropper. Do not use eyedrops that have changed color; if more than one type of eyedrop is used, wait 5 min between administration.

Ointment
Wash hands thoroughly before administering; hold tube between hands for several minutes to warm the ointment; discard the first cm of ointment when opening the tube for the first time; tilt head backward or lie down and stare upward; gently pull out lower lid to form pouch; place 0.25–0.5 in of ointment inside the lower lid; have patient close eyes for 1–2 min and roll eyeball in all directions; remove any excess ointment from around eye. If using more than one kind of ointment, wait 10 min between administration.

Drug Specific Teaching Points
Teach patient the proper administration technique for the ophthalmic agent ordered; caution patients that transient stinging or burning may occur and that blurring vision may also occur—appropriate safety measures should be taken; sensitivity to sun will occur with mydriatic agents which cause pupils to dilate, sunglasses may be needed; report severe eye discomfort, palpitations, nausea, headache.

Adverse effects in *Italics* are most common; those in **Bold** are life-threatening.

Ophthalmic Agents

Drug	Brand Names	Usage	Special Considerations
apraclonidine	*Lopidine*	To control or prevent postsurgical elevations of IOP in patients after argon-laser eye surgery.	Monitor for the possibility of vasovagal attack; do not give to patients with allergy to clonidine.
carbachol	*Miostat* *Isopto Carbachol*	Direct acting miotic; for treatment of glaucoma; for miosis during surgery.	Surgical dose a one-use only portion; 1–2 gt up to tid as needed for glaucoma.
cyclopentolate	*Cyclogyl*	Mydriasis/cycloplegia in diagnostic procedures.	Individuals with dark pigmented irides may require higher doses; compress lacrimal sac for 1–2 min after admin. to decrease any systemic absorption.
dapiprazole	*Rev-Eyes*	Miotic: iatrogenically induced mydriasis produced by adrenergic or parasympathetic agents	Not for use to reduce IOP; do not use if constriction is undesirable. Do not use more than once a week.
demecarium	*Humorsol*	Treatment of glaucoma and strabismus; cholinesterase inhibitor.	If response is not adequate in first 24h, consider another drug. Do not use more often than necessary—1–2 gt/wk up to 1–2 gt/d have been used.
echothiopate	*Phospholine Iodide*	Treatment of glaucoma; irreversible cholinesterase inhibitor; long-acting. Accommodative esotropia.	Given only once a day because of long action; tolerance may develop with prolonged use, usually responds to a rest period.
fluorometholone	*Fluor-op, FML*	Topical corticosteroid used for treatment of inflammatory conditions of the eye.	Improvement should occur within several days, discontinue if no improvement is seen. Discontinue if swelling of the eye occurs.
homatropine	*Isopto-Homatropine* *Homatropine HBr*	Long-acting mydriatic and cycloplegic used for refraction and treatment of inflammatory conditions of the uveal tract.	Individuals with dark pigmented irides may require larger doses; 5–10 min is usually required for refraction.
idoxuridine (IDU)	*Herplex*	Antiviral; used to treat herpes simplex keratitis	Transient burning and stinging may occur; reconsider drug if improvement is not seen within 7–8 d. Do not administer for longer than 21 d at a time. Protect drug from light; do not mix with other medications.

(Continued)

Ophthalmic Agents (Continued)

Drug	Brand Names	Usage	Special Considerations
levocabastine	*Livostin*	Relief of allergic conjunctivitis	Treatment may be needed for up to 2 wk. Do not wear soft contact lenses during use of this drug. Shake well before use and do not use any discolored solution.
lodoxamide	*Alomide*	Treatment of vernal conjunctivitis and keratitis	Patients should not wear contact lenses while using this drug; discontinue if stinging and burning persist after instillation.
metipropranolol	*OptiPranolol*	Beta blocker; used in treating chronic open-angle glaucoma and ocular hypertension.	Concomitant therapy may be needed; caution patient about possible vision changes.
natamycin	*Natacyn*	Antibiotic used to treat fungal blepharitis, conjunctivitis and keratitis; drug of choice for *Fusarium sotani* keratitis.	Shake well before each use; store at room temp.; failure to improve in 7–10 d suggests a nonsusceptible organism, re-evaluate.
pilocarpine	*Pilocar Piloptic Pilostat Ocu-Carpine Akarpine*	Chronic and acute glaucoma; treatment of mydriasis caused by drugs; direct acting miotic agent.	Can be stored at room temp. for up to 8 wk, then discard. 1–2 gt up to 6 times/d may be needed, based on patient response.
physostigmine	*Eserine, Isopto Eserine*	Miotic, cholinesterase inhibitor; used only for reduction of IOP in primary glaucoma.	Headache may occur and may be unresponsive to analgesics; avoid night driving or performing tasks in low light.
rimexolone	*Vexal*	Corticosteroid; postop ocular surgery and for treatment of anterior uveitis.	Monitor for signs of steroid absorption.
suprofen	*Profenal*	NSAID; used to inhibit intraoperative miosis	Local burning may occur; monitor patient for any cross sensitivities to other NSAIDs.
trifluridine	*Viroptic*	Antiviral; used to treat primary keratoconjunctivitis and recurrent epithelial keratitis due to herpes simplex virus types 1 & 2	Transient burning and stinging may occur; reconsider drug if improvement is not seen within 7 d. Do not administer for longer than 21 d at a time.

APPENDIX L: Drug Compatibility Guide

1244 ■ Appendix L

	aminophylline	amphotericin B	ampicillin	atropine	calcium gluconate	carbenicillin	cefazolin	cimetidine	clindamycin	diazepam	dopamine	epinephrine	erythromycin	fentanyl	furosemide	gentamicin	glycopyrrolate	heparin sodium	hydrocortisone	hydroxyzine	levarterenol	lidocaine	meperidine	morphine	nitroglycerin	pentobarbital	potassium chloride	sodium bicarbonate	tetracycline	vancomycin	verapamil	vitamin B & C complex
aminophylline	*	N	Y		Y	N	N		N		Y	N	N			N		Y	Y	N	N	Y	N	N	Y	Y	Y	Y	N	N	Y	N
amphotericin B	N		N		N	N		N			N		N			N		Y	Y			N					N		N		N	
ampicillin	Y	N	*	N	N	Y	Y		N		N		N					Y	N			Y					Y	Y	N		Y	Y
atropine			N	*				Y				N		Y			Y	N		Y		Y	Y	Y		N	Y	N			Y	Y
calcium gluconate	Y	N	N		*			N		N	Y	N	Y					Y	Y	Y	N	Y					Y	N	N		Y	Y
carbenicillin	N	N	Y			*		Y	Y		Y	N	N		Y	N			Y		Y	Y				N	Y	N	N		Y	Y
cefazolin	N		Y				*	N					N			N			Y		N	N				N	Y		N		Y	N
cimetidine		N		Y	N	Y	N	*	Y			Y	Y		Y	Y		Y	Y		Y	Y	Y		Y		Y		Y	Y	Y	Y
clindamycin	N		N		N	Y		Y	*						N	Y		Y				N		N		N	Y	Y			Y	Y
diazepam	Y		N							*		N					Y	N	Y			N					N				Y	Y
dopamine	Y	N	N		Y	Y					*		N			N		N				Y					N				Y	Y
epinephrine	N		N	N	N	N		Y		N		*	N														Y	Y			Y	Y
erythromycin	N		N		Y	N	N	Y			N	N	*														Y	N	N	Y	Y	Y
fentanyl				Y										*						Y			Y	Y		N						

Appendix L — 1245

furosemide					Y						Y		*		Y			N		Y	Y
gentamicin	N											N							Y	Y	Y
glycopyrrolate		Y																Y			Y
heparin sodium	Y	Y	Y		Y	Y	N		Y	Y	N	Y		Y	Y	*	N	Y	Y	Y	Y
hydrocortisone	Y	Y	Y	N	N	N					Y				Y	Y	Y	N	Y	*	Y
hydroxyzine	N		Y	N	Y				N	Y						N			Y	Y	Y
levarterenol	N			N		N	Y		N	N		Y			*	*	Y	Y	N	N	N
lidocaine	Y	Y		Y	Y	Y	Y	Y	Y	Y	*	Y	Y	Y	Y		Y	Y		Y	Y
meperidine	N	Y	Y	Y	Y	Y			N	N		Y			*		Y	N	Y	*	Y
morphine	N		Y	Y	Y		Y	Y	N	N		Y			N	*	N	N		Y	Y
nitroglycerin	Y					Y											*				Y
pentobarbital	Y	N		N	Y				N	N		Y	Y		N	Y	Y	N	N	Y	Y
potassium chloride	Y	Y	Y	Y	Y	Y	N	Y	N			Y	Y		Y	Y	Y	Y	Y	Y	Y
sodium bicarbonate	Y	Y	N	N	Y	N	N	Y				Y	Y		Y	Y	Y	N	Y	*	Y
tetracycline	N		N	N	N	N	*	N				N	Y	N		N	Y		N	Y	N
vancomycin	N		Y	Y	Y	Y		Y	Y			Y	Y	Y	N		Y		Y	Y	Y
verapamil	Y	Y	Y	Y	Y	Y	Y	Y	Y	Y	Y	Y	Y	Y		Y	Y	Y	Y	*	Y
vitamin B & C complex	N	Y	Y	Y	Y	N	N	Y	Y	Y	Y	Y	Y	Y	N	Y	Y	N	Y	Y	*

NOTE: Because the compatibility of two or more drugs in solution depends on several variables such as the solution itself, drug concentration and the method of mixing (bottle, syringe, or Y-site), this table is intended to be used solely as a guide to general drug compatibilities. Before mixing any drugs, the health-care professional should ascertain if a potential incompatibility exists by referring to an appropriate information source.

KEY:
Y = Compatible
N = Incompatible
Blank space = Information about compatibility was not available

(Reprinted from Malseed, R.T., Goldstein, F.J. & Balkon, N. (1995). *Pharmacology: Drug Therapy and Nursing Management* (4th ed) Philadelphia: JB Lippincott Co. Used with permission.)

APPENDIX M: Quick Check: Compatibility of Drugs in Syringe

	atropine	butorphanol	chlorpromazine	cimetidine	dimenhydrinate	dimenhydramine	fentanyl	glycopyrrolate	heparin	hydroxyzine	meperidine	metoclopramide	midazolam	morphine	nalbuphine	pentazocine	pentobarbital	prochlorperazine	promethazine	ranitidine	secobarbital	thiopental
atropine		Y	Y	Y	M	M	M	Y	M	Y	Y	M	Y	M	Y	M	M	M	M	Y		
butorphanol	Y		Y	Y	N	Y	Y			Y	M		Y	Y		Y	N	Y	Y			
chlorpromazine	Y	Y		N	N	M	M	Y	N	M	M	M	Y	M		M	N	Y	M	Y		N
cimetidine	Y	Y	N			Y	Y	Y	Y	Y	Y		Y	Y	Y	Y	N	Y	Y		N	
dimenhydrinate	M	N	N			M	M		M	N	M	M	N	M		M	N	N	N			N
dimenhydramine	M	Y	M	Y	M		Y			M	M	M	Y	M		M	N	M	M	Y		N
fentanyl	M	Y	M	Y	M	Y				Y	M	Y	Y	M		M	N	Y	Y	Y		
glycopyrrolate	Y		Y	Y						Y	Y		Y	Y		Y	N	Y	Y	Y		
heparin	M		N	Y	M		M				N	M	Y	N		N	N		N	Y	N	N

Appendix M

drug																
hydroxyzine	Y	Y	M	Y	N	Y	M	Y	Y	M	Y	M	N	M		
meperidine	Y	M	M	Y	M	Y	Y	M	Y	Y	Y	N	M	Y		N
metoclopramide	M		M	M	Y	M	Y	N	Y	M	M	M	M	Y		
midazolam	Y	Y	Y	N	Y	Y	Y	Y	Y	Y	Y		N	M		N
morphine	M	Y	M	M	Y	M	Y	M	Y	Y	Y	N	M	Y		
nalbuphine	Y	Y		Y		Y	Y	Y	Y	Y	Y	N	Y	M		
pentazocine	M	Y	M	M	Y		M	Y	M	Y	Y	N	M	Y		
pentobarbital	M	N	N	Z	M	N	M		M	N	N	Y	N	Y		Y
prochlorperazine	M	Y	Y	M	Y	Y	M	N	Y	M	M	N	M	M		
promethazine	M	M.	M	Y	Y	Y	M	N	M	Y	Y	N	M	Y		
ranitidine	Y	Y	Y	Y	Y		Y	Y	Y	Y	Y		Y	Y		
secobarbital			N												Y	
thiopental		N		N		Y		Y	N	N	N		Y	N		Y

KEY:
Y = Compatible in syringe
M = Moderately compatible, inject immediately after combining
N = Incompatible, do not mix in syringe
Blank space = Information about compatibility is not currently available

Bibliography

Drug evaluations subscription (1994). Chicago: American Medical Association.

Carpenito, L.J. (1995). *Nursing diagnosis* (6th ed.). Philadelphia: J.B. Lippincott Company.

Drug facts and comparisons (1994). St. Louis, MO: J.B. Lippincott Company.

Tatro, D.S. (Ed.). (1994). *Drug interaction facts.* St. Louis, MO: J.B. Lippincott Company.

Gilman, A.G., Goodman, L.S., Rall, T.W., and Murad, F. (Eds.). (1993) *Goodman and Gilman's the pharmacological basis of therapeutics* (8th ed.) New York: MacMillan.

Handbook of adverse drug interactions. (1994). New Rochelle, NY: The Medical Letter.

Katzung, B.G. (1987). *Basic and clinical pharmacology* (3rd ed.). Norwalk, Connecticut: Appleton and Lange.

Levine R.R. (1993). *Pharmacology: Drug actions and reactions (3rd ed.).* Boston: Little, Brown.

Lindberg, J. et al. (1989). *Introduction to Nursing.* Philadelphia: J.B. Lippincott Company.

Malseed, R. (1995). *Textbook of pharmacology and nursing care.* Philadelphia: J.B. Lippincott Company.

PDR for nonprescription drugs. (1994). Oradell, NJ: Medical Economics Company.

PDR for ophthalmology. (1994). Oradell, NJ: Medical Economics Company.

Physicians' desk reference (41st ed.). Oradell, NJ: Medical Economics Company.

Professionals guide to patient drug facts. (1994). St. Louis, MO: J.B. Lippincott Company.

Rodman, M.J., Karch, A.M., Boyd, E.H., and Smith, D.W. (1985). *Pharmacology and drug therapy in nursing* (3rd ed.). Philadelphia: J.B. Lippincott Company.

Smeltzer, S.C., & Bare, B.G. (1992). *Brunner and Suddarth's textbook of medical-surgical nursing* (7th ed.). Philadelphia: J.B. Lippincott.

Spencer, Nichols, Waterhouse, et al. (1993). *Clinical pharmacology and nursing management.* Philadelphia: J.B. Lippincott Company.

The medical letter on drugs and therapeutics (1994). New Rochelle, NY: Medical Letter.

Griffiths, M.C. (Ed.). (1987) *USAN 1987 and the USP dictionary of drug names.* Rockville, MD: United States Pharmacopeial Convention.

Index

Index

Official generic names are shown in **bold**. Brand names of drugs are shown in *italics*, followed by the generic name in parentheses. Brand names of drugs that are Canadian are followed by (CAN). Chemical or nonofficial names appear in plain print. Drug Classes appear in **BOLD CAPITALs** with the drugs that fall in that class listed as official names under the class heading.

A

A (vitamin A): 1208
Abbokinase (urokinase): 1125
Abbokinase Open-Cath (urokinase): 1125
ABORTIFACIENTS
   carboprost: 215
   dinoprostone: 395
absorbable gelatin: 1215
Accupril (quinapril): 964
Accurbron (theophylline): 1056
Accutane (isotretinoin): 610
acebutolol hydrochloride: 57
Acel-Imune (diphtheria and tetanus toxoids and acellular pertussis vaccine): 1160
Aceon (perindopril): 874
Acephen (acetaminophen): 58
Aceta (acetaminophen): 58
Ace-Tabs (CAN) (acetaminophen): 58
acetaminophen: 58
Acet-Amp (CAN) (theophylline): 1056
acetazolamide: 60
acetohexamide: 62
acetohydroxamic acid: 63
acetophenazine maleate: 64
acetylcycsteine: 66
Aches-N-Pain (ibuprofen): 576
Achromycin Ophthalmic (tetracycline):1052
Achromycin V (tetracycline): 1052
aclometasone dipropionate: 1217
Aclovate (aclometasone): 1217
ACNE PRODUCTS
   isotretinoin: 610
ACT (dactinomycin): 342
ACTH (corticotropin): 321
Acthar (corticotropin): 321
ACTHIB-DTP (diphtheria and tetanus toxoids and pertussis vaccine with haemophilus influenzae b vaccine): 1161
Actidose-Aqua (charcoal): 256
Actidose with Sorbital (charcoal): 256
Actigall (ursodiol): 1127
Actimmune (interferon gamma-1b): 596
actinomycin D (dactinomycin): 342
Activase (alteplase): 83
Activated Charcoal (charcoal): 256
ACU-dyne (povidone iodine): 1213
Acular (ophthalmic) (keterolac): 619
acycloguanosine (acyclovir): 69
acyclovir: 69
acyclovir sodium: 69
Adalat (nifedipine): 793
adenocorticotropin (corticotropin): 321
adenosine: 70
adenosine arabinoside (vidarabine): 1136
Adenocard (adenosine): 70
Adipex-P (phentermine): 1152
Adipost (phentermine): 1152
ADJUNCTS TO ANESTHETICS (see page 1238)
   atracurium: 1239
   doxacurium: 1239
   gallamine: 1239
   metocurine iodide: 1239
   mivacurium: 1239
   pancuronium: 1239
   pipercuronium: 1239
   rocuronium: 1239
   succinylcholine: 1239
   tubocurarine: 1239
   vecuronium: 1239
ADR (doxorubicin): 413
adrenaline (epinephrine): 430
Adrenaline Chloride (epinephrine): 430

1254 ■ Index

ADRENAL CORTICAL HORMONES
  cortisone: 323
  hydrocortisone: 561
ADRENAL CYTOTOXIC DRUGS
  mitotane: 754
ADRENERGIC AGONISTS
  alpha
    dopamine: 405
    metaraminol: 700
    phenylephrine: 888
  alpha and beta
    epinephrine: 430
    norepinephrine: 802
  beta
    albuterol: 73
    bitolterol: 178
    dobutamine: 404
    dopamine: 405
    isoetharine: 602
    isoproterenol: 605
    metaproterenol: 699
    pirbuterol: 902
    ritodrine: 983
    salmeterol: 985
    terbutaline: 1045
ADRENERGIC BLOCKERS
  alpha (see page 8)
    doxazosin: 409
    phenoxybenzamine: 884
    phentolamine: 887
    prazosin: 916
    terazosin: 1044
  alpha and beta
    amiodarone: 102
    bretylium: 181
    guanadrel: 542
    guanethidine: 542
    labetalol: 620
    rauwolfia: 975
  beta (see page 26)
    acebutolol: 57
    atenolol: 135
    betaxolol: 170
    bisoprolol: 176
    carteolol: 219
    esmolol: 443
    metrolol: 737
    nadolol: 766
    penbutolol: 854
    pindolol: 897
    propranolol: 947
    sotalol: 1008
    timolol: 1076

ADRENERGIC NEURON BLOCKERS
  bretylium: 181
  guanadrel: 542
  guanethidine: 542
  rauwolfia: 975
Adriamycin (doxorubicin): 413
Adrin (nylidrin): 1206
Adrucil (fluorouracil): 500
Advil (ibuprofen): 576
A-E-R (hamamelis water): 1212
Aerobid (flunisolide): 499
Aerodine (povidone iodine): 1213
Aeroid (thimersol): 1213
Aerolate (theophylline): 1056
Aeroseb-Dex (dexamethasone): 358, 1219
Aerosporin (polymyxin B): 907
Afrin (oxymetazoline): 833
Afrin Repetabs (pseudoephedrine): 954
Aftate (tolnaftate): 1214
Agoral Plain (mineral oil): 1204
AHA (acetohydroxamic acid): 63
AHF (antihemophilic factor): 124
A-hydroCort (hydrocortisone): 561
a-2-interferon (interferon alfa-2b): 591
Airbron (CAN) (acetylcysteine): 66
Akarpine (pilocarpine): 1242
AK-Dex (dexamethasone): 358
AK-Dex Ophthalmic (dexamethasone): 358
AK-Dilate (phenylephrine): 888
Akineton (biperiden): 173
AK-Mycin (erythromycin): 440
AK-Nefrin (phenylephrine): 888
Akne-mycin (erythromycin): 440
AK-Pred (prednisolone): 918
AK-Tate (prednisolone): 918
AK-Tracin (bacitracin): 151
albumin, human: 72
Albuminar-5 (albumin): 72
Albuminar-25 (albumin): 72
Albutein 5% (albumin): 72
Albutein 25% (albumin): 72
albuterol: 73
albuterol sulfate: 73
Alcomicin (CAN) (gentamycin): 525
Alcon-efrin (phenylephrine): 888
Aldactazide (spironolactone and
        hydrochlorothiazide): 1198
Aldactone (spironolactone): 1012
aldesleukin: 75
Aldomet (methyldopa): 723
ALDOSTERONE ANTAGONIST
  spironolactone: 1012

Index ■ 1255

Aleve (naproxen): 778
Alferon N (interferon alfa-N3): 593
alglucerase: 77
Alka-Seltzer (aspirin): 131
Alkeran (melphalan): 680
ALKYLATING AGENTS (see page 7)
    busulfan: 194
    carboplatin: 213
    carmustine: 217
    chlorambucil: 259
    cisplatin: 291
    cyclophosphamide: 331
    ifosfamide: 579
    lomustine: 649
    mechlorethamine: 670
    melphalan: 680
    streptozocin: 1020
    thiotepa: 1067
    uracil mustard: 1121
Allerest 12 Hour Nasal (oxymetazoline): 833
Allerest Nasal (phenylephrine): 888
allopurinol: 78
Alomide (lodoxamide): 1242
Alophen Pills (phenolphthalein): 1204
Alpha-Baclofen (CAN) (baclofen): 152
Alphamid (castor oil): 1203
alpha1-proteinase inhibitor: 79
alpha-1-PL (alpha 1 proteinase inhibitor): 79
Alpha-Tamoxifen (CAN)(tamoxifen): 1040
Alphatrex (betamethasone): 167
alprazolam: 80
alprostadil: 82
Altace (ramipril): 972
Alterna GEL (aluminum): 86
alteplase, recombinant: 83
altretamine: 85
Alu-Cap (aluminum): 86
aluminum acetate: 1212
aluminum carbonate gel: 86
aluminum hydroxide gel: 86
aluminum phosphate gel: 86
Alupent (metaproterenol): 699
Alurate (aprobarbital): 127
Alu-Tab (aluminum): 86
ALZHEIMER'S DRUG
    tacrine: 1037
amantadine hydrochloride: 88
Ambien (zolpidem): 1149
AMEBICIDES
    chloroquine: 265
    iodoquinol: 598
    metronidazole: 739
    paromomycin: 849

ambenonium chloride: 89
amcinonide: 1217
Amcort (triamcinolone): 1093
Amen (medroxyprogesterone): 674
Amersol (CAN) (ibuprofen): 576
amethopterin (methotrexate): 714
Amicar (aminocaproic acid): 96
Amidate (etomidate): 1155
Amigesic (salsalate): 986
Amikacin (amikacin): 91
amikacin sulfate: 91
Amikin (amikacin): 91
amiloride hydrochloride: 93
Aminess (amino acids): 94
amino acids: 94
aminocaproic acid: 96
aminoglutethimide: 97
AMINOGLYCOSIDES (see page 9)
    amikacin: 91
    gentamicin: 525
    kanamycin: 614
    neomycin: 782
    netilmicin: 786
    streptomycin: 1018
    tobramycin: 1079
Amino-Opti-C (vitamin P): 1210
Amino-Opti-E (vitamine E): 1209
aminophylline: 99
4-AMINOQUINOLONES
    chloroquine: 265
    hydroxychlorquine: 570
8-AMINOQUINOLONES
    primaquine: 922
5-aminosalicylic acid (mesalamine): 694
Aminosyn (amino acids): 94
amiodarone hydrochloride: 102
amitriptyline hydrochloride: 104
amlodipine: 106
AMMONIA REDUCTION AGENT
    lactulose: 622
ammonia spirit, aromatic: 108
ammoniated mercury: 1213
ammonium chloride: 108
amobarbital: 109
amobarbital sodium: 109
Amoline (aminophylline): 99
amoxapine: 112
amoxicillin: 114
Amoxil (amoxicillin): 114
AMPHETAMINE
    dextroamphetamine: 367
Amphojel (aluminum): 86

amphotericin B: 116
ampicillin: 118
ampicillin sodium: 118
Ampicin (CAN) (ampicillin): 118
amrinone lactate: 120
amylbarbitone (amobarbital): 109
amyl nitrate: 121
Amyl Nitrate Aspirols (amyl nitrate): 121
Amyl Nitrate Vaporole (amyl nitrate): 121
Amytal Sodium (amobarbital): 109
ANABOLIC STEROIDS
  nandrolone: 777
  oxandrolone: 824
  oxymetholone: 835
  stanozolol: 1014
Anadrol 50 (oxymetholone): 835
Anafranil (clomipramine): 303
ANALEPTICS
  caffeine: 200
  doxapram: 408
ANALGESICS, NARCOTIC AGONISTS
  codeine: 315
  dezocine: 371
  hydromorphone: 567
ANALGESICS, NON-NARCOTIC
  acetaminophen: 58
  aspirin: 131
  choline magnesium trisalicylate: 282
  choline salicylate: 283
  diclofenac: 577
  diflunisal: 384
  etodolac: 469
  fenoprofen: 481
  flurbiprofen: 510
  ibuprofen: 576
  ketoprofen: 618
  ketorolac: 619
  mefenamic acid: 676
  methotrimeprazine: 716
  nabumetone: 766
  naproxen: 778
  oxaprozin: 826
  salsalate: 986
  sodium thiosalicylate: 1005
Anamid (CAN) (kanamycin): 614
Anapolon 50 (CAN) (oxymetholone): 835
Anaprox (naproxen): 778
Anaprox DS (naproxen): 778
Ancef (CAN) (cefazolin): 225
Ancobon (flucytosine): 494
Ancotil (CAN) (flucytosine): 494
Andro-cyp (testosterone): 1050

Andro-cyp 100 (testosterone): 1050
ANDROGEN HORMONE INHIBITOR
  finasteride: 487
ANDROGENS
  danazol: 344
  fluoxymestrone: 504
  testolactone: 1049
  testosterone: 1050
Android-F (fluoxymesterone): 504
Andro L.A. (testosterone): 1050
Androlone-D (nandrolone): 777
Andronaq (testosterone): 1050
Andronaq L.A. (testosterone): 1050
Andronate (testosterone): 1050
Andropository (testosterone): 1050
Andryl 200 (tetracycline): 1052
Anectine (succinylcholine): 1239
Anergan (promethazine): 941
Anestacon (lidocaine): 636
ANGIOTENSIN CONVERTING ENZYME INHIBITORS (ACE INHIBITORS) (see page 11)
  benazepril: 155
  captopril: 207
  enalapril: 424
  fosinopril: 517
  lisinopril: 643
  quinapril: 964
  perindopril: 874
  ramipril: 972
  spirapril: 1011
Anicort (triamcinolone): 1093
anistreplase: 123
anisoylated plasminogen streptokinase activator complex (anistreplase): 123
Anorex (phendimetrazine): 1152
ANOREXIANTS (see page 1151)
  dextroamphetamine: 367
  diethylpropion: 1151
  fenfluramine: 1151
  mazindol: 1152
  phendimetrazine: 1152
  phentermine: 1152
Ansaid (flurbiprofen): 510
Antabuse (disulfiram): 402
ANTACIDS
  aluminum: 86
  calcium salts: 204
  dihydroxyaluminum: 390
  magaldrate: 660
  magnesium salts: 661
  sodium bicarbonate: 999

ANTERIOR PITUITARY HORMONE
corticotropin: 321
ANTHELMINTICS
mebendazole: 667
niclosamide: 789
oxamniquine: 823
piperazine: 900
praziquantel: 915
pyrantel: 956
quinacrine: 962
thiabendazole: 1060

Anthra-Derm (anthralin): 1213
anthralin: 1213
ANTIALCOHOLIC AGENT
disulfiram: 402
ANTIALLERGIC DRUG
cromolyn: 326
nedocromil: 780
ANTIANDROGEN
flutamide: 511
ANTIANGINAL DRUGS
amlodipine: 106
amyl nitrate: 121
bepridil: 165
diltiazem: 392
dipyridamole: 399
erythrityl: 438
isosorbide dinitrate: 609
nadolol: 767
nicardipine: 788
nifedipine: 793
nitroglycerin: 797
propranolol: 947
verapamil: 1134
ANTIANXIETY DRUGS
alprazolam: 80
amoxapine: 112
buspirone: 193
chlordiazepoxide: 263
chlorpromazine: 272
clorazepate: 309
diazepam: 372
doxepin: 410
halazepam: 541
hydroxyzine: 575
lorazepam: 654
meprobamate: 691
mesoridazine: 696
oxazepam: 827
prazepam: 914
prochlorprazine: 932
thioridazine: 1064

trifluoperazine: 1101
triflupromazine: 1103
ANTIARRHYTHMICS (see page 12)
acebutolol: 57
adenosine: 70
amiodarone: 102
bretylium: 181
disopyramide: 401
flecainide: 489
lidocaine: 636
mexiletine: 742
moricizine: 760
procainamide: 928
propafenone: 943
propranolol: 947
quinidine: 969
sotalol: 1008
tocainamide: 1081
verapamil: 1134
ANTIASTHMATIC DRUGS
albuterol: 73
bitolterol: 178
cromolyn: 326
ephedrine: 428
epinephrine: 430
isoetharine: 602
isoproterenol: 605
metaproterenol: 699
nedocromil: 780
pirbuterol: 902
salmeterol: 985
terbutaline: 1045
ANTIBACTERIALS
cinoxacin: 288
ciprofloxacin: 289
enoxacin: 426
lomefloxacin: 647
methenamine: 708
metronidazole: 739
nalidixic acid: 773
nitrofurantoin: 795
norfloxacin: 806
ofloxacin: 814
paromomycin: 849
trimethoprim: 1113
ANTIBIOTICS (see also aminoglycosides, penicillins, cephalosporins, lincosamides, macrolides, sulfonamides, tetracycline)
azetreonam: 148
bacitracin: 151

1258 ■ Index

ANTIBIOTICS (*continued*)
benzalkonium: 158
capreomycin: 206
chloramphenicol: 261
cycloserine: 333
metronidazole: 739
nafcillin: 770
polymyxin B: 907
rifabutin: 978
rifampin: 979
spectinomycin: 1010
vancomycin: 1130

ANTIBIOTICS, ANTINEOPLASTIC
bleomycin: 179
dactinomycin: 342
daunorubicin: 350
doxorubicin: 413
idarubicin: 578
mitomycin: 753
mitoxantrone: 756
pentostatin: 870
plicamycin: 905

ANTIBIOTICS, TOPICAL
mupirocin: 1213

ANTICHOLINERGICS
atropine: 138
buclizine: 186
i1glycopyrrolate: 534
cyclizine: 329
dicyclomine: 379
dimenhydrinate: 393
glycopyrrolate: 534
ipratropium: 600
meclizine: 672
methscopolamine: 719
oxyphencyclimine: 838
propantheline: 944
scopolamine: 989

ANTICOAGULANTS (see page 13)
daltepirin: 342
enoxapirin: 427
heparin: 551
warfarin: 1142

ANTICONVULSANTS
amobarbital: 109
magnesium sulfate: 662
paramethadione: 848
pentobarbital: 868
phenacemide: 877
phenobarbital: 882
secobarbital: 992
trimethadione: 1109

ANTIDEPRESSANTS
bupropion: 192
fluoxetine: 503
maprotiline: 665
nefazodone: 781
paroxetine: 850
phenelzine: 879
sertraline: 996
tranylcypramine: 1087
trazodone 1091
venlafaxine: 1133

ANTIDIABETIC AGENTS (see page 15)
acetohexamide: 62
chlorpropamide: 276
glipizide: 527
glyburide: 531
insulin: 587
metformin: 702
tolazamide: 1082
tolbutamide: 1085

ANTIDIARRHEAL DRUGS
bismuth subsalicylate: 175
loperamide: 650
opium: 819

ANTIDOTES
acetylcysteine: 66
atropine: 138
charcoal: 256
deferoxamine: 352
digoxin immune fab: 387
dimercaprol: 394
edetate disodium: 420
edrophonium: 421
flumazenil: 498
mesna: 695
methylene blue: 725
neostigmine: 784
pralidoxime: 911
pyridostigmine: 957
succimer: 1021

ANTIEMETICS
benzquinamide: 160
buclizine: 186
chlorpromazine: 272
cyclizine: 329
diphenidol: 398
dronabinol: 416
granisetron: 540
hydroxyzine: 575
meclizine: 672
metoclopramide: 734
ondansetron: 817

perphenazine: 875
prochlorperazine: 932
promethazine 941
triethylperazine: 1062
triflupromazine: 1103
trimethobenzamide: 1112
ANTIEPILEPTIC DRUGS
acetazolamide: 60
carbamazepine: 209
clonazepam: 305
clorazepate: 309
diazepam: 372
ethosuximide: 465
ethotoin: 467
gabapentin: 520
lamotrigine: 623
mephenytoin: 687
mephobarbital: 689
methsuximide: 720
phenobarbital: 882
phensuximide: 885
phenytoin: 892
primidone: 923
valproic acid: 1128
ANTIESTROGEN DRUG
tamoxifen: 1040
ANTIFLATULENT
simethicone: 997
ANTIFUNGALS (see page 17)
amphotericin B: 116
butoconazole: 198
clotrimazol: 311
fluconazole: 492
flucytosine: 494
itraconazole: 613
ketoconazole: 616
miconazole: 745
nystatin: 811
ANTIFUNGALS, TOPICAL
clotrimazole: 1214
econazole: 1214
gentian violet: 1214
naftitine: 1214
oxiconazole: 1214
terbinafine: 1214
tolnaftate: 1214
ANTIGLAUCOMA AGENTS
acetazolamide: 60
betaxolol: 170
epinephrine: 430
methazolamide: 705
timolol: 1076

ANTIGOUT DRUGS
allopurinol: 78
colchicine: 317
probenecid: 925
sulfinpyrazone: 1031
ANTIHEMOPHILIC AGENTS
antihemophilic factor: 124
factor IX complex: 473
antihemophilic factor: 124
ANTIHISTAMINES (see page 18)
astemizole: 134
azatadine: 144
brompheniramine: 185
buclizine: 186
chlorpheniramine: 271
clemastine: 296
cyclizine: 329
cyproheptadine: 336
dexchlorpheniramine: 362
dimenhydrinate: 393
diphenhydramine: 397
hydroxyzine: 575
loratidine: 652
meclizine: 672
methdilazine: 706
promethazine: 941
terfenadine: 1047
trimeprazine: 1108
tripelennamine: 1118
triprolidine: 1119
ANTIHYPERCALCEMIC DRUG
gallium: 521
ANTIHYPERLIPIDEMIC AGENTS
cholestyramine: 281
clofibrate: 301
colestipol: 319
dextrothyroxine: 370
etoposide: 470
fenofibrate: 479
fluvastatin: 512
gemfibrozil: 524
lovastatin: 656
pravastatin: 913
probucol: 927
simvastatin: 998
ANTIHYPERTENSIVE DRUGS
acebutolol: 57
amlodipine: 106
atenolol: 135
benazeprin: 155
betaxolol: 170
bisoprolol: 176

ANTIHYPERTENSIVE DRUGS (*continued*)
- captopril: 207
- carteolol: 219
- clonidine: 307
- diazoxide: 375
- diltiazem: 391
- doxazosin: 409
- enalapril: 424
- felodipine: 478
- fosinopril: 515
- guanabenz: 541
- guanadrel: 542
- guanethidine: 544
- guanfacine: 546
- hydralazine: 557
- isradipine: 612
- labetalol: 620
- lisinopril: 643
- mecamylamine: 668
- methyldopa: 723
- metoprolol: 737
- minoxidil: 750
- nadolol: 767
- nicardipine: 788
- nifedipine: 793
- nitroprusside: 800
- penbutolol: 854
- perindopril: 874
- pindolol: 897
- prazosin: 916
- propranolol: 947
- quinapril: 964
- ramipril: 972
- rauwolfia: 975
- spirapril: 1011
- terazosin: 1044
- timolol: 1076
- tolazoline: 1084
- trimethaphan: 1110
- verapamil: 1134

ANTI-INFECTIVES
- benzalkonium: 158

ANTI-INFLAMMATORY AGENTS
- aspirin: 131
- diclofenac: 377
- diflunisal: 384
- flurbiprofen: 510
- mesalamine: 694
- olsalazin: 815
- salsalate: 986
- sodium thiosalicylate: 1005

ANTILITHIC DRUG
- cellulose: 245

ANTIMANIC DRUG
- lithium: 645

ANTIMALARIALS
- chloroquine: 265
- hydroxychloroquine: 570
- mefloquine: 677
- primaquine: 922
- pyrimethamine: 959
- quincrine: 962
- quinine: 970

ANTIMETABOLITES (see page 20)
- cytaraban: 338
- floxuridine: 491
- fludarabine: 495
- fluorouracil: 500
- mercaptopurine: 693
- methotrexate: 714
- thioguanine: 1063

ANTIMIGRAINE DRUGS
- dihydroergotamine: 389
- ergotamine: 437
- methysergide: 732
- sumatriptan: 1036
- *Antimith* (pyrantel): 956

ANTI-MOTION SICKNESS AGENTS
- buclizine: 186
- cyclizine: 329
- dimenhydrinate: 393
- diphenhydramine: 397
- meclizine: 672
- promethazine: 941
- scopolamine: 989

ANTIMUSCARINIC DRUGS
- atropine: 138
- dicyclomine: 379
- glycopyrrolate: 534
- ipratropium: 600
- methscopolamine: 719
- oxyphencyclimine: 838
- propantheline: 944
- scopolamine: 989

ANTIMYASTHENIC DRUGS
- ambenonium: 89
- neostigmine: 784
- pyridostigmine: 957

ANTINEOPLASTIC DRUGS
- aldesleukin: 75
- altretamine: 85
- aminoglutethimide: 97
- asparaginase: 129

Index ■ 1261

bleomycin: 179
busulfan: 194
carboplatin: 213
carmustine: 217
chlorambucil: 259
cisplatin: 291
cladribine: 293
cyclophosphamide: 331
cytarabine: 338
dacarbazine: 340
dactinomycin: 342
daunorubicin: 350
doxorubicin: 413
estramustine: 449
etoposide: 470
floxuridine: 491
fludarabine: 495
fluorouracil: 500
goserelin: 539
hydroxyurea: 573
idaruabicin: 578
ifosfamide: 579
interferon alfa-2a: 589
interferon alfa-2b: 591
interferon alfa-n3: 593
leuprolide: 625
levamisole: 626
lomustine: 649
mechlorethamine: 670
medroxyprogesterone: 674
megestrol: 679
melphalan: 680
mercaptopurine: 693
methotrexate: 714
mitomycin: 753
mitotane: 754
mitoxantrone: 756
paclitaxel: 843
pegasparagase: 851
pentostatin: 870
plicamycin: 905
procarbazine: 930
streptozocin: 1020
teniposide: 1042
testolactone: 1049
thioguanine: 1063
thiotepa: 1067
trimetrexate: 1114
uracil mustard: 1121
vinblastine: 1138
vincristine: 1139
vinorelbine: 1141

ANTIPARKINSONISM AGENTS
amantadine: 88
atropine: 138
benztropine: 163
biperidin: 173
bromocriptine: 182
diphenhydramine: 397
levodopa: 627
pergolide: 873
procyclidine: 934
selegiline: 994
trihexyphenidyl: 1106
ANTIPEPTIC AGENTS
sucralfate: 1022
ANTIPLATELET DRUGS
aspirin: 131
dispyridamole: 399
sulfinpyrazone: 10
toclopidine: 1075
ANTIPROTOZOALS
atovaquone: 137
metronidazole: 739
pentamidine: 864
quinacrine: 962
ANTIPSORIATIC AGENT
etretinate: 471
ANTIPSORIATICS, TOPICAL
ammoniated mercury: 1213
anthralin: 1213
calcipotriene: 1214
ANTIPSYCHOTIC DRUGS
acetophenazine: 64
chlorpromazine: 272
chlorprothixene: 277
clozapine: 314
fluphenazine: 506
haloperidol: 548
loxapine: 657
mesoridazine: 696
molindone: 757
perphenazine: 875
pimoxide: 896
prochlorperazine: 932
promazine: 938
resperidone: 982
thioridazine: 1064
thiothixene: 1068
trifluoperazine: 1101
triflupromazine: 1103
ANTIPYRETIC DRUGS
acetaminophen: 58
aspirin: 131

1262 ■ Index

ANTIPYRETIC DRUGS (*continued*)
- choline magnesium trisalicylate: 282
- choline salicylate: 283
- diclolfenac: 377
- diflunisal: 384
- etodolac: 469
- oxaprozin: 826
- salsalsate: 986
- sodium thiosalicylate: 1005

ANTIRHEUMATIC AGENTS
- aspirin: 131
- auranofin: 141
- aurothioglucose: 142
- gold: 535
- hydroxychloroquine: 570
- penicillamine: 855
- salsalate: 986
- sodium thiosalicylate: 1005

ANTISEBORRHEICS
- chloroxine: 1214
- selenium: 1214

ANTISECRETORY AGENTS
- omeprazole: 816

ANTISEPTICS
- benzalkonium: 1213
- chlorhexidine: 1213
- hexachloraphene: 1213
- iodine: 1213
- povidone iodine: 1213
- sodium hypochlorite: 1213
- thimersol: 1213

Antispas (dicyclomine): 379

ANTISPASMODICS
- dicyclomine: 379
- glycopyrrolate: 534
- methscopolamine: 719
- oxyphencyclimine: 838
- propantheline: 944

antithrombin: 125

ANTITHYROID DRUGS
- methimazole: 711
- propylthiouracil: 950

ANTITUBERCULOUS DRUGS
- capreomycin: 206
- cycloserine: 333
- ethambutol: 462
- ethionamide: 464
- isoniazid: 604
- pyrazinamide: 957
- rifabutin: 978
- rifampin: 979
- streptomycin: 1018

Anti-Tuss (guaifenesin): 541

ANTITUSSIVES
- benzonatate: 160
- codeine: 316
- dextromethorphan: 369
- hydrocodone: 560
- terpin hydrate: 1048

Antivert (meclizine): 672

antivenin (crotalidae) polyvalent: 1179

Antivenin (Latrodectus maclans) (Black Widow spider species antivenin): 1179

antivenin (micrurus fulvius): 1179

ANTIVERTIGO DRUG
- diphenidol: 398
- thiethylperazine: 1062

ANTIVIRAL DRUGS (see page 21)
- acyclovir: 69
- amantadine: 88
- didanosine: 380
- famciclovir: 475
- foscarnet: 515
- ganciclovir: 522
- ribavirin: 977
- rimantadine: 981
- stavudine: 1015
- vidarabine: 1136
- zalcitabine: 1146
- zidovudine: 1147

Antrizine (meclizine): 672
Anturan (CAN) (sulfinpyrazone): 1031
Anturane (sulfinpyrazone): 1031
Anusol-HC (hydrocortisone): 1221
Anxanil (hydroxyzine): 575
A.P.L. (chorionic gonadotropin): 284
Apo-Acetazolamide (CAN) (acetazolamide): 60
Apo-Allopurinal (CAN) (allopurinol): 78
Apo-Alpraz (CAN) (alprazolam): 80
Apo-Amoxi (CAN) (amoxicillin): 114
Apo-Ampi (CAN) (ampicillin): 118
Apo-Asa (CAN) (aspirin): 131
Apo-Atenol (CAN) (atenolol): 135
Apo-Benztropine (CAN) (benztropine): 163
Apo-Capto (CAN) (captopril): 207
Apo-Carbamazepine (CAN) (carbamazepine): 209
Apo-Cephalex (CAN) (cephalexin): 249
Apo-Chlorodiazepoxide (CAN) (chlorodiazepoxide): 263
Apo-Chlorpropamide (CAN) (chlorpropamide): 276
Apo-Chlorthalidone (CAN) (chlorothalidone): 279

Index ■ 1263

Apo-Clonidine (CAN) (clonidine): 307
Apo-Clorazepate (CAN) (clorazepate): 309
Apo-Cloxi (CAN) (cloxicillin): 313
Apo-Diazepam (CAN) (diazepam): 372
Apo-Diltiaz (CAN) (diltiazem): 391
Apo-Doxy (CAN) (doxycycline): 415
Apo-Fluphenazine (CAN) (fluphenazine): 506
Apo-Haloperidol (CAN) (haloperidol): 548
Apo-Imipramine (CAN) (imipramine): 581
Apo-Indomethacin (CAN) (indomethacin): 585
Apo-Lorazepam (CAN) (lorazepam): 654
Apo-Meprobamate (CAN) (meprobamate): 691
Apo-Metronidazole (CAN) (metronidazole): 739
Apo-Naproxen (CAN) (naproxen): 778
Apo-Oxazepam (CAN) (oxazepam): 827
Apo-Perphenazine (CAN) (perphenazine): 875
Apo-Piroxicam (CAN) (piroxicam): 903
Apo-Prazo (CAN) (prazosin): 916
Apo-Prednisone (CAN) (prednisone): 921
Apo-Primidone (CAN) (primidone): 923
Apo-Propranolol (CAN) (propranolol): 947
Apo-Tamoxifen (CAN) (tamoxifen): 1040
Apo-Thioridazine (CAN) (thioridazine): 1064
Apo-Trifluoperazine (CAN) (trifluoperazine): 1101
Apo-Trihex (CAN) (trihexyphenidyl): 1106
APPG (pencillin G procaine): 861
apraclonidine: 1241
Apresoline (hydralazine): 557
aprobarbital: 127
aprotinin: 128
APSAC (anistreplase): 123
Aquacare (urea): 1212
Aquachloral Supprettes (chloral hydrate): 258
Aquamox (CAN) (quienthazone): 967
Aquaphylline (theophylline): 1056
Aquasol A (vitamin A): 1208
Aquasol E (vitamin E): 1209
Aquatensen (methylclothiazide): 721
Ara-A (vidarabine): 1136
Ara-C (cytarabine): 338
Aralen Hydrochloride (chloroquine): 265
Aralen Phosphate (chloroquine): 265
Aralen Phosphate with Primaquine Phosphate (chloroquine and primaquine): 1196
Aramine (metaraminol): 700

Aredia (pamidronate): 844
Arduan (pipercuronium): 1239
Arfonad (trimethaphan): 1110
Argesic (salsalate): 986
8-arginine-vasopressin (vasopressin): 1132
Aristocort (triamcinolone): 1093, 1222
Aristocort Intralesional (triamcinolone): 1093
Aristopsan Intra-Articular (triamcinolone): 1093
Aristospan Intralesional (triamcinolone): 1093
Arlidin (nylidrin): 1206
Arm-a-Med Isoetharine Hydrochloride (isoetharine): 602
Armour Thyroid (thyroid dessicated): 1070
Arrestin (trimethobenzamide): 1112
Artane (trihexyphenidyl): 1106
Arthra-G (salsalate): 986
Arthropan (choline salicylate): 283
Articulose (prednisolone): 918
Articulose LA (triamcinolone): 1093
5-ASA (mesalamine): 694
Asacol (mesalamine): 694
Ascendin (amoxapine): 112
ascorbic acid: 1208
asparaginase: 129
Ascriptin (aspirin): 131
Asmalix (theophylline): 1056
Aspergum (aspirin): 131
aspirin: 131
astemizole: 134
Asthma Haler (epinephrine): 430
AsthmaNefrin (epinephrine): 430
Astramorph PF (morphine): 762
Atarax (hydroxyzine): 575
atenolol: 135
Atesol (CAN) (acetaminophen): 58
Atgam (lymphocyte immune globulin): 1178
Ativan (lorazepam): 654
Atnativ (antithrombin): 125
atovaquone: 137
atracurium besylate: 1239
Atromid S (clofibrate): 301
atropine sulfate: 138
Atropine Sulfate S.O.P. (atropine): 138
Atriposol (CAN) (atropine): 138
Atrovent (ipratropium): 600
A/T/S (erythromycin): 440
Attenuvax (measles virus vaccine): 1169
Augmetin (amoxicillin with clavulanic acid): 1191

1264 ■ Index

auranofin: 141
aurothioglucose: 142
Aventyl (nortriptyline): 809
Avitene (microfibrillar collagen): 1216
Avlosulfan (CAN) (dapsone): 348
Axid Pulvules (nizatidine): 801
Ayercillin (CAN) (pencillin G procaine): 861
Aygestin (norethindrone): 804
Azactam (aztreonam): 148
azatadine maleate: 144
azathioprine: 145
azidothymidine (zidovudine): 1147
azithromycin: 147
Azmacort ((triamcinolone): 1093
Azo-Standard (phenazopyridine): 878
AZT (zidovudine): 1147
aztreonam: 148
Azulfidine (sulfasalazine): 1029

B

BAC (benzalkonium): 158
bacampicillin: 150
Baciguent (bacitracin): 151
BACI-IM (bacitracin): 151
Bacitin (CAN) (bacitracin): 151
bacitracin: 151
baclofen: 152
Bactine Hydrocortisone (hydrocortisone): 1220
Bactocil (oxacillin): 822
Bactrim (co-trimoxazole): 1192
Bactroban (mupirocin): 1213
BAL in Oil (dimercaprol): 394
Banflex (orphenadrine): 820
BARBITURATES (see page 22)
    amobarbital: 109
    aprobarbital: 127
    butabarbital: 196
    mephobarbital: 686
    pentobarbital: 868
    phenobarbital: 882
    secobarbital: 992
Baridium (phenazopyridine): 878
Basaljel (aluminum): 86
Bayer (aspirin): 131
Baylocaine (lidocaine): 636
BCG: 1179
BCNU (carmustine): 217
Beclodisk (CAN) (beclomethasone): 154
Becloforte Inhaler (beclomethasone): 154
beclomethasone dipropionate: 154
Beclovent (beclomethasone): 154
Beclovent Rotocaps (CAN) (beclomethasone): 154
Beconase AQ Nasal Spray (beclomethasone): 154
Beepen VK (penicillin V): 862
Beesix (pyridoxine): 1210
Beldin (diphenhydramine): 397
BELLADONNA ALKALOID
    atropine: 138
    scopolamine: 989
Bell/ans (sodium bicarbonate): 999
Bemote (dicyclomine): 379
Benadryl (diphenhydramine): 397
Benahist (diphenhydramine): 397
benazepril hydrochloride: 155
bendroflumethiazide: 157
Benemid (probenecid): 925
Benoject (diphenhydramine): 397
Bentyl (dicyclomine): 379
Bentylol (CAN) (dicyclomine): 379
Benylin Cough (diphenhydramine): 397
Benylin DM (dextramethorphan): 369
Benza (benzalkonium): 158, 1213
benzalkonium chloride: 158, 1213
BENZISOXAZOLES
    risperidine: 982
benzocaine: 1158
BENZODIAZEPINES (see page 24)
    alprazolam: 80
    chlordiazepoxide: 263
    clonazepam: 305
    clorazepate: 309
    diazepam: 372
    estazolam: 444
    flurazepam: 509
    halazepam: 547
    lorazepam: 654
    oxazepam: 827
    prazepam: 914
    quazepam: 961
    temazepam: 1041
    triazolam: 1097
BENZODIAZEPINE RECEPTOR ANTAGONISTS
    flumazenil: 498
benzonatate: 160
benzquinamide hydrochloride: 160
benzthiazide: 161
benztropine mesylate: 163
Bepen (CAN) (betamethasone): 167, 1217

Apo-Clonidine (CAN) (clonidine): 307
Apo-Clorazepate (CAN) (clorazepate): 309
Apo-Cloxi (CAN) (cloxicillin): 313
Apo-Diazepam (CAN) (diazepam): 372
Apo-Diltiaz (CAN) (diltiazem): 391
Apo-Doxy (CAN) (doxycycline): 415
Apo-Fluphenazine (CAN) (fluphenazine): 506
Apo-Haloperidol (CAN) (haloperidol): 548
Apo-Imipramine (CAN) (imipramine): 581
Apo-Indomethacin (CAN) (indomethacin): 585
Apo-Lorazepam (CAN) (lorazepam): 654
Apo-Meprobamate (CAN)(meprobamate): 691
Apo-Metronidazole (CAN) (metronidazole): 739
Apo-Naproxen (CAN) (naproxen): 778
Apo-Oxazepam (CAN)(oxazepam): 827
Apo-Perphenazine (CAN)(perphenazine): 875
Apo-Piroxicam (CAN)(piroxicam): 903
Apo-Prazo (CAN)(prazosin): 916
Apo-Prednisone (CAN)(prednisone): 921
Apo-Primidone (CAN)(primidone): 923
Apo-Propranolol (CAN)(propranolol): 947
Apo-Tamoxifen (CAN)(tamoxifen): 1040
Apo-Thioridazine (CAN)(thioridazine): 1064
Apo-Trifluoperazine (CAN) (trifluoperazine): 1101
Apo-Trihex (CAN)(trihexyphenidyl): 1106
APPG (pencillin G procaine): 861
apraclonidine: 1241
Apresoline (hydralazine): 557
aprobarbital: 127
aprotinin: 128
APSAC (anistreplase): 123
Aquacare (urea): 1212
Aquachloral Supprettes (chloral hydrate): 258
Aquamox (CAN) (quienthazone): 967
Aquaphylline (theophylline): 1056
Aquasol A (vitamin A): 1208
Aquasol E (vitamin E): 1209
Aquatensen (methylclothiazide): 721
Ara-A (vidarabine): 1136
Ara-C (cytarabine): 338
Aralen Hydrochloride (chloroquine): 265
Aralen Phosphate (chloroquine): 265
Aralen Phosphate with Primaquine Phosphate (chloroquine and primaquine): 1196
Aramine (metaraminol): 700
Aredia (pamidronate): 844
Arduan (pipercuronium): 1239
Arfonad (trimethaphan): 1110
Argesic (salsalate): 986
8-arginine-vasopressin (vasopressin): 1132
Aristocort (triamcinolone): 1093, 1222
Aristocort Intralesional (triamcinolone): 1093
Aristopsan Intra-Articular (triamcinolone): 1093
Aristospan Intralesional (triamcinolone): 1093
Arlidin (nylidrin): 1206
Arm-a-Med Isoetharine Hydrochloride (isoetharine): 602
Armour Thyroid (thyroid dessicated): 1070
Arrestin (trimethobenzamide): 1112
Artane (trihexyphenidyl): 1106
Arthra-G (salsalate): 986
Arthropan (choline salicylate): 283
Articulose (prednisolone): 918
Articulose LA (triamcinolone): 1093
5-ASA (mesalamine): 694
Asacol (mesalamine): 694
Ascendin (amoxapine): 112
ascorbic acid: 1208
asparaginase: 129
Ascriptin (aspirin): 131
Asmalix (theophylline): 1056
Aspergum (aspirin): 131
aspirin: 131
astemizole: 134
Asthma Haler (epinephrine): 430
AsthmaNefrin (epinephrine): 430
Astramorph PF (morphine): 762
Atarax (hydroxyzine): 575
atenolol: 135
Atesol (CAN) (acetaminophen): 58
Atgam (lymphocyte immune globulin): 1178
Ativan (lorazepam): 654
Atnativ (antithrombin): 125
atovaquone: 137
atracurium besylate: 1239
Atromid S (clofibrate): 301
atropine sulfate: 138
Atropine Sulfate S.O.P. (atropine): 138
Atriposol (CAN) (atropine): 138
Atrovent (ipratropium): 600
A/T/S (erythromycin): 440
Attenuvax (measles virus vaccine): 1169
Augmetin (amoxicillin with clavulanic acid): 1191

auranofin: 141
aurothioglucose: 142
Aventyl (nortriptyline): 809
Avitene (microfibrillar collagen): 1216
Avlosulfan (CAN) (dapsone): 348
Axid Pulvules (nizatidine): 801
Ayercillin (CAN) (penicillin G procaine): 861
Aygestin (norethindrone): 804
Azactam (aztreonam): 148
azatadine maleate: 144
azathioprine: 145
azidothymidine (zidovudine): 1147
azithromycin: 147
Azmacort (triamcinolone): 1093
Azo-Standard (phenazopyridine): 878
AZT (zidovudine): 1147
aztreonam: 148
Azulfidine (sulfasalazine): 1029

B

BAC (benzalkonium): 158
bacampicillin: 150
Baciguent (bacitracin): 151
BACI-IM (bacitracin): 151
Bacitin (CAN) (bacitracin): 151
bacitracin: 151
baclofen: 152
Bactine Hydrocortisone (hydrocortisone): 1220
Bactocil (oxacillin): 822
Bactrim (co-trimoxazole): 1192
Bactroban (mupirocin): 1213
BAL in Oil (dimercaprol): 394
Banflex (orphenadrine): 820
BARBITURATES (see page 22)
    amobarbital: 109
    aprobarbital: 127
    butabarbital: 196
    mephobarbital: 686
    pentobarbital: 868
    phenobarbital: 882
    secobarbital: 992
Baridium (phenazopyridine): 878
Basaljel (aluminum): 86
Bayer (aspirin): 131
Baylocaine (lidocaine): 636
BCG: 1179
BCNU (carmustine): 217
Beclodisk (CAN) (beclomethasone): 154
Becloforte Inhaler (beclomethasone): 154

beclomethasone dipropionate: 154
Beclovent (beclomethasone): 154
Beclovent Rotocaps (CAN) (beclomethasone): 154
Beconase AQ Nasal Spray (beclomethasone): 154
Beepen VK (penicillin V): 862
Beesix (pyridoxine): 1210
Beldin (diphenhydramine): 397
BELLADONNA ALKALOID
    atropine: 138
    scopolamine: 989
Bell/ans (sodium bicarbonate): 999
Bemote (dicyclomine): 379
Benadryl (diphenhydramine): 397
Benahist (diphenhydramine): 397
benazepril hydrochloride: 155
bendroflumethiazide: 157
Benemid (probenecid): 925
Benoject (diphenhydramine): 397
Bentyl (dicyclomine): 379
Bentylol (CAN) (dicyclomine): 379
Benylin Cough (diphenhydramine): 397
Benylin DM (dextramethorphan): 369
Benza (benzalkonium): 158, 1213
benzalkonium chloride: 158, 1213
BENZISOXAZOLES
    risperidine: 982
benzocaine: 1158
BENZODIAZEPINES (see page 24)
    alprazolam: 80
    chlordiazepoxide: 263
    clonazepam: 305
    clorazepate: 309
    diazepam: 372
    estazolam: 444
    flurazepam: 509
    halazepam: 547
    lorazepam: 654
    oxazepam: 827
    prazepam: 914
    quazepam: 961
    temazepam: 1041
    triazolam: 1097
BENZODIAZEPINE RECEPTOR ANTAGONISTS
    flumazenil: 498
benzonatate: 160
benzquinamide hydrochloride: 160
benzthiazide: 161
benztropine mesylate: 163
Bepen (CAN) (betamethasone): 167, 1217

bepridil hydrochloride: 165
beractant: 166
Beta-2 (isoetharine): 602
Betabloc (CAN) (metoprolol): 602
Betacort (CAN) (betamethasone): 168, 1218
Betaderm (CAN) (betamethasone): 168, 1218
Betadine (povidone iodine): 1213
Betagen (povidone iodine): 1213
betamethasone: 168
betamethasone benzoate: 167, 1218
betamethasone dipropionate: 167, 1218
betamethasone sodium phosphate: 167
betamethasone sodium phosphate and acetate: 167
betamethasone valerate: 167, 1218
Betapace (sotalol): 1008
Betapen -VK (penicillin V): 862
Betaseron (interferon beta 1b): 594
Betatrex (betamethasone): 168, 1218
Beta-Val (betamethasone): 168, 1218
betaxolol hydrochloride: 170
bethanechol chloride: 172
Betnesol (CAN) (betamethasone): 168
Betnovate (CAN) (betamethasone): 168, 1218
Betoptic (betaxolol): 170
Biamine (thiamine): 1211
Biaxin Filmtabs (clarithromycin): 294
Bicillin L-A (penicillin G benzathine): 857
BiCNU (carmustine): 217
BILE ACID SEQUESTRANTS
  cholestyramine: 281
  colestipol: 319
Biltricide (praziquantel): 915
Bio Aerola C (vitamin P): 1210
Biocal (calcium): 204
Biocef (cephalexin): 249
Bioflavonoids (vitamin P):
biperiden hydrochloride: 173
biperiden lactate: 173
bisacodyl: 1203
bisacodyl tannex: 1203
Bisco-Lax (bisacodyl): 1203
bismuth subsalicylate: 175
bisoprolol fumarate: 176
bitolterol mesylate: 178
Black Draught (senna): 1205
Black Widow spider species antivenin: 1179
Blenoxane (bleomycin): 178
bleomycin sulfate: 178
BLM (bleomycin): 178

Blocadren (timolol): 1076
BLOOD PRODUCTS
  albumin: 73
  alpha 1 proteinase inhibitor: 79
  factor IX complex: 473
  plasma protein fraction: 904
Bluboro Powder (Burow's solution): 1212
Bonamine (CAN) (meclizine): 672
Bontril (phendimetrazine): 1152
Bonine (meclizine): 672
boric acid ointment: 1212
Borofax (boric acid): 1212
Boropak Powder (aluminum acetate): 1212
Branch Amin (amino acid): 94
Breonesin (guaifenesin): 541
Brethaire (terbutaline): 1045
Brethine (terbutaline): 1045
Bretylate (CAN) (bretylium): 181
bretylium tosylate: 181
Bretylol (bretylium): 181
Brevibloc (esmolol): 443
Brevicon (combo. OC): 1199
Brevital (methohexital): 1153
Bricanyl (terbutaline): 1045
British Anti-Lewisite (dimercaprol): 394
bromocriptine mesylate: 182
Bromphen (brompheniramine): 185
brompheniramine maleate: 185
BRONCHODILATORS
  albuterol: 73
  aminophylline: 99
  bitoterol: 178
  dyphylline: 418
  ephedrine: 428
  epinephrine: 430
  isoetharine: 602
  isoproterenol: 605
  metaproterenol: 699
  oxtriphylline: 828
  pirbuterol: 902
  terbutaline: 1045
  theophylline: 1056
Bronitin (epinephrine): 430
Bronkaid Mist (epinephrine): 430
Bronkodyl (theophylline): 1056
Bronkometer (isoetharine): 602
Bronkosol (isoetharine): 602
Bucladin-S Softabs (buclizine): 186
buclizine hydrochloride: 186
budenoside: 188
Buffaprin (aspirin): 131
Bufferin (aspirin): 131

1266 ■ Index

bumetanide: 189
Bumex (bumetanide): 189
Buminate 5% (albumin): 72
Buminate 25% (albumin): 72
bupivacaine: 1158
Buprenex (buprenorphine): 190
buprenorphine hydrochloride: 190
bupropion hydrochloride: 191
BURN PREPARATIONS
 mafenide: 1216
 nitrofurazone: 1216
 silver sulfadiazine: 1216
Burow's solution: 1212
BuSpar (buspirone): 193
buspirone hydrochloride: 193
busulfan: 194
butabarbital sodium: 196
butamben picrate: 1158
Butesin Picrate (butamben): 1158
Butisol Sodium (butabarbital): 196
butoconazole nitrate: 198
butorphanol tartrate: 198
BUTYROPHENONE
 haloperidol: 548
Byclomine (dicyclomine): 379
Bydramine (diphenhydramine): 379

C

Cafergot (ergotamine and caffeine): 1197
caffeine: 200
Caffedrine (caffeine): 200
Caine-2 (lidocaine): 1158
Calamatum (calamine lotion): 1212
Calamox (calamine lotion): 1212
calamine lotion: 1212
Calan (verapamil): 1134
Calan SR (verapamil): 1134
Calcedrol (calcidediol): 1208
Calcibind (cellulose): 248
Calciday (calcium): 204
calcifediol: 1208
Calcijex (calcitriol): 203
Calcilean (CAN) (heparin): 551
Calcimar (calcitonin): 201
Calciparine (heparin): 551
calcipotriene: 1214
Calcisorb (CAN) (cellulose): 248
calcitonin, human: 201
calcitonin, salmon: 201

calcitriol: 203, 1208
calcium carbonate: 204
CALCIUM CHANNEL BLOCKERS (see page 28)
 amlodopine: 106
 bepridil: 165
 diltiazem: 391
 felodopine: 478
 isradipine: 612
 nicardipine: 768
 nifedipine: 793
 nimodipine: 794
 verapamil: 1134
calcium chloride: 204
Calcium Disodium Versenate (edetate calcium): 420
calcium EDTA (edetate calcium): 420
calcium gluceptate: 204
calcium gluconate: 204
calcium lactate: 204
CALCIUM REGULATORS
 calcitonin: 201
 calcitriol: 203
 pamidronate: 844
Caldecort (hydrocortisone): 1221
Calm-X (dimenhydrinate): 393
CALORIC AGENTS
 amino acids: 94
 fat emulsion: 477
Caltrate (calcium): 204
Campain (CAN) (acetominophen): 58
Camphorated Tincture of Opium (opium): 819
Canesten (CAN) (clotrimazole): 311
cantharidin: 1215
Cantharone (cantharidin): 1215
Capastat Sulfate (capreomycin): 206
Capitrol (chloroxine): 1214
Capoten (captopril): 207
Capozide (hydrochlorothiazide and captopril): 1195
capreomycin: 206
capsaicin: 1216
captopril: 207
Carafate (sucralfate): 1022
carbachol: 1241
carbamazepine: 209
carbapenem: 1192
carbenicillin indanyl sodium: 212
Carbocaine (mepivocaine): 1159
Carbolith (CAN) (lithium): 645

CARBONIC ANHYDRASE INHIBITOR
   acetazolamide: 60
   methazolamide: 705
carboplatin: 213
carboprost tromethamine: 215
Cardene (nicardipine): 788
Cardene IV (nicardipine): 788
Cardene SR (nicardipine): 788
CARDIAC GLYCOSIDE
   digoxin: 386
CARDIAC STIMULANTS
   epinephrine: 430
   norepinephrine: 802
Cardilate (erythrityl): 438
Cardioquin (quinidine): 969
CARDIOTONIC DRUGS
   amrinone: 120
   digoxin: 386
   milrinone: 747
Cardizem (diltiazem): 391
Cardizem CD (diltiazem): 391
Cardizem SR (diltiazem): 391
Cardura (doxazosin): 409
carisoprodol: 216
Carmol (urea): 1212
carmustine: 217
carteolol hydrochloride: 219
Cartrol (carteolol): 219
cascara: 1203
castor oil: 1203
Cataflam (diclofenac): 377
Catapres (clonidine): 307
Catapres TTS (clonidine): 307
CATECHOLAMINES
   epinephrine: 430
   norepinephrine: 802
CATION
   cellulose: 248
CCNU (lomustine): 649
CdA (cladribine): 293
CDDP (cisplatin): 291
Cebid (ascorbic acid): 1208
Ceclor (cefaclor): 221
CeeNu (lomustine): 649
cefaclor: 221
cefadroxil: 222
Cefadyl (cephapirin): 252
cefamandole nafate: 223
Cefanex (cephalexin): 249
cefazolin sodium: 225
cefixime: 227
Cefizox (ceftizoxime): 242
cefmetazole: 228

Cefobid (cefoperazone): 231
cefonicid: 230
cefoperazone sodium: 231
Cefotan (cefotetan): 235
cefotaxime sodium: 233
cefotetan disodium: 235
cefoxitin sodium: 236
cefpodoxime proxetil: 238
cefprozil monohydrate: 239
Cefracycline (CAN)(tetracycline): 1052
ceftazidime: 241
Ceftin (cefuroxime): 246
ceftizoxime sodium: 242
ceftriaxone sodium: 244
cefuroxime axetil: 246
cefuroxime sodium: 246
Cefzil (cefprozil): 239
Celestoderm (CAN)(betamethasone): 1218
Celestone (betamethasone): 167
Celestone Phosphate (betamethasone): 167
cellulose sodium phosphate: 248
Celontin Kapseals (methsuximide): 720
Cel-U-Jec (betamethasone): 167
Celestoderm (CAN) (betamethasone): 167
Celestone Soluspan (betamethasone): 167
Cenafed (pseudoephedrine): 954
Cena-K (potassium): 910
Cenocort A-40 (triamcinolone): 1093
Cenocort Forte (triamcinolone): 1093
CENTRAL NERVOUS SYSTEM STIMULANTS
   dextroamphetamine: 367
   methylphenidate: 727
   pemoline: 852
Centrax (prazepam): 914
cephalexin: 249
cephalexin hydrochloride monohydrate: 249
CEPHALOSPORINS (see page 29)
   cefaclor: 221
   cefadroxil: 222
   cefamandole: 223
   cefazolin: 225
   cefixime: 227
   cefmetazole: 228
   cefonicid: 230
   cefoperazone: 231
   cefotaxime: 233
   cefotetan: 235
   cefoxitin: 236
   cefpodoxime: 238
   cefprozil: 239

1268 ■ Index

CEPHALOSPORINS (*continued*)
   ceftazidime: 241
   ceftizoxime sodium: 242
   ceftriaxone sodium: 244
   cefuroxime: 246
   cephalexin: 249
   cephalothin: 250
   cephapirin: 252
   cephradine: 254
   loracarbef: 651
cephalothin sodium: 250
cephapirin sodium: 252
cephradine: 254
Cephulac (lactulose): 622
Ceredase (alglucerase): 77
Cerespan (papaverine): 1206
Cerubidine (daunorubicin): 350
C.E.S. (CAN) (estrogens, conj.): 450
CESTICIDE
   paromomycin: 849
Cetane (ascorbic acid): 1208
Cevalin (ascorbic acid): 1208
Cevi-Bid (ascorbic acid): 1208
Charcoaid (charcoal): 256
charcoal, activated: 256
Charcolate (CAN) (charcoal): 256
CHELATING AGENTS
   deforoxamine: 352
   dimercaprol: 394
   penicillamine: 855
   succimer: 1021
   trientine: 1100
Chemet (succimer): 1021
chenodiol: 256
chenodeoxycholic acid (chenodiol): 256
chloral hydrate: 258
chlorambucil: 259
chloramphenicol: 261
chloramphenicol palmitate: 261
chloramphenicol sodium succinate: 261
chlordiazepoxide hydrochloride: 263
chlorhexidine gluconate: 1213
2-chlorodeoxyandenosine (cladribine): 293
Chloromycetin Kapseals (chloramphenicol): 261
Chloromycetin Ophthalmic (chloramphenicol): 261
Chlormycetin Otic (chloramphenicol): 261
Chloromycetin Pamlitate (chloramphenicol): 261
Chloromycetin Succinate (chloramphenicol): 261

chloroprocaine: 1158
Chloroptic Ophthalmic (chloramphenicol): 261
chloroquine hydrochloride: 265
chloroquine phosphate: 265
chlorothiazide: 266
chlorothiazide sodium: 266
chlorotrianisene: 268
chloroxine: 1214
Chlorphen (CAN) (chlorpheniramine): 271
chlorphenesin carbamate: 270
chlorpheniramine maleate: 271
Chlor-Pro (chlorpheniramine): 271
chlorpromazine hydrochloride: 272
chlorpropamide: 276
chlorprothixene hydrochloride: 277
chlorprothixene lactate: 277
Chlorspan (chlorpheniramine): 271
Chlortab (chlorpheniramine): 271
chlortalidone: 278
Chlor-Trimeton (chlorpheniramine): 271
Chlor-Tripolon (CAN) (chlorpheniramine): 271
chlorzoxazone: 280
Cholac (lactulose): 622, 1204
cholecalciferol: 1208
Choledyl (oxtriphylline): 828
Choledyl A (oxtriphylline): 828
cholera vaccine: 1179
cholestyramine: 281
choline magnesium trisalicylate: 282
choline salicylate: 283
CHOLINESTERASE INHIBITORS
   ambenonium: 89
   edrophonium: 421
   neostigmine: 784
   pyridostigmine: 957
   tacrine: 1037
choline theophyllinate (oxytriphylline): 828
Choloxin (dextrothyroxine): 370
Cholybar (cholestyramine): 281
Chooz (calcium): 204
Chorex (chorionic gonadotropin): 284
Chorigon (chorionic gonadotropin): 284
chorionic gonadotropin: 284
Choron 10 (chorionic gonadotropin): 284
Chronulac (lactulose): 622, 1204
Chymodiactin (chymopapain): 285
chymopapain: 285
Cibacalcin (calcitonin): 201
Cidomycin (CAN) (ganciclovir): 525
Cilaxin (CAN) (ciprofloxacin): 289

cimetidine: 286
Cinobac Pulvules (cinoxacin): 288
cinoxacin: 288
Cin-Quin (quinidine): 969
Cipro (ciprofloxaxin): 289
ciprofloxacin hydrochloride: 289
cisapride: 291
cisplatin: 291
13-cis-retinoic acid isotretinoin 610
Citanest (prilocaine): 1159
Citrate of Magnesia (magnesium): 661, 1204
Citro-Flav 2000 (vitamin P): 1210
Citro-Nesia (magnesium citrate): 1204
citrovorum factor (leucovorin): 624
cladribine: 293
Claforan (cefotaxime): 233
clarithromycin: 294
Claritin (loratidine): 652
clemastine fumarate: 296
Cleocin (clindamycin): 297
Cleocin Pediatric (clindamycin): 297
Cleocin Phosphate (clindamycin): 297
Cleocin T (clindamycin): 297
Climesterone (CAN) (estrotens, ester.): 453
clindamycin hydrochloride: 297
clindamycin palmitate hydrochloride: 297
clindamycin phosphate: 297
Clinoril (sulindac): 1034
clobetasol propionate: 1218
clocortolone pivalate: 1218
Cloderm (clocortolone): 1218
clofazimine: 299
clofibrate: 301
Clomid (clomiphene): 302
clomiphene citrate: 302
clomipramine hydrochloride: 303
clonazepam: 305
clonidine hydrochloride: 307
clorazepate dipotassium: 309
Clotrimaderm (CAN) (clotrimazole): 311
clotrimazole: 311, 1214
cloxacillin sodium: 313
Cloxapen (cloxacillin): 313
clozapine: 314
Clozaril (clozapine): 314
Clysodrast (bisacodyl):
COAGULATION INHIBITOR
  antithrombin: 125
codeine phosphate: 315
codeine sulfate: 315
Codimal-A (brompheniramine): 185

Cogentin (benztropine): 163
Cognex (tacrine): 1037
Colace (docusate): 1203
colaspase (asparaginase): 129
colchicine: 317
Colestid (colestipol): 319
colestipol hydrochloride: 319
colfosceril palmitate: 320
Collylirium Fresh Eye Drops (tetrahydrolozine): 1055
COLONY STIMULATING FACTOR
  filgrastin: 486
  sargramostim: 988
Combantrin (CAN) (pyrantel): 956
Combipres (chlorthalidone and clonidine): 1196
Compazine (prochlorperazine): 932
Compound S (zidovudine): 1147
Compoz (diphenhydramine): 397
Concentraid (desmopressin): 356
Condylox (podofilox): 1215
Congespirin for Children (dextramethorphan): 369
Constant T (theophylline): 1056
Constilac (lactulose): 622, 1204
Constulose (lactulose): 1204
CONTRACEPTIVES (see page 1199)
  levonorgestrel: 631
Cophene-B (brompheniramine): 185
Cordarone (amiodarone): 102
Cordran (flurandranolide): 1220
Corgard (nadolol): 767
Coricidin (phenylephrine): 888
CortaGel (hydrocortisone): 1221
Cortaid (hydrocortisone): 1221
Cortaid with Aloe (hydrocortisone): 1221
Cort-Dome (hydrocortisone): 1220
Cortef (hydrocortisone): 561
Corticaine (hydrocortisone): 1221
CORTICOSTEROIDS
  beclomethasone: 154
  betamethasone: 167
  budenoside: 188
  cortisone: 323
  dexamethasone: 358
  fludrocortisone: 496
  flunisolide: 499
  hydrocortisone: 561
  methylprednisolone: 728
  prednisolone: 918
  prednisone: 921
  triamcinolone: 1093

corticotrophin (corticotropin): 321
corticotropin injection: 321
corticotropin repository injection: 321
cortisone acetate: 323
Cortizone 5 (hydrocortisone): 1220
Cortizone 10 (hydrocortisone): 1221
Cortone Acetate (cortisone): 323
Cortrosyn (cosyntropin): 325
Cosmegan (dactinomycin): 342
cosyntropin: 325
Cotazym (pancreatic enzymes): 845
Cotrim (co-trimoxazole): 1192
co-trimoxazole: 1192
COUGH SUPPRESSANT
  diphenhydramine: 397
Coumadin (warfarin): 1142
COUMARIN DERIVATIVE
  warfarin: 1142
Creon Capsules (pancreatic enyzmes): 845
cromoglicic acid (cromolyn): 326
cromoglycic acid (cromolyn): 326
cromolyn sodium: 326
crotamiton: 1215
Crystapen (CAN)(penicillin G sodium): 859
Crysticillin (penicillin G procaine): 861
C.S.D. (CAN) (estrogens, conj.): 450
CSP (cellulose): 248
Cuprimine (penicillamine): 855
Curretab (medroxyprogesterone): 674
Cutivate (fluticasone): 1220
cyancobalamin: 1209
Cyclan (cyclandelate): 1206
cyclandelate: 1206
cyclizine: 329
cyclobenzaprine hydrochloride: 330
Cyclocort (amcinonide): 1217
Cyclogyl (cyclopentolate): 1241
Cyclomen (CAN) (danazol): 344
cyclopentolate: 1241
cyclophosphamide: 331
cyclopropane: 1153
cycloserine: 333
Cyclospasmol (cyclandelate): 1206
cyclosporin A (cyclosporine): 334
cyclosporine: 334
Cylert (pemoline): 852
cyproheptadine hydrochloride: 336
Cystagon (cysteamine): 337
cysteamine: 337
CYSTIC FIBROSIS DRUG
  dornase: 407
Cytadren (aminoglutethemide): 97

cytarabine: 338
cytomegalovirus immunoglobulin: 1178
Cytomegalovirus Immunoglobulin Intravenous (cytomegalovirus immune globulin): 1178
Cytomel (liothyronine): 640
Cytosar-U (cytarabine): 338
cytosine arabinoside (cytarabine): 338
Cytotec (misoprostol): 752
Cytovene (ganciclovir): 522
Cytoxan (cyclophosphamide): 331

D

D (vitamin D): 1209
dacarbazine: 340
dactinomycin: 342
Dakin's (sodium hypochlorite): 1213
Dalacin C (CAN) (clindamycin): 297
Dalalone (dexamethasone): 358
Dalcaine (lidocaine): 636
Dalgan (dezocine): 371
Dalmane (flurazepam): 508
dalteparin: 343
D'Amp (ampicillin): 118
danazol: 344
Danocrine (danazol): 344
dantrolene sodium: 346
Dantrium (dantrolene): 346
dapiprazole: 1241
dapsone: 348
Daricon (oxphencyclimine): 838
Darvocet-N (propoxyphene): 946
Darvon (propoxyphene): 946
Darvon-N (propoxyphene): 946
daunomycin (daunorubicin): 350
daunorubicin hydrochloride: 350
Daypro (oxaprozin): 826
Dazamide (acetazolamide): 60
DCF (pentostatin): 870
DDAVP (desmopressin): 356
ddC (zalcitabine): 1146
ddI (didanosine): 380
DDPC (beractant): 166
DDS (dapsone): 348
1-deamino-8-D-arginine vasopressin (desmopressin):356
Decaderm (dexamethasone): 358, 1219
Decadrol (dexamethasone): 358

Index ■ 1271

Decadron (dexamethasone): 358
Decadron L.A. (dexamethasone): 358
Decadron Phosphate
 (dexamethasone): 358, 1219
Decadron Phosphate Ophthalmic
 (dexamethasone): 358
Decadron Phosphate Respihaler
 (dexamethasone): 358
Deca-Durabolin (nandrolene): 777
Decaject (dexamethasone): 358
Decameth (dexamethasone): 358
Decaspray (dexamethasone): 358, 1219
Declomycin (demeclocycline): 353
Decofed (pseudoephedrine): 954
deferoxamine mesylate: 352
Dehist (brompheniramine): 185
Delalone (dexamethasone): 358
Deladiol (estradiol): 446
Delatest (testosterone): 1050
Delatestryl (testosterone): 1050
Delestrogen (estradiol): 446
Delsym (dextramethorphan): 369
Delta-Cortef (prednisolone): 918
Delta-D (cholecalciferol): 1208
Deltalin Gelseals (ergocaliferol): 1209
Deltasone (prednisone): 921
delta-9-tetrahydrocannabinol (dronabinol): 416
delta-9-THC (dronabinol): 416
Del-Vi-A (vitamin A): 1208
Demadex (torsemide): 1087
demecarium: 1241
democlocycline hydrochloride: 353
Demer-Idine (CAN) (meperidine): 683
Demerol HCl (meperidine): 683
demethylchlortetracycline hydrochloride: 353
 (demeclocycline): 353
Demo-Cineal (CAN) (dextromethorphan): 369
Demser (metyrosine): 741
Demulen 1/35 (combo OC): 1199
Demulen 1/50 (combo OC): 1199
2'-deoxycoformycin (pentostatin): 870
Depakene (valproic acid): 1128
Depakote (valproic acid): 1128
depAndro (testosterone): 1050
Depen (penicillamine): 855
depGynogen (estradiol): 446
dep Medalone (methylprednisilone): 728
Depo-Estradiol Cypionate (estradiol): 446
Depogen (estradiol): 446
Depoject (methylprednisilone): 728
Depo-pred (methylprednisilone):728
Depo-Provera (medroxyprogesterone): 674
Depotest (testosterone): 1050
Depo-Testosterone (testosterone): 1050
Dermabet (betamethasone): 168, 1218
Dermatop (prednicarbate): 1222
Dermolate (hydrocortisone): 1220
Dermoplast (benzocaine): 1158
Dermovate (CAN) (clobetasol): 1218
Dermtex HC (hydrocortisone): 1220
DES (diethylstilbestrol): 383
Desferal (deferoxamine): 352
desflurane: 1154
desipramine hydrochloride 354
desmopressin acetate: 356
Desogen (combo OC): 1199
desonide: 1218
DesOwen (desonide): 1218
desoximetasone: 1218
Desxasone-L.A. (dexamethasone): 358
Desyrl (trazodone): 1091
Dexacen-4 (dexamethasone): 358
dexamethasone: 358, 1219
dexamethasone acetate: 358
dexamethasone sodium phosphate: 358, 1219
Dexasone (dexamethasone): 358
Dexasone L.A. (dexamethasone): 358
dexchlorpheniramine maleate: 362
Dexchlor (dexchlorpheniramine): 362
Dexedrine (dextroamphetamine): 367
Dexone (dexamethasone): 358
Dexone-L.A. (dexamethasone): 358
dexpanthenol: 363, 1212
dextropantothenyl alcohol (dexpanthenol): 363
Dextran 40 (dextran, low): 365
Dextran 70 (dextran, high): 364
Dextran 75 (dextran, high): 364
dextran, high molecular weight: 364
dextran, low molecular weight: 365
dextroamphetamine sulfate: 367
dextramethorphan hydrobromide: 369
dextropropoxyphene (propoxyphene): 946
dextrothyroxine sodium: 370
Dey Dose Isoproterenol Hydrochloride
 (isoproterenol): 605
dezocine: 371
D.H.E. 45 (dihydroergotamine): 389
DHPG (ganciclovir): 522
DHT (dihydrotachysterol): 1209
Diabenese (chlorpropamide): 276
DiaBeta (glyburide): 531

1272 ■ Index

DIAGNOSTIC AGENTS
  atropine: 138
  corticotropin: 321
  cosyntropin: 325
  edrophonium: 421
  glucagon: 529
  gonadorelin: 537
  mannitol: 664
  naloxone: 774
  phentolamine: 887
  scopolamine: 989
  thyrotropin: 1072
Diamine T.D. (brompheniramine): 185
Diamox (acetazolamide): 60
Diamox Sequels (acetazolamide): 60
diaphenylsulfone (dapsone): 348
Diapid (lypressin): 658
Diazemuls (CAN) (diazepam): 372
diazepam: 372
diazoxide: 375
Dibent (dicyclomine): 379
Dibenzyline (phenoxybenzamine): 884
dibucaine: 1158
Dicarbosil (calcium): 204
diclofenac sodium: 377
diclofenac potassium: 377
dicloxacillin sodium: 378
dicyclomine hydrochloride: 379
didanosine: 380
dideoxycytidine (zalcitabine): 1146
dideoxyinosine (didanosine): 380
dienestrol: 382
diethylpropion hydrochloride: 1151
diethylstilbestrol diphosphate: 383
diflorasone diacetate: 1219
Diflucan (flurazepam): 492
diflunisal: 384
DIGESTIVE ENZYMES
  pancreatic enzymes: 845
  pancreatin: 845
Digibind (digoxin immune fab): 387
digoxin: 386
digoxin immune fab: 387
digoxin specific antibody fragments (digoxin immune fab): 387
dihydroergotamine mesylate: 389
Dihydroergotamine Sandoz (CAN) (dihydroergotamine): 389
dihydrotachysterol: 1209
dihydroxyaluminum sodium carbonate: 390

1,25-dihydroxycholecalciferol (calcitriol): 203
dihydroxyproply theophyllin (diphylline): 48
diiodohydroxyquinoline (iodoquinol): 598
Dilacor XR (diltiazem): 391
Dilantin (phenytoin): 892
Dilaudid (hydromorphone): 567
Dilocaine (lidocaine): 636, 1158
Dilor (diphylline): 418
Dilosyn (CAN) (methdilazine): 706
diltiazem hydrochloride: 391
Dimelor (CAN) (acetohexamide): 62
dimenhydrinate: 393
Dimentabs (dimenhydrinate): 393
dimercaprol: 394
Dimetane Extentabs (brompheniramine): 185
Dimetane-Ten (brompheniramine): 185
Dinate (dimenhydrinate): 393
dinoprostone: 395
Diochloram (CAN) (chloramphenicol): 261
Diocto C (docusate): 1203
Diodoquin (CAN) (iodoquinol): 598
Dioptic's Atropine (CAN) (atropine): 138
Dioval (estradiol): 446
dipalmitoylphosphatidylcholine (colfosceril): 320
Dipentum (olsalazine): 815
Diphenacen (diphenhydramine): 397
Diphen Cough (diphenhydramine): 397
diphenhydramine hydrochloride: 397
diphenidol: 398
DIPHENYLBUTYLPIPERDINE
  pimozide: 896
diphenylhydantoin (phenytoin): 892
diphtheria antitoxin: 1178
diphtheria and tetanus toxoids and acellular pertussis vaccine, adsorbed: 1160
diptheria and tetanus toxoids and pertussis vaccine, adsorbed with haemophilus b conjugated vaccine: 1161
diphtheria and tetanus toxoids and whole cell pertussis vaccine, adsorbed: 1157
diphtheria and tetanus toxoids and whole cell pertussis vaccine with haemophilus influenzae b conjugates vaccine: 1162

diphtheria and tetanus toxoids, combined, absorbed: 1157
Diprivan (propofol): 1155
Diprolene (betamethasone): 167
Diprosone (betamethasone): 167
dipyridamole: 399
Disalcid (salsalate): 986
disodium cromoglycate (cromolyn): 326
d-isoephedrine hydrochloride
   (pseudoephedrine): 954
Disonate (docusate): 1203
disopyramide phosphate: 401
Disotate (edetate): 420
Dispos-A-Med Isoproterenol Hydrochloride
   (isoproterenol): 605
Ditropan (oxybutynin): 830
Diucardin (hydroflumethiazide): 565
Diuchlor H (CAN) (hydroclorothiazide): 559
Diurigen (chlorothiazide): 266
Diuril (chlorothiazide): 266
Diuril Sodium (chlorothiazide): 266
disulfiram: 402
Diurese (trichlormethiazide): 1098
DIURETICS (see also specific type and see also page 31)
   acetazolamide: 60
   amiloride: 93
   methazolamide: 705
divalproex sodium (valproic acid): 1128
Dixarit (CAN) (clonidine): 307
Dizmiss (meclizine): 672
Dizymes Capsules (pancreatic enzymes): 845
Dnase (dornase): 407
DNR (daunorubicin): 350
dobutamine: 404
Dobutrex (dobutamine): 404
docusate: 1203
DOK (docusate): 1203
Doktors (phenylephrine): 888
Dolanex (acetaminophen): 58
Dolene (propoxyphene): 946
Dolobid (diflunisal): 384
Dolophine (methadone): 703
Domeboro Powder (aluminum acetate): 1212
Donnazyme (pancreatic enzymes): 845
Dopamet (CAN) (methyldopa): 723
dopamine hydrochloride: 405
DOPAMINE RECEPTOR AGONISTS
   bromocriptine: 182

DOPAMINERGIC BLOCKING DRUGS
   acetophenazine: 64
   chlorpromazine: 272
   chlorprothixene: 277
   clozapine: 314
   dopamine: 405
   fluphenazine: 506
   haloperidol: 548
   loxapine: 657
   mesoridazine: 696
   methdilazine: 706
   metoclopramide: 734
   molindone: 757
   perphenazine: 875
   prochlorperazine: 932
   promazine: 938
   promethazine: 941
   thioridazine: 1064
   thiothixene: 1068
   trifluoperazine: 1101
   triflupromazine: 1103
   trimeprazine: 1108
Dopar (levodopa): 627
Dopram (doxapram): 408
Doral (quazepam): 961
Dorcol Pediatric Formula
   (pseudoephedrine): 954
Dormarex 2 (diphenhydramine): 397
dornase alfa: 407
Doryx (doxycycline): 415
DOS Softget (docusate): 1203
Dovonex (calcipotriene): 1214
doxacurium chloride: 1239
doxapram hydrochloride: 408
doxazosin mesylate: 409
doxepin hydrochloride: 410
Doxinate (docusate): 1203
doxorubicin hydrochloride: 413
Doxy-Caps (doxycycline): 415
1-doxycoformycin (pentostatin): 870
Doxychel Hyclate (doxycycline): 415
Doxycin (CAN) (doxycycline): 415
doxycycline: 415
Dozamide (acetazolamide): 60
DPPC (colfosceril): 320
Dramamine (dimenhydrinate): 393
Dramanate (dimenhydrinate): 393
Dramocen (dimenhydrinate): 393
Dramoject (dimenhydrinate): 393
Dr. Caldwell Senna (senna): 1205

Drisdol drops (ergocalciferol): 1209
Dristan Long Lasting (oxymetazoline): 833
Drithocreme (anthralin): 1213
dronabinol: 416
droperidol: 1155
D-S-S (docusate): 1203
DTIC (dacarbazine): 340
DTIC-Dome (dacarbazine): 340
DT (diphtheria and tetanus toxoids, combined, adsorbed): 1157
DTaP (diphtheria and tetanus toxoids and acellular pertussis vaccine): 1160
DTwP (diphtheria and tetanus toxoids and whole cell pertussis vaccine, adsorbed): 1157
DTwP-HIB (diphtheria and tetanus toxoids and whole cell pertussis vaccine with *haemophilus influenzae* b conjugates vaccine): 1162
Dulcagen (bisacodyl): 1203
Dulcolax (bisacodyl): 1203
Dull-C (ascorbic acid): 1208
Duo-K (potassium): 910
Duo-Trach Kit (lidocaine): 636
Duphalac (lactulose): 622, 1204
Durabolin (nandrolone): 777
Dura-Estrin (estradiol): 446
Duragen (estradiol): 446
Duragesic (fentanyl): 482
Duralith (lithium): 645
Duralone (methylprednisolone): 728
Duralutin (hydroxyprogesterone): 572
Duramist Plus (oxymetazoline): 833
Duramorph (morphine): 762
Duranest HCl (etidocaine): 1158
Duraquin (quinidine): 969
Duratest-100 (testosterone): 1050
Durathate-200 (testosterone): 1050
Duration Mild (phenylephrine): 888
Duretic (CAN)(methyclothiazide): 721
Duricef (cefadroxil): 222
Duvoid (bethanechol): 172
DV (dienestrol): 382
Dyazide (triamterene and hydrochlorothiazide): 1198
Dycil (dicloxacillin): 378
Dyflex (diphylline): 418
Dymelor (acetohexamide): 62
Dymenate (dimenhydrinate): 393
DynaCirc (isradipine): 612

Dyna-Hex (chlorhexidine): 1213
Dynapen (dicloxacillin): 378
Dy-Phyl-Lin (diphylline): 418
dyphylline: 418
Dyrenium (triamterene): 1096
Dyrexan-OD (phendimetrazine): 1152

E

E (vitamin E): 1209
EACA (aminocaproic acid): 96
Easprin (aspirin): 131
echothiopate: 1241
E-Complex (vitamin E): 1209
econazole nitrate: 1214
Econopred (prednisolone): 918
Ecotrin (aspirin): 131
Edecrin (ethacrynic acid): 460
edetate calcium disodium: 420
edetate disodium: 420
edrophonium chloride: 421
E.E.S. (erythromycin): 440
Effexor (venlafaxine): 1133
Efudex (fluorouracil): 500
Elase (fibrinolysin): 485
Elavil (amitriptyline): 104
Eldepryl (selegiline): 994
ELECTROLYTES
   ammonium chloride: 108
   calcium carbonate: 204
   calcium chloride: 204
   calcium gluconate: 204
   calcium lactate: 204
   magnesium sulfate: 662
   potassium: 910
   sodium bicarbonate: 999
   sodium chloride: 1001
Elimite (permethrin)): 1215
Elixomin (theophylline): 1056
Elixophyllin (theophylline): 1056
Elixophyllin SR (theophylline): 1056
Elocon (mometasone): 1221
Elspar (asparaginase): 129
Eltor (CAN) (pseudoephedrine): 954
Eltroxin (CAN) (levothyroxine): 634
Emcyt (estramustine): 449
Emersal (ammoniated mercury): 1213
Emete-Con (benzquinamide): 160
EMETIC AGENT
   ipecac syrup: 599
Eminase (anistreplase): 123

EMOLLIENTS
- boric acid: 1212
- dexpanthenol: 1212
- glycerin: 1212
- lanolin: 1212
- urea: 1212
- vitamin A & D: 1212
- zinc oxide: 1212

Empirin (aspirin): 131
Empirin with Codeine (aspirin with codeine): 1191
Emulsoil (castor oil): 1203
E-Mycin (erythromycin): 440
enalapril maleate: 424
enalaprilat: 424
Endep (amitriptyline): 104
Endrate (edetate): 420
Enduron (methyclothiazide): 721
Ener-B (cyanocobalamin): 1209
enflurane: 1154
Engerix-B (hepatitis B vaccine): 1165
Enlon (edrophonium): 421
Enovid 5 mg (combo OC): 1199
Enovid-E 21 (combo OC): 1199
Enovil (amitriptyline): 104
enoxacin: 426
enoxaprin: 427
Entacyl (CAN) (piperazine): 900
Enthrane (enflurane): 1154
Entozyme (pancreatic enzymes): 845
Entrophen (CAN) (aspirin): 131
Enulose (lactulose): 622, 1204

ENZYME INHIBITOR
- disulfiram: 402
- metyrosine: 741

ENZYMES
- alglucerase: 75
- chymopapain: 286
- fibrinolysin: 485
- hyaluronidase: 555

ephedrine sulfate: 428
Epifrin (epinephrine): 430
Epimorph (CAN) (morphine): 762
Epinal (epinephrine): 430
epinephrine: 430
epinephrine bitartrate: 430
epinephrine borate: 430
epinephrine hydrochloride: 430
EpiPen AutoInjector (epinephrine): 430
EpiPen AutoInjector Jr. (epinephrine): 430
Epival (CAN) (valproic acid): 1128
EPO (epoetin): 434

epoetin alfa: 434
Epogen (epoetin): 434
Eppy (epinephrine): 430
epsom salt granules (magnesium sulfate): 662
Epsom Salts (magnesium sulfate): 1204
Equalactin (polycarbophil): 1205
Equanil (meprobamate): 691
Equilet (calcium): 204
Eramycin (erythromycin): 440
Ergamisol (evamisole): 626
ergocalciferol: 1209
ergonovine maleate: 436
Ergostat (ergotamine): 437
ergotamine tartrate: 437

ERGOT DERIVATIVES
- bromocriptine: 182
- dihydroergotamine: 389
- ergotamine: 437

Ergotrate Maleate (ergonovine): 436
Eryc (erythromycin): 440
Eryderm (erythromycin): 440
Erymax (erythromycin) : 440
EryPed (erythromycin) : 440
Ery-Tab (erythromycin): 440
erythrityl tetranitrate: 438
Erythromid (CAN)(erythromycin): 440
erythromycin base: 440
erythomycin estolate: 440
erythromycin ethlysuccinate: 440
erythromycin gluceptate: 440
erythromycin lactobionate: 440
erythromycin stearate: 440

ERYTHROPOETIN
- epoetin alfa: 434

Eserine (physostigmine): 1242
Esidrix (hydrochlorothiazide): 559
Eskalith (lithium): 645
esmolol hydrochloride : 443
ESPA (thiotepa): 1067
Espotabs (phenolphthalein): 1204
estazolam: 444
Estrace (estradiol): 446
Estra-D (estradiol): 446
Estraderm (estradiol): 446
estradiol cypionate in oil: 446
estradiol oral: 446
estradiol transdermal: 446
estradiol valereate in oil: 446
Estra-L 40 (estradiol): 446
estramustine phosphate sodium: 449
Estratab (estrogens, esterified): 453

Estro-Cyp (estradiol): 446
estrogenic substance (estrone): 455
ESTROGENS
 chlorotrianisene: 268
 dienestrol: 382
 diethylstilbestrol: 383
 estradiol: 446
 estramustine: 449
 estrogens, conjugated: 450
 estrogens, esterified: 453
 estrone: 455
 estropipate: 458
 quinestrol: 965
estrogens, conjugated: 450
estrogens, esterified: 453
Estroject L.A. (estradiol): 446
Estromed (CAN) (estrogens, esterified): 453
estrone: 455
Estronol LA (estradiol): 446
estropipate: 458
Estrovis (quinestrol): 965
ethacrynic acid: 460
ethacrynate sodium (ethyacrynic acid): 460
ethambutol hydrochloride: 462
Ethaquin (ethaverine): 1206
Ethatab (ethaverine): 1206
ethaverine: 1206
Ethavex (ethaverine): 1206
ethchlorvynol: 463
ethionamide: 464
Ethmozine (moricizine): 760
Ethon (methyclothiazide): 721
ethosuximide: 465
ethotoin: 470
ethylene: 1153
Etibi (CAN) (ethambutol): 462
etidocaine: 1158
etodolac: 469
etomidate: 1155
etoposide: **470**
Etrafon (perphenazine with amitriptyline): 1194
etretinate: 471
Eulexin (flutamide): 511
Eurax (crotamiton): 1215
Evac-U-Gen (phenolphthalein): 1204
Everone (testosterone): 1050
E-Vista (hydroxyzine): 575
Excedrin IB (ibuprofen): 576
Exdol (CAN) (acetaminophen): 58
Exidine (chlorhexidine): 1213

Ex-Lax (phenolphthalein): 1204
Exna (benzthaizide): 161
Exosurf Neonatal (colfosceril): 320
EXPECTORANTS
 guaifenesin: 541
 terpin hydrate: 1048
Exsel (selenium): 1214
Eyesine (tetrehydrolozine): 1055

F

Factor VIII (antihemophilic factor): 124
factor IX complex: 473
Factrel (gonadorelin): 537
Falapen (CAN) (penicillin G potassium): 859
famciclovir sodium: 475
famotidine: 476
Famvir (famciclovir): 475
Fansidar (sulfadoxine and pyrimethamine): 1197
Fastin (phentermine): 1152
fat emulsion, intravenous: 477
5-FC (flucytosine): 494
Feen-a-Mint (phenolphthalein): 1204
Feldene (piroxicam): 903
felodipine: 478
Femazole (metronidazole): 739
Femogen (CAN) (estrone): 455
Femstat (butoconazole): 198
fenfluramine hydrochloride: 1151
fenofibrate: 479
fenoprofen: 481
fentanyl: 482
Fentanyl Oralet (fentanyl): 482
Feosol (ferrous sulfate): 483
Feostat (ferrous fumarate): 483
Fergon (ferrous gluconate): 483
Fer-In-Sol (ferrous sulfate): 483
Fer-Iron (ferrous sulfate): 483
Fero-Gradumet Filmtabs (ferrous sulfate): 483
Ferospace (ferrous sulfate): 483
Ferralet (ferrous gluconate): 483
Ferralyn Lanacaps (ferrous sulfate, exsiccated): 483
ferrous fumarate: 483
ferrous gluconate: 483
ferrous sulfate: 483
ferrous sulfate exsiccated: 483
Fersamal (CAN) (ferrous fumarate): 483

FERTILITY DRUGS
clomiphen: 302
menotropins: 681
urofollitropin: 1124

Fertinic (CAN) (ferrous gluconate): 483
Fesofor (CAN) (ferrous sulfate): 483
Fiberall (polycarbophil): 1205
Fiberall Natural (psyllium): 1205
Fiber Con (polycarbophil): 1205
Fiber-Lax (polycarbophil): 1205
fibrinolysin and desoxyribonuclease: 485
filgrastin: 486
finasteride: 487
FK506 (tacrolimus): 1038
Flagyl (metronidazole): 739
Flatulex (simethicone): 997
Flavons-500 (vitamin P): 1210
Flavorcee (ascorbic acid): 1208
flavoxate hydrochloride: 488
Flaxedil (gallamine): 1239
flecainide hydrochloride: 489
Fleet Babylax (glycerin): 532, 1203
Fleet Flavored Castor (castor oil): 1203
Fleet Lax (bisacodyl): 1203
Fletcher's Castoria (senna): 1205
Flexeril (cyclobenzaprine): 330
Flexoject (orphenadrine): 820
Floricet C Codeine (acetaminophen, caffeine, butabarbital): 1191
Florinal with Codeine (aspirin, caffeine, utabarbital): 1191
Florinef Acetate (fludrocortisone): 496
Florone (diflorasone): 1219
Florone E (diflorasone): 1219
Floxin (ofloxacin): 814
floxuridine: 491
fluconazole: 492
flucytosine: 494
fludarabine: 495
Fludara (fludarabine): 495
fludrocortisone acetate: 496
Flu-Immune (influenza virus vaccine): 1168
Flumadine (rimantidine): 981
flumazenil: 498
flunisolide: 499
fluocinolone acetonide: 1219
fluocinonide: 1220
Fluogen (influenza virus vaccine): 1168
Fluonex (fluocinonide): 1220
Fluonid (fluocinolone): 1219
Fluor-A-Day (CAN) (sodium fluoride): 1002

5-fluoragtosine (flucytosine): 494
5-fluorocystosine (flurocytosine): 494
Fluoritab (sodium fluoride): 1002
5-fluorocytosine (flucytosine): 494
fluorometholone: 1241
Fluoro-op (fluorometholone): 1241
Fluoroplex (fluorouracil): 500
FLOUOROQUINOLONES (see page 32)
ciprofloxacin: 289
enoxacin: 426
lomefloxacin: 647
norfloxacin: 806
ofloxacin: 814
fluorouracil: 500
5-fluorouracil: 500
Fluothane (halothane): 1154
Fluotic (CAN) (sodium fluoride): 1002
fluoxetine hydrochloride: 503
fluoxymesterone: 504
fluphenazine decanoate: 506
fluphenazine enanthate: 506
fluphenazine hydrochloride: 506
Flura (sodium fluoride): 1002
Flura-Loz (sodium fluoride): 1002
flurandrenolide: 1220
flurazepam: 508
flurbiprofen: 510
Fluro-Drops (sodium fluoride): 1002
Fluorsyn (fluocinolone): 1219
Flu-Shield (influenza virus vaccine): 1168
flutamide: 511
Flutex (triamcinolone): 1093, 1222
fluticasone propionate: 1220
fluvastatin: 512
fluvoxamine maleate: 513
Fluzone (influenza virus vaccine): 1168
FML (fluorometholone): 1221
Foile (benzocaine): 1158
FoilleCort (hydrocortisone): 1221
folacin (folic acid): 514
folate (folic acid): 514
Folex PFS (methotrexate): 714
FOLIC ACID
folic acid: 514
folic acid: 514
FOLIC ACID ANTAGONISTS
purimethamine: 959
trimetrexate: 1114
FOLIC ACID DERIVATIVE
leucovorin: 624
folinic acid (leucovorin): 624
Follutein (chorionic gonadotropin): 284

1278 ■ Index

Folvite (folic acid): 514
Forane (isoflurane): 1154
Formula Q (quinine): 970
Formulex (CAN) (dicyclomine): 379
Fortaz (ceftazidime): 241
foscarnet sodium: 515
Foscavir (foscarnet): 515
fosinopril sodium: 517
Fragmin (dalteparin): 343
FreAmine (amino acids): 94
5-FU (fluorouracil): 500
FUDR (floxuridine): 491
Fumasorb (ferrous fumarate): 483
Fumerin (ferrous fumarate): 483
Fungizone (amphotericin B): 116
Fungizone Intravenous (amphotericin B): 116
Furacin (nitrofurazone): 1216
Furadantin (nitrofurantoin): 795
Furanite (nitrofurantoin): 795
furosemide: 518

G

gabapentin: 520
gallamine triethiodide: 1239
gallium nitrate: 521
GALLSTONE SOLUBILIZING AGENTS
   chenodiol: 256
   monoctanoin: 759
   ursodiol: 1127
Gamastan (immune globulin IM): 1166
Gamimune (immune globulin IV): 1166
Gammagard (immune globulin IV): 1166
Gamma Globulin (immune globulin IM): 1166
Gammar (immune globulin IM): 1166
Gammar-IV (immune globulin IV): 1166
Gamulin Rh (RH immune globulin): 1175
ganciclovir sodium: 522
GANGLIONIC BLOCKER
   mecamylamine: 668
   trimethaphan: 1110
Ganite (gallium): 521
Gantanol (sulfamethoxazole): 1028
Gantrisin (sulfisoxazole): 1032
Garamycin (gentamicin): 525
Gardenal (CAN) (phenobarbital): 882
Gas Relief (simethicone): 1032
Gastrocrom (cromolyn): 326

Gas-X (simethicone): 1032
G-CSF (filgastrin): 486
Gelfoam (absorbable gelatin): 1215
gemfibrozil: 524
Genabid (papaverine): 1206
Genasal (oxymetazoline): 833
Genaspor (tolnaftate): 1214
Genatuss (guaifenesin): 541
Gen-Cefazolin (CAN) (cefazolin): 325
Genebs (acetaminophen): 58
GENERAL ANESTHETICS (see page 1152)
   cyclopropane: 1152
   desflurane: 1154
   droperidol: 1155
   enflurane: 1154
   ethylene: 1153
   etomidate: 1155
   halothane: 1154
   isoflurane: 1154
   ketamine: 1155
   methohexital: 1153
   methoxyflurane: 1154
   midazolam: 1154
   nitrous oxide: 1153
   propofol: 1155
   thiamylal: 1153
   thiopental: 1153
Gen-K (potassium): 910
Genoptic (gentamicin): 525
Genora 1/35 (combo OC): 1200
Genora 1/50 (combo OC): 1200
Genova 0.5/35 (combo OC): 1199
Genpril (ibuprofen): 576
Genprin (aspirin): 131
Gen-Salbutamol Strinebs (CAN) (albuterol): 73
Gentacidin (gentamicin): 525
Gentamicin Liposome Injection (gentamicin): 525
Gentak (gentamicin): 525
gentamicin sulfate: 525
gentian violet: 1214
Gentlax (senna): 1205
Gentran 75 (dextran, high): 364
Gentran 40 (dextran, low): 365
Gen-Xene (cloazepate): 309
Geocillin (carbenicillin): 212
Geopen Oral (CAN) (carbenicillin): 212
Geridium (phenazopyridine): 878
Gesterol 50 (progesterone): 936
GG-Cen (guaifenesin): 541

GI DRUGS
cisapride: 291
GI STIMULANT
dexpanthenol: 363
methscopolamine: 719
metoclopramide: 734
Glaucon (epinephrine): 430
glipizide: 527
Glaucon (epinephrine): 430
glucagon: 529
GLUCOCORTICOIDS
beclomethasone: 154
betamethasone: 167
dexamethasone: 358
flunisolide: 499
hydrocortisone: 561
methylprednisolone: 728
prednisolone: 918
prednisone: 921
triamcinolone: 1093
Glucophage (metformin): 702
GLUCOSE ELEVATING AGENTS
diazoxide: 375
glucagon: 529
Glucotrol (glipizide): 527
Glukor (chorionic gonadotropin): 284
glutethimide: 530
Glyate (guaifenesin): 541
glyburide: 531
glycerin: 532, 1203, 1212
glycerol: 532
glycopyrrolate: 534
GM-CSF (sargramostin): 988
GnRH (gonadorelin): 537
GnRH (gonadotropic-releasing hormone)
gonadorelin: 537
nafarelin: 768
GnRH ANTAGONIST
histrelin: 554
GOLD COMPOUNDS
auranofin: 141
aurothioglucose: 142
gold sodium thiomalate: 535
gold sodium thiomalate: 535
gonadorelin acetate: 537
gonadorelin hydrochloride: 537
Gonic (chorionic gonadotropin): 284
Gormel (urea): 1212
goserelin acetate: 539
granisetron hydrochloride: 540
granulocyte colony-stimulating factor (filgrastin): 486

granulocyte macrophage colony-stimulating factor (sargramostin): 988
Gravol (CAN) (dimenhydrinate): 393
guaifenesin: 541
Guaitussin (guaifenesin): 541
guanabenz acetate: 541
guanadrel sulfate: 542
guanethidine monosulfate: 544
guanfacine hydrochloride: 546
G-Well (lindane): 1215
Gynecort (hydrocortisone): 1221
Gyne-Lotrimin (clotrimazole): 311
Gynergen (CAN) (ergotamine): 430
Gynogen L.A. 20 (estradiol): 446

H

Habitrol (nicotine transdermal): 792
halazepam : 547
halcinonide: 1220
Halcion (triazolam): 1097
Haldol (haloperidol): 548
Haldol Deconoate (haloperidol): 548
Haldol LA (CAN) (haloperidol): 548
halobetasol propionate: 1220
Halofed (pseudoephedrine): 954
Halog (halcinonide): 1220
haloperidol: 548
haloperidol decanoate: 548
haloperidol lactate: 548
Halotestin (fluoxymesterone):504
halothane: 1154
Halotussin (guaifenesin): 541
Haltran (ibuprofen): 576
hamamelis water: 1212
HBIG (hepatitis immune globulin): 1164
H-BIG (hepatitis immune globulin): 1164
HCG (human chorionic gonadotropin): 284
HDCV (rabies vaccine): 1180
Hemabate (carboprost): 215
Hemocyte (ferrous fumarate): 483
Hemofil-M (antihemophilic factor): 124
hemophilus b conjugate vaccine: 1163
HEMORHEOLOGIC DRUG
pentoxifylline: 872
HEMOSTATIC AGENTS
absorbable gelatin: 1215
microfibrillar collagen: 1216
thrombin: 1216
Hepalean (CAN) (heparin): 551

1280 ■ Index

HEPARIN ANTAGONIST
   protamine sulfate: 951
heparin calcium injection: 551
Heparin Lock Flush (heparin): 551
heparin sodium injection: 551
heparin sodium and 0.9% sodium chloride: 551
heparin sodium lock flush solution: 551
hepatitis B immune globulin: 1164
hepatitis B vaccine: 1165
Hep-B-Gammagee (hepatitis B immune globulin): 1164
Hep-Lock (heparin): 551
Heptamine (amino acids): 94
Herplex (idoxuridine): 1241
HES (hetastarch): 553
Hespan (hetastarch): 553
hetastarch: 553
hexachlorophene: 1213
Hexadrol (dexamethasone): 338
Hexadrol Phosphate (dexamethasone): 338
Hexalen (altretamine): 85
hexamethylamine (altretamine): 85
Hibiciens (chlorohexidine): 1213
Hibistat (chlorhexidine): 1213
HibTITER (hemophilus b vaccine): 1163
Hip-Rex (CAN)(methenamine): 708
Hiprex (methenamine): 708
Hismanal (astemizole): 134
Histaject (brompheniramine): 185
HISTAMINE 2 ANTAGONISTS (see page 34)
   cimetidine: 286
   famotidine: 476
   nizatadine: 801
   ranitidine: 973
Histanal (CAN) (promethazine): 941
Histerone (testosterone): 1050
histrelin acetate: 554
Hivid (zalcitabine): 1146
HMG CoA INHIBITORS (see page 35)
   fluvastatin: 512
   lovastatin: 656
   pravastatin: 913
   simvastatin: 998
HN2 (mechlomethamine): 670
Hold (dextramethorphan): 369
homatropine: 1241
Homatropine HBr (homatropine): 1241
Hondrocil Instant (psyllium): 1205
Honvol (CAN) (diethylstilbesterol): 383

HORMONES
   beclomethasone: 154
   betamethasone: 167
   calcitonin: 201
   chlorotrianisene: 268
   chorionic gonadotropin: 284
   clomiphene: 302
   cortisone: 323
   danazol: 344
   desmopressin: 356
   dexamethasone: 358
   dienestrol: 382
   diethylstilbestrol: 383
   estradiol: 446
   estramustine: 449
   estrogens, conjugated: 450
   estrogens, esterified: 453
   estrone: 456
   estropipate: 458
   fludrocortisone: 496
   flunisolide: 499
   fluoxymesterone: 504
   glucagon: 529
   gonadorelin: 537
   goserelin: 539
   hydrocortisone: 561
   hydroxyprogesterone: 572
   insulin: 587
   leuprolide: 625
   levonorgestrel: 631
   lypressin: 659
   medroxyprogesterone: 674
   megestrol: 679
   menotropins: 681
   methylprednisolone: 728
   nafarelin: 768
   nandrolone: 777
   norethindrone: 804
   norgestrel: 807
   octreotide: 812
   oxandrolone: 824
   oxymetholone: 835
   oxytocin: 841
   prednisolone: 918
   prednisone: 921
   progesterone: 936
   quinestrol: 965
   somatrem: 1006
   somatropin: 1007
   stanozolol: 1014
   testolactone: 1049
   testosterone: 1050

thyrotropin: 1072
triamcinolone: 1093
urofollitropin: 1124
vasopressin: 1132
HORMONE ANTAGONIST
aminoglutethemide: 97
H.P. Acthar Gel (corticotropin): 321
human chorionic gonadotropin (chorionic gonadotropin): 284
Humibid Sprinkle (guaifenesin): 541
Humate-P (antihemophilic factor): 124
Humatin (paramomycin): 849
Humatrope (somatropin): 1007
Humorsol (demecarium): 1241
Humulin N (insulin-NPH): 587
Humulin R (insulin) : 587
hyaluronidase: 555
Hybolin Decanoate (nandrolone): 777
Hybolin Improved (nandrolone): 777
Hycodon (hydrocodone): 560
Hycort (CAN) (hydrocortisone): 561, 1221
HYDANTOINS
ethotoin: 467
mephenytoin: 687
phenytoin: 892
Hydeltra (prendisolone): 918
Hydeltrasol (prednisolone): 918
hydralazine hydrochloride: 557
Hydrate (dimenhydrinate): 393
Hydrea (hydroxyurea): 573
Hydrobexan (hydroxocobalamin): 569
hydrochlorothiazide: 559
Hydrocil (psyllium): 1205
hydrocodone bitartrate: 560
hydrocortisone: 1220
hydrocortisone acetate: 1221
hydrocortisone butyrate: 561, 1221
hydrocortisone cypoinate: 561
Hydrocortisone Phosphate (hydrocortisone): 561
hydrocortisone sodium phosphate: 561
hydrocortisone sodium succinate: 561
hydrocortisone valerate: 561, 1221
Hydrocortone (prednisolone): 918
Hydro-Crysti 12 (hydroxocobalamin): 569
Hydro DIURIL (hydrochlorothiazide): 559
hydroflumethiazide: 565
Hydromox (quinethazone): 967
hydromorphone hydrochloride: 567
Hydro-Par (hydrochlorothiazide): 559
HydroTEX (hydrocortisone): 1220

Hydroxacen (hydroxyzine): 575
hydroxocobalamin crystalline: 569
hydroxychloroquine sulfate: 570
hydroxyethyl starch (hetastarch): 553
hydroxymagnesium aluminate (magaldrate): 660
hydroxyprogesterone caprate in oil: 572
hydroxyurea: 573
hydroxyzine hydrochloride: 575
hydroxyzine pamoate: 575
Hydrozide (CAN) (hydrochlorothiazide): 559
Hygroton (chlorthalidone): 279
Hylorel (guanadrel): 542
Hylutin (hydroxyprogesterone): 572
hyoscine Hbr (scopolamine): 989
Hyperab Imogam (rabies immune globulin): 1178
HyperHep (hepatitis immune globulin): 1164
Hyperstat (diazoxide): 375
Hyper-Tet (tetanus immune globulin): 1175
HYPNOTICS (see Sedative/Hypnotics)
HypRho-D (RH immune globulin): 1175
HypRho-D Mini Dose (RH immune globulin micro-dose): 1175
Hyprogest (hydroxyprogesterone): 572
Hytakerol (dihydrotachysterol): 1209
Hytone (hydrocortisone): 1221
Hytress 2X (guaifenesin): 541
Hytrin (terazosin): 1044
Hyzine (hydroxyzine): 575

I

ibuprofen: 576
Ibuprin (ibuprofen): 576
Ibuprohm (ibuprofen): 576
Ibu-Tab (ibuprofen): 576
Idamycin (idarubicin):578
idarubicin hydrochloride: 578
idoxuridine: 1241
IDU (idoxuridine): 1241
IFLrA (interferon alfa 2a): 589
IFN-alpha 2 (interferon alfa 2b): 592
ifosfamide: 579
Ifex (ifosfamide): 579
IG (immune globulin intramuscular): 1166
IGIV (immune globulin intravenous): 1166
IL-2 (aldesleukin): 75
Iletin PZI (CAN) (insulin): 587

1282 ■ Index

Ilopan (dexpanthenol): 363
Ilosone (erythromycin): 440
Ilotycin (erythromycin): 440
Ilotycin Gluceptate (erythromycin): 440
Ilotycin Ophthalmic (erythromycin): 440
Ilozyme (pancreatic enzymes): 845
imidazole carboxamide (dacarbazine): 340
imipramine hydrochloride: 581
imipramine pamoate: 581
Imitrex (sumatriptan):1036
Immune Globulin (immune globulin IM):
immune globulin intramuscular: 1166
immune globulin intravenous: 1166
IMMUNOSUPPRESSANTS
    azathioprine: 145
    cyclosporine: 334
    muromonab-CD 3: 764
    tacrolimus: 1038
Imodium (loperamide): 650
Imodium A-D (loperamide): 650
Imovax Rabies (rabies vaccine): 1180
Impril (CAN) (imipramine): 581
Imuran (azathioprine): 145
Inapsine (droperidol): 1155
indapamideL: 583
Inderal (propranolol): 947
Inderide (hydrochlorothiazide and
    propranolol): 1196
Indocin (indomethacin): 585
Indocin-IV (indomethacin): 585
Indocin-SR (indomethacin): 585
Indo-Lemmon (indomethacin): 585
Indometh (indomethacin): 585
indomethacin: 585
indomethacin sodium trihydrate: 585
In FeD (iron dextran): 600
Inflamase (prednisolone): 918
influenza virus vaccine: 1168
Infumorph (morphine): 762
INH (isoniazid): 604
Inocid (CAN) (indomethacin): 585
Inocor (amrinone): 120
Insulatard NPH (insulin): 587
insulin: 587
insulin zinc suspension: 587
insulin zinc suspension, extended: 587
insulin zinc suspension, prompt (semilente): 587
Intal (cromolyn): 326
INTERFERONS
    interferon alfa 2a: 589

    interferon alfa 2b: 591
    interferon alfa n3: 593
    interferon beta 1b: 594
    interferon gamma 1b: 596
interferon alfa 2a: 589
interferon alfa 2b: 591
interferon alfa n3: 593
interferon beta 1b: 594
interferon gamma 1b: 596
Interleukin-2 (aldesleukin): 75
Intralipid 10% (fat emulsion): 477
Intralipid 20% (fat emulsion): 477
Intron-A (interferon alfa 2b): 589
Intropin (dopamine): 405
Inversine (mecamylamine): 668
Iodex (povidone iodine): 1213
iodine: 1213
iodine thyroid products: 597
iodoquinol: 598
Ionamin (phentermine): 1152
Iopidine (apraclonidine): 1214
ipecac syrup: 599
IPOL (poliovirus vaccine, inactivated): 1174
IPV (poliovirus vaccine, inactivated): 1174
ipratropium bromide: 600
Ircon (ferrous fumarate): 483
iron dextran: 600
IRON PREPARATIONS
    ferrous fumarate: 483
    ferrous gluconate: 483
    ferrous sulfate: 483
    ferrous sulfate excissated: 483
    iron dextran: 600
ISG (immune globulin IM): 1166
Ismelin (guanethidine): 544
Ismotic (isosorbide): 608
Iso-Bid (isosorbide dinitrate): 609
Isocaine (mepivocaine): 1159
isoetharine hydrochloride: 602
isoetharine mesylate: 602
isoflurane: 1154
isomeprobamate (carisoprodol): 216
isoniazid: 604
isonicotinic acid hydrazide (isoniazide): 604
isophane insulin suspension (NPH): 587
isoproterenol hydrochloride: 605
isoproterenol sulfate: 605
Isoptin (verapamil): 1134
Isopto-Atropine Ophthalmic (atropine): 138
Isopto Carbachol (carbachol): 1241
Isopto Eserine (physostigmine): 1242

Isopto Frin (phenylephrine): 888
Isopto Homatropine (homatropine): 1241
Isopto Hyoscine Ophthalmic (scopolamine): 989
Isordil (isosorbide dinitrate): 609
isosorbide: 608
isosorbide dinitrate: 609
Isotamine (CAN) (isoniazid): 604
Isotrate Timecelles (isosorbide dinitrate): 609
isotretinoin: 610
Isovex (isoxsuprine): 1206
isoxsuprine hydrochloride: 1206
isradipine: 612
Isuprel (isoproterenol): 605
Itch-X (promaxine): 1159
itraconazole: 613
Iveegam (immune globulin intravenous): 1166

J

Janest-28 (combo OC): 1201
Janimine (imipramine): 581
Japanese encephalitis vaccine: 1180
Jenamicin (gentamicin): 525
JE-VAX (Japenese encephalitis vaccine): 1180

K

Kabikinase (streptokinase): 1016
kanamycin sulfate : 614
Kantrex (kanamycin): 614
Kaochlor (potassium): 910
Kaon-Cl (potassium): 910
Kaopectate (loperamide): 650
Karidium (sodium fluoride): 1002
Kato (potassium): 910
Kay Ciel (potassium): 910
Kayexalate (sodium polystyrene sulfonate): 1003
Kaylixir (potassium): 910
Keflex (cephalexin): 249
Keflin (cephalothin): 250
Keftab (cephalexin): 249
Kefzol (cefazolin): 225
Kefurox (cefuroxime): 246
Kemadrin (procycildine): 934
Kenacort (triamcinolone): 1093
Kenaject (triamcinolone): 1093

Kenalog (triamcinolone): 1093, 1222
KERATOLYTICS
   cantharidin: 1215
   podophyllium resin: 1215
   podofilox: 1215
Kerlone (betaxolol): 170
Kestrone S (estrone): 455
Ketalar (ketamine): 1155
ketamine: 1155
ketoconazole: 616
ketoprofen: 618
ketorolac tromethamine: 618
Key-Pred (prednisolone): 918
K-G Elixir (potassium): 910
Kidrolase (CAN) (asparaginase): 129
Klonopin (clonazepam): 305
K-Lor (potassium): 910
Klor-Con (potassium): 910
Klorvess (potassium): 910
Klotrix (potassium): 910
K-Lyte/Cl (potassium): 910
Koate-HP (antihemophilic factor): 124
Koate-HS (antihemophilic factor): 124
Koffex (CAN) (dextramethorphan): 369
Kolyum (potassium): 910
Kondon's Nasal (ephedrine): 428
Kondremul Plain (mineral oil): 1204
Konsyl (psyllium): 1205
Konyne-HT (factor IX): 473
Ku-Zyme HP Capsules (pancreatic enzymes): 845
Kwell (lindane): 1215
Kybernin (antithrombin): 125
Kytril (granisetron): 540

L

LA-12 (hydroxocabalamin): 569
labetalol hydrochloride: 620
lactulose: 622, 1204
Lamictal (lamotrigine): 623
Lamisil (terbinafine): 1214
lamotrigine: 623
Lamprene (clofazimine): 299
Lanacane (benzocaine): 1158
Lanacort 5 (hydrocortisone): 1221
Lanaphilic (urea): 1212
Laniazid (isoniazide): 607
lanolin: 1212
Lanophyllin (theophylline): 1056

Lanoxicaps (digoxin): 386
Lanoxin (digoxin): 386
Lanvis (CAN) (thioguanine): 1063
Larodopa (levodopa): 627
Largactil (CAN) (chlorpromazine): 272
Lariam (mefloquine): 677
Lasan (anthralin): 1213
Lasix (furosemide): 518
LAXATIVES (see page 1202)
  bisacodyl: 1203
  cascara: 1203
  castor oil: 1203
  docusate: 1203
  glycerin: 532, 1203
  lactulose: 622, 1204
  magnesium citrate: 1204
  magnesium hydroxide: 1204
  magnesium salts: 661, 1204
  magnesium sulfate: 662, 1204
  mineral oil: 1204
  phenolphthalein: 1204
  polycarbophil: 1205
  psyllium: 1205
  senna: 1205
Lax Pills (phenolphthalein): 1204
L-Caine (lidocaine): 630
LCR (vincristine): 1139
L-Deprenyl (selegiline): 994
Ledercillin VK (penicillin V): 862
Legatrin (quinine): 970
Lente Insulin (insulin): 587
LEPROSTATIC DRUGS
  clofazimine: 299
  dapsone: 348
Lescol (fluvastatin): 512
leucovorin calcium: 624
Leukeran (chlorambucil): 259
Leukine (sargramostin): 988
leuprolide acetate: 625
Leustatin (cladribine): 293
levamisole hydrochloride: 626
levarterenolol (norephinephrine): 802
Levate (CAN) (amitriptyline): 104
Levatol (penbutolol): 854
Levlen (combo OC): 1199
levocabastine: 1242
levodopa: 627
Levo-Dromoran (levorphanol): 633
levomethadyl acetate hydrochloride: 629
levonorgestrel: 631
Levophed (norephinephrine): 802

Levoprome (methotrimeprazine): 716
Levora (combo OC): 1199
levorphanol sulfate: 633
Levothroid (levothyroxine): 634
levothyroxine sodium: 634
Libritabs (chlordiazepoxide): 263
Librium (chlordiazepoxide): 263
Lidex (fluocinonide): 1220
lidocaine hydrochloride: 636, 1158
lidocaine hydrochloride in 5% dextrose: 636
lidocaine hydrochloride without preservatives: 636
Lidoject (lidocaine): 636
LidoPen Auto-Injector (lidocaine): 636
Limbitrol (chlordiazepoxide and amitriptyline): 1195
Lincocin (lincomycin): 639
lincomycin hydrochloride: 639
Lincorex (lincomycin): 639
LINCOSAMIDE ANTIBIOTICS
  clindamycin: 297
  lincomycin: 639
lindane: 1215
Lioresal (baclofen): 152
liothyronine sodium: 640
liotrix: 642
Lipidil (fenofibrate): 479
Lipo-Hepin (heparin): 551
Liposyn II 10% (fat emulsion): 477
Liposyn II 20% (fat emulsion): 477
Liposyn III 10% (fat emulsion): 477
Liposyn III 20% (fat emulsion): 477
Liquaemin Sodium (heparin): 551
Liqui-Char (charcoal): 256
Liquid Pred (prednisone): 921
Liquiprin (acetaminophen): 58
lisinopril: 643
Lithane (lithium): 645
lithium carbonate: 645
lithium citrate: 645
Lithizine (CAN)(lithium): 645
Lithonate (lithium): 645
Lithostat (acetohydroxamic acid): 63
Lithotabs (lithium): 645
Livostin (levocabastine): 1242
10% LMD (dextran, low): 365
LOCAL ANESTHETICS (see page 1156)
  benzocaine: 1158
  bupivacaine: 1158
  butamben: 1158
  chloroprocaine: 1158

dibucaine: 1158
etidocaine: 1158
lidocaine: 636, 1158
mepivocaine: 1159
prilocaine: 1159
procaine: 1159
promaxine: 1159
tetracaine: 1159
Locoid (hydrocortisone): 561, 1221
Lodine (etodolac): 469
lodoxamide: 1242
Loestrin 21 1/20 (combo OC): 1200
Loestrin 21 1.5/30 (combo OC): 1199
Logen (diphenoxylate and atropine): 1195
Lomanate (diphenoxylate and atropine): 1195
lomefloxacin hydrochloride: 647
Lomotil (diphenoxylate and atropine): 1195
lomustine: 649
Lonox (diphenoxylate and atropine): 1195
LOOP DIURETICS (see page 31)
 bumetanide: 189
 ethacrynic acid: 460
 furosemide: 518
 torsemide: 1087
Lo/Ovral (combo OC): 1200
Loniten (minoxidil): 750
loperamide hydrochloride: 650
Lopid (gemfibrozil): 524
Lopidine (apraclonidine): 1241
Lopresor (CAN) (metoprolol): 737
Lopressor (metoprolol): 737
Lopurin (allopurinol): 78
Lorabid (loracarbef): 651
loracarbef: 651
loratidine: 652
lorazepam: 654
Lorelco (probucol): 927
Lotensin (benazepril): 155
Lotrimin (clotrimazole): 311, 1214
lovastatin: 656
Lovenox (enoxaparin): 427
Lowsium (magaldrate): 550
Loxapac (CAN) (loxapine): 657
loxapine hydrochloride: 657
loxapine succinate: 657
Loxitane (loxapine): 657
Loxitane-C (loxapine): 657
Lozol (indapamide): 583
L-PAM (melphalan): 680
L-thyroxine (levothyroxine): 634
Ludiomil (maprotiline): 665

Lufyllin (dyphylline): 418
Lugol's Solution (iodine thyroid): 597
Luminol Sodium (phenobarbital sodium): 882
LUNG SURFACTANTS
 beractant: 166
 colfosceril: 320
Lupron (leuprolide): 625
Lupron Depot (leuprolide): 625
Lupron Depot-Ped (leuprolide): 625
Luride Lozi Tablets (sodium fluoride): 1002
Lutrepulse (gonadorelin): 537
Lutrizine (CAN) (lithium): 645
Luvox (fluvoxamine): 513
L-sarcolysin (melphalan): 680
Lyderm Cream (CAN) (fluocinonide): 1220
lymphocyte, immune globulin: 1178
lypressin: 658
8-lysine vasopressin (lypressin): 658
Lysodren (mitotane): 754

M

Maalox Anti-Diarrheal Caplets (loperamide): 650
Macrodantin (nitrofurantoin): 795
Macrodex (dextran, high): 364
MACROLIDE ANTIBIOTICS (see page 36)
 azithromycin: 147
 clarithryomycin: 294
 erythromycin: 440
mafenide: 1216
magaldrate: 660
magnesium citrate: 661, 1204
magnesium hydroxide: 661, 1204
magnesia: 661
magnesium oxide: 661, 1204
magnesium sulfate: 662
Mag-Ox (magnesium): 661
Major-Con (simethicone): 997
Mallazine Eye Drops (tetrahydrolozine): 1055
Mallergan (promethazine): 941
Malotuss (guaifenesin): 541
Mandelamine (methenamine): 708
Mandol (cefamandole): 223
mannitol: 664
Maolate (chlorphenesin): 270
Maox (magnesium): 661

1286 ■ Index

maprotiline hydrochloride: 665
Marcaine (bupivacaine): 1158
Marezine (cyclizine): 329
Marinol (dronabinol): 416
Matulane (procarbazine): 930
Maxair (pirbuterol): 902
Maxaquin (lomefloxacin): 647
Maxeran (CAN) (metoclopramide): 734
Maxidex Ophthalmic (dexamethasone): 358
Maxiflor (diflorasone): 1219
Maxivate (betamethasone): 167, 1218
Maxolon (metoclopramide): 734
Maxzide (traimterene and hydrochlorothiazide): 1198
Mazanor (mazindol): 1152
mazindol: 1152
measles, mumps, rubella vaccine: 1170
measles (rubeola) virus vaccine: 1169
Mebaral (mephobarbital): 689
mebendazole: 667
mecamylamine: 668
mechlorethamine hydrochloride: 670
meclizine hydrochloride: 672
meclofenamate sodium: 673
Meclomen (meclofenamate): 673
Medicycline (CAN) (tetracycline): 1052
Medihaler-Epi (epinephrine): 430
Medihaler-Iso (isoproterenol): 605
Medilax (phenolphthalein): 1205
Medimet (CAN) (methyldopa): 723
Medipren (ibuprofen): 576
Mediquell (dextromethorphan): 369
Medralone (methylprednisolone): 728
Medrol (methylprednisolone): 728
Medrol Acetate (methylprednisolone): 728
medroxyprogesterone acetate: 674
mefenamic acid: 676
mefloquine hydrochloride: 677
Mefoxin (cefoxitin): 236
Megace (megestrol): 679
Megacillin (CAN) (penicillin G potassium): 859
megestrol acetate: 679
Mellaril (thioridazine): 1064
melphalan: 680
menadiol sodium diphosphate: 1209
Menest (estrogens, ester.): 453
meningococcal polysaccharide vaccine: 1179
Menomune-A/C/Y/W-135 (meningococcal vaccine): 1179
menotropins: 681

meperedine hydrochloride: 683
Mephaquin (mefloquine): 677
mephentermine sulfate: 686
mephenytoin: 687
mephobarbital: 689
Mephyton (phytonadione): 1210
mepivocaine: 1159
meprobamate: 691
Mepron (atovaquone): 137
Meprospan (meprobamate): 691
Meravil (CAN) (amitriptyline): 104
mercaptopurine: 693
6-mercaptopurine (mercaptopurine): 693
Mersol (thimersol): 1213
Meruvax II (rubella virus vaccine): 1176
mesalamine: 694
Mesantoin (mephytoin): 687
mesna: 695
Mesnex (mesna): 695
mesoridazine besylate: 696
Mestinon (pyridostigmine): 957
Metahydrin (trichlormethaizide): 1098
metaminodiazepoxide hydrochloride (chlordiazepoxide): 263
Metamucil (psyllium): 1205
Metaprel (metaproterenol): 699
metaproterenol sulfate: 699
metaraminol bitartrate: 700
metformin: 702
methadone hydrochloride: 703
methazolamide: 705
methdilazine hydrochloride: 706
methenamine: 708
methenamine hippurate: 708
methenamine mandelate: 708
Methergine (methylergonovine): 726
methicillin sodium: 709
methimazole: 711
methocarbamol: 712
methohexital sodium: 1153
methotrexate: 714
methotrimeprazine hydrochloride:716
methoxsalen: 717
methoxyflurane: 1154
methscopolamine bromide: 719
methsuximide: 720
methychlothiazide: 721
methyldopa: 721
methyldopate hydrochloride: 723
methylene blue: 725
methylergonovine maleate: 726
methylphenidate hydrochloride: 727

methylprednisolone: 728
methylprednisolone acetate: 728
methylprenisolone sodium succinate: 728
methyprylon: 731
methysergide maleate: 732
Meticorten (prednisone): 921
metipropranolol: 1242
metoclopramide: 734
metocurine iodide: 1239
metolazone: 736
metoprolol tartrate: 737
Metreton (prednisolone): 918
Metrodin (urofollitropin): 1124
MetroGel (metronidazole): 739
Metro I.V. (metronidazole): 739
metronidazole: 739
Metronidazole Redi-Infusion (metronidazole): 739
metyrosine: 741
Mevacor (lovastatin): 656
mevinolin (lovastatin): 656
mexiletine hydrochloride: 742
Mexitil (mexilitine): 742
Mezlin (mezlocillin): 743
mezlocillin sodium: 743
Miacalcin (calcitonin): 210
Miacalcin Nasal Spray (calcitonin): 210
Micatin (miconazole): 745
miconazole: 745
miconazole nitrate: 745
MICRho-GAM (RH immune globulin): 1175
microfibrillar collagen: 1216
Micronase (glyburide): 531
microNefrin (epinephrine): 430
Midamor (amiloride): 93
midazolam hydrochloride: 1155
Midol (ibuprofen): 576
MIH (procarbazine): 930
Milkinol (mineral oil): 1204
Milk of Magnesia (magnesium): 661, 1204
Milontin Kapseals (phensuximide): 885
Milophene (clomiphene): 302
milrinone lactate: 747
Miltown (meprobamate): 691
MINERALOCORTICOIDS
  fludrocortisone: 496
  hydrocortisone: 561
mineral oil: 1204
MINERALS
  sodium fluoride: 1002
  zinc: 1148

Mini-Gamulin Rh (RH immune globulin): 1175
Minims (CAN) (atropine): 138
Minims (CAN) (chloramphenicol): 261
Minipress (prazosin): 916
Minocin (minocycline): 748
minocycline hydrochloride: 748
minoxidil: 750
Mintezol (thiabendazole): 1060
Minthracin (plicamycin): 905
Miostat (carbachol): 1241
mithramycin (plicamycin): 905
misoprostol: 752
mitomycin: 753
mitomycin C (mitomycin): 753
mitotane: 754
MITOTIC INHIBITORS
  etoposide: 470
  teniposide: 1042
  vinblastine: 1138
  vincristine: 1139
  vinorelbine: 1141
mitoxantrone hydrochloride: 756
Mitran (chlordiazepoxide): 263
Mitrolan (polycarbophil): 1205
Mivacron (mivacurium): 1239
mivacurium chloride: 1239
Mixtard (insulin): 587
M-KYA (quinine): 970
M-M-R II (measles, mumps, rubella vaccine): 1170
Moban (molindone): 757
Mobenol (CAN) (tolbutamide): 1085
Moctanin (monoctanoin): 759
Modane (phenolphthalein): 1205
Modecate Deconate (CAN) (fluphenazine): 506
Modicon (combo OC): 1199
Moditen Enanthate (CAN) (fluphenazine): 506
Moditen Hydrochloride (fluphenazine): 506
Modoine Soft (docusate): 1203
Moduretic (amiloride and hydrochlorothiazide):
Moi-stir (saliva): 985
molindone hydrochloride: 757
Mol-Iron (ferrous sulfate): 483
MOM (milk of magnesia): 1204
mometasone furoate: 1221
Monistat 3 (miconazole): 745
Monistat 7 (miconazole): 745
Monistat-Derm (miconazole): 745

1288 ■ Index

Monistat Dual Pak (miconazole): 745
Monistat i.v. (miconazole): 745
Monitan (CAN) (acebutolol): 57
MONOAMINE OXIDASE INHIBITORS (MAO Inhibitors)
  phenelzine 879
  tranylcypromine: 1089
MONOBACTAM ANTIBIOTICS
  aztreonam: 148
Monocid (cefonicid): 230
Monoclate-P (antihemophilic factor): 124
monoctanoin: 759
Mono-Gesic (salsalate): 986
Monopril (fosinopril): 517
8-MOP (methoxsalen): 717
moricizine hydrochloride: 760
morphine sulfate: 762
Motrin (ibuprofen): 576
6-MP (mercaptopurine): 693
M-Prednisol (methylprednisolone): 728
MS Contin (morphine): 762
MSIR (morphine): 762
MTC (mitomycin): 753
MTX (methotrexate): 714
MUCOLYTICS
  acetylcysteine: 66
Mucomyst (acetlycysteine): 66
Mucosal (acetylcysteine): 66
Multipax (CAN) (hydroxyzine): 575
Mumpsvax (mumps virus vaccine): 1175
mumps virus vaccine, live: 1175
mupirocin: 1213
Murine (tetrahydrolozine): 1055
muromonab-CD3: 764
Muromyst (acetylcysteine): 66
Mustargen (mechlorethamine): 670
Mutamycin (mitomycin): 753
Myambutol (ethambutol): 462
Mycelex (clotrimazole): 311
Mycelex-G (clotrimazole): 311, 1214
Mycifradin (CAN) (neomycin): 782
Mycifradin Sulfate (neomycin): 782
Myciguent (neomycin): 782
Myclo (CAN) (clotrimazole): 311
Mycobutin (rifabutin): 978
Mycostatin (nystatin): 811
Mydfrin (phenylephrine): 888
MYDRIATICS
  epinephrine: 430
Myidil (triprolidine): 1119
Mykrox (metolazine): 736
Mylanta Gas (simethicone): 997
Mylceon (simethicone): 997
Myleran (busulfan): 194
Myochrysine (gold): 535
Myotonachol (bethanechol): 172
Mysoline (primidone): 923
Mytelase Caplets (ambenonium): 89
Mytussin (guaifenesin): 541

N

nabumetone: 766
N-acetylcysteine (acetylcysteine): 66
N-acetyl-P-aminophenol (acetaminophen): 58
nadolol: 767
Nadopen-V (CAN) (pencillin V): 862
Nadostine (CAN) (nystatin): 811
nafarelin acetate: 768
Nafcil (nafcillin): 770
nafcillin sodium: 770
naftifine hydrochloride: 1214
Naftine (naftifine): 1214
nalbuphine hydrochloride: 771
Naldecon-EX (guaifenesin): 541
Nalfon (fenoprofen): 481
nalidixic acid: 773
Nallpen (nafcillin): 770
naloxone hydrochloride: 774
naltrexone hydrochloride: 775
Nandrobolic (nandrolone): 777
nandrolone decanoate: 777
nandrolone phenpropionate: 777
Naprosyn (naproxen): 778
naproxen: 778
naproxen sodium: 778
Naqua (trichlormethiazide): 1098
Narcan (naloxone): 774
NARCOTIC AGONIST ANALGESICS (see page 37)
  codeine: 315
  fentanyl: 482
  hydrocodone: 560
  hydromorphone: 567
  levomethadyl: 629
  levorphanol: 633
  meperidine: 683
  methadone: 703
  morphine: 762
  opium: 819
  oxycodone: 832

oxymorphone: 836
propoxyphene: 946
sufentanil: 1023
NARCOTIC AGONIST-ANTAGONISTIC ANALGESICS
buprenorphine: 190
butorphanol: 198
dezocine: 371
nalbupine: 771
pentazocine: 866
NARCOTIC ANTAGONISTS
naloxone: 774
naltrexone: 775
Nardil (phenelzine): 879
Nasahist B (brompheniramine): 185
Nasalcrom (cromolyn): 326
NASAL DECONGESTANTS
ephedrine: 428
epinephrine: 430
oxymetazoline: 833
phenylephrine: 888
pseudoephedrine: 954
tetrahydrozoline: 1055
xylometazoline: 1145
Nasalide (flunisolide): 499
Natacyn (natamycin): 1242
natamycin: 1242
Natulan (CAN) (procarbazine): 930
natural lung surfactant (beractant): 166
Naturetin (bendroflumethiazide): 157
Nausetol (CAN) (dimenhydrinate): 393
Navane (thiothixene): 1068
Navelbine (vinorelbine): 1141
Naxen (CAN) (naproxen): 778
ND-Stat (brompheniramine): 185
Nebcin (tobramycin): 1079
NebuPent (pentamidine): 864
nedocromil sodium: 780
N.E.E. 1/35 (combo OC): 1200
nefazodone hydrochloride: 781
Neg Gram (nalidixic acid): 773
Nelova 0.5/35 (combo OC): 1199
Nevola 1/50 M (combo OC): 1200
Nelova 10/11 (combo OC): 1201
Nelova 35 (combo OC): 1200
Nembutal (pentobarbital): 868
Nembutal Sodium (pentobarbital): 868
Neocin (CAN) (neomycin): 782
Neo-Codema (CAN) (hydrochlorothiazide): 559
Neo-Cultol (mineral oil): 1204
Neo-Durabolic (nandrolone): 777

Neofed (pseudoephedrine): 954
Neolid (castor oil): 1203
neomycin sulfate: 782
Neopap (acetaminophen): 58
Neoquess (dicyclomine): 379
Neosar (cyclophosphamide): 331
neostigmine bromide: 784
neostigmine methylsulfate: 784
Neo-Synephrine (phenylephrine): 888
Neo-Synephrine (oxymetazoline): 833
Neo-Tetrine (CAN) (tetracycline): 1052
Neothylline (dyphylline): 418
Neo-Tran (meprobamate): 691
Neo-Tric (CAN) (metrondiazole): 739
Nephramine (amino acids): 94
Nephron (epinephrine): 430
Nephronex (CAN) (nitrofurantoin): 795
Neptazane (methazolamide): 705
Nervine (diphenhydramine): 397
Nervocaine (lidocaine): 636, 1158
Nesacaine (chloroprocaine): 1158
Nestrex (pyridoxine): 1210
netilmicin sulfate: 786
Netromycin (netilmicin): 786
Neupogen (filgrastin): 486
Neurontin (gabapentin): 520
Neut (sodium bicarbonate): 999
Neutrexin (trimetrexate): 1114
niacin: 1210
Niacor (niacin): 1210
nicardipine hydrochloride: 788
N'Ice Vitamin C Drops (ascorbic acid): 1208
Niclocide (niclosamide): 788
niclosamide: 788
Nicoderm (nicotine transdermal): 792
Nicolar (niacin): 1210
Nicorette (nicotine polacrilex): 790
Nicorette DS (nicotine polacrilex): 790
nicotinamide: 1210
nicotine polacrilex: 790
nicotine resin complex: 790
nicotine transdermal: 792
Nictonic Acid (niacin): 1210
Nicotrol (nicotine transdermal): 792
nifedipine: 793
Nilstat (nystatin): 811
nimodipine: 794
Nimotop (nimodipine): 794
Nipent (pentostatin): 870
Nirflex (orphenadrine): 820
NITRATES (see age 40)
amyl nitrate: 121

1290 ■ Index

NITRATES (*continued*)
erythrityl: 438
isosorbide dinitrate: 609
nitroglycerin: 797
Nitro-Bid (nitroglycerin): 797
Nitro-Bid IV (nitroglycerin): 797
Nitrodisc (nitroglycerin): 797
Nitro-Dur (nitroglycerin): 797
Nitrofan (nitrofurantoin): 795
nitrofurantoin: 795
nitrofurantoin macrocrystals: 795
nitrofurazone: 1216
Nitrogard (nitroglycerin): 797
nitrogen mustard (mechlorethamine): 670
NITROGEN MUSTARDS
cyclophosphamide: 331
ifosfamide: 579
uracil mustard: 1121
nitroglycerin, intravenous: 797
nitroglycerin, sublingual: 797
nitroglycerin, sustained release: 797
nitroglycerin, topical: 797
nitroglycerin, transdermal: 797
nitroglycerin, translingual: 797
nitroglycerin, transmucosal: 797
Nitroglyn (nitroglycerin): 797
Nitrol (nitroglycerin): 797
Nitrolingual (nitroglycerin): 797
Nitrong (nitroglycerin): 797
Nitropress (nitroprusside): 800
nitroprusside sodium: 800
Nitrostat (nitroglycerin): 797
Nitrostat IV (nitroglycerin): 797
nitrous oxide: 1153
Nix (permethrin): 1215
nizatidine: 801
Nizoral (isoniazid): 616
N-methylhydrazine (procarbazine): 930
NMJ BLOCKERS (see page 42)
atracurium: 1239
doxacurium: 1239
gallamine: 1239
metocurine: 1239
mivacurium: 1239
pancuronium: 1239
pipercuronium: 1239
rocuronium: 1239
tubocurarine: 1239
vecuronium: 1239
Nobesin (CAN) (diethylpropion): 1151
NoDoz (caffeine): 200
Nolvadex (tamoxifen): 1040

NONSTEROIDAL ANTI-INFLAMMATORY DRUGS (NSAIDs) (see page 43)
aspirin: 131
choline magnesium trisalicylate: 282
choline salicylate: 283
diclofenac: 377
diflunisal: 383
etodolac: 469
fenoprofen: 481
flurbiprofen: 520
ibuprofen: 576
indomethacin: 585
ketoprofen: 618
ketorolac: 619
meclofenamate: 673
mefenamic acid: 676
nabumetone: 766
naproxen: 778
oxaprozin: 826
piroxicam: 903
salsalate: 986
sodium thiosalicylate: 1005
sulindac: 1034
tolmetin: 1086
Norcuron (vecuronium): 1239
Nordette (combo OC): 1199
norepinephrine bitrate: 802
norethindrone: 804
norethindrone acetate: 804
Norethrin 1/35 E (combo OC): 1200
Norethrin 1/50 (combo OC): 1200
Norflex (orphenadrine): 820
norfloxacin: 806
norgestrel: 807
Norinyl 1 + 35 (combo OC): 1200
Norinyl 1 + 50 (combo OC): 1200
Norlestrin 21 2.5/50 (combo OC): 1200
Norlutate (norethindrone): 804
Norlutin (norethindrone): 804
normal serum albumin (albumin): 72
Normodyne (labetolol): 620
Noroxin (norfloxacin): 806
Norpace (disopyramide): 401
Norpace CR (disopyramide): 402
Norplant System (levonorgestrel): 631
Norpramin (desipramine): 354
Nor-Pred (prednisolone): 918
Nor-Tet (tetracycline): 1052
nortriptyline hydrochloride: 809
Norvasc (amlodipine): 106
Norwich (aspirin): 131

Nosalide (flunisolide): 499
Nostril (phenylephrine): 888
Nostrilla (oxymetazoline): 833
Novafed (pseudoephedrine): 954
Novamine (amino acids): 94
Novamobarb (CAN) (amobarbital): 109
Novamoxin (CAN) (amoxicillin): 114
Novasen (CAN) (aspirin): 131
Novo-Alprozol (CAN) (alprazolam): 80
Novo-Ampicillin (CAN) (ampicillin): 118
Novantrone (mitoxantrone): 756
Novo-Atenol (CAN) (atenolol): 135
Novobutamide (CAN) (tolbutamide): 1085
Novocain (procaine): 1159
Novo-Captopril (CAN) (captopril): 207
Novo-Carbamaz (CAN) (carbamazepine): 209
Novo-Cimetine (CAN) (cimetidine): 286
Novo-Clopate (CAN) (clorazepate): 309
Novo-Cloxin (CAN) (cloxacillin): 313
Novo-Digoxin (CAN) (digoxin): 386
Novo-Diltazem (CAN) (diltiazem): 391
Novo-Doxepin (CAN) (doxepin): 410
Novoferrogluc (CAN) (ferrous gluconate): 483
Novoferrosulfa (CAN) (ferrous sulfate): 483
Novofolacid (CAN) (folic acid): 514
Novofumar (CAN) (ferrous fumarate): 483
Novofuran (CAN) (nitrofurantoin): 795
Novohydrazide (CAN) (hydrochlorothiazide): 559
Novo-Lexin (CAN) (cephalexin): 249
Novolin L (insulin): 587
Novolin N (insulin): 587
Novolin R (insulin): 587
Novolorazem (CAN) (lorazepam): 654
Novomedopa (CAN) (methyldopa): 723
Novomepro (CAN) (meprobamate): 691
Novomethacin (CAN) (indomethacin): 585
Novoperidol (CAN) (haloperidol): 548
Novopheniram (CAN) (chlorpheniramine): 271
Novo-Pirocam (CAN) (piroxicam): 903
Novopramine (CAN) (imipramine): 581
Novopranol (CAN) (propranolol): 947
Novo-Prazin (CAN) (prazosin): 916
Novoprednisolone (CAN) (prednisolone): 918
Novoprednisone (CAN) (prednisone): 921
Novonaprox (CAN) (naproxen): 778
Novonidazol (CAN) (metronidazole): 739
Novopentobarb (CAN) (pentobarbital): 868
Novopen VK (CAN) (pencillin v): 862

Novoquindin (CAN) (quinidine): 969
Novorythro (CAN) (erythromycin): 440
Novo-Salmol (CAN0 (albuterol): 73
Novosecobarb (CAN) (secobarbital): 992
Novosemide (CAN) (furosemide): 518
Novosoxazole (CAN) (sulfisoxazole): 1032
Nova-Tamoxifen (CAN) (tamioxifen): 1040
Novotetra (CAN) (tetracycline): 1052
Novotriptyn (CAN) (amitriptyline): 104
Novoxapam (CAN) (oxazepam): 827
Nozinan (CAN) (methotrimeprazine): 716
NSAIDs (see Non-Steroidal Anti-Inflammatories)
Nu-Alpraz (CAN) (alprazolam): 80
Nu-Amoxi (CAN) (amoxicillin): 114
Nu-Ampi (CAN) (ampicillin): 118
Nubain (nalbuphine): 771
Nubicaine (lidocaine): 1158
Nu-Capto (CAN) (captopril): 207
Nu-Capto (CAN) (captopril): 207
Nu-Cephalex (CAN) (cephalexin): 249
Nu-Cimet (CAN) (cimetidine): 286
Nu-Clonidine (CAN) (clonidine): 307
Nu-Cloxi (CAN) (cloxacillin): 313
Nu-Diltiaz (CAN) (diltiazem): 391
Nulicaine (lidocaine): 1158
Numorphan (oxymorphone): 836
Nupercainal (dibucaine): 1158
Nu-Prazo (CAN) (prazosin): 916
Nuprin (ibuprofen): 576
Nuromax (doxacurium): 1239
Nutraplus (urea): 1212
Nutropin (somatropin): 1007
Nydrazid (isoniazid): 607
nylidrin hydrochloride: 1206
nystatin: 811
Nystex (nystatin): 811
Nytol (diphenhydramine): 397

O

Obalan (phendimetrazine): 1152
Obe-Nix (phentermine): 1152
Obephen (phentermine): 1152
Occulcort (CAN) (betamethasone): 167
Octamide PFS (metoclopramide): 734
octereotide acetate: 812
Octocaine (lidocaine): 1158
Ocu-Carpine (pilocarpine): 1242
Ocufen (flurbiprofen): 520

1292 ■ Index

Ocuflox (ofloxacin): 814
ofloxacin: 814
Ogen (estropipate): 458
1,25 [OH]2-D3 (calcitriol): 203
olsalazine sodium: 815
omeprazole: 816
Omnipen (ampicillin): 118
Omnipen-N (ampicillin): 118
Oncaspar (pegasparagase): 851
Oncovin (vincristine): 1139
ondansetron hydrochloride: 817
o.p'-DDD (mitotane): 754
opium preparations: 819
OPHTHALMIC AGENTS (see page 1240)
    apraclonidine: 1241
    carbachol: 1241
    cyclopentolate: 1241
    dapirrazole: 1241
    demarcarium: 1241
    echothiopate: 1241
    fluorometholone: 1241
    homatropine: 1241
    idoxuridine: 1241
    levocabastine: 1242
    lodoxamide: 1242
    metipropranolol: 1242
    natamycin: 1242
    pilocarpine: 1242
    physostigmine: 1242
    suprofen: 1242
    trifluridine: 1242
OPTHALMIC-VASOCONSTRICTOR/ MYDRIATICS
    phenylephrine: 888
    tetrahydrolozine: 1055
Opticrom 4% (cromolyn): 326
Optigene 3 (tetrahydrozoline): 1055
Optimine (azatadine): 144
OptiPranolol (metipropranolol): 1242
OPV (polio virus vaccine): 1173
ORAL ANTICOAGULANT
    warfarin: 1142
ORAL CONTRACEPTIVES (see appendix A, Combination Drugs)
    norgestrel: 807
Oramide (tobutamide): 1085
Orap (pimozide): 896
Oraphen (CAN) (acetaminophen): 58
Orasone (prednisone): 921
Orazinc (zinc): 1148
Orbenin (CAN) (cloxacillin): 313

Oretic (hydrochlorothiazide): 559
Orex (saliva): 985
Orimune (poliovirus vaccine): 1173
Orinase (tobutamide): 1055
ORLAAM (levomethadyl): 629
Ormazine (chlorpromazine): 272
orphenadrine citrate: 820
Ortho-Cept (combo OC): 1199
Orthoclone OKT3 (muromonab-CD3): 764
Ortho Dienestroool (dienestrol): 382
Ortho-Est (estropipate): 458
Ortho-Novum 1/35 (combo OC): 1200
Ortho-Novum 1/50 (combo OC): 1200
Ortho-Novum 7/7/7 (combo OC): 1201
Ortho-Novum 10/11 (combo OC): 1201
Ortho Tri-cyclen (combo OC): 1201
Orudis (ketoprofen): 618
Oruvail SR (ketoprofen): 618
Os-Cal (calcium): 204
Osmitrol (mannitol): 664
Osmoglyn (glycerin): 532
OSMOTIC DIURETICS (see page 31)
    glycerin: 532
    isosorbide: 608
    mannitol: 664
    urea: 1123
Otrivin Nasal Drops N Spray (xylometazoline): 1145
Otrivin Pediatric Nasal Drops (xylometazoline): 1145
Otrivin with M-D Pump (CAN) (xylometazoline): 1145
Oval (CAN) (simethicone): 997
Ovcon-35 (combo OC): 1200
Ovral (combo OC): 1200
Ovrette (norgestrel): 997
oxacillin sodium: 822
oxamniquine: 823
Oxandrin (oxandrolone): 824
oxandrolone: 824
oxaprozin: 826
oxazepam: 827
oxiconazole: 1214
Oxistat (oxiconazole): 1214
Ox-Pam (CAN)(oxazepam): 827
oxytriphylline: 828
oxybutynin chloride: 830
oxycodone hydrochloride: 832
oxymetazoline: 833
oxymetholone: 835
oxymorphone hydrochloride: 836
oxyphencyclimine hydrochloride: 838

oxytetracycline: 840
OXYTOCICS
  ergonovine: 436
  methylergonovine: 726
  oxytocin: 841
oxytocin: 841
Oyst-Cal (calcium): 204
Oystercal (calcium): 204

P

P (vitamin P): 1210
paclitaxel: 843
PAIN RELIEVER, TOPICAL
  capsaicin: 1216
Palafer (CAN) (ferrous fumarate): 483
PAM (melphalon): 680
PAM (pralidoxime): 911
Pamelor (nortriptyline): 809
pamidronate disodium: 844
Pamine (methscopolamine): 719
Pamprin-IB (ibuprofen): 576
Panadol (acetaminophen): 58
Panasol (prednisone): 921
Pan C-500 (vitamin P): 1210
Pancrease Capsules (pancreatic enzymes): 845
pancreatic enzymes: 845
pancreatin: 845
4X Pancreatin (pancreatic enzymes): 845
8X Pancreatin (pancreatic enzymes): 845
Pancreatin Enseals (pancreatic enzymes): 845
pancrelipase: 845
Pancrezyme (pancreatic enzymes): 845
pancuronium bromide: 1239
Panectyl (CAN) (trimeprazine): 1108
Panex (acetaminophen): 58
Panmycin (tetracycline): 1052
Panthoderm (dexpanthenol): 1212
Panwarfarin (warfarin): 1142
papaverine hydrochloride: 1206
parabromdylamine maleate (brompheneramine): 185
Paradione (paramethadione): 848
Paraflex (chlorzoxazone): 280
Parafon Forte DSC (chlorzoxazone): 280
Paral (paraldehyde): 846
paraldehyde: 846
paramethadione: 848

Paraphen (CAN) (acetaminophen): 58
Paraplaten (carboplatin): 213
PARASYMPATHOLYTICS
  atropine: 138
  dicyclomine: 379
  flavoxate: 488
  glycopyrrolate: 534
  ipratropium: 600
  methscopolamine: 719
  oxyphencyclimine: 838
  propantheline: 944
  scopolamine: 989
PARASYMPATHOMIMETICS
  ambenonium: 89
  bethanechol: 172
  neostigmine: 784
Paregoric (opium): 819
Parlodel (bromocriptine): 182
Parnate (tranylcypromine): 1089
paromomycin sulfate: 849
paroxetine: 850
Pathocil (dicloxacillin): 378
Pavabid (papaverine): 1206
Pavased (papaverine): 1206
Pavasule (papaverine): 1206
Pavatine (papaverine): 1206
Pavulon (pancuronium): 1239
Paxil (paroxetine): 850
Paxipam (halazepam): 547
PBZ (tripelennamine): 1118
PDF (CAN) (sodium fluoride): 1002
Pediacare (dextramethorphan): 369
Pediacare (pseudoephedrine): 954
Pediaflor (sodium fluoride): 1002
PediaProfen (ibuprofen): 576
Pediaxole (erythromycin, sulfisoxazole): 1193
PEDICULOCIDES/SCABICIDES:
  crotamiton: 1215
  lindane: 1215
  permethrin: 1215
Pedi-Boro Soak (aluminum acetate): 1212
Pedident (CAN) (sodium fluoride): 1002
PedvaxHIB (hemophilus b vaccine):
Peganone (ethotoin): 467
pegasparagase: 851
PEG-L (pegasparagase): 851
pemoline: 852
Penbec V (CAN) (penicillin V): 862
Penbritin (CAN) (ampicillin): 118
penbutolol sulfate: 854
Penetrex (enoxacin): 426
Penglobe (CAN) (bacampicillin): 150

penicillamine: 855
**PENICILLIN ANTIBIOTICS
(see page 44)**
  amoxicillin: 114
  ampicillin: 118
  bacampicillin: 150
  carbenicillin: 212
  mezlocillin: 743
  penicillin G benzathine: 857
  penicillin G potassium: 859
  penicillin G procaine: 861
  penicillin G sodium: 862
  penicillin V: 862
  piperacillin: 898
  ticarcillin: 1073
**PENICILLINASE RESISTANT
PENICILLINS**
  cloxacillin: 313
  dicloxacilliln: 378
  methicillin: 709
  nafcillin: 770
  oxacillin: 822
penicillin G (aqueous) (penicillin G potassium): 859
penicillin G (aqueous) (penicillin G potassium,sodium): 859
penicillin G benzathine: 857
penicillin G potassium: 859
penicillin G procaine: 861
penicillin G procaine, aqueous: 861
penicillin G sodium: 859
penicillin V: 862
penicillin V potassium: 862
Pentam 300 (pentamidine): 864
pentamidine isoethionate: 864
Pentazine (promethazine): 941
pentazocine lactate: 866
pentazocine hydrochloride with noloxone hydrochloride: 866
Penthrane (methoxyflurane): 1154
pentobarbital: 868
pentobarbital sodium: 870
pentostatin: 872
Penthothal (thiopental): 1153
pentoxifylline: 872
Pen-Vee-K (penicillin V): 862
Pepcid (famotidine): 476
Pepto-Bismol (loperamide): 650
Peptol (CAN) (cimetidine): 286
Percocet (oxycodone with acetaminophen): 1191
Percodan (oxycodone with aspirin): 1191

pergolide mesylate: 873
Pergonal (menotropins): 681
Periactin (cyproheptadine): 336
Peridin C (vitamin P): 1210
Peridol (CAN) (haloperidol): 548
perindopril erbumine: 874
**PERIPHERAL VASODILATORS
(see page 1202)**
  cyclandelate: 1202
  ethaverine: 1202
  isoxsuprine: 1202
  nylidrin: 1202
  papaverine: 1202
Perles (benzonatate): 160
Permapen (pencillin G benzocaine): 857
Permax (pergolide): 873
permethrin: 1215
Permitril (fluphenazine): 506
perphenazine: 875
Persantin (dipyridmole): 399
Persantin IV (dipyridmole): 399
Pertofrane (desipramine): 354
Pertussin (dextramethorphan): 369
pethidine (meperidine): 683
Pfizerpen (penicillin G potassium): 859
Pfizerpen-AS (penicillin G procaine): 861
PGE 1 (alprostadil): 82
Pharmaflur (sodium fluoride): 1002
Phazyme (simethicone): 997
Phazyme 55 (CAN)(simethicone): 977
phenacemide: 877
Phenaphen (acetaminophen): 58
Phenazine (promethazine): 941
Phenazine (CAN)(perphenazine): 875
Phenazo (CAN)(phenazopyridine): 878
Phenazodine (phenazopyridine): 878
phenazopyridine hydrochloride: 878
Phencen (promethazine): 941
phendimetrazine titrate: 1152
phenelzine sulfate: 879
Phenergan (promethazine): 941
Phenetron (chlorpheniramine): 271
phenobarbital: 882
phenobarbital sodium: 882
Phenoject-500 (promethazine): 941
Phenolax (phenolphthalein): 1205
phenolphthalein: 1204
PHENOTHIAZINES (see page 46)
  acetophenazine: 64
  chlorpromazine: 272
  fluphenazine: 506
  mesoridazone: 696

methdilazine: 706
methotrimeprazine: 716
perphenazine: 875
prochlorperazine: 932
promazine: 938
promethazine: 941
thioridazine: 1064
trifluoperazine: 1101
triflupromazine: 1103
trimeprazine: 1108
phenoxybenzamine hydrochloride: 884
phensuximide: 885
phentermine hydrochloride: 1152
phentolamine mesylate: 887
Phenurone (phenacemide): 877
Phenylalamine Mustard (melphalon): 680
phenylazo-diaminopyridine hydrochloride (phenazopyramide): 878
phenylephrine hydrochloride: 888
phenytoin: 892
phenytin sodium: 892
Phicon (promaxine): 1159
pHisoHex (hexachlorophene): 1213
Phillip's MOM (magnesium hydroxide): 1204
Phos-Flur (sodium fluoride): 1002
Phosphaljel (aluminum): 86
Phospholine Iodide (echothiopate): 1241
Phyllocontin (aminophylline): 99
physostigmine: 1242
phytonadione: 1210
Pilocar (pilocarpine): 1242
pilocarpine: 1242
Piloptic (pilocarpine): 1242
Pilostat (pilocarpine): 1242
pimozide: 896
pindolol: 897
piperacillin sodium: 898
piperazine citrate: 900
piperazone estrone sulfate (estropipate): 458
pipercuronium bromide: 1239
Pipracil (piperacillin): 898
pirbuterol acetate: 902
piroxicam: 903
Pitocin (oxytocin): 841
Pitressin Synthetic (vasopressin): 1132
Placidyl (ethchlovynol): 463
plague vaccine: 1179
Plaquenil Sulfate (hydroxychloroquine): 570
Plasbumin-5 (albumin): 72
Plasbumin-25 (albumin): 72
Plasmanate (plasma protein fraction): 904

Plasma-Plex (plasma protein fraction): 904
plasma protein fraction: 904
Plasmatein (plasma protein fraction): 904
PLASMA VOLUME EXPANDERS
  dextran, high molecular weight: 364
  dextran, low molecular weight: 365
  hetastarch: 553
PLASMA PROTEINS
  albumin: 72
  plasma protein fraction: 904
Platinol (cisplatin): 291
Platinol AQ (cisplatin): 291
Plegine (phendimetrazine): 1152
Plenfil (felodipine): 478
plicamycin B sulfate: 905
PMS-ASA (CAN) (aspirin): 131
PMS Benztropine (CAN) (benztropine): 163
PMS Bethanecol Chloride (CAN) (bethanechol): 172
PMS Bisacodyl (CAN) (bisacodyl)
PMS Cyroheptadine (CAN) (cyproheptadine): 336
PMS Metronidazole (CAN) (metronidazole): 739
PMS-Prochlorperazine (CAN): (prochlorperazine): 932
PMS-Procyclidine (CAN) (procyclidine): 934
PMS-Promethazine (CAN) (promethazine): 941
PMS-Propranolol (CAN) (propranolol): 947
PMS-Pyrazinamide (CAN) (pyrazinamide): 956
pneumococcal vaccine, polyvalent: 1172
Pneumovax 23 (pneumococcal vaccine): 1172
Pnu-Imune 23 (pneumococcal vaccine): 1172
Pod-Ben-25 (podophylliium): 1215
Podocon-25 (podophyllium): 1215
podofilox: 1215
Podofin (podophyllium): 1215
podophyllium resin: 1215
Poladex (dexchlorpheniramine): 362
Polaramine (dexchlorpheniramine): 362
Poliovax (poliovirus vaccine, inactivated): 1174
poliovirus vaccine, inactivated: 1175
poliovirus vaccine, live, oral, trivalent: 1173
Polocaine (mipivocaine): 1159
polycarbophil: 1205

1296 ■ Index

Polycillin (ampicillin): 118
Polycillin N (ampicillin): 118
Polymax (amoxicillin): 114
polymyxin b sulfate: 907
Polymyxin B Sulfate Sterile Ophthalmic (polymyxin B): 907
polythiazide: 908
Ponderal (CAN) (fenfluramine):
Pondimin (fenfluramine): 1151
Ponstan (CAN) (mefenamic acid): 676
Ponstel (mefenamic acid): 676
Pontocaine (tetracaine): 1159
Potachlor (potassium): 910
Potasalan (potassium): 910
potassium acetate: 910
potassium chloride: 910
potassium gluconate: 910
potassium iodide (iodine thyroid): 597
POTASSIUM REMOVING RESIN
 sodium polystyrene sulfonate: 1003
POTASSIUM SPARING DIURETICS (see page 31)
 amiloride: 93
 spironolactone: 1012
 triamterene: 1096
povidone iodine: 1213
pralidoxime chloride: 911
PrameGel (promaxine): 1159
Pravachol (pravastatin): 913
pravastatin: 913
Prax (promaxine): 1159
prazepam: 914
praziquantel: 915
prazosin hydrochloride: 916
Predaject (prednisolone): 918
Predcor (prednisolone): 918
Predcor-TBA (prednisolone): 918
Pred-Forte (prednisolone): 918
Pred Mild (prednisolone): 918
prednicarbate: 1222
Prednicen M (prednisone): 921
prednisolone: 918
prednisolone acetate: 918
prednisolone acetate and sodium phosphate: 918
prednisolone sodium phosphate: 918
prednisolone tebutate: 918
Prednisol TBA (prednisolone): 918
prednisone: 921
Prednisone Intensol (prednisone): 921
Pregenyl (chorionic gonadotropin): 284
Prelone (prednisolone): 918

Prelu 2 (phendimetrazine): 1152
Premarin (estrogens, conj.): 450
Premarin Intravenous (estrogens, conj.): 450
Prepidil Gel (CAN) (dinoprostone): 395
Pretz-D (ephedrine): 428
Prevex B (CAN) (betamethasone): 168, 1218
prilocaine: 1159
Prilosec (omeprazole): 816
Primaclone (CAN) (primidone): 923
Primacor (milrinone): 747
primaquine phosphate: 922
Primatene Mist (epinephrine): 430
Primaxin (carbapenem): 1192
primidone: 923
Principen (ampicillin): 18
Prinivil (lisinopril): 643
Priscoline (tolazoline): 1084
Pro-50 (promethazine): 941
Probalan (probenecid): 925
Pro-Banthine (CAN) (propantheline): 944
probenecid: 925
probucol: 927
procaine: 1159
procainamide hydrochloride: 928
Procal Amine (amino acids): 94
Procan SR (procainamide): 928
procarbazine hydrochloride: 930
Procardia (nifedipine): 793
Procardia XL (nifedipine): 793
prochlorperazine: 932
prochlorperazine edisylate: 932
prochlorperazine maleate: 932
Procrit (epoetin): 434
Procyclid (CAN) (procyclidine): 934
procyclidine: 934
Procytox (CAN) (cyclophosphamide): 331
Profasi HP (chorionic gonadotropin): 284
Profenal (suprofen): 1242
Profilate HP (antihemophilic factor): 124
Profilnine Heat Treated (factor IX): 473
Progestasert (progesterone): 936
progesterone: 936
progesterone aqueous: 936
progesterone in oil: 936
progesterone powder: 936
Progestilin (progesterone): 936
PROGESTINS
 hydroxyprogesterone: 572
 levonorgestrel: 631
 medroxyprogesterone: 674
 megestrol: 679

Index ■ 1297

norethindrone: 804
norgestrel: 807
progesterone: 936
Prograf (tacrolimus): 1038
Proglycem (diazoxide): 375
ProHIBIT (hemophilus b vaccine): 1163
Prokine (sargramostim): 988
PROKINETIC AGENTS
   cisapride: 291
Prolastin (alpha 1-proteinase inhibitor): 79
Prolet (phenophthalein): 1205
Proleukin (aldesleukin): 75
Prolixin (fluphenazine): 506
Prolixin Decanoate (fluphenazine): 506
Prolixin Enanthate (fluphenazine): 506
Proloprim (trimethoprim): 1113
promaxine: 1159
promazine hydrochloride: 938
promethazine hydrochloride: 941
Promith (promethazine): 941
Pronestyl (procainamide): 928
Pronestyl SR (procainamide): 928
propafenone hydrochloride: 943
propantheline bromide: 944
Proplex T (factor IX): 473
PROPIONIC ACID DERIVATIVES
   fenoprofen: 481
   ibuprofen: 576
propofol: 1155
Propoint (CAN) (diethylpropion): 1151
propoxyphene hydrochloride: 946
propoxyphene napsylate: 946
propranolol hydrochloride: 947
Propranolol Intensol (propranolol): 947
Propulsid (cisapride): 291
propylthiouracil: 950
Propyl-Thyracil (CAN) (propylthiouracil): 950
Prorex (promethazine): 941
Proscar (finasteride): 487
Pro-Sof (docusate): 1203
ProSom (estazolam): 444
prostaglandin E 2 (dinoprostone): 395
PROSTAGLANDINS
   alprostadil: 82
   carboprost: 215
   dinoprostone 395
   misoprostol: 752
Prostaphlin (oxacillin): 822
ProStep (nicotine transdermal): 792
Prostigmin (neostigmine): 784
Prostin E2 (dinoprostone): 395
Prostin VR Pediatric (alprostadil): 82

protamine sulfate: 951
Protamine Zinc Suspension (NPH) (insulin): 587
Protenate (plasma protein fraction): 904
PROTEIN SUBSTRATE
   amino acids: 94
Protilase (pancreatic enzymes): 845
Protopam Chloride (pralidoxime): 911
Protophylline (CAN) (dyphylline): 418
Protostat (metronidazole): 739
protriptyline hydrochloride: 954
Protropin (somatrem): 1006
Provera (medroxyprogestrone): 674
Proventil (albuterol): 73
Prozac (fluoextine): 503
Prozine-50 (promazine): 938
pseudoephedrine hydrochloride: 954
pseudoephedrine sulfate: 954
PSORALEN
   methoxsalen: 717
Psorcon (diflorasone): 1219
psyllium: 1205
pteroylglutamic acid (folic acid): 514
PTU (propylthiouracil): 950
Pulmozyme (dornase): 407
Purge (castor oil): 1203
Purinethol (mercaptopurine): 693
Purinol (CAN) (allopurinol): 79
pyrantel pamoate: 956
pyrazinamide: 956
Pyridiate (phenazopyridine): 878
Pyridium (phenazopyridine): 878
pyridostigmine bromide: 957
pyridoxine hydrochloride: 1210
pyrimethamine: 959
Pyronium (phenazopyridine): 878
PZI (insulin): 587

Q

quazepam: 961
Quelicin (succinylcholine): 1239
Questran (cholestryamine): 281
Quibron-T Dividose (theophylline): 1056
Quibron-T/SR Dividose (theophylline): 1056
Quick Pep (caffeine): 200
Quiess (hydroxyzine): 575
quinacrine hydrochloride: 964
Quinaglute Dura-Tabs (quinidine): 969
Quinamm (quinine): 970

1298 ■ Index

quinapril hydrochloride: 964
Quinate (quinidine): 969
Quinatime (quinidine): 969
quinestrol: 965
quinethazone: 967
Quinidex Extentabs (quinidine): 969
quinidine gluconate: 969
quinidine polygalacturonate: 969
quinidine sulfate: 969
quinine sulfate: 970
Quinora (quinidine): 969
Quin-Release (quinidine): 969
Quiphile (quinine): 970
Q-vel (quinine): 970

R

rabies immune globulin: 1178
rabies vaccine: 1180
Rabigesic (CAN) (acetaminophen): 58
Rabimycin (erythromycin): 440
ramipril: 972
ranitidine: 973
Raudixin (rauwolfia): 975
rauwolfia derivatives: 975
recombinant human deoxyribonuclease (dornase): 407
recombinant human erythropoietin (epoetin): 434
recombinant tissue plasminogen activator (alteplase): 83
Recombivax-HB (hepatits B vaccine): 1165
Reese's Pinworm (pyrantel): 956
Regibon (CAN) (diethylpropion): 1151
Regitine (phentolamine): 887
Reglan (metoclopramide): 734
Regonal (pyridostigmine): 957
Regular Iletin I (insulin): 587
Regular Iletin II U-500 (insulin): 587
Regutol (docusate): 1203
Relafen (nambutemone): 766
Remular-S (chlorzoxazone): 280
RenAmin (amino acids): 94
Renese (polythiazide): 908
Renormax (spirapril): 1011
Reposans-10 (chlordiazepoxide): 263
Resectisol (mannitol): 664
Reserfia (CAN) (reserpine): 975
reserpine: 975
RESIN EXCHANGE AGENT
cellulose: 248

Resinol (calamine lotion): 1212
Respbid (theophylline): 1056
RESPIRATORY AND CARDIAC STIMULANT
ammonia spirit, aromatic: 108
Restoril (temazepam): 1041
Retrovir (zidovudine): 1147
Rev-Eyes (dapirrazole): 1241
Revia (naltrexone): 776
Revimine (CAN) (dopamine): 405
Rexolate (sodium thiosalicylate): 1005
RH (D) immune globulin: 1175
RH (D) immune globulin micro-dose: 1175
Rheomacrodex (dextran 10): 365
Rhesonativ (RH immune globulin): 1175
Rheumatrex Dose Pak (methotrexate): 714
Rhinall (phenylephrine): 888
Rhinocort (budenoside): 188
RhoGAM (RH immune globulin): 1175
Rholosone (CAN) (betamethasone): 168, 1218
Rhoprosone (CAN) (betamethasone): 1218
Rhospirosone (CAN) (betamethasone): 167
Rhotral (CAN) (acebutolol): 57
ribavirin: 977
riboflavin: 1211
Ridaura (auranofin): 141
rifabutin: 978
Rifadin (rifampin): 979
rifampin: 979
rIFN-A (interferon alfa 2a): 589
rIFN-a2 (interferon alfa 2b): 591
rIFN-B (interferon beta 1B): 594
Rimactane (rifampin): 979
rimantidine hydrochloride: 981
rimexolone: 1242
Rimifon (CAN) (isoniazid): 607
Riopan (magaldrate): 660
risperidone: 982
Risperdal (risperidone): 982
Ritalin (methylphenidate): 727
ritodrine hydrochloride: 983
Rivotril (CAN) (clonazepam): 305
RMS (morphine): 762
R.O. Atropine (CAN) (atropine): 138
Robaxin (methocarbamol): 712
Robicillin VK (penicillin V): 862
Robidex (CAN) (dextramethorphan): 369
Robidrine (CAN) (pseudoephedrine): 954
Robigesic (acetaminophen): 58
Robimycin (erythromycin): 440
Robinul (glycopyrrolate): 534

Robitet (tetracycline): 1052
Robitussin (guaifenesin): 541
Rocaltrol (calcitriol): 203, 1208
Rocephin (ceftriaxone): 244
rocuronium bromide: 1239
Rofact (CAN) (rifampin): 979
Roferon-A (interferon alfa 2a): 589
Rogaine (minoxidil): 750
Rogitine (CAN) (phentolamine): 887
Rolaids Antacid (dehydroxyaluminum): 390
Romazicon (flumazenil): 498
Rounox (CAN)(acetaminophen): 58
Rowasa (mesalamine): 694
Roxanol (morphine): 762
Roxanol SR (morphine): 762
Roxicodone (oxycodone): 832
rt-PA (alteplase): 83
rubella virus vaccine, live: 1176
Rufen (ibuprofen): 576
Rum K (potassium): 910
Ru-Vert-M (meclizine): 672
Rynacron (CAN) (cromolyn): 326
Rythmodan (CAN) (disopyramide): 401
Rythmol (propafenone): 943

S

S-2 (epinephrine): 430
Sabin (poliovirus vaccine): 1173
Saint Joseph's Aspirin Free (acetaminophen): 58
Saint Joseph's Cough (dextramethorphan): 369
Salbutamol (CAN) (albuterol): 73
Saleto-200 (ibuprofen): 576
Salfex (salsalate): 986
SALICYLATES
 aspirin: 131
 choline magnesium trisalicylate: 282
 choline salicylate: 283
 salsalate: 996
 sodium thiosalicylate: 1005
salicylsalicyclic acid (salsalate): 986
Salium (chlordiazepoxide): 263
SALIVA SUBSTITUTE
 saliva substitute: 985
saliva substitute
Salivart (saliva substitute): 985
Salk (polio virus vaccine, inactivated): 1174
salmeterol: 985

salsalate: 986
Salsitab (salsalate): 986
Saluron (hydroxyflumethiazide): 565
Sandimmune (cyclosporine): 334
Sandoglobulin (immune globulin intravenous): 1166
Sandostatin (octreotide): 812
Sani-Supp (glycerin): 532, 1203
Sanorex (mazindol): 1152
Sansert (methysergide): 732
sargramostim: 988
Sarisol No. 2 (butabarbital): 196
Scabene (lindane): 1215
Scopolamine Hbr (scopolamine): 989
scopolamine hydrobromide: 989
Scot-tussin Expectorant (guaifenesin): 541
secobarbital: 992
secobarbital sodium: 992
Seconal Sodium (secobarbital): 992
secubutabarbital (butabarbital): 196
secubarbiton (butabarbital): 196
Sectral (acebutolol): 57
SEDATIVE/HYPNOTICS
 amobarbital: 109
 aprobarbital: 127
 butabarbital: 196
 chloral hydrate: 258
 diphenhydramine: 397
 estazolam: 444
 ethchlorvynol: 463
 furazepam: 508
 glutethimide: 530
 lorazepam: 654
 mephobarbital: 689
 methylprylon: 731
 paraldehyde: 846
 pentobarbital: 868
 phenobarbital: 882
 promethazine: 941
 quazepam: 961
 secobarbital: 992
 temazepam: 1041
 triazolam: 1097
 zolpidem: 1149
Sedatuss (CAN) (dextramethorphan): 369
Seldane (terfenadine): 1047
SELECTIVE SEROTONIN REUPTAKE INHIBITORS (SSRIs)
 fluoxetine: 503
 fluvoxamine: 513
 sertraline: 996
 sumatriptan: 1036
 trazodone: 1091

selegiline hydrochloride: 994
selenium sulfide: 1214
Selestoject (betamethasone): 167
Selsun Blue (selenium): 1214
Semilente Iletin I (insulin): 587
Semilente Insulin (insulin): 587
SEMI-SYNTHETIC ERGOT DERIVATIVE
  bromocriptine: 182
  methysergide: 732
senna: 1205
Senna-Gen (senna): 1205
Senokot (senna): 1205
Senokot-xtra (senna): 1205
Sensorcaine (bupivacaine): 1158
Septisol (hexochlorophene): 1213
Septopal (gentamicin): 525
Septra (co-trimaxazole): 1192
Serax (oxazepam): 827
Serentil (mesoridazine): 696
Serevent (salmeterol): 985
Seromycin Pulvules (cycloserine): 333
Serophene (clomiphene): 302
sertraline hydrochloride: 996
Serzone (nefazodone): 781
SHOCK, DRUGS USED IN
  dobutamine: 404
  dopamine: 405
  ephedrine: 428
  epinephrine: 430
  isoproterenol: 605
  metaraminol: 700
Silfoton (phenobarbital): 882
silver sulfadiazine: 1216
Silvadene (silver sulfadiazine): 1216
simethicone: 997
Simron (ferrous gluconate): 483
simvastatin: 998
Sinarest Nasal (phenylephrine): 888
Sinemet (carbidopa and levodopa): 1197
Sinequan (doxepin): 410
Sinex Long Lasting (oxymetazoline): 833
Sinutabs Sinus Spray (CAN)(xylometazoline): 1145
SKELETAL MUSCLE RELAXANTS, CENTRALLY ACTING
  baclofen: 152
  carisoprodol: 216
  chlorphenesin: 270
  chlorzoxazone: 280
  cyclobenzaprine: 330
  diazepam: 372
  methocarbamol: 712
  orphenadrine: 820

SKELETAL MUSLCE RELAXANTS, DIRECT ACTING
  dantrolene: 346
  quinine: 970
Sleep Eze 3 (diphenhydramine): 397
Slo-bid Gyrocaps (theophylline): 1056
Slo-Phyllin (theophylline): 1056
Slo-Phyllin Gyrocaps (theophylline): 1056
Slo-Salt (sodium chloride): 1001
Slow FE (ferrous sulfate excissated): 483
Slow-K (potassium): 910
SMOKING DETERRENTS
  nicotine polacrilex 790
  nicotine transdermal: 792
Soda Mint (sodium bicarbonate): 999
sodium bicarbonate: 999
sodium chloride: 1001
Sodium Chloride Injection (sodium chloride): 1001
Sodium Edecrin (ethacrynic acid): 460
sodium fluoride: 1002
sodium hypochlorite: 1213
sodium iodide (iodine): 597
sodium polystyrene sulfonate: 1003
sodium thiosalicylate: 1005
sodium valproate (valproic acid): 1128
Sofarin (warfarin): 1142
Solarcaine (lidocaine): 1159
Solfoton (phenobarbital): 882
Solganal (aurothioglucose): 142
Solium (CAN)(chlordiazepoxide): 263
Solu-Cortef (hydrocortisone): 561
Solu-Medrol (methylprednisolone): 728
Solurex (dexamethasone): 358
Solurex L.A. (dexamethasone): 358
Soma (carisoprodol): 216
somatrem: 1006
somatropin: 1007
Sominex (diphenhydramine): 397
Somnal (CAN) (flurazepam): 508
Sopamycetin (CAN) (chloramphenicol): 261
Sorbitrate (isosorbide dinitrate): 609
sotalol hydrochloride: 1008
Span C (vitamin P): 1210
Sparine (promazine): 938
Spasmoject (dicyclomine): 379
Spectazole (econazole):
spectinomycin hydrochloride: 1010
Spectrobid (bacampicillin): 150
spirapril: 1011
spironolactone: 1012
Spirozide (spironolactone and hydrochlorothiazide): 1198

Sporanox (itraconazole): 613
SPS (sodium polystyrene sulfonate): 1003
S-P-T (thyroid dessicated): 1070
SsF Cream (silver sulfadiazine): 1216
Stadol (butorphanol): 198
Stadol NS (butorphanol): 198
stanozolol: 1014
Staphcillin (methicillin): 709
Staticin (erythromycin): 440
stavudine: 1015
Stelazine (trifluoperazine): 1101
Stemitil (CAN) (prochlorperazine): 932
Sterine (CAN) (methenamine): 708
Stilphostrol (diethylstilbesterol): 383
Stimate (desmopressin): 356
Streptase (streptokinase): 1016
streptokinase: 1016
streptomycin sulfate: 1018
streptozocin: 1020
strong iodine solution (iodine): 597
Sublimaze (fentanyl): 482
succimer: 1021
SUCCINIMIDES
   ethosuximide: 465
   methsuximide: 720
   phensuximide: 885
succinylcholine chloride: 1239
Sucostrin (succinylcholine chloride): 1239
sucralfate: 1022
Sucrets Cough Control (dextramethorphan): 369
Sudafed (pseudoephedrine): 954
Sudrin (pseudoephedrine): 954
Sufenta (sufentanil): 1023
sufentanil citrate: 1023
Sulcrate (CAN) (sulcralfate): 1022
sulfadiazine: 1025
sulfamethizole: 1026
Sulfamethoprim (co-trimoxazole): 1192
sulfamethoxazole: 1028
Sulfamylon (mafenide): 1216
sulfasalazine: 1029
Sulfatrim (co-trimoxazole): 1192
sulfinpyrazone: 1031
sulfisoxazole: 1032
SULFONAMIDES, BACTERIOSTATIC (see page 48)
   sulfadiazine: 1025
   sulfamethizole: 1026
   sulfamethoxazole: 1028
   sulfasalazine: 1029
   sulfisoxazole: 1031

SULFONAMIDES, NONBACTERIOSTATIC
   acetazolamide: 60
   methazolamide: 705
SULFONYLUREAS
   acetohexamide: 62
   chlorpropamide: 276
   glipizide: 527
   glyburide: 531
   tolazamide: 1082
   tolbutamide: 1085
sulindac: 1034
sumatriptan succinate injection: 1036
Sumycin (tetracycline): 1052
Supeudol (CAN) (oxycodone): 832
Supprelin (histrelin): 554
Suprane (desflurane): 1154
Suprax (cefixime): 227
suprofen: 1242
SURFACE ACTIVE AGENT
   benzalkonium: 158
Surital (thiamylal): 1153
Surmontil (trimipramine): 1115
Survanta (beractant): 166
Sus-Phrine (epinephrine): 430
Symadine (amantadine): 88
Symmetrel (amantadine): 88
SYMPATHOLYTICS, CENTRALLY ACTING
   clonidine: 307
   guanabenz: 541
   guanfacine: 546
   methyldopa: 723
SYMPATHOMIMETICS
   albuterol: 73
   bitolterol: 178
   dobutamine: 404
   dopamine: 405
   ephedrine: 428
   epinephrine: 430
   isoetharine: 602
   isoproterenol: 605
   mephentermine: 686
   metaproterenol: 699
   metaraminol: 700
   norepinephrine: 802
   phenylephrine: 888
   pirbuterol: 902
   pseudoephedrine: 954
   ritodrine: 983
   terbutaline: 1045
Synacthen Depot (CAN) (cosyntropin): 325

1302 ■ Index

Synalar (fluocinolone): 1219
Synarel (nafarelin): 768
Syn-Captopril (CAN) (captopril): 207
Syn-Diltiazem (CAN) (diltiazem): 391
Synemol (fluocinolone): 1219
Synkayvite (menadiol): 1209
synthetic lung surfactant (colfasceril): 320
Synthroid (levothyroxine): 634
Syntocinon (oxytocin): 841
Syprine (trientine): 1100
SYSTEMIC ALKALINIZERS
   sodium bicarbonate: 999
   tromethamine: 1120
SYSTEMIC HEMOSTATIC AGENTS
   aminocaproic acid: 96
   aprotinin: 128

T

T 3 (liothyronine): 640
T 4 (levothyroxine): 634
Tacaryl (methdilazine): 706
TACE (chlorotrianisene): 268
tacrine hydrochloride: 1037
tacrolimus: 1038
Tagamet (cimetidine): 286
Talwin (pentazocine): 866
Talwin NX (pentazocine): 866
Tambocor (flecainide): 489
Tamofen (tamoxifen): 1040
Tamone (CAN) (tamoxifen): 1040
Tamoplex (tamoxifen): 1040
Tamovate (clobetasol): 1218
tamoxifen citrate: 1040
Tapazole (methimazole): 711
Taro-Sone (CAN) (betamethasone): 167
Tavist (clemastine): 296
Tavist-1 (clemastine): 296
Tavist-D (phenylpropanolamine and clemastine): 1202
Taxol (paclitaxel): 843
Tazicef (ceftazidime): 241
Tazidine (ceftazidime): 241
Td (diptheria and tetanus toxoids, combined, adsorbed): 1157
Tebamide (trimethobenzamide): 1112
Tebrazide (CAN) (pyrazinamide) : 956
Tegison (etretinate): 471
Tegopen (cloxacillin): 313
Tegretol (carbamazepine): 209

Tegrin-HC (hydrocortisone): 1221
Teject-20 (trimethobenzamide): 1112
Telachor (chlorpheniramine): 271
Teladar (betamethasone): 1218
Temaril (trimeprazine): 1108
temazepam: 1041
Tempra (acetaminophen): 58
Tenex (guanfacine): 546
teniposide: 1042
Ten K (potassium): 910
Tenormin (atenolol): 135
Tensilon (edrophonium): 421
Tenuate (diethylpropion): 1151
Tepavil (diethylpropion): 1151
terazosin hydrochloride: 1044
terbinafine: 1214
terbutaline sulfate: 1045
terfenadine: 104
Ternovate (clobetasol): 1218
terpin hydrate: 1048
Terramycin (oxytetracycline): 840
Teslac (testolactone): 1049
Tessalon (benzonatate): 160
Testa-C (testosterone): 1050
Testamone (testosterone): 1050
Testex (testosterone): 1050
Testoderm (testosterone): 1050
Testoject (testosterone): 1050
Testoject 50 (testosterone): 1050
Testoject-LA (testosterone): 1050
testolactone: 1049
testosterone: 1050
testosterone cypionate: 1050
testosterone enanthate: 1050
testosterone propionate: 1050
Testone LA (testosterone): 1050
Testrin PA (testosterone): 1050
tetanus antitoxin: 1178
tetanus immune globulin: 1178
tetracaine: 2259
Tetracap (tetracycline): 1052
TETRACYCLINE ANTIBIOTICS (see page 49)
   democlocycline: 353
   doxycycline: 415
   minocycline: 748
   oxytetracycline: 840
   tetracycline : 1052
tetracycline hydrochloride: 1052
tetrahydroaminoacridine (tacrine): 1037
tetrahydrozoline hydrochloride: 1055
Tetralan (tetracycline): 1052

Tetralean (CAN) (tetracycline): 1052
Tetram (tetracycline): 1052
Tetramune (diptheria and tetanus toxoids and whole cell pertussis vaccine with haemophilus influenzae b conjugates): 1162
Tetrasine (tetrahydrozaline): 1055
TG (thioguanine): 1063
T-Gen (trimethobenzamide): 1112
THA (tacrine): 1037
Thalitone (chlorthalidone): 279
Tham (tromethamine): 1120
Tham E (tromethamine): 1120
Theelin Aqueous (estrone): 455
Theo-24 (theophylline): 1056
Theobid (theophylline): 1056
Theoclear-80 (theophylline): 1056
Theoclear LA (theophylline): 1056
Theocron (theophylline): 1056
Theo-Dur (theophylline): 1056
Theo-Dur Sprinkle (theophylline): 1056
Theolair (theophylline): 1056
Theolair-SR (theophylline): 1056
theophylline: 1056
theophylline ethylenediamine (aminophylline): 99
theophylline sodium glycinate: 1056
Theospan-SR (theophylline): 1056
Theostat 80 (theophylline): 1056
Theovent Long Acting (theophylline): 1056
Thermazene (silver sulfadiazine): 1216
thiabendazole: 1060
Thiamilate (thiamine): 1211
thiamine hydrochloride: 1211
thiamylal sodium: 1153
THIAZIDE DIURETICS (see page 31)
   bendroflumethiazide: 157
   benzthiazide: 161
   chlorothiazide: 266
   hydrochlorothiazide: 559
   hydroflumethiazide: 565
   methyclothiazide: 721
   polythiazide: 908
   trichlormethiazide: 1098
THIAZIDE-LIKE DIURETICS (see page 31)
   chlorthalidone: 279
   indapamide: 583
   metolazone: 736
   quinethazone: 967
THIAZIDE, NONDIURETIC
   diazoxide: 375

thiethylperazine maleate: 1062
thimersol: 1213
thioguanine: 1063
6-thioguanine: 1063
THIOL COMPOUND
   tiopronin: 1078
Thiola (tiopronin): 1078
thiopental sodium: 1153
thioridazine hydrochloride: 1064
thiotepa: 1067
thiothixene: 1068
thiothixene hydrochloride: 1068
THIOXANTHINES
   chlorprothioxene: 277
   thiothixene: 1068
Thorazine (chlorpromazine): 272
Thrombate III (antithrombin): 125
thrombin: 1216
Thrombinaire (thrombin): 1216
THROMBOLYTIC AGENTS
   alteplase: 83
   anistreplase: 123
   streptokinase: 1016
   urokinase: 1125
Thrombostat (thrombin): 1216
Thyrar (thyroid dessicated): 1070
Thyro-Block (iodine thyroid): 597
thyroid dessicated: 1070
THYROID HORMONES
   levothyroxine: 634
   liothyronine: 640
   liotrix: 642
   thyroid dessicated: 1070
thyroid stimulating hormone (thyrotropin): 1072
Thyroid Strong (thyroid dessicated): 1070
THYROID SUPPRESSANTS
   iodine thyroid: 597
Thyrolar (liotrix): 642
Thytropar (thyrothropin): 1072
thyrotropin: 1072
Tibsazid (CAN) (pyrazinamide): 956
Ticar (ticarcillin): 1073
ticarcillin disodium: 1073
TICE BCG (BCG): 1179
Ticlid (ticlopidine): 1075
ticlopidine hydrochloride: 1075
Ticon (tremethobenzamide): 1112
Tigan (trimethobenzamide): 1112
Tiject 20 (trimethobenzamide): 1112
Tildale (nedocromil): 780
Timentin (piperacillin and tazobactam): 1194

timolol maleate: 1076
Timoptic (timolol): 1076
Tinactin (tolnaftate): 1214
Tindal (acetophenazine): 64
Ting (tolnaftate): 1214
tiopronin: 1078
Tipramine (imipramine): 581
Tirend (caffeine): 200
TMP (trimethoprim): 1113
TMP-SMZ (co-trimaxazole): 1192
tobramycin sulfate: 1079
Tobrex Ophthalmic (tobramycin): 1079
tocainide hydrochloride: 1081
TOCOLYTIC AGENTS
 ritodrine: 983
 terbutaline: 1045
Tofranil (imipramine): 581
Tofranil-PM (imipramine): 581
tolazamide: 1082
tolazoline hydrochloride: 1084
tolbutamide: 1085
Tolectin (tolmetin): 1086
Tolectin DS (tolmetin): 1086
Tolinase (tolazamide): 1082
tolmetin sodium: 1086
tolnaftate: 1214
Tonocard (tocainide): 1081
TOPICAL CORTICOSTEROIDS
 aclometasone: 1217
 amcinonide: 1217
 betamethasone benzoate: 1217
 betamethasone dipropionate: 1218
 betamethasone dipropionate, augmented: 1218
 betamethasone valerate: 1218
 clobetasol: 1218
 clocortolone: 1218
 desonide: 1218
 desoximetasone: 1218
 dexamethasone: 1219
 dexamethasone sodium phosphate: 1219
 diflorasone: 1219
 fluocinolone: 1219
 fluocinonide: 1220
 flurandrenolide: 1220
 fluticasone: 1220
 halcinonide: 1220
 halobetasol: 1220
 hydrocortisone: 1220
 hydrocortisone acetate: 1221
 hydrocortisone butyrate: 1221
 hydrocortisone valerate: 1221
 mometasone: 1221
 prednicarbate: 1222
 triamcinolone: 1222
TOPICAL LOTIONS AND SOLUTIONS
 Burow's solution: 1212
 aluminum acetate: 1212
 calamine lotion: 1212
 hamamelis water: 1212
Topicort (desoximetasone): 1218
Topicycline (tetracycline): 1052
Toprol XL (metoprolol): 737
TOPV (poliovirus vaccine, live): 1173
Topsyn Gel (CAN)(flucinonide): 1220
Toradol (ketorolac): 619
Torecan (thiethylperazine): 1062
Tornalate (bitolterol): 178
torsemide: 1087
Totacillin (ampicillin): 118
Totacillin N (ampicillin): 118
TPA (alteplase): 83
Tracrium (atracurium): 1239
Trandate (labetalol): 620
Transderm-Nitro (nitroglycerin): 797
Transderm-Scop (scopolamine): 989
tranylcypromine sulfate: 1089
Tranxene (clorazepate): 309
Trasylol (aprotinin): 128
Travasol (amino acids): 94
Travel Aid (CAN) (dimenhydrinate): 393
Travel Eze (CAN) (dimenhydrinate): 393
Travel Tabs (CAN) (dimenhydrinate): 393
trazodone hydrochloride: 1091
Trecator S.C. (ethionamide): 464
Trendar (ibuprofen): 576
Trental (pentoxifylline): 872
Triacet (triamcinolone): 1093, 1222
Triadapin (CAN) (doxepin): 410
triamcinolone: 1093
triamcinolone acetonide: 1093, 1222
triamcinolone diacetate: 1093
triamcinolone hexacetonide: 1093
Triam Forte (triamcinolone): 1093
Triamonide (triamcinolone): 1093
Triamolone 40 (triamcinolone): 1093
triamterene: 1096
Triavil (perphenazine and amitriptyline): 1194
triazolam: 1097
trichlormethiazide: 1098
Tricosal (choline magnesium trisalicylate): 282

TRICYCLIC ANTIDEPRESSANTS (TCAs) (see page 51)
    amotriptyline: 104
    amoxapine: 112
    clomipramine: 303
    desipramine: 354
    doxepin: 410
    imipramine: 581
    nortriptyline: 809
    protriptyline: 952
    trimipramine: 1115
Triderm (triamcinolone): 1093, 1222
Tridesilon (desonide): 1218
Tridil (nitroglycerin): 797
Tridione (trimethadione): 1109
trientine hydrochloride: 1100
triethylenethiophosphoramide (thiotepa): 1067
trifluoperazine hydrochloride: 1101
triflupromazine hydrochloride: 1103
trifluridine: 1242
trihexyphenidyl hydrochloride: 1106
Trihexy (trihexyphenidyl): 1106
Tri-Immunol (diptheria and tetanus toxoids and whole cell pertussis vaccine): 1157
triiodithyronine (liothyronine): 640
Tri-K (potassium): 910
Trikacide (CAN)(metronidazole): 739
Trikates (potassium): 910
Trilafon (perphenazine): 875
Tri-Levlen (combo OC): 1201
Trilisate (choline magnesium trisalicylate): 282
Trilone (triamcinolone): 1093
Trimazide (trimethobenzamide): 1112
trimeprazine tartrate: 1108
trimethadione: 1109
trimethaphan camsylate: 1110
trimethobenzamide hydrochloride: 1112
trimethoprim: 1113
trimetrexate glucuronate: 1114
trimipramine maleate: 1115
Trimox (amoxicillin): 114
Trimpex (trimethoprim): 1113
Trinalin (azatidine and pseudoephedrine): 1202
Tri-Norinyl (combo OC): 1201
Triostat (liothyronine): 640
Tripedia (diphtheria and tetanus toxoids and acellular pertussis vaccine): 1160
tripelennamine hydrochloride: 1118
Triphasil (combo OC): 1201
triprolidine hydrochloride: 1119
Tristoject (triamcinolone) 1093
Triptil (CAN) (protriptylline): 952
Triptone (scopolamine): 989
Trobicin (spectinomycin): 1010
tromethamine: 1120
Tronothane (promaxine): 1159
TrophAmine (amino acids): 94
Truphylline (aminophylline): 99
TSH (thyrotropin) 1072
TSPA (thiotepa): 1067
T-Stat (erythromycin): 440
tubocurarine chloride: 1239
Tucks (hamemalis water): 1212
Tums (calcium): 204
Turbinaire Decadron Phosphate (dexamethasone): 358
Tusal (sodium thiosalicylate): 1005
Twice-A-Day (oxymetazoline): 833
Twin-K (potassium): 910
Tylenol (acetaminophen): 58
Tylenol with Codeine (acetaminophen with codeine): 1177
Tyzine (tetrahydrozoline): 1055
Tyzine Pediatric (tetrahydrozoline): 1055

U

U-Cort (hydrocortisone): 1221
Ultracef (cefadroxil): 222
Ultralente Insulin (insulin): 587
ULtrase MT 8 (pancreatic enzymes): 845
ULtrase MT 12 (pancreatic enzymes): 845
ULtrase MT 20 (pancreatic enzymes): 845
ULtrase MT 24 (pancreatic enzymes): 845
ULtravate (halobetasol): 1220
Unasyn: (piperacillin and tazobactam): 1194
Unguentin (benzocaine): 1158
Unipen (nafcillin): 770
Uniphyl (theophylline): 1056
Uni-tussin (guaifenesin): 541
Urabeth (bethanechol): 172
Uracil Mustar (uracil mustard): 1121
uracil mustard: 1121
urea: 1123, 1212
Ureacin (urea):1212
Ureaphil (urea): 1123
Urecholine (bethanechol): 172

Index

Urex (methenamine): 708
URICOSURIC DRUGS
  probenecid: 925
  sulfinpyrazone: 1031
URINARY ACIDIFIER
  ammonium chloride: 108
URINARY ALKALINIZER
  sodium bicarbonate: 999
URINARY ANALGESICS
  phenazopyridine: 878
URINARY ANTISPASMODIC
  flavoxate 488
  oxybutynin: 830
URINARY IRRIGANT
  mannitol: 664
URINARY TRACT AGENTS
  acetohydroxamic acid: 63
  cysteamine: 337
  neostigmine: 784
URINARY TRACT ANTI-INFECTIVE
  cinoxacin: 288
  methenamine: 708
  methylene blue: 725
  nalidixic acid: 773
  nitrofurantoin: 795
  norfloxacin: 806
Urispas (flavoxate): 488
Uri-Tet (oxytetracycline): 840
Uritol (CAN) (furosemide): 518
Urobak (sulfamethoxazole): 1028
Urodine (phenazopyridine): 878
urofollitropin: 1124
urokinase: 1125
Urolene Blue (methylene blue): 725
Uro-Mag (magnesium): 661
Uroplus (co-trimaxazole): 1192
Urozide (CAN) (hydrochlorothiazide): 559
ursodeoxycholic acid (ursodiol): 1127
ursodiol: 1127
Ursofalk (CAN) (ursodiol): 1127
Uticort (bethamethasone): 167, 1217

V

Valergen (estradiol): 446
Valisone (betamethasone): 168, 1218
Valium (diazepam): 372
valproic acid: 1128
Valrelease (diazepam): 372
Vancenase Nasal Inhaler (beclomethasone): 154
Vanceril (beclomethasone): 154
Vancocin (vancomycin): 1130
Vancoled (vancomycin): 1130
vancomycin hydrochloride
Vansil (oxamniquine): 823
Vantin (cefpodoxime): 238
Vaponefrin (epinephrine): 430
varicella-zoster immune globulin: 1178
Vascor (bepridil): 165
Vaseretic (enalapril and hydrochlorothiazide):1196
Vasoderm (flucinonide): 1220
Vasodilan (isoxsuprine): 1206
VASODILATORS
  hydralazine: 557
  minoxidil: 750
  nitroprusside: 800
  tolazoline: 1084
vasopressin: 1132
VASOPRESSORS
  ephedrine: 428
  epinephrine: 430
  metaraminol: 700
  norepinephrine: 802
  phenylephrine: 888
Vasotec (enalapril): 424
Vasotec IV (enalapril): 424
V-Cillin K (penicillin V): 862
VCR (vincristine): 1139
vecuronium bromide: 1239
Veetids (pencillin V): 862
Velban (vinblastine): 1138
Velbè (CAN) (vinblastine): 1138
Velosef (cephradine): 254
Velosulin (insulin): 587
venlafaxine: 1133
Venoglubulin-I (immune globulin IV): 1166
Ventodisk (CAN) (albuterol): 73
Ventolin (albuterol): 73
VePesid (etoposide): 470
verapamil hydrochloride: 1134
Verazinc (zinc): 1148
Verelan (verapamil): 1134
Vermox (mebendazole): 667
Verr-Canth (cantharidin): 1215
Versed (midazolam): 1155
Vesprin (triflupromazine): 1103
Vexol (rimexolone): 1242
V-Gan (promethazine): 941
Vibramycin (doxycycline): 415
Vibra-Tabs (doxycycline): 415
Vicks V9-Tro-Nol Nose Drops (ephedrine): 428

vidarabine: 1136
Videx (didanosine): 380
vinblastine sulfate: 1138
Vincasar PFS (vincristine): 1139
vincristine sulfate: 1139
vinorelbine tartrate: 1141
Viokase (pancreatic enzymes): 845
Vira-A (vidarabine): 1136
Virazole (ribavirin): 977
Viroptic (trifluridine): 1242
Viscerol (CAN) (dicyclomine): 379
Visine (tetrahydrozoline): 1055
Visken (pindolol): 897
Vistacon (hydroxyzine): 575
Vistaject (hydroxyzine): 575
Vistaquel (hydroxyzine): 575
Vistaril (hydroxyzine): 575
Vita-C (ascorbic acid): 1208
vitamin A metabolite (isotretinoin): 610
vitamin A & D: 1212
vitamin B 12a (hydroxycabalamin): 569
VITAMINS (see page 1206)
  A: 1208
  ascorbic acid (C): 1208
  calcifediol: 1208
  calcitriol: 203, 1208
  cholecalciferol: 1208
  cyanocobalamin: 1209
  D: 1209
  dihydrotachysterol: 1209
  E: 1209
  ergocalciferol: 1209
  hydroxocabalamin: 569
  menadiol sodium diphosphate: 1209
  niacin: 1210
  nictinamide: 1210
  P: 1210
  phytonadione: 1210
  pyridoxine hydrochloride: 1210
  riboflavin: 1211
  thiamine hydrochloride: 1211
VITAMIN METABOLITE
  isotretinon: 610
Vita-Plus B Softgels (vitamin E): 1209
Vivactil (protripylline): 952
Vivarin (caffeine): 200
Vivoli (CAN) (diazepam): 372
VLB (vinblastine): 1138
VM-26 (teniposide): 1042
Volmax (CAN) (beclomethasone): 154
Voltaren (diclofenac): 377
Vontrol (diphenidol): 398
Voxsuprine (isoxsuprine): 1206

VP-16-213 (etoposide): 470
Vumon (teniposide): 1042

W

warfarin sodium: 1142
Warfilone (CAN)(warfarin): 1142
Warnerin (CAN)(warfarin): 1142
Wehgen (estrone): 455
Web-less (phendimetrazine): 1152
Wellbutrin (bupropion): 191
Wellcovorin (leucovorin): 624
Westcort (hydrocortisone): 561, 1221
whole root rauwolfia (reserpine): 975
Winpred (CAN) (prednisone): 921
Winstrol (stanozolol): 1014
Witch Hazel (hamamelis water): 1212
Wyamine (mephentermine): 686
Wycillin (penicillin G procaine): 861
Wydase (hyaluronidase): 555
Wymox (amoxicillin): 114
Wytensin (guanabenz): 541

X

Xanax (alprazolam): 80
XANTHINES
  aminophylline: 99
  caffeine: 200
  dyphylline: 418
  oxtriphylline: 828
  pentoxifylline: 872
  theophylline: 1056
Xero-Lube (saliva): 985
Xylocaine (lidocaine): 636, 1158
Xylocaine HCl (lidocaine): 636
Xylocaine HCl IM for Cardiac Arrhythmias
  (lidocaine): 636
Xylocaine HCl IV for Cardiac Arrhythmias
  (lidocaine): 636
xylometazoline hydrochloride: 1145

Y

yellow fever vaccine: 1180
YF-Vax (yellow fever vaccine): 1180
Yodoxin (iodoquinol): 598
Yutopar (ritodrine): 983

Z

zalcitabine: 1146
Zanosar (streptozocin): 1020
Zantac (ranitidine): 973
Zapex (CAN) (oxazepam): 827
Zarontin (ethosuximide): 465
Zaroxolyn (metolazone): 736
Zartan (cephalexin): 249
Zebeta (bisoprolol): 176
Zefazone (cefmetazole): 228
Zemuron (rocuronium): 1239
Zephiran (benzalkonium): 158, 1213
Zerit (stavudine): 1015
Zestril (lisinopril): 643
Zetran (diazepam): 372
Ziac (bisoprolol and hydrochlorothiazide): 1196

zidovudine: 1147
Zinacef (cefuroxime): 246
zinc: 1148
zinc oxide: 1212
Zincate (zinc): 1148
zinc gluconate: 1148
zinc sulfate: 1148
Zithromax (azithromycin): 147
Zocor (simvastatin): 998
Zofran (ondanestron): 817
Zoladex (goserelin): 539
Zolicef (cefazolin): 225
Zoloft (sertraline): 996
zolpidem tartrate: 1149
ZORprin (aspirin): 131
Zostrix (capsaicin): 1216
Zovirax (acyclovir): 69
Zyloprim (allopurinol): 78